AMYLOIDOSIS

AMYLOIDOSIS

EDITED BY

GEORGE G. GLENNER
University of California, San Diego
La Jolla, California

ELLIOTT F. OSSERMAN
Columbia University
New York, New York

EARL P. BENDITT
University of Washington
Seattle, Washington

EVAN CALKINS
State University of New York at Buffalo
Buffalo, New York

ALAN S. COHEN
Boston University School of Medicine
Boston, Massachusetts

AND

DOROTHEA ZUCKER-FRANKLIN
New York University School of Medicine
New York, New York

PLENUM PRESS • NEW YORK AND LONDON

Library of Congress Cataloging in Publication Data

International Symposium on Amyloidosis: The Disease Complex (4th: 1984: Columbia University)
   Amyloidosis.

   ''Proceedings of the Fourth International Symposium on Amyloidosis: The Disease Complex, held November 9–12, 1984, at Columbia University, New York, New York''—T.p. verso.
   Includes bibliographies and index.
   1. Amyloidosis—Congresses. I.Glenner, George G., 1927–   . II. Osserman, Elliott F., 1925–   . III. Title. [DNLM: 1. Amyloid—congresses. W3 IN916AAm 4th 1984a/WD 205.5.A6 I612 1984a]
RC632.A5I58   1984   616.8'3   86-4889
ISBN-13:978-1-4612-9292-0   e-ISBN-13:978-1-4613-2199-6
DOI: 10.1007/978-1-4613-2199-6

\

Proceedings of the Fourth International Symposium on Amyloidosis:
The Disease Complex, held November 9–12, 1984, at Columbia University,
New York, New York

© 1986 Plenum Press, New York
Softcover reprint of the hardcover 1st edition 1986

A Division of Plenum Publishing Corporation
233 Spring Street, New York, N.Y. 10013

" There is no such thing as death.
In nature nothing ever dies.
From each sad remnant,
new forms of precious life arise. "

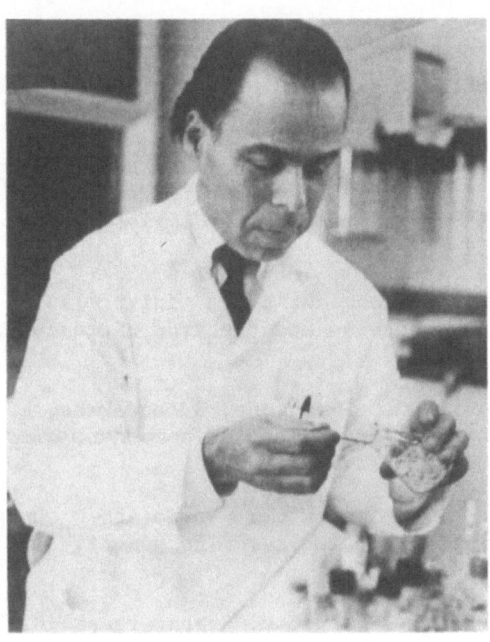

EDWARD C. FRANKLIN, M.D.

Dr. Edward C. Franklin died on February 20, 1982. Ed was a close friend and an esteemed scientific colleague to many of us. He was an active participant in the second (Helsinki, 1974) and third (Porto, 1978) Amyloidosis Symposia and would have played a key role in the organization of our present meeting.

Without question, Ed was a major contributor to amyloid research starting in 1968 (1) with the publication of the now standard "Pras-Franklin" method for the preparation of purified amyloid fibrils from tissues using distilled water extraction (1, 2); to this date, this procedure is employed by virtually all laboratories. The contributions of Ed and his colleagues in the ensuing years included the demonstration of intracellular amyloid by fluorescence and electron microscopy (3), the sequencing of human AA, the identification of its serum precursor (SAA) and delineation of its role as an acute phase reactant (5, 6), the demonstration of the probable role of a defect in monocyte-macrophage serine protease in the pathogenesis of AA amyloidosis (7) and the demonstration of a variant of prealbumin in an Israeli with FAP (8).

Ed entered the field of amyloid research after many years of highly productive investigation in basic and clinical immunology. He was possessed of a keen mind, rigorous discipline and consummate skill with the most sophisticated methods in protein research. As further evidence of Ed's continuing influence, many of his collaborators in amyloid research are participants in this meeting. These collaborators include Mordechai Pras, Blas Frangione, Julian Rosenthal, Reinhold Linke, Joel Buxbaum, Peter Gorevic, Gad Lavie and, to be sure, Ed's most important, full-time, lifetime collaborator, Dorothea Zucker-Franklin.

In recognition of both past and present contributions of Ed Franklin's research team, we dedicate this Symposium to his memory.

1. Pras, M., Schubert, M., Zucker-Franklin, D., Rimon, A. and Franklin, E.C.: The characterization of soluble amyloid prepared in water. J. Clin. Invest. 47: 924, 1968.

2. Pras, M., Zucker-Franklin, D., Rimon, A. and Franklin, E.C.: Physical chemical and ultrastructural studies of water-soluble human amyloid fibrils: Comparative analyses of nine amyloid preparations. J. Exp. Med. 130: 777, 1969.

3. Zucker-Franklin, D and Franklin, E.C.: Intracellular localization of human amyloid by fluorescence and electron microscopy. Am. J. Path. 59: 23, 1970.

4. Levin, M., Franklin, E.C., Frangione, B. and Pras, M.: The amino acid sequence of a major non-immunoglobulin component of some amyloid fibrils. J. Clin. Invest. 51: 2773-2776, 1972.

5. Rosenthal, C.J. and Franklin, E.C.: Variation with age and diseases of an amyloid A protein-related serum component. J. Clin. Invest. 55: 746, 1975.

6. Gorevic, P.D., Levo, Y., Frangione, B. and Franklin, E.C.: Polymorphism of tissue and serum amyloid A (AA and SAA) proteins. J. Immunol. 121: 138-140, 1978.

7. Lavie, G., Zucker-Franklin, D. and Franklin, E.C.: The degradation of serum amyloid A protein by peripheral blood monocytes. J. Exp. Med. 148: 1020-1031, 1978.

8. Pras, M., Franklin, E.C., Pirelli, F. and Frangione, B.: A variant of prealbumin from amyloid fibrils in Familial Polyneuropathy of Israeli origin. J. Exp. Med. 154: 989, 1981.

Elliott F. Osserman, M.D.

INTRODUCTION

From a process that from the days of Virchow and Rokitansky, primarily
stimulated the relatively narrow interest of pathologists, amyloidosis has
risen full-blown as one of the most important of disease complexes. Its
presence dominates the lesions of Alzheimer's disease, a disease affecting
an estimated 2.5 million people in the U.S.A. and thereby closely rivaling
stroke as the third most common cause of death. If, as it has been described, Alzheimer's disease is the "Disease of the Century," then amyloidosis is the Disease Complex of the Ages. It affects in one or more of
its manifestations every organ of the body, and is at least as old as the
afflicted Egyptian mummies of the pyramids. With an increasing percentage
of older individuals amyloid of the senior population becomes increasingly
more frequent.

The subjects covered in this Symposium range through almost every
clinical medical specialty. From an average of one paper in each of the
past three Symposiums, the explosive interest in cerebral amyloidosis has
led to the presentation of 12 papers on this subject in the present volume.
The genetically predisposed familial amyloidotic processes, such as the
polyneuropathies and familial Mediterranean fever have also stimulated extensive and intriguing investigations which have revealed the striking
effect of a single amino acid substitution in transforming a normal protein
into a lethal "amyloidogenic" one.

This Symposium clearly depicts the advances since the first amyloid
fibril protein was definitively identified and defined 14 years ago. Since
all amyloid fibril proteins so far described are variants of normal proteins,
attention to gene abnormalities now becomes a significant focus as well as
the pathogenic sequences which lead in these cases to twisted β-pleated
sheet (amyloid) fibril formation. Tentative concepts such as the "amyloidogenic protein precursor of the fibril," "proteolysis as one mechanism
of fibril formation," "Congo red birefringence as a marker for the twisted
β-pleated sheet protein" are now substantiated by recurring confirmation.
Even a prophylactic treatment for one of the amyloidotic conditions, familial Mediterranean fever, is now available. Predictably, as the pathogeneses
of the amyloid diseases are individually deciphered, highly specific and directed therapies will evolve to treat their devastated victims.

Amyloidosis is no longer an exotic mystery wrapped in a conundrum, but
rather a substantive source of information in defining the underlying causative abnormality in a variety of disease states. It is no longer the dark
tunnel of knowledge, but rather the light at the end.

Under the best of circumstances, to organize an International Symposium
of this diversity and magnitude requires energy and determination. It is,
however, not often that it also requires courage. It is therefore appro-

priate to acknowledge herein the intrepid fortitude in the face of debil-
itating illness that has characterized the Chairman of this Symposium,
Dr. Elliott Osserman, and his supportive family and to whom we all owe this
volume.

George G. Glenner, M.D.
Senior Editor

CONTENTS

A. SAA, AA AND AP PROTEINS

B. EXPERIMENTAL MODELS

C. IN VITRO SYNTHESIS

D. DEGRADING FACTORS

E.   HEREDITARY AND FAMILIAL (AF) AMYLOIDOSIS

H. AGING AND AMYLOIDOSIS

I. CEREBRAL AMYLOIDOSIS AND ALZHEIMER'S DISEASE

A. SAA, AA, AND AP PROTEINS

PROTEIN AA AND ASSOCIATED PROTEINS IN TYPE-AA

AMYLOID SUBSTANCE

Nils Eriksen and Earl P. Benditt

Department of Pathology
University of Washington
Seattle, Washington 98195

ABSTRACT

Type-AA amyloid substance was isolated from human amyloidotic liver by the water-extraction method of Pras. Pellet material collected by 10^5 g centrifugation of the water extracts was dialyzed against water and lyophilized. The lyophilized product was extracted with 6 M urea at pH 3, and the soluble portion was fractionated by passage through a Sephadex G-100 column in the acid-urea solvent. The intact pellet material, the acid-urea-insoluble portion, and the chromatographic fractions were subjected to SDS/polyacrylamide gel electrophoresis, electrotransfer of the electrophoretically resolved samples to nitrocellulose, and subsequent reaction with antibodies to human AA, AP, prealbumin, albumin, fibronectin and kappa and lambda L-chains.

The bulk of the amyloid substance consisted of monomeric AA, and higher-molecular-weight, AA-related entities that survived heating in SDS plus β-mercaptoethanol. AP was found, but in an amount that casts doubt on its essentiality in the structure of the amyloid fibril. Polyclonal IgG and a trace of fibronectin were found, but appeared to be adventitious constituents. ApoSAA (11.5 kD), prealbumin, and albumin were not found. Other, unrecognized constitutents of the pellet material may be necessary for fibril formation.

INTRODUCTION

The existence of different chemical classes of amyloid substance is now generally recognized, each type having a characteristic, major protein. Recent descriptions of amyloid substance are likely to convey the impression that the amyloid fibril is a homopolymer of the characteristic protein, with no requirement for other subunits. Presumably, then, such diverse proteins as AA, IgG light-chain fragments, and prealbumin can aggregte with themselves to produce fibrils that have identical morphological and tinctorial properties. If a pure fibril preparation is attainable, a complete analysis of its composition would test the validity of the idea.

The insolubility of amyloid substance in nondegrading media imposes great difficulty on its purification, if indeed there exists a single entity (e.g., the fibril) that is representative of the whole amyloid deposit. The water-extraction procedure of Pras et al. [1] is probably the most widely used method for isolating fibrils from amyloidotic tissue, but the purity of the product is difficult to assess. Centrifugation combined

3

with gentle washing conditions appears to be the only suitable method of purification available at present. With this limitation in mind, we present here some findings about the composition of a type-AA amyloid substance isolated from human tissue.

MATERIALS AND METHODS

Fibril-rich material was obtained, as previously described [2], from saline-washed amyloidotic liver tissue by serial extraction (5×) with water, differential centrifugation at 70,000 and 100,000 g, suspension of the 10^5 g pellets in water, recentrifugation at 10^5 g, dialysis against water, and lyophilization.

Samples of lyophilized 10^5 g pellet material from the 2nd, 3rd, and 4th water extractions were pooled, then extracted overnight at 4°C with 6 M urea△0.01 M HCOONa/HCOOH, pH 3.0. The suspension in acid-urea was centrifuged for 30 min at 35,000 g and the clarified extract was passed through a Sephadex G-100 column in the acid-urea medium. The acid-urea-insoluble material was washed twice more by centrifugation with acid-urea, suspended in water, dialyzed against water, and lyophilized.

Pooled effluent fractions representing the four components separated by the Sephadex G-100 chromatography were dialyzed against distilled water and lyophilized. Lyophilized material from the major component (peak IV) was dissolved in acetic acid at pH 3.3 and passed through a Sephadex G-50 column in 0.05 M acetic acid. A pool of fractions representing the rechromatographed peak IV material was titrated with 5 M NaOH to incipient precipitation (pH 5.3), dialyzed against distilled water, and lyophilized.

Samples of lyophilized 10^5 g pellet material and its acid-urea-insoluble and chromatographically separated fractions were examined by electrophoresis in 11% acrylamide/SDS/urea slab gels as previously described [3]. Before application to the gel, samples were heated for 2 min at 100°C with sufficient sample buffer to provide a several-fold excess of SDS over protein. When reduction of samples was desired, β-mercaptoethanol was added (5% v/v) to the sample buffer before heating. Gels were stained with 0.25% Coomassie blue R-250.

Electrophoretically separated constituents were further characterized by electrotransfer to nitrocellulose paper ("Western" blotting) [4] and identification by use of rabbit antisera to human AA, amyloid P component (AP), albumin, prealbumin, fibronectin, and kappa and lambda L-chains, as previously described [3]. The antiserum to human AA was prepared in our laboratory [5] and purified by immunoaffinity chromatography on Sepharose 4 B to which AA was covalently bound. The antiserum to human AP was a gift from Dr. Martha Skinner and the other antisera were from commercial sources. ^{125}I-Staphylococcal protein A was used to detect the antigen/antibody complexes by autoradiography.

RESULTS

The chromatographic profile of the soluble portion (first acid-urea extract) of 400 mg of 10^5 g pellet material in 6 M urea at pH 3 is shown in Fig. 1. An SDS-gel electrophoretic pattern of the whole pellet material is superimposed on the profile, with the respective principal components made to coincide. Electrophoretic bands are seen to coincide approximately with chromatographic peaks II and III. Peaks Ia and Ib are represented by electrophoretic bands too faint to reproduce well and material too large to enter the polyacrylamide gel. The recoveries of lyophilized product repre-

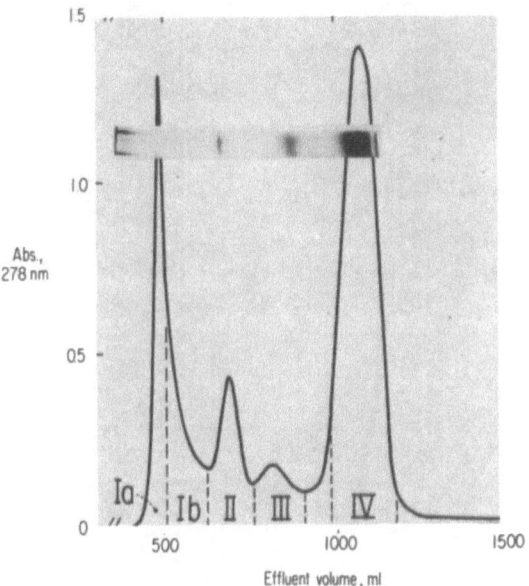

Fig. 1.   Sephadex G-100 chromatography of
          acid-urea extract of amyloid sub-
          stance in 6 M urea/0.01 M HCOONa/
          HCOOH, pH 3.   Column dimensions,
          5 × 88 cm; sample volume, 12 ml;
          flow rate, 47 ml/h.   Overlay:
          SDS-polyacrylamide gel electro-
          phoretic pattern of whole amy-
          loid substance, with principal
          component made to coincide with
          principal chromatographic com-
          ponent.

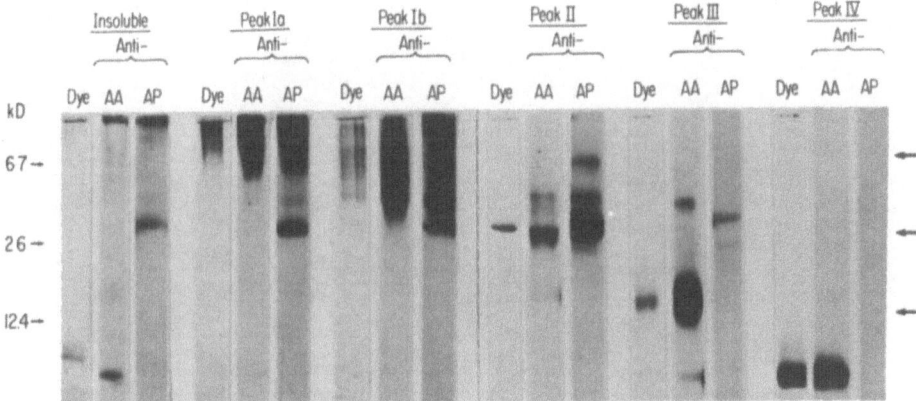

Fig. 2.   SDS/acrylamide gel gelectrophoresis and immunoblotting of
          chromatographic components and acid-urea-insoluble portion of
          amyloid substance.   Sample loadings: ∿10 μg of peaks II,
          III, IV; ∿20 μg of other samples.   Part of reaction at ori-
          gin of samples of peaks Ia and Ib due to IgG (see text and
          Fig. 3).

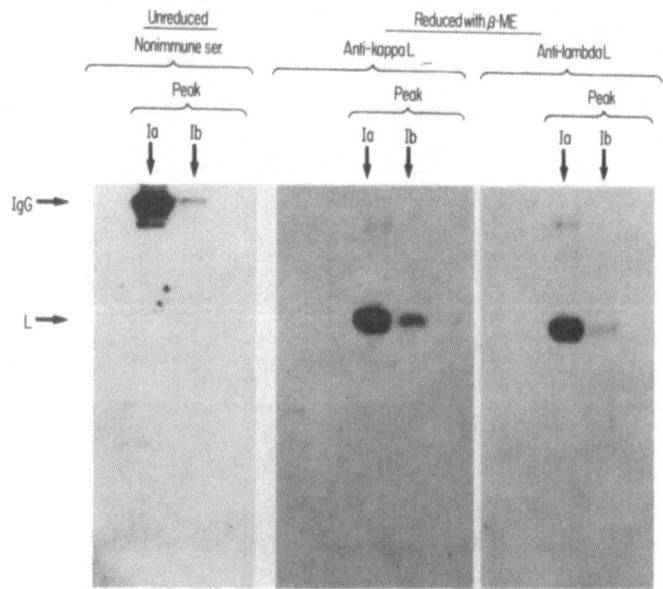

Fig. 3. Immunoblotting of peaks Ia and Ib after SDS/ acrylamide gel electrophoresis, showing L- chains derived from IgG by reduction with β-mercaptoethanol. Samples loadings: ∿20 μg.

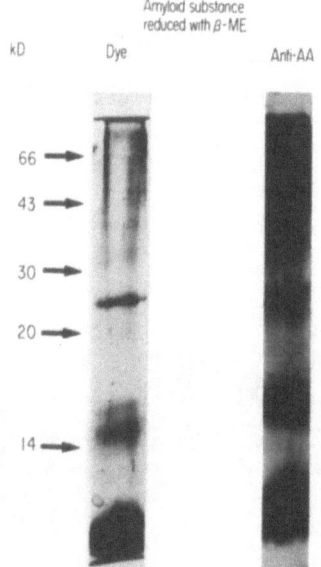

Fig. 4. SDS/acrylamide gel electrophoresis and immunoblotting of whole amyloid sub- stance reduced with β-mercaptoethanol. Sample loadings: ∿50 μg.

TABLE 1. Immunological Identification of Constituents in Fractions of Amyloid Substance (Qualitative; boxed + indicates main location)

Constituent	Insol.	Peak Ia	Peak Ib	Peak II	Peak III	Peak IV
AA	+	+			+	[+]
"(AA)$_2$"	+				[+]	
"(AA)$_3$"	+	+	+	[+]		
"(AA)$_x$"	+	+	[+]			
AP	+	+	+	[+]	+	
IgG		[+]	+			
Fibronectin		tr.				

Albumin and prealbumin sought but not found.
No indication of apoSAA (11.5 kD) in peak III.

senting chromatographic components Ia, Ib, II, III, and IV (rechromatographed) were 33, 23, 20, 11, and 52 mg, respectively. The lyophilized acid-urea-insoluble portion of the starting material weighed 153 mg.

Examples of SDS-gel electrophoretic patterns and corresponding immunological identification of the 10^5 g-pellet fractions are shown in Fig. 2. Peak IV consists almost exclusively of the 8.5-kilodalton (kD) protein AA. The principal constituent of peak III has the earmarks of an AA dimer, exceeding in size the 11.5-kD apoSAA [6]. Peak II is a mixture of protein AP and what could be a trimer of AA; the dye-binding capacity of this putative trimer is weak, but its reaction with anti-AA is relatively intense. Peaks Ia and Ib and the insoluble fraction are quite heterogeneous, but all show immunoreactivity against anti-AA and anti-AP. IgG was detected in peak Ia, and to a slight extent in peak Ib, without recourse to any immunoreaction, simply by the interaction between the Fc portion and staphylococcal protein A. Kappa and lambda L-chains were detected in these peaks after reduction of samples with β-mercaptoethanol (Fig. 3). A trace of fibronectin was detected in peak Ia, but albumin and prealbumin were not detected in any of the fractions. The immunological identifications are summarized in Table 1.

Figure 4 shows an SDS-gel electrophoretic pattern and the corresponding AA-immunoreactivity of a sample of 10^5 g-pellet material reduced with β-mercaptoethanol in SDS-containing sample buffer. In spite of this usually effective combination of degrading agents, the distribution of higher-molecular-weight entities with AA-immunoreactivity was similar to that shown by the unreduced samples of the chromatographic fractions.

The effect of extraction with EDTA on the SGS-gel electrophoretic pattern and AP-immunoreactivity of the 10^5 g-pellet material is shown in Fig. 5. A 2.5% suspension of the material in 0.05 M Na$_2$EDTA/0.01 M Tris, pH 8.0, was stirred for 6 h at 5°C and centrifuged at 1500 rpm. The pellet was resuspended in the initial volume of EDTA solution, stirred for 16 h, centrifuged, washed by centrifugation with 0.1 volume of water, and compared with a non-extracted sample by the electrophoresis/immunoblotting technique. According to the amount of dye bound, all components appeared to be diminished after extraction with EDTA, but densitometric scanning of the stained gel patterns revealed that the AA and AP monomers were diminished relatively more than the other components. The mole ratio of AP to

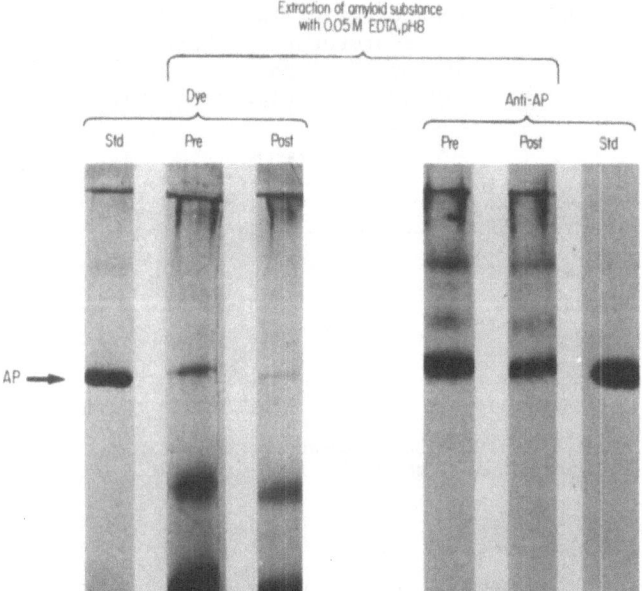

Fig. 5. SDS/acrylamide gel electrophoresis and immunoblotting of whole amyloid substance before (Pre) and after (Post) extraction with
EDTA. Standard is AP prepared by ion-exchange chromatography of pH-8 extract of
saline-washed amyloidotic liver. Sample
loadings: standard, ∿10 μg; preextraction
amyloid substance, ∿50 μg; post-extraction
amyloid substance, residue of 50 μg amyloid
substance after EDTA extraction.

AA estimated from dye binding was approximately 0.03 before and after extraction. This figure is probably an over-estimate because in the system
used AP is not completely resolved from the aforementioned component that
could be an AA trimer.

DISCUSSION

The most prominent constituent of the amyloid substance described
herein is monomeric AA. Other AA-immunoreactive constituents, whether
homologs, multimers, or heteropolymers of AA, contribute substantially to
the total amount of material. Some of the AA-immunoreactive constituents
of molecular mass 17 kD or greater may represent AA multimers or heteropolymers covalently bound, for example, by ε-(γ-glutamyl)lysyl linkages, as
in fibrin [7]. Such elements could stabilize the fibrils and account for
their resistance to degradation. From the results of studies on bovine
AA-type amyloid fibrils, it has been concluded that non-AA proteins are required for the spontaneous formation of AA amyloid fibrils [8]. The necessary structural element was found in a mixture of 19- and 23-kD proteins
that showed no immunological relationship to AA; curiously, the amino acid
composition of this mixture was strikingly similar to that of bovine AA
(about 10 kD). Our peak III material (∿17 kD) has an amino acid composition

closely resembling that of AA [9] and an N-terminal sequence, determined through 30 residues, identical to that of AA (L. H. Ericsson and K. A. Walsh, unpublished data).

The consistent occurrence of AP in amyloid deposits suggests that it could be an essential part of the fibril structure. Hock et al. [10] found that about 20% of the total protein in a fibril preparation from a case of primary amyloidosis was a protein homologous with AP, and that this protein was released only after dissociation and reduction of the fibrils in 6 M guanidine/0.001 M EDTA/0.1 M dithiothreitol; this close association was considered strong evidence that AP is an integral part of the amyloid substance. A contrary view has been taken by Skinner et al. [11], who found that an isolation procedure for amyloid fibrils which uses a mild calcium-chelating buffer (0.05 M sodium citrate in Tris-buffered saline, pH 8.0) completely frees the fibrils (type AL or type AA) of AP; how rigorously the fibrils were examined for residual AP was not stated. We found evidence for residual AP in EDTA-extracted amyloid substance, but the amount of monomeric AP that remained, compared to AA on a molar basis, seems inadequate to infer an essential role for AP in fibril formation. We did observe a parallel diminution of AP and AA monomers as a result of the extraction with EDTA, and noted the presence of higher-molecular-weight forms of AP after as well as before extraction. Whether these pieces of evidence, coupled with uncertainties attributable to unequal dye-binding capacities in the densitometric determination of AA and AP, warrant considering AP as an integral part of the fibril is difficult to decide.

No evidence was found for the presence of monoclonal IgG L-chains in any of the chromatographic fractions or the insoluble portion of the amyloid substance. Both kappa and lambda L-chains were detected in peak Ia, and to a slight extent in peak Ib, after reduction of the samples with β-mercaptoethanol. We conclude that polyclonal IgG was present adventitiously in the amyloid substance.

It has been suggested that amyloid fibrils are complexes of a variety of macromolecules, including the characteristic protein (e.g., AA or AL), fibronectin, and a noncollagenous component of reticulin [12]. The trace of fibronectin that we detected in our peak Ia appears to us to have been adventitous, but we recognize that substances for which we did not test (e.g., other proteins, carbohydrate, lipid, nucleic acid) may be present, although probably not in large amounts. If type-AA amyloid fibrils are composed exclusively of AA and its homopolymers, the amino acid compositions of the fibrils and AA should be identical. In fact, the amino acid compositions of the amyloid substance described herein and of its chromatographic components Ia, Ib, and II, although showing the flavor of AA, differ significantly from the amino acid composition of AA [9]. It follows that other proteins are present, either as essential ingredients or as contaminants.

The problem of determining the composition of amyloid fibrils can be approached in two ways. One is by analysis, as we and others have attempted, but the difficulty of this approach is in ascertaining the purity of the preparation being analyzed. The other is by formation of fibrils from basic ingredients. Such an attempt has been made with fragments of Bence Jones proteins [13]. The results obtained are suggestive but not entirely convincing evidence that a single protein can make authentic amyloid fibrils. The nagging question remains: Is there another ingredient required in the formation of the fibrils, e.g., a central core or framework? A model might be the RNA filament found in tobacco mosaic virus [14]. An analogous structural element in combination with a particular form of the major protein could be what is required for the creation of the true amyloid fibril. Other combinations of molecules can be envisioned that could enter into or condition the native structure of amyloid fibrils.

REFERENCES

1. M. Pras, M. Schubert, D. Zucker-Franklin, A. Rimon, and E. C. Franklin, J. Clin. Invest., 47, 924 (1968).
2. E. P. Benditt and N. Eriksen, Am. J. Pathol., 65, 231 (1971).
3. N. Eriksen and E. P. Benditt, Clin. Chim. Acta, 140, 139 (1984).
4. W. N. Burnette, Anal. Biochem., 112, 195 (1981).
5. E. P. Benditt and N. Eriksen, Proc. Natl. Acad. Sci. U.S.A., 74, 4025 (1977).
6. N. Eriksen and E. P. Benditt, Proc. Natl. Acad. Sci. U.S.A., 77, 6860 (1980).
7. J. J. Pisano, J. S. Finlayson, and M. J. Peyton, Biochemistry, 8, 871 (1969).
8. P. R. Hol, J. P. M. Langeveld, E. W. van Beuningen-Jansen, J. H. Veerkamp, and E. Gruys, Scand. J. Immunol., 20, 53 (1984).
9. E. P. Benditt and N. Eriksen, Lab. Invest., 26, 615 (1972).
10. M. Holck, G. Husby, K. Sletten, and J. B. Natvig, Scand. J. Immunol., 10, 55 (1979).
11. M. Skinner, T. Shirahama, A. S. Cohen, and C. L. Deal, Prep. Biochem., 12, 461 (1983).
12. D. L. Scott, G. Marhaug, and G. Husby, Clin. Exp. Immunol., 52, 693 (1983).
13. G. G. Glenner, D. Ein, E. D. Eanes, H. A. Bladen, W. Terry, and D. L. Page, Science, 174, 712 (1971).
14. A. Klug, Fed. Proc., 31, 30 (1972).
15. This work was supported by National Institutes of Health Grant HL-03174.

HETEROGENEITY OF HUMAN AMYLOID PROTEIN AA AND SAA

B. Skogen,* K. Sletten,†
T. Lea*, and J. B. Natvig*

*Institute of Immunology and Rheumatology
 Rikshospitalet
 The National Hospital, and

†Department of Biochemistry
 University of Oslo
 Oslo, Norway

ABSTRACT

The heterogeneity of SAA and AA was studied. Both proteins could be separated into several fractions by ion exchange chromatography. Amino acid analysis of the ion exchange chromatographed fractions of AA showed that the main difference was in the length of the polypeptide. Thus, it seems as the original AA preparation consists of a mixture of AA proteins with length ranging from 66 to 78 amino acid residues. Although AA seems to be as heterogeneous as SAA, it is not excluded that AA may be derived from one or a restricted number of SAA forms. The molecular weight heterogeneity of AA and the possibility of deamidation of asparagine residues may explain that one SAA variant can be transformed to a heterogeneous mixture of AA proteins.

INTRODUCTION

The amyloid protein AA usually has a molecular weight of about 8600 dalton [1]. However, some patients have amyloid AA proteins with lower molecular weight, and in one patient an AA protein with a molecular weight of 13000 dalton has been found [2, 3, 4]. Also within the same patient molecular weight heterogeneity of the AA protein has been observed [4]. In most AA preparations sequenced, a part of the protein lack arginine in position 1 and starts with serine [4, 5, 6]. A microheterogeneity in the C-terminal region has also been observed in amyloid preparations [1]. By amino acid sequence analysis of mouse AA, isoleucine was found in position 6, whereas both valine and isoleucine were identified at the same position in SAA [7, 8, 9]. In subsequent studies with ion exchange chromatography, several forms of SAA have been identified [10, 11]. In this investigation the heterogeneity of both SAA and AA was studied.

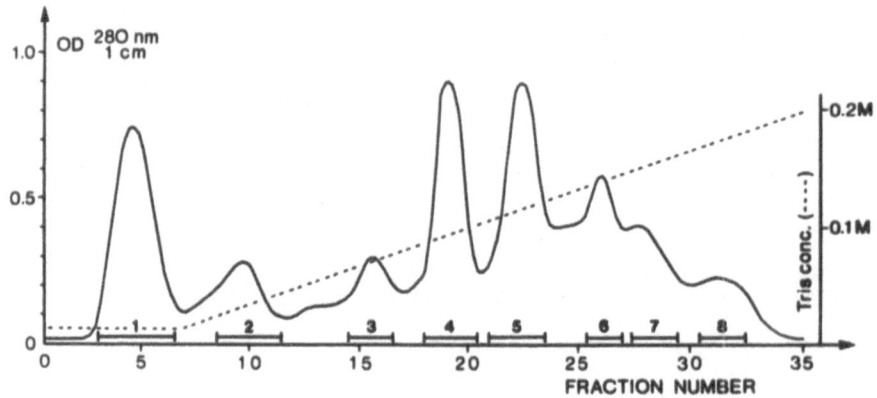

Fig. 1. Ion exchange chromatography of purified protein SAA. The solid lines show the pooled fractions analyzed in DI and SDS-PAGE. The broken line shows the Tris gradient.

MATERIALS AND METHODS

Isolation of SAA and AA

Protein SAA-containing sera from two theumatoid arthritis patients were pooled, and SAA was isolated by gel filtration in 10% formic acid [12]. Protein AA was isolated from water extracted fibrils by gel filtration on Sepharose CL 4 B under dissociating conditions [13, 14].

Ion Exchange Chromatography

Isolated SAA or AA was dissolved in 0.01 M Tris-HCl buffer, pH 8.2, with 6 M urea, and applied to DEAE-Sephacel (Pharmacia AB, Uppsala, Sweden) equilibrated with the same buffer. A 300 ml linear gradient, 0.01 M-0.2 M Tris-HCl, pH 8.2, with 6 M urea, was used to elute the proteins [10]. The proteins were desalted by passing through Sephadex G 25 equilibrated with 10% formic acid.

Double Immunodiffusion (DI)

DI was performed in 1% agarose gel in 0.025 M barbital buffer, pH 8.6. Anti-human SAA was raised in sheep [15]. In DI the antiserum gives a reaction of complete identity between SAA and AA. Isolated SAA and AA was dissolved in 0.1 M NaHCO$_3$, pH 8.3, at a concentration of 1 mg/ml and used as controls.

Sodium Dodecyl Sulfate-Polyacrylamide Gel Electrophoresis (SDS-PAGE)

SDS-PAGE of proteins was performed as described [16]. For DI analysis of proteins in polyacrylamide gels, these were washed for 30 min in PBS, 1 mm slices were cut and placed on glass plates, and 1% agarose was poured onto the glas plates around the gel slices.

Enzymatic Degradation of SAA

SAA from three of the peaks obtained in ion exchange chromatography was desalted, lyophilized and dissolved in 0.1 M NaHCO$_3$, at a concentration of 1.0 mg/ml. Kallikrein (K-8000, Sigma Chemical Co., St. Louis, Mo., USA) from porcine pancreas was dissolved in PBS at 10 micrograms/ml. SAA and enzyme were mixed at a weight ratio 100:1, incubated at 37°C for 20 min, and subjected to SDS-PAGE [17].

Amino Acid Analysis

Amino acid composition of the proteins was determined on 24 h acid hydrolysates as otherwise described [1]. N-terminal analysis was performed in an automatic sequence analyzer, JAS-47K [18]. C-terminal was made by digesting the protein with carboxypeptidase A and B [18]. As test samples, peptides C-2 and T-(5 + 6) obtained from AA were used [1].

RESULTS

Ion Exchange Chromatography of SAA

Purified SAA was subjected to ion exchange chromatography. The protein was eluted in several peaks (Fig. 1). The recovery was about 60%. Fractions of the eluted protein were pooled as indicated by horizontal bars. DI analysis showed that SAA was present in all eight fractions. SDS-PAGE of the protein was also compatible with the presence of SAA in each fraction. No material reacting with the anti-SAA antiserum was eluted from the column after increasing the Tris concentration in the eluant to 0.4 M.

Digestion of SAA with Kallikrein

SAA from the ion exchange chromatography fractions 4-6 was degraded with kallikrein. SDS-PAGE of the incubated protein solutions showed that SAA from all three fractions was transformed to fragments with molecular weight similar to AA. DI analysis showed that the degradation fragments of SAA in fractions 4-6 reacted as identical to AA.

Characterization of Purified AA

Amyloid fibrils were solubilized in 8 M urea and gel filtered under dissociating conditions (Fig. 2). The eluted AA protein was pooled in two main fractions, I and II. SDS-PAGE showed that the protein in fraction I migrated as one single band, whereas the protein in fraction II gave two distinct bands. In addition to the protein with mobility similar to the single band in fraction I, fraction II also contained a band with lower mobility. The molecular weight of this additional protein was about 10000 dalton. DI analysis of the proteins fractionated in SDS-PAGE was performed. Both proteins in fraction II reacted with the antiserum to AA, as did the protein in fraction I. All three proteins showed reactions of complete identity with AA. N-terminal analyses of the purified protein AA resulted in a rather low yield, but the sequence of the first six residues confirmed that of protein AA, and showed that about 90% of the polypeptides started with arginine and about 10% with serine.

Ion Exchange Chromatography of AA

Purified AA was fractionated in several peaks when subjected to ion exchange chromatography (Fig. 3). The recovery was about 70%. The fractions were pooled as indicated by the horizontal bars. DI analysis and SDS-PAGE showed that AA was present in all the pooled fractions.

Amino Acid Analyses of AA Subfractions

Amino acid composition of the subfractions, together with that of protein AA [1] is shown in Table 1. Fraction 1 seems to be a rather inhomogeneous fraction that contained threonine and a higher content of leu-

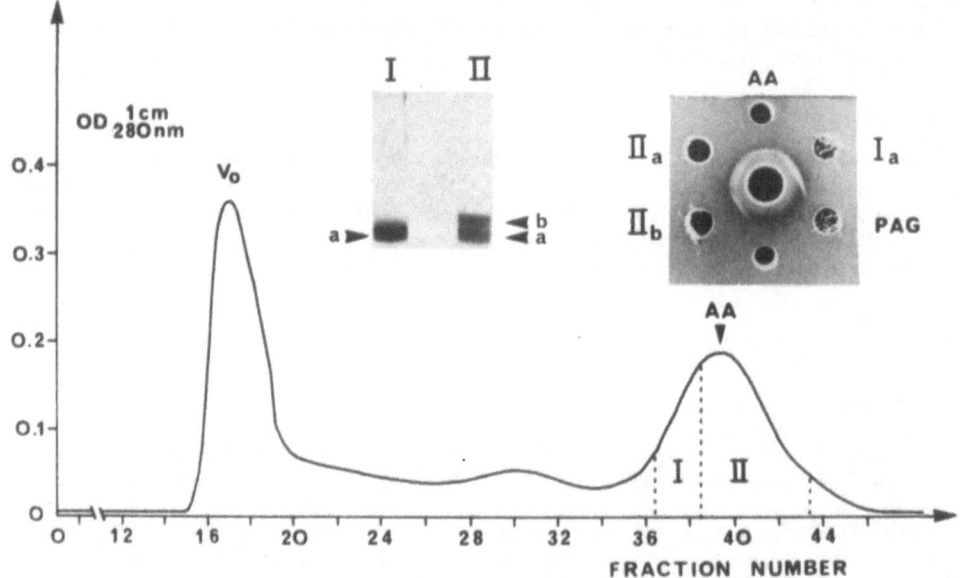

Fig. 2. Gel filtration of amyloid proteins on a Sepharose CL 6 B column equilibrated with 0.01 M Tris-HCl buffer, pH 8.6, containing 8 M urea and 1 mM Na₂-EDTA. The elution position of protein AA is indicated by an arrow. The AA protein was collected in two main fractions, I and II. The figure also shows the polyacrylamide gels after electrophoresis of AA-fractions I and II. Results from double immunodiffusion analysis of proteins in gel slices corresponding to the bands I_a, II_a, and II_b are shown. Protein AA was used as positive control, and polyacrylamide gel without protein (PAG) as negative control.

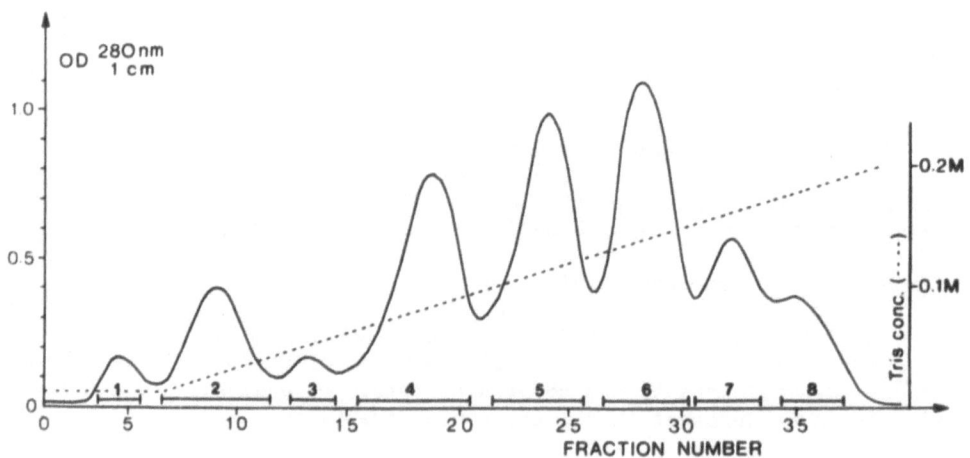

Fig. 3. Ion exchange chromatography of purified protein AA (A pool of Fraction I and II in Fig. 1). The solid lines show the pooled fractions analyzed in DI and SDS-PAGE. The broken line shows the Tris gradient.

TABLE 1. Amino Acid Composition of Fractions Obtained after Ion Exchange Chromatography of Protein AA. Residue Numbers in Parentheses are Those According to the Sequence [1]. ND: Not determined.

Residues per molecule

	Fr.1	Fr.2	Fr.3	Fr.4	Fr.5	Fr.6	Fr.7	Fr.8	Protein AA(1)
Aspartic acid	6.2	9.1(9)	10.0(10)	9.1(9)	10.3(10)	10.0(10)	10.0(10)	10.0(10)	(10)
Threonine	0.8	0.2(0)	0.3(0)	0.1(0)	0.1(0)	0.1(0)	0.1(0)	0.2(0)	(0)
Serine	3.6	4.9(5)	5.0(5-6)	4.6(5)	5.1(5-6)	5.6(5-6)	4.6(5)	4.8(5)	(6)
Glutamic acid	5.7	5.6(6)	7.6(6)	5.7(5)	6.7(7)	6.5(6)	6.3(6)	7.4(6)	(6)
Proline	1.5	1.1(1)	1.1(1)	1.1(1)	0.9(1)	0.9(1)	0.9(1)	1.0(1)	(1)
Glycine	7.0	8.7(9)	9.3(9)	7.7(7)	8.8(9)	8.5(9)	8.2(9)	8.3(9)	(9)
Alanine	7.6	12.9(12)	13.3(13)	12.1(11)	12.8(12)	12.8(12)	12.3(12)	11.6(12)	(12)
Valine	1.6	1.3(1)	1.4(1)	1.1(1)	1.1(1)	1.2(1)	1.3(1)	1.0(1)	(1)
Methionine	1.1	1.9(2)	1.8(2)	1.9(2)	2.9(2)	2.0(2)	1.9(2)	1.8(2)	(2)
Isoleucine	1.7	2.8(3)	3.2(3)	2.3(3)	2.7(3)	2.9(3)	2.9(3)	2.9(3)	(3)
Leucine	2.0	1.2(1)	1.8(2)	1.2(1)	1.3(1)	1.1(1)	1.2(1)	1.3(1)	(1)
Tyrosine	2.2	3.9(4)	4.2(4)	3.7(4)	3.9(4)	3.7(4)	3.6(4)	3.4(4)	(4)
Phenylalanine	3.5	6.0(7)	6.8(7)	5.5(5)	6.4(7)	6.4(7)	6.1(7)	5.9(7)	(7)
Histidine	0.8	1.2(2)	1.5(2)	1.1(1)	1.4(2)	1.4(2)	1.4(2)	1.3(2)	(2)
Lysine	2.1	2.0(2)	1.7(2)	1.8(2)	1.8(2)	1.4(2)	1.4(2)	1.3(2)	(2)
Tryptophan	ND	ND	ND	ND	ND	ND	ND	ND	
Arginine	4.9	7.3(7-8)	8.4(8)	6.8(7)	7.5(8)	7.4(8)	6.9(7)	6.6(7)	(8)
Positions		1-75	1-78	1-66	1-76	1-76	2-75	2-75	1-76

		52				57	58	Ref.

Human SAA:　$-^{Ala}_{Val}$-Trp-Ala-Ala-Glu-$^{Val}_{Ala}$-$^{Ile}_{Leu}$-　(20)

Human SAA:　-Ala-Trp-Ala-Ala-Glu-Val-Ile-　(24)

Human SAA:　-Val-Trp-Ala-Ala-Glu-Ala-Ile-　(24)

Human AA:　-Ala-$^{Trp}_{Arg}$-Ala-Ala-Glu-Val-Ile-　(22)

Human AA:　-Val-Trp-Ala-Ala-Glu-Ala-Ile-　(1)

Human AA:　-Val-Trp-Ala-Ala-Glu-Ala-Ile-　(4)

Human AA:　$-^{Val}_{Ala}$-$^{Trp}_{Arg}$-Ala-Ala-Glu-Ala-Ile-　(21)

Fig. 4.　Partial amino acid sequence of human SAA and AA
proteins. Isoleucine and leucine are found at
position 58 in SAA, whereas only isoleucine is
present at the same position in AA.

cine than other proteins so far analyzed. However, the protein material in
this peak amounted to less than 5% of the total yield. Fraction 2 has an
amino acid composition almost identical to protein AA, and six steps of
Edman degradation revealed Arg-Ser-Phe-Phe-Ser-Phe as the N-terminal sequence. Fraction 3 gave a N-terminal sequence identical to Fraction 2.
However, the amino acid composition showed that this protein AA seemed to
consist of 78 residues. Fraction 4 has an amino acid composition almost
identical to the residues 1 through 66 of protein AA. This was confirmed
by an N-terminal sequence of Arg-Ser-Phe-Phe-Ser-Phe and a C-terminal sequence of Ile-Gln-Arg. Both Fractions 5 and 6 have an amino acid composition almost identical to protein AA consisting of 76 residues. N-terminal
analyses revealed that the protein in both fractions started with Arg-Ser-
Phe-Phe-Ser-Phe. Fractions 7 and 8 have very similar amino acid composition and compared to protein AA seemed to consist of residues 2 through 75.
This was also confirmed by N-terminal analyses of Fraction 7 which showed
that the main part of the protein started with Ser-Phe-Phe-Ser-Phe-Leu, but
that a smaller amount started with arginine.

DISCUSSION

Heterogeneity in the N-terminal region of SAA has been observed.
Anders et al., found that mouse SAA had either valine or isoleucine at position 6, whereas the corresponding AA protein had only isoleucine [7, 8].
This might indicate that only a selected population of several different
SAA proteins can be transformed to AA and deposited as fibrils. Recently
it has been shown by several investigators that SAA can be separated into
several fractions by ion exchange chromatography [10, 11]. In our study
pooled human SAA was separated in at least eight fractions by the same
method. Individual differences between the SAA proteins from different
patients might explain some of the heterogeneity, but can not account for
all SAA variants, as SAA protein from only two patients was pooled. The
presence of other proteins in some of the ion exchange chromatography fractions of SAA has been described [11]. This "contamination" is expected to
be very small [7, 12], and does not influence our results, as we have
shown that all chromatographic fractions react with antiserum to SAA. SAA
from three of those fractions was subjected to proteolytic degradation with
kallikrein. Sufficient material was not present to do a kinetic study of

the enzymatic activity on SAA. It was, however, observed that by degradation of SAA from the analyzed fractions, a fragment similar to AA in molecular weight and antigenic properties was formed. This might indicate
that the origin of protein AA is not restricted to one form of SAA. Heterogeneity in the length of the polypeptide has been found in the N-terminal
of most AA protein preparations, with either arginine or serine in the first
position, and also in the C-terminal part [4, 5, 6]. Two proteins with different molecular weight have been identified in an amyloid fibril preparation
extracted from a human liver. Both reacted antigenically identical with
protein AA [4]. Essentially the same observation was made in this investigation. In addition to the formerly described 8600 dalton AA protein, our
fibril preparation also contains an AA protein with a molecular weight of
about 10000 daltons. Ion exchange chromatography showed an even higher degree of heterogeneity of protein AA, as at least eight subfractions could
be distinguished. Amino acid analyses of the different subfractions revealed that protein AA consisted of polypeptides varying in length from
about 66 to 78 amino acid residues. Fractions 5 plus 6, and 7 plus 8 seem
to be pairs consisting of 76 and 74 residues, respectively, that were well
separated by the ion exchange chromatography. The charge differences could
in this case be due to deamidated forms of protein AA. The protein contains three asparagine residues in positions 23, 60, and 75, which may be
deamidated [1]. The low content of threonine, which is expected to be absent in the AA protein, indicates that the subfractions of AA has been isolated in a pure form. The results indicate that a microheterogeneity of
protein AA in this case, showed to be less than that observed earlier as
compared to several other sequenced AA proteins [1]. An explanation for
the heterogeneity in the length of the polypeptide is that several enzymes
may attack SAA proteins within a limited area, susceptible to proteolysis,
and depending on the specificity of the enzyme, AA proteins with small differences in molecular weights are formed [15, 17]. This would then be in
accordance with our previous observation that several serine proteases are
able to transform SAA to fragments with molecular weights very similar to
AA [17]. Recently it was found that the AA protein is homogeneous in size,
as judged from gel filtration, polyacrylamide gel electrophoresis and amino
acid composition [19]. Based on this observation, and the observation that
AA consists of several proteins with different isoelectric points, it was
concluded that AA is probably not derived from one or a restricted number
of the different SAA forms. From our analysis of the AA protein, we can
not draw the same conclusion, as evidence for a molecular weight heterogeneity of AA was obtained from both SDS-PAGE and amino acids analysis.
This, in addition to the possibility of deamidation of asparagine residues,
do not exclude the probability that AA may be derived from a very restricted number of SAA forms. By amino acid sequence analysis of human SAA from
two individuals, Sletten et al., found heterogeneity at three positions,
52, 57, and 58 [20]. Both valine and alanine were detected at positions
52 and 57. At position 58 leucine and isoleucine were found in both SAA
preparations. This is interesting as in all human AA proteins sequenced,
only isoleucine is found at this position [1, 4, 21, 22]. This might mean
that only those SAA variants with isoleucine in position 58 are incorporated in amyloid fibrils. Isoleucine is supposed to be a "helix breaker"
because of the methyl group in beta position [23]. Therefore the SAA variant with isoleucine may have a different tertiary structure that makes it
more amyloidogenic. As to the heterogeneities at positions 52 and 57, it
seems as alanine in one position is associated with valine in the other,
and both variants occur in AA proteins. A similar alanine-valine association was found by Parmelee and coworkers in a human SAA protein [24]. In
the sequence of this SAA protein only isoleucine was found at position 58.
This protein was, however, a pure apoSAA$_1$ preparation, whereas the SAA
preparation sequenced by Sletten's group consisted if at least two of the
most abundant SAA variants. Further work is in progress to find out whether
one or a few SAA variants are more amyloidogenic than others.

REFERENCES

1. Sletten, K., and Husby, G., Eur. J. Biochem., 41, 117 (1974).
2. Ein, D., Kimura, S., Terry, W. D., Magnotta, J., and Glenner, G. G., J. Biol. Chem., 247, 5653 (1972).
3. Isobe, T., Husby, G., and Sletten, K., in: Amyloid and Amyloidosis, (G. G. Glenner, P. P. Costa, and F. de Freitas, eds.), Excerpta Medica. Amsterdam, Oxford, Princeton, pp. 331 (1980).
4. Sletten, K., Husby, G., and Natvig, J. B., Biochem. Biophys. Res. Commun., 69, 19 (1976).
5. Benditt, E. P., Eriksen, N., Hermodsson, M. A., and Ericsson, L. H., FEBS Letters, 19, 169 (1971).
6. Franklin, E. C., Pras, M., Levin, M., and Frangione, B., FEBS Letters, 22, 121 (1972).
7. Anders, R. F., Natvig, J. B., Sletten, K., Husby, G., and Nordstoga, K., J. Immunol., 118, 339 (1977).
8. Hoffman, J. S., Ericsson, L. H., Eriksen, N., Walsh, K. A., and Benditt, E. P., J. Exp. Med., 159, 641 (1984).
9. Gorevic, P. D., Levo, Y., Frangione, B., and Franklin, E. C., J. Immunol., 121, 138 (1978).
10. Bausserman, L. L., Herbert, P. N., and McAdam, K. P. W. J., J. Exp. Med., 152, 641 (1980).
11. Marhaug, G., and Husby, G., Clin. Exp. Immunol., 45, 97 (1981).
12. Anders, R. F., Natvig, J. B., Michaelsen, T. E., and Husby, G., Scand. J. Immunol., 4, 397 (1975).
13. Harada, M., Isersky, C., Cuatrecasas, P., Page, D., Bladen, H. A., Eanes, E. D., Keiser, H. R., and Glenner, G. G., J. Histochem. Cytochem., 19, 1 (1971).
14. Pras, M., Schubert, M., Zucker-Franklin, D., Rimon, A., and Franklin, E. C., J. Clin. Invest., 47, 924 (1968).
15. Skogen, B., Thorsteinsson, L., and Natvig, J. B., Scand. J. Immunol., 11, 533 (1980).
16. Swank, R. T., and Munkres, K. D., Analyt. Biochem., 39, 462 (1971).
17. Skógen, B., and Natvig, J. B., Scand. J. Immunol., 14, 391 (1981).
18. Sletten, K., Natvig, J. B., Husby, G., and Juul, J., Biochem. J., 195, 561 (1981).
19. Westermark, P., Biochem. Biophys. Acta., 701, 19 (1982).
20. Sletten, K., Marhaug, G., and Husby, G., Hoppe-Seyler's Z. Physiol. Chem., 364, 1039 (1983).
21. Møyner, K., Sletten, K., Husby, G., and Natvig, J. B., Scand. J. Immunol., 11, 549 (1980).
22. Levin, M., Franklin, E. C., Frangione, B., and Pras, M., J. Clin. Invest., 51, 2773 (1972).
23. Dickerson, R. E., and Geis, I., in: The Structure and Action of Proteins, Harper & Row, Publishers, New York—Evanston—London, p. 21 (1969).
24. Parmelee, D. C., Titani, K., Ericsson, L. H., Eriksen, N., Benditt, E. P., and Walsh, K. A., Biochemistry, 21, 3298 (1982).

VASCULAR AA AMYLOIDOSIS IS CHARACTERIZED

BY SPECIAL PROTEIN AA SUBSPECIES

Per Westermark and Gunilla T. Nilsson

Institute of Pathology
University Hospital
S-751 85 Uppsala
Sweden

ABSTRACT

Amyloid protein AA is a mixture of closely related polypeptides which can be separated by their different isoelectric points. Usually AA subspecies with pI 5.1 and 5.5 predominate. In a variant of reactive amyloidosis, in which mainly vessels are affected, the fibrils contain AA variants, with pI 4.6 and 4.9. These are slightly larger than other AA-proteins and diverge from them in amino acid composition. Amyloid fibrils containing these AA-variants have a remarkable resistance to degradation by serum.

INTRODUCTION

Amyloid fibrils in reactive (secondary) amyloidosis consist mainly of a low molecular weight protein AA [1-3]. This protein, which contains about 76 amino acid residues has under certain circumstances in vitro a spontaneous tendency to aggregate in amyloid-like fibrils [4, 5] but the mechanism of fibril formation in vivo is unknown. The amyloid deposition in reactive amyloidosis is believed to be a dynamic event in which not only new amyloid fibrils are formed from the serum precursor serum AA (SAA) but also already deposited fibrils are degraded to a certain extent. Only when fibril formation overwhelms degradation, does amyloidosis occur.

In a previous paper the occurrence of two distinctively different patterns of amyloid deposition in the kidneys was described in reactive (secondary) amyloidosis: one common with deposits in glomeruli and vessels, and one more rare saving the glomeruli but with a extensive infiltration in and around the vessels [6]. The existence of these two patterns has been confirmed by others [7]. Intermediates between these two extremes are common. The gel filtration pattern of amyloid fibrils dissolved in strong denaturing agents differed between the two variants [6]. A double AA peak was typical of cases with the vascular pattern.

The present study shows that each of the two patterns of amyloid deposition is characterized by certain protein AA species, which can be distinguished between their isoelectric points. Some peculiar properties of the fibrils and of protein AA in vascular amyloidosis are also shown.

MATERIAL AND METHODS

Kidney and splenic tissues from patients with systemic amyloidosis in association with rheumatoid arthritis were removed at autopsy and stored at -20°C until used. Tissues from 3 patients with vascular pattern of amyloidosis, 7 patients with glomerular pattern and 5 with mixed pattern were used in this study.

Protein Purification Methods

Amyloid fibrils were extracted with distilled water according to Pras et al. [18]. Amyloid fibrils were defatted, dissolved in 6 M guanidine HCl in 0.1 M Tris HCl buffer, pH 8.0 containing 0.2% EDTA and 0.1 M dithio-threitol. After centrifugation, the dissolved material was gel filtered on a Sepharose 6 B CL (Pharmacia, Uppsala, Sweden) column equilibrated with 8 M urea in 0.01 M sodium citrate buffer, pH 3.0 and eluted with this solution. The protein AA containing fractions were pooled, dialyzed exhaustively against distilled water and lyophilized. The subspecies of protein AA were partially purified by preparative isoelectric focusing as described [9].

Protein Analyses

Proteins were analyzed by gradient (10-15%) polyacrylamide gel electrophoresis in the presence of sodium dodecyl sulfate (SDS-PAGE) [10] and by analytic isoelectric focusing [9]. Amino acid analysis was performed after hydrolysis in 6 N HCl at +110°C.

Fibril Degradation

Water extracted fibrils from patients MB, 798, 860, and 182 were suspended in water and mixed with an agarose solution with a final concentration of 0.25% amyloid fibrils in 1% agarose - 0.05 M Tris HCl buffer, pH 7.4 containing 0.15 M NaCl. The mixtures were heated and poured on glass plates in a 1.3 mm thick layer. After cooling, wells with a diameter of 4.4 mm were cut in the agar and filled with serum. Serum from five normal blood donors were tested. The diameter of the lysed area was measured after incubation at room temperature for 18 h.

RESULTS

Gel Filtration

Gel filtration of dissolved amyloid fibrils from patients with the glomerular pattern of kidney amyloidosis resulted in one major retarded peak containing protein AA. This peak was symmetric or slightly asymmetric. When amyloid from tissues with the vascular pattern of amyloidosis, the major retarded AA peak (AA_1) was followed by another but considerably smaller one (AA_2). Gel filtration of amyloid from patients with mixed type of amyloid deposition revealed one clearly asymmetric AA peak.

Electrophoretic Analyses

Analytical isoelectric focusing of protein AA from kidneys with glomerular pattern of amyloid deposits showed major bands at pH 5.1 and 5.5 [9]. AA species with both higher and lower isoelectric points usually occurred. In protein AA_1 of kidneys with vascular amyloid pattern, acidic peptides predominated with major bands at pH 4.6 and 4.9, respectively, while the peptides with pI 5.1 and 5.5 occurred in low concentrations (Fig. 1). In AA_2 more basic peptides predominated.

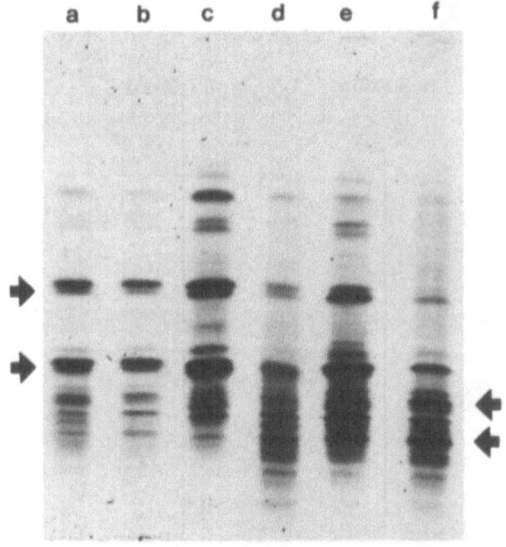

Fig. 1. Analytical isoelectric focusing, pH 3.5-9.5 of protein AA from six different individuals. In case a-c AA-species with pI 5.1 and 5.5 (arrows) predominate. These patients had pronounced glomerular amyloid deposits. In case f, AA-species with pI 4.6 and 4.9 (arrow) occur in high concentration and this patient had predominantly vascular amyloid deposits in the kidneys. In d and e AA from cases with intermediate type of amyloid deposition is shown. Anode is down.

SDS-PAGE of dissolved amyloid fibrils from cases MB (vascular pattern) and 182 (glomerular pattern) is shown in Fig. 2. Protein AA in 182 shows one band while in MB, three AA-bands are seen, two corresponding to AA_1 and one to AA_2. A SAA-like protein is seen only in case 182. Addition of reducing agent to the sample solution resulted in stronger bands indicating that S-S bonds might be of importance for the stability of the fibril. SDS-PAGE of protein AA_1 of the two tested cases MB and 350 showed that this protein consists of the two closely situated bands, both moving a little slower than most other AA proteins and only slightly faster than SAA and the SAA-like amyloid fibril protein [11]. Their estimated molecular weights were 10,000 and 11,000 daltons, respectively.

Further Characterization of AA_1

The subspecies of AA_1 were partially purified by preparative isoelectric focusing (Fig. 3) and the amino acid composition of proteins eluted in peak 1 and peak 2 material are shown in Table 1. The peak 2 material, eluted at pH 4.9 and corresponding to the fast AA_1 band in SDS-PAGE has an amino acid composition comparable with that of SAA [12, 13]. The peak 1 material, eluted at pH 4.6 and corresponding to the slow AA_1 band has a slightly different amino acid composition with considerable amounts of half-cystine.

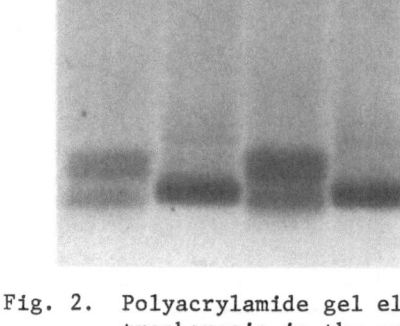

Fig. 2. Polyacrylamide gel elec-
         trophoresis in the pres-
         ence of sodium dodecyl-
         sulfate of patient MB
         with vascular pattern of
         kidney amyloidosis (a,
         c) and patient 182 with
         glomerular pattern of
         kidney amyloidosis (b, d).
         In 182 protein AA shows
         one fast distinct band
         followed by a faint band
         corresponding to the SAA-
         like protein. Protein AA
         of MB consists of three
         bands, one fast moving
         corresponding to AA_2 and
         two slower bands corre-
         sponding to AA_1. In c and
         d dithiothreitol was added
         to the sample solution re-
         sulting in stronger bands
         in both cases but espe-
         cially in MB, indicating
         that disulfide bridges
         might be of importance
         for the stability of the
         AA-fibril.

TABLE 1. Amino Acid Composition of the Two Main Fractions of Protein AA₁ of Patient MB Obtained by Column Isoelectric Focusing (Fig. 3), Compared to a 76 Amino Acid Residues Protein AA (TH) (A). In B, Peak Material, Calculated as Residues/90 Residues (since tryptophan is destroyed), is Compared to SAA₁. Position 2 through 93.

| | A. Residues/100 residues | | | | B. Residues/molecule | |
	Peak 1	Peak 2	TH[1]	SAA[2]	Peak 2	SAA, pos 2 - 93
Asx	12.4	16.6	13.2	13.5	14.8	14
Thr	2.5	0.8	-	-	0.7	-
Ser	7.9	7.0	7.9	6.7	6.2	7
Glx	11.0	9.5	7.9	8.7	8.4	8
Pro	3.2	2.2	1.3	3.8	1.9	2
Gly	11.4	11.4	11.8	11.5	10.1	11
Ala	13.4	16.1	15.8	15.4	14.3	15
1/2 Cys	1.4[3]	0.5[3]	-	-	0.4	-
Val	3.0	1.7	1.3	1.0	1.6	1
Met	2.0[3]	2.4[3]	2.6	1.9	2.1	2
Ile	4.1	3.7	3.9	2.9	3.3	2
Leu	5.0	3.2	1.3	2.9	2.9	3
Tyr	4.4	4.7	5.3	4.8	4.2	4
Phe	6.1	7.5	9.2	7.7	6.7	7
His	2.2	2.2	2.6	2.9	2.0	2
Lys	3.3	2.6	2.6	3.8	2.4	3
Arg	6.8	7.9	10.5	9.6	7.0	8
Trp	ND[4]	ND	2.6	2.9	ND	3

1) Sletten and Husby, 1974 (14)

2) Sletten et al., 1983 (12)

3) Determined in oxidized sample
4) ND = not determined

Protein AA from the Spleen and the Kidney

In 8 individuals, protein AA was purified from both the spleen and the kidney. The analytical isoelectric focusing pattern varied only slightly when AA purified from different tissues in one individual was used and considerably less compared to the pattern of protein AA purified from different patients. Thus, protein AA both from the kidney and the spleen of patient MB who had mainly vascular amyloidosis, was dominated by acidic AA species. However, generally protein AA of the kidney contained slightly less quantities of the more basic (pI > 5.1) AA species.

TABLE 2. The Effect of Serum from Five Normal Blood Donors on Amyloid
Fibrils from Patients with Different Amyloid Deposition Pattern

Amyloid fibrils from patient	Pattern of kidney amyloidosis	Diameter of cleared area in 0.1 mm. Mean $\pm$ SEM
860	glomerular	48.4 ± 2.0
182	glomerular	50.2 ± 1.2
798	intermediate	26.0 ± 1.2
MB	vascular	0.0

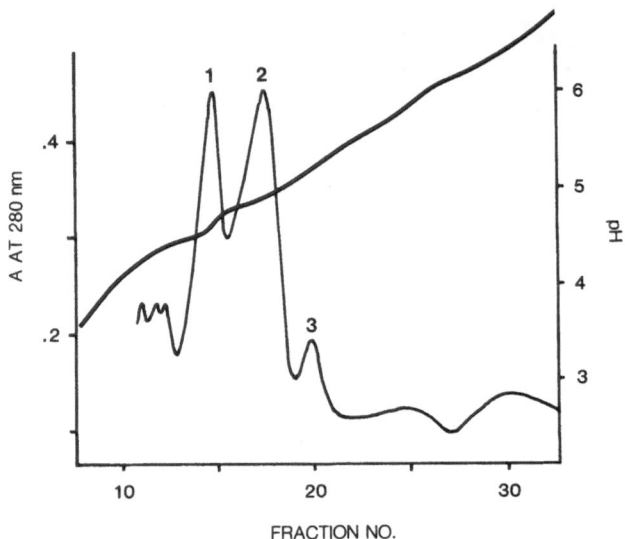

Fig. 3. Elution profile after column isoelectric
focusing of protein AA_1, of patient MB.
Two peaks, eluted at pH 4.6 and 4.9, respectively, predominate.

Fibril Degradation

The results of the degradation in agar gel is shown in Table 2. In
gels containing fibrils from patients 860, 182 (glomerular pattern) and 798
(mixed pattern) an area of lysis occurred around wells containing human
serum. The diameter of this area was significantly smaller in case 798 as
compared to that of the two others. In case MB (vascular pattern), no lysis
at all was seen.

DISCUSSIONS

This study shows that amyloid fibrils in the vascular variant of AA
amyloidosis are dominated by other AA subspecies than found in the common
type of AA amyloidosis. Protein AA is probably formed by an enzymatic
cleavage of a plasma acute phase reactant, the apolipoprotein serum AA (SAA),

of which a C-terminal piece is cut off. A heterogeneous C-terminal in protein AA seems to be formed by varying cleavage points on the SAA molecule, and AA species with length varying between 45 and 83 amino acid residues have been described [2, 3, 14-16], although most protein AA's have been said to consist of 76 residues [3, 14]. Also the N-terminal part of protein AA varies a little, since some of the protein lacks the N-terminal arginine [3, 16, 17]. This N-terminal variability is also seen in SAA [12, 13, 18]. AA_1 in the vascular type of amyloidosis contains at least two AA-forms, which both are larger than most AA-proteins. AA_1 of patient MB has previously been shown to have the N-terminal amino acid sequence Ser-Phe-Phe-Ser [6]. The amino acid composition of the 10 kd AA_1 subspecies reveals that it may correspond to SAA, positions 2-92 [12, 13]. This is the first evidence that variations in amyloid deposition in reactive (AA) amyloidosis are correlated to variations in the cleavage position of SAA. If differences in the amino acid sequence also occurs is unknown. Not only the "pure" vascular type of AA amyloidosis contained the acid and large variant of AA. Similar variants were found in varying amounts also in the mixed type of amyloid infiltration.

Several investigators have shown that amyloid fibrils in reactive amyloidosis can be degraded by human serum [19-21]. The fibril degrading activity is decreased in rheumatoid arthritis [20-21] and in other inflammatory conditions [24]. An inadequate degradation activity has been proposed to contribute in the pathogenesis of reactive amyloidosis and in fact, the most pronounced decrease of the fibril degrading activity is seen in that condition [19-21]. The finding that the amyloid fibrils in the vascular type of reactive amyloidosis are much more resistant to degradation of serum shows that putative important differences in the properties of amyloid fibrils exist within this disease. It seems probable that the fibrils vascular amyloid are less prone to resolution, which has been shown to occur in reactive amyloidosis [22]. A greater lability of the parenchymatous amyloid as compared to the vascular amyloid has in fact been noted histologically on sequential rectal biopsies [23].

REFERENCES

1. E. P. Benditt, N. Eriksen, M. A. Hermodson, and L. H. Ericsson, FEBS Lett., 19, 169 (1971).
2. E. Ein, S. Kimura, and W. D. Terry, J. Biol. Chem., 247, 5653 (1972).
3. M. Levin, E. C. Franklin, B. Frangione, and M. Pras, J. Clin. Invest., 51, 2773 (1972).
4. A. Zuckerberg, J. Gazith, A. Rimon, T. Reshef, and J. Gafni, Eur. J. Biochem., 28, 161 (1972).
5. M. Pras and T. Reshef, Biochim. Biophys. Acta, 271, 193 (1972).
6. P. Westermark, K. Sletten, and M. Eriksson, Lab. Invest., 41, 427 (1979).
7. H. M. Falck, T. Tönroth, and O. Wegelius, Clin. Nephrol., 19, 137 (1983).
8. M. Pras, M. Schubert, D. Zucker-Franklin, A. Rimon, and E. C. Franklin, J. Clin. Invest., 47, 924 (1968).
9. P. Westermark, Biochim. Biophys. Acta, 701, 19 (1982).
10. G. Blobel and B. Dobberstein, J. Cell. Biol., 67, 835 (1975).
11. P. Westermark and K. Sletten, Clin. Exp. Immunol., 49, 725 (1982).
12. K. Sletten, G. Marhaug, and G. Husby, Hoppe-Seyler's Z. Physiol. Chem., 364, 1039 (1983).
13. D. C. Parmelee, K. Titani, L. H. Ericsson, N. Eriksen, E. P. Benditt, and K. A. Walsh, Biochemistry, 21, 3298 (1982).
14. K. Sletten and G. Husby, Eur. J. Biochem., 41, 117 (1974).
15. K. Møyner, K. Sletten, G. Husby, and J. B. Natvig, Scand. J. Immunol., 11, 549 (1980).

16. K. Sletten, G. Husby, and J. B. Natvig, Biochem. Biophys. Res. Commun., 69, 19 (1976).
17. B. Skogen, K. Sletten, T. Lea, and J. B. Natvig, Scand. J. Immunol., 17, 83 (1983).
18. L. L. Bausserman, P. N. Herbert, and K. P. W. J. McAdam, J. Exp. Med., 152, 641 (1980).
19. I. Kedar, M. Ravid, and E. Sohar, in: Amyloid and Amyloidosis (G. G. Glenner, P. P. Costa, and F. de Freitas, eds.), Excerpta Medica, Amsterdam (1968), p. 60.
20. C. P. J. Maury, A.-M. Teppo, and O. Wegelius, in: Amyoidosis E.A.R.S. (C. R. Tribe and P. A. Bacon, eds.), John Wright and Sons, Bristol (1983), pp. 73-76.
21. P. Maddison, P. A. Bacon, A. F. Strachan, and C. R. Tribe, in: Amyloidosis E.A.R.S. (C. R. Tribe and P. A. Bacon, eds.), John Wright and Sons, Bristol (1983), pp. 124-127.
22. H. M. Falck, T. Törnroth, B. Skrifvars, and O. Wegelius, Acta Med. Scand., 205, 651 (1979).
23. C. R. Tribe, P. A. Bacon, and J. C. Mackenzie, in: Amyloidosis E.A.R.S. (C. R. Tribe and P. A. Bacon, eds.), John Wright and Sons, Bristol (1983), pp. 183-186.

ACKNOWLEDGEMENTS

Supported by the Swedish Medical Research Council (Project No. 5941) and the Research Fund of King Gustaf V.

THE PHYSICO-CHEMICAL, ANTIGENIC, AND FUNCTIONAL

HETEROGENEITY OF HUMAN SERUM AMYLOID A

M. E. Martin, C. J. Rosenthal,
and A. Huq

Department of Medicine
Downstate Medical Center-SUNY
450 Clarkson Avenue
Brooklyn, N. Y. 11203

ABSTRACT

In the present study we attempted to develop a rapid method to isolate serum amyloid A isomers (SAA is.) and to determine whether this physico-chemical heterogeneity corresponds to an antigenic and functional one. Pure human low molecular SAA (SAAL) was prepared from the serum of 6 patients (pts.) using standard techniques. Preparative isoelectric focusing in agarose/sephadex gels was used to separate SAAL is. Monoclonal antibodies (m. abs.) to SAAL and to AA were prepared by hybridization of P3XU-1 nonsecretory murine myeloma cells with murine spleen cells from Balb/c mice immunized with pooled SAAL and AA respectively. Four distinctly migrating SAAL isomers with PI's of 4.9, 5.8, 6.6, and 7.2 were isolated from 6 pts. while only three isomers were separated from the pt. with myasthenia gravis. Four m. abs. to SAAL, one to AA, six m. abs. to SAAL-2 is. and one to SAAL-1 is. were generated in murine ascitic fluid. Dishes coated with the four human SAA is., human AA, various mammalian and human proteins as well as with serum from 31 pts. with metastatic Ca. and 23 pts. with inflammatory diseases (ID) were reacted with the m. abs. The amount of binding was determined using ^{125}I labelled goat antimouse serum. The m. abs. to SAA were found specific for human SAA recognizing two different patterns in relationship to the intensity of binding to SAA is. One of them (7A2-43) had a greater affinity for SAA from pts with ID, while the other (5A6-5) reacted stronger with SAA from pts with metastatic Ca. In addition, the m. ab. 7A2-43 consistently blocked SAA suppression of IgG production by human B lymphocytes while three others (4C1-1, 103-1, and 1A1-5) blocked SAA inhibition of EAC rosetting. Thus, it appears that the m. abs. to SAA are able to distinguish at least two antigenically different SAA is. which appear to also have different functions and to circulate in the serum at different levels in distinct pathogenetic states.

INTRODUCTION

Serum Amyloid A (SAA) the precursor of tissue amyloid deposits in patients with Reactive Systemic Amyloidosis (RSA) and Familial Mediteranean Fever (FMF) was found to be heterogeneous at its NH_2 terminus (1, 2, 3) since its early purification as a 12,000 dalton low molecular weight protein by sephadex chromatography in formic acid.

When Benditt and Eriksen [4] discovered that SAA is an apolipoprotein transported in the serum in association with the second subfraction of plasma high density lipoprotein (HDL_2) it was also noted that some of the SAA immunoreactivity was identified in two other fractions indicating again that apo SAA was heterogeneous. In recent studies Hoffman and Benditt [5] found that after delipidation of HDL of plasma from BALB/c mice which recevied intraperitoneal endotoxin two major apo SAA isotypes were separated by isoelectric focusing and two dimensional gel electrophoresis: apo SAA_1 and apo SAA_2, which have close, but distinct, molecular weights and isoelectric points. Four other minor bands were clearly distinguishable by analytical isoelectric focusing only in the serum of mice receiving Salmonella typhosa endotoxin. In parallel studies Bausserman et al. [6] isolated six polymorphic forms of SAA with different electrophoretic mobilities but similar molecular weights. They are obtained by DEAE cellulose chromatography in urea containing buffers after discarding the major HDL apoproteins by molecular sieve chromatography from human serum. Some differences in the NH_2 terminal composition of two of these isomers, SAA_4 and SAA_5, were also noted but no antigenic differences could be found among these six polymorphs. They were all detected by an immunoassay using polyclonal antihuman AA antibody.

In an attempt to better define possible structural and functional differences among these SAA isomers (polymorphs) we decided to produce, in this study, a number of distinct monoclonal antibodies to SAA after mouse immunization with pooled human SAA purified by gel filtration chromatography as well as with two of the four SAA isomers isolated by preparative isoelectric focusing following a rapid technique. Among the monoclonal antibodies produced some were capable of detecting elevation of the SAA level during the acute phase reaction accompanying specific disorders and to block only certain in vitro effects that SAA was found to have on various subpopulations of leukocytes [7].

METHODS

1. Purification of low molecular weight serum amyloid A (SAAL) isomers. Sufficient amounts of SAA were separated from the serum of six patients with high SAA serum levels (above 5 μd/dl); two had metastatic carcinoma of the ovary and breast respectively; three had chronic inflammatory diseases (rheumatoid arthritis, tuberculosis, and chronic osteomyelitis) while the last one had more than two years of myasthenia gravis accompanying a thymoma. After signing appropriate consent these patients underwent plasmapheresis, which permitted the removal of 500 to 1000 ml plasma while an equal amount of fresh frozen plasma was infused back to the patient. SAAL was then purified by molecular sieve chromatography through 2 successive Sephadex columns in 10% formic acid following a method devised by us [8] and others [9]. The chromatographic fractions enriched in SAA and ultimately containing pure SAA were detected by a liquid phase RIA with polyethylene glycol precipitation of the formed immune complexes as previously reported [2]. The purity of the extracted SAAL was tested by SDS polyacrylamide (10%) gel electrophoresis following Weber and Osborn's technique [10].

Analytical isoelectric focusing (IEF) of the pure SAAL was then performed in a flat bed system in a gel composed of 5% polyacrylamide, 10% glycerol and 2.5% carrier ampholytes (pH 3-10) (Pharmacia, Piscataway, N.J.). Two hundred microgram samples of SAAL were applied to the gel surface flanked by markers proteins of known pI (pI Calibration Kit, Pharmacia). Focusing (for approx. 1.7 hr) was performed using 0.04 M aspartic acid as the anolyte and 0.1 M NaOH at the cathode at 30 watts constant power and 2000 volts; the gel was then fixed in 10% TCA and 5% sulfosalicylic acid stained in 0.2% Comassie Brilliant Blue for 3 hours and destained. The pI's of separated proteins were extrapolated from a graph where the distance of migration of marker proteins was plotted against their known pI's.

In order to purify the isomers identified by analytical IEF preparative isoelectric focusing was then performed according to Manrique and Lasky [11]. In brief, 30 mg pure SAAL was incorporated in the gel made of 0.5% agarose, 2.5% sephadex G-200SF and 3% ampholytes. The proteins separated after focusing for 3 hours at 15 watts, 2000 volt-hours, were then detected by the "replica" technique by applying a Whatman IMM paper to the gel surface, which was then stained in 0.2% Comassie Brilliant Blue. Thereafter, following the replica indications the protein bands were excised from the gel, ground to a paste; their content (protein mixed with ampholytes) was extracted in 0.1 M NaCl followed by centrifugation. The amplolytes were then discarded by chromatography in phenyl-Sepharose 4B (Pharmacia).

2. Production of monoclonal antibodies to SAAL and AA. Monoclonal antibodies were produced following a modification [12] of Kohler and Milstein's technique [13].

In brief three Balb/c female mice were immunized with pure SAAL obtained by gel filtration chromatography, AA extracted from the liver of a patient with RSA [14] and two of the SAA isomers obtained by preparative IEF. Two hundred microgram of antigen was injected subcutaneously twice at one week intervals then intraperitoneally; three days later the animals were sacrificed and 2×10^7 cell from their minced spleen was fused with 1×10^8 nonsecretory murine myeloma cells of the P3xU-1 cell line in HAT selective medium [12]. The clones producing antibodies were then selected applying the limiting dilution technique [13]. The reaction of the m. abs. with SAAL or AA as well as with the serum of 31 patients with advanced metastatic carcinoma and 23 patients with chronic or acute inflammatory diseases was detected by a "sandwich" double antibody solid phase RIA [13]. Fifty lambdas of the serum to be tested or of the antigen solution (1 mg/ 1 ml of PBS) were first absorbed into the wells of a 96 well U bottom polyvinyl chloride plate (Falcon Plastics) usually by keeping the plate for 2 h at 37°C. The monoclonal antibody to be tested is added to the wells and kept for 1 h at 37°C then discarded. The plates are washed several times with PBS.

Finally, a radioinated ^{125}I goat F (ab)'$_2$ antimouse gamma globulin serum is added to the wells for 1 h and then discarded. The plates are thoroughly washed, and individual wells counted in a gamma counter.

3. Studies on the impact monoclonal antibodies to SAAL have on some of the effects of SAA on circulating leukocytes. The effect of various monoclonal antibodies to SAA and AA was tested first in in vitro experiments in which partial suppression by SAA of complement mediated sheep red cell rosettes (EAC rosettes) formed by B lymphocytes was previously demonstrated [7]. Various populations of leukocytes were first separated by discontinuous Ficoll-Hypaque gradient centrifugation [15] and ammonium chloride lysis of red cells. EAC rosette formation by lymphocytes was performed according to Bianco et al. [16] in the presence and absence of 1 µg SAA in 10 λ PBS. Each of the m. abs. to SAA was also added (50 λ of undiluted antibody in ascitic form) to the mixture of triplicate chambers containing SAA, and compared to the results of the three chambers to which no monoclonal antibody was added. In other experiments Moretta's technique [17] of separating T suppressor, T helper and B lymphocytes was applied and the effect of m. ab. to SAA and AA on the immunoglobulin production by B lymphocytes was tested, as extensively described in a previous paper [18]. Fifty λ of each of the produced monoclonal antibodies in ascitic form was added

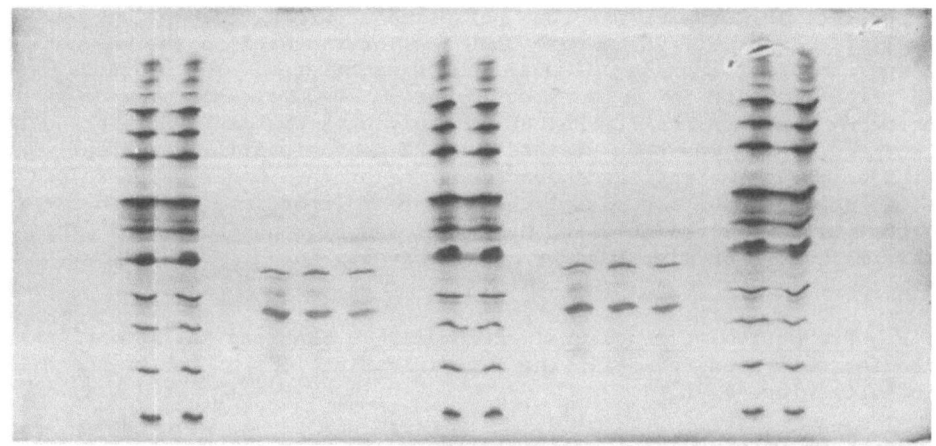

Fig. 1. Analytic isoelectric focusing of SAAL extracted from three patients
with high SAA levels (two with inflammatory diseases and one with
metastatic cancer). The four bands resulting from the repetitive
separation of the three SAAL samples are flanked by bands of
proteins with known pIs serving as markers.

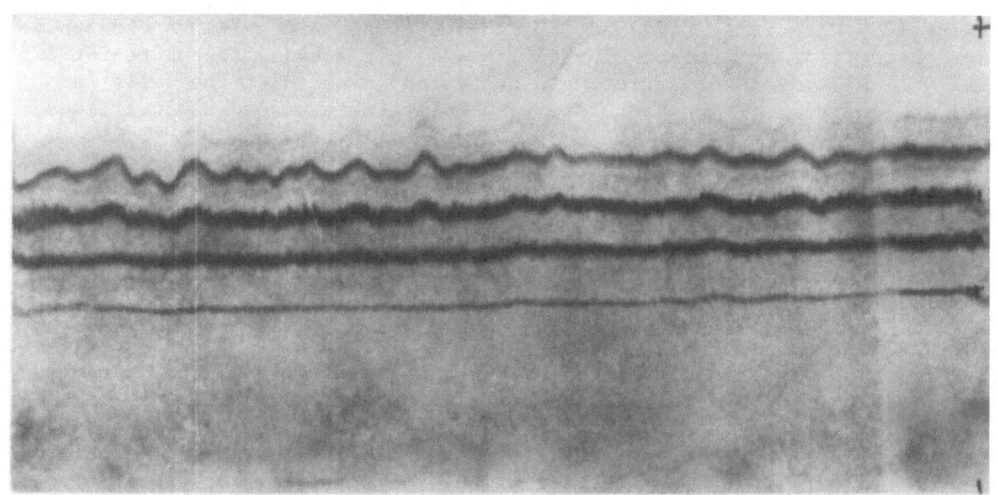

Fig. 2. Preparative isoelectric focusing of SAAL from one of the two cases
with inflammatory diseases in which four isomers were noted by
analytical IEF.

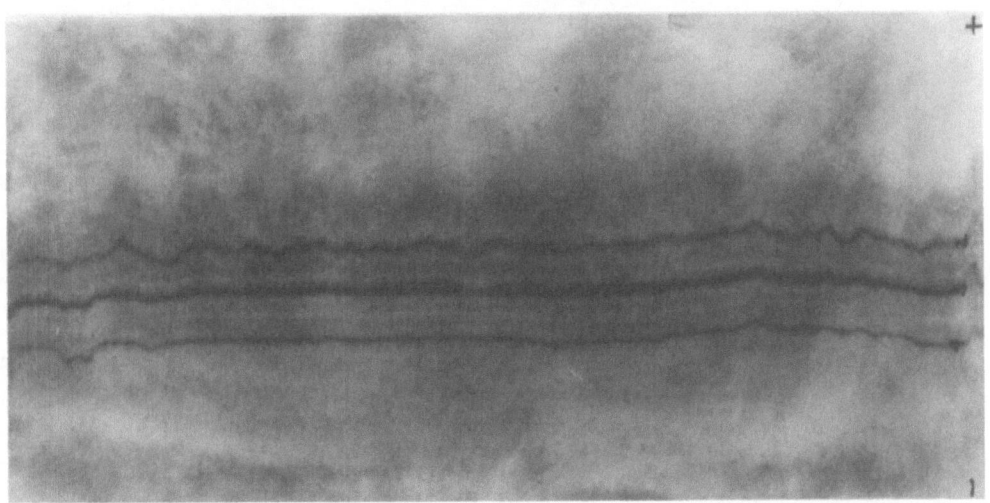

Fig. 3.   Preparative isoelectric focusing of SAAL from a patient with myasthenia gravis and thymoma.

to triplicate cultures containing a mixture of 5×10^5/ml B lymphocytes, 1×10^5/ml Tμ (helper) lymphocytes and 2×10 Tγ suppressor lymphocytes, 10 μg pokeweed mitogen/ml and 1 μg SAA/ml and compared to triplicate cultures with SAA but without anti SAA m. ab. and other triplicate cultures without SAA nor anti-SAA antibody. The amount of polyclonal human immunoglobulin (produced by the PWM-stimulated B lymphocytes) contained in each culture was determined by a "sandwich" RIA using a rabbit antihuman immunoglobulin antibody and a radioiodinated sheep anti-rabbit immunoglobulin anti-serum.

Finally, the binding affinity of m. abs. to SAA and AA to various peripheral human blood leukocytes was tested using an indirect immunofluorescent staining technique [19]. Separated subsets of leukocytes were first incubated with normal mouse serum to block nonspecific binding sites. After washing they were incubated for 30 min at 4°C with the m. ab. to be tested at an optimal dilution (between 1:20 to 1:200). After washing with PBS, pH 7.2 they were incubated with fluorescein conjugated goat antimouse immunoglobulin at dilutions ranging from 1:10 to 1:50.

RESULTS

1. Separation of human SAA isomers. The technique described applied to SAA extraction from six donors showed that the allegedly homogeneous SAA protein (as revealed by SDS-PAGE) resulting from molecular sieve chromatography separation in 10% formic acid consists, in fact, of four molecular species with different isoelectric points of 4.9, 5.8, 6.6, and 7.2 as seen by analytical (Fig. 1) as well as preparative (Fig. 2) isoelectric focusing of five of the six SAAL preparations we separated. The sixth SAA extracted from the patient with myasthenia gravis consistently gave only three isomers (Fig. 3) by IEF (the SAAL with pI of 4.9 was missing).

The molecular weights of all these 4 isolated SAA isomers appear similar by SDS-PAGE (11.800 daltons) with a possible minimal difference for the SAAL₂ isomer preparation from three donors.

31

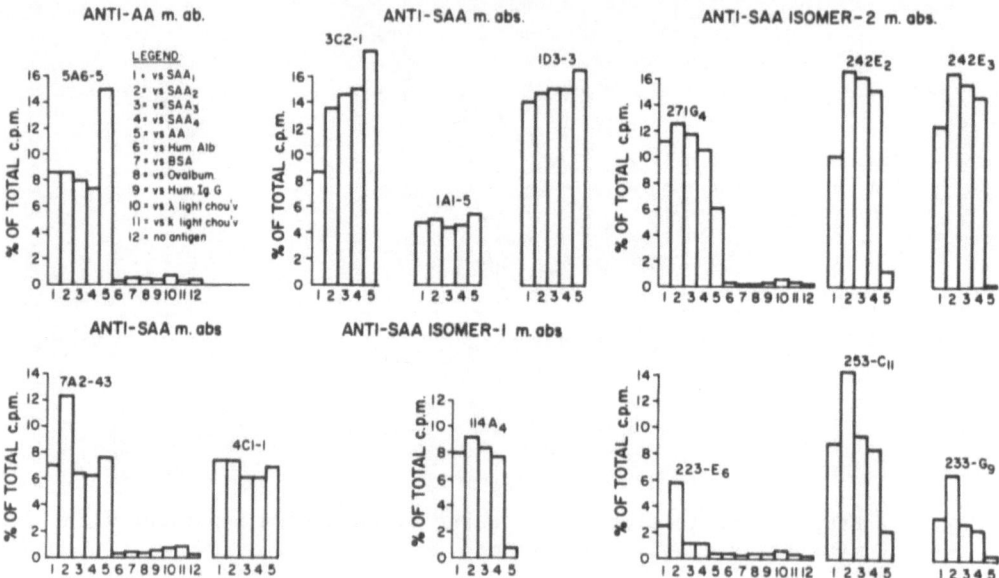

Fig. 4. Reaction of monoclonal antibodies (m. abs.) to human SAA and AA
with SAA isomers, AA and other proteins. 1) Reaction against (vs)
SAA_1 (isomer 1), 2) vs SAA_2, 3) vs SAA_3, 4) vs SAA_4, 5) vs AA, 6)
vs human albumin, 7) vs ovalbumin, 8) vs human IgG, 9) vs λ light
chain, 10) vs k light chain, 12) vs no antigen.

All SAA isomers were soluble in water and acid solutions but had a
tendency to precipitate in alkaline solutions (pH > 8.5).

    2. Production of monoclonal antibodies to human SAA and AA. The ini-
tial fusion of SAAL immunized spleen cells resulted in 18 immunoglobulin
secreting, transferable clones, five of which were selected (due to better
antibody titers) and inoculated in the peritoneal cavity of BALB/c mice
resulting in the production of antibody rich ascitic fluid (m. abs. 7A2-43,
4C1-1, 3C2-1, 1A1-5, and 1D3-3). Similarly, among the 3 m. abs. to AA
protein one was produced in murine ascitic fluid (5A6-5). Finally six m.
abs. to the SAA-2 isomer and one against the SAA-1 isomer were also selected
(among a total of 12 initial clone derived antibodies) for large scale production in the supernatant of cultures maintained for more than 6 months
and in murine ascitic fluid.

    None of the produced monoclonal antibodies reacted with any protein
other than SAAL, AA, and the SAAL isomers (Fig. 4). Their monoclonality
was demonstrated in the ascitic fluid by the presence of an IgG band with
restricted heterogeneity on electrophoresis.

    All the selected m. abs. were found to be IgG antibodies when tested
with a panel of class specific goat antimouse immunoglobulin antibodies.
Among the originally selected 28 clones which secreted immunoglobulins two
produced an IgM m. ab. to SAAL and $SAAL_2$ respectively. They were, however,
much weaker than the m. abs. we selected for production in ascitic fluid.

    None of the produced m. abs. gave precipitin reactions in Ouchterlony
immunodiffusion gels. Their reactions with SAA and AA molecules were easily
detected by a solid phase radioimmunoassay used also for their selection
(see methods). All the produced m. abs. were stable when kept at low temperature up to -70°C but did not react with AA nor SAA if kept at tempera-

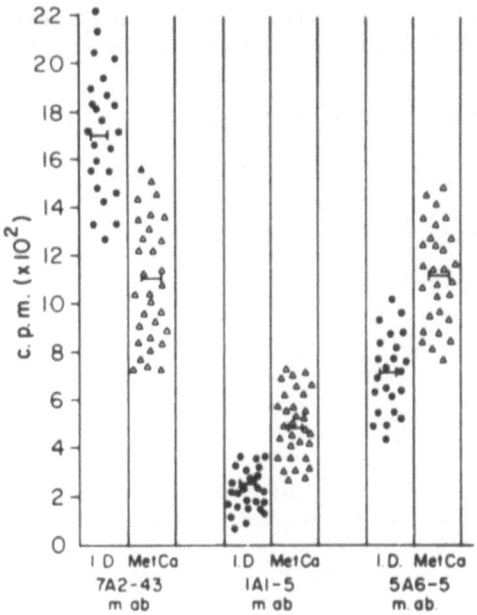

Fig. 5. Reaction of monoclonal antibodies to SAA and AA with
sera of patients with metastatic cancer and inflammatory diseases. ● — ID) Inflammatory and infectious
diseases, Δ — Met. Ca.) meta-
static carcinoma, |—|) mean
value, m. ab.) monoclonal
antibody.

ture higher than 56°C more than 10 min. The reaction of m. abs. to SAAL,
AA, and the four SAAL isomers presented two major patterns: one of an almost equally strong reaction with all SAA isomers and with AA (as for m.
abs. 4C1-1, 3C2-1, 2A2-5, 1D3-3). The other, seen only with m. ab. 7A2-43,
was twice as strong with SAAL isomer-2 than with the other SAAL isomers
and AA (Fig. 4).

The m. ab. to SAA isomer 1 and three of the m. abs. to SAA isomer 2
(242 E_2, 242 E_3, 271 G_4) did not react (or had minimal reaction) with AA
and reacted equally well with all SAAL isomers (Fig. 4). The other three
m. abs. to SAAL isomer 2 (223-E_6, 253-C11, and 233)G_9) similarly did not
react with AA but had a stronger reaction with $SAAL_2$ than the other SAAL
isomers.

When tested against sera of two groups of patients with acute phase
reaction accompanying metastatic cancer in 31 patients and acute inflammatory and infectious processes in 23 patients it was found that among five
m. abs. used in the solid phase RIA (see methods) one of them, 7A2-43, appeared to react differently from the other monoclonal antibodies: it had a
higher affinity with the SAA of patients with inflammatory and infectious
diseases (mean 1724.79 ng/ml ± 266) than with the SAA of patients with metastatic cancer (mean 1118.67 mg/μl ± 265). On the contrary, the m. abs.
1A1-5 and 5A6-5 tested against some sera had a higher affinity for SAA from
patients with metastatic cancer (mean 486.1 ± 139 and 1126.2 ± 209.3 respectively) than for SAA from patients with inflammatory diseases (mean 229.1 ±
and 729.1 ± 159 respectively) (Fig. 5).

TABLE 1. Percentage of Lymphocytes Forming EAC Rosetting in the
Presence of SAA and of Various m. abs. to SAA

Monoclonal Antibodies	% EAC s̄ SAA	% EAC c̄ SAA	% EAC c̄ SAA m. ab.
7A2-43	122±8.2	5.6 ±1.8	6.0 ±2.2
4C1-1	13.6±3.1	6.1 ±2.2	13.6±2.1
1D3-1	14.2±3	5.8 ±1.2	13.8±2.6
1A1-5	12.8±2.8	6.3 ±1.8	12.5±3.1

TABLE 2. Immunoglobulin Production by Lymphocytes Stimulated by PWM in the
Presence of SAA and of Various m. abs. to SAA (ng/1 × 10^6 cells)

Monoclonal Antibodies	B*+T_h**	B+T_h+T_s+	B+T_h+T_s+SAA	B+T_h+T_s+ SAA+m. ab.
7A2-43	1720±310	840±150	1530+425	830±402
4C1-1	1850±380	755±220	1620±328	1550±360
1D3-3	1530±260	620±310	1510±240	1480±230
1A1-5	1680±310	560±210	1620±320	1650±340

*B = B lymphocytes; **T_h = Tμ helper lymphocytes; +T_s = Tγ suppressor
lymphocytes.

3. Modulation by monoclonal antibodies to SAAL of the in vitro effects
of SAAL on circulating human leukocytes. The in vitro experiments previously described were carried on, to date, only in the presence of monoclonal antibodies to SAAL. Among the four m. abs. tested on their ability
to interfere with the inhibitory effect that SAAL was found to have on EAC
rosetting by B lymphocytes, three of them (Table 1) 4C1-1, 1D3-1, and 1A1-5
were able to block this effect while 7A2-43 did not have any effect.

Opposite results were noted when we assessed the effect of the same
four m. abs. on the SAAL ability to block the inhibitory effect of T suppressor lymphocytes on the immunoglobulin secretion by PWM stimulated B
lymphocytes we previously observed [7]. The 7A2-43 m. ab. was the only one
capable of reversing the blocking effect of SAAL (Table 2).

All four m. abs. used in these in vitro experiments were able to bind
to human circulating granulocytes when tested by indirect immunofluorescent
staining. No staining of lymphocytes was noted, while that of monocytes
was very faint, likely nonspecific.

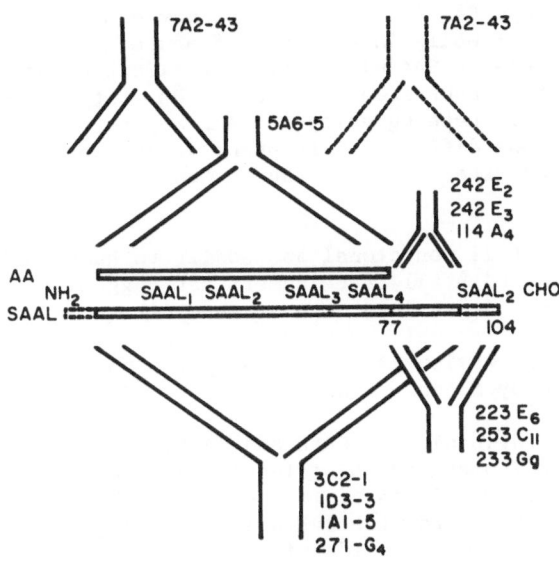

Fig. 6. Hypothetical recognition of different
portions of the SAAL molecule by the
produced monoclonal antibodies to
human SAAL and AA. The recognition of
various segments of the SAAL and AA
molecules by various m. abs. listed
aside of each of the schematically
depicted antibody molecules was derived from the intensity of m. abs.
reactions with various SAA isomers
and AA.

DISCUSSION

The studies described confirm the previously noted physico-chemical
heterogeneity of human and murine SAA molecule and amply demonstrate its
antigenic and functional heterogeneity. Using a relatively rapid isoelectric focusing technique [11] it was consistently found that the apparently
homogeneous SAAL molecule extracted from human sera by gel filtration chromatography in 10% formic acid (giving one band on SDS-PAGE) was, in fact,
heterogeneous, consisting of 4 isomers with different electrical mobilities
(pI of 4.9, 5.8, 6.6, and 7.2). One one occasion the SAAL extracted from
patient A. S. was found to have 6 isoelectric polymorphs of SAAL when the
serum was collected while patient was suffering of an infection in addition to her chronic rheumatoid arthritis. These data are similar to those
reported by Hoffman and Benditt [5] on murine apo SAA which was found to
have two isomers with different electrical charge and slightly different
molecular weight in all mice and 4 other isomers in mice who had received
intraperitoneal endotoxin; six polymorphs with different electrical charges
were also found by Bausserman for apo SAA extracted from two donors during
an acute phase reaction caused by etiocholanolone injection [6]. Of interest is the fact that the SAAL extracted from one of our patients with myasthenia gravis had only three isomers identified by IEF (Fig. 3). These
data suggest that the SAAL isoelectric microheterogeneity may be due to
different cellular origins of the proteins; for instance, the missing SAAL
isomer 1 may originate primarily in the thymus, the organ affected by a
malignant tumor in our myasthenia gravis patient while the isomers 2 and 3
which consistently have the largest bands are likely released by the liver,

the major source of apo SAA [20, 21]. $SAAL_4$ may come from polymorphonucleated leukocytes [22] while in the peak of acute phase reaction other
tissues could also release SAA with different electric charge, accounting
for the additional two bands seen in these cases. It is also possible that
some of the isoelectric heterogeneity of SAAL may be due to NH_2-terminal
differences found among different SAAL preparations obtained in initial
studies by us [2] and others [3] and found among SAA isomers separated by
Bausserman [6].

The production of 11 monoclonal antibodies to human SAAL and of one
m. ab. to AA reacting with all SAAL isomers has suggested the existence of
structural differences in at least one of the SAAL isomers, the $SAAL_2$ and
the other three isomers as well as between the SAAL isomers and AA, heterogeneity that has been previously suggested by two monoclonal antibodies to
SAA isomers produced by McAdam et al. [23].

The monoclonal antibodies to SAAL and AA have significant cross reactivity with the SAAL isomers and AA molecules due to the recognition of
identical determinants within these molecules, which have a very similar
chemical structure [24]. From the intensity of their reaction with various SAAL isomers and AA, one can identify five groups of m. abs., each of
which recognizes a different segment of the SAA molecule as depicted schematically in Fig. 6. First, there is the group including m. abs. 3C2-1,
1D3-3, 1A1-5, and 271 G_4, which in view of their reaction of equal intensity
with all these antigens, recognizes the common core of amino acid residues
present in all SAAL isomers as well as in AA. Then there is the 5A6-5 m.
ab. produced against AA which has a reaction of equal intensity with all
SAAL isomers but reacts more strongly with AA suggesting that at least the
AA we extracted from the liver of a patient with RSA may have some heter-
geneity at its NH_2 terminal when compared to that of SAAL isomers.

Another group of m. abs. (242 B_2, 242 E_3, and 114-A_4) recognize the
amino acid residues common only to all SAAL isomers based upon their equally
intense reaction with these isomers and their lack of reaction with AA.
Another group of m. abs. (223 E_6, 253-C_{11}, and 233-G_9) highly suggest the
existence of unique groups of amino acid residues present only in the $SAAL_2$
isomer, likely present at its NH_2-terminal in view of the much more intense
reaction of these m. abs. with $SAAL_2$ which suggests that $SAAL_2$ could have
a different NH_2 terminus from the other SAAL isomers as well as from AA.
These data seem to indicate that the $SAAL_2$ isomer heterogeneity may be due
to a few extra amino acid residues which should increase the molecular
weight of this isomer; this increase, however, is not significant enough
to permit the detection of $SAAL_2$ in SDS-PAGE as a distinct band. This data
is consistent with those concerning murine SAA for which the two major
isomers identified as apo SAA and apo SAA_2, have also a slight difference
in their molecular weight which can be seen on SDS-PAGE.

Our data also suggest that during the acute phase reaction accompanying various diseases, the levels of all SAAL isomers are not equally increased) this suggests again the likelihood of different tissue origin.
The stronger reaction of the 7A2-43 m. ab. with SAA from patients with inflammatory diseases than with those with metastatic cancer and the opposite
results noted with the 5A6-5 and 1A1-5 m. abs. might find clinical applications in discriminating SAA elevations due to an infection in patients with
metastatic cancer; this could make the measurement of SAAL level in patients
with cancer the best monitor of their disease activity. It is possible that
when other groups of m. abs. are used in this assay their discriminatory
power between the SAA elevation in inflammatory diseases and malignancies
may be even more significant, perhaps to the point of eliminating any overlapping values; this could make the RIA for SAA a valuable tool for the
early detection of cancer.

Finally, our studies have revealed functional heterogeneity between various SAAL isomers. It is likely that the $SAAL_2$ isomer which is the only one recognized by 7A2-43 m. ab. among the antibodies so far tested, is the only isomer responsible for the suppression by SAA of the T suppressor lymphocyte inhibition of immunoglobulin secretion by B lymphocytes while one or all of the other SAAL isomers are responsible for the partial inhibition by SAA of EAC rosette formation; this, in view of the fact that this function was blocked by m. abs. with reactivity to the portion of the SAA molecule common to all isomers.

These data also indicate that the various m. abs. produced could be used in affinity chromatography columns to separate various portions of the SAA molecule identified by these antibodies as well as in DNA recombinant studies as probes for the product of SAA gene(s). Our study as well as that of Hoffman and Benditt [5] suggest the existence of two genetic determinants for SAA: one for the extra piece present in $SAAL_2$ and the other for the common structure of all SAAL isomers.

ACKNOWLEDGEMENTS

We gratefully acknowledge the excellent assistance of Ms. S. Amrani in preparing this manuscript.
This study was supported, in part, by NIH Grant #5R01AM2008006.

REFERENCES

1. M. Levin, E. C. Franklin, B. Frangione, and M. Pras, J. Clin. Invest., 51:2773 (1972).
2. C. J. Rosenthal, E. C. Franklin, J. Clin. Invest., 55:746 (1975).
3. R. F. Anders, J. B. Natvig, K. Sletten, G. Husby, and K. Nordstoga, J. Immunol., 118:229 (1977).
4. E. P. Benditt and Eriksen, Proc. Natl. Acad. Sci. USA, 74:4025 (1977).
5. J. S. Hoffman and E. P. Benditt, J. Biol. Chem., 257:10510 (1982).
6. L. L. Bausserman, P. N. Herbert, and K. P. W. J. McAdam, J. Exp. Med., 152:641 (1980).
7. C. J. Rosenthal, Clinic Res., 25:366 (1977).
8. C. J. Rosenthal, E. C. Franklin, B. Frangione, and J. Greenspan, J. Immunol., 116:1415 (1976).
9. R. F. Anders, J. B. Natvig, T. E. Michaelson, and G. Husby, Scand. J. Immunol., 4:397 (1975).
10. K. Weber and M. Osborn, J. Biol. Chem., 244:4406 (1969).
11. A. Manrique and M. Lasky, Electrophoresis, 2:315 (1981).
12. J. M. Bastin, J. Kirkly, and A. J. McMichael, in: Monoclonal Antibodies in Clinical Medicine (A. J. McMichael and J. W. Fabre, eds.), Acad. Press, London—New York—Paris, p. 503 (1982).
13. G. Kohler and G. Milstein, Nature, 256:495 (1975).
14. M. Pras and T. Reshef, Biochim. et Bioph. Acta, 271:258 (1972).
15. A. Boyum, Scand. J. Clin. Lab. Invest. (Suppl. 97), 21:9 (1968)-
16. C. Biano, R. Patrick, and V. Nussenzweig, J. Exp. Med., 132:702 (1970).
17. L. Moretta, M. Ferrarin, M. C. Mingari, A. Moretta, and S. R. Webb, J. Immunol., 117:217 (1970).
18. C. J. Rosenthal, C. A. Noguera, A. Coppola, and S. N. Kapelner, Cancer, 49:2305 (1982).
19. T. H. Weller and A. H. Coons, Proc. Soc. Exp. Biol. Med., 86:789 (1954).
20. M. D. Benson, in: C-Reactive Protein and the Plasma Protein Response to Tissue Injury (I. Kushner, J. E. Volanakis, and H. Gewurz, eds.), N. Y. Acad. Sci., New York, p. 116 (1982).
21. J. S. Hoffman and E. P. Benditt, J. Biol. Chem., 257:10518 (1982).

22. C. J. Rosenthal and L. J. Sullivan, Clin. Invest., 62:1181 (1978).
23. K. P. W. J. McAdam, J. H. Knowles, H. T. Foss, C. A. Dinarello, in: C-Reactive Protein and the Plasma Protein Response to Tissue Injury (I. Kushner, J. E. Volanakis, and H. Gewerz, eds.), N. Y. Acad. Sci., New York, p. 126 (1982).
24. C. Milstein, in: Monoclonal Antibodies in Clinical Medicine (A. J. McMichael and J. W. Dabre, eds.), Acad. Press, London—New York—Paris, p. 3 (1982).

REAGGREGATION OF BOVINE AMYLOID A FIBRIL COMPONENTS

TO β-PLEATED SHEET FIBRILLAR STRUCTURES*

A. C. J. van Andel†, P. R. Hol†,
J. H. van der Maas‡, E. T. G. Lutz‡,
H. Krabbendam**, and E. Gruys†

†Department of Veterinary Pathology
 State University of Utrecht, Utrecht

‡Department of Analytical Chemistry
 State University of Utrecht, Utrecht

**Department of General Chemistry
  State University of Utrecht, Utrecht

ABSTRACT

   Amyloid fibrils were isolated from renal papillae of cows with spontaneous AA-amyloidosis. The fibrils were solubilized with guanidine-HCl and
subjected to gel filtration. Reaggregation studies were performed by dialyz-
ing the fractions obtained, separately or in combinations, against acetic
acid. Protein AA alone appeared not to precipitate. Dialysis of total
solubilized amyloid fibrils led to reformation of amyloid fibrils. The
precipitate obtained by dialysis of the combined retarded peaks (without the
V_o-peak) showed fine curvilinear amyloid-like fibrillar structures, indicating that non-protein AA components are necessary for the formation of AA
amyloid fibrils.

   Infrared spectroscopy and preliminary X-ray studies on the original
fibrils and reaggregates were performed. The results from these studies
showed the presence of β-pleated sheet conformation and also α-helix/coil
conformation as known in amyloid. From the low amount of β conformation
found in protein AA and the occurrence of different conformations besides
the β-pleated sheet in the reaggregates and amyloid fibrils, it is suggested
that the intrafibrillar protein AA has little β-conformation. A modification of the twisted antiparallel β-pleated sheet concept of the amyloid
fibril in which α-helix/coil moieties extend from β-pleated sheets, is given.

*These investigations were supported by the Foundation for Medical Research
 Fungo (Grant Nr. 13-48-119) and by the Netherlands League against Rhema-
 tism (Nr. 84CR18).

INTRODUCTION

Amyloid protein AA has been described as the major amyloid protein in secondary amyloid fibrils, and idiopathic amyloid fibrils obtained from patients with a secondary distribution pattern of amyloid [1]. Protein AA is thought to be derived from the larger and partly homologous serum protein SAA by proteolytic cleavage. Definite proof, however, is still lacking. Our experiments with proteolytic digestion of bovine SAA rich serum fractions revealed small quantities of Congophilic fibrils [2, 3]. These low results might be explained by the occurrence of different types of SAA, the one being more amyloidogenic than the other, as recently was found in mice [4]. Moreover, in quantitative amyloid formation other components, like protein SAP and tissue factors, may be involved. Reconstitution experiments using bovine AA fibrils revealed an apparently non-protein SAP and non-protein AA fibril component to be necessary for the reaggregation of protein AA into Congophilic fibrils [5, 6].

On studying the reaggregation of protein AA into fibrils, the protein conformation and fibril structure become important. Electron microscopic studies showed the amyloid fibrils to be rigid, non-branching and approximately 10 nm wide [7]. On negative contrast staining they appeared as pairs of twisting filaments [2, 7]. On positive contrast staining cross-sections of the fibrils showed circular and oval structues with a "hollow" core [2a, 7] and two opposite electron dense areas [2a]. Infrared spectroscopical and X-ray diffraction studies of amyloid fibrils published by several groups of investigators [8, 9, 10, 11] revealed the cross anti-parallel β-pleated sheet as the major conformation. Staining with Congo red and subsequent green birefringence is thought to depend on the presence of this conformation [12]. After these papers further studies revealed theoretical ideas of the molecular structure of these fibrils [13, 14] and led to the concept of the twisted β-pleated sheet conformation for the whole amyloid fibril [13, 14, 15]. Concerning the amino acid composition, for protein AL indeed a high β-potential was computed. Protein AA, however, showed a low β-potential [16]. Furthermore, from circular dichroism studies and a computer search it was concluded that protein AA contains stretches of amphipatic α-helices [17]. These findings suggest the presence of non-β-structures in protein AA amyloid fibrils. To investigate this possibility the molecular conformation of bovine protein AA, reaggregates and fibrils was studied using infrared spectroscopy and X-ray diffraction.

MATERIALS AND METHODS

Amyloid Fibril Preparations

Amyloid fibrils were isolated from the renal papillae of 5 cows with spontaneous AA-amyloidosis [18]. The Skinner et al. [19] modification of the water extraction method was used, in which citrate is added to the saline washes to remove protein AP.

Purification of Amyloid Fibril Proteins

Amyloid fibril prpearations were solubilized (8 mg/ml) for 18 h at room temperature with 6 M guanidine-HCl in 0.55 M Tris-HCl buffer, pH 8.5, containing 0.1 mM ethylenediaminetetraacetic acid and 0.1 mM dithiotreitol (Gu-HCl-TED buffer). After centrifugation for 30 min at 20,000 g, 5 ml aliquots were gel filtered on a Sephacryl S 200 column in 4 M Guanidine-HCl, 0.55 M Tris, pH 7.0, revealing 4 peaks (Fig. 1) as described [5]. Separate peaks or combined peaks from a single run were rechromatographed on the same column after concentration using an Amicon YM 5 filter membrane. Fractions were concentrated as above, dialyzed against 1 M acetic acid and distilled water and finally lyophilized.

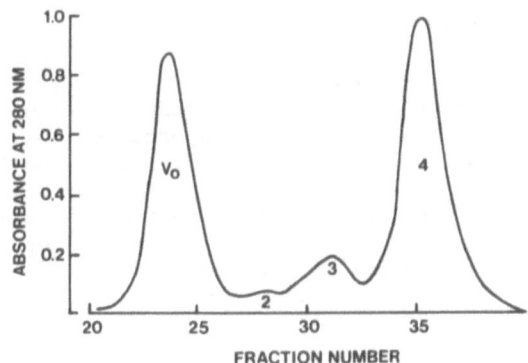

Fig. 1. Gel filtration profile of bovine
amyloid fibrils on a Sephacryl
S 200 column (96 × 2.6 cm) in 4
M Gu-HCl, 0.55 M Tris-HCl, pH
7.0.

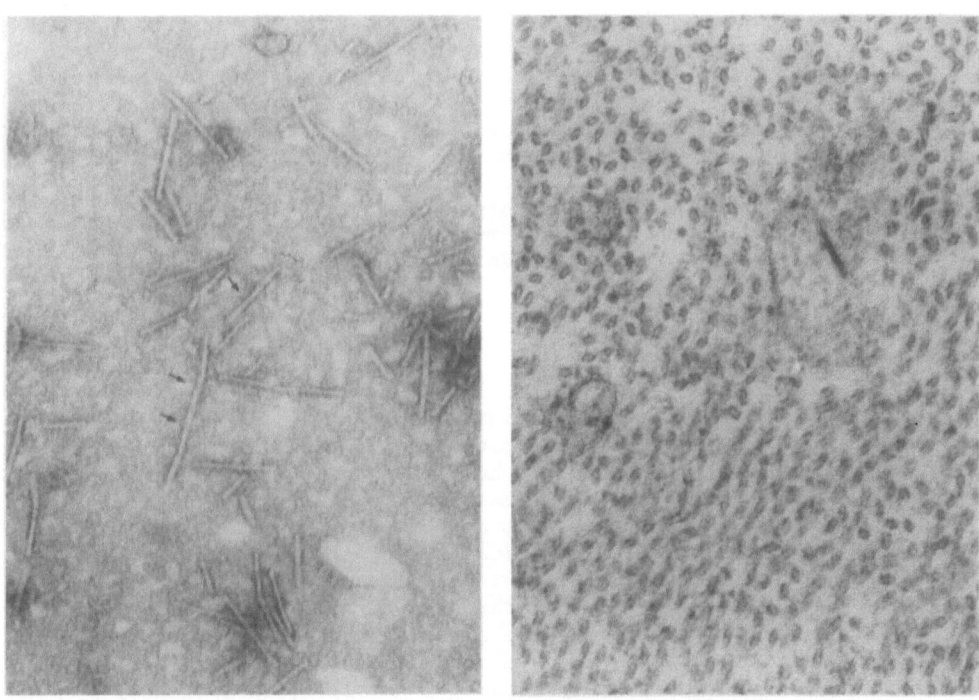

A   **B**

Fig. 2. Electron micrographs of amyloid fibrils from bovine renal papillae.
Panel A: Negatively stained with 2% phosphotungstic acid
(×65,000). Note the indication of twisting filaments (arrows).
Panel B: On cross-section in subendothelial renal interstitial
areas stained with uranyl acetate and lead citrate (×171,000).
Note the circular and oval structures with "hollow" cores and two
opposite electron dense areas.

Reaggregation Experiments

In a first experiment amyloid fibrils from cows 1, 2, and 3 were solubilized (15 mg/ml) in Gu-HCl-TED buffer. These solutions were centrifuged for 30 min at 20,000 g. Aliquots of the supernatants were diluted with the same buffer, to protein concentrations of 15, 10, 5, and 1 mg/ml and dialyzed at room temperature against 1 M acetic acid with and without the addition of 4 mM $CaCl_2$. In a second experiment using material derived from all 5 cows, amyloid fibril protein fractions obtained by gel filtration were solubilized in Gu-HCl-TED buffer to the final concentration of 15 mg/ml and dialyzed at room temperature against 1 M acetic acid.

Electron Microscopy

Electron microscopy was performed as described [2, 2a, 5].

X-Ray Diffraction

Lyophilized samples without orientation were examined by X-ray diffraction with CuK_α radiation using a Debye-Scherer powder camera. Photographs obtained were scanned with a microdensitometer. The standard deviation in the d values of the principal reflections is 0.03 Å for d = 4.7 Å and 0.15 Å for d = 10 Å.

Infrared Spectroscopy

Infrared spectra were run on a Perkin Elmer 580 B connected to a Perkin Elmer 3600 data station. Spectra were recorded using an integrated scan mode 4-A-DB: region 4000-700 cm^{-1}, data interval 1.0 cm^{-1}, maximal resolution of 2.3 cm^{-1}, relative noise 0.15% T, abcissa accuracy: ±1 cm^{-1} from 2000 to 700 cm^{-1}, ordinate accuracy ±0.3% T. After background correction (Irtran resp. Zn Se) the spectra were plotted in the absorbance range: 0-0.5. The read out abscissa accuracy was dependent on the bandshape. Samples (0.8 mg) were cast as a film on an Irtran or a Zn Se window and dried in air or _in vacuo_ above phosphorpentoxide. No significant differences were observed between these two methods. Lyophilized amyloid fibrils were also examined in potassium bromide pellets, pressed at ca. $6 \cdot 10^3$ kg/cm^2.

RESULTS AND DISCUSSION

Electron micrographs of the original bovine amyloid fibril preparations showed the typical rigid, non-branching twisting fibrils with varying length and a diameter of about 12 nm with a hollow core on cross-section (Fig. 2) as described [2, 2a]. Examination of the fibrils with X-ray crystallography revealed a strong diffraction line at 4.71 Å and a broad ring at 10.2 Å (Fig. 3). This is typical for proteins containing the β-pleated sheet conformation [20, 21]. In addition, weak diffuse lines were observed at 4.2 Å and 3.8 Å. The infrared spectra of amyloid fibrils cast as a film on a window, revealed in the amide 1 band a strong absorption at 1635 cm^{-1} and in some cases a very weak shoulder at approximately 1695 cm^{-1}. The 1635 cm^{-1} peak indicates the presence of parallel, antiparallel or mixed parallel/antiparallel β-pleated sheets [22, 23, 25]. The intensity of the absorption at 1695 cm^{-1} gives an indication of the quantity of antiparallel β-strands [25], although β-turns also can give an absorption at this position [24]. The very low intensity of the shoulder at 1695 cm^{-1} thus suggest the presence of at most mixed sheets in bovine AA-amyloid. The broad absorption at ca. 1655 cm^{-1} indicates the presence of α-helix and/or coil [22]. The observed absorption maximum in the amide 2 band at 1543 cm^{-1} is also compatible with the presence of α-helix/coil conformations. Spectra

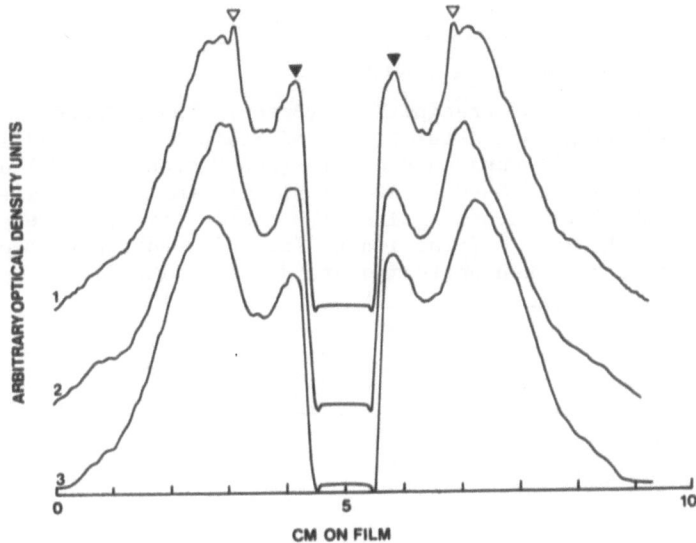

Fig. 3.   Microdensitometer scans of the X-ray diffrac-
          tion photographs of 1) bovine amyloid fibrils,
          2) reaggregate formed by dialysis of solu-
          bilized amyloid fibrils (15 mg/ml) against 1 M
          acetic acid, 3) acetic acid treated protein AA.
          Note the 10.2 Å (closed arrow) and 4.71 Å
          d-spacing (open arrow) in the amyloid fibrils.

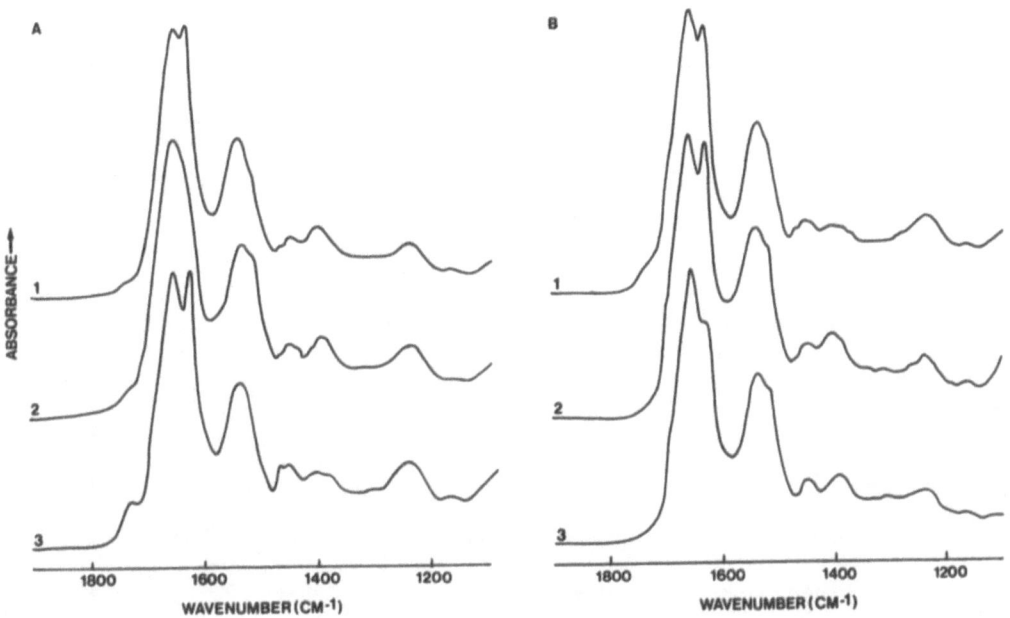

Fig. 4.   Infrared spectra of: Panel A, 1) amyloid fibrils cast as a film
          on a window, 2) amyloid fibrils pressed in a potassium bromide
          pellet, and 3; a film of a reaggregate formed by dialysis of solu-
          bilized amyloid fibrils (15 mg/ml) against 1 M acetic acid. Panel
          B, 1) a film of solubilized V_0 material dialyzed against 1 M acetic
          acid, 2) a film of the precipitate formed by the combined peaks 2,
          3, and 4, and 3) a film of the acetic acid treated protein AA.

TABLE 1. Formation of Precipitates (Prec.), Their Green Birefringence after Congo Red Staining (CR), and Their Fibrillar Appearance on Electron Microscopy (EM) after Dialysis of Gu-HCl-TED Solubilized Amyloid Fibrils and Fibril Fractions Against 1 M Acetic Acid (Samples on which X-ray diffraction and/or infrared spectroscopy (IR) has been performed are denoted with *)

Material derived from:	Prec.	CR	EM	X-ray	IR
Cow 1					
Peak 4	-	-	-		*
Peak 3	-	-	-		*
V_o-peak	++	-	-	*	*
Combined peaks 2,3 and 4	+	++	++		*
Total fibrils	+++	+++	++	*	*
Cow 2					
Peak 4	-	-	-		*
Total fibrils	+++	+++	++		*
Cow 3					
Peak 4	-	-	-		*
V_o-peak	++	-	-		*
Combined peaks 2,3 and 4	+	++	++		*
Total fibrils	+++	+++	+++		
Cow 4					
Peak 4	-	-	-		*
Peak 3	+	-	-		*
V_o-peak	++	-	-		*
Combined peaks 2,3 and 4	+	++	++		*
Cow 5					
Peak 4	-	-	-	*	*
V_o-peak	++	-	-	*	*

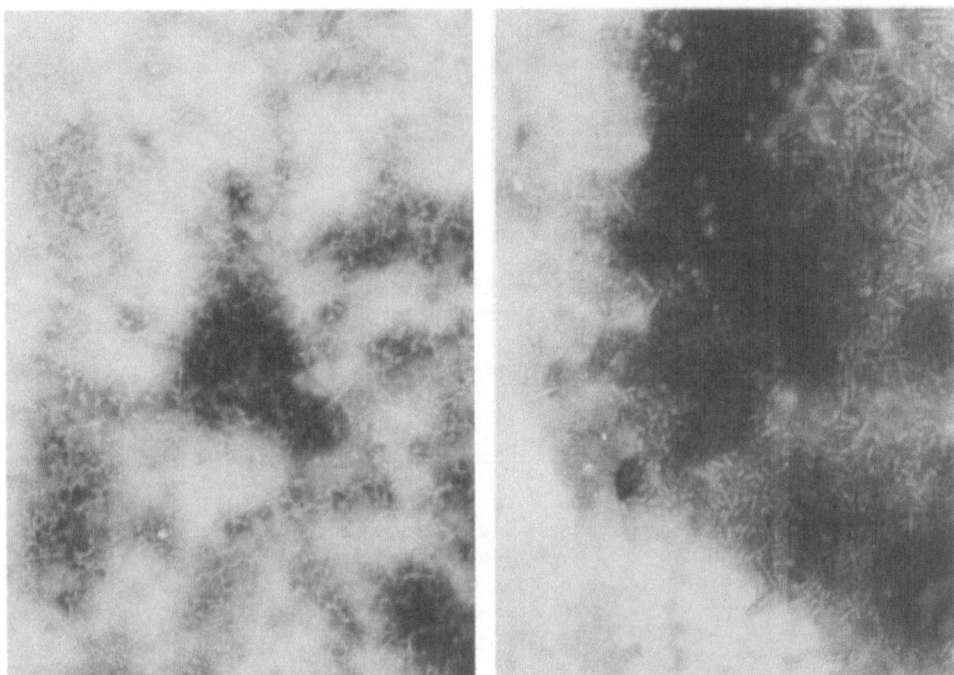

A   B

Fig. 5.   Panel A: Electron micrograph of the reaggregate formed by the com-
          bined peaks 2, 3, and 4.   Panel B: Electron micrograph of the re-
          aggregate formed by dialysis of solubilized amyloid fibrils (15
          mg/ml), obtained from cow 3, against 1 M acetic acid (both ×54,000).

of the same fibrils pressed in potassium bromide pellets showed a broad absorption maximum at 1655 cm^{-1} and a shoulder at 1635 cm^{-1} (Fig. 1) indicating the potassium bromide method to be inferior to the window method.

Reaggregation of Solubilized Amyloid Fibrils

Precipitates were formed in all cases, when solubilized amyloid fibrils
(15, 10, 5, and 1 mg/ml) were dialysed against 1 M acetic acid (Table 1).
Smears of these precipitates showed green birefringence after Congo red
staining.   The precipitates obtained by dialysis of the more concentrated
fibril solutions, however, showed larger and more numerous areas of green
birefringent material.   Electron microscopical examination revaled fibrillar
structures in all samples (Fig. 5) with features of amyloid fibrils in some
areas (cows 2 and 3).   The reaggregates gave an X-ray diffraction pattern
in which the 4.60 Å line was close to the 4.71 Å line of the original
fibrils (Fig. 3).   Furthermore, a sharp and a diffuse line were observed
at 4.11 and 10.3 Å respectively.   The infrared spectra showed two strong
absorbance maxima, at 1653 cm^{-1} and 1627 cm^{-1} respectively, and a medium
shoulder at ca. 1695 cm^{-1} in the amide 1 region (Fig. 4).   The absorption
peak at 1627 cm^{-1} coupled with a shoulder at 1695 cm^{-1} indicates the presence of an antiparallel-β-pleated sheet conformation in the reaggregates.
The shift of the absorption peak at 1635 cm^{-1} in the original amyloid
fibrils to 1627 cm^{-1} in the reaggregates reflects a change within the conformation of the β-sheets.   The absorption at 1695 cm^{-1} appeared to be
stronger in the reaggregates.   This may have been caused by either an increase in the ratio of antiparallel/parallel chains in the sheet [25] or by
an increase in the number and/or a change in the types of β-turns present
[24].   No significant change was observed of the infrared spectra of reaggregates formed in the presence of 4 mM calcium chloride.

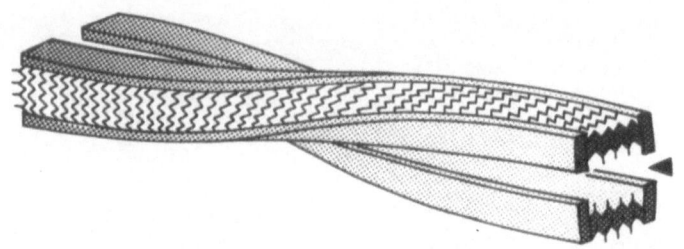

Fig. 6. Proposed model for AA-amyloid fibrils. Note
the hollow core (arrow) formed in between the
twisting filaments and the non-β areas on the
lateral sides of the filaments (shaded area).

Reaggregation of Purified Amyloid Fibril Proteins

Dialysis of solubilized peak 4 (protein AA) against 1 M acetic acid
resulted in a transient appearance of a precipitate. Smears of the lyophilized protein did not show any green birefringence after Congo red staining or definite electron microscopical fibrils. This is in accordance with
previous results showing that protein AA does not form fibrillar precipitates in 1 M acetic acid [5]. The X-ray diffraction pattern of protein AA
lacked specific diffraction lines, thus indicating the presence of amorphous structures (Fig. 3). The amide 1 band of the infrared spectrum showed
a strong absorption maximum at 1653 cm^{-1} accompanied by medium and weak
shoulders at resp. 1627 and 1695 cm^{-1} (Fig. 4). Hence it follows that only
a small part of protein AA has a β-pleated sheet conformation. Dialysis of
peak 3 (cows 1 and 4) and the V_o-peak (cows 1, 2, 3, and 4) resulted in the
formation of precipitates (Table 1). Smears of the precipitates showed no
green birefringence after Congo red staining. All precipitates appeared
amorphous on electron microscopy. Peak 3 (cows 1 and 4) appeared to contain a higher A_{1627}/A_{1653} ratio than peak 4 (protein AA), indicating a
higher content of β-conformation in peak 3 proteins. The infrared spectrum
of V_o-material (cows 1, 3, 4, and 5) showed peaks with varying intensities
at 1627 cm^{-1}. The X-ray diffraction pattern of the V_o-material showed diffuse bands with a weak line at 4.55 Å overlaying a diffuse halo at 4.0 Å
and a broad and less intense ring at 10.1 Å, indicating the presence of
some non-amorphous material with a β-like conformation. Reaggregation of
combined peaks 2, 3, and 4 (quantitative weight ratio 2:5:30 as calculated
from O.D. 280;, resulted in the formation of precipitates which showed green
birefringence after Congo red staining (cows 1, 3, and 4). On electron microscopy evident fine fibrillar curvilinear structures were observed in all
cases (Fig. 5). The infrared spectra of these samples showed them to contain more β-conformation than peak 4 (protein AA) as judged from the ratio
A_{1627}/A_{1653} (Fig. 4).

CONCLUSIONS

The infrared and X-ray data on whole fibrils were in agreement with
those presented by others [8, 9, 11], indicating the presence of a β-
pleated sheet conformation in the amyloid fibrils. However, also coil and/
or α-helic conformations were definitely present as indicated by the infrared spectra. Moreover, infrared spectroscopy showed that the antiparallel β-pleated sheet constitutes a minor conformation in acetic acid
treated protein AA. Dialysis of the combined retarded peaks resulted in
the formation of curvilinear aggregates showing Congo red staining characteristics and β-conformation like amyloid. Dialysis of the total material (V_o + retarded peaks) resulted in the formation of amyloid fibrils.

This indicates that non-protein AA low molecular weight components are necessary for the aggregation of protein AA, and V_0 material will be involved in the final morphogenesis of amyloid fibrils. From the low amount of β-conformation found in isolated protein AA and the occurrence of other conformations in addition to the β-pleated sheet in the reaggregates and original fibrils, it is suggested that the intrafibrillar protein AA has little β-conformation. Further studies on the observed phenomena are in progress. From the present findings, however, a preliminary modification of the twisted β-pleated sheet concept [15] can be given for the AA-amyloid fibrils (Fig. 6), in which α-helix/coil moieties extend from β-pleated sheets.

ACKNOWLEDGEMENT

We thank Dr. A. M. F. Hezemans for making the microdensitometer scans of the X-ray photographs.

REFERENCES

1. M. H. van Rijswijk, Amyloidosis, PhD. Thesis Groningen (1980).
2. E. Gruys, Bovine renal amyloidosis. A comparative study of secondary amyloidosis, PhD. Thesis Utrecht (1979).
2a. E. Gruys, Vet. Pathol., 12, 94 (1975).
3. E. Gruys, H. F. J. Timmermans, in: Proc. 7th ICLAS Symp. Utrecht 1979 (A. Spiegel, E. Erichson, and H. A. Solleveld, eds.), Gustav Fisher Verlag, Stuttgart, New York (1980), p. 139.
4. J. S. Hoffman, L. H. Ericson, N. Eriksen, K. A. Walsh, and E. P. Benditt, J. Exp. Med., 159, 641 (1984).
5. P. R. Hol, J. P. M. Langeveld, E. W. van Beuningen-Jansen, J. H. Verrkamp, and E. Gruys, Scand. J. Immunol., 20, 53 (1984).
6. P. R. Hol, E. W. van Beuningen-Jansen, and J. Gruys, in: Amyloidosis E.A.R.S. (C. R. Tribe and P. A. Bacon, eds.), J. Wright and Sons, Ltd., Bristol (1983), p. 158.
7. E. C. Franklin, D. Zucker-Franklin, Adv. Immunol., 15, 249 (1972).
8. J. D. Termine, E. D. Eanes, D. Ein, and G. G. Glenner, Biopolymers, 11, 1103 (1972).
9. E. D. Eanes and G. G. Glenner, J. Histochem. Cytochem., 16, 673 (1968).
10. L. Bonar, A. S. Cohen, and M. Skinner, Proc. Soc. Exp. Biol. Med., 131, 1373 (1969).
11. U. E. Shmueli, J. Gavni, E. Sohar, and Y. Ashkenazi, J. Mol. Biol., 41, 309 (1969).
12. G. G. Glenner, E. D. Eanes, and D. L. Page, J. Histochem. Cytochem., 20, 821 (1972).
13. J. H. Gooper, Lab. Invest., 31, 232 (1974).
14. J. H. Cooper, in: Amyloidosis E.A.R.S. (C. R. Tribe and P. A. Bacon, eds.), J. Wright and Sons, Ltd., Bristol (1983), p. 31.
15. G. G. Glenner, New Engl. J. Med., 302, 1283 (1980).
16. T. J. Muckle and C. H. Goldsmith, in: Amyloidosis E.A.R.S. (G. G. Glenner, P. P. Costa, and A. F. Freitas, eds.), Exerpta Medica, Amsterdam (1980), p. 274.
17. J. P. Segrest, H. J. Pownall, R. L. Jackson, G. G. Glenner, and P. S. Pollock, Biochem., 15, 3187 (1976).
18. E. Gruys and H. J. F. Timmermans, Vet. Sci. Commun., 3, 21 (1979).
19. M. Skinner, T. Shirahama, A. S. Cohen, and C. L. Deal, Prep. Biochem., 12, 461 (1982).
20. L. Pauling and R. B. Corey, Proc. Natl. Acad. Sci. USA, 39, 253 (1953).
21. G. N. Ramachandran and V. Sasisekharan, in: Adv. Protein Chem., 23, 283 (1968).

22. T. Miyazawa and E. Blout, J. Am. Chem. Soc., 83, 712 (1961).
23. S. Krimm, J. Mol. Biol., 4, 528 (1962).
24. S. Krimm and J. Bandakar, Biopolymers, 19, 1 (1980).
25. Yu. N. Chirgadze and N. A. Nevskaya, Biopolymers, 15, 627 (1976).

ANALYSIS OF X-RAY SCATTERING BY HUMAN AA FIBRILS

USING SECONDARY STRUCTURE PREDICTIONS OF HUMAN SAA$_1$

W. G. Turnell[1], R. Sarra[1],
I. D. Glover[1], J. O. Baum[1],
D. Caspi, M. L. Baltz,
and M. B. Pepys

MRC Acute Phase Protein Research Group
Immunological Medicine Unit
Department of Medicine
Royal Postgraduate Medical School
DuCane Road
London W12 OHS, and

[1]Department of Crystallography
Birkbeck College
University of London
Malet Street
London WC1, United Kingdom

ABSTRACT

The complete sequence of human SAA has recently been reported and we have devised a consensus prediction of the secondary structure of SAA$_1(\alpha)$ using computer programs based upon two different techniques. These show that SAA$_1(\alpha)$ may include three α-helices and one β-hairpin. Position 76 is predicted to be between secondary structural elements. In view of the close homology between the first 76 residues of SAA$_1$ and AA sequences, we have used the predicted secondary structure to account for the X-ray scattering which we have obtained from AA fibrils and the results reported by other workers. Our present observations are not consistent with the structure of AA fibrils previously proposed by others, that is stacks of anti-parallel β sheets. Differences from the previous reports can be accounted for by differences in the degree of hydration of the AA fibril gel preparations.

We propose that inter-fibril packing is the source of the Astbury "cross-β" X-ray scattering pattern that has previously been thought to be characteristic of individual AA fibrils. Furthermore, we suggest that the AA molecule is a globular protein, and contains a small, well-ordered β-sheet, probably of only two strands. In the AA fibril, these β-strands run perpendicular to the fibril axis, and comparison of results from wet and previously reported dry gels suggests that they form part of the surface of the fibril.

INTRODUCTION

The pathogenesis of AA amyloidosis is not well understood, in particular the mechanisms underlying the deposition of AA fibrils and their persistence in vivo. The generally accepted concept of amyloid fibrils as stacks of peptide chains arrayed in anti-parallel β sheets has been considered responsible for many of the pathophysiological and histochemical properties of amyloid. However, the primary structures of AA proteins from several vertebrates show sequences typical of globular proteins, with amino acid compositions suggesting α as well as β content. The present of amphiphatic helical structures, originally suggested by Segrest et al. [1], may depend on hydrophobic residues in positions which are conserved between species, as indicated by Waalen et al. [2]. There is very close homology between AA and the first 75 residues of SAA [3, 4] and analysis of the secondary structure of SAA, based on the recently published complete sequence [4] should therefore help to elucidate the structure of AA fibrils.

We report here detailed predictions of the secondary structure of $SAA_1(\alpha)$ derived by the use of computer programs based on statistical comparison with known protein structures and on patterns of hydrophobicity in the amino acid sequence. We have also re-examined X-ray scattering by human AA amyloid fibrils since these are not particularly resistant to proteolysis in vitro, as might be expected of the silk-like β structures proposed by Glenner et al. [5]. Together with the beading of negatively stained fibrils, and the nature of the AA sequences, this lack of resistance suggests that the structure of the principal fibril component is more typical of small globular proteins than has been suggested by previous models.

METHODS

Secondary Structure Prediction

Most methods for the prediction of secondary structures from amino acid sequences can be placed into two broad categories: probabilistic and physicochemical. Those of the first category start with an estimate of the propensity for helix or sheet formation for individual amino acids or groups of residues along the sequence, usually in groups of 2 to 4. Of this type we have used the programs of Nagano et al. [6], Chou and Fasman [7], and Burgess et al. [8]. The latter program also uses helix forming propensities based on an empirical energy function. The more recent method of Garnier et al. [9] was also used. This program is distinctly different in its mathematical approach, using elements of information theory in its prediction routines.

Prediction programs of the second class exploit, to differing extents, patterns in the 'hydrophobicities' of residues along the amino acid sequence. From this category we have used the program by Lim [10] and the method of Finer-Moore and Stroud [11]. The latter approach uses Fourier analysis of hydrophobic residue distributions, as has also been employed by Johnson et al. [12]. McLachlan has discussed such methods as a means of identifying periodic properties of amino acid sequences [13].

X-Ray Scattering from a Gel of AA Fibrils

All electron micrographs of AA fibrils recorded to date show straight or nearly straight rods. While the large variations in length are not a feature in common with preparations of tobacco mosaic virus (TMV) [14], the apparent lack of flexibility is. We were therefore encouraged to design our gel-making experiments along the lines of the pioneering work on TMV of Bernal and Fankuken [15]. We have, however, made a simple cylindrical gel not employed by earlier workers.

Species	Human $SAA_1(\alpha)$		Monkey AA		Mink AA		Duck AA	
No. or residues	104(76)		76		64		81	
Percentage α or β	α	β	α	β	α	β	α	β
Nagano et al.	37(41)	8(11)	33	12	44	6	40	0
Chou et al.	40(45)	0(0)	57	0	44	0	32	0
Burgess et al.	13(12)	4(5)	18	0	11	0	5	5
Garnier et al.	30(32)	11(13)	36	14	30	7	23	20
Lim	8(8)	18(18)	11	21	13	9	5	11

Amyloid AA Fibrils

Amyloid fibrils were extracted in water [16] from the spleen of a patient with long-standing rheumatoid arthritis and known AA amyloidosis which had been confirmed by the permanganate test [17] and by immunohistochemical staining with specific anti-AA antibodies. Stock solutions of 2 mg/ml of AA protein in distilled water were stored at -20°C after the addition of 0.01 M azide as an anti-bacterial agent.

Gel Preparation

The sum of 0.2 ml of a concentrated, 10 mg/ml, solution of AA fibrils was drawn up into a 0.7 mm diameter borosilicate glass capillary tube. The water in the sample was allowed to partially evaporate slowly, by suspending the tube overnight at 5°C in a 250 ml sealed conical flask that contained a few drops of water to maintain humidity. Once the gel had formed the tube was sealed with wax at both ends to prevent further drying.

RESULTS AND DISCUSSION

Secondary Structure Prediction

Table 1 shows that the programs based upon statistically weighted probability for secondary structure formation predict that SAA and AA are predominantly α helical, to a degree that could not be deduced from the X-ray scattering from human splenic AA fibrils [20]. The programs of Burgess et al. [8] and Lim [10], however, weight down the amount of α helix enormously. The percentage of β predicted remained low with the program of Burgess et al. [8] but increased to a significant proportion with Lim. Indeed with Lim's program β predominated over α in all except the mink sequence.

The prediction results using the program of Garnier et al. [9] (unweighted) are midway between the extremes predicted by the programs of Chou and Fasman [7] and Lim [16]. The Garnier program predicts structures with α helices but with significant β content.

Rather than evaluate a collective secondary structure prediction consisting of an unweighted average of several individual predictions [18] we

51

TABLE 2.   Summary of Concensus Secondary Structure Prediction of Human
           SAA$_1$(α) using Garnier and Fourier Transformation Methods

Residues	Predicted structure	Comments
1-5	Weak strand	Fourier transform
6-11	Random coil	Prediction unavailable
12-21	α-Helix	
22-25	Random coil	
26-37	β-Strand	
38-41	β-Turn	Residue 40 is glycine and is highly conserved
42-47	β-Strand	
48-49	Undetermined	Highly conserved pro49
50-55	Undetermined	Hydrophobic region
56-66	α-Helix	High potential only for central 7 residues
67-76	Undetermined	Residues 74 to 76 are polar and expected to be in a surface loop as residue 76 is a putative cleavage point to form AA
77-85	α-Helix	Garnier-predicted helix terminates at residue 85
86-92	Weak helix	Conflicting Garnier potentials (for turn and coil). The Fourier transform suggests that trp85, gly86, and gly89 could still contribute to the apolar side of a helix.
93-96	Weak strand	Fourier transform prediction unavailable
97-104	Undetermined	Low Garnier potential. Residues 102-104 are polar, and expected to be on surface.

have arrived at a consensus prediction derived from the results obtained by
the two radically different methods of Finer-Moore and Stroud [11] and
Garnier et al. [9]. A summary of our prediction of the secondary structure
of SAA$_1$(α) is presented in Table 2.

Nearly all the sites of variations between AA and partial SAA sequences
obtained from different sources lie away from, or towards the ends of, predicted hydrogen bonded regions (i.e., the α helices, and the β hairpin of
residues 31 to 48). The exception is position 15 where Arg of human SAA$_1$
and primate AA's is substituted by Trp in mink and duck, and by Gly in
murine SAA and AA sequences (this is position 14 in the murine sequences
reported by Hoffman et al. [19]).

The X-ray scattering pattern from the wet gel shows the expected effects
due to gelation from the solution: the broad central ring covering 1.4 nm
to 0.7 nm due to protein super-secondary structural interactions predomin-
ates over the background water curve. The central region of the scattering
pattern shows two small equatorial arcs at reciprocal spacings of 1.67 nm
(marked 2 in Fig. 1), well inside the super-secondary structure ring. These
arcs we take to be Bragg reflections from stacked microlayers of AA fibrils
making up the wet gel, and we suggest that they are the second order of the
protein:protein distance within each layer. This would make each protein
molecule 3.3 nm across, in close agreement with the diameter of the lightly
staining globular units seen in electron micrographs. That this is the correct interpretation of the equatorial arcs is reinforced by the presence of
the corresponding first order peaks at a reciprocal spacing of between 3.5
and 3.2 nm each side of the beam stop (marked 1 in Fig. 1A).

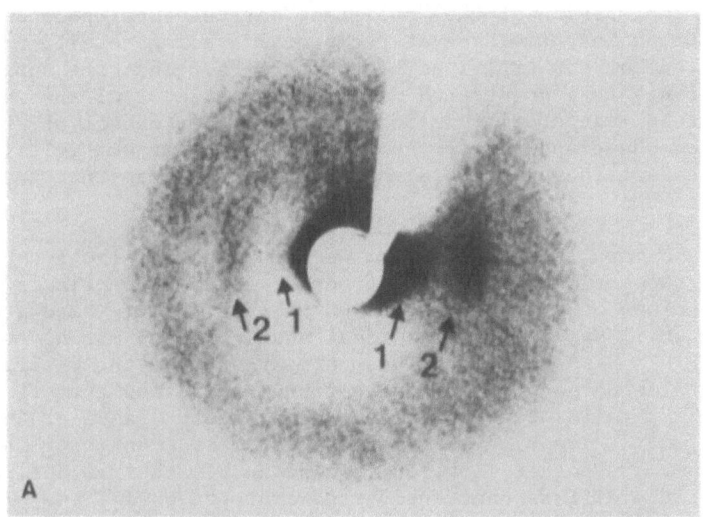

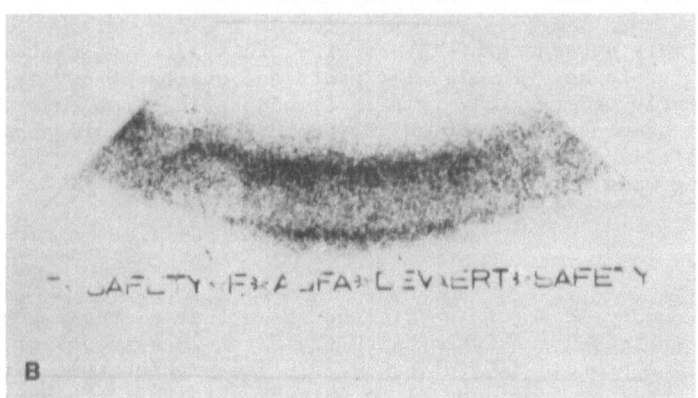

Fig. 1.   A. Enlargement of the central region of
the X-ray scattering pattern from the wet
gel. The higher scattering to the right
of the beam stop corresponds to scattered
beam paths through the flat gel/air interface. Equatorial arcs marked 1 and 2 are
centered upon reciprocal spacings of 3.3
and 1.67 nm respectively, the outer ring
on 1.1 nm. Camera length 89.0 nm.   B.
The meridional arc scattered from the
cylindrical wet gel showing splitting
into two fine arcs at reciprocal spacings of 0.468 nm and 0.408 nm.   Camera
length 142.0 mm.

Further support for our interpretation is provided by the X-ray scattering from air dried lamellae of human amyloid fibrils reported by previous workers, e.g., Fig. 3 of Eanes et al. [20]. Here the inner arcs have "moved out" to a reciprocal spacing of 1.3 nm which would be caused by compaction of the fibrils during drying, as occurs with TMV gels [15]. This provides an explanation of the "splitting" of the super-secondary structural scattering into two arcs at reciprocal spacings of 1.3 nm and 0.98 nm as reported but not explained by the authors. That the super-secondary structural ring has concentrated into diffuse equatorial arcs at 0.98 nm to give a "cross-β" pattern is, we suggest, a further effect of drying, as no such oriented sheet:sheet interaction is seen in our wet gels (Fig. 1A) in spite of the fact that we record sharp meridional arcs that are due to inter β-strand spacings.

Using a camera length of 142 mm we have measured the reciprocal spacings of the two meridional arcs that border the 0.45 nm ring to be at reciprocal spacings of 0.468 nm and 0.408 nm (Fig. 1B). These are within 1% of the side chain spacings of the ideal anti-parallel strand:strand interactions within a β-sheet [21]. These arcs show that the β-strands within each β-sheet lie perpendicular to the fibril axis, and that the axis lies approximately parallel to the plane of each sheet. Pairs of sheets within a molecular would give rise to equatorial arcs from an inter-sheet spacing of about 1 nm. We do not, however, record such arcs from our wet gel. Instead we see the diffuse unoriented ring centered on 1.1 nm. Thus we suggest that there be only one sheet per AA molecule.

The primary sequences of AA proteins are typical of globular rather than fibrous proteins. In globular proteins, sheets of several strands are not sufficiently ordered to give rise to scattering from such idealized inter-strand spacings as 0.468 and 0.408 nm. We therefore propose that the observed splitting of the 0.45 nm meridional arc is indicative of the single β-sheet being made up from very few strands.

CONCLUSIONS

Our secondary structure prediction shows that a single β-hairpin per AA molecule is indeed consistent with the first 76 residues of the human serum amyloid A protein SAA$_1$(α) sequence. The amphiphathic nature of this part of the sequence (residues 31 to 48) suggests that the antiparallel strands would form part of the surface of each molecule, and therefore possibly of the fibril. We propose that close proximity of surface β-hairpins from adjacent fibrils could give rise to the X-ray pattern scattered from dry gels reported by previous authors.

REFERENCES

1. J. P. Segrest, H. J. Pownall, R. L. Jackson, G. G. Glenner, and P. S. Pollack, Biochemistry, 15, 3187 (1976).
2. K. Waalen, K. Sletten, G. Husby, and K. Nordstoga, Europ. J. Biochem., 104, 407 (1980).
3. G. Marhaug, K. Sletten, and G. Husby, in: Amyloid and Amyloidosis (G. G. Glenner, P. Pinho e Costa, and A. Falcao de Freitas, eds.), Excerpta Medica, Amsterdam (1980), p. 337.
4. D. C. Parmelee, K. Titani, L. H. Ericsson, N. Eriksen, K. P. Benditt, and K. A. Walsh, Biochemistry, 21, 3298 (1982).
5. G. G. Glenner, New Engl. J. Med., 302, 1283, and 1333 (1980).
6. K. Nagano, J. Mol. Biol., 75, 401 (1973).
7. P. Y. Chou and G. D. Fasman, Biochemistry, 13, 222 (1974).
8. A. W. Burgess, P. K. Ponnuswamy, and H. A. Scheraga, Israel J. Chem., 12, 239 (1974).

9. J. Garnier, D. J. Osguthorpe, and B. Robson, J. Mol. Biol., 120, 97 (1978).
10. V. I. Lim, J. Mol. Biol., 88, 857 (1974).
11. J. Finer-Moore and R. M. Stroud, Proc. Natl. Acad. Sci. USA, 81, 155 (1984).
12. P. Johnson and R. R. Williams, Biochim. Biophys. Acta, 747, 1 (1983).
13. A. D. McLachlan and J. Karn, J. Mol. Biol., 164, 605 (1983).
14. G. E. Schulz, C. D. Barry, J. Friedman, P. Y. Chou, G. D. Fasman, A. V. Finkelstein, V. I. Lim, O. B. Ptitsyn, E. A. Kabat, T. T. Wu, M. Levitt, B. Robson, and K. Nagano, Nature, 250, 140 (1974).
15. J. S. Hoffman, L. H. Ericsson, N. Eriksen, K. A. Walsh, and E. P. Benditt, J. Exp. Med., 159, 641 (1984).
16. R. W. G. Wyckoff, Biochem. Biophys. Acta, 1, 139 (1947).
17. J. D. Bernal and I. Fankuken, J. Gen. Phys., 25, 111 (1941).
18. M. M. Pras, Schubert, D. Zucker-Franklin, A. Rimon, and E. C. Franklin, J. Clin. Invest., 47, 924 (1969).
19. J. R. Wright, E. Calkins, and R. L. Humphrey, Lab. Invest., 36, 274 (1977).
20. E. D. Eanes and G. G. Glenner, J. Histochem. Cytochem., 16, 673 (1968).
21. L. Pauling and R. B. Corey, Proc. Natl. Acad. Sci. USA, 7, 729 (1951).

CHARACTERIZATION OF TWO DISTINCT SERUM AMYLOID A GENE

PRODUCTS DEFINED BY THEIR COMPLEMENTARY DNAs

J. D. Sipe*, P. Woo†,
G. Goldberger†, A. S. Cohen*,
and A. S. Whitehead†

*Arthritis Center
 Boston University School of Medicine
 K5, 71 East Concord Street
 Boston, MA 02118

†Division of Cell Biology
 Childrens Hospital
 Department of Pediatrics
 Harvard Medical School
 Boston, MA 02115

ABSTRACT

Two distinct serum amyloid A specific complementary DNA clones have been isolated from a human adult liver library. One clone contains coding information for the alpha form of apoSAA1. The other shares substantial sequence homology, but differs, however, in that it lacks a Pst I restriction site present in its homologue. Both cDNA clones hybridize to an SAA genomic clone.

INTRODUCTION

Two major isotypes, apoSAA1 and apoSAA2, and four minor variants of human SAA have been described in studies of the chemical and physical properties of purified serum amyloid A (SAA) [1, 2]. The variant apoSAA1 has been found to consist of two forms, the alpha form with valine at position 52 and alanine at position 57, and the beta form with alanine at 52 and valine at position 57 [3].

To facilitate the study of these variants of SAA, complementary DNA clones were isolated from a human acute phase liver library. One clone, pA1, has been completely sequenced and contains a Pst I restriction enzyme recognition site spanning the nucleotide sequence coding for residues 54-56 [4]. Another SAA specific cDNA clone, pA10 differs from pA1 in that it lacks the internal Pst I recognition site. Clone pA10 was analyzed by DNA sequence analysis and by Southern blot hybridization with a human genomic DNA clone in order to determine its coding information and how the gene product it specified differs from apoSAA1 alpha. This is a preliminary report of the results of that study.

MATERIALS AND METHODS

SAA specific cDNA clones have been isolated from a human acute phase liver cDNA library [4]. SAA specific plasmid DNA was isolated from bacteria by the cleared lysate method of Clewell and Helinski [5]. Complementary DNA was excised from plasmids by Pst I digestion and purified by agarose electrophoresis. DNA sequence analysis was carried out both by the chemical cleavage method of Maxam and Gilbert [6] and by the chain termination method of Sanger et al. [7].

A 20 Kb human genomic SAA clone was isolated from a partial SaII human genomic library (gift of S. K. Karanthanasis) by the method of Benton and Davis [8]. A 3.5 Kb Hind III fragment containing SAA coding sequence was subcloned into the cosmid vector PTCF. DNA restriction fragments were analyzed by Southern blot hybridization [9] under standard conditions [10].

RESULTS AND DISCUSSION

The SAA specific cDNA clone pA1 contains the entire coding sequence for mature SAA and an additional 30 nucleotides that specify 10 amino acids of the 18 residue signal peptide [4]. The pA1 clone also includes a 70 nucleotide long 3' untranslated region and approximately 120 bases of the poly A tail. The derived amino acid sequence of pA1 is identical to the alpha form of apoSAA1 with valine specified at position 52 and alanine at position 57. A recognition site for the restriction endonuclease Pst I spans residues 54-56 (-AAE-) of the derived amino acid sequence of pA1. We have designated the 5' Pst I fragment pA1a and the 3' Pst I fragment pA1b. The size of pA10 is similar to pA1, about 550 base pairs. The 5' end of the clone encodes 10 residues of the signal peptide followed by the entire coding sequence for mature SAA, a 3' untranslated region and a poly A tail. Its nucleotide and derived amino acid sequence is idential to pA1 between residues 2 and 47; however, it lacks the Pst I recognition site spanning residues 54-56. Studies are in progress to complete the nucleotide sequence analysis of pA10.

The amino acid sequence from residues 33-45 is conserved in human [3, 11], monkey [12], guinea pig [13], mouse [14, 15], mink [16], and duck [17] SAA and AA. The nucleotide sequences of pA1 and pA10 are identical in this region. Furthermore, the nucleotide sequences specified by these clones are identical to that reported by others [18, 19] for mouse SAA mRNA in this invariant region. This is in contrast to the substantial differences between mouse and human SAA mRNA which are apparent in other regions.

Southern blot hybridization of pA1 and pA10 to a 3.5 Kb Hind III fragment of an SAA specific genomic clone was performed. This fragment, which contains the entire SAA coding sequence, was digested with the restriction endonuclease PsT I, giving rise to subfragments of 2.9 Kb and 0.6 Kb. Radiolabelled pA10 hybridized to both PsT subfragments whereas pA1a hybridized only to the 0.6 Kb subfragment and pA1b hybridized only to the 2.9 Kb subfragment (Fig. 1). This result indicates that the genomic clone shares the internal Pst I site present in pA1 and establishes that the 3' end of clone pA10 shares sufficient homology with the corresponding region of pA1 to allow hybridization to the 3' end of the gene.

Thus, we have defined two distinct SAA gene products. It is to be determined whether pA1 and pA10 are derived from mRNAs transcribed from allelic variants of the same gene or from the mRNA products of two different genes.

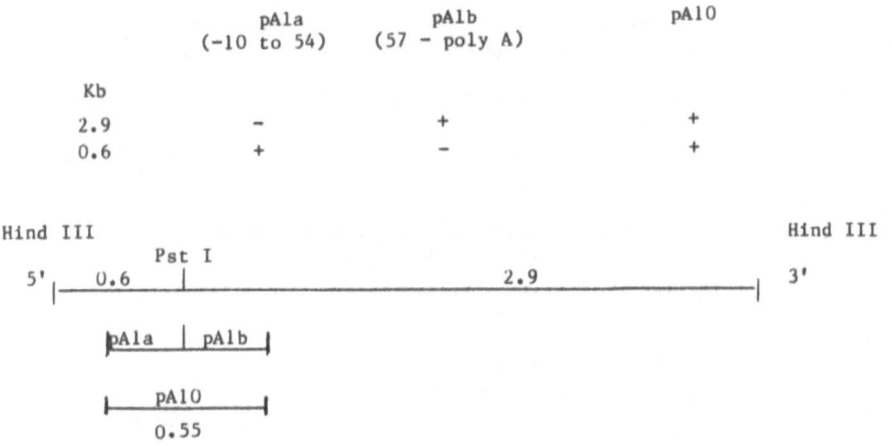

Fig. 1. Position of pAla, pAlb, and pAl0 relative to the 3.5 Kb
Hind III fragment of a human genomic SAA clone based on
Southern hybridization experiments. +) Indicates probe
hybridizers; −) indicates probe does not hybridize.

Like pA1, pAl0 contains only a portion of the signal peptide sequence.
Human acute phase liver mRNA is about 600 nucleotides in length [4] and it
directs synthesis of preSAA (14,000 M_r) in a cell free translation system.
In a Xenopus oocyte translation system, preSAA is synthesized and processed
to the mature 12,000 M_r product [4]. The complete 18 amino acid signal peptide sequence of preSAA was derived from sequencing the 5' end of the cDNA
clone and by primer extension of the SAA mRNA. The leader sequence is typical in that it begins with an N-terminal methionine and contains 12 hydrophobic residues.

The cDNA fragment pAla, which includes the region coding for residues
33 to 45, cross hybridizes with mouse and rabbit acute phase mRNA while
pAlb does not [4]. In preliminary studies (G. Goldberger et al., unpublished observations) liver SAA mRNA increased markedly in rabbits injected
with turpentine oil. The elevation was maximal after one day and declined
over a period of 6 days. The increase in SAA mRNA was due at least, in
part, to an increase in transcription. This series of experiments indicates
that maximal induction of SAA mRNA occurs earlier than that of C-reactive
protein, the other inducible acute phase protein in humans.

The SAA specific cDNA probes pAla, pAlb, and pAl0 will permit future
studies of genomic structure, extrahepatic SAA synthesis, regulation of SAA
mRNA and will permit a detailed examination of the fine tuning of SAA synthesis in acute and chronic inflammation.

REFERENCES

1.   E. P. Benditt, J. S. Hoffman, N. Eriksen, and K. A. Walsh, Ann. N. Y.
     Acad. Sci., 389:183 (1982).
2.   L. L. Bausserman, A. L. Saritelli, P. N. Herbert, K. P. W. J. McAdam,
     and R. S. Shulman, Biochem. Biophys. Acta, 702:556 (1982).
3.   D. C. Parmelee, K. Titani, L. H. Ericsson, N. Eriksen, E. P. Benditt,
     and K. A. Walsh, Biochemistry, 21:3298 (1982).

4. J. D. Sipe, A. S. Whitehead, G. Goldberberger, P. Woo, M. D. Edge, B. F. Tack, R. M. Kay, A. S. Cohen, and H. R. Colten, Biochemistry, in press (1985).

5. D. B. Clewell and D. R. Helsinki, Proc. Natl. Acad. Sci., 69:1159 (1969).

6. A. Maxam and W. Gilbert, Proc. Natl. Acad. Sci., 74:560 (1977).

7. F. Sanger, S. Nicken, and A. R. Coulson, Proc. Natl. Acad. Sci., 74: 5463 (1977).

8. M. D. Benton and R. W. Davis, Science, 196:180 (1977).

9. E. M. Southern, J. Mol. Biol., 98:503 (1975).

10. A. J. Jeffreys and R. A. Flavell, Cell, 12:429 (1977).

11. K. Sletten, G. Marhaug, and G. Husby, Hoppe-Seyle's Z. Physiol. Chem. Bd., 364:1039 (1983).

12. M. A. Hermodson, R. W. Kuhn, K. A. Walsh, H. Neurath, N. Eriksen, and E. P. Benditt, Biochemistry, 11:2934 (1972).

13. M. Skinner, E. S. Cathcart, A. S. Cohen, and M. D. Benson, J. Exp. Med., 140:871 (1974).

14. P. D. Gorevich, Y. Levo, B. Frangione, and E. C. Franklin, J. Immunol., 121:131 (1978).

15. J. S. Hoffman, L. H. Ericsson, N. Eriksen, K. A. Walsh, and E. P. Benditt, J. Exp. Med., 159:641 (1984).

16. K. Waalen, K. Sletten, G. Husby, and K. Nordstoga, Eur. J. Biochem., 104:407 (1980).

17. P. D. Gorevic, M. Greenwald, B. Frangione, M. Pras, and E. C. Franklin, J. Immunol., 118:1113 (1977).

18. J. F. Morrow, R. S. Stearman, C. G. Peltzman, and D. A. Potter, Proc. Natl. Acad. Sci., 78:4718 (1981).

19. R. S. Stearman, C. A. Lowell, W. R. Pearson, and J. F. Morrow, Ann. N. Y. Acad. Sci., 389:106 (1982).

HUMAN SERUM AMYLOID GENES —

MOLECULAR CHARACTERIZATION

George H. Sack, Jr. and John J. Lease

Departments of Medicine
Biological Chemistry, Orthopedics, and Pediatrics
The John Hopkins University School of Medicine and
The John F. Kennedy Institute
Baltimore, Maryland

ABSTRACT

Three clones containing human genes for serum amyloid A protein (SAA) have been isolated and characterized. Each of two clones, GSAA 1 and 2 (of 12.8 and 15.9 kilobases, respectively), contains two exons, accouting for amino acids 12-58 and 58-103 of mature SAA; the extreme 5' termini and 5' untranslated regions have not yet been defined but are anticipated to be close based on studies of murine SAA genes. Initial amino acid sequence comparisons show 78/89 identical residues. At 4 of the 11 discrepant residues, the amino acid specified by the codon is the same as the corresponding residue in murine SAA. Identification of regions containing coding regions has permitted use of selected subclones for blot hybridization studies of larger human SAA chromosomal gene organization. The third clone, GSAA 3 also contains SAA coding information by DNA sequence analysis but has a different organization which has not yet been fully described.

We have reported the isolation of clones of human DNA hybridizing with pRS48 - a plasmid containing a complementary DNA (cDNA) clone for murine serum amyloid A (SAA; 1, 2). We now present more detailed data confirming the identity and defining some of the organizational features of these clones.

MATERIALS AND METHODS

Restriction endonucleases and DNA polymerase-Klenow fragment were purchased from International Biochemical Industries. DNA polymerase, 17 base pair sequencing primer fragment oligomer and T4 DNA polymerase were purchased from New England Biolabs. ^{32}P nucleotides were purchased from New England Nuclear. Deoxy- and dideoxyribonucleoside triphosphates were purchased from PL Biochemicals.

Vertical slab gel electrophoresis in agarose or polyacrylamide was performed as described [1, 3] and photography was made following staining with ethidium bromide. Fragment molecular weights were determined by reference to known restriction fragments run in a separate lane [3]. DNA transfers to nitrocellulose were made using the technique of Southern [4].

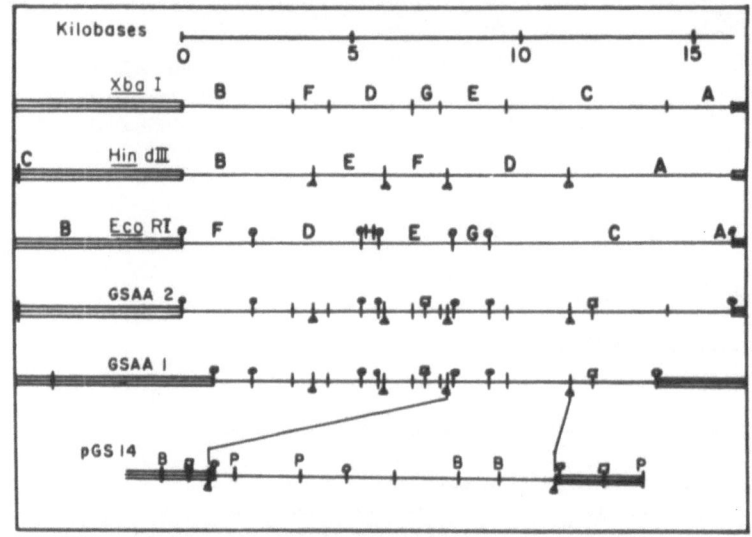

Fig. 1. Restriction endonuclease cleavage maps of recombinant human DNA library phase GSAA 1 and 2 showing the derivation of subclones pGS1 and pGS14,
respectively. Sizes indicated in kilobases. Symbols for restriction endonucleases are: Xba I)
|; Hin dIII) ⅃; Eco RI) ↑; Hpa II) ᵠ; Pst I) ᵖ;
Bam HI) ᴮ|. Orientation places 5' gene regions on
the left. Single horizontal lines indicate human
DNA; multiple lines are vector DNA. Letters
designate fragments in order of decreasing size
for each digestion reaction.

DNA sequence determination was performed on DNA cloned into bacteriophage M13 using the Klenow fragment of DNA polymerase I to direct polymerization from an oligonucleotide primer in the presence of selected dideoxy-
nucleoside triphosphates and ^{32}P-labeled dATP [5, 6]. Three additions of
reaction aliquots were made to a 15% polyacrylamide/urea gel permitting
275-350 bases to be read per reaction.

Reiteration frequency determinations were performed according to the
method of Zasloff and Santos [7]. Terminally labeled restriction fragments
were separated by gel electrophoresis and then blotted onto filters to which
total human cellular DNA was covalently bound; the strength of the resulting
autoradiographic signal was then proportional to the frequency of the sequences represented by the fragment within the entire genome. All signals
were standardized to results from a human β globulin cDNA plasmid which was
the kind gift of Dr. H. Kazazlan.

RESULTS

Initial hybridization with $5 \cdot 10^5$ phage plaques from a recombinant human DNA library [8] disclosed 4 clones, two of which appeared identical by
restriction endonuclease cleavage patterns. Thus, three clones have been
designated GSAA 1, 2, and 3. Figure 1 shows that GSAA 1 and GSAA 2 are
very similar, differing only in flanking Eco RI cleavage sites; we anticipate that these clones contain alleles. GSAA 3 differs completely from the
others and the map (Fig. 2) shows the relatively few restriction endonuclease sites which it contains.

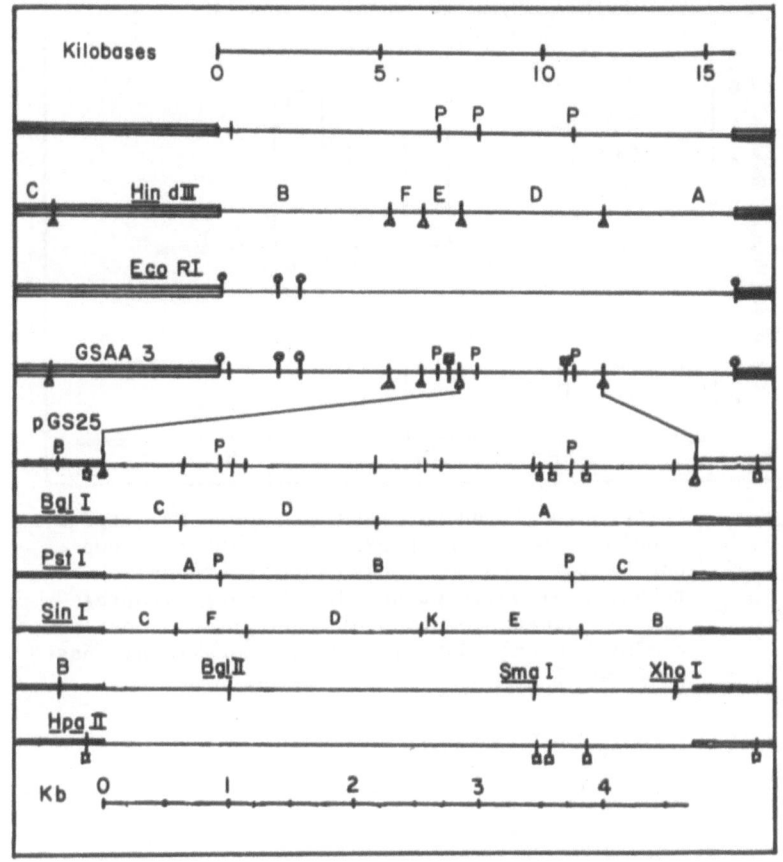

Fig. 2. Restriction endonclease cleavage map for recombinant human DNA library phage GSAA 3 and its subclone pGS25. Sizes indicated in kilobases. Symbols for restriction endonucleases are: Xba I) |; Pst I) P; Hin dIII) $\triangle$; Eco RI) Υ; Hpa II) $\Box$. Sites on pGS25 are presented without all distinctions for clarity. Orientation places 5' gene region on the left. Single horizontal lines indicate human DNA; multiple lines are vector DNA. Letters designate fragments in order of decreasing size for each digestion reaction.

As shown earlier [1] hybridization of pRS48 to restriction endonuclease fragments of the library isolates showed high specificity to single Hin dIII and overlapping Hpa II fragments from each phage. The Hin dIII fragments were subcloned into pBR322 to simplify detailed analysis. Figures 1 and 2 also show cleavage maps for these subclones (designated pGS1, pGS14, and pGS25 for derivatives of GSAA 1, 2, and 3, respectively).

The direction of transcription was determined for each putative gene by hybridizing ^{32}P-labeled 5', middle, and 3' regions of pRS48 to nitro-cellulose transfers [4] of restriction endonuclease cleavage fragment arrays from the subclones. Figures 1 and 2 present clone maps in the conventional 5' to 3' orientations.

Further evaluation of the nature of the nucleic acid sequences in the putative gene regions was made by comparing the hybridization of terminally

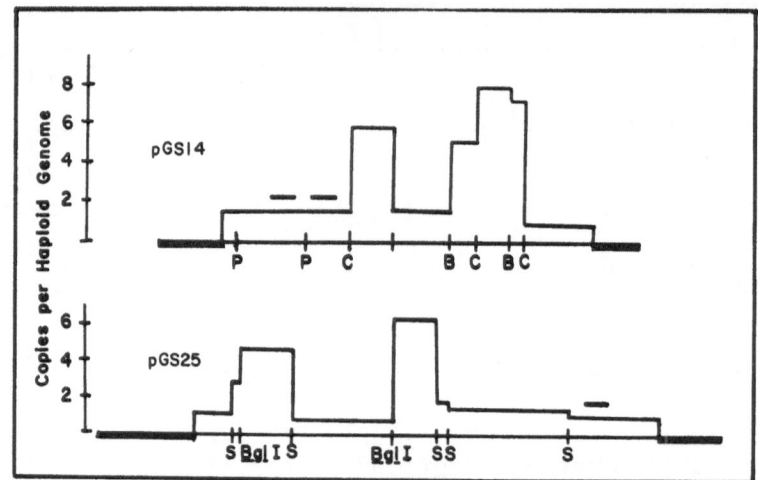

Fig. 3. Reiteration frequency maps for human SAA region subclones pGS14 and pGS25. The number of copies per haploid genome is based on reference to internal β globulin standard. Heavy horizontal lines indicate location of identified exons in coding region. Restriction map details are based on Figs. 1 and 2.

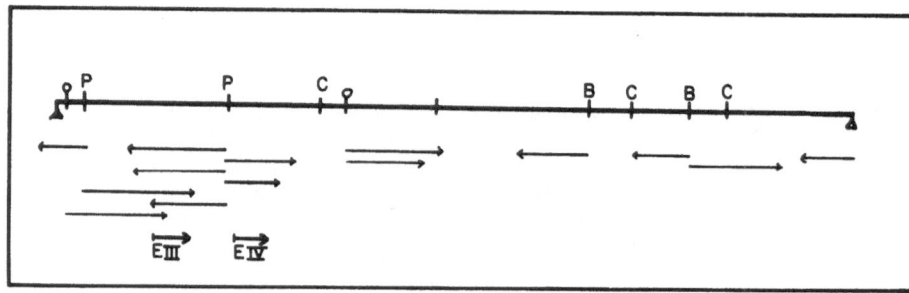

Fig. 4. Sequencing strategy for clones pGS1 and pGS14. Small arrows indicate direction and extent of reading of sequence data from individual M13 phage subclones with positions of exons 3 and 4 shown. No further coding information was found between the 5' end of the third exon and the left Hin dIII cloning site. Restriction enzyme symbols as shown in Fig. 1 with the addition of Hin dII) C.

^{32}P-labeled restriction endonuclease fragments of the subclones to filters containing a uniform layer of fragments of the entire human genome as described [7]. Figure 3 shows the reiteration frequencies thus determined for subclones pGS14 and pGS25 and indicates regions of apparently low and multiple copy number. No very highly repetitive DNA domains were detected in these relatively short regions. These data have been useful in devising sequencing strategies and planning mapping studies as discussed below.

Unequivocal identification of these clones has been established through direct DNA sequence determination. The data were compared with reported

pGS14

289 TCA CAC ATG GTA TTA ACA AAG TAA TAA CAG AAC TTA GAA TGG AAT GAA 336

337 ACA GAA TGA AAA TTA CAC CAA GTA CAA TTC TCA TTA CAT TAA CCC AGA 384

395 GAA GTG AAA AGT AGA AGA ATA TTT ATT TCA AGC CAT ATT AAT TTC CAA 432

433 GGG CTT TGT TGA AGG CTG AAT CTT CGG GAG GAA AGT AGT GAG AAG AAA 480

481 CTG TTA CTT CCT CTA TTT CCC AGT ATA TAA TTG TTT GAT CAT TTC TTC 528
                                                         acceptor

         splice
529 CTT CCA GGG GCT AAA GAC ATG TGG AGA GCC TAC TCT GAC ATG AAA GAA 576
         Gly Ala Lys Asp MET Trp Arg Ala Tyr Ser Asp MET Lys Glu
         12   15   20   25

577 GCC AAT TAC AAA AAT TCA GAC AAA TAC TTC CAT GCT CGG GGG AAC TAT 624
    Ala Asn Tyr Lys Asn Ser Asp Lys Tyr Phe His Ala Arg Gly Asn Tyr
                  30   35   40

625 GAT GCT GCA ACA AGA GGG CCT GGG GGT GCT TGG GCT ACA GAA GTG ATC 672
    Asp Ala Ala Thr Arg Gly Pro Gly Gly Ala Trp Ala Thr Glu Val Ile
        splice   45   50   55

673 AGG TAA TGC ACA TTC CTG ATG TTG CCA GGA ATG AGT GAG CAG AGC TTG 720
    Ser donor

    58
721 GAC TGC CTT GGA CAG TCA GGA GAG AGG TAA GCT CCT TGC AGA GAA GTT 768

769 AGA GCT GCA G, 778. . . . .
         Pst I

pGS1
. . . . CAG AGC CTC ACT TGA AAT GAG AGA ATG GGA AGT GGG CGT GTG CTC ACT

                                                  splice
    GCC TGT ATT AAG TCC TTG CGT TGC CTG GAC TAC AGC GAT GCC AGG GAA
                                     acceptor Ser Asp Ala Arg Glu
                                               58   60

    AAC GTC CAG AGA CTC ACA GGA AGG ACT GCA GAG GAT TCG CTG GCT GAC
    Asn Val Gln Arg Leu Thr Gly Arg Thr Ala Glu Asp Ser Leu Ala Asp
            65   70   75

    CAG GCT ACG AAC AAA TGG GGC CAG AGT GGC AAA GAC CCC AAT CAC TTC
    Gln Ala Thr Asn Lys Trp Gly Gln Ser Gly Lys Asp Pro Asn His Phe
        80   85   90

    CGA CCT GCT GGC CTG CCA GAG AAA TAC TGA GCT TCC TTT TCA ATC TGC
    Arg Pro Ala Gly Leu Pro Glu Lys Tyr *   3' untranslated region
    95   100

    TCT CAG AGG ACC TGC TGT GAC GCC CTG AGG GCA GGG ACA TTT GTT GAC
                                                          Hin cII

    CTA CAG TTA CTT GAA TTC
              Eco RI

Fig. 5. Combined DNA sequence data showing third exon region of pGS14 and
         fourth exon region of pGS1. Numbers in pGS14 region indicate base
         pairs from the left Hin dIII site of subcloning. Basic location
         of exons is also shown in Figs. 3 and 4. Consensus sequences for
         splice donor and acceptor sites are indicated.

pGS14/1   [12]Gly Ala Lys Asp Met Trp Arg Ala Tyr Ser Asp Met Lys Glu Ala Asn Tyr Lys

human   Gly Ala Arg Asp Met Trp Arg Ala Tyr Ser Asp Met Arg Glu Ala Asn Tyr Ile

mouse   Gly(Ala/Ser)(Gly/Arg)Asp Met Trp(Arg/Lys)Ala Tyr(Thr/Ser)Asp Met Lys(Glu/Lys)Ala(Asn/Gly)Trp Lys

pGS14/1   [30]Asn Ser Asp Lys Tyr Phe His Ala Arg Gly Asn Tyr Asp Ala Ala Thr Arg Gly

human   Gly Ser Asp Lys Tyr Phe His Ala Arg Gly Asn Tyr Asp Ala Ala Lys Arg Gly

mouse   (Asn/Asp)(Ser/Gly)Asp Lys Tyr Phe His Ala Arg Gly Asn Tyr Asp Ala Ala(Gln/Arg)Arg Gly

                                                    exon 3 | exon 4

pGS14/1   [48]Pro Gly Gly Ala Trp Ala Thr Glu Val Ile Ser Asp Ala Arg Glu Asn Val Gln

human   Pro Gly Gly(Val/Ala)(Trp/Arg)Ala Ala Glu(Val/Ala)Ile Ser(Asp/Asn)Ala Arg Glu Asn Ile Gln

mouse   Pro Gly Gly(Val/Ala)Trp Ala Ala(Glu/Lys)(Val/Lys)Ile Ser Asp(Gly/Ala)Arg Glu(Ala/Asn)(Phe/Val)Gln

pGS14/1   [66]Arg Leu Thr Gly Arg Thr Ala Glu Asp Ser Leu Ala Asp Gln Ala Thr Asn Lys

human   Arg(Phe/Leu)Thr Gly(Arg/His)Gly(Ala/His)Glu Asp Ser Leu Ala Asp Gln Ala Ala Asn Glu

mouse   (Glu/Lys)Phe(Phe/Thr)Gly(Arg/His)Gly(Ala/His)Glu Asp(Thr/Ser)(Ile/Met/Arg)Ala Asp Gln(Glu/Phe)Ala Asn(Arg/Glu)

pGS14/1   [84]Trp Gly Gln Ser Gly Lys Asp Pro Asn His Phe Arg Pro Ala Gly Leu Pro Glu

human   Trp Gly Arg Ser Gly Lys Asp Pro Asn His Phe Arg Pro Ala Gly Leu Pro Glu

mouse   (His/Trp)Gly Arg Ser Gly Lys Asp Pro Asn(Tyr/His)(Tyr/Phe)Arg Pro(Pro/Ala)Gly Leu Pro(Asp/Ala/Lys)

pG 14/1   [102]Lys Tyr *

human   Lys Tyr *

mouse   (Lys/Arg)Tyr *

Fig. 6.   Combined data for amino acids specified by pGS1 and pGS14 with
          published data for human [9-15] and murine [16-18] SAA proteins.
          Sites of more than one amino acid indicated by brackets.

human SAA amino acid sequences [9-15] as well as the corresponding murine
sequencies [16-18] and the base sequence of the murine cDNA clone pRS48
[19]. Selected restriction endonuclease fragments were subcloned in bacteriophage M13 and sequence data were obtained by primer extension and dideoxy chain termination [5, 6]. Figure 4 shows the cloning and sequencing
strategies used for pGS1 and pGS14.

    Figure 5 shows sequence data for the critical regions of pGS1 and
pGS14; several features are apparent. 1) Two exons are present corresponding to amino acids 12-58 and 58-103 of known human SAA, respectively. Based
on studies in the murine system, where two additional exons have been found
at the 5' end, these have been designated exons "3" and "4." 2) Transcription orientation corresponds to that predicted from studies cited above and

summarized in Figs. 1 and 2. 3) There are authentic 15 and 6 base pair splice acceptor sites and a 9 base pair donor sequence compatible with the compilation of Mount [20]. 4) The exon-intron boundary positions are identical to those found in corresponding murine genes [21]. 5) No other 5' coding sequences are found in the 500 base pairs to the 5' end of exon 3 in the subclones and the ultimate 5' ends of the human SAA genes have thus not yet been identified. This is consistent with hybridization of pGS1 and pGS14 to pRS48 which was, itself, a cDNA clone. 6) The 3' end includes an authentic termination codon – UGA – followed by an untranslated region whose length has not yet been determined. No unequivocal polyadenylation signal has yet been found 3' to the coding region of exon 4.

Figure 6 compares the 92 amino acids corresponding to the exons in these clones with reported data for human and murine SAA proteins [9–18]. As noted above, splicing occurs at identical positions. The amino acid sequences show a close relationship to those reported from human and murine SAA isolates. However, these are discrepancies are amino acids 14, 24, 29, 30, 45, 54, 64, 71, 81, 83, 86. In several – 24, 29, 30, 64 – the codon found specifies an amino acid differing from that reported for human SAA but identical to the corresponding residues for murine SAA. Studies of base sequences for pGS25 have been more difficult because of difficulties in finding suitable restriction endonuclease sites for subcloning. However, sequences corresponding to the 4th exon have been found at the position indicated in Fig. 3 which are consistent with the transcription orientation shown in Fig. 2.

Current studies are extending these sequences data into neighboring 5' regions in order to permit complete comparisons between human and murine SAA genes. These also should establish whether 5' coding heterogeneity exists compatible with reported variation in human SAA [12]. They will also identify 5' untranslated regions and, presumably, those sequences critical to control of human SAA gene expression.

Identification of the SAA coding regions has permitted the use of our recombinants for studies of SAA gene structure and expression in human tissues. As we will report elsewhere, signals in blotting studies provide evidence for human chromosomal gene organization as well as transcription, and are consistent with GSAA 1, 2, and 3 representing all human SAA loci.

Our findings are compatible with considerable conservation of human and murine SAA gene loci. Emerging data should provide more information regarding recognized structural polymorphisms of SAA as well as pathophysiologic correlations and features of expression control.

ACKNOWLEDGEMENTS

We are delighted to acknoledge the important contributions of David Potter, John Tower, and Rodney Owen in some of these experiments and the valuable collaborations with Dr. John Morrow and his coworkers Robert Stearman and Clifford Lowell. We are grateful for support from the Garrett Fund and the Kroc Foundation and generous gifts from Mr. and Mrs. William M. Griffin and Mr. Daniel M. Kelley. George H. Sack, Jr. is a Joseph P. Kennedy, Jr. Foundation scholar.

REFERENCES

1. G. H. Sack, Jr., Gene 21, 19 (1983).
2. J. F. Morrow, R. S. Stearman, C. G. Peltzman, and D. A. Potter, Proc. Natl. Acad. Sci. U.S.A., 78, 4718 (1981).

3. K. J. Danna, G. H. Sack, Jr., and D. Nathans, J. Mol. Biol., 78, 363 (1973).
4. E. M. Southern, J. Mol. Biol., 98, 503 (1975).
5. P. H. Schreier and R. Cortese, J. Mol. Biol., 129, 169 (1979).
6. A. J. H. Smith, in: Methods in Enzymology (L. Grossman and K. Moldave, eds.), New York (1980), p. 65, 560.
7. M. Zasloff and T. Santos, Proc. Natl. Acad. Sci. U.S.A., 77, 5668 (1980).
8. R. M. Lawn, E. F. Fritsch, R. C. Parker, G. Blake, and T. Maniatis, Cell, 15, 1157 (1978).
9. E. P. Benditt, N. Eriksen, M. A. Hermodson, and L. H. Ericsson, FEBS Lett., 19, 169 (1971).
10. D. Ein, S. Kimura, W. D. Terry, J. Magnotta, and G. G. Glenner, J. Biol. Chem., 247, 5653 (1972).
11. M. Levin, E. C. Franklin, B. Frangione, and M. Pras, J. Clin. Invest., 51, 2773 (1972).
12. L. L. Bausserman, P. N. Herbert, and K. P. W. J. McAdam, J. Exp. Med., 152, 641 (1980).
13. G. Husby and K. Sletten, in: Amyloid and Amyloidosis (G. G. Glenner, P. P. e Costa, and A. F. de Freitas, eds.), Amsterdam (1980), p. 266.
14. G. Marhaug and G. Husby, Clin. Exp. Immunol., 46, 97 (1981).
15. P. Westermark, Biochim. Biophys. Acta, 701, 19 (1982).
16. K. Sletten and G. Husby, Eur. J. Biochem., 41, 117 (1974).
17. R. F. Anders, J. B. Natvig, K. Sletten, G. Husby, and K. Nordstoga, J. Immunol., 118, 229 (1977).
18. P. C. Gorevic, Y. Levo, B. Frangione, and E. C. Franklin, J. Immunol., 121, 138 (1978).
19. R. S. Stearman, C. A. Lowell, W. R. Pearson, and J. F. Morrow, Ann. N. Y. Acad. Sci., 389, 106 (1982).
20. S. M. Mount, Nucl. Acids Res., 10, 459 (1982).
21. C. A. Lowell, J. F. Morrow, personal communication.

KINETICS OF HUMAN SERUM AMYLOID A

C. J. Rosenthal, N. Solomon
and M. E. Martin

Departments of Medicine and Radiology
Downstate Medical Center-SUNY
Brooklyn, New York

ABSTRACT

In order to better understand the pathogenetic role of serum amyloid A (SAA) we studied the kinetics of ^{131}I radiolabelled pure SAA, extracted from 400 ml serum of a human volunteer. 50 μCi of ^{131}I SAA and 15 μCi ^{125}I labelled sodium iodide were administered i.v. on two occasions at 6 month intervals. Serum and plasma samples were collected at 10-20 min intervals × 10, then once daily × 10; lymphocytes were separated from monocytes and granulocytes. Counts per minute of ^{131}I and ^{125}I were measured in each sample in the serum, in serum precipitates resulting after addition of a rabbit anti-SAA antibody and of TCA and in various cell subpopulations as well as in the whole urine and TCA precipitated urine from each micturition. The ^{131}I disappearance curves from the plasma and serum precipitates were semilogarithmically plotted; cumulative ^{131}I cpm in plasma, cells and urine at various intervals were determined. Body scanning was performed at 2, 16, and 48 h. The results of the two experiments were very similar. The curve of ^{131}I SAA in plasma TCA precipitates indicated the existence of 4 compartments likely due to uptake of ^{131}I SAA by some plasma proteins, circulating cells and other tissues; later release from tissues started at 6 h. The ^{131}I SAA half-life time in these compartments was found to be 35, 170, 255, and 550 min, respectively. Tissue binding of ^{131}I was also suggested by a rising of the ^{125}I:^{131}I ratio with time and by a 26% release of ^{131}I in the urine at 15 h which could not account for its plasma disappearance. Scanning, except for ^{131}I uptake in the spleen at 2 h likely due to blood activity, showed no organ concentration. 92% of the injected ^{131}I was found in the urine but only 6.2% of ^{131}I SAA was accounted for in urine precicipitates.

INTRODUCTION

Serum Amyloid A (SAA), the serum precursor of amyloid fibrils was found to be a normal component of human serum [1], to behave as an acute phase reactant protein [2] which rises during inflammatory and infectious processes [1], after trauma or surgery [2] as well as in patients with disseminated malignancies [3]. It circulates in plasma as a low molecular weight protein (of approximately 12,000 daltons) with the HDL portion of the plasma lipoprotein [4] forming a larger molecule of 180,000 daltons. While the chemical structure of apo SAA or SAAL has been elucidated [5, 6, 7, 8] little is known about its function and metabolic fate.

Since 1977 it was noted in mice [9] that endogenously generated SAA (after casein or bovine serum albumin injection) was cleared from the plasma 24-48 h after SAA reached its peak level.

In other experiments Benditt et al. [10], administering ^{125}I radio-labelled enriched SAA plasma into the tail vein of mice, noted that the plasma half-life of SAA is approximately 38 min; its disappearance was much faster than the diphasic clearance of the normal plasma HDL. Recently, Bausserman [11] confirmed the rapid clearance of SAA from high density lipoproteins. The fact that the endogenously produced and the exogenously radiolabelled SAA showed similar disappearance time makes unlike the possibility that this is due to SAA degradation by proteases at the surface of circulating monocytes [12] or by the amyloid degrading activity of the serum [13]. The occurrence of significant SAA degradation in human serum and the complexity of the analysis of radiolabelled SAAL distribution have discouraged studies on SAA turnover in humans.

In order to improve our understanding concerning the pathogenetic role of SAA and our knowledge concerning its body distribution and its excretion we performed this study on the kinetics of [131]Iodide radiolabelled human SAA; the data obtained confirmed the rapid SAA clearance from the plasma but also revealed its early binding to circulating proteins, circulating cells and various tissues followed by its relatively slow release and rapid excretion in the urine in an almost completely degraded form.

METHODS

Preparation of Radioiodinated SAAL for Turnover Studies

Apo SAA (SAAL) was extracted from 400 ml serum of a normal volunteer collected by plasmapheresis (Hemonetics, Braintree, Massachusetts). Pure SAAL, as demonstrated by the presence of one band in SDS-PAGE gels at 12,000 daltons-molecular weight level, was obtained by gel filtration chromatography in 10% formic acid using a method previously described by us [6] and others [5].

Purified SAAL (apo SAA) was iodinated with [131]Iodide, a stronger gamma emiter than [125]Iodide, which was necessary to permit scanning of organs potentially retaining radiolabelled SAAL. Iodination was performed by the procedure of Greenwood, Hunter, and Glover [14] through chloramine T oxidation of the protein. 2 mCi [131]Iodine as NaI in 0.1 Na OH (New England Nuclear, Boston, Massachusetts) was mixed with 200 µg of SAAL dissolved in 0.2 M barbital buffer pH 8.0.50 µg chloramine T in 0.1 M barbital buffer, pH 8.0 (2 mg/ml) was added. Oxidation was stopped after 30 sec with 60 µg sodium metabisulfite in 0.1 M barbital buffer (1.2 mg/ml). The labelled SAAL was separated from the free [131]Iodine by gel filtration through a small Sephadex G-25 column (0.7 × 30 cm) pretreated with 30 ml of 1% bovine serum gamma globulin (BSG) in 0.1 M barbital buffer in order to minimize absorption of ^{131}I-SAAL. The most radioactive fraction collected in the first eluted peak was stored mixed 1:1 with BSG at -20°C for SAA kinetic studies.

Turnover Studies. Two turnover studies at 6 month intervals were carried out in the same normal y.o. male who donated the plasma for SAAL extraction - after appropriate permit was secured from the N.Y. State Commission on human radioactive experiments and appropriate consent form was signed.

The proband received 0.5 ml of a saturated solution of potassium iodide every 8 h for two days prior to iodide administration and during the
monitoring of [131]Iodine distribution. Approximately 50 µg of radioiodinated
SAAL containing 50 µCi of ^{131}I was administered intravenously from a calibrated syringe along with 15 µCi of ^{125}I labelled sodium iodide (New England
Nuclear). The latter was used to determine the parameters of iodide metabolism. Fifteen milliliters of heparinized blood samples were collected at
10 and 24, 40 and 60 min $1^1/_2$ h, $3^1/_2$, $6^1/_2$, 9 h then daily throughout the
study. Red cells were separated by slow centrifugation (150 G) in 5% Dextran; plasma, granulocytes and mononuclear cells were then separated from
each sample by Ficoll-Hypaque discontinuous gradient centrifugation [15].

Urine was collected in 3 h lots during the first 24 h of study and
then in 24 h lots until the study was terminated.

0.1 mg ε-amino caproic acid (ε-ACA) per ml was added to all samples in
order to prvent in vitro degradation of SAAL.

Measurement of Radioactivity

In each sample obtained, the following measurements of ^{131}I and [125]I
radioactivities were performed: the total radioactivity, the non protein-
bound radioactivity after precipitation of protein with 10% trichloracitic
acid (TCA) and the SAA-bound radioactivity. The latter was determined by
a liquid phase radioimmunoassay devised by one of the authors [1] in which
the antigen-antibody complexes were precipitated by 30% polyethylene glycol
(Sigma). In all other samples the radioactivity was counted in an automatic gamma-ray well counter with appropriate standards to a counting accuracy of ±3%.

Whole body scanning was also performed with a Picker 4-15 Auger gamma
scanner apparatus at 2, 16, and 48 h after the injection of radiolabelled
[131]I SAAL.

Proband's thyroid scanning and his plasma radioactivity were tested at
10, 20, and 30 days after the radioactive injection in order to assess any
residual radioactivity; none was found.

Methods for Calculating the Fractional Catabolic Rate (FCR)
of SAAL, Determining Its Disappearance Curve and the Plasma
Half Times of Its Various Fractions

There are two mathematical methods for calculating the FCR for a plasma
protein [16], the two tracers plasma urine (2T-PU) and the two tracers-
plasma (2T-P), and a graphic one in which various parameters of the FCE are
derived from plotting the plasma disappearance of the respective plasma
protein and of the free iodide tracer on semilogarithmic graph paper. Using
both mathematical methods the FCR of SAAL was determined from the plasma
disappearance curve of the labelled SAAL and the appearance curve of the
iodide from SAAL catabolism; this latter function was measured from urinary
collection in the 2T-PU method or directly in plasma samples by separation
of the inorganic activity by gel filtration chromatography in the 2T-P
method. In both methods the iodide kinetics were determined by simultaneous injection of differentially labelled sodium iodide [16] which permits
one to take into account the distribution and excretion of iodide released
from protein catabolism. Two basic assumptions are implicit in both methods: 1) the site of protein degradation is in rapid equilibrium with the
plasma compartment; 2) the behavior of iodide released from SAAL breakdown
and of the free, directly injected iodide is the same [16].

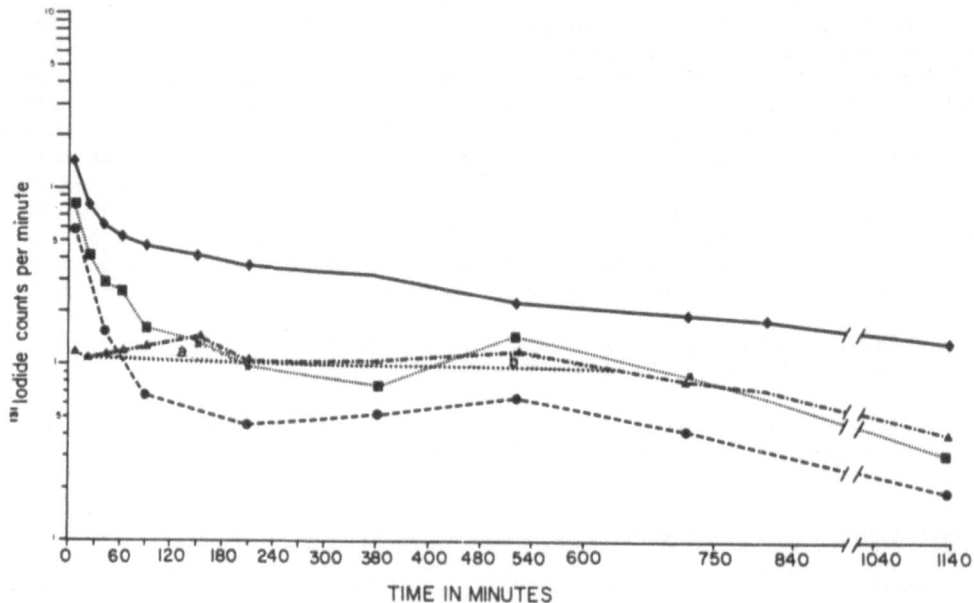

Fig. 1.   Disappearance curves of ^{131}I SAAL from various human blood components. Legend: ♦–♦) Free ^{131}Iodide in plasma; ■--■) protein
bound ^{131}Iodide in TCA precipitated plasma; ▲–·–▲) ^{131}I SAAL in
circulating granulocytes; ●--●) ^{131}I SAAL in plasma detected by
RIA.

The most rapid way to calculate the SAA-FCR is that of applying the
following formula using results derived from the 2T-P method: IA (t) =
FCR·P(t)·VP·I(t)DI in which IA (t) = plasma concentration of ^{131}I released
from ^{131}I SAAL breakdown (c.p.m./ml); P (t) = plasma concentration of ^{131}I
labelled SAAL (c.p.m./ml); I (t) = plasma concentration of free ^{125}I
(c.p.m./ml); DI = dose of free ^{125}I (c.p.m.); VP = DA (dose of ^{131}I labelled SAAL)/P (0) (plasma volume).

The graphic method permitted the analysis of the disappearance curves
[17] of the ^{131}I labelled SAAL, of the ^{131}I SAAL bound to circulating cells,
of the free ^{131}I resulting from the degradation of SAA and of ^{131}I bound to
plasma proteins not recognized by anti SAAL or anti AA antibody (after its
degradation).

The half-time disappearance from the apparent blood compartments of
the ^{131}I SAAL, resulting from the "breaking" of the disappearance curves,
was then calculated by "peeling" the desired curve and defining the various
compartments [18]. The value of each compartmental half-time was found on
the abscissa by a perpendicular line from a point crossed on the projected
straight line of the compartment by a parallel with the abscissa starting
at the half of c.p.m. value on the ordinate (defined by the compartmental
straight line).

RESULTS

The results of both experiments carried out at 6 month intervals were
very similar. As can be seen in Fig. 1 the plasma disappearance curve of
^{131}I SAAL determined by the liquid phase RIA, which does not reflect the degraded SAAL, runs parallel with the plasma disappearance curve of ^{131}I

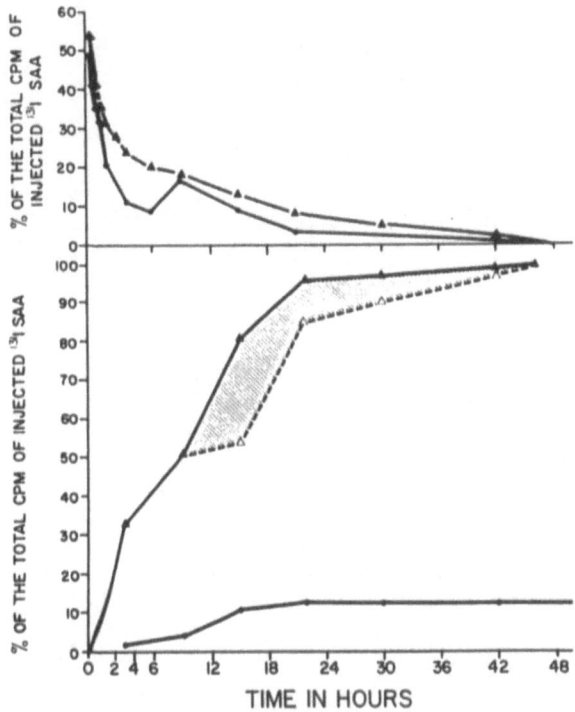

Fig. 2. Plasma disappearance and cumulative
         urinary excretion rates of free [131]Iodide
         and TCA precipitated ^{131}I SAAL after the
         i.v. administration of ^{131}I SAAL.

SAAL in TCA precipitated plasma, which accounts also for degraded SAA. Both
curves suggest the existence of 4 compartments (detailed in Fig. 3) and con-
cur in indicating the presence of a late release of ^{131}I SAAL in plasma from
extravascular tissues (approximately 9 h after the injection of ^{131}I SAAL).
This late release is less evident on the free [131]Iodide disappearance curve;
because of it, however, this curve tapers off at a much slower pace than the
comparative curve of free [125]Iodide tracer which was rapidly and completely
cleared in the urine within 36 h with only a slight delay due to transient
protein binding (curve not shown in Fig. 2) as previously noted by others
[19]. Of interest is the disappearance curve of ^{131}I SAAL bound to circulating granulocytes (separated by Ficoll-Hypaque gradient centrifugation).
It shows two moments of increased uptake by polymorphonucleated cells suggesting phagocytosis or binding of ^{131}I SAAL to their surface, initially
within 2 h of ^{131}I SAAL injection and seven hours later, when the release
of ^{131}I SAA from extravascular tissues in the vessels reaches it peak.

     When plasma disappearance curves of free [131]Iodide and of ^{131}I SAAL in
TCA precipitated plasma were compared with the cumulative excretion curves
of free [131]Iodide and of ^{131}I SAA in TCA precipitated urine (Fig. 2) it was
found that all plasma [131]Iodide was accounted for in the urine. In fact,
starting with the 10th hour after the ^{131}I SAAL injection and peaking in
the 15th hour post injection, approximately 26% of the ^{131}I counts per minute
in the urine were in excess of the direct decrease of [131]Iodide in the
plasma; this was likely due to their release from the extravascular tissues.
The analysis of the curve of ^{131}I SAAL in TCA precipitated plasma (Fig. 2,
upper graph) indicate an initial, rapid disappearance within 30 min of approximately 80% of the radiolabelled SAAL and its complete disappearance

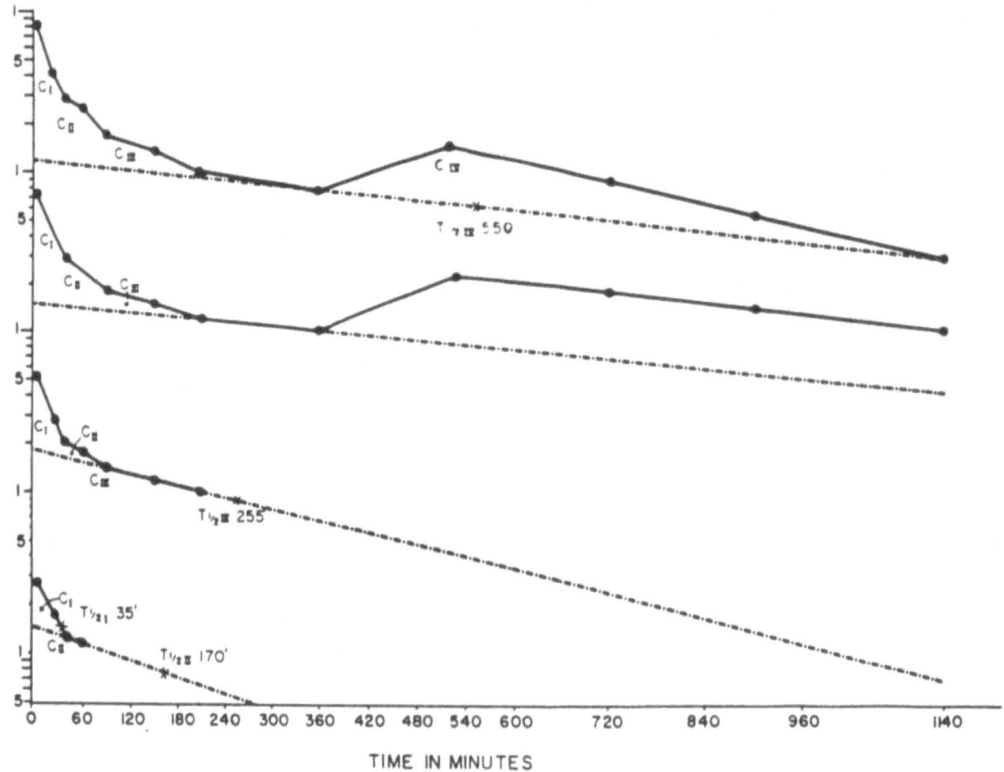

TIME IN MINUTES

Fig. 3. Compartmental distribution of ^{131}I SAAL. (It is derived from the disappearance curve of ^{131}I SAAL precipitated by TCA: "curve peeling" procedure.) Legend: C) Compartment of distribution; $(x)T^1/_2$) half-life time of ^{131}I SAAL in the respective compartment.

from the plasma by the end of the second day. In the urine, however, very little ^{131}Iodide can be detected in the TCA precipitated material (Fig. 2, bottom graph) likely due to the complete degradation of SAAL before it reaches the urine.

A more detailed analysis of the disappearance curve of ^{131}I SAAL in TCA precipitated plasma permitted the detection of compartmental distribution of ^{131}I SAAL and the calculation of ^{131}I SAAL plasma half-life time $(T^1/_2)$ by "peeling" the disappearance curve (see Methods).

Four compartments were defined by this method (Fig. 3). Their respective plasma half-life times were: 35, 170, 255, and 550 min (Fig. 3).

Finally, the ratio of the two Iodide tracers used was determined in the volunteer's plasma at various time intervals (Table 1) and was found to progressively rise, up to the 9th h, and to fall thereafter.

Whole body CT scanning of the subject on study was performed at 2, 16, and 36 h after the injection of ^{125}I SAAL. It showed a slightly increased uptake of the radioactive material over the spleen at 2 h; however, the obtained image was more than 30% smaller than the splenic image obtained after the injection of 99-m Technetium colloid being likely caused by the blood accumulated in the sinusoids of the splenic medulla. No increased uptake over any part of the body was seen at 16 and 48 h following the injection of ^{131}I SAAL.

DISCUSSION

    The analysis of the turnover studies of exogenous radiolabelled ^{131}I SAAL we carried out in a human volunteer showed the feasibility of such investigation despite the presence of an intensive SAA degradation activity in human and mammalian blood and confirmed previous experimental data which indicated rapid clearance (within 12-24 h) of casein induced SAA in a CBA/J mouse model [9] as well as a relatively rapid half-life time (40 to 60 min) for apo SAA in Balb/c mice after surgical removal of a segment of their small bowel [10]. Our data showed an overall half-life time of SAAL of 45 min (Fig. 2) which is much faster than the clearance rate of any other plasma apolipoprotein. However, the detailed analysis of the disappearance curve of ^{131}I SAAL in TCA precipitated plasma indicates that, in fact, this clearance does not follow an exponential curve; it has a rather parabolic shape and it permits the distinction of four compartments with plasma half-life times of 35, 270, 255, and 550 min (Fig. 3). Similar compartments could be recognized following the disappearance curve of ^{131}I SAAL detected by the liquid phase RIA. This curve, however, does not keep into account the SAA degradation in proteic fragments that even though no longer recognized by an anti AA antibody, remained radiolabelled and are precipitated by TCA. For this reason, in order to study the clearance from plasma of SAAL and its metabolites we derived the disappearance half-life time values of ^{131}I SAAL from the curve of ^{131}I SAAL in TCA precipitated plasma.

    The analysis of the various compartments of ^{131}I SAAL disappearance permits some speculations on the fate of SAAL in the human body. As shown on Fig. 2 (upper graph) 50% of the injected ^{131}I SAA disappeared within the first 5 min representing, likely, the SAAL which, in view of its low molecular weight, is rapidly cleared by the kidney before its binding or distribution in other compartments occur; this part of the curve, due to its steepness, was not depicted on the graph showing the fragmentation of the ^{131}I SAA disappearance curve by the so called "curve peeling" procedure (Fig 3) which permits an indirect analysis of the distribution of SAAL. The first two compartments (CI and CII) of ^{131}I SAAL distribution have a half-life time of 35 and 170 min respectively and probably represents SAAL binding to various plasma components, likely to the apolipoprotein fraction (from which apo SAA was previously shown [10] to disappear within 40 min) and to albumin to which SAA was previously found to bind non-covalently [19].

    The third compartment of the ^{131}I SAA disappearance curve with a half-life time of 255 min results likely from binding of SAAL to circulating cells primarily granulocytes (Fig. 1) as found after Ficoll-Hypaque gradient separation of various cellular components, as well as following immuno-fluorescent staining studies reported elsewhere [20].

    Finally, the fourth compartment with a half-life time of 550 min is highly suggestive of ^{131}I SAAL binding and retention by extravascular tissues from which SAAL is then released once more in the circulating blood; this release occurs from most of the tissues over a relatively short period of time reaching its peak at 9 h; from other few tissues, however, this release is likely to occur slowly which explains the tail of the plasma disappearance curve of ^{131}I SAAL reaching the abscissa only after 48 h (Fig. 2, upper graph).

    The analysis of the urinary excretion curve (Fig. 2, bottom graph) indicates first that only 10-12% of the originally injected ^{131}I SAAL reaches the urine in a form in which ^{131}I is still bound to SAA or one of its degradation proteic products. Half of this (6.2%) was still detectable by the RIA for SAA. 90% of the injected radioactive material reaches, however, the urine as free [131]Iodide indicating that the urinary route is indeed the main

TABLE 1. Plasma Ratio of ^{125}I ^{131}I

Time in minutes	$^{125}I:^{131}I$
1	72.5
10	0.91
25	1.12
40	1.08
60	1.41
90	1.22
150	1.51
210	1.48
360	1.77
540	2.4
1140	1.13

route of excretion of ^{131}I SAA which, however, reaches the urine so degraded that very little ^{131}I is still bound to any portion of its molecule.

The urinary excretion curve of ^{131}I SAAL and its comparison with the plasma disappearance curve (Fig. 2) confirms the existence of the previously described compartments especially of the retention and late release of ^{131}I SAA from tissues. The hatched area on the bottom graph on Fig. 2 depicts the amount of ^{131}I present in the urine that cannot be accounted by its plasma disappearance at the respective time, suggesting its release from extravascular tissues. This release appears to start 9 h after the ^{131}I SAAL injection and to continue to the end of the disappearance period of ^{131}I SAAL from the plasma indicating that, indeed, the release of ^{131}I SAA from the tissues is responsible for the tail of its plasma disappearance. Tissue binding of ^{131}I SAA was also suggested by a rising of the $^{125}I:^{131}I$ ratio in time up to the 9th hour following the ^{131}I SAAL administration.

Finally, the absence of ^{131}Iodide uptake detectable by a scanning camera in any of the tissues and organs of the subject on study indicates that ^{131}I SAA is not significantly engulfed or bound by reticulo-endothelial cells nor by myofibrils which is somewhat contrary to previous reports.

The data herein presented contribute to our understanding of the pathogenetic events leading to the formation and deposition of amyloid. The clear indication that SAAL is retained by and thereafter released from extravascular tissues suggests that the pathogenetic events leading to the deposition of amyloid occur at the level of tissues where amyloid is deposited rather than in the blood.

REFERENCES

1. C. J. Rosenthal and E. C. Franklin, J. Clin. Invest., 55:746 (1975).
2. P. D. Gorevic, C. J. Rosenthal, and E. C. Franklin, Clin. Immun. Immunopath., 6:83 (1976).
3. C. J. Rosenthal and L. Sullivan, Ann. Int. Med., 91:383 (1979).
4. E. P. Benditt and N. Eriksen, Proc. Natl. Acad. Sci. USA, 74:4025 (1977).
5. R. D. Anders, J. B. Natvig, T. F. Michaelson, and G. Husby, Scand. J. Immunol., 4:397 (1975).

6. C. J. Rosenthal, E. C. Franklin, B. Frangione, and J. Greenspan, J. Immunol., 116:1415 (1976).

7. R. P. Linke, J. D. Sipe, P. S. Pollock, T. F. Ignaczak, and G. G. Glenner, Proc. Natl. Acad. Sci. (Wash.), 272, 1473 (1975).

8. E. P. Benditt, J. S. Hoffmann, N. Eriksen, et al., in: c-Reactive Protein and the Plasma Protein Response to Tissue Injury (I. Kushner, J. E. Volanakis, and H. Gerwurtz, eds.), p. 183 (1982).

9. M. D. Benson, M. A. Scheinberg, T. Shirahama, E. S. Cathcart, and M. Skinner, J. Clin. Invest., 59:412 (1972).

10. E. P. Benditt, N. Eriksen, and J. S. Hoffmann, in: Amyloid and Amyloidosis (G. G. Glenner, P. Coast, and F. de Freitas, eds.), Experta Medica, Amsterdam-Oxford-Princeton, p. 397 (1980).

11. L. Bausserman, Biochem. Biophys. Acta, 792:186 (1984).

12. G. Lavie, D. Zucker-Franklin, and E. C. Franklin, J. Exp. Med., 148:1020 (1978).

13. I. Kedar, E. Sohar, and J. Gafni, Proc. Soc. Exp. Biol. Med., 145:343 (1974).

14. F. C. Greenwood, W. M. Hunter, and J. S. Glover, Biochem. J., 89:114 (1963).

15. A. Boyum, Scand. J. Clin. Lab. Invest., Suppl. 97, 21:9 (1968).

16. R. Bianchi, G. Mariani, A. Pilo, M. G. Toni, and L. Donato, in: Protein Turnover - Ciba Foundation Symposium - Elsevier-Experta Medica, Amsterdam-London-New York, p. 47 (1973).

17. B. Nosslin, in: Protein Turnover - Ciba Foundation Symposium - Elsevier Experta Medica, Amsterdam-London-New York, p. 113 (1973).

18. K. L. Zierler, Circ. Res., 12:464 (1973).

19. C. J. Rosenthal and E. C. Franklin, J. Immunol., 119:630 (1984).

20. M. E. Martin, C. J. Rosenthal, and A. Huq, Proceed. IVth International Sympos. in Amyloidosis

21. We gratefully acknowledge the excellent assistance of Ms. S. Amrani in preparing this manuscript.

22. This study was supported, in part, by NIH Grant No. 5R01AM2008006.

ULTRASTRUCTURAL IDENTIFICATION OF AA-TYPE AMYLOID

FIBRILS USING POLYCLONAL AND MONOCLONAL ANTIBODIES*

Reinhold P. Linke†   and Dieter Huhn‡

†Institut für Immunologie der Universität
 Schillerstrasse 42
 8000 Munich 2, Federal Republic of Germany

‡Abteilung für Klinische Hämatologie im Institut für
 Hämatologie der Gesellschaft für Strahlen-
 und Umweltforschung
 Landwehrstrasse 61
 8000 Munich 2, Federal Republic of Germany

ABSTRACT

Monoclonal and polyclonal antibodies against amyloid-A fibril protein (AA) were used to identify the respective amyloid fibrils in plastic embedded ultrathin sections. Binding was visualized by electron microscopy using the protein-A colloidal gold technique.

The results demonstrated that, in spite of the embedding procedure, polyclonal and monoclonal anti-AA antibodies bind to amyloid fibrils present in ultrathin sections. No binding to endothelial, epithelial, or red blood cells, or staining of normal basement membrane and collagen was observed. Control experiments showed a specific immunoelectron microscopic reaction. Consequently, minute amounts of amyloid could be identified that may not be visible with light microscopy.

Due to the extremely low background, the staining quality with monoclonal antibodies was superior to that with polyclonal antibodies. Monoclonal antibodies, therefore, would seem to be well-suited for early detection of amyloid by electron microscopy.

INTRODUCTION

Recent biochemical and immunochemical studies have demonstrated the existence of amyloid classes based on different chemistry which, in many cases, correlate with the clinical classification and agree with the permanganate reaction [1]. To recognize these chemically defined amyloid classes in patients, antibodies against the different amyloid fibril proteins were prepared and applied on tissue sections using immunofluorescence [2] and immunoperoxidase [3-5] methods.

---

*This study was supported by Sonderforschungsbereich, LP-12, Munich.

The respective amyloid fibrils were also distinguished in ultrathin tissue sections by extending this approach to the ultrastructural level using the protein-A colloidal gold (pAg) technique and affinity purified antibodies directed against amyloid-A fibril protein (AA) and against amyloid fibril proteins of λ- and κ-immunoglobulin light chain origin [7]. In this report, autopsy specimens with chemically or immunochemically typed amyloid fibrils, but with poorly preserved ultrastructure, were used.

We have now extended these studies to include well-preserved specimens and use monoclonal antibodies to identify amyloid fibrils on the ultrastructural level.

MATERIAL AND METHODS

1. Tissues

A kidney biopsy from a patient with recurrent fibril episodes was fixed for 8 h at 4 C in 1.5% paraformaldehyde diluted with PBS (0.01 M phosphate, 0.85% NaCl, pH 7.2). The control specimen was a kidney biopsy without amyloid. Small tissue fragments were embedded in either paraffin or Maraglas [8]. 4 μ-thick paraffin and 1 μ-semithin sections etched with sodium ethoxide were immunohistochemically stained with anti-AA antibodies [12]. A moderate amount of AA-type amyloid was identifiable in all glomeruli. Blocks from semithin sections with glomeruli were trimmed, and the ultrathin sections mounted on Pioloform F-coated 150-mesh nickel grids.

2. Preparation of Protein-A Gold Particles

A monodisperse suspension of colloidal gold (particle size, approx. 15 nm in diameter) was prepared as described by Frens [9]; adsorption of protein A (Pharmacia, Uppsala/Sweden) onto the colloidal gold particles carried out according to Roth et al. [10].

3. Immunoelectron Microscopic Staining

The staining procedure was basically performed as described elsewhere [7]. After etching with 10% H_2O_2 for 15 min, washing in PBS for 10 min, and exposure to 0.1% ovalbumin in PBS for 30 min, antibodies were applied for 2 h. These antibodies included a murine IgG 2aκ monoclonal immunoglobulin with specificity for protein AA [11] and affinity purified rabbit anti-AA polyclonal immunoglobulins at 10 to 30 μg/ml in PBS [6]. After washing with PBS for 10 min, the sections were exposed to the protein-A gold complex (diluted 10 times) for 30 min and washed as described above. The sections were contrasted with either 5% uranyl acetate for 10 min [10] or as described by Reynolds [8]. The sections were inspected and photographed with a Siemens Elmiscope I electron microscope at 80 kW.

RESULTS

Electron microscopic inspection of uncontrasted or weakly contrasted (uranyl acetate) sections with AA-type amyloid immunohistochemically stained with anti-AA antibodies revealed agglomerated gold particles in well-defined areas of tissue (Figs. 1, 2). Representing background staining, pAg was randomly and thinly distributed on the tissue-free Pioloform membrane and on tissues which were apparently free of amyloid, e.g., cytoplasm (Fig. 1, left half). When polyclonal antibodies were employed, the particles in these areas were frequently organized in rows, like strings of pearls, or in groups (see Fig. 1). With the monoclonal antibody mc 20, however, agglomeration was less dense, rows of particles were rare, and the background was virtually free of pAg particles (Fig. 2).

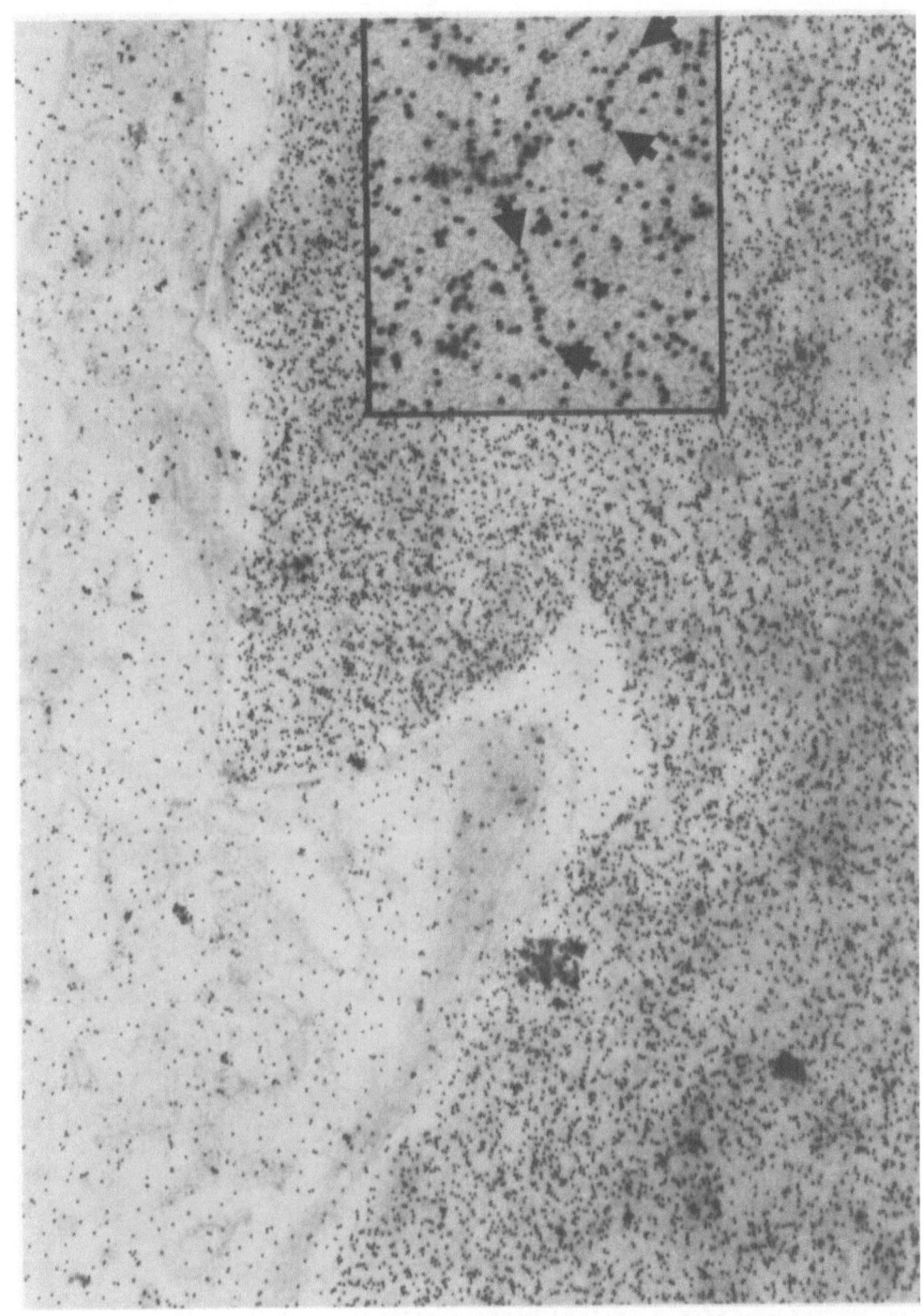

Fig. 1. Kidney biopsy stained with polyclonal anti-AA and pAg particles
(uranyl acetate). Magnification: 37,200 ×. A) Amyloid deposit
with numerous threaded beads. Inset: Amyloid fibrils slightly
stained with uranyl acetate. pAg beads are 15 nm in diameter.
◄   = Two of several threaded pAg particles. Magnification:
83,000 ×.

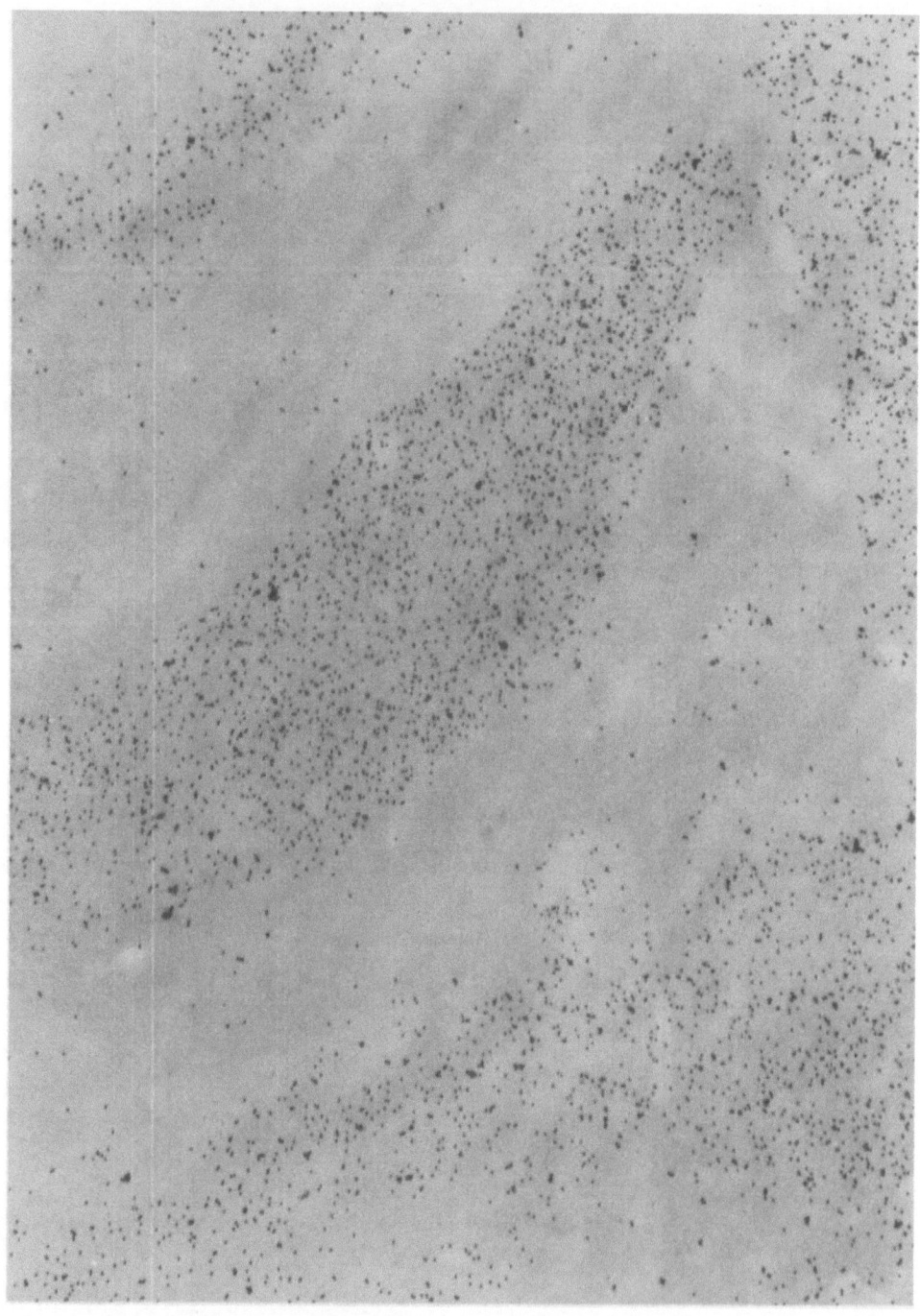

Fig. 2. Kidney biopsy stained with monoclonal antibody mc20 and pAg par-
         ticles (not contrasted). Note well-defined areas with agglomer-
         ated pAg particles that are not well organized in rows. Magnifi-
         cation: 31,000 ×.

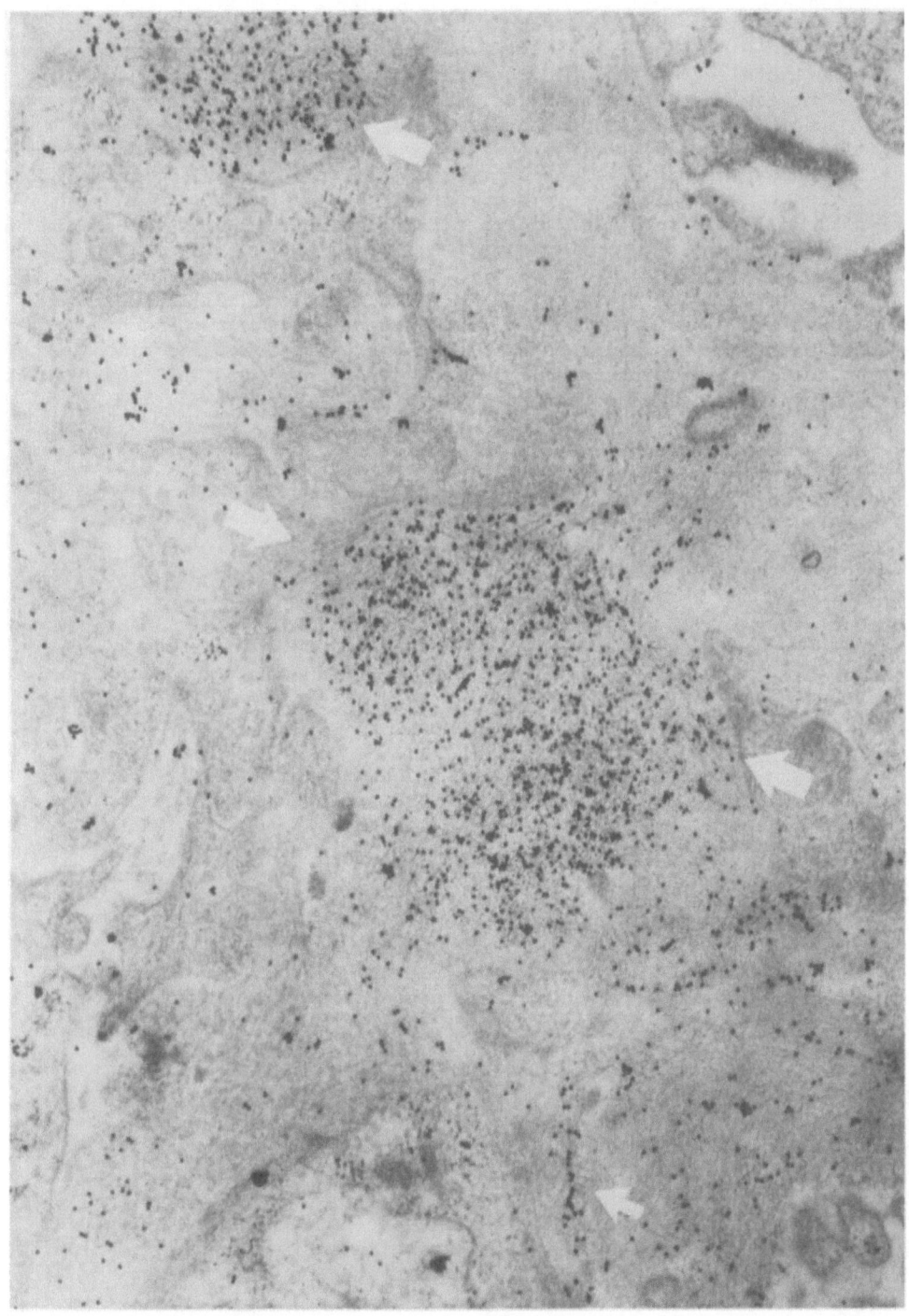

Fig. 3. Kidney biopsy stained with monoclonal antibody mc20 and pAg particles (optimally contrasted with uranyl acetate).
⟵ = typical amyloid deposits labeled with pAg particles,
⟵ = bundle of parallel amyloid fibrils.
Magnification: 46,500 ×.

The contrasted sections showed which tissue structures were labeled with pAg. In Fig. 3, pAg is located on fine fibrillar extracellular material with the size, morphologic appearance, and localization of amyloid fibrils. In Fig. 3, larger deposits are labeled by large white arrows; a small deposit with parallel amyloid fibrils, by a small white arrow. Epithelial cell processes are visible in the upper right corner of the figure. One thickened basement membrane penetrated by small amounts of amyloid fibrils can be seen adjacent to the epithelial cell processes. An (endothelial?) cell with invaginations containing stained fibrils is visible on the far left.

Mesangial, endothelial, epithelial, and red blood cells as well as their rough entoplasmic reticulum, when present, were not stained. Normal basement membranes and collagen bundles along extraglomerular blood vessels and control sections without amyloid were also negative. Only those thickened basement membranes containing amyloid were stained (Fig. 3).

Comparison of uranyl acetate and contrasting according to Reynolds showed that uranyl acetate is to be preferred (see Fig. 3) because lead citrate frequently leads to precipitation [10].

DISCUSSION

Our study, which was carried out on a kidney biopsy with AA-type amyloid that was identified by immunohistochemical typing on paraffin- and Maraglas-embedded semithin sections, shows that the pAg technique with polyclonal and monoclonal antibodies can be used for antigenic identification of amyloid fibrils in ultrathin sections.

The fact that more densely agglomerated and threaded pAg which appeared to be located along amyloid fibrils was visible when polyclonal antibodies were used indicates that more antigenic determinants are available for these antibodies. As was to be expected, staining with monoclonal antibodies was less intense than with polyclonal antibodies. mc20-Antigenic determinants, therefore, are considerably less available. That they are still available at all is astonishing enough!

The fact that the organelles of cells adjacent to amyloid deposits are not stained indicates that these cells probably do not synthesize the AA-precursor molecules.

The advantage of monoclonal antibodies for immunoelectron optical identification of AA-type amyloid is obvious. This reagent ensures specific staining with almost no background, is more reproducible, and has the demonstrated advantages of monoclonal antibodies, i.e., monospecificity and the potential of unlimited supply.

These reagents and this electron microscopic technique, therefore, seem well suited for diagnostic application in early glomerular dysfunction, in high-risk patients, and in other amyloid-induced impairments.

ACKNOWLEDGEMENTS

We would like to thank Mss. H. Darsow and S. Steudinger for their expert technical assistance, Ms. A. Werner for her help with the photography, and Drs. W. Volker and J. Rauterberg for their suggestions concerning the protein-A gold technique.

REFERENCES

1. G. G. Glenner, New Engl. J. Med., 302:1283, 1333 (1980).
2. G. G. Cornwell, III, G. Husby, P. Westermark, J. B. Natvig, T. E.
    Michaelson, and B. Skogen, Scand. J. Immunol., 6:1071 (1977).
3. Y. Levo, N. Livni, and A. Laufer, in: Amyloid and Amyloidosis (G. G.
    Glenner, P. P. Costa, and F. de Freitas, eds.), Excerpta Medica,
    Amsterdam, pp. 35 (1980).
4. S. Fujihara, J. E. Balow, J. C. Costa, and G. G. Glenner, Lab. Invest.,
    43:358 (1980).
5. R. P. Linke and W. B. J. Nathrath, Münch. Med. Wschr., 122:1772 (1980).
6. R. P. Linke, W. B. J. Nathrath, and P. D. Wilson, Ultrastruct. Path.,
     4:1 (1983).
7. B. O. Spurlock, V. C. Kattine, and J. A. Freeman, J. Cell. Biol., 17:
    203 (1963).
8. E. S. Reynolds, J. Cell Biol., 17:208 (1963).
9. G. Frens, Nature Phys. Sci., 241:20 (1973).
10. J. Roth, M. Bendayan, and L. Orci, J. Histochem. Cytochem., 26:1074
    (1978).
11. R. P. Linke, J. Histochem. Cytochem., 32:322 (1984).
12. B. P. Lane and D. L. Europa, J. Histochem. Cytochem., 13:579 (1965).

HUMAN SERUM AMYLOID P-COMPONENT (SAP) AS AN ACUTE PHASE

REACTANT IN THE FEMALE

Shunsuke Migita*, Shigeru Hashimototo†,
Haruo Hisazumi‡, Mine Harada**,
and Hiroaki Okabe††

*Department of Molecular Immunology
 Cancer Research Institute
 Kanazawa University

†Department Gynecology and Obstetrics
 Kanazawa University Medical School

‡Department of Urology
 Kanazawa University Medical School

**Third Department of Internal Medicine
 Kanazawa University Medical School

††Department of Clinical Pathology
 Yooikuin Hospital
 Tokyo, Japan

ABSTRACT

SAP levels in the serum of 531 healthy Japanese from newborn to 95 years old were measured by single radial immunodiffusion method. The mean SAP concentration in males of 15 to 60 years old, 41 + 11 µg/ml, was significantly higher than that in females of corresponding ages, 20 + 8 µg/ml. The effect of sex hormones on the serum SAP level was examined during hormonal therapy in 21 patients suffering from climacteric syndrome. The average increase in the SAP level per week caused by dehydroepiandrone was 5.5 µg/ml.

In order to confirm that SAP is an acute phase protein, SAP levels were measured after surgical operation in 8 patients (3 males and 5 females). A significant increase in the SAP level was observed only in the females with the peak occurring three days after operation. However, SAP levels following experiment may explain a part of the discrepancy. Blood samples were obtained simultaneously both from kidney arteria and vena during kidney operations. In 20 cases, the arterial SAP levels were higher than the venous SAP levels, with a mean difference of 4.8 µg/ml. Such differences in relative concentration were not observed for the other 35 components of serum protein.

---

*Kanazawa University, Kanazawa, 920, Japan.

INTRODUCTION

SAP (serum amyloid pentagonal component) was first described as 9.5S α_1-glycoprotein by Haupt et al., [1]. This was later identified as a protein that had been extracted from amyloid tissues [2, 3] and had been seen as a pentagonal molecule by electron microscopy, suggesting a pentameric structure [4, 5]. Another pentagonal protein composed of a pentamer is CRP, a typical acute phase protein in the human [6]. However, CRP in the mouse does not belong to any of the acute phase proteins, though SAP is an acute phase protein in the mouse [7].

SAP and CRP have a 70% homology in primary structure and belong to the same gene family. Pepys proposed the name "pentaxin 1 and 2" instead of CRP and SAP [6]. Another member of this gene family is hamster female protein (FP). Concentration of FP in the serum of the hamster was high in the adult female and was very low in the adult male. It was confirmed that the concentration was suppressively controlled by testosterone [8].

A concentration difference for SAP in human serum between the sexes was also reported by Pepys [9]. However, age dependent changes of SAP concentration in the sera of normal human have not reported and effects of sex hormones on the SAP concentration have also not been clarified.

Is SAP in the human an acute phase protein? An increase in SAP level in the serum after the surgical operation was observed only in the female. However, a rapid decrease of SAP in the serum during renal blood flow indicated that a high level of SAP as an acute phase protein could not be maintained due to rapid catabolism, even though the synthesis of SAP may increase as an acute phase protein.

MATERIALS AND METHODS

Normal Human Sera

The sum of 531 human serum samples from healthy Japanese of various age and from both sexes were collected for 6 years from various sources, such as from the Department of Gynecology and Obstetrics and the Department of Pediatrics, Kanazawa University Hospital, for the sera of younger aged persons. The Blood Transfusion Unit of the same hospital supplied sera for adult specimens. Yooikuin Hospital in Tokyo supplied sera from older aged persons.

Patient Sera

Patient sera were collected in the Department of Medicine, the Department of Gynecology and Obstetrics, the Department of Dermatology, and the Department of Urology in this University Hospital. Serial sera obtained during hormonal treatment in climacteric women, serial sera obtained during and after surgical laparotomy, and the other sera obtained simultaneously from arteria and vena of the kidney during operation on the kidney were submitted for SAP measurement.

Serum Amyloid P-Component (SAP)

SAP was purified from normal human sera with Sepharose column chromatography according to Pepys [9], and its purity was confirmed by SDS polyacrylamide gel electrophoresis revealing a single band of 30,000 dalton without Ca ion. The concentration of SAP was measured by UV absorption with OD 280 in 1% solution, 18.2.

Single Radial Immunodiffusion

SAP was measured by the single radial immunodiffusion method on a microscale. Anti-SAP or anti-9.5S α_1-glycoprotein was presented by Dr. G. Schwick, Bering Institute, West Germany and by Dr. M. B. Pepys, Royal Postgraduate Medical School, London. The same specificity of both anti-SAP antisera was confirmed by the Ouchterlony test. QS sera, a pooled and lyophilized mixture of over 2000 normal adult human sera, Hechst Japan Co., was used as the standard concentration of SAP, that was previously confirmed with purified SAP. The concentration of SAP measured in 18 lots of QS sera in 8 years was relatively constant at 33 to 38 µg/ml, i.e., from 94 to 108%. One tenth diluted antiserum mixed with 1% agarose was solidified in plates of 1 mm thickness. Eight-tenth µl of standard and sample sera were put in each hole of 1 mm diameter by a Hamilton microsyringe and a Repeating Dispensor. The concentrations of serum protein components, other than SAP, were also measured by the single radial immunodiffusion method on a microscale, using each specific antiserum of Behringwerke. The diameter of the precipitin ring, enlarged 10 times, was read by a Profile Projector Model 6C, Nikon Co., Japan. The data was analyzed with FACOM M-170F electric computer using "SAS (Statistical Analysis System)" in Data Processing Center, Kanazawa University.

RESULTS

Normal Level of SAP in the Serum

The normal level of SAP in the serum of 531 healthy Japanese is shown in Fig. 1. The SAP concentration in the male was significantly higher for the age group of 15 to 60 years than for the female of corresponding ages $(0.01 > P > 0.005)$. The mean level and standard deviation of SAP in the adult serum were $117 \pm 31\%$ in 87 males, and those were $58 \pm 23\%$ in 75 females. The SAP concentration was shown by the percentage of QS sera as a standard. The values can exchange for concentration of µg/ml at a rate of $35 \times$ percentage. However, this sex difference was not significant in the sera of normal individuals younger than 14 years of age. In the sera of those older than 61 years, the mean concentration of SAP was still higher in the male than in the female. Statistical analysis showed that the differences between the sexes was not significant $(0.2 > P > 0.1)$ in these aged population.

Effect of Sex Hormones on SAP Level in the Serum

The SAP level difference between the sexes was examined to see which sex hormone is responsible for the higher SAP concentration in the male. The SAP level in the serum was measured every week throughout the hormonal therapy of 21 patients suffering from climacteric syndrome. The results were shown in Fig. 2. When we include the entire treatment period, the average increase of SAP and the standard error of the mean by dehydroepiandrone per week was $7.5 \pm 3.2\%$, and the average decrease of SAP by conjugated estrogen per week was $-5.4 \pm 3.1\%$. However, when we take into account the SAP change during the first week of therapy, the average increase by dehydroepiandrone was $15.7 \pm 2.8\%$, and the average decrease by conjugated estrogen was $-13.4 \pm 5.2\%$. In both estimations, the increase by the male hormone was statistically significant, and the effect of the female hormone was less significant. The change during the first week was larger than that of the later period of the hormonal administration.

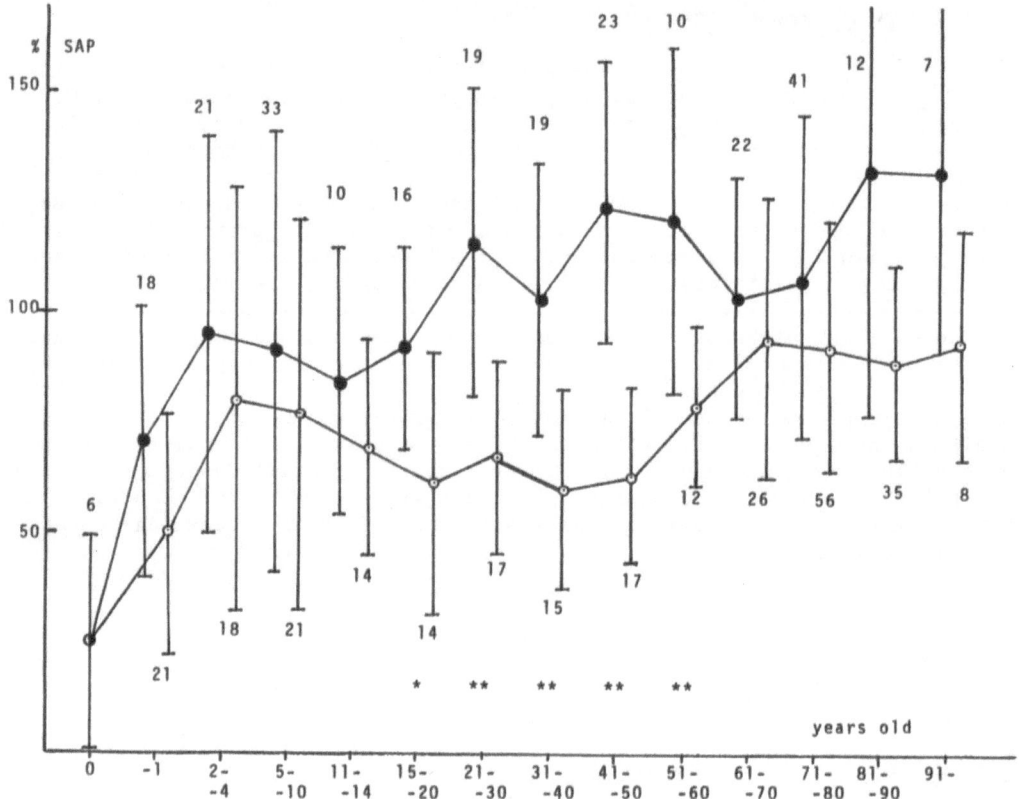

Fig. 1. Changes upon aging of normal serum SAP levels and its differences between the sexes. SAP levels are expressed as the means and standard deviations. ●) Male, ○) female, *) significant difference between the sexes. SAP was measured by the single radial immunodiffusion method with specific anti-SAP antiserum and expressed as percentage of the concentration of SAP in QS standard sera. The SAP concentration in a lot of QS sera (35 μg/ml) was measured using a purified SAP as standard sample.

Changes in the SAP Level in Patient Sera

SAP level in the sera of patients with bladder cancer, kidney cancer, pyoderma and erythema nodosum was measured, and the means and the standard errors of the means are shown in Table 1. Though increases of α_1-antitrypsin, α_1-acid glycoprotein, α_1-antichymotrypsin and haptoglobin as acute phase proteins were noted in these diseases, increases of SAP were less extensive. Increases of the above acute phase proteins were generally lower in the aged persons over 61 years than those in young persons under 60 years. Increase of SAP is similar with those of the acute phase proteins in this point. The difference of SAP level in normal persons between the sexes was uncertain in these patients sera.

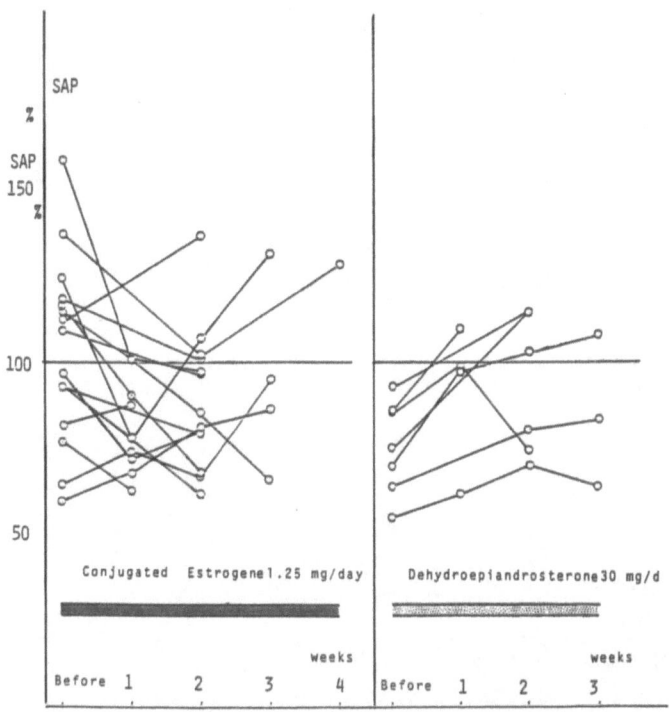

Fig. 2. Effects of sex hormones on serum SAP concentrations. Twenty-one patients with
climacteric syndrome were treated with
daily doses of 1.25 mg of conjugated estrogen or 30 mg of dehydroepiandrone. SAP
levels in the sera were measured in weekly
intervals before and during the treatment.

TABLE 1. Concentrations of SAP and 4 Acute Phase
Proteins in the Sera of the Patients
Suffering from Cancer or Chronic Inflammation. [The concentrations are expressed
as percentage of QS sera (pooled and
lyophilized standard sample of healthy
adults)]

	n	α1AT %	α1AG %	α1X %	Hp %	SAP %
Bladder cancer	16	164±5	260±29	193±16	183±25	130±18
Kidney cancer	45	148±7	167±21	158±14	203±16	120±8
Pyoderma	10	124±16	163±12	153±20	224±29	112±13
Erythema nodosum	14	179±12	181±14	238±32	241±31	140±12
Age>61	39	142±7	174±15	145±11	165±11	115±9
Age<60	45	159±8	190±13	184±15	239±17	131±8
<60, m	22	156±12	196±23	158±19	238±28	134±12
<60, f	23	163±10	184±13	205±21	241±22	130±11

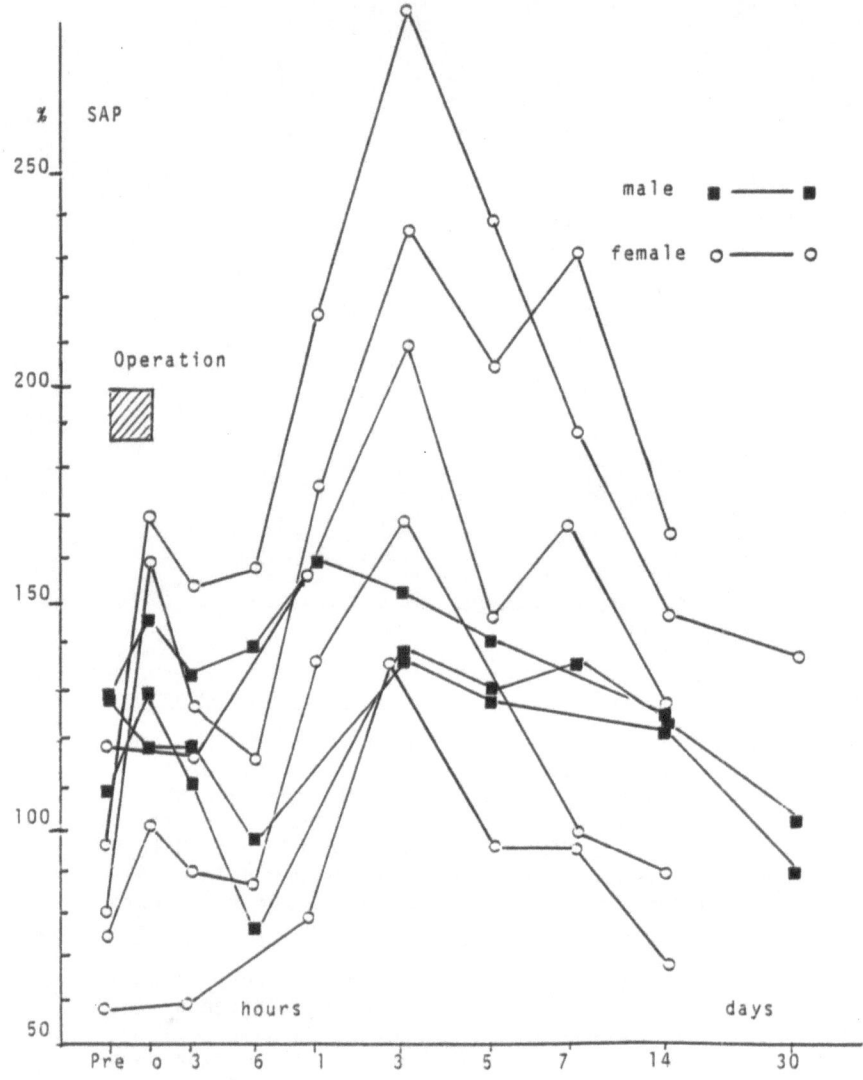

Fig. 3.   Changes of SAP concentration during and after surgical op-
          eration.   In 8 patients (3 males and 5 females) with kid-
          ney stone, ovarian cyst, myoma uteri, and other non-severe
          diseases undergoing laparotomy, the SAP leves were measured
          sequencially by SRID.

Changes in the SAP Level after Surgical Operation

     We wondered whether SAP is an acute phase protein or not. The SAP
level in the serum was periodically measured after surgical operation.

     Eight selected patients (3 males and 5 females), 16 to 57 years of age,
suffered from ovarian cyst, kidney stone, myoma uteri, or dermoid cyst, and
had a relatively normal pattern for serum protein before the laparotomy.
As shown in Fig. 3, the SAP level before the operation was higher in the
males (mean 123%) than that in the females (mean 84%).

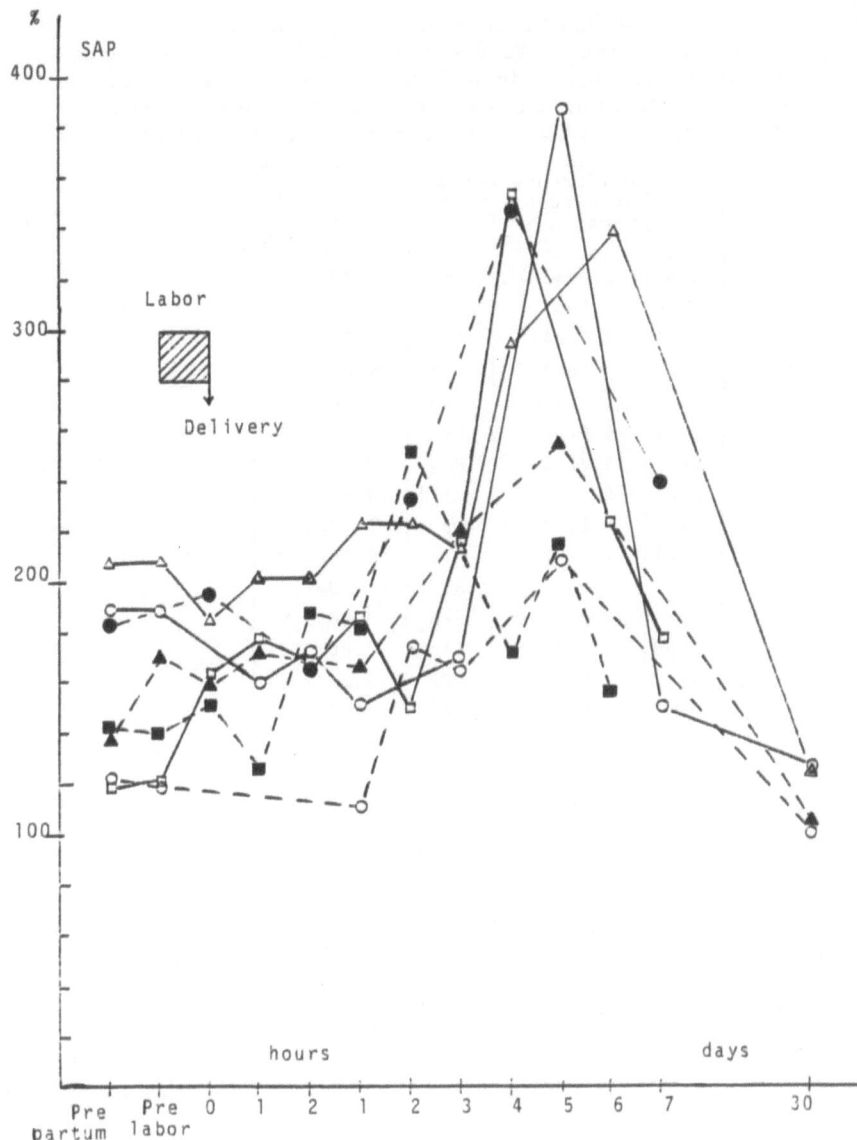

Fig. 4. Changes in SAP concentration before, during, and after deliveries. The levels of SAP increased as an acute phase protein at 3 to 5 days after delivery.

However, a significant increase in the SAP level was observed in the female patients with the peak appearing 3 days after the operation and with the average increase of 2.5 times to the initial level. On the other hand, SAP level did not change in the male sera after the operation.

Changes in the Serum SAP Level in Mothers After Delivery

Changes in the serum protein concentration of 8 components before and after the delivery in 7 females of 20 to 28 years old were examined. Changes in the serum SAP level are shown in Fig. 4.

TABLE 2. Differences in the Protein Concentrations between the Kidney Arterial and Venous Blood. [The values are means of 20 sets of the specimens obtained simultaneously at the time of operation of the kidney and the standard errors of the means. Significant differences are marked with *.]

Proteins	Difference in concent.	Proteins	Difference in concent.
	%		%
$\alpha 1AT$	2.60±3.7	C4	1.40±4.0
$\alpha 1AG$	2.95±3.6	IgM	4.68±2.4
$\alpha 1B$	2.42±4.6	IgG	1.89±2.9
$\alpha 1X$	4.50±4.8	IgA	4.84±5.8
Hp	4.84±10.8	IgD	9.50±5.5
$Zn\alpha 2$	-14.67±13.9	C9	-0.80±3.3
Cp	5.75±3.6	Pmg	0.35±3.6
$\alpha 2M$	6.47±2.5*	ATII	1.10±2.7
Hx	5.53±3.1	C5	7.93±3.9
$\beta 2II$	1.42±2.8	C1s	3.50±3.0
Alb	2.00±2.3	αL	-1.60±2.7
Pre	1.00±2.6	RPB	0.80±3.1
$\alpha 2HS$	3.70±3.4	C1q	2.06±3.2
Tf	2.80±2.0	CRP	-15.33±23.1
βL	4.83±2.7	SAP	13.70±4.2**
$\beta 2I$	5.73±5.3	$\alpha 2PI$	3.45±5.1
Bf	6.74±2.3	P	1.50±3.7
C3	6.50±3.3	FN	-1.55±7.3
C6	6.82±3.3		

The peaks of the protein concentration appeared at different intervals, namely 2 to 5 days after delivery depending upon the individual processes. Serum obtained from patients at the stage of pre-partum, pre-labor, just after the delivery, 1 hour, 2 hours, and 1 day after the delivery, showed a relatively constant concentration of SAP. The SAP levels were generally increased by pregnancy and showed individual differences. The mean increase of SAP at post-partum as an acute phase protein is 2.0 times the SAP concentration at pre-partum.

Changes in the SAP Level in the Sera of Arteria and Venous Blood

Blood samples were obtained from the kidney arteria and vena simultaneously by syringe during surgical procedure carried out on 20 patients with kidney diseases. The mean differences in protein concentration in these sera (the protein levels of the arterial sera minus those of the venous sera) and the standard errors of the means were listed as shown in Table 2.

The changes in the SAP concentration was noted in all cases, with the mean being 13.7%, i.e., 4.8 µg/ml during the blood flow of the kidney.

The difference was statistically significant ($0.0025 > P > 0.0005$). α_1-Macroglobulin also showed a significant decrease, 6.5%, i.e., 163 µg/ml and $0.0125 > P > 0.001$. The affinity of SAP to the kidney tissue are suspected. Such differences in protein concentration were not observed for the other 35 serum components.

DISCUSSION

The normal level for SAP in human sera reported by Pepys is 43 ± 14 µg/ml in the adult males and 30 ± 10 µg/ml in the adult females [9]. A difference in the SAP level between the sexes have been described. However, further studies have not yet been carried out.

We measured SAP levels of large number of normal individuals of various ages and both sexes. The ontogeny of SAP from placenta blood to the sera of normal persons over 95 years old has been reported here. The mean of SAP level and SD was 8.8 ± 8.6 µg/ml, in placent blood, and gradually increased to 27 ± 9.8 µg/ml at an age of 14 years. No difference in SAP levels between the sexes was noted in the serum from new born up to 14 years old. However, the difference became significant and was observed all the way from puberity to climacterium. The average and SD for SAP in the adult male was 41 ± 11 µg/ml, and that in female was 20 ± 8 µg/ml.

The difference in SAP level between the sexes was not significant in the serum of normal aged persons over 60 years old, 37 ± 11 µg/ml in 82 men and 32 ± 10 µg/ml in 125 women. A difference in normal serum components between the sexes has been noted: α_2-macroglobulin, IgM and possibly α_1-antitrypsin are higher in the female, while C4 are higher in the male. However, we had reported in 1979 that the SAP sex difference was the most significant among 35 serum components in 232 normal individuals [12]. The results are confirmed here with data from an additional 256 normal individuals.

In the previous paper [12], the difference in SAP level between the sexes was insignificant in the persons aged 11 to 20. In thia paper, we separated into two age groups of these specimens and added 35 new samples. The sera obtained from normal persons in the Clinic of the Department of Pediatrics, in this university, aged from 11 to 14 years, are the first group. Those from blood donors in the Blood Transfusion Unit, aged from 15 to 20 are the second group. A significant difference in SAP level between the sexes was noted in the second group, but not in the first group. to 20 are the second group. A significant difference in SAP level betweeen the sexes was noted in the second group, but not in the first group.

The effect of sex hormone on the SAP level in the serum was examined in patients of climacteric syndrome who were treated with either conjugated estrogen, 1.25 mg per day for 3 to 4 weeks, or dehydroepiandrone, 30 mg per day for three weeks. A mean and the standard error of the mean of changes in the SAP concentration in the serum per week were 5.5 ± 1.3 µm/ml in seven cases for the male hormone and -4.6 ± 1.9 µg/ml in 14 cases for female hormones. The effect of the male hormone on the SAP level was statistically significant and that of female hormones were less significant. Coe et al., have reported a hamster female protein that belongs to the same pentaraxin gene family as SAP and CRP [13]. The level of this protein in the serum was significantly higher in adult females than that in adult males. This protein in the hamster decreased in the adult female with daily injection of testosterone, and increased in adult males after castration. However, no effects were observed in cases of castration in adult females. Administration of diethyl stilbestrol to adult male hamsters consistently resulted in the prolonged appearance of female protein in the serum [8]. These data indicate that testosterone has a suppressor effect on the level of serum female protein. Human SAP is the opposite of the situation for hamster female protein because of a higher serum level in the male and the positive effect of the male hormone.

After surgical operations, the SAP level in the female increased significantly as an acute phase protein with its peak on the third day. However, the SAP level in the male did not change, though the level of SAP before the operation was higher in the male than in the female. We reported a part of this result previously [14] and confirmed it here with an additional three cases. In order to observe the acute phase response in the human, a preferable condition is as follows: the serum protein profile of the patient before the operation should be relatively normal, and the operation should include laparotomy as a stimulation. Cases selected here are cystoma ovary, kidney stone, myoma utery, and so on. Pepys reported that an increase in SAP after the surgical operation was not significant. However, sex and diagnostic discriminations of the patients were not described in his report [15]. Here, an increase in SAP as an acute phase protein was observed only in the female. The increase in serum SAP level in the female was 2 to 2.5 times of the normal level, while the normal SAP concentration in the male is about 2 times higher than that in the female.

The increase of SAP concentration in human males may not be distinct, because of a high normal level. A difference of acute phase response between the sexes observed here, was also reported in hamster female protein [14] and mouse C4 response [17]. In the latter, the increase of C4 level after turpentine injection was greater in females, while normal level of C4 was higher in males than that in females.

Acute phase protein has been characterized by an increase in the concentration of certain plasma proteins, which starts within hours or days of most forms of acute tissue damage or inflammation, and persists with chronic inflammation and malignant neoplasia [7]. Mouse SAP belongs to one of the acute phase proteins, but human SAP does not [16]. This is because human SAP does not satisfy the later half of the above criteria as shown in Table 1. This situation was solved with a prompt accumulation of SAP probably in the glomerular basement membrane, and possibly in other connective tissue [18] that may be related to accumulation on amyloid fibril in amyloidosis [19]. Pepys reported that SAP is a constituent of normal human glomerular basement membrane by immunofluorography, immunoelectron microscopy, and also by chemical detection of the eluted protein [20]. Calcium dependent polymerization of SAP may be included in this process of accumulation [21].

REFERENCES

1. H. Haupt, N. Heimberger, T. Kranz, and S. Baudner, Hoppe-Seyler's Z. Physio. Chem., 352:1841 (1972).
2. M. Skinner, A. S. Cohen, T. Shirahama, and E. S. Cathart, J. Lab. Clin. Med., 84:604 (1974).
3. M. D. Benson, M. Skinner, T. Shirahama, and A. S. Cohen, Arthr. Rheum., 19:749 (1976).
4. H. A. Bladen, M. U. Nylen, and G. G. Glenner, J. Ultrastructure Res., 14:449 (1966).
5. A. P. Osmand, B. Friedenson, H. Gewurz, R. H. Painter, T. Hoffmann, and E. Shelton, Proc. Natl. Acad. Sci., 74:739 (1977).
6. M. B. Pepys and M. L. Baltz, Ad. Immunol., 34:141-212 (1983).
7. M. B. Pepys, M. Baltz, K. Gomer, A. J. S. Davies, and M. Doenhoff, Nature, 278:259 (1979).
8. J. E. Coe, J. Exper. Med., 74:730 (1977).
9. M. B. Pepys, A. C. Dash, R. E. Markham, H. C. Thomas, B. D. Williams, and A. Petrie, Clin. Exptl. Immunol., 32:119 (1978).

10. M. B. Pepys, A. C. Dash, E. A. Munn, A. Feinstein, M. Skinner, A. S. Cohen, H. Gewurz, A. P. Osmand, and R. H. Painter, Lancet, 14:1029 (1977).
11. M. B. Pepys, F. C. de Beer, C. P. Milstein, J. F. March, A. Feinstein, N. Butress, J. R. Clamp, J. Taylor, C. Brutin, and T. C. Fletcher, Biochim. Biophys. Acta, 704:123 (1982).
12. S. Migita, in: Plasma Protein (C. Hirayma and S. Migita, eds.), Ishiyaku Pub. Co., Tokyo, pp. 239:254 (1979).
13. J. E. Coe, S. S. Margossian, H. S. Slayter, and J. A. Sogn, J. Exper. Med., 153:977-991 (1981).
14. S. Hashimoto, S. Migita, Acta Haematol., Japan, 42:47 (1979).
15. M. B. Pepys, M. L. Baltz, R. F. Dyck, F. C. de Beer, D. J. Evans, J. Feinstein, C. P. Milstein, E. A. Munn, N. Richardson, J. F. March, T. C. Fletcher, A. J. S. Davies, K. Gomer, A. S. Cohen, M. Skinner, and G. G. B. Klaus, in: Amyloid and Amyloidosis (G. Glenner, P. Costa, and F. Freitas, eds.), 373-383 (1979).
16. J. E. Coe and M. J. Ross, J. Exper. Med., 157:1421-1433 (1983).
17. S. Migita, unpublished observation.
18. G. G. Glenner, E. D. Eanes, H. A. Bladen, R. P. Linke, and J. D. Termine, J. Histochem. and Cytochem., 22:1141-1158 (1974).
19. M. B. Pepys, R. F. Dyck, F. C. de Beer, M. Skinner, and A. S. Cohen, Clin. Exp. Immunol., 38:284-293 (1979).
20. R. F. Dyck, G. M. Lockwood, M. Kershow, N. McHugh, V. C. Duance, M. L. Baltz, and E. B. Pepys, J. Exper. Med., 152:1162 (1980).
21. M. L. Baltz, F. C. de Beer, A. Feinstein, and M. B. Pepys, Biochem. Biophys. Acta, 701:229-236 (1982).

B. EXPERIMENTAL MODELS

PATHOGENETIC MECHANISMS AND PRECURSOR PRODUCT

RELATIONSHIPS IN MURINE AMYLOIDOSIS

M. L. Baltz, D. Caspi,
I. F. Rowe, C. R. K. Hind,
D. J. Evans*, and M. B. Pepys

MRC Acute Phase Protein Research Group
Immunological Medicine Unit
Department of Medicine, and

*Department of Histopathology
 Royal Postgraduate Medical School
 Du Cane Road
 London W12 OHS, United Kingdom

ABSTRACT

Intravenous injection of ^{125}I-labeled isolated mouse serum amyloid P component (SAP) into mice with systemic AA amyloidosis led to specific deposition of the labeled proetin in mayloidotic organs. The amount correlated with the quantity of amyloid present and localized in the same distribution within the organs as the amyloid deposits. Human SAP, when injected intravenously into amyloidotic mice, also localized specifically to the amyloid deposits. These observations establish directly that circulating SAP is the precursor of the amyloid P component (AP) found associated with amyloid deposits. In addition to elucidating one aspect of the pathogenesis of amyloid deposition, these results suggest a means for selective targeting of diagnostic traces and/or effector agents to amyloid deposits in vivo.

INTRODUCTION

In all forms of localized and systemic amyloidosis with the exception of the intracerebral plaques in Alzheimer's diseases and senile dementia [1], amyloid P component (AP) is found associated with the fibrillar amyloid deposits [2, 3]. AP, a nonfibrillar glycoprotein, is found in amounts up to 15% of the mass of the amyloid deposits [4]. AP is apparently identical to a normal plasma protein, serum amyloid P components (SAP) as judged by immunochemical testing, by polyacrylamide gel electrophoresis performed either in the presence of sodium dodecyl sulfate or under non-denaturing conditions, by partial amino acid sequence analysis and by appearance in the electron microscope [2, 3]. Thus it has been assumed, although never directly demonstrated, that AP is derived from circulating SAP. It is not known however, whether SAP or AP play a role in the deposition and persistence of amyloid.

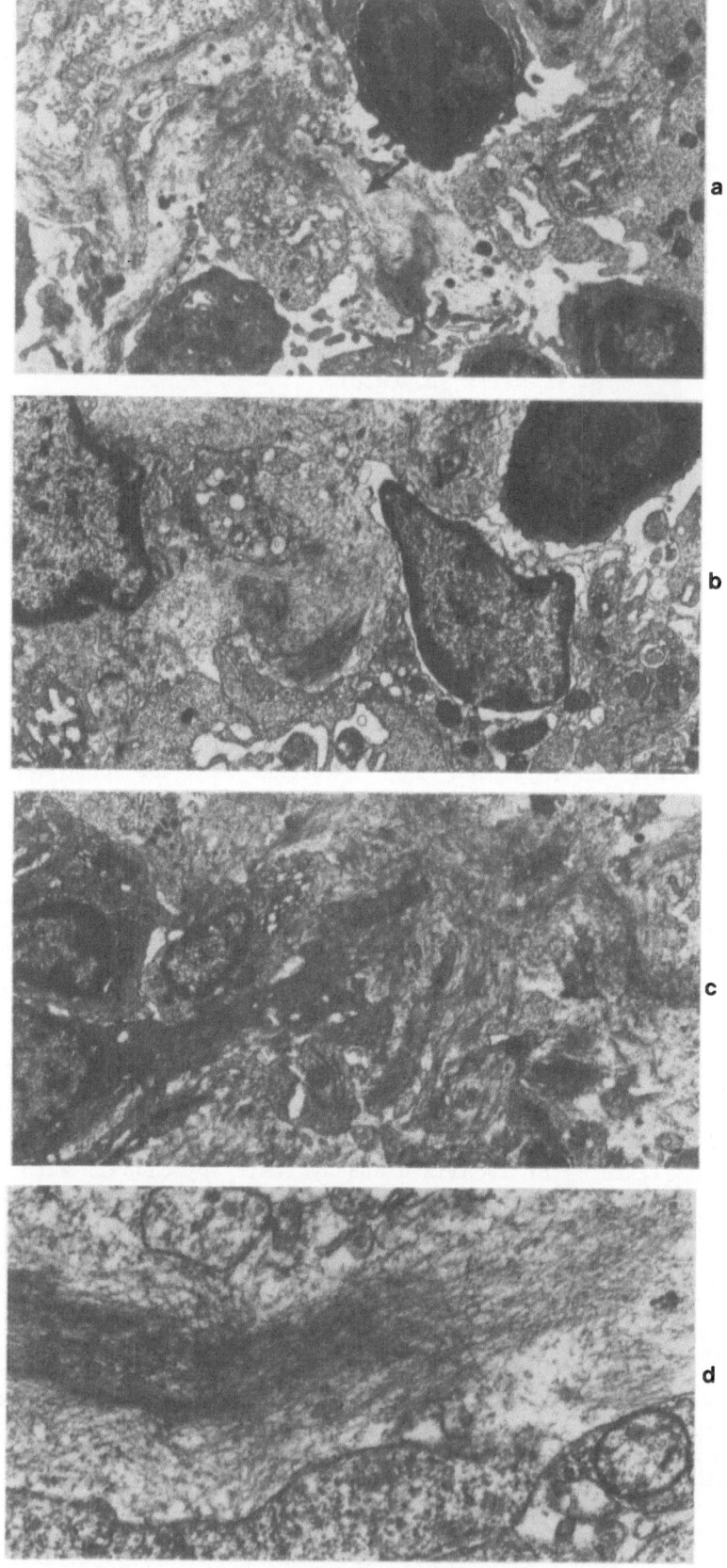

102

We report here a direct demonstration that in murine models of AA amyloidosis, both in the long-term model induced by repeated casein injection [5] and the accelerated model induced by amyloid enhancing factor (AEF) [6] SAP from the circulation is indeed the precursor of AP in the amyloid deposits. Furthermore, intravenous injection of human SAP results in its deposition in the murine amyloid. These findings elucidate one aspect of the pathogenesis of amyloidosis and have implications for its diagnosis and management.

MATERIALS AND METHODS

Amyloid Induction

In the casein-induced model, CBA/ca and C57/B16 mice were injected daily with casein for 4-6 weeks [7]. In the accelerated model, CBA/ca mice were injected intravenously (i.v.) with 0.5 ml amyloid enhancing factor (AEF) [6] (extracted from amyloid laden spleen) and subcutaneously (s.c.) with 2% w/v AgNO$_3$ in distilled water. Mice were killed at times as indicated in Results.

Histo- and Immuno-chemical Staining

Tissue sections were stained for amyloid by the alkaline Congo red method as previously described [7]. The presence of specific proteins in the amyloid deposits was sought by immunofluorescent staining as described previously [7] except that 0.01 M Tris-saline, pH 8.0 containing 2 mM calcium was used in all washing steps. For the direct staining technique, the reagents used were fluorescein-isothiocyanate (FITC) coupled IgG$_1$ fraction of sheep anti-human SAP [8], FITC-IgG fraction of rabbit anti-human C-reactive protein (CRP) and FITC-F(ab')$_2$ sheep anti-mouse SAP [7]. For the indirect staining technique, rabbit anti-human serum albumin (HSA) and FITC-goat anti-rabbit IgG (Miles Scientific, Slough, U.K.) were used. The antisera were monospecific and the specificity of the positive staining was established by its abolition when the antiserum was absorbed before use with the relevant pure antigen.

Electron Microscopy

One mm^3 tissue blocks were fixed in phosphate buffered 3.4% v/v glutaraldehyde, postfixed in 1% w/v Millonig's osmium tetroxide, dehydrated and embedded in TAAB resin (TAAB Laboratories Ltd., Reading, U.K.). Thin sections were cut and stained with alcoholic uranyl acetate and Reynold's lead citrate.

Proteins

Mouse SAP, human SAP and human CRP were purified as previously described [9, 10]. HSA was obtained commercially (Sigma London Chemical Co.

Fig. 1. Electron micrographs of spleen after AEF and AgNO$_3$ administration. a) Day 1, scanty deposit of amyloid seen as extracellular fibrils (arrowed) (×9450); b) day 2, substantial increase in amyloid deposition (×9450); c) day 3, extensive amyloid deposits present (×9450); d) detail of amyloid fibrils (×37,500) taken from a day 2 spleen but similar appearances were present at all times.

Ltd., Poole, U.K.). For injection, proteins were dialyzed into phosphate buffered saline, pH 7.4 (PBS). Pure mouse SAP was radiolabeled with ^{125}I using carrier-free Na-[125]I (IMS30, Amersham Plc, Amersham, U.K.) by the Iodogen method (Pierce and Warriner U.K. Ltd., Chester, U.K.) [11]. The labelled material was tested for purity as described previously [12].

RESULTS

Kinetics of Amyloid Deposition in the AEF Model

Mice were injected with AEF and AgNO₃ and killed 24, 48, 72, or 96 h later. Although there was some splenic uptake of Congo red at 24 h, no green birefringence was seen under polarized light. Unequivocal Congophilia and green birefringence was present in a perifollicular distribution in the spleen at 48 h and increased out to 96 h. At the electron microscope level, extracellular amyloid fibrils were present at 24 h and increased in amount thereafter (Fig. 1).

The presence of murine SAP in the deposits could be demonstrated at 24 h by immunofluorescent staining. Although initially only weak perifollicular staining was seen, it increased in intensity and at 96 h resembled the appearance of anti-SAP staining in deposits in early casein induced amyloid [7]. Neither amyloid nor SAP was detected in normal spleens or in spleens of mice injected with AgNO₃ only.

Localization and Persistence of Circulating ^{125}I-Mouse SAP in AEF Induced Amyloid

Groups of mice were injected with AEF and AgNO₃ or AgNO₃ alone (control). On day 0, 1, 2, or 3 after injection, mice in each group were injected i.v. with 3.3 µg of ^{125}I-mouse SAP ($5 \cdot 10^6$ cpm). On day 4 all mice were killed, the spleens counted for radioactivity and processed for histochemical staining. A greater amount of ^{125}I-mouse SAP localized to the spleens of mice receiving AEF and AgNO₃ (amyloid present) compared to control spleens (no amyloid present) (Fig. 2). The amount of ^{125}I-mouse SAP localized to the spleen correlated with the quantity of amyloid present. Furthermore, the distribution of ^{125}I-mouse SAP, detected by autoradiography, corresponded precisely with the perifollicular zones containing amyloid as detected by Congo red and anti-mouse SAP staining.

Although dramatically more than in control spleens, the amount of ^{125}I-mouse SAP that localized to the amyloid deposits represented only a small percentage of the injected dose, indicating that only a fraction of the total intravascular pool is involved. This corresponds with the failure to detect an acceleration in the plasma clearance of SAP (T 1/2 = 7.2-8.0 h) in amyloid laden mice compared to normal mice [12].

When mice were examined 12 or 29 days after injection of ^{125}I-mouse SAP, less than 10% of the amounts of radioactivity shown in Fig. 2 were found in the spleen, indicating that there was a relatively rapid turnover of AP despite persistence or even increase in the quantity of Congophilic amyloid.

Localization and Persistence of ^{125}I-Mouse SAP in Casein-Induced Amyloid

Mice with established casein-induced amyloid were injected i.v. with 3.3 µg ($5 \cdot 10^6$ cpm) of ^{125}I-mouse SAP, and were then killed at intervals thereafter, their spleens removed and counted for radioactivity. One day after ^{125}I-mouse SAP injection, there was a significant splenic localiza-

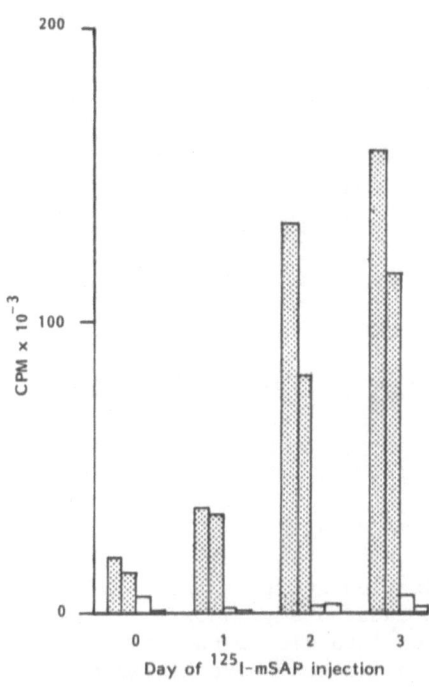

Fig. 2. Localization of circulating
^{125}I-mouse SAP in splenic
amyloid deposits. Mice were
treated with AEF + AgNO$_3$
(stippled bars) or AgNO$_3$
only (open bars) on day 0.
^{125}I-mouse SAP was injected
on day 0, 1, 2, or 3. Mice
were killed on day 4 and
spleens counted for radioactivity. Each bar repre-
sents an individual mouse.
The amount of radioactivity
corresponds to 0.028-0.32%
of the injected dose for
amyloidotic mice (stippled
bias) and 0.001-0.013% for
the control mice (open bars).

tion of the labelled material with a greater proportion of the injected dose
localizing than seen in the AEF model (Fig. 3). This difference correlated
with the greater extent of the amyloid deposits seen in the casein model.
The amount of label in the spleen decreased rapidly, reaching 50% after
about 3 days and declining slowly thereafter. However, there was no change
in the amount of amyloid present over this time.

Similar correlations were observed between the amount of ^{125}I-mouse SAP
initially localizing to the liver and kidneys and the quantity of amyloid
present. The radioactivity localized to these organs decreased at the same
rate as in the spleen.

Localization of Human SAP to Deposits of Murine Amyloid

Groups of mice were injected with AEF and AgNO$_3$, AgNO$_3$ only or nothing.
Three days later, mice of each group were injected i.v. with 1) isolated

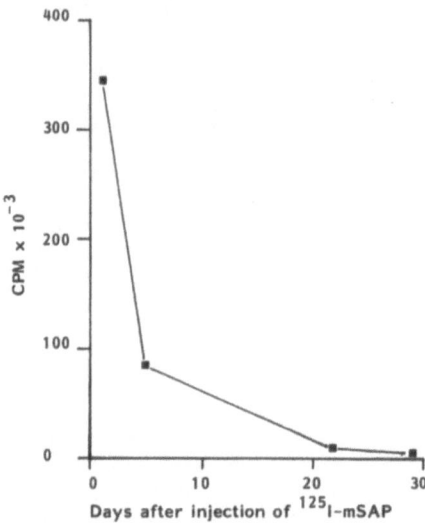

Fig. 3.   Localization and persistence of ^{125}I-mouse SAP in
casein-induced amyloidosis. ^{125}I-mouse SAP was
injected into mice with established casein induced
amyloidosis. Mice were killed at intervals thereafter and the spleens counted for radioactivity.
Each point represents the mean of two mice. The
amount of radioactivity in the spleen at day 1 after injection represents 0.79% of the total injected dose. Counts were corrected for decay of
the isotopes.

pure human SAP (100 μg^{-1} mg), 2) normal human serum (0.5 ml containing 25 μg
of human SAP), 3) pure human CRP (300 μg), or 4) HSA (300 μg). Mice were
killed one day later, the spleens removed and processed for Congo red staining and immunofluorescent staining for detection of specific proteins. Mice
with established casein induced amyloidosis were also injected with the same
proteins as indicated above, killed one day later and the spleen, liver, and
kidney processed for staining.

When either isolated human SAP or whole human serum was administered
to mice with amyloid, human SAP localized specifically to the amyloid deposits (Fig. 4) with the intensity of staining corresponding to the amount
of amyloid present as determined by Congo red staining. There was less
staining in the kidney and liver than in the spleen. No human SAP was detected in spleens of normal or $AgNO_3$ treated mice without amyloid. No
staining for the other injected proteins, CRP and HSA, was seen in any mice,
establishing the specificity of the SAP deposition. If amyloidotic mice
were killed at longer intervals after human SAP injection, SAP could still
be detected 30 days later, although the intensity of staining decreased

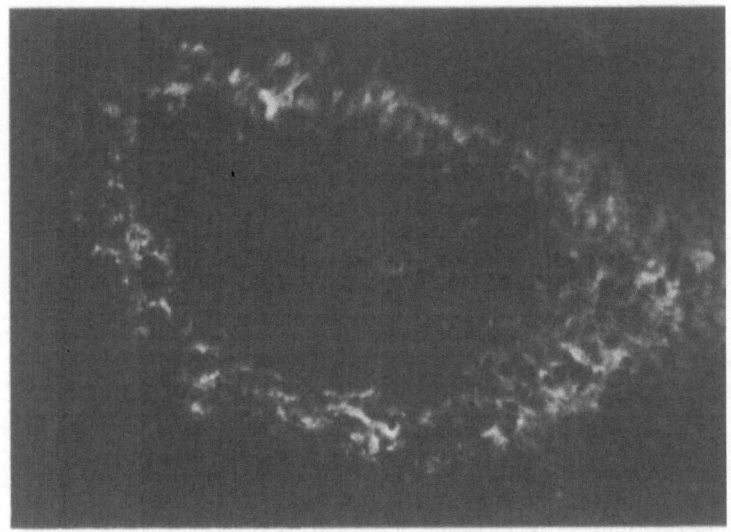

Fig. 4. Direct immunofluorescence staining with anti-human
         SAP of spleen from a mouse which had received pure
         human SAP by i.v. injection 3 days after AEF and
         AgNO₃ and 1 day before being killed. A single
         follicle with characteristic perifollicular stain-
         ing is shown (×430).

steadily from its peak at day 1. There was not a significant change in the
amount of amyloid present as the amount of human SAP associated with it declined. Positive staining with anti-human SAP persisted longer in mice
with casein-induced amyloid than in those with AEF induced amyloid, probably corresponding to the greater amount of amyloid present.

DISCUSSION

These results establish that circulating SAP is deposited as AP in
tissue amyloid. Although the initial SAP deposition is rapid, the persistence is not prolonged, probably as a result of replacement of existing AP
molecules from the pool of circulating SAP. The demonstration that human
SAP can be deposited in murine amyloid reinforces the only known in vivo
pathophysiological function of SAP, its propensity to deposit with amyloid
fibrils. These observations have two important potential applications.
Firstly, amyloid deposits are not completely inert in vivo which may allow
for therapeutic mobilization. Secondly, production of "chimeric" amyloid,
that is, xenogeneic AP associated with autologous AA fibrils, suggests the
possibility of application in the diagnosis and management of human amyloid.
This could include use of isologous or heterologous SAP as a diagnostic
probe for determining the presence and distribution of amyloid deposits in
man and the effect of the sustained presence in amyloid deposits of xeno-
genic (immunogenic) AP on the persistence and effects of the amyloid fibrils.

ACKNOWLEDGEMENTS

This work was supported by Medical Research Council program Grant
G979/51 to M. B. Pepys. C. R. K. Hind is the receipient of a MRC training
research fellowship.

REFERENCES

1. P. Westermark, T. Shirahama, M. Skinner, A. Brun, R. Cameron, and
    A. S. Cohen, Lab. Invest., 46, 457 (1982).
2. M. B. Pepys, M. Baltz, F. C. de Beer, R. F. Dyck, S. Holford, S. M.
    Breathnach, M. M. Black, C. R. F. Tribe, D. J. Evans, and A. Feinstein,
    Ann. N. Y. Acad. Sci., 389, 286 (1982).
3. M. B. Pepys and M. L. Baltz, Adv. Immunol., 34, 141 (1983).
4. M. Skinner, M. B. Pepys, A. S. Cohen, L. M. Heller, and J. B. Lian, in:
    Amyloid and Amyloidosis (G. G. Glenner, P. P. e Costa, and A. Falcao
    de Freitas, eds.), Excerpta Medica, Amsterdam (1980), p. 384.
5. D. T. Janigan, Am. J. Pathol., 47, 159 (1965).
6. M. A. Axelrad, R. Kisilevsky, J. Willmer, S. J. Chen, and M. Skinner,
    Lab. Invest., 47, 139 (1982).
7. M. L. Baltz, R. F. Dyck, and M. B. Pepys, Immunology, 41, 59 (1980).
8. R. F. Dyck, D. J. Evans, C. M. Lockwood, A. J. Rees, D. Turner, and
    M. B. Pepys, Lancet ii, 606 (1980).
9. M. B. Pepys, Immunology, 37, 637 (1979).
10. F. C. de Beer and M. B. Pepys, J. Immunol. Meth., 50, 17 (1982).
11. P. R. P. Salacinski, C. McLean, J. E. C. Sykes, V. V. Clement-Jones,
    and P. J. Lowry, Analyt. Biochem., 117, 137 (1981).
12. M. L. Baltz, R. F. Dyck, and M. B. Pepys, Clin. Exp. Immunol. (1985),
    in press.

A POSSIBLE EFFECT OF ORAL TOLERANCE IN CASEIN

INDUCED MURINE AMYLOIDOSIS?

Ronald I. Carr *,
Judith Katilus †, and D. Petty †

*Department of Medicine
 Victoria General Hospital
 Dalhousie University Faculty of Medicine
 Halifax, Nova Scotia, Canada, and

†The National Jewish Hospital and Research Center
 Denver, Colorado 80206

ABSTRACT

Mice raised on a normal mouse chow diet have a low immune response to immunization with casein. In addition, attempts to experimentally induce oral tolerance with casein in mice raised on a normal diet failed. Normal mouse chow contains substantial casein as a protein source. However, when mice were raised on a casein free diet and immunized with casein they had 4-5× the immune response of the normal diet mice. If such casein free mice were fed casein experimentally and then immunized the immune response was markedly suppressed. Thus mice raised on normal mouse chow are orally tolerized by the casein it contains, and this accounts for the low immune responses to casein previously reported. There are conflicting reports regarding the effect of neonatal parenterally induced tolerance to casein on susceptibility to amyloidosis, but no reports have ever considered a possible role of dietary induced tolerance in interpreting the results, a phenomenon which might well be a variable in different studies. In fact we found that one of the so called "tolerizing" protocols actually immunized the mice and prevented the development of oral tolerance due to the dietary casein. This raises the intriguing possibility that oral tolerance may be a susceptibility factor in amyloidosis.

INTRODUCTION

The phenomenon of the systemic tolerance induced by enteric exposure to antigens was first described at the turn of the century by Besredka who found that guinea pigs fed milk became unresponsive to subsequent parenteral milk challenge, and Wells and Osborne who found that guinea pigs fed corn as part of their diet could not be anaphylactically sensitized with a protein constituent of corn [1]. The phenomenon was "rediscovered" in the 1970's and both the nature of the phenomenon and its possible significance is now under intense investigation [2]. We have been studying immune response to dietary antigens for a number of years, among them bovine casein. When we attempted to induce systemic anti-casein antibodies in mice by feeding we were unsuccessful. In view of the above we decided to determine if casein was an oral tolerogen, which could account for our failure to induce IgG casein antibodies by feeding.

MATERIALS AND METHODS

Mice

The mice used were BDF₁ (C57B1/6 × DBA/2) females, raised in our mouse colony.

Normal Diet

The normal diet the C57B1/6 female parents were on at mating, during gestation and while nursing was Wayne Breeder Blox (Allied Mills, Inc., Chicago, Illinois). Prior to weaning the BDF₁ progeny were therefore also exposed to the breeder blox. After weaning the mice were maintained on Wayne Lab. Blox.

Detection of Circulating Antibodies to Casein

One hundred μl of ¹²⁵I-Casein at 0.25 μg protein/ml diluted in 1:100 normal rabbit serum, were added to 100 μl dilutions of test sera in borate buffer (0.125 M sodium borate-boric acid, 0.075 M NaCl, pH 8.3). Then 200 μl of 20% polyethylene glycol 6000 (PEG) in borate buffer was immediately added and the tubes were vortexed. After overnight incubation at 4°C, they were centrifuged for 30'. They were then decanted, drained, and washed once with 1 ml of 10% PEG. After recentrifugation and draining they were counted. Results were calculated as percentage of TCA precipitable counts bound by the test serum, corrected forthe radioactivity in the precipitate of a normal control serum [3].

Oral Tolerizing Protocol

We assessed 3 different tolerizing protocols. The mice were given 20 mgm of casein by i.g. tube 1×, 4×, on consecutive days, or at 1 mg/ml in their drinking water for 28 days. To assess the induction of tolerance, one week after casein feeding was completed they received 500 μg casein in CFA i.p. and 14 days later they were boosted. After another 7 days they were bled. Antibodies to casein were assessed using a radio immunoassay and the antigen binding capacity (ABC₃₃) in μg of casein bound per ml of undiluted serum determined.

Statistical analyses were performed using the Mann-Whitney "U" test.

RESULTS

As can be seen from Table 1, our initial attempts to produce orally induced tolerance with casein in BDF₁ mice failed, suggesting that casein was not an oral tolerogen. However, the antibody levels were relatively low, and we had come across the statement in one of Clerici's papers on the possible role of the immune system in casein induced amyloidosis, that "the mouse...is such a poor producer of anti-casein antibodies that they are hardly, if at all, detectable in the serum..." [4]. Thus it occurred to us that if there was casein in normal mouse chow, all mice raised on normal chow might be "pretolerized" by the dietary exposure. Indeed, we discovered that both Wayne Breeder Blox and Wayne Lab Blox contained substantial casein as a protein source. Therefore we repeated the experiments, but this time with mice that had been bred and raised in such a way that

TABLE 1. Casein Antibodies after i.p. Immunization of Mice Raised on a
          Normal Diet

Pretreatment	Post 2 i.p. immunizations	
IG saline 1×	2.8 ± 1.1	
IG casein 1×	2.6 ± 1.6	p > .5
IG saline 4×	1.9 ± 1.7	
IG casein 4×	2.2 ± 1.6	p > .5
None	2.2 ± 1.1	
Casein in drinking water for 28 days	1.5 ± 0.9	p > .05

they had no oral exposure to bovine casein. To achieve this, parental mice
were put on a chow free of bovine casein one month prior to mating (Special
diet #838, Bioserve, Frenchtown, New Jersey). During gestation and nursing
the casein free diet was maintained. Post weaning, and throughout the experiment the BDF$_1$ progeny were maintained on the same casein free diet.
These mice were thus never exposed to bovine casein and will be referred
to as casein free mice. (Clearly, there was no way we could avoid exposure
to murine casein in the maternal milk. However, we found that purified
murine casein showed no cross reactivity with bovine casein.)

The mice were tested with the same tolerizing protocols as above and
the results were obtained (Table 2). The antibody response to casein in
mice raised casein free prior to parenteral immunization was 4-5 fold
higher than in mice raised on the normal diet. In addition, when casein
free mice were fed casein experimentally they did develop orally induced
tolerance and became as suppressed as the mice raised on the normal diet.
Thus two things were evident. First, casein is a good oral tolerogen, and
second, mice raised on normal mouse chow containing casein are orally tolerized by their dietary exposure.

These findings raised some interesting questions with respect to a
possible role of oral tolerance in the casein model of amyloidosis. In
1957 Grayzel et al., had found that mice raised on a milk protein free
diet were significantly less susceptible to casein induced amyloidosis than
mice on the normal diet [5]. They suggested this resistance might have
been due to protein deprivation. In 1965, Clerici et al., induced tolerance to casein by subcutaneous injection of neonatal mice and found that
such tolerance had no effect on susceptibility to the disease [6]. However, they did not specify the diet and it is reasonably probable that both
experimental and control mice were raised on casein containing mouse chow,
thus both groups would have been orally tolerized, a phenomenon they would
not have considered.

It was also of considerable interest that in 1966 Letterer and Kretschmer reported results which apparently conflicted with Clerici's [7]. They
injected neonatal mice with a casein-Complete Freund's Adjuvant mixture to
induce tolerance, and found that such animals were resistant to casein induced amyloidosis. They interpreted their results as indicating that tolerance to casein decreased susceptibility. However, they did not verify
that their mice were actually tolerant. We decided to determine if their
protocol really induced tolerance, or if it immunized the mice instead.

111

TABLE 2. Casein Antibodies after i.p. Immunization of Mice Raised on a Casein Free Diet

Pretreatment	Post 2 i.p. immunizations	
IG saline 1×	13.8 ± 3.4	p > .5
IG casein 1×	10.3 ± 3.8	
IG saline 4×	10.9 ± 4.5	p < .02
IG casein 4×	3.2 ± 1.5	
None	11.0 ± 1.8	p < .002
Casein in drinking water for 28 days	2.8 ± 1.1	

TABLE 3

	Time from "First" immunization		After booster
	7 days	14 days	7 days
CFA alone	0	0	1.9 1.5
Casein + CFA	8.9 ± 5.6	10.6 ± 4.8	24.9 ± 14.5

Neonatal mice were injected with 0.03 ml of 4% casein in CFA s.c. and the injections were repeated at 12 and 24 days of age. Seven days after this "tolerizing protocol" the mice received a "primary immunization" of 500 μg of casein in CFA as usual. They were bled 7 and 14 days after the immunization, boosted and bled 7 days later. The antibody response (ABC$_{33}$ in μg/ml) obtained is presented in Table 3.

As can be seen, the mice injected only with CFA had no detectable response to the primary immunization with casein, and only a low response to the secondary immunization, results compatible with a state of orally induced tolerance since the mice in these experiments were raised on normal mouse chow. In striking contrast, the mice treated with the Letterer and Kretschmer "tolerizing protocol" showed a very good response to the "primary" immunization, even at 7 days, and there was no significant difference in their response between 7 and 14 days post immunization. These results are typical of a secondary response and indicate that the so-called "tolerizing" protocol actually immunized the mice. It has previously been shown, that the induction of oral tolerance in a previously primed animal is very difficult, thus the dietary exposure in the mice immunized at birth would not have been expected to tolerize them, and it did not.

CONCLUSIONS

All the results discussed are compatible with the possibility that oral tolerance is a susceptibility factor in the casein induced model of amyloidosis. Thus, Grayzel's result might have been due to the lack of maintenance of oral tolerance when he took the mice off dietary casein, rather than due to protein depletion. Clerici's failure to demonstrate a difference in susceptibility in control mice compared to mice parenterally tolerized as neonates, might have been due to both groups of animals having been tolerized orally. Conversely, the apparently conflicting results of Letterer and Kretschmer might be accounted for because their "tolerizing" protcol actually immunized the mice and prevented the developed of oral tolerance.

Clearly, the possibility that oral tolerance is a susceptibility factor in casein induction is still theoretical and further studies are now underway in our laboratory to assess it.

ACKNOWLEDGEMENT

This study was supported in part by NIH grant No. AM-30434

REFERENCES

1. Besredka, A., Ann. Inst. Pasteur Lille, 23:166 (1909); Wells, H. G., and Osborne, T. B., J. Infect. Dis., 8:66 (1911).
2. Thomas, H. C., and Parrott, D. M. V., immunology, 27:631 (1974); Richman, L. K., Chiller, J. M., Brown, W. R., Hanson, D. G., and Vaz, N. M., J. Immunol., 121:2429 (1978); McDonald, T. T., Eur. J. Immunol., 12:767 (1982); Mattingly, J. A. Ann. N.Y. Acad. Sci., 409:204 (1983); Mattingly, J. A., Cell Immunology, 86:46 (1984).
3. Minden, P., and Farr, R. S., Ammonium sulfate method to measure antigen binding capacity, in: Handbook of Experimental Immunology, Vol. I, Immunochemicstry (D. M. Weir, ed.), 3rd Edition, Blackwell Scientific Publications, London, P. 131 (1978).
4. Clerici, E., and Schechter, I., Int. Arch. Allergy Appl. Immunol., 38: 554 (1970).
5. Grayzel, H. G., Grayzel, D. M., Miller, P., Cohen, H., and Akst, P., Lab. Invest., 6:148 (1957).
6. Clerici, E., Pierpaoli, W., and Romussi, M., Path. Microbiol., 28:806 (1965).
7. Letterer, E., and Kretschmer, Nature, 210:390 (1966).

ISOLATION AND CHARACTERIZATION OF AMYLOID

ENHANCING FACTOR (AEF)

M. L. Baltz, D. Caspi,
C. R. K. Hind, A. Feinstein*,
and M. B. Pepys

MRC Acute Phase Protein Research Group
Immunological Medicine Unit
Department of Medicine
Royal Postgraduate Medical School
Du Cane Road
London W12 OHS, and

*AFRC Institute of Animal Physiology
 Babraham
 Cambridge, United Kingdom

ABSTRACT

   Injection into mice of extracts of amyloid laden or of normal organs
at the same time as a single potent inflammatory stimulus induces the extremely rapid deposition of systemic AA amyloid. This activity has been
designated amyloid enhancing factor (AEF) and we report here a preliminary
characterization of the material which confirms and extends previous work.
AEF activity was extractable from normal murine organs as well as from
amyloid laden tissues but in very much smaller amounts, and it was also
present in normal or amyloidotic tissues of man, dog, and hamster. AEF
extracts are very potent in vivo, as little as 0.002 A_{280} units being
effective. AEF activity was not inhibited by proteinase inhibitors, by nuclease or periodate treatment, by lipid extraction, or by low pH. It was,
however, inactivated by proteolytic digestion or by alkaline pH treatment.
Gel filtration indicated that the activity resided in a species of apparent molecular weight around 400,000. These findings suggest that AEF depends on a protein component possibly associated with non-protein material.
Interestingly preparations of isolated human or murine AA fibrils had the
same effect in vivo as AEF.

INTRODUCTION

   The ability to transfer or accelerate the deposition of amyloid in experimental animals by injection of cells or tissue extracts has been reported by numerous workers [1-4]. A material called amyloid enhancing factor (AEF) has been described which when injected intravenously (i.v.) into
mice results in rapid amyloid deposition provided an inflammatory stimulus
is also given [5]. Amyloid deposits can be detected as early as 24 h after
injection [6] and these deposits increase dramatically with time [5, 6].

AEF was originally extracted from pre-amyloidotic organs but such activity was also found in amyloid laden and normal tissue [5]. To date, AEF has been incompletely characterized. It is thought to be glycoprotein of high molecular weight, soluble in 0.5 M KCl or 4 M glycerol but which precipitates in physiological buffer [5].

Elucidation of the biochemical nature of AEF and determination of its mode of action may make a fundamental contribution to an understanding of the pathogenesis of amyloidosis.

MATERIALS AND METHODS

Source of Amyloid and Normal Organs

Systemic AA amyloid was induced in mice by repeated casein injection [7]. Human amyloidotic (AA) spleen was obtained at autopsy from a patient with long-standing rheumatoid arthritis. Kidneys were obtained from a dog and Syrian hamster with spontaneously developing amyloid.

Extraction of AEF from Organs

AEF was extracted from amyloid laden or normal organs using 4 M glycerol, 10 mM Tris, pH 7.4 (4 M glycerol) as described by Axelrad et al. [5], except that the homogenized material was centrifuged at 100 K × g. The supernatant was dialyzed into 0.01 M phosphate buffered saline, pH 7.4. For homogenization 8 ml were used per gram spleen and 4 ml were used per gram of liver, kidney, heart, or lung.

Extraction of AEF from Isolated Cells

AEF was extracted from isolated cells using the general procedure as described above for extraction from organs.

Normal human skin fibroblasts: cells were grown to confluency using standard techniques and detached from the flasks by trypsin-EDTA treatment. After washing in PBS, AEF was extracted from approximately 2×10^6 cells using 0.5 ml 4 M glycerol.

Human peripheral blood mononuclear cells and red blood cells (RBC): mononuclear cells were isolated from normal human peripheral blood [8]. The isolated mononuclear cell layer and the red blood cell pellet were collected separately and washed in Hank's balanced salt solution. The sum of 10^7 cells were homogenized with 1 ml 4 M glycerol.

Murine splenic mononuclear cells and peritoneal exudate cells (PEC): a single cell suspension was prepared from amyloid-laden or normal spleens and mononuclear cells were isolated [8]. After separation, a portion of the isolated cells was allowed to adhere to plastic Petri dishes for 18 h. Adherent and non-adherent cell populations were harvested, washed in PBS and homogenized in 4 M glycerol, using 0.5 ml per 10^6 cells. PEC's were induced by injection of 1 ml 10% proteose peptone broth 3 days earlier. Cells were isolated and AEF extracted as described above for spleen cells.

Isolation of AA Fibrils

AA fibrils from amyloid laden murine or human spleen was isolated by the method of Pras et al. [9].

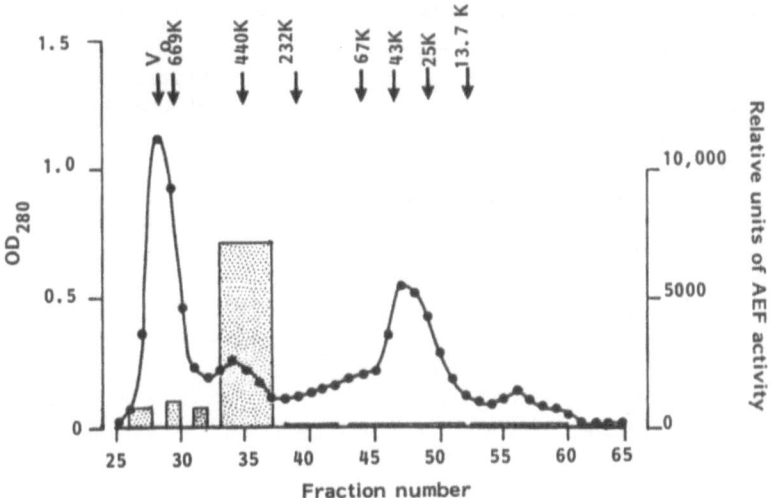

Fig. 1. Gel filtration profile on Sephacryl S-300 of AEF
extract in 10 mM Tris, 0.5 M KCl, pH 7.4. Arrows
indicate positions of marker proteins of known
molecular weight.

In-vivo Assay for AEF Activity

Mice were injected i.v. with 0.1 ml AEF extract, followed by a subcutaneous injection of 0.5 ml AgNO$_3$ (2% in distilled water). AEF activity
was titrated by injection of the neat extract and 10 fold serial dilutions
out to 1:10^4 of the neat material. Mice were killed 4 days later and spleen
sections processed for Congo red staining [7].

Inactivation of AEF Activity

AEF was treated in-vitro with the reagents indicated in Table 3. Reagents were obtained from the following suppliers: trypsin type IX from
bovine pancreas (Sigma London Chemical Co., Ltd., Poole, U.K.); DNase and
RNase from bovine spleen (Koch-Light Laboratories, Ltd., Suffolk, U.K.);
pronase from S. griseus (Boehringer Manheim, Boehringer Corporation, Ltd.,
Lewes, U.K.); NaIO$_4$ (Sigma); ascorbic acid (Hoffman-La Roche, Basel, Switzerland); Aprotinin (Traysolol) (Bayer U.K. Ltd., Newbury, U.K.); phenylmethylsulfonylfluoride (PMSF), soybean trypsin inhibitor (SBT1) and α$_1$-proteinase
inhibitors (α$_1$-Pl) (Sigma).

AEF extract was treated with 1.6% sodium dodecyl sulfate (SDS) containing 0.04% 2-mercaptoethanol (2 ME) and boiled for 10 min. Cold meth-
anol:ether (1:3) was used to extract lipid from AEF. For pH stability, the
pH of the AEF extract was altered by addition of 0.1 M HCl or 0.1 M NaOH
(final concentration) and the mixture was allowed to stand at room temperature for 15 min. The pH of the AEF extract was brought back to neutrality
by addition of NaOH or HCl, respectively.

Gel Filtration of AEF Extract on Sephacryl S-300

The sum of 5 ml of AEF extracted from amyloid laden mouse spleen were
dialized into 10 mM Tris, 0.5 M KCl, pH 7.4 [5] and gel filtered in the
same buffer on a Sephacryl S-300 (Pharmacia G. B. Ltd., Milton Keynes,
U.K.) column (2.5 × 100 cm) calibrated with marker proteins of known molecular weight (Pharmacia). The sum of 6.1 ml fractions were collected.

117

TABLE 1.   Sources of AEF Activity Extracted with 4 M Glycerol

Species	Extract	Presence of amyloid	AEF activity
Mouse	Amyloid spleen	+	+
	liver	+	+
	kidney	+	+
	heart	−	+
	lung	−	−
	Normal spleen	−	+
	liver	−	+
	kidney	−	+
	heart	−	+
	lung	−	−
Human	Amyloid spleen	+	+
Dog	Amyloid kidney	+	+
Hamster	Amyloid kidney	+	+
Mouse	Isolated AA fibrils		+
	EDTA washed AA fibrils		+
Human	Isolated AA fibrils		+
	EDTA washed AA fibrils		+
Human	Fibroblasts		+
	RBC		−
	Peripheral blood mononuclear cells		+
Mouse	Peritoneal exudate cells		+
	Spleen cells		+
	adherent cells		+
	non-adherent cells		+

Protein peaks were pooled, concentrated using an Amicon PM30 membrane (Amicon Ltd., Woking, U.K.) and dialyzed into PBS prior to in-vivo titration. Relative units of AEF activity for each pool were calculated as follows:

$$\frac{OD_{280} \text{ units/ml} \times 100}{\text{Endpoint dilution}}$$

RESULTS

Sources of AEF Activity

AEF activity could be extracted from either amyloid laden or normal murine organs (Table 1). Spleen, liver, kidney, and heart all contained AEF activity while lung did not. However, extracts from normal organs contained much less AEF activity than amyloid-laden organs when titrated in-vivo (Table 2). Furthermore, organs with heavier amyloid deposits contained proportionately more AEF activity. Extracts of amyloid-laden tissue from a

TABLE 2. In-vivo Titration of AEF Activity Extracted from Amyloid-Laden or Normal Mouse Spleen

O.D.$_{280}$ units injected	Splenic amyloid deposits induced by	
	Amyloid AEF	Normal AEF
2.100	++++	+++
0.2100	+++	++
0.0210	+++	+
0.0021	+	-

TABLE 3. In-vitro Inactivation of AEF Activity. AEF Extracted from Amyloidotic Mouse Spleen was Treated at 37°C for 1 h and Dialyzed into PBS Prior to Injection

Treatment	Concentration	AEF activity
Pronase	1% w/v	±
Trypsin	1% w/v	++
DNase	1% w/v	++++
RNase	1% w/v	++++
Soybean trypsin inhibitor	5 mg/ml	++++
α_1-Proteinase inhibitor	5 mg/ml	++++
Aprotinin	10^3 units	++++
Ascorbic acid	55 mg/ml	++++
PMSF	5 mM	++++
NaIO$_4$	100 mM	++++
Nil	-	++++

TABLE 4. In vitro Inactivation of AEF Activity. AEF Extracted from Amyloidotic Mouse Spleen was Treated and Dialyzed into PBS Prior to Injection

Treatment	AEF activity
100°/10 min	+
SDS-2ME/100°/10 min	-
0.22 µM filtered	-
Lipid extraction	++++
Low pH	++++
High pH	-
Nil	++++

dog, hamster, and man also contained AEF activity when assayed in the murine model (Table 1).

AEF activity was present in isolated cells as well as in the intact organ (Table 1). Isolated mononuclear cells, derived from either normal or amyloid-laden murine spleen or peritoneal exudate cells, contained AEF activity. AEF activity could also be extracted from isolated human peripheral blood mononuclear cells or cultured skin fibroblasts but not from RBC's. This suggests the activity is associated with a component of nucleated cells.

Isolated AA fibrils obtained from human and murine spleen mimicked the effect of AEF (Table 1). Washing the AA fibrils with EDTA prior to i.v. injection did not abolish this effect. The AEF-like activity was not due to splenic uptake of the AA fibrils as human AA fibrils could not be detected in the spleen when stained immunochemically using rabbit anti-human AA serum. Furthermore, mice injected with AA fibrils only and not receiving $AgNO_3$ failed to develop amyloid.

Since these preparations of AA fibrils contained traces of other proteins when run on SDS-PAGE, it is not clear whether the AEF activity residues in the AA fibrils themselves or in a co-isolating material.

In-vitro Inactivation of AEF Activity

AEF activity appears to depend upon a protein component as it was sensitive to pronase treatment and partially sensitive to trypsin treatment (Table 3). DNase or RNase treatment or lipid extraction had no effect. The activity did not appear to depend on glycosylation since it was not affected by $NaIO_4$, although inactivation of AEF by $NaIO_4$ has been previously reported by others [10]. The AEF activity was not affected by a variety of agents including SBT1, α_1-Pl, Aprotinin, PMSF, or ascorbic acid.

In-vivo Activity of AEF

AEF activity is very potent, injection of as little as 0.002 units of OD_{280} absorbing material produces amyloid (Table 2). Once injected, an inflammatory stimulus (e.g., $AgNO_3$) is required for amyloid deposition although this can be given as long as 41 days after AEF injection and still result in amyloid deposition within 4 days. This long-lived in-vivo effect has been reported previously [5] and suggests either that the AEF itself has a long in-vivo half life or that once injected, its effect is long lasting. Once AEF and $AgNO_3$ were injected, amyloid deposition was not affected by daily injection of SBT1 (2 mg), α_1-Pl (1 mg), Eglin (0.2 mg) (a gift of Dr. H. P. Schnebli, Ciba Geigy, Basel, Switzerland) or ascorbic acid (0.5 mg). If the reticuloendothelial system was blockaded with dextran sulfate [11] prior to AEF and $AgNO_3$ injection, amyloid is still deposited.

Gel Filtration of AEF Extract on Sephacryl S-300

When AEF extract was gel filtered on Sephacryl S-300 in a high salt buffer (10 mM Tris, 0.5 M KCl, pH 7.4) most of the AEF activity localized to a peak eluting with an apparent molecular weight of 440,000 (Fig. 1). Although AEF activity is apparently soluble in 0.5 M KCl [5] it is possible that microaggregates formed giving an erroneously high apparent molecular weight. When this pool was run on 4-30% w/v SDS-PAGE under reducing conditions, no discrete protein staining band could be detected.

ACKNOWLEDGEMENTS

This work was supported by Medical Research Council programme grant G979/51 to M. B. Pepys. C. R. K. Hind is the recipient of a MRC training research fellowship.

REFERENCES

1. F. Hardt and P. Ranlov, Int. Rev. Exp. Path., 16:273 (1976).
2. I. Keizman, A. Rimon, E. Sohar, and J. Gafni, Act. Path. Microbiol. Scand., Section A, 233:172 (1972).

3. I. Kedar and M. Ravid, Eur. J. Clin. Invest., 10:63 (1980).

4. J. T. Willerson, J. K. Gordon, N. Talal, and W. F. Barth, Arth. Rheum., 12:232 (1969).

5. M. A. Axelrad, R. Kisilevsky, J. Willmer, S. J. Chen, and M. Skinner, Lab. Invest., 47:139 (1982).

6. M. L. Baltz, D. Caspi, I. F. Rowe, C. R. K. Hind, D. J. Evans, and M. B. Pepys, this volume.

7. M. L. Baltz, R. F. Dyck, and M. B. Pepys, Immunology, 41:59 (1980).

8. A. Boyum, Scand. J. Clin. Lab. Invest., 21, Suppl. 97 (1968).

9. M. Pras, M. Schubert, D. Zucker-Franklin, A. Rimon, and E. C. Franklin, J. Clin. Invest., 47:924 (1962).

10. M. A. Axelrad and R. Kisilevsky, in: Amyloid and Amyloidosis (G. G. Glenner, P. P. e Costa, and F. Falcao de Freitas, eds.), Excerpta Medica, Amsterdam (1980), p. 527.

11. L. E. Retegui, N. Moguilevsky, C. F. Costracane, and P. L. Masson, Lab. Invest., 50:323 (1984).

ENHANCEMENT OF AMYLOID DEGRADATION BY ASCORBIC ACID:

IN VIVO EVIDENCE IN A MURINE MODEL

M. Ravid, B. Chen,
and I. Kedar

Heller Institute of Medical Research, and
Department of Medicine
Sackler School of Medicine
Tel-Aviv University
Tel-Aviv, Israel

ABSTRACT

In vitro experiments have shown that the amyloid degrading activity of amyloidotic sera could be restored by ascorbic acid, citric acid and by EDTA. It was therefore decided to test the influence of Vitamin C on experimental murine amyloidosis. Amyloidosis was induced during 14 days in three groups of 60 animals each. The first group received Vitamin C in the drinking water, as 3.5% solution, throughout the entire experimental period. Vitamin C was given to the second group after the induction of amyloidosis, while the control group received water alone. On the tenth, 17th, and 20th post induction days, 15 mice of each group were sacrificed. Their spleens were examined for the presence of amyloid. On the 17th day no amyloid was found in nine mice (out of 15) of the first group and in eight of the second. Small deposits were observed in five and three animals respectively. However, in the control groups giant deposits of amyloid were found in ten out of 15 animals. Amyloid degrading activity (ADA) of murine serum was examined in untreated, amyloidotic and Vitamin C treated animals. In healthy animals the ADA is unaffected by Vitamin C. In amyloidotic mice which have very low ADA initially, the addition of Vitamin C significantly increases the ADA. These results may possibly indicate that the in vitro effect of Vitamin C on amyloidotic sera is also expressed in an in vivo experimental model.

INTRODUCTION

Systemic amyloidosis is an incurable disease [1]. Current evidence, based on animal experiments and human studies, indicates that certain amyloidoses may be prevented by continuous colchicine treatment [2-4]. Under specific experimental or clinical conditions regression of amyloidosis was observed on long term treatment with dimethylsulfoxide [5-7]. However, for the patient with far advanced systemic amyloidosis no cure and no relief are as yet available.

In vitro experiments have demonstrated an amyloid degrading activity of normal human serum. This activity is lost in patients with amyloidosis due to the presence of a specific inhibitor of the amyloid degrading factor. The addition of ascorbic acid, citric acid and EDTA to amyloidotic serum restores the amyloid degarding activity [8].

The present experiments were designed in order to find whether the addition of Vitamin C to the diet of amyloidotic experimental animals would result in any appreciable degree of regression of the amyloid deposits, and in any change in the amyloid degarding activity of murine serum.

MATERIALS AND METHODS

White Swiss mice, 6-8 weeks old and weighing approximately 30 gm each, were used. They were fed a standard Purina diet ad libitum. Amyloidosis was induced by 14 consecutive, daily injections of 0.5 ml 13% vitamin free casein (NBC, Cleveland, Ohio) in 0.05 mole NaOH. The presence of amyloidosis was determined by polarization microscopy of Congo red stained slides.

Amyloidosis was induced in 180 animals which were allocated into three groups equal in number as follows: The first was a control. Ascorbic acid (as 3.5% sodium ascorbate) in a dose of 5 gm/kg body weight was added to the drinking water of the second group animals from the 15th post-induction day onwards. The animals of the third group were given the ascorbic acid from the first day of the experiment. Fifteen animals of each group were sacrificed on days 25, 32, and 35. Congo red stained histological sections of the spleen were examined by an independent observer who was not aware of the details of the experimental procedure. The results were classified into three categories: first - no amyloid, second - sporadic microdeposits only around blood vessels, and third - diffuse deposition of amyloid. Eight mice of the first group, eight of the second, and twelve of the third group died during this experiment. These experiments were repeated with 2% and 5% concentrations of ascorbic acid, and the animals were sacrificed on day 35.

On day 35 of the experiment mice were bled through a tail cut. The serum was tested for amyloid degrading activity on human AA amyloid by radial diffusion in agar as previously described [8].

Serum was obtained from ten non treated mice, ten control amyloidotic mice, ten animals which were given 5% ascorbic acid, and ten non-amyloidotic mice which drank water with 5% ascorbic acid. The sum of 0.01 ml of mouse serum were placed in wells (5 mm in diameter) in amyloid containing agar and the amyloid degrading activity was expressed as the diameter of the halo at 24 h and as the volume of the agar under the halo.

RESULTS

All 15 control animals sacrificed on day 25 showed abundant splenic amyloidosis. Microdeposits of amyloid were found in one control animal on day 32 and in three animals on day 35. Diffuse deposits were seen in all the rest.

Among the sacrificed animals of the second group the spleen slides were free of amyloid in two animals on day 25, in eight on day 32 and in four on day 35. Microdeposits were seen in two mice on day 25, in two on day 32 and in six on day 35. On days 32 and 35 there was also a significant decrease in the degree of amyloid deposition in the other animals as compared to the control group. Altogether diffuse amyloid deposition was observed in 21 animals of this group and in 41 controls.

TABLE 1. Splenic Amyloidosis in Control and in Vitamin C Treated Animals. There is a Gradual Time Dependent Decrease in the Number of Mice with Diffuse Amyloidosis. This Decline is Significantly Augumented by Vitamin C (Chi square test)

| | Amyloidosis | | | | | | |
| | day 25 | | day 32 | | day 35 | | |
Group	diffuse	micro-dep. or none	diffuse	micro-dep. or none	diffuse	micro-dep. or none	significance vs. control
Control	15	0	14	1	12	3	
Vit. C 3.5% days 15-35	11	4	5	10	5	10	p < 0.05
Vit. C 3.5% days 1-35	10	5	1	14	2	13	p < 0.001
Vit. C 5%					12	3	p < 0.001
Vit. C 2%					7	8	p < 0.05

TABLE 2. Amyloid Degrading Activity (ADA) of Murine Serum. Treatment with Vitamin C Seems to Increase the ADA of Amyloidotic Murine Serum

	Mean diameter, mm	Vol. of agar cleared of amyloid, mm^3
NHS	16	272
NMS	13	169
AMS	9.0	66*
AMS + Vitamin C	10.0	91*
NMS + Vitamin C	12.2	146

NHS) Normal human serum; NMS) normal murine serum; AMS) amyloidotic murine serum; *) the difference in degrading activity of amyloidotic murine serum with and without Vitamin C is significantly different from NMS ($p < 0.001$). The difference between ADA of AMS + Vitamin C and AMS is of borderline significance ($p < 0.05$).

On day 25 of the experiment diffuse amyloid deposits were present in ten animals of the third group, and no amyloid was found in the remaining five. On day 32 diffuse amyloidosis was detected in only one animal and on day 35 the spleens of 10 out of 15 mice were amyloid free, and additional three showed microdeposits. These results are summarized in Table 1.

The amyloid degrading activity of the murine sera was as follows:

The mean diameter of untreated non-amyloidotic mice was 13 mm (range 12-14), while the diameter of the control amyloidotic animals was 9 mm (range 8–11). The serum of non-amyloidotic animals which were given as-corbic acid showed a mean diameter of 12.2 mm (range 10–14), the amyloidotic Vitamin C treated mice showed a mean diameter of 10.1 mm (range 9–11). At the same experimental conditions the degrading activity of normal human serum was 16 mm. The mean halo diameter and the calculated volume of agar which was rendered amyloid free are given in Table 2. The thickness of the agar plate was 1.5 mm.

DISCUSSION

In vitro experiments revealed the presence of two factors relevant to the pathogenesis of AA amyloidosis [8]. Both normal human serum and serum of amyloidotic patients contain an amyloid degrading factor. The serum of amyloidotic patients contains, in addition, an inhibitor of the amyloid de-grading factor. Accumulation of amyloid may therefore become possible upon the depression of the degrading factor by the inhibitor. Ascorbic acid, together with two other agents, was found to neutralize the inhibiting fac-tor, thus partially restoring the initial amyloid degrading activity of the tested serum. The possible therapeutic implications of these findings prompted the animal experiments described in this paper.

Since murine amyloid is of the AA type [9], one may expect ascorbic acid to be effective also in the murine model. Likewise, murine serum was expected to contain the ability to degrade human AA amyloid. A review of the histopathological findings of the control amyloidotic animals, on a time scale suggests that upon termination of the amyloidogenic stimulus some de-gree of spontaneous regression of amyloidosis does occur. However, the pace of amyloid degradation was markedly enhanced in the animals provided with ascorbic acid in their drinking water.

Table 1 clearly shows the decrease in the number of mice with diffuse deposits of amyloid in the treated groups and the increase in the number of amyloid free specimens. Thirty-five days after the beginning of induction, 12 of 15 control mice showed diffuse splenic amyloidosis as opposed to 5 animals among those which received ascorbic acid since the 15th day and only 2 mice among the group in which the vitamin was started on the first day of the experiment.

The increase of the concentration of ascorbic acid in the animals' drinking water from 3.5 to 5% did not further enhance amyloid degradation. These animals lost apetite and the mortality among them was somewhat higher. It seems therefore, that 3.5% is the highest tolerated concentration of as-corbic acid in this model. The decrease of ascorbic acid concentration to 2% resulted in a clearly reduced effect. The results, however, still dif-fered significantly from the control, demonstrating the unequivocal effect of ascorbic acid on amyloid degradation in vivo.

Human AA amyloid was degraded by murine serum though the activity was somewhat lower as compared to human serum. This may further prove the al-ready described homology of human AA and murine amyloid. Sera of amyloid-otic mice showed a markedly decreased degrading activity which, in turn, could be partially restored by addition of Vitamin C to the diet of the amyloidotic animals. These experiments do not shed further light on the mechanism of action of ascorbic acid. They only confirm previous observa-tions on a human in vitro model and strengthen the assumption that Vitamin C may have a therapeutic effect on clinical amyloidosis.

REFERENCES

1. Gorevic, P. D., and Franklin, E. C., Ann. Rev. Med., 32:261 (1981).
2. Kedar (Keizman), I., Greenwald, M., and Ravid, M., Brit. J. Exp. Path., 57:686 (1976).
3. Kedar (Keizman), I., Ravid, M., Sohar, E., and Gafni, J., Isr. J. Med. Sci., 19:787 (1974).
4. Shirahama, T., and Cohen, A. S., J. Exp. Med., 140:1102 (1974).
5. Kedar (Keizman), I., Greenwald, M., and Ravid, M., Eur. J. Clin. Invest., 7:149 (1977).
6. Hanai, N., Ishihara, T., Uchino, F., and Imada, N., Virchows Arch. Anat., and Histol., 384:45 (1979).
7. Ravid, M., Shapira, J., Lang, R., and Kedar, I., Ann. Rheum. Dis., 41:587 (1982).
8. Kedar, I., Sohar, E., and Ravid, M., Clin. Lab. Med., 99:693 (1982).
9. Eriksen, N. L., Ericcson, H., Pearsail, N., Languoff, D., and Beneditt, E. P., Proc. Natl. Acad. Sci., 73:964 (1976).

EFFECT OF COLCHICINE ON THE ACUTE PHASE SERUM AMYLOID A PROTEIN RESPONSE AND SPLENIC AMYLOID DEPOSITION DURING EXPERIMENTAL MURINE INFLAMMATION

Sydney R. Brandwein*, J. D. Sipe†,
Martha Skinner†, and Alan S. Cohen†

*Rheumatic Disease Unit
 Montreal General Hospital
 McGill University
 Montreal, Quebec, Canada

†Arthritis Center
 Boston University School of Medicine
 Boston, Massachusetts, U.S.A.

ABSTRACT

We investigated the effects of colchicine on the acute phase serum amyloid A protein (SAA) response and splenic amyloid A protein (AA) deposition in CBA/J mice undergoing chronic inflammatory stimulation with silver nitrate ($AgNO_3$), and on accelerated amyloid deposition induced by amyloid-enhancing factor (AEF). Colchicine (10 µg daily) significantly lowered splenic AA levels after 25 days of inflammation, as determined by radioimmunoassay. Pretreatment (3 days) with colchicine decreased SAA levels 24 h after $AgNO_3$. It was (unexpectedly) observed that brief pretreatment (12 h) with colchicine augmented the acute phase SAA response to $AgNO_3$ at 24 h. Colchicine stimulated production of both the SAA inducer and lymphocyte-activating factor (LAF) activities of interleukin 1 (IL 1) by macrophages. Decreased SAA levels did not appear to be the mechanism by which colchicine inhibited amyloidosis, since SAA levels fell both in colchicine-treated and control mice after 25 days of inflammation. Colchicine only partially lowered AA deposition after injection of AEF. This effect could be explained by decreased acute phase SAA levels. It is postulated that colchicine inhibits amyloidosis in the pre-deposition period by altering the production of factors (e.g., AEF) required in the deposition phase.

INTRODUCTION

Experimental (secondary) amyloid deposits are composed of a nonimmunoglobulin polypeptide with a unique amino acid sequence termed amyloid A protein (AA) (Benditt and Eriksen, 1971). Tissue AA is believed to be derived from a larger antigenically-related precursor, serum amyloid A protein (SAA) (Linke et al., 1975), which is an apoprotein of high density lipoprotein (HDL) (Benditt et al., 1979).

The pathogenesis of amyloidosis during chronic inflammation can be conveniently divided into two stages (Kisilevsky, 1983). The first stage in amyloid induction involves the acute phase response, in which the concentration of SAA is markedly elevated (McAdam and Sipe, 1976). SAA is synthesized by hepatocytes (Benson and Kleiner, 1980; Selinger et al., 1980) stimulated by a soluble macrophage-derived factor originally termed "SAA inducer" (Sipe et al., 1979). SAA inducer activity has been found in purified preparations of interleukin 1 (IL 1) (Sztein et al., 1981). IL 1 induces thymocyte proliferation in vitro (hence, its earlier name "lymphocyte activating factor" of LAF) and the acute phase SAA response when injected into mice (Sztein et al., 1981). Although acute phase increases in SAA levels are believed to be necessary in order to provide substrate for conversion to tissue AA, increased SAA concentration per se is not a sufficient precondition for the development of amyloidosis. Tissue amyloid is not deposited immediately following an acute phase SAA response in animals, but rather requires a prolonged course of chronic inflammation (Benson et al., 1977). Furthermore, amyloidosis occurs rarely in humans with chronic inflammatory diseases, in spite of persistantly elevated SAA levels (Brandwein et al., 1984a). Thus, other factors are believed to arise during the late stages of chronic inflammation which are of pathogenetic importance in amyloid fibril deposition.

The second phase of amyloid formation is believed to involve the partial degardation of SAA to AA, which is then deposited in tissues. The conversion of SAA to AA is mediated via the proteolytic activity of peripheral blood monocyte surface serine proteases in vitro (Lavie et al., 1978), however, it is not known whether this occurs in vivo as well. While the precise mechanism regulating tissue deposition of AA is unclear, a factor termed amyloid-enhancing factor (AEF) may play an essential role in this process (Axelrad et al., 1975; Kisilevsky et al., 1977; Axelrad et al., 1980). AEF is a glycoprotein (Axelrad et al., 1980) distinct from either of the two known secondary amyloid proteins, AA and P-component (AP) (Axelrad et al., 1982). The appearance of AEF in preamyloidotic mouse spleen or liver 48 h prior to the histologic detection of amyloid supports the hypothesis that AEF has pathogenetic importance (Kisilevsky et al., 1983).

Colchicine has previously been demonstrated to inhibit amyloidosis induced by chronic antigenic stimulation with casein, as determined by semiquantitative histologic assessment (Shirahama and Cohen, 1974). Using a sensitive radioimmunoassay to accurately determine tissue concentrations of protein AA, we have evaluated the effectiveness of colchicine in blocking amyloidosis induced by inflammatory stimulation with the nonantigenic irritant silver nitrate ($AgNO_3$). Two possible mechanisms of action of colchicine were investigated in the present study. The effects of colchicine on SAA levels during acute and chronic inflammation in vivo and on production of IL 1 by macrophages in vitro were determined. Also, the possible role of colchicine in blocking accelerated amyloid deposition induced by AEF was investigated. The 2 experimental models presented here differ distinctly from each other. One model involves chronic inflammatory stimulation, allowing for production of both SAA and other factors (including AEF) involved in the pathogenesis of amyloidosis. The other model involves an acute inflammatory episode resulting in SAA production, to which is added a preformed product of chronic inflammation (AEF), thus bypassing the long latent period of amyloid induction.

MATERIALS AND METHODS

Animals

Female CBA/J mice (aged 8-32 weeks) and C3H/HeJ mice (aged 4-6 weeks) were obtained from Jackson Laboratories, Bar Harbor, Maine. C3H/HeCR mice (aged 6-10 weeks' were obtained from Charles River Laboratories, Wilmington, Massachusetts.

Reagents

Endotoxin (lipopolysaccharide, LPS) from E. coli K235 was a gift of Dr. Stefanie N. Vogel (U.S.U.H.S., Bethesda, Maryland). AgNO₃ (Fisher Scientific Co., Fairlawn, New Jersey) was prepared as a 0.2% or 2% solution in endotoxin-free water. Colchicine (Sigma Chemical Co., St. Louis, Missouri) was dissolved in endotoxin-free water or obtained as injectable ampules (Eli Lilly and Co., Indianopolis, Indiana). RPMI 1640 medium (containing 25 mM Hepes and 2 mM glutamine) and fetal bovine serum were obtained from MA Bioproducts, Walkersville, Maryland. Phytohemagglutinin (PHA) was obtained from Burroughs-Wellcome, Research Park, North Carolina and tritiated thymidine (^{3}H-TdR, 6.7 Ci/mmol) from New England Nuclear, Boston, Massachusetts.

Induction of Acute and Chronic Inflammation

CBA/J mice were injected with 0.2% AgNO₃ (0.5 ml) s.c. daily for 21 days of a 25 day course. Test mice received, in addition, a single daily injection of 10 µg colchicine i.p., starting 3 days before AgNO₃ and throughout the full 25 day course. Control mice were given a daily injection of 0.5 ml endotoxin-free water i.p. An additional group of mice were pretreated with 10 µg colchicine 12 h and 1 h before AgNO₃. Mice were bled serially via the retro-orbital venous plexus and sera stored at -20°C in phosphate buffered saline (PBS), pH 7.2 for determination of SAA content.

Production of AEF

AEF was isolated from the spleens of CBA/J mice that had undergone chronic inflammatory stimulation with 10% casein, as previously described (Kisilevsky and Boudreau, 1983; Brandwein et al., 1985).

Induction of Amyloid Deposition of AEF

Accelerated amyloidosis was induced as previously described (Brandwein et al., 1985). CBA/J mice were given a single injection of 500 µg AEF via the lateral tail vein, followed by a single injection of 2% AgNO₃ (0.5 ml) s.c. Test mice received 10 µg colchicine i.p. daily starting 2 days prior to injection of AEF and continuing for 2 days afterwards. Control mice were given a daily injection of saline i.p. Mice were sacrificed 48 h after administration of AEF and sera and splenic tissue stored at -20°C.

Production and Measurement of SAA Inducer Activity

Thioglycollate-induced C3H/HeCR (LPS-sensitive) mouse peritoneal macrophage monolayers were stimulated to produce SAA inducer (IL 1) activity in vitro by LPS (10 µg/ml), as previously described (Brandwein et al., 1984b). The effects of colchicine ($2.5 \cdot 10^{-5}$ M) on SAA inducer production were determined in the presence or absence of LPS. SAA inducer activity was determined by injecting 1 ml of cell-free macrophage culture supernatant into C3H/HeJ mice (LPS-resistant). These mice were bled 18 h later and SAA levels determined as a measure of "SAA inducer" capacity.

IL 1 (LAF) Measurements

Pooled macrophage culture supernatants were dialyzed extensively against PBS to remove colchicine. IL 1 (LAF) activity was determined as the ability of test supernatants to augment the proliferation (^{3}H-TdR uptake) of C3H/HeJ thymocytes in the presence of a suboptimal concentration of PHA, as previously described (Brandwein et al., 1984b).

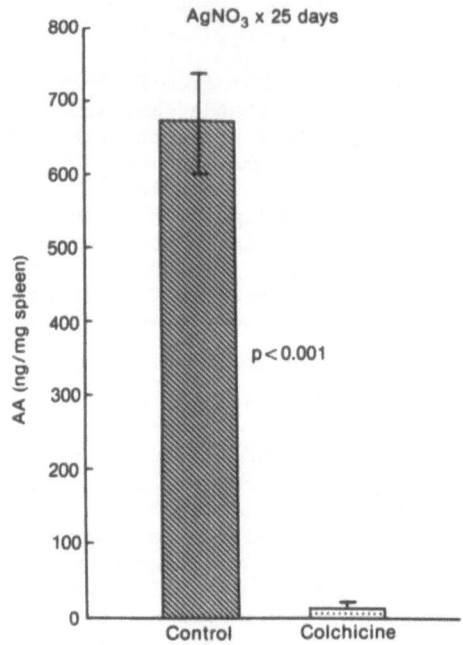

Fig. 1. Splenic AA concentrations
(mean ± S. E.; ng/mg spleen
after 25 days of inflammation
induced by 0.2% $AgNO_3$ (0.5 ml)
s.c. daily. Colchicine-
treated mice received 10 µg
(0.5 ml) i.p. daily. Control
mice received injectable water
(0.5 ml) i. p. daily.

Determination of SAA and Splenic AA

SAA concentration was measured by solid phase radioimmunoassay, as previously described (Sipe et al., 1976). SAA concentrations were expressed
as µg/ml serum (mean ± S.E.) and results compared using a Student's t test.
Tissue AA levels were determined in formic acid-denatured (10% formic acid,
12 h, 37°C) splenic homogenates by radioimmunoassay, as previously described (Brandwein et al., 1985). AA concentrations in pooled splenic
homogenates were expressed as ng protein AA/mg spleen.

RESULTS

Effect of Colchicine on Splenic AA Levels in Chronic Inflammation

Chronic inflammation was induced in CBA/J mice by daily injection of
0.2% $AgNO_3$. Control mice (n = 20) received endotoxin-free water (0.5 ml)
i.p. daily. The concentration of AA in splenic homogenates was determined
after 25 days in the remaining mice (Fig. 1). Treatment with colchicine
lowered AA levels to 12 ± 68 ng/mg spleen in $AgNO_3$-stimulated control mice
$p < 0.001$).

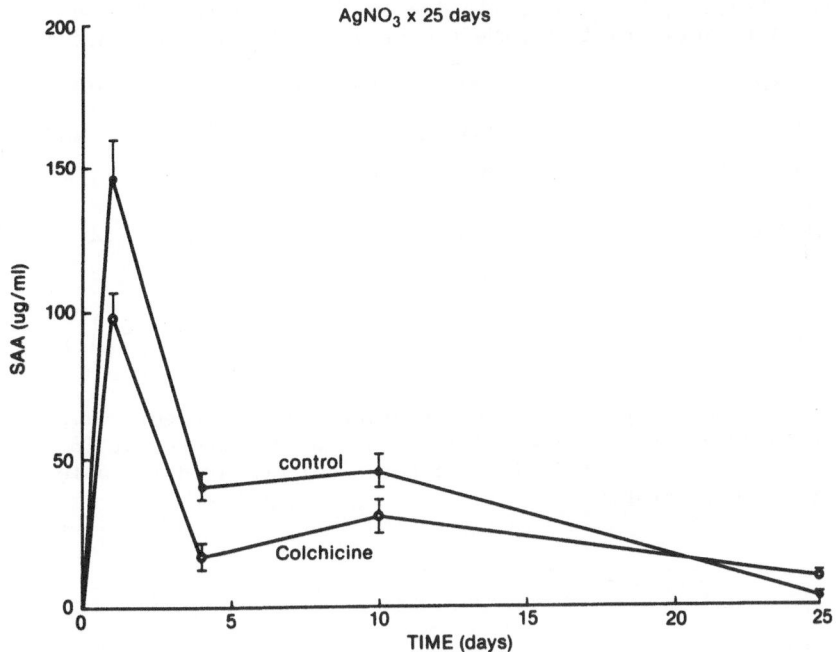

Fig. 2.   SAA concentrations (mean ± S.E.; μg/ml) during chronic
          inflammation induced by injection of 0.2% AgNO₃ (0.5
          ml) s.c. daily. Colchicine-treated mice (open circles)
          received 10 μg i.p. daily. Control mice (closed circles)
          received injectable water (0.5 ml) i.p. daily.

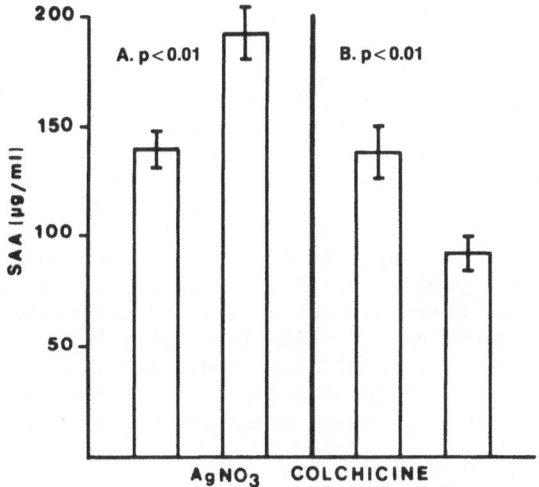

Fig. 3.   Effect of colchicine on SAA concen-
          trations 24 h after injection of
          0.2% AgNO₃ (0.5 ml) s.c.   A) Pre-
          treatment with 10 μg colchicine 12
          and 1 h before AgNO₃.   B) Pretreat-
          ment with 10 μg colchicine 72, 48,
          24, and 1 h before AgNO₃.   Control
          mice received injectable water
          (0.5 ml).

TABLE 1. Effect of LPS and Colchicine on IL 1 (SAA Inducer and
ALF) Activity in C3H/HeCR Macrophage Culture Supernatants

Test Group	SAA Inducer *	LAF**
	(SAA ug/ml)	(U/ml)
Control	21.9 ± 4.8	17.8
Colchicine	56.7 ± 13.8	32.9
LPS	79.3 ± 10.3	135.7
LPS + Colchicine	91.3 ± 11.9	178.6

*C3H/HeCR macrophage culture supernatants (1 ml) injected i.p.
 into C3H/HeJ mice and SAA μg/ml (mean ± SEM) measured at 18 h.
**IL 1 (LAF) activity (^{3}H-TdR incorporation) measured in pooled
 culture supernatants.

Effect of Colchicine on SAA Levels

SAA kinetics were compared in colchicine-treated and control $AgNO_3$-
stimulated mice (Fig. 2). Pretreatment (3 days) with colchicine suppressed
the acute phase SAA response 24 h after $AgNO_3$ injection compared to control
mice ($p < 0.01$). While SAA levels fell in the colchicine-treated mice during the course of chronic inflammation, a marked decline in SAA concentrations was also (unexpectedly) observed in control $AgNO_3$-stimulated mice.
The effect of colchicine on the acute phase SAA response was found to be
dependent on the duration of pretreatment with colchicine prior to injection of $AgNO_3$. Administration of 10 μg colchicine 12 h and 1 h prior to
$AgNO_3$ resulted in unexpected augmentation of the $AgNO_3$-induced acute phase
SAA response (n = 8, $p < 0.01$) (Fig. 3). It is noted that a single injection of 10 μg colchicine only (without $AgNO_3$) did not significantly stimulate SAA production, resulting in an SAA level of 1.8 ± 0.9 μg/ml (n = 4)
at 18 h compared to 1.2 ± 0.3 μg/ml after injection of endotoxin-free water
($p > 0.10$). Stimulation of SAA production by colchicine was not caused by
endotoxin contamination of colchicine preparations (Brandwein et al., 1984b).

Effect of Colchicine on IL 1 Production

In order to investigate the mechanism by which colchicine alters SAA
levels in vivo, we examined the effect of colchicine on production of IL 1
by macrophages in vitro. Colchicine alone (without LPS) stimulated a 2-3
fold increase in IL 1 production by C3H/HeCR macrophages ($p < 0.05$) (Table
1). The stimulation by LPS was more marked than by colchicine, however,
the effects of LPS and colchicine in combination appeared to be additive.

TABLE 2. Effect of Colchicine on Accelerated Amyloid Deposition
Test substance

AEF	AgNO$_3$	Colchicine	Saline	SAA (μg/ml)	AA (ng/mg spleen)
+	+	−	+	451 ± 46*	974 ± 46**
+	+	+	−	236 ± 22*	578 ± 91**
−	+	−	+	475 ± 21	7 ± 0.3
+	−	−	+	6 ± 1	2 ± 0.7
−	−	−	−	0.5 ± 0.1	4 ± 1

*p = 0.0065
**p < 0.02

AEF = 500 μg IV at time 0; AgNO$_3$ = 0.5 ml of 2% solution s.c. at time 0;
colchicine = 10 μg i.p. every 24 h starting 48 h prior to AEF + AgNO$_3$ and
for 48 h afterwards; saline = 0.5 ml every 12 h. SAA and splenic AA determined 48 h after injection of AEF + AgNO$_3$.

Effect of Colchicine on AEF-Accelerated Amyloidosis

The effects of colchicine on SAA and splenic AA levels induced by injection of AgNO$_3$ and preformed AEF are summarized in Table 2. Colchicine
partially blocked splenic AA deposition. However, this effect may have
been the result of blunted acute phase SAA levels, rather than due to direct inhibition of AA deposition. It is noted as well that AgNO$_3$ (without
AEF) resulted in insignificant splenic AA levels in the presence of marked
acute phase SAA levels, indicating the lack of significant splenic seques-
tration of SAA.

DISCUSSION

The results presented in the present study (Fig. 1) indicate that colchicine effectively blocks experimental amyloisosis induced by chronic nonantigenic inflammatory stimulation with AgNO$_3$, as has been demonstrated in
several laboratories for antigenic substances like casein and azocasein
(Shirahama and Cohen, 1974; Kisilevsky et al., 1983). Quantitative analysis
of AA in tissue homogenates by radioimmunoassay has previously been determined to compare well with the amount of tissue amyloid observed histologically (Sipe et al., 1978).

Two general mechanisms may be postulated to explain the inhibition of
amyloidosis by colchicine. Firstly, attenuation of the acute phase SAA
response would lead to diminished availability of substrate for conversion
to AA. Alternatively, colchicine could inhibit the deposition phase at a
number of specific points: the conversion of SAA to AA; the aggregation of
AA subunits into fibrils; or the production of other factors (such as AEF)
required for amyloid deposition.

Colchicine has previously been demonstrated to modulate the acute phase
SAA response 24 h after injection of LPS or casein (Benson and Kleiner,
1980; Selinger et al., 1980), possibly via inhibition of hepatic protein
secretion (Redman et al., 1975) or protein synthesis (Tatsuta et al., 1984).
This has suggested that colchicine prevents amyloid deposition primarily by

lowering SAA levels. The massive doses of colchicine (100-1000 µg/mouse) used previously were in the lethal range and the effects of colchicine in the chronic phase of amyloid deposition were not evaluated (Benson and Kleiner, 1980; Selinger et al., 1980). In the present study, pretreatment with colchicine significantly suppressed the acute phase SAA response 24 h after AgNO₃ injection (Fig. 2). The smaller dose of colchicine (10 µg/mouse) was well-tolerated during long-term administration. SAA levels fell progressively in colchicine-treated mice during the course of inflammatory stimulation, in spite of repeated daily injections of AgNO₃ (Fig. 2). It was (unexpectedly) observed that repeated daily injections of AgNO₃ (in the absence of colchicine treatment) were accompanied by a decline in acute phase SAA levels, which approached baseline at 25 days. The tendency of SAA levels to fall as part of the normal chronic inflammatory response in this model system suggests that suppression of acute phase SAA levels may not be the primary mechanism by which colchicine inhibits amyloidosis.

Prolonged pretreatment with colchicine in the present study (72 h, cumulative dose 40 µg) diminished the acute phase SAA response 24 h after AgNO₃ injection, presumably due to hepatic effects of the drug. The effects of colchicine, however, appeared to be dependent on the dose and duration of pretreatment. Colchicine (12 h, cumulative dose 20 µg) unexpectedly augmented the in vivo acute phase SAA response to AgNO₃ (Fig. 3). The simulatory effect of colchicine in vivo was evident as an augmented SAA response to another inflammatory stimulus (AgNO₃), while colchicine alone did not stimulate an acute phase SAA response in vivo. In order to investigate the augmentation of SAA levels observed in vivo, the effect of colchicine on the monokine-mediated (IL 1) control mechanism for SAA production was studied. Colchicine directly stimulated production of both the SAA inducer and LAF activates of IL 1 and augmented the IL 1 response to another inflammatory stimulus, LPS, in vitro (Table 1).

The injection of preformed AEF (isolated from the spleens of chronically inflamed mice) into recipient mice undergoing acute inflammatory stimulation, results in rapid tissue deposition of AA (Table 2). It is thus possible to set up a specific model system which bypasses the long latent period of amyloidosis and focuses on the deposition step by which AA is laid down in tissues. Using this model, we tested the hypothesis that colchicine specifically blocks the action of AEF, thus preventing accelerated AA deposition. We observed, however, that colchicine was only partially effective in blocking AEF-induced amyloidosis (Table 2). The suppression of splenic AA levels by colchicine in the AEF model may have been related to a parallel decreases observed in acute phase SAA levels. The marked potency of colchicine in blocking amyloidosis in the model of chronic inflammation, and its relative lack of efficacy in inhibiting amyloidosis induced by administration of AEF, suggests that colchicine exerts it effects during the latent (predeposition) stage. It is postulated that colchicine inhibits the production of factors (e.g., AEF) during the latent period, which regulate the conversion of SAA to AA and/or the aggregation of AA subunits into amyloid fibrils.

ACKNOWLEDGEMENTS

This work was supported by research grants from the U.S. Public Health Service, National Institute of Arthritis, Metabolism and Digestive Diseases (AM04599 and AM07014), from the General Clinical Research Centers Branch of the Division of Research Resources, National Institutes of Health (AM20613), The Arthritis Foundation, the Kroc Foundation and The Arthritis Society of Canada.

REFERENCES

Axelrad, M. A., and Kisilevsky, R., in: Amyloid and Amyloidosis (G. G. Glenner, P. P. Costa, A. F. de Freitas, eds.), Excerpta Medica, Amsterdam (1980), pp. 527-533.

Axelrad, M. A., Kisilevsky, R., and Beswetherick, S., Am. J. Pathol., 78, 277 (1975).

Axelrad, M. A., Kisilevsky, R., Willmer, J., Chen, S. J., and Skinner, M., Lab. Invest., 47, 139 (1982).

Benditt, E. P., and Eriksen, N., Am. J. Pathol., 65, 231 (1971).

Benditt, E. P., Eriksen, and Hanson, R. H., Proc. Natl. Acad. Sci., U.S.A., 76, 4092 (1979).

Benson, M. D., and Kleiner, E., J. Immunol., 128, 495 (1980).

Benson, M. D., Scheinberg, Shirahama, T., Cathcart, E. S., and Skinner, M., J. Clin. Invest., 59, 412 (1977).

Brandwein, S. R., Medsger, T. A., Jr., Skinner, M., Sipe, J. D., Rodnan, G. P., and Cohen, A. S., Ann. Rheum. Dis., 43, 586 (1984).

Brandwein, S. R., Sipe, J. D., Tatsuta, E., Skinner, M., and Cohen, A. S., J. Rheumatol., 11, 597 (1984).

Brandwein, S. R., Sipe, J. D., Skinner, M., and Cohen, A. S., Lab. Invest., (1985), in press.

Kisilevsky, R., Lab. Invest., 49, 391 (1983).

Kisilevsky, R., Axelrad, M., Corbett, W., Brunet, S., and Scott, F., Lab. Invest., 37, 544 (1977).

Kisilevsky, R., and Boudreau, L., Lab. Invest., 48, 53 (1983).

Kisilevsky, R., Boundareau, and Foster, D., Lab. Invest., 48, 60 (1983).

Lavie, G., Zucker-Franklin, D., and E. C. Franklin, J. Exp. Med., 148, 1020 (1978).

Linke, R. P., Sipe, J. D., Pollock, P. S., Ignaczak, T. F., and Glenner, G. G., Proc. Natl. Acad. Sci., U.S.A., 72, 1473 (1975).

McAdam, K. P. W. J., and Sipe, J. D., J. Exp. Med., 144, 1121 (1976).

Redman, C. M., Banerjee, D., Howell, K., and Palade, G. E., J. Cell Biol., 66, 42 (1975).

Selinger, M. J., McAdam, K. P. W. J., Kaplan, M., Sipe, J. D., Rosenstreich, D., and Vogel, S. N., in: Amyloid and Amyloidosis (G. G. Glenner, P. P. Costa, and A. F. de Freitas, eds.), Excerpta Medica, Amsterdam (1980), pp. 486-490.

Shirahama, T., and Cohen, A. S., J. Exp. Med., 140, 1102 (1974).

Sipe, J. D., Ignaczak, T. F., Pollock, P. S., and Glenner, G. G., J. Immunol., 116, 1151 (1976).

Sipe, J. D., McAdam, K. P. W. J., and Uchino, F., Lab. Invest., 38, 110 (1978).

Sipe, J. D., Vogel, S. N., Ryan, J. L., McAdam, K. P. W. J., and Rosenstreich, D. L., J. Exp. Med., 150, 597 (1979).

Sztein, M. B., Vogel, S. N., Sipe, J. D., Murphy, P. A., Mizel, S. B., Oppenheim, J. J., and Rosenstreich, D. L., Cell Immunol., 63, 164 (1981).

Tatsuta, E., Sipe, J. D., Shirahama, T., Skinner, M., and Cohen, A. S., Arthritis Rheum., 27, 349 (1984).

SERUM AMYLOID A PROTEIN (SAA) FROM MINK, HORSE, AND MAN:

A COMPARATIVE STUDY

G. Marhaug*, A. Husebekk*,
G. Husby*, K. Sletten†,
A. L. Børresen‡, B. Lium**,
and K. Nordstoga**

*Institute of Clinical Medicine
 University of Tromsø

†Institute of Biochemistry
 University of Oslo

‡Institute of Medical Genetics
 University of Oslo

**Norwegian College of Veterinary Medicine
  Oslo, Norway

ABSTRACT

    Serum amyloid A protein (SAA) was isolated from mink, horse, and human
serum by ultracentrifugation and gel filtration and characterized by two-
dimensional gel electrophoresis, Western blotting followed by autoradiography and N-terminal amino acid analysis. SAA was found in similar quantities in the high density lipoprotein (HDL) fraction of serum from a patient suffering from systemic juvenile rheumatoid arthritis (JRA) and mink
stimulated with lipopolysaccharide (LPS), and in somewhat smaller quantities in serum from horses stimulated with Escherichia coli cultures.
Only very small quantities were present in normal human controls and not
detectable in normal mink and horse. Striking similarities were found between human and mink SAA with respect to molecular weight, isoelectric
point and degree of heterogeneity, while the molecular weight of horse SAA
seemed to be somewhat lower, and no obvious heterogeneity could be demonstrated in this protein using two-dimensional gel electrophoresis. Immunologic cross-reactivity between SAA from the three species was not
found. In contrast to human and horse HDL, mink HDL was found not to contain apoA-II and only minute amounts of apoC proteins. Normal horse HDL
also contained additional apoproteins not present in HDL from the other
species. N-terminal amino acids analysis of SAA from mink and horse demonstrated the same similarity with the corresponding AA protein as previously
reported for human SAA/AA.

INTRODUCTION

Amyloid-related serum protein (SAA) is a newly described protein which behaves like an acute phase reactant [1, 2], and is the putative precursor of the amyloid fibril protein AA present in some forms of amyloid disease [3]. SAA was detected in serum of both man [3, 4], mouse [5, 6], rabbit [7], and mink [8, 9], because of its antigenic cross-reactivity with protein AA from the same species. SAA is larger (mol. wt. 11,500), but otherwise structurally identical to protein AA (mol. wt. 8600) [10, 11]. Its physiological role is not characterized, but it may act as a regulator of certain immune functions [12], and may have some importance in the handling of endotoxin [13]. SAA is produced by hepatocytes [14], after stimuli from activated macrophages [15], probably mediated by a monokine, SAA-stimulating factor. The major portion of SAA is present in the high density lipoprotein (HDL) fraction of serum (apoSAA) in man, mouse, and rabbit [7, 16, 17]. The covalente structure of mink AA has shown marked homology with AA from other species [18].

The purpose of this study was to compare apoSAA from the three phylogenetically distant species man, horse, and mink with respect to acute phase response, binding proteins in serum, molecular weight, isoelectric point, possible molecular polymorphism and N-terminal amino acid sequence.

MATERIALS AND METHODS

Reagents

Acrylamide, bisacrylamide, biolyte (ampholines pH 3-10) and glycine (all electrophoresis purity reagents) was purchased from Bio-Rad, California, USA, urea and SDS from BDH Chemicals Ltd., England; Tris and Coomassie brillinat blue R 250 from Sigma Chemicals Co., USA and N,N,N^1,N^1-tetramethylene-diamine (TEMED) from Eastman Kodak Company, USA; Non-idet-NP-40 from Shell Company, USA. Nitrocellulose was from Schleicer and Shull, West-Germany, ^{125}I-protein A from Amersham, England, and Sephadex G-100 from Pharmacia Fine Chemicals, Sweden.

The Sources of apoSAA

Plasma rich in SAA was obtained from a patient with systemic juvenile rheumatoid arthritis (JRA) without amyloidosis. Pooled sera from 20 healthy normal blood donors were used as control. Mink (Mustela vision) were injected subcutaneously with lipopolysaccharide (4 mg LPS from Escherichia coli 026:B6 purchased from Difco, Detroit, Mich.) and exanguinated 24 h later. Pooled sera from healthy, non-stimulated mink were used as control. Two horses (Equus caballus) were injected with Escherichia coli cultures (5×10^{10} bacterias/horse) and blood samples drawn after 24 h. Serum from a normal horse was used as control. These three sera were investigated separately.

Preparative Ultracentrifugation

Human, horse, and mink serum were subjected to ultracentrifugation for isolation of HDL (d = 1.09-1.21 g/ml) following the method of Havel et al. [19]. Centrifugation was done in a Beckman, Model L3-50 ultracentrifuge (Beckman Instruments, Inc., USA) using a Beckman 60Ti rotor for 21 h at 4°C at 40,000 rpm. Supernatants were aspirated, and the HDL fraction was washed twice by recentrifugation in a solution of KBr and NaCl with density 1.21 g/ml.

Delipidation of the HDL fraction was done with methanol and diethyl ether (1:3) at -10°C, followed by centrifugation and washing in anhydrous ether [20].

Gel Filtration

The apoproteins of HDL were dissolved in 5 M guanidine/0.1 M acetic acid, and gel filtered on a 5 × 100 cm column of Sephadex G-100.

Two-dimensional polyacrylamide gel electrophoresis of purified HDL, apoHDL and gel filtration fractions was carried out essentially as described by O'Farrell [21], with modifications as described by Børresen and Berg [22]. The samples were prepared by adding 50 μl of a 2% sodium dodecyl sulfate (SDS) solution containing 2% dithiothreitol (DDT) and 10% glycerol to 25-100 μg of lyophilized fractions. The solutions were heated at 95°C for 5 min. After cooling to room temperature, solid urea was added until saturation was reached. The samples were submitted to electrofocusing in 6.7% acrylamide for a total of 10,000 Vh, and submitted to gel electrophoresis in the second dimension in gel slabs (20 × 20 cm) with 10-20% gradient acrylamide at 1.3 A for 4 h. Proteins were visualized by staining gel slabs overnight in 50% methanol containing 12% acetic acid and 0.2% Coomassie brilliant blue. Destaining was performed in ethanol/acetic acid. Silver staining was performed after Coomassie brilliant blue staining using the commercial available silver stain from Bio-Rad derived from the method of Merril et al. [23].

Western Blotting

Electrophoretic transfer of the proteins from the SDS polyacrylamide gels to nitrocellulose followed by radiographic detection with anti-SAA and radioiodinated protein A was performed as described by Burnette [24]. The electrophoretic transfer was performed using 25 mM Tris-HCl buffer, pH 8.3, containing 192 mM glycine and 20% methanol overnight at 0.1-0.2 A. The nitrocellulose sheets were immediately after transfer put in a solution containing 0.9% NaCl, 10 mM Tris-HCl, pH 7.4 (Tris-saline) and 3% bovine serum albumin (BSA), and incubated at 37°C on a rocking platform. The sheets were transferred to a fresh solution of Tris-saline with 5% BSA containing antiserum against human SAA (20 mg/ml), incubated overnight at 37°C, then washed 5 × 10 min in 0.9% NaCl and emersed in fresh Tris-saline with 5% BSA containing 5×10^5 cpm of ^{125}I-labelled protein A. Binding of protein A was allowed to occur for 30 min at room temperature. This radioactive solution was pipetted off and the nitrocellulose sheets again rinsed in saline several times. The sheets were then dried and exposed at -70αC to Kodak X-ray film.

Immunological Analyses

Antisera to horse AA, mink AA, human AA, and human SAA were prepared as described before [5, 25]. Double diffusion in 1% agarose gel, pH 8.6 and ionic strength 0.025 was used for detection of mink, horse, and human SAA. In addition, a second antibody precipitation radioimmunoassay (RIA) [26], was used to detect low concentrations of human SAA, and to evaluate eventual cross reactivity between mink and human SAA when tested against antibodies to human AA and SAA. Quantitative immunological analysis of apoA-I and apoB was performed as described by Børresen and Berg [27].

RESULTS

SAA in Mink, Horse, and Human Sera

By using the RIA technique it was shown that serum from the patient
with JRA contained 1500 mg/l of SAA. This represents an extremely increased
serum level since mean + 2 SD of 100 normal healthy blood donors has been
estimated to 3 mg/l [26]. Normal mink and horse serum showed no precipitation in double immunodiffusion against anti mink or anti horse AA, while
serum from LPS-treated mink showed a strong precipitin reaction against the
same antibody, indicating increase of SAA after stimulation. Serum from
the LPS-treated horses showed no precipitation when tested against anti
horse AA, probably due to the low concentrations of SAA in these sera.

Yield of apoHDL and apoSAA

After delipidation of HDL the yield of proteins from normal serum was
300 mg/l and patient serum 417 mg/l. Normal amounts of apoA-I (111 mg/100
ml) was found both in the patients serum and the normal control serum. The
yield of proteins after delipidation of HDL from mink serum was considerably
higher, 2700 mg/l, with no measurable difference between normal and LPS-
treated animals. Delipidation of horse HDL yielded 300 mg protein/l serum,
with no difference between normal and stimulated animals.

Gel Filtration

Gel filtration profiles of apoHDL from normal human and patient serum
are shown in Fig. 1a, and from normal and LPS-treated mink in Fig. 1b, and
from normal and E. coli-treated horse in Fig. 1c. SAA antigenic material
was eluted from the G-100 column corresponding to a molecular weight of
approximately 12,000 daltons both from the patient, the normal human serum
pool and LPS-treated mink serum (Fig. 1a and b, peak 4), whereas no antigenic reactivity could be found at this position in material from normal
mink serum with the method used. SAA in horse serum eluted together with
the apoC-proteins corresponding to a somewhat lower molecular weight than
human and mink SAA. The protein from the normal human serum eluted in peak
4 comprised 7% of the apoHDL applied to the column, in the patient 25%, in
normal mink 0-1% and in LPS-treated mink 12%, respectively, and in normal
and E. coli-treated horse approximately 10% (Fig. 1). In normal human
serum peak 4 is known to consist mainly of apoC proteins [28], so the relative amount of apoC in mink HDL is less than that of normal human HDL (Fig.
1a and b). Thus, the amount of protein eluted in peak 4 appeared to be
largely determined by the concentration of SAA in the different sera.
Double immunodiffusion did not detect SAA in the peak 4 material from normal mink and horse serum, while the corresponding material from normal human
serum gave a positive precipitation reaction and inhibition in RIA (Fig. 1a
and b). Protein eluted corresponding to apoA-II in human serum (peak 3,
Fig. 1a) could not be detected in normal or LPS-treated mink. The elution
profile of delipidated horse HDL showed an additional peak with mol. wt.
14,000 daltons, not present in HDL from the other two species.

Two-dimensional polyacrylamide gel electrophoresis of the HDL fraction
from the JRA patient (Fig. 2a) contained several additional peptides when
compared with HDL from normal human serum. The two main "extra" spots in
HDL from the patient had pI 5.6 and 6.0, and molecular weight of approximately 11,000 daltons, and Sephadex G-100 fraction 4 contained a variety of
protein components in addition to the normal apoC-proteins (Fig. 2b).
Silver staining of the gel (not shown) confirmed these results, showing not
only a variety of peptides with the same molecular weight and different pI,
but also some heterogeneity with respect to molecular weight. However,
Western blotting of the gels using anti SAA showed that the SAA peptides

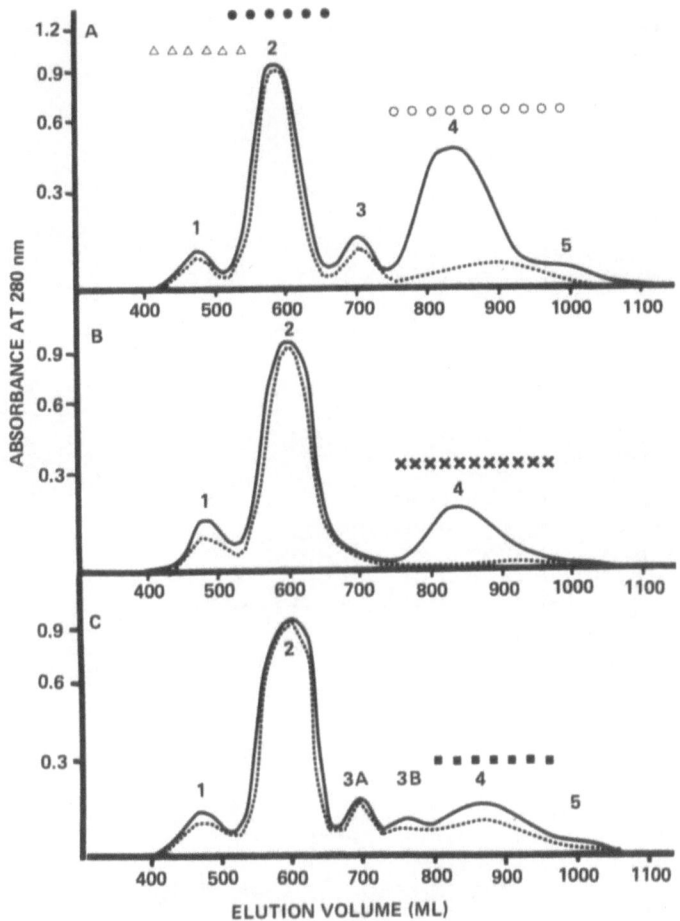

Fig. 1. Gel-filtration of delipidated HDL on a 5 × 10
cm Sephadex G-100 in 5 M guanidine/0.1 M acetic
acid. Samples: 300 mg apoproteins in 30 ml
eluent. a) ApoHDL from human serum. Patient
with JRA: ——. Normal controls: -----.
b) ApoHDL from mink serum. Endotoxin-treated
mink: ——. Normal controls: -----. c)
ApoHDL from horse serum. E. coli-treated
horse: ——. Normal controls: -----. Reactivity with antisera to: human albumin)
△△△△△; human apoA-I) ●●●●●; human apoSAA)
○○○○○; mink AA) ×××××; horse AA) ■■■■■.

with antigenic activity had isoelectric points varying from approximately
4.5 to 8.0, i.e., a very high degree of charge heterogeneity, but the same
molecular weight (results not shown).

Two-dimensional polyacrylamide gel electrophoresis of normal mink HDL
gave no protein spots in the area where SAA was expected to be found (Fig.
2c). ApoA-I from mink was found to be heterogeneous, apoA-II was lacking,
and only three very faint protein spots were found in the position of apoC.
In contrast, HDL from LPS-treated mink showed at least two additional protein components with pI 6.0 and 7.4 respectively (Fid. 2d). Sephadex G-
100 fraction 4 from LPS-treated mink HDL (Fig. 1b), which by N-terminal

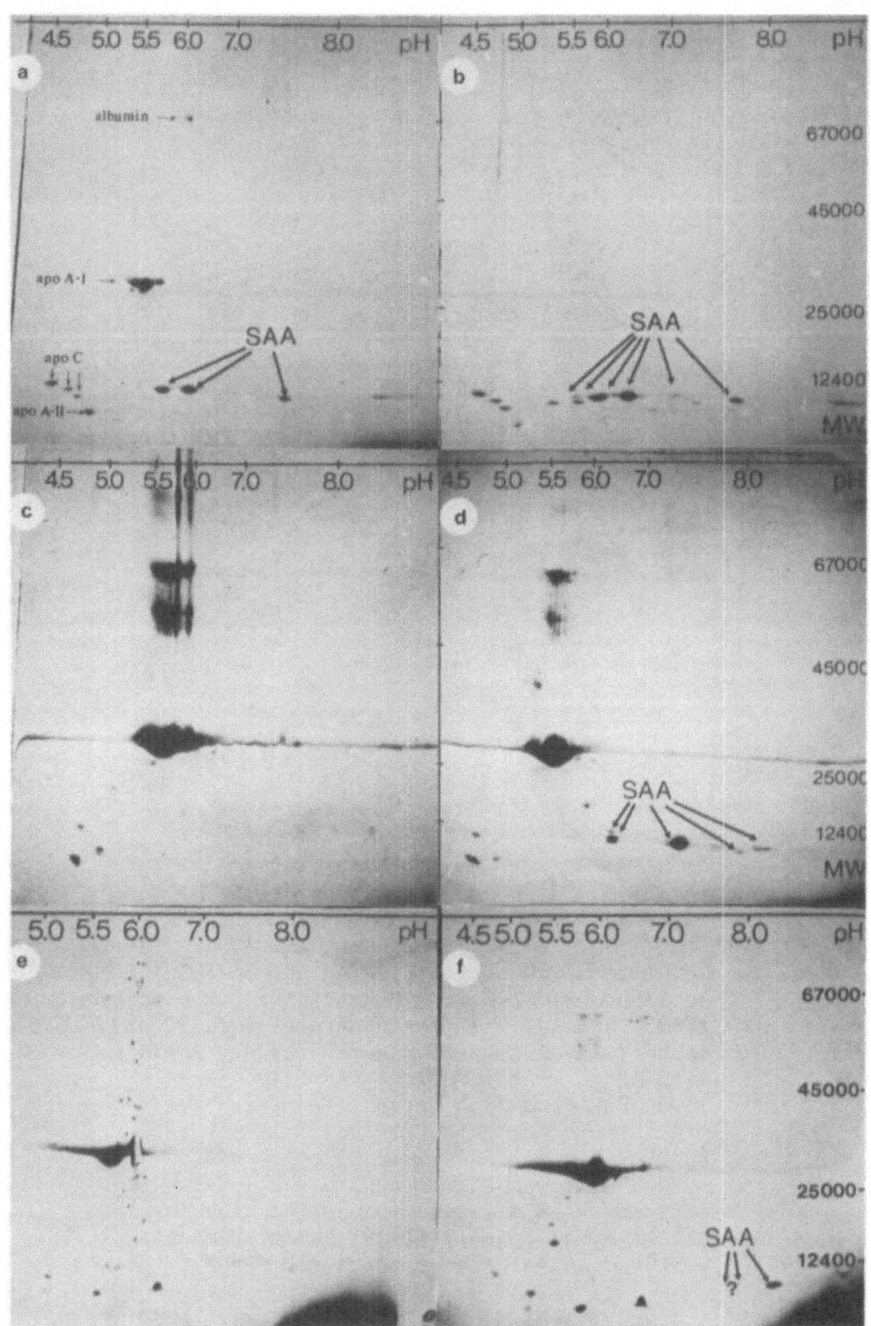

Fig. 2. Two-dimensional polyacrylamide gel electrophoresis of a) HDL from
the JRA patient, showing the two main subspecies of human apoSAA
b) Sephadex G-100 fraction 4 (Fig. 1a) from the same patient, showing several SAA subspecies. c) apoHDL from normal mink serum where
no apoSAA, apoA-II and only minor amounts of apoC is present. d)
apoHDL from endotoxin-treated mink, demonstrating the two main
subspecies of apoSAA. e) HDL from normal horse showing an apoprotein pattern quite different from human HDL, and only a faint
SAA spot with a very high pI. f) HDL from E. coli-treated horse
showing an increase in the SAA content.

amino acid analysis was found to be almost completely pure SAA, was found to contain a variety of protein spots, representing SAA molecules with the same molecular weight of approximately 11,000 daltons, but with a profound electric charge heterogeneity with a pI range from 5.5 to 8.0 (results not shown). HDL from stimulated horse showed an increase in SAA compared with normal horse HDL (Fig. 2e and 2f), but no heterogeneity could be demonstrated.

Antigenic Properties of SAA

Serum from LPS-treated mink, HDL from the same serum and purified mink SAA was tested in the second antibody precipitation RIA technique against anti human AA and anti human SAA, and no cross-reactivity could be found with human SAA. Horse SAA was tested against anti human SAA in immunodiffusion without signs of cross-reactivity.

Amino Acid Analyses

The results of the N-terminal amino acid analyses of mink and human SAA preparations were compared with the N-terminal amino acid sequence of the respective AA proteins, and the results are shown in Table 1.

DISCUSSION

The biological significance of SAA is not well understood, but it is phylogenetically a conservative protein [5], and should therefore be of importance for the survival of the species. This conservatism was confirmed in this study where striking similarities for human, horse, and mink SAA are observed. In these three species SAA occurred as a peptide in the HDL-fraction in increased amounts during an inflammatory response to disease or after stimulation with LPS. SAA from mink, horse, and man had approximately the same molecular weight, as determined by electrophoresis, and mink and man SAA were very heterogeneous with respect to electric charge. Both groups of SAA contained two major molecular species, in addition to several minor subspecies of SAA molecules. Horse SAA seemed to be more homogeneous, but this apparent lack of heterogeneity could be due to the low response to E. coli. The amounts of horse SAA applied to the gels were therefore low, and consequently heterogeneities were difficult to detect.

Our findings are in good agreement with other reports of the presence of SAA in the HDL fraction of both mouse and rabbit serum [6, 7, 17]. Heterogeneity has also been demonstrated for mouse [6] and human SAA [28, 29]. The observed heterogeneity of mink SAA is very similar to that of human SAA, and, since a similar heterogeneity is characteristic of the phylogenetically rather distant species mink and man, this property of SAA may be involved in its biological function. Also, since SAA is so well conserved, and since it responds to inflammatory stimuli, an important function in tissue damage and repair could be suggested.

There was a striking lack of antigenic cross-reactivity, particularly in view of the structural homology which has been demonstrated for human and mink AA, and which is also the case for SAA from these three species (to be published). This has previously been described for SAA from other species [5]. The inter-species cross-reactivity reported by others [30] may probably be explained by insufficient specificity of the antisera used.

SAA was detected in normal human serum but not in normal mink serum. This apparent lack of SAA in normal mink may be explained by the less sensitive methods used to trace mink SAA. One would assume that SAA is a normal protein also in mink and horse, being present in small amount in a non-

TABLE 1. Partial N-Terminal Amino Acid Sequence of Human SAA/AA and Mink SAA/AA

	Residue number					
	1	2	3	4	5	6
Human SAA/AA	Arg	Ser	Phe	Phe	Ser	Phe
Mink SAA/AA	PCA	Trp	Tyr	Ser	Phe	

stimulated state. The two-dimensional gel electrophoresis could indicate the presence of SAA in normal horse HDL, but this could not be verified by immunological methods.

The two-dimensional gel electrophoresis gave also some additional information of the other mink apoproteins. ApoA-I is heterogeneous in mink, like it is in man [31], while apoA-II is lacking in mink as has been shown also in the rabbit [32]. ApoC proteins are present in mink HDL in only very minute quantities, or even lacking. Horse HDL also contained several until now unidentified proteins in addition to apoA-I, apoA-II, apoC, and apoSAA.

The studies of SAA from species other than man could give new informations leading to the understanding of the phylogenesis and the biological function of this protein. Presently we are performing extended studies of mink and horse SAA, which includes its complete amino acid sequence. SAA is the putative precursor of reactive (secondary) amyloid fibrils in man an in spontaneous and experimentally induced amyloid in animals [14, 33]. Knowledge about its phylogenesis and biological functions can also provide information about the development of these forms of amyloid disease.

ACKNOWLEDGEMENTS

This work has been supported by grants from Anders Jahres Foundation for Promotion of Science and from The Norwegian Research Council for Science and the Humanities.

REFERENCES

1. K. P. W. J. McAdam, R. J. Elin, J. D. Sipe, and S. M. Wolff, J. Clin. Invest., 61, 390 (1978).
2. I. Kushner and H. Gewurz, J. Lab. Clin. Med., 97, 739 (1981).
3. G. Husby and J. B. Natvig, J. Clin. Invest., 53, 1054 (1974).
4. M. Levin, M. Pras, and E. C. Franklin, J. Exp. Med., 138, 373 (1973).
5. R. F. Anders, J. B. Natvig, K. Sletten, G. Husby, and K. Nordstoga, J. Immunol., 118, 229 (1977).
6. P. D. Gorevic, Y. Levo, B. Frangione, and E. C. Franklin, J. Immunol., 123, 138 (1978).
7. B. Skogen, A. L. Børresen, J. B. Natvig, K. Berg, and T. E. Michaelsen, Scand. J. Immunol., 10, 39 (1979).
8. G. Husby, J. B. Natvig, K. Sletten, K. Nordstoga, and R. F. Anders, Scand. J. Immunol., 4, 811 (1975).
9. R. F. Anders, K. Nordstoga, J. B. Natvig, and G. Husby, J. Exp. Med., 143, 678 (1976).
10. D. C. Parmelee, K. Titani, L. H. Ericsson, N. Eriksen, E. P. Benditt, and K. A. Walsh, Biochemistry, 21, 3298 (1982).

11. K. Sletten, G. Marhaug, and G. Husby, Hoppe-Seyler's Z. Physiol. Chem., 364, 1039 (1982).
12. M. A. Aldo-Benson and M. D. Benson, J. Immunol., 126, 2390 (1982).
13. P. S. Tobias, K. P. W. J. McAdam, and J. Ulevitch, J. Immun., 128, 1420 (1882).
14. M. D. Benson and E. Kleiner, J. Immunol., 124, 495 (1980).
15. M. B. Sztein, S. N. Vogel, J. D. Sipe, P. A. Murphy, S. B. Mizel, J. J. Oppenheim, and D. L. Rosenstreich, Cell Immun., 63, 164 (1981).
16. E. P. Benditt and N. Eriksen, Proc. Natl. Acad. Sci. USA, 74, 4025 (1977).
17. E. P. Benditt, N. Eriksen, and R. H. Hanson, Proc. Natl. Acad. Sci. USA, 76, 4092 (1979).
18. K. Waalen, K. Sletten, G. Husby, and K. Nordstoga, Eur. J. Biochem., 104, 407 (1980).
19. R. J. Havel, H. A. Eder, and J. H. Bragdon, J. Clin. Invest., 34, 1345 (1955).
20. A. M. Scanu, Biochim. Biophys. Acta, 265, 471 (1972).
21. P. H. O'Farrell, J. Biol. Chem., 250, 4007 (1975).
22. A. L. Børresen and K. Berg, Clin. Genet., 20, 438 (1981).
23. C. R. Merril, D. Goldman, S. A. Sedman, and M. H. Ebert, Science, 211, 1437 (1981).
24. W. N. Burnette, Analytical Biochemistry, 112, 195 (1981).
25. G. Marhaug and G. Husby, Clin. Exp. Immunol., 45, 97 (1981).
26. G. Marhaug, Scand. J. Immunol., 18, 329 (1983).
27. A. L. Børresen and K. Berg, Artery, 7, 139 (1980).
28. G. Marhaug, K. Sletten, and G. Husby, Clin. Exp. Immunol., 50, 382 (1982).
29. L. L. Bausserman, P. N. Herbert, and K. P. W. J. McAdam, J. Exp. Med., 152, 641 (1980).
30. N. Livni, A. Laufer, and Y. Levo, J. Pathology, 132, 343 (1980).
31. G. Thompson and Soutar, Nature Lond., 301, 658 (1980).
32. A. L. Børresen, J. Immunogen., 3, 73 (1976).
33. R. Kisilevski, M. D. Benson, M. A. Axelrad, and L. Boudreau, Lab. Invest., 41, 206 (1979).

THE TIME RELATIONSHIP BETWEEN AMYLOID DEPOSITION AND GLYCOSAMINOGLYCAN

ACCUMULATION DURING EXPERIMENTAL AMYLOIDOSIS

A. Snow and R. Kisilevsky

Department of Pathology
Queen's University
Kingston, Ontario
Canada K7L 3N6

ABSTRACT

The temporal relationship between glycosaminoglycan (GAG) accumulation and amyloid deposition was examined in two models of amyloid induction.

In the first model amyloid was induced rapidly by injections of amyloid enhancing factor (AEF) and $AgNO_3$ (the inflammatory stimulus). Animals were killed at 24, 36, 48, and 72 h and the spleens, livers, and kidneys were taken for histology. In the second model amyloid was induced slowly by daily subcutaneous injections of azocasein. Animals were sacrificed daily from 1 to 14 days.

Congo red staining was used to detect amyloid. The presence of GAGs was shown either by (1) the sulfated Alcian blue (SAB) method or (2) Alcian blue (pH 5.7) with various amounts of $MgCl_2$. The latter method was used to distinguish between sulfated and carboxylated GAGs.

In the rapid model amyloid and GAG deposition occurred only in mice receiving both AEF + $AgNO_3$. Amyloid was first detected, at 36 h, in the spleen. The initial presence of GAGs was also seen at 36 h in the exact locale where amyloid was found. By 48 h amyloid deposition had extended to most perifollicular areas in the spleen and was now present in the walls of the central veins in the liver. GAG staining showed a similar increase in intensity in the spleen and onset of deposition in the liver. It was seen in the same areas where amyloid deposition was taking place. Sections stained with Alcian blue (pH 5.7) at 0.3-0.7 $MgCl_2$ indicated the accumulation of sulfated GAGs primarily. Positive staining with Alcian blue at 1 M $MgCl_2$ indicated small amounts of keratan sulfate. The results at 72 h were similiar to those at 48 h but more exaggerated.

In the model utilizing azocasein, amyloid was first seen at 6-7 days in the perifollicular areas of the spleen. Again glycosaminoglycans appeared coincidentally with and in the same locale as the amyloid.

The present studies show that amyloid-associated GAGs appear in the tissues coincidentally with the amyloid protein deposit. The appearance of GAGs is not a function of the nature of the inflammatory stimulus, nor its length of action, nor the tissue of deposition, but appears to be part of the process involved in the laying down of the AA protein.

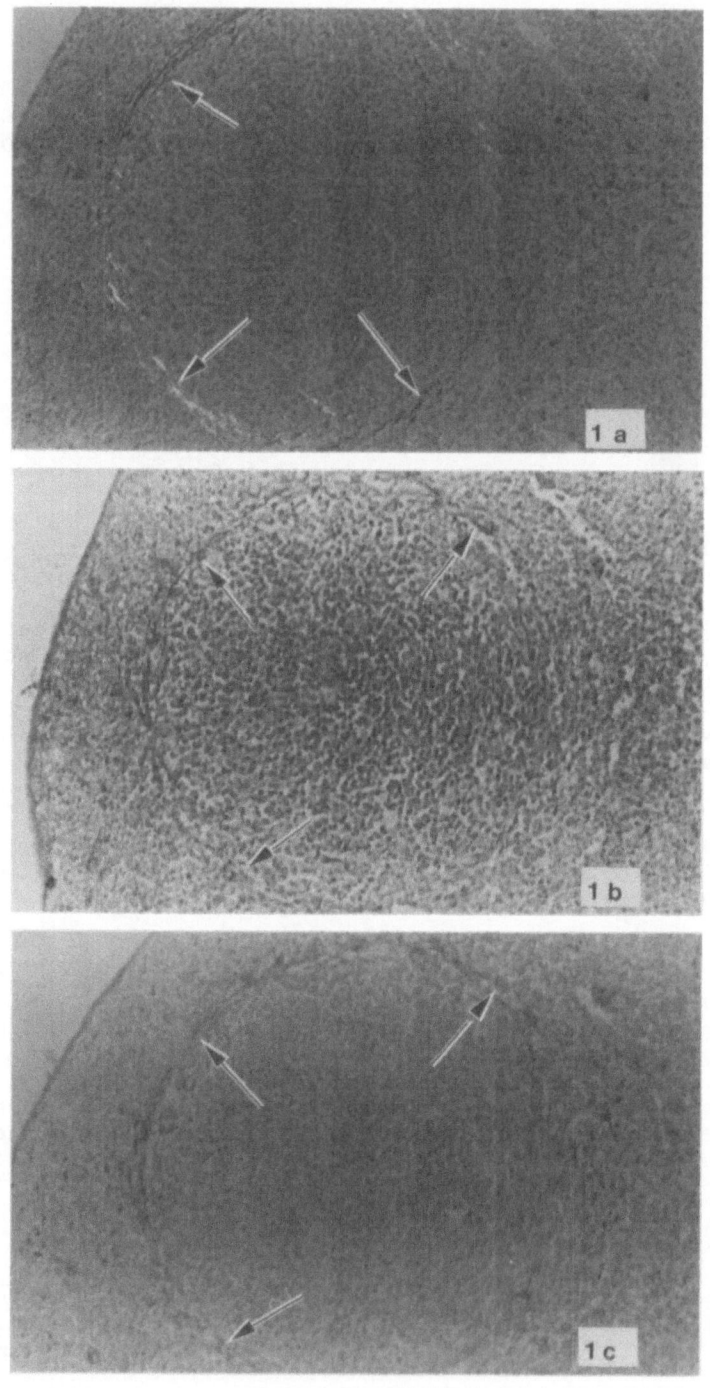

INTRODUCTION

Amyloid, as the name implies, is more than simply a tissue protein deposit. The demonstration by Virchow of positive iodine staining of amyloid deposits clearly indicated the presence of a carbohydrate moiety, which subsequent investigators have shown to be glycosaminoglycans (GAG) [1-6]. Isolation and electrophoresis of these GAGs have shown them, in most cases, to be heparan sulfate [1, 2, 4, 6]. These latter investigations were done in the late 1960s and early 1970s. Most investigations since then have focussed primarily upon the protein component of amyloid.

The presence of GAGs may however indicate that they play an important role in the deposition of the amyloid protein. To be implicated in such a role there must be an appropriate temporal relationship between the deposition of the protein and the GAGs. The GAGs should clearly not be deposited after the protein, but may be deposited before or concurrent with the protein.

The present investigations were undertaken to explore the time sequence of AA protein and GAG deposition. Two different experimental protocols were used. The first, a rapid induction protocol, involved CBA/J mice given amyloid enhancing factor (AEF), and $AgNO_3$ (0.5 ml of a 2% solution subcutaneously) as an inflammatory stimulus [7]. Animals were sacrificed over a 72 h period at varying intervals following injections. Controls consisted of uninjected mice and those given only AEF, or $AgNO_3$, sacrificed at identical time points as those receiving AEF + $AgNO_3$. The second, a traditional protocol, utilized daily subcutaneous injections of azocasein (0.5 ml of a 7% solution in $NaHCO_3$) [8]. In this second protocol animals were killed daily from 1 to 14 days.

Spleens, livers, and kidneys were taken from all animals and fixed in 90% ethanol: 10% formaldehyde. Serial sections were prepared and stained with one of the following procedures.

a) Alkaline Congo red [9] for the demonstration of amyloid;

b) sulfated Alcian blue (SAB) [10, 11] for the demonstration of GAGs;

c) Alcian blue (pH 5.7) with varying concentrations of $MgCl_2$ to distinguish between sulfated and carboxylated GAGs [12].

AEF and azocasein were prepared in the same manner as previously described [7, 8].

Fig. 1. Appearance of amyloid deposits and GAG accumulation in the spleen at 36 h. These animals received AEF + $AgNO_3$. Serial sections were stained with Congo red, SAB, or Alcian blue (pH 5.7) with $MgCl_2$ added at various concentrations - (0.1 M, 0.3 M, or 0.7 M). A) Splenic amyloid (arrows) in a perifollicular area as shown by Congo red staining under polarized light using a green filter and Kodak Tri X-pan film. Magnification 141×. B) Positive SAB staining (arrows) in the exact perifollicular area as the amyloid deposits. Photographed under a yellow filter using Kodak Plus X-pan film. Magnification 141×. C) Alcian blue (pH 5.7) staining at 0.3 M $MgCl_2$. Glycosaminoglycans (arrows) are stained in the same locale as amyloid staining. Positive staining was also seen at 0.7 M $MgCl_2$ indicating that primarily sulfated GAGs are present. Photographed under a yellow filter using Kodak Plus X-pan film. Magnification 141×.

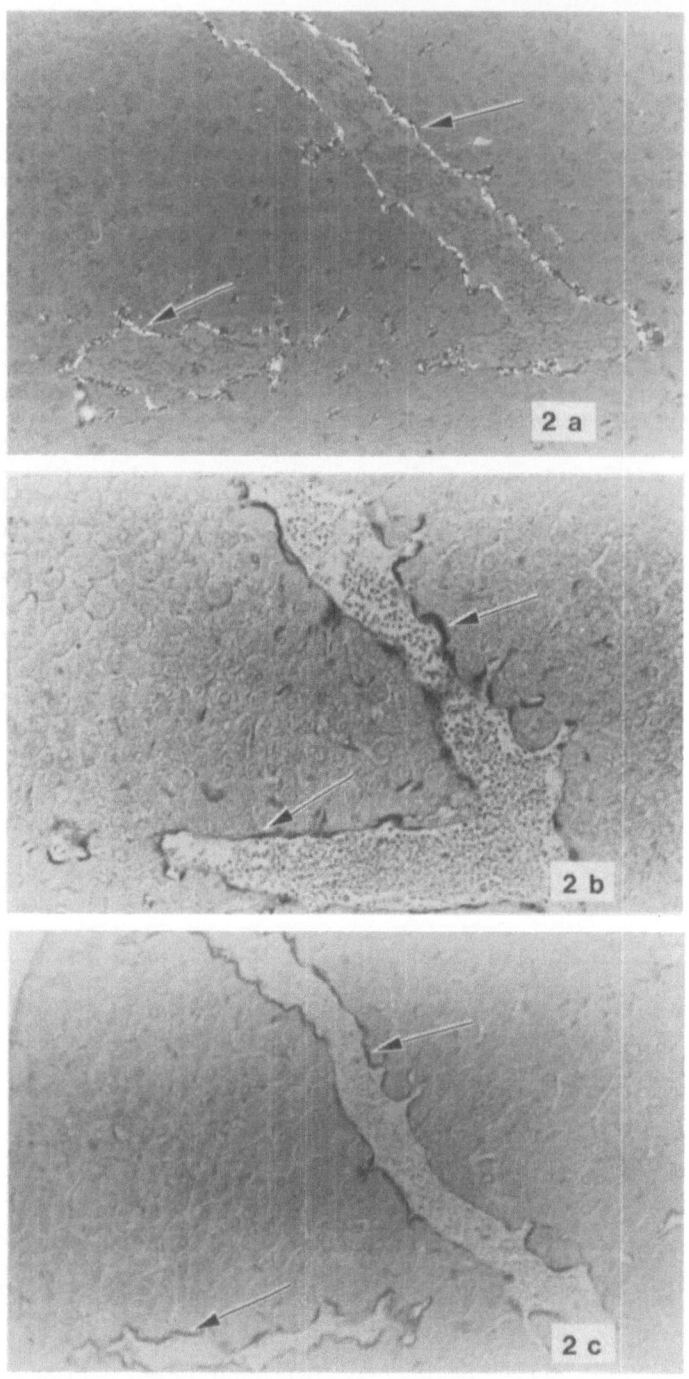

Fig. 2. Glycosaminoglycan and amyloid accumulation in the liver at 48 h.
These animals received AEF + AgNO₃. Serial sections were stained
and photographed as in Fig. 1. A) Amyloid deposits (arrows are
seen around central veins. Magnification 141×. B) Positive SAB
staining (arrows) in exact areas as amyloid deposits. Magnification 141×. C) Positive Alcian blue staining (arrows) in same
areas as amyloid. Positive staining was also seen at 0.7 M and
to a lesser extent at 1.0 M MgCl₂. Magnification 141×.

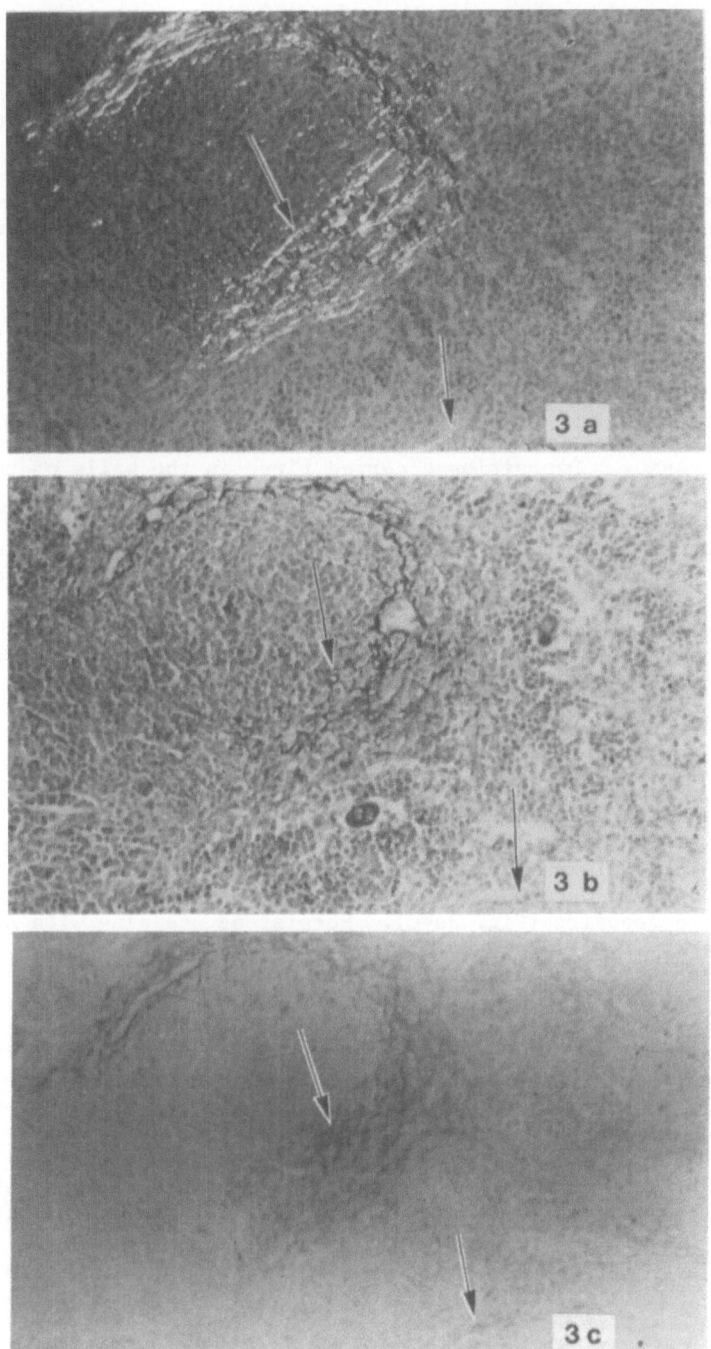

Fig. 3. The appearance of amyloid and glycosaminoglycan deposits in the spleen of animals receiving daily azocasein injections (day 7). A) Amyloid deposits (arrows) in a perifollicular location in the spleen. Magnification 141×. B) SAB positive areas (arrows) in the same areas as Congo red positivity. Magnification 141×. C) Alcian blue (pH 5.7) positive areas (arrows) correspond to the Congo red positive areas. Magnification 141×.

RESULTS

Rapid Induction Model

During the rapid induction protocol none of the control groups (uninjected, AEF alone, $AgNO_3$ alone), nor the AEF + Agno3 24 h group, showed any
amyloid or GAG deposition in any organ. At 36 h splenic amyloid was visible
in a few perifollicular areas only in the group receiving $AgNO_3$ + AEF (Fig.
1A). Adjacent serial sections stained with the SAB (Fig. 1B), and Alcian
blue (Fig. 1C) techniques showed the presence of GAGs accumulating in the
same local as the amyloid. Staining for GAGs with the Alcian blue technique persisted at $MgCl_2$ concentrations higher than 0.3 M and indicated
that primarily sulfated GAGs were being deposited. At subsequent time
periods (48 and 72 h) the quantity of splenic perifollicular amyloid and
GAG accumulation increased in parallel.

Amyloid did not appear in the liver until 48 h after its induction
with AEF and $AgNO_3$. Deposition occurred first in the walls of the central
veins (Fig. 2A) and subsequently extended along the sinusoids radiating into
the parenchyma [11]. Staining of adjacent sections with the SAB method
(Fig. 2B) and with the Alcian blue - $MgCl_2$ method (Fig. 2C) again demonstrated the coincidental accumulation of sulfated GAGs at the same locale.

In this 3 day experiment the kidney did not show any amyloid or GAG
staining in any of the four groups. However previous work [11] has indicated that renal amyloid subsequently does occur approximately two weeks
into this protocol.

Induction with Azocasein

Using daily injections of azocasein Congo red positive amyloid deposits
were first seen in the splenic perifollicular area at 6 to 7 days. The SAB
and Alcian blue staining techniques of adjacent serial sections again demonstrated the deposition of GAGs appearing at the same time and same locale
as the amyloid deposits (Fig. 3A-C). Persistent staining with Alcian blue
at high molarity $MgCl_2$ again indicated that sulfated GAGs were the primary
GAGs accumulating at the sites of amyloid deposition.

While in this model there was some animal to animal variation in exactly when amyloid actually appeared in the spleen, in no case did Congo
red positively appear without concomitant SAB or Alcian blue positivity,
nor vice-versa. Animals remaining on this protocol for longer periods of
time (8-14 days) demonstrated increased staining intensity with all three
techniques. Renal amyloid was again not seen until approximately two weeks
into this protocol. This appeared first in the renal papillae which again
correlated with the coincidental deposition of SAB and Alcian blue positive
material at the same locale (data not shown).

DISCUSSION

Using histochemical techniques and light microscopy the present study
assessed the temporal relationship of AA and GAG deposition in two separate
models. A comparison of GAG and AA deposition in these two models allowed
us to examine:

1) when GAG accumulation takes place in relation to AA deposition;

2) where, anatomically the GAGs accumulate in relation to AA deposition, and

3) whether the nature of the inflammatory stimulus influences GAG deposition.

In both models amyloid deposition takes place together with GAG deposition. This was true regardless of the nature of the tissue examined, be it spleen, liver, or kidney. Though amyloid consistently appeared later in some tissues than others (e.g., first in spleen followed by liver and then kidney) in no case was there a dissociation of Congo red staining from GAG positivity, nor vice-versa.

The present results also show that GAG deposition not only occurs at the same time but in the same locale as the AA deposits. This was again true regardless of tissue type.

Neither the nature of the inflammatory stimulus (AgNO₃ vs. azocasein) nor the length of inflammation (36 h vs. 7 days) altered the coincident deposition of the AA protein and GAGs.

This temporal and anatomic coincidence of AA and GAG deposition suggests that GAGs may play a significant role in the genesis of the AA deposits. The present study also reconfirms that the deposited GAGs are predominantly sulfated.

ACKNOWLEDGEMENTS

This work was supported by Grant MT-3153 of the Medical Research Council of Canada. The authors express their appreciation to Mrs. B. Latimer for her secretarial assistance.

REFERENCES

1. Bitter, T., and Muir, H., Mucopolysaccharides of whole human spleens in generalized amyloidosis, J. Clin. Invest., 45:963 (1966).
2. Dalferes E. R., Radhakrishnamurthy, B., and Berenson, G. S., Acid mucropolysaccharides of amyloid tissue, Arch. Biochem. Biophys., 118:284 (1967).
3. Dalferes, E. R., Radhakrishnamurthy, B., and Berenson, G. S., Glycoaminoglycans in experimental amyloidosis, Proc. Soc. Exp. Biol. Med., 127:925 (1968).
4. Pennock, C. A., Association of acid mucopolysaccharides with isolated amyloid fibrils, Nature, 217:753 (1968).
5. Pennock, C. A., Burns, J., and Massarella, G., Histochemical investigation of acid mucosubstances in secondary amyloidosis, J. Clin. Path., 21:578 (1968).
6. Pras, M., Nevo, Z., Schobert, M., Rotman, J., and Matalon, R., The significance of mucropolysaccharides in amyloid, Histochem. Cytochem., 19:443 (1971).
7. Kisilevsky, R., and Boudreau, L., Kinetics of amyloid deposition. I. The effects of amyloid enhancing factor and splenectomy, Lab. Invest., 48:53 (1983).
8. Janigan, D. T., and Druet, R. L., Experimental amyloidosis: role of antigenicity and rapid induction, Am. J. Pathol., 48:1013 (1966).
9. Puchtler, H., Sweat, F., and Levine, M., On the binding of Congo red by amyloid, J. Histochem. Cytochem., 10:355 (1962).
10. Mowry, R. W., and Scott, J. E., Observations on the basophilia of amyloids, Histochemie, 10:8 (1967).
11. Scott, J. E., and Dorling, J., Differential staining of acid glycosaminoglycans (Mucopolysacchiardes) by Alcian blue in salt solutions, Histochemie, 5:221 (1965).

12.   Lendrum, A. C., Sidders, W., and Fraser, S., Renal hyalin. A study
      of amyloidosis and diabetic fibrinous vasculosis with new staining
      methods, J. Clin. Path., 25:373 (1972).

KINETICS OF SELECTIVE DEPOSITION OF ApoSAA$_2$

DURING DEVELOPMENT OF AMYLOIDOSIS IN MICE

Rick L. Meek, Jeffrey S. Hoffmann,
and Earl P. Benditt

Department of Pathology
University of Washington
Seattle, Washington 98195

ABSTRACT

The major murine serum amyloid proteins (apoSAA$_1$, apoSAA$_2$) have been identified, of which only one (apoSAA$_2$) shares amino acid sequence identity with tissue protein AA. To examine the mechanism of this apparent isotype-specific amyloid protein deposition, we have studied apoSAA metabolism at the levels of gene expression and plasma content during amyloidogenesis. In CBA mice, daily intraperitoneal casein administration resulted in a linear increase in splenic amyloid content, beginning within 10 days and reaching approximately 30% of the organ volume at 20 days. Hepatic apoSAA mRNA content, estimated by in vitro translation, was highest at day 1 (3% of total mRNA) and declined thereafter (to 1%, day 20). The relative content of apoSAA$_2$ mRNA compared with that of apoSAA$_1$ was unchanged throughout amyloid induction. Simultaneously, a 2-3 fold drop in total serum apoSAA levels was observed with, by contrast, a 10-fold reduction in the serum ratio of apoSAA$_2$/apoSAA$_1$. These results are consistent with the hypothesis that murine tissue protein AA accumulates by selective deposition of apoSAA$_2$ from the serum.

INTRODUCTION

The pathophysiology of amyloid fibril deposition remains obscure despite recent advances in our knowledge of serum amyloid protein (apoSAA) structure and metabolic regulation. Although it seems likely that protein AA fibrils are formed from circulating apoSAA, no direct evidence has, in fact, been obtained to support this hypothesis. Recent studies which indicate the existence of two or more sub-species of apoSAA in man [1, 2] and other mammals [3] suggest another question: Are some apoSAA isotopes more amyloidogenic than others?

The possibility that protein AA might be related to a subset of circulating apoSAA's was originally proposed by Gorevic et al. [4], based upon a comparison of murine amyloid protein AA and apoSAA NH$_2$-terminal sequences. At that time, the purification of apoSAA subspecies had not been accomplished. Subsequently we showed that two major murine apoSAA isotypes exist [5] and that of these only one, namely apoSAA$_2$, has NH$_2$-terminal sequence identity with tissue protein AA [6]. Morrow and collaborators [7], using recombinant DNA techniques, have identified a third, quantitatively minor, apoSAA isotype. It appears, then, that the murine serum amyloid proteins are a multigene family of which only one contributes to the formation of AA deposits.

Recent work in our laboratory has been aimed at studying the deposition of murine protein AA vis a vis the plasma content of apoSAA isotypes. Two mechanisms can be invoked to explain the selective accumulation of apoSAA$_2$-derived protein AA during amyloidogenesis. Differential gene expression might favor the production of apoSAA$_2$ during chronic inflammation such that amyloid deposition is a reflection of the high apoSAA$_2$ levels during this period. (We note that during acute inflammation serum apoSAA$_1$ and apoSAA$_2$ levels are nearly equal.) Alternatively, the selective deposition of apoSAA$_2$-derived protein AA might be due to properties intrinsic to the polypeptide, resulting in AA altered metabolism relative to apoSAA$_1$. Our approach to this problem was to measure and compare circulating levels of murine apoSAA$_1$ and apoSAA$_2$, as well as tissue mRNA levels in CBA mice during the progression of amyloidosis.

METHODS

Tissue content of amyloid substance was estimated morphometrically. Total serum apoSAA content was measured by radioimmunoassay, and the relative content of apoSAA$_1$ and apoSAA$_2$ estimated by densitometric anlysis of isoelectric focusing patterns obtained from HDL apoproteins recovered by centrifugation of serum [5]. Likewise, densitometric measurement of apoSAA mRNA levels was made following SDS-polyacrylamide gel electrophoresis of pre-apoSAA polypeptides quantitatively immunoprecipitated from the in vitro translation products of total liver mRNA [8].

RESULTS

The well-documented susceptibility of CBA mice to amyloid induction by daily casein administration is illustrated in Fig. 1. Splenic accumulation of amyloid substance was apparent by Congo red staining within 5-10 days and increased linearly through 20 days of intraperitoneal casein administration. Hepatic and renal amyloid deposition at day 20 was, by comparison, negligible.

Serum apoSAA levels (Fig. 2) during amyloid induction showed a rapid rise on day 1 to >250 g/ml, followed by a decline to approximately 120 μg/ml on days 15 and 30. Concurrent with these changes a striking drop in apoSAA$_2$ content was observed relative to that of apoSAA$_1$. The molar apo-

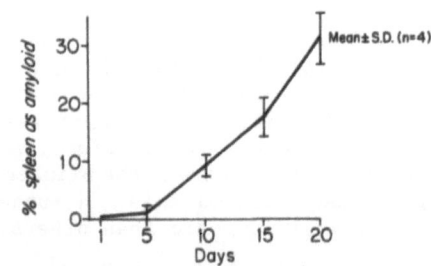

Fig. 1. Time course of splenic amyloid deposition. CBA mice were administered 0.5 ml of 10% casein in H_2O, daily. Points and bars represent the mean cross-sections areas ±S.D. (n = 4) occupied by amylid substance as measured morphometrically.

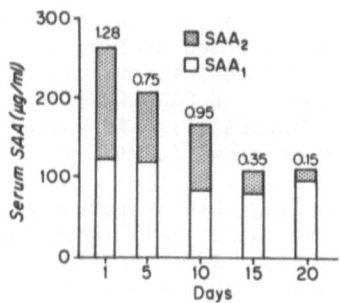

Fig. 2. Serum apoSAA levels
during amyloid induc-
tion. Bars represent
mean serum apoSAA
values for eight mice.
Numbers above bars
indicate the mean
apoSAA$_2$/apoSAA$_1$ ratio.

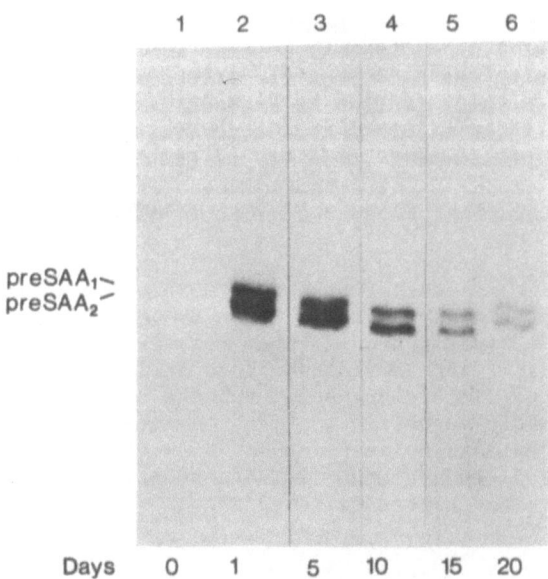

Fig. 3. Immunoprecipitation of cell-free hepatic mRNA translation products during
amyloid induction. Total RNA isolated from murine liver was translated in the presence of [^{35}]methion-
ine and antibody precipitated. Shown
is an autoradiogram of SDS/urea polyacrylamide gel patterns from untreated
(day 0) and casein-induced mice after
1, 5, 10, 15, and 20 days of casein
injections.

$SAA_2/apoSAA_1$ ratio dropped from an initial value of 1.28 on day 1 to 0.15 on day 20. In summary, the observed decline in circulating apoSAA levels during the course of amyloid deposition was in part accounted for by the apparent selective depletion of $apoSAA_2$ from the pool of circulating apo-SAA. By comparison, plasma $apoSAA_1$ levels showed a relatively small net decline during this period as shown in Fig. 2.

To examine the possibility that differential gene expression favors hepatic $apoSAA_1$ synthesis during amyloid induction, in vitro ^{35}S-labeled translation products, from total liver mRNA obtained during amyloid induction, were immunoprecipitated with anti-murine A antiserum and examined by SDS-polyacrylamide gel electrophoresis. Two immunoreactive bands with estimated molecular weights of 13.0 and 12.2 kd were observed (Fig. 3). Translation in the presence of microsomes resulted in the of two additional bands (11.2 kd and 10.6 kd) which comigrated with purified $apoSAA_1$ and $apoSAA_2$ respectively (not shown), indicating that the larger molecular weight bands are preproteins with intact signal peptides.

During the course of amyloid induction, the hepatic content of apoSAA mRNA dropped three fold, accounting for approximately 3% of the TCA-precipitable ^{35}S-translation product at day 1 and 1% of the total labeled protein at day 20. However, the relative intensities of the pre-apoSAA bands showed only minor variation with time (Fig. 3). Fluctuations in the relative serum levels of apoSAA isotypes during the course of amyloid deposition could not, therefore, be accounted for by differential gene expression, although an overall drop in liver apoSAA mRNA levels may in part account for the declining serum apoSAA levels during amyloidogenesis.

In addition to these experiments, we similarly studied the secretion of apoSAA isotypes in vitro by hepatocytes harvested from CBA mice after 1 and 20 days of casein administration. Consistent with the results obtained by in vitro translation, no differences were observed in the relative secretion of [35] and $apoSAA_2$ by cells. At these times, therefore, the observed shift in plasma $apoSAA_2/apoSAA_1$ ratios during amyloidogenesis could not be explained either by differential gene expression or by post-translational events favoring the secretion of $apoSAA_1$ during chronic inflammation.

A quantitative assessment of apoSAA metabolism during amyloidogenesis will require further study, with focus on the clearance kinetics of $apoSAA_1$ and $apoSAA_2$. As a first approximation, however, these data give support to the hypothesis that murine amyloid protein AA is derived from serum $apoSAA_2$, as reflected by the diminishing serum content of the latter protein during the period of amyloid deposition. It seems likely that structural features intrinsic to the $apoSAA_2$ polypeptide may be necssary prerequisites for fibril formaton, and thus account for its relative depletion from the serum during amyloidosis as compared with $apoSAA_1$.

ACKNOWLEDGEMENTS

We thank Marlene Wambach for technical support and Virginia Wejak for help in preparing the manuscript. This work was supported in part by Grants HL-03174, HL-07312, and GM-15731 from the National Institutes of Health.

REFERENCES

1. N. Eriksen and E. P. Benditt, Proc. Natl. Acad. Sci., U.S.A., 77, 6860 (1980).
2. L. L. Bausserman, P. N. Herbert, and K. P. W. J. McAdam, J. Exp. Med., 152, 641 (1980).
3. R. F. Anders, J. B. Natvig, K. Sletten, G. Husby, and K. Nordstoga, J. Immunol., 118, 229 (1977).
4. P. D. Gorevich, Y. Levo, B. Frangione, and E. C. Franklin, J. Immunol., 121, 138 (1978).
5. J. S. Hoffman and E. P. Benditt, J. Biol. Chem., 257, 10510 (1982).
6. J. S. Hoffman, L. H. Ericsson, N. Eriksen, K. A. Walsh, and E. P. Benditt, J. Exp. Med., 159, 641 (1984).
7. R. S. Stearman, C. A. Lowell, W. R. Pearson, and J. F. Morrow, Ann. N.Y. Acad. Sci., 389, 106 (1982).
8. R. L. Meek, L. D. Lonsdale-Eccles, and B. A. Dale, Biochemistry, 22, 4867 (1983).

IN VIVO RADIOIMMUNODETECTION OF AMYLOID

DEPOSITS IN EXPERIMENTAL AMYLOIDOSIS

John Marshall*, William McNally†,
Dan Muller*, George Meincken‡,
Irwin Fand†, S. C. Srivastava‡, Harold Atkins‡,
David D. Wood**, and Peter D. Gorevic*

*Department of Medicine and
†Long Island Research Institute
 SUNY at Stony Brook, New York 11794

**Ayerst Laboratories
  Princeton, New Jersey 08540, and

‡Brookhaven National Laboratories
 Upton, New York, 11973

ABSTRACT

    Two rat IgG monoclonal antibodies (MAbs) to mouse AA protein have been
used as reagents for an ELISA assay for SAA, for the demonstration of tissue
deposits by the immunoperoxidase method, and for the definition of AA polymorphs in solubilized amyloidotic tissue specimens run onto two-dimensional
(2D) gels and probed as Western Blots. Both MAbs localize to tissue deposits in vivo when labelled (MAb*) with I^{125} or I^{123} and injected into
colchicine-pretreated amyloidotic mice, assessed by (a) whole-body autoradiography (WBAR) (b) external photoscanning (c) tissue autoradiography
of perfused organs. Serum t 1/2 of MAb* in amyloidotic animals was greatly
accelerated compared to controls, and sustained concentration of label was
found in spleen, liver, and kidney quantitated by organ counts up to 96 h
post injection. MAb* label copurified with amyloid fibrils up to 10-fold
over saline-soluble proteins and residue following homogenization in distilled water and acid extraction; purified fibrils contained AA protein and
MAb* heavy and light chain visualized on 2D gels and by autoradiography.
Animals were also injected with a mixture of the two MAbs, one labeled with
$Indium^{111}$-DTPA (126 µCi), the other with I^{125} (6 µCi) and serially scanned
over a 48 h period. Fractionation of serum taken after injection showed
both isotopes to be present as uncomplexed IgG in blood. WBAR was performed at 48 h and at a time at which I^{125}/In^{111} radioactivity was calculated to be 127/1; autoradiograms were similar and confirmed localization
of both isotopes to tissue deposits in amyloidotic animals. These studies
provide evidence that MAbs to amyloid subunit proteins may be useful reagents for the in vivo radioimmunodetection of some of the amyloid diseases.

INTRODUCTION

    Monospecific antibodies to amyloid fibril subunit proteins have proven
to be useful reagents for the immunohistological definition of the different forms of amyloidosis in tissue section [1] and for the design of sensi-

TABLE 1. Monoclonal Antibodies—Clinical Applications

Diagnostic

Imaging of neoplasms and metases
    Lymphoscintigraphy
Detection and definition of vascular lesions
    Antimyosin antibodies for myocardial infarction
Definition of foci of infectious disease
    Organism-specific antibodies

Therapeutic

Tumor therapy by conjugation to
    Alpha emitters
    Chemotherapeutic agents
    Bacterial or plant toxins
Abrogation of allograft rejection

tive radio-, enzyme-linked immunoabsorbent and other assays for the quantitation of amyloid-related proteins in serum, other body fluids, and in tissue extracts [2]. Interest has also developed recently in exploring the utility of monoclonal antibodies (MAbs) to amyloid subunit proteins as a means of defining specific isotopes of the polymorphic forms of these proteins, as more precise reagents for immunohistological and assay studies, and to identify variant molecules that may be important in the pathogenesis of some amyloid diseases. Such antibodies have been reported to SAA, AA protein and prealbumin and may provide molecular probes for examining significant domains of these molecules, as well as for more precise biosynthetic studies in cell free systems [3].

Over 20 years of clinical and experimental research has examined the potential of labeled antibodies for the diagnostic imaging of carcinomas, and much current work is examining the efficacy of MAbs as therapeutic reagents in the treatment of hematological and solid malignancies [4]. Other clinical applications that have been examined include as reagents for the in vivo imaging of intravascular clot formation, in the diagnosis and treatment of infectious diseases and for the diagnostic imaging of myocardial infarcts (Table 1) [5]. Results obtained with MAbs are reproducible because of the availability of large quantities of material of uniform quality and monospecificity. Specifically, the homogeneity of MAbs ensures that radiolabelling will not introduce isotope into the host via extraneous molecules, as is the case for polyclonal antisera. Disadvantages of MAbs include the fact that single epitope specificity may result in variable binding in the face of heterogeneities in expression of antigenic determinants and that only a limited number of species (mouse, rat, and to some extent, human) are currently available as sources for fusions.

Applicability of this methodology to the study of amyloidosis was suggested by (a) the utility of such antibodies for in vitro studies, possibly reflecting high epitope density of antigenic determinants in fibrils and (b) the extracellular location of amyloid deposits and their proximity to Congophilic angiopathy. The latter might be expected in turn to enhance accessibility of deposits to such antibodies from the vascular space, perhaps augmented nonspecifically by increased vascular permeability in amyloidosis [6]. Casein-induced amyloidosis in mice provided a model system biochemically analogous to human secondary amyloidosis, and we utilized two rat MAbs to mouse AA protein as reagents for study.

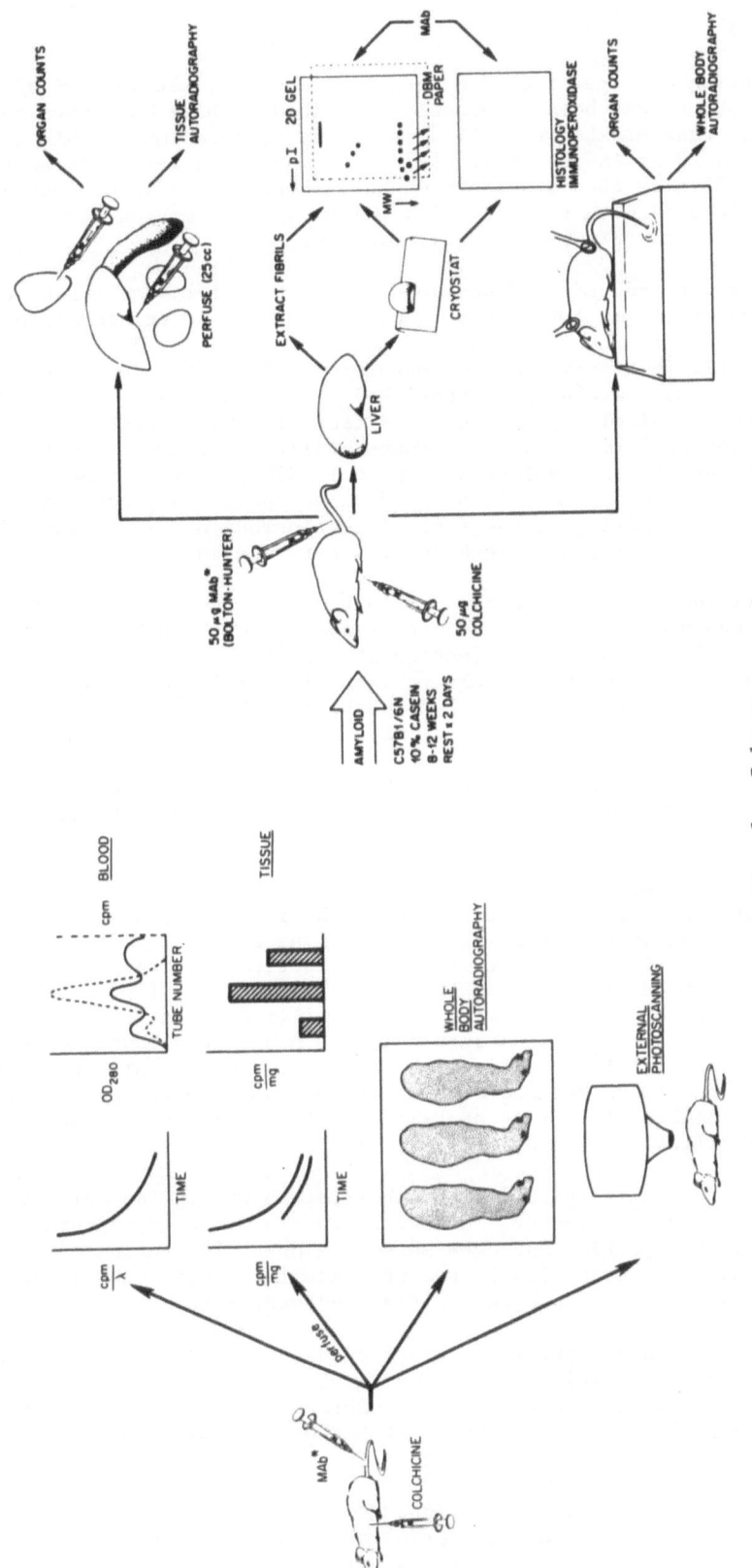

Fig. 1. Schema.

METHODS (Fig. 1)

The production and specificity of 5F8-11 and 4B7-4, rat anti-AA MAbs of the IgG_1k isotype, has been previously described. These MAbs have been also utilized as reagents for an ELISA assay that measures murine SAA to a sensitivity below 10 ng AA-reactivity [7]. Each antibody was purified to homogeneity by affinity chromatography on an AA-Sepharose immunoabsorbent and gave a single band with the molecular weight of rat immunoglobulin G when run unreduced on a 7% SDS-polyacrylamide gel.

Amyloidosis was induced in 8 week old C57Bl/6N mice by daily subcutaneous injections of 0.5 ml 10% casein in 0.3 N $NaHCO_3$. In our laboratory, this regimen results in the appearance of splenic amyloid by 3-4 weeks, followed by hepatic (6-8 weeks) and glomerular (10-12 weeks) deposits. The presence of tissue AA protein was established by immunohistological and biochemical studies of animals sacrificed at different time points. Immunoperoxidase studies of formalin-fixed tissues utilized either of the two anti-AA rat MAbs as primary antisera at up to 1:1000 dilution, biotinylated anti-rat immunoglobulin, and avidin peroxidase-antiperoxidase conjugates [8]. Because of variability in the rate of development of tissue amyloid between individual animals, 8-12 week animals were chosen for study.

Casein amyloidotic mice were allowed to rest two days to permit a decrease of SAA levels toward normal and then injected with 50 µg colchicine intraperitoneally 3 h before the injection of MAb [9]. This pretreatment resulted in a depression of SAA levels in control animals to the lower limits of detection by ELISA assay that lasted about 24 h. MAb was iodinated with I^{125}-labeled Bolton-Hunter reagent, with each animal receiving 50 µg (10-20 µCi) by tailvein injection. Prior to injection, antibody was centrifuged at 100,000 g for two hours to remove aggregates. In control studies, commercially available (Sigma) rat polyclonal immunoglobulin (pIg) was similarly labeled.

Anti-AA MAb was labeled with I^{123} produced at the Brookhaven Linac Isotope Producer (BLIP) facility at Brookhaven National Laboratories using the chloramine-T procedure, resulting in a labeling efficiency of 40-70%. MAb was also coupled to diethylenetriamine-pentacetic acid (DTPA) by the cyclic anhydride method at ratios of 10-100/1 DTPA antibody [10]. DTPA-antibody conjugates were labelled with Indium-111 (medi-physics) with about 80% efficiency; prior to injection into animals, nonprotein bound activity was removed by passage through a Biogel P-6 column. For scanning studies, each animal received 10 µg MAb and a total of 100-200 µCi radioactivity. Specificity of labelled MAb for AA protein was established by western blot analysis of solubilized amyloidotic tissue [11].

Immediately following injection of labelled MAb or pIg, animals were bled from the retroorbital plexus. This serum sample was used to establish the completeness of injection and as a zero time point for serial measurements of the disappearance of label from the vascular space; subsequent time points are expressed as percent initial radioactivity.

Whole body radioautography was performed on animals sacrificed at various time points following injection as previously described [12]. Sections were cut at 50 µm on an LKB model 2258 cryomicrotome, dried on scotch tape and then exposed on the emulsion surface of LKB ultrofilm. Exposure time for I^{125} were 7 days, whereas 5 h was sufficient for Indium-111.

At various times following injection, groups of animals were sacrificed by exsanguination, followed by perfusion with saline through the left ventricle and hepatic portal vein. Organs were weighed, counted and the concentration of label in individual organs expressed as percent total

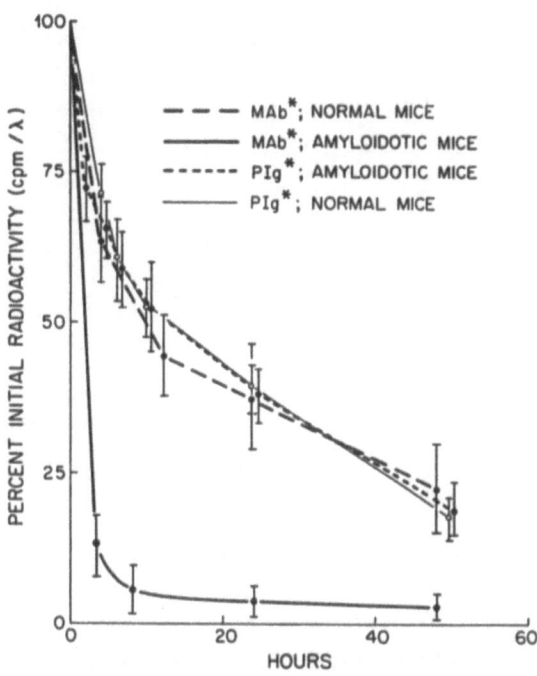

Fig. 2.   Persistence in serum of monoclonal
          immunoglobulin (pIg*) in normal
          and amyloidotic mice.   Each time
          point represents the mean of five
          animals.   At each time point,
          >99% of counts were precipitable
          in 10% trichloroacetic acid.

counts (dpm) per gram wet weight of tissue ×10^{-3}.   Portions of livers, kidneys, and spleens were fixed in formalin for histological studies and for
tissue autoradiography.   For the latter, 10 μm sections on albumin subbed
slides were dipped into Kodak NTB-2 emulsion, and exposed at 4°C for three
days [13].

Amyloid fibrils were extracted from involved organs by the water flotation method followed by acid extraction in dilute hydrochloric acid [14].
AA protein was visualized by two dimensional gel electrophoresis in pur-
fied material, as well as in solubilized frozen sections of individual organs using the Anderson ISODALT System [15].

External photoscanning following injection of I^{123} or In^{111}-labelled
MAb was performed with a General Electric data gamma camera with pinhole
collimation using a small-bore pinhole (I^{123}-159 KeV; In^{111}-172 KeV; 20%
window).   Scans were analyzed on a Digital Electronics Corporation (DEC)
computer using Gamma-11 software.

Serum Studies and Tissue Washout

The disappearance curve of I^{125}-labelled MAb (MAb*) from serum was
strikingly different when groups of amyloidotic and control mice were compared (Fig. 2).   Loss of label from the circulation of control mice, as
well as amyloidotic and control mice injected with pIg*, was biphasic, with
a rapid fall-off followed by a slower equilibration phase, falling to 10-

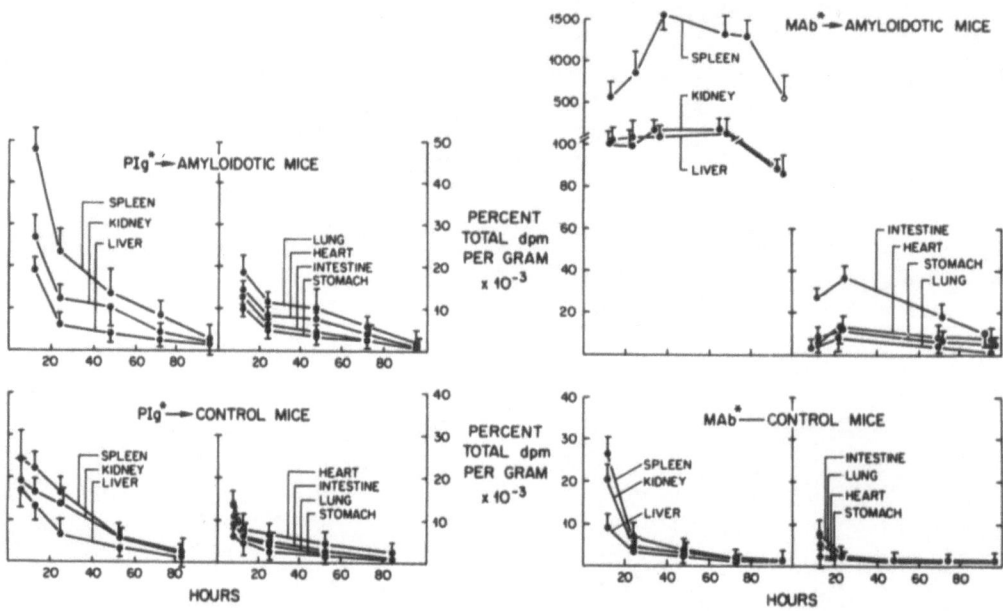

Fig. 3. Loss of radioactivity expresssed as percent injected counts per
gram wet weight of perfused tissue ×10⁻³ at different time points
following injections of radiolabeled MAb* or pIg*. Counts are
normalized for a 20 gram mouse; each time point is the mean of
3-5 animals.

15% initial levels by 48 h. Similar biphasic disappearance curves have been
reported by other investigators following injection of labeled heterologous
immunoglobulin in both rodents and other mammalian species [16]. By contrast, the disappearance curve of MAb* in amyloidotic animals was much more
rapid, in some groups of animals dropping to levels below 10% by one hour
following injection. In a small sampling, the slope of the initial drop
appeared to vary with the degree of amyloid involvement assessed by histological stains.

Tissue distribution studies showed that MAb* was taken up in a selective and sustained manner by involved organs (spleen, liver, kidney) of amyloidotic animals (Fig. 3). Control groups included amyloidotic animals injected with pIg* and animals matched as to age and size that did not receive casein and had no evidence of amyloidosis histologically. All groups
showed early "nonspecific" label in these organs, which largely washed out
by 24 h post injection. Even during early time points, however, the percent label retained in these organs in amyloidotic animals injected with
MAb* exceeded by 10-20 fold that achieved in a comparable group of animals
injected with equivalent amounts of pIg*. This difference became more
striking at later time points and was apparent in the MAb*-injected amyloidotic animals in studies extending out to 96 h (Fig. 3).

Size fractionation of zero time point sera on Sephadex G-200 columsn
showed both MAb* and pIg* to be present in the circulation uncomplexed,
comigrating with monomeric IgG. Consequently, more rapid clearance of MAb*
in the affected animals is unlikely to be due to the formation of complexes
with low levels of SAA or other cross-reacting material in the circulation.

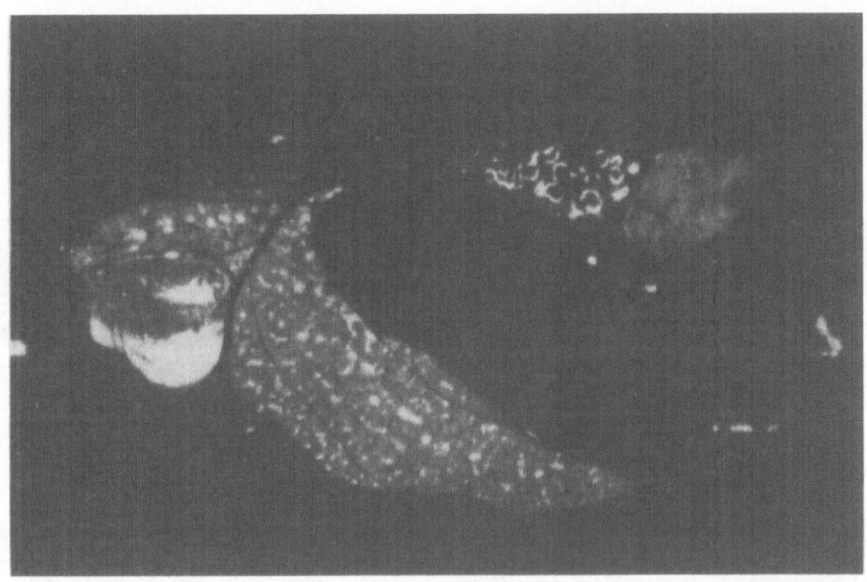

Fig. 4. Whole body autoradiogram of amyloidotic mouse showing predominantly perifollicular uptake of label in spleen and
periportal uptake in liver blood. Background in this
early time point is seen in heart and lungs.

Autoradiography

Specific uptake of label over amyloid deposits was confirmed by whole-
body (WBAR) and tissue autoradiography. WBAR done on amyloidotic animals
found to have early splenic amyloid involvement clearly showed the characteristically perifollicular pattern of the deposits (Fig. 4), closely approximating that revealed by immunoperoxidase staining using the same MAb
(Fig. 5, top). Whereas the early washout of label from the liver in control groups was diffuse, in the amyloidotic mice hepatic involvement was
revealed as predominantly periportal (Fig. 4), and in animals with renal
amyloid, a clearcut glomerular pattern could be seen. Animals with renal
involvement also often were found to have intense uptake over the adrenal
glands, confirmed by histological stains to be due to amyloid deposition.

Localization of label to amyloid deposits was also seen at the light
microscopic level in tissue autoradiograms of perfused livers, spleens, and
kidneys collected at varous time points up to 96 h post injection (Fig. 4,
middle). These studies confirm the close correlation between amyloid deposition revealed by Congo red staining, immunohistology and injected label.

Copurification of MAb* with Amyloid Fibrils

Amyloid fibrils were isolated from involved organs of animals injected
with MAb* by water flotation; following saline homogenization, additional
radioactivity, as well as AA protein, could be obtained by acid extraction
of the residue remaining after water extraction [14]. MAb* label copurified with fibrils up to 10 fold over saline-soluble proteins. Purified
fibrils contained AA protein and MAb* heavy and light chain when solubilized
in dissociating buffer and visualized by two dimensional gel electrophoresis
[15]. AA protein was apparent as a series of six major chain-length and
charge polymorphs that are seen on coomassie or silver stains (Fig. 6A),
while MAb* could be seen on autoradiograms of the same gel exposed for suf-

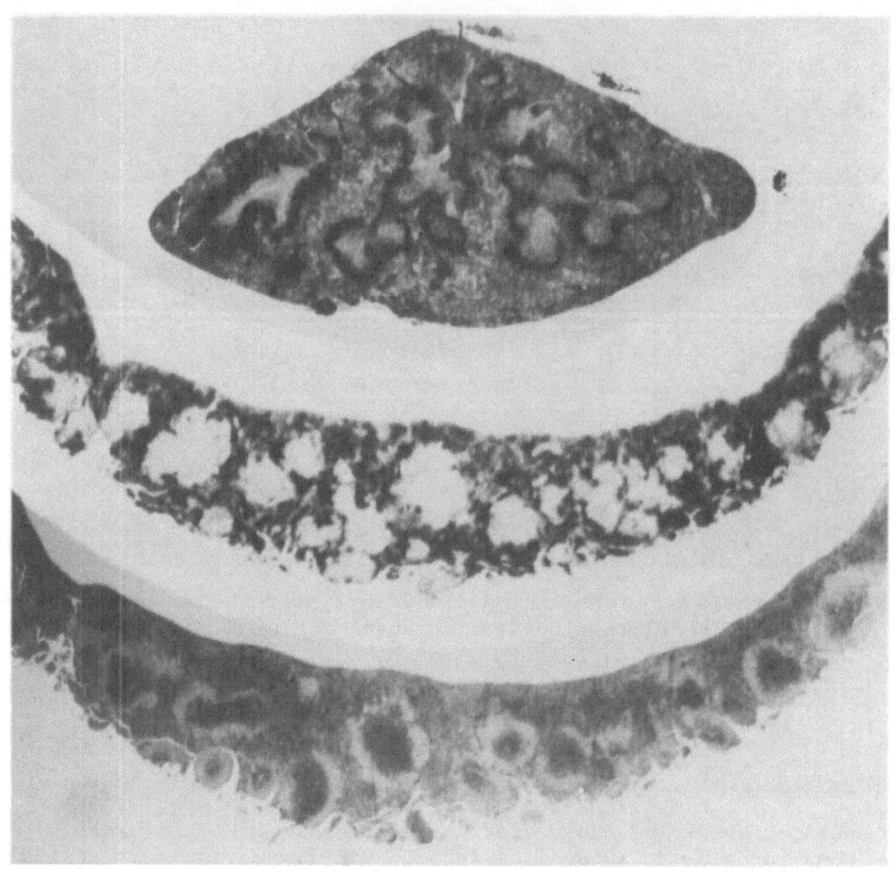

Fig. 5. Composite low power view showing amyloidotic spleen with perifollicular amyloid by hematoxylin and eosin stain (bottom), localization of radiolabel in a parallel section exposed for tissue autoradiography (middle) and immunoperoxidase-stained with MAb (1:1000) and biotinylated anti rat antibody (top).

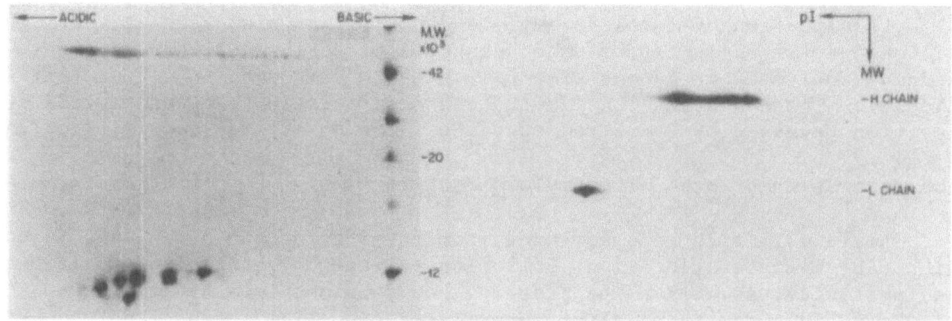

Fig. 6. Two dimensional (2D) gel electrophoretogram (A) of purified amyloid fibrils, isolated by water flotation and acid extraction, from amyloidotic mice injected with MAb*, (B) autoradiogram showing copurification of MAb heavy (H) and light (L) chains with AA protein.

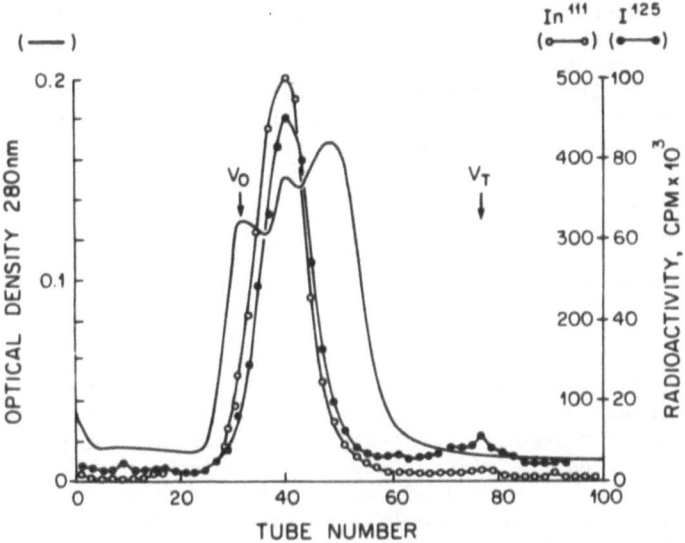

Fig. 7. Fractionation of serum from an amyloidotic mouse collected immediately following injection of a mixture of two MAb*, one labelled with iodine-125 and the other indium-111. Serum was fractionated on Sephadex G-200, counted immediately for indium, and then again at 12 half-lives for iodine-125.

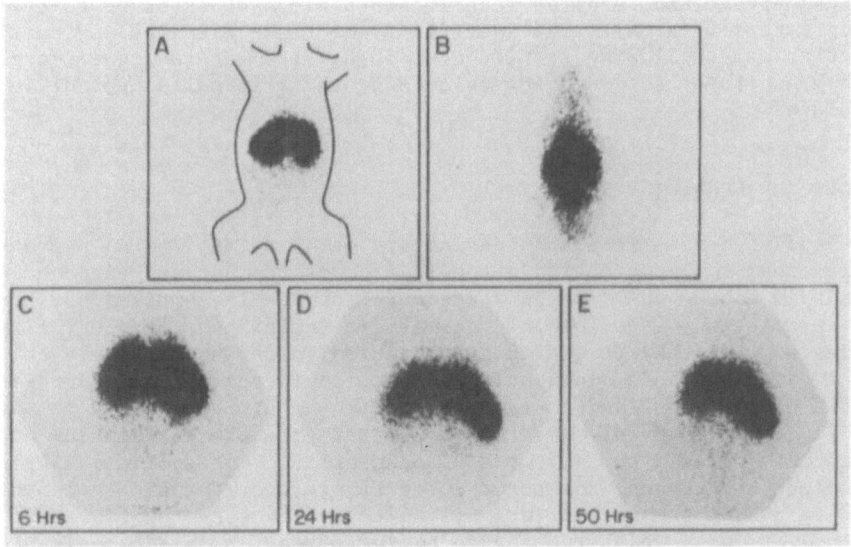

Fig. 8. Serial scans of amyloidotic (A, C, D, E) and control (B) animals over a 50 h period post injection of indium-111-labeled MAb.

ficient periods to pick up the label (Fig. 6B). These observations confirm that at least some of the MAb* is able to reach amyloid deposits in vivo without degradation or apparent modification, even during purification of fibrils from tissue. They also appear to exclude co-localization of label with amyloid deposits that might result from the reticuloendothelial hyperplasia that is known to accompany the early stages of tissue deposition [17].

Gamma Scintigraphy

These findings suggested that MAb* might be optimally visualized at time points at least 12-24 h post injection to minimize "nonspecific" washout in control animals. Isotopes suitable for gamma camera imaging are technetium-99m (t 1/2 of 6 h), iodine-123 (t 1/2 of 13 h) and indium-111 (t 1/2 of 2.8 h) [18]. Initial studies were carried out with iodine-123, which provided external photoscans showing sharp resolution of livers and spleens of amyloidotic animals, the relative intensity of which could be correlated with Congo red staining of livers and spleens of these animals examined histologically at the end of each experiment (Fig. 5, bottom). Gamma scintigraphy was not sufficiently sensitive to detect renal involvement because of the size of the animals, the resolution attained with the crystal and collimator employed for these studies, and the superimposition of enlarged livers and spleens of amyloidotic animals on the renal outlines. Iodine-123 studies demonstrated that specific uptake to amyloidotic organs could be seen with as little as 10 µg MAb* per animal, labelled to high specific activity (100-200 µCi per animal) by the harsher chloramine-T method.

Four animals (2 amyloidotic; 2 controls) were injected with 50 µg of a mix of 5F8-11 and 4B7-4 in a ratio of 10:1 by weight. The former was labelled with indium-111 following conjugation to DTPA (∿125 µCi) and the latter with I^{125} by Bolton-Hunter acylation (∿5 µCi). Following injection, both isotopes were found to circulate uncomplexed in the circulation (Fig. 7). Serial photoscans of the two amyloidotic animals showed specific and sustained uptake of label over spleens and livers in the amyloidotic animals up to 50 h post injection. By contrast, the control animals showed only diffuse uptake and required much longer periods of exposure to attain comparable images (Fig. 8). The specificity of these findings was confirmed by WBAR of animals following sacrifice at 50 h, with autoradiograms exposed immediately and then at time point calculated to be 12 half lives of Indium-111 later.

CONCLUSIONS AND CURRENT PROBLEMS

Our studies demonstrate the feasibility of using MAb* to AA protein for the in vivo radioimmunodetection of amyloid deposits in casein-induced AA amyloidosis in mice. The disappearance curve of labeled anti-AA antibody from the circulation of amyloidotic animals is reminiscent of older clinical studies showing that Congo red dye injected intravenously could be used to similar advantage as a diagnostic reagent, could reach tissue deposits through the circulation, and could be demonstrable histologically in tissue sections [19]. To study disappearance of label from the circulation and tissue washout, we used sufficient MAb to swamp low levels of circulating SAA that might be present, further reduced by pretreatment with colchicine. Results obtained by gamma scintigraphy indicate that much lower amounts of these MAbs, labeled to higher specific activity, may in fact be suitable for imaging. However, each run needs to be monitored by fractionation studies to check for nonspecific aggregation of antibody, degradation, or the presence of free isotope or DTPA-conjugates in the injected material and in the circulation. It is also not clear that maintaining low levels of circulating SAA is a prerequisite for successful localization of label, as studies of similar design utilizing antibodies to carcinoembryonic antigen for the localization of colonic carcinomas have clearly demonstrated specific uptake of label to tumor masses in spite of high levels of circulating antigen [20]. An alternative approach would be the design of MAb that recognize conformational determinants unique to the fibril and which have little binding affinity for the circulating cross-reactive serum protein.

Results were obtained in animals with established and sometimes massive amyloid deposits primarily in spleen, liver, and kidney. The ability of such reagents to demonstrate small deposits in other organs, or to recognize the so-called "preamyloid" phase of tissue deposition [17] remains to be shown. Lastly, prolonged (at least to 96 h) retention of MAb* in tissue deposits, and the copurification of intact heavy and light chains with AA protein in fibrils, suggests that specific antibody might engender an immune and/or inflammatory response to the fibril in the host that could speed resorption and have therapeutic potential. These possibilities are currently under investigation.

ACKNOWLEDGEMENTS

Work funded by NIH Grants AG01973 and GM31866 and the HOR Foundation. The authors gratefully acknowledge the secretarial support of Ms. Karen Abramowski.

REFERENCES

1. S. Fujihara, J. E. Balow, J. C. Costa, and G. G. Glenner, Lab. Invest., 43:358 (1980); T. Shirahama, M. Skinner, and A. S. Cohen, Histochemistry, 72:161 (1981).
2. J. D. Sipe, T. F. Ignaczak, P. S. Pollock, and G. G. Glenner, J. Immunol., 116:1151 (1976); G. Marhaug, Scand. J. Immunol., 18:329 (1983); M. J. M. Saraiva, P. P. Costa, and D. S. Goodman, J. Lab. Clin. Med., 102:590 (1983).
3. K. P. W. J. McAdam, et al., Ann. N.Y. Acad. Sci., 389:126 (1982); G. Marhaug, et al., Clin. Exp. Immunol., 50:390 (1982); R. Linke, J. Histochem. Cytochem., 32:322 (1984); C. J. Rosenthal, A. Huq, and M. E. Martin, Routh Intl. Symposium of amyloidosis, November 9-12, 1984.
4. D. Pressman, Cancer Res., 40:2960 (1980); R. W. Baldwin, M. J. Embleton, and M. R. Price, Molec. Aspects Med., 4:329 (1980); Tumor Imaging (S. E. Burchiel, R. A. Rhodes, and B. E. Friedman, eds.), Masson, New York (1982); R. Levy and R. A. Miller, Fed. Proc., 42: 2650 (1983).
5. B. A. Khaw et al., J. Clin. Invest., 58:439 (1976); J. Nucl. Med., 23: 1011 (1982); N. C. Engleberg and B. I. Eisenstein, New Engl. J. Med., 311:892 (1984).
6. R. T. Schultz, Amer. J. Pathol., 86:321 (1977).
7. D. D. Wood, M. Gammon, and M. J. Staruch, J. Immunol. Meth., 55:19 (1982).
8. J.-L. Guesdon, T. Ternynck, and S. Avrameas, J. Histochem. Cytochem., 27:1131 (1979).
9. M. D. Benson, et al., J. Clin. Invest., 59:412 (1977); M. D. Benson and E. Kleiner, J. Immunol., 124:495 (1980); M. J. Selinger, et al., Nature, 285:498 (1980).

10. W. C. Eckelman, S. M. Karesh, and R. C. Reba, J. Pharm. Sci., 64:704 (1975); G. E. Krejcarek and K. Tucker, Biochim. Biophys. Res. Comm., 77:581 (1977); D. A. Scheinberg, M. Strand, and O. A. Ganslow, Science, 215:1511 (1982); J. Powe, et al., Cancer Drug Delivery, 1:125 (1984).

11. P. D. Gorevic, A. B. Cleveland, and D. D. Wood, Arth. Rheum., 25:S141 (1982).

12. I. Fand and W. P. McNally, in: Current Trends in Morphological Techniques (J. E. Johnson, Jr., ed.), CRC Press, Inc., Boca Raton, Florida, Vol. 2, p. 1 (1981).

13 A. Henrickson, in: Current Trends in Morphological Techniques (J. E. Johnson, Jr., ed.), CRC Press, Inc., Boca Raton, Florida, Vol. 2, p. 29 (1981).

14. M. Pras, et al., J. Clin. Invest., 47:924 (1968); M. Pras and T. Reshef, Biochim. Biophys. Acta, 271:193 (1972).

15. N. G. Anderson and N. L. Anderson, Anal. Biochem., 85:331 (1978); 85: 312 (1978); P. D. Gorevic, et al., Amer. J. Ophth., 98:216 (1984).

16. H. L. Spiegelberg and W. D. Weigle, J. Exp. Med., 121:323 (1965); T. W. Smith, B. L. Lloyd, N. Spicer, and E. Haber, Clin. Exp. Immunol., 36:384 (1979); S. J. Nelson and D. D. Manning, J. Immunol., 175:2339 (1980); S. W. Burchiel, et al., in: Tumor Imaging (S. W. Burchiel and B. A. Rhodes, eds.), Masson Publishing, New York, p. 128 (1982).

17. G. Telium, Acta. Pathol. Microbiol. Scand., 61:21 (1964).

18. W. F. Bale, M. A. Contreras, and E. D. Grady, Cancer Res., 40:2965 (1980); W. C. Eckelman, C. H. Paik, and R. C. Reiba, Cancer Res., 40: 3036 (1980).

19. E. Calkins and A. S. Cohen, Bull. Rheum. Dis., 10:215 (1960); H. Benhold and H. Steilner, in: Protides of the Biological Fluids (H. Peeters, ed.), Pergamon Press, Oxford (1973), p. 113.

20. D. M. Goldenberg, et al., New Engl. J. Med., 298:1384 (1978); J. P. Mach, et al., Immunol. Today, 2:239 (1981).

PROSTACYCLIN AND THROMBOXANE PRODUCTION FROM MACROPHAGES OF AMYLOID RESISTANT AND SENSITIVE MICE*

Crystal A. Leslie, Antonio Lazzarri,
and Edgar S. Cathcart

E.N.R.M. Veterans Administration Hospital
200 Springs Road
Bedford, Massachusetts 01730, and

Biochemistry Department
Boston University School of Medicine
80 East Concord Street
Boston, Massachusetts 02118

ABSTRACT

Peritoneal macrophages from amyloid resistant A/J mice produced more prostacyclin (PGI_2) and protaglandin E (PGE_2) and less thromboxane A_2 (TXA_2) into the incubation medium than similarly prepared macrophages from CBA/J mice. When CBA/J mice were given injections of azocasein sufficient to produce amyloid in the spleen, the amount of PGI_2, but not PGE_2 or TXA_2 found in the medium from incubated macrophages was significantly decreased. This inhibition of PGI_2 synthetase (and/or augmentation of PGI_2 catabolism) was also found in the macrophages from azocasein treated A/J mice and to a lesser extent in water injected CBA/J and A/J mice. However, this inhibition of PGI_2 synthetase in response to azocasein injections occurred much more slowly in the A/J macrophages than in the CBA/J macrophage. It is suggested that in the presence of elevated serum AA an altered arachidonic acid metabolism by cells of the mononuclear phagocytitic system may contribute to a susceptibility to amyloidosis.

INTRODUCTION

Amyloidosis is characterized by the deposition of a variety of extra-cellular proteins with specific physical properties. One of these proteins known as AA is thought to be a catabolic product of a structurally related serum protein with similar antigenic properties but higher molecular weight than AA. SAA which is a normal constituent of serum, increases dramatically in response to an inflammatory or immune stimulus [1]. While the consensus is that this is an appropriate homeostatic response to injury, the deposition of AA is clearly a pathologic one.

---

*This work was supported by the Veterans Administration and US PHS Grant #AM 32588.

175

Recent evidence implicating the macrophage in this pathologic process suggests that either the altered release of a factor necessary for the degradation of SAA or inappropriate SAA uptake and degradation within the macrophage, may be responsible. First there is the historical observation that amyloid is often laid down in close association with the reticulo-endothelial system [2]. Second, enzymes of monocytic origin have been shown to degrade serum amyloid [3] and thirdly, it is well established that the in vivo environment of the macrophage is the main determinant of its activation and secretory products [4].

In general, the arachidonate products, i.e., prostaglandins (PG's), and thromboxanes (TX's) are potent regulators of cellular metabolism and are proposed as intercellular mediators of the immune and inflammatory response [5]. They appear to act primarily in the cells in which they are synthesized often by changing intracellular cyclic nucleotide levels [6]. Since monocytes and macrophages, of all the cells in the immune response, appear to a major source of these products [7], we set out to determine if macrophages of amyloid sensitive and resistant strains of mice showed differences in their arachidonate metabolism either before, during, or after production of amyloid.

METHODS

Animals

Six to eight week old, female CBA/J (amyloid sensitive) and age, sex matched A/J (amyloid resistant) mice obtained from Jackson Labs, Maine, were used. One group from each strain was injected daily with 0.3 ml of sterile distilled water and the other with the same volume of 10% azocasein (the amyloidogenic agent). In some experiments a group of mice were left untreated. Four to five animals were used in each group.

Macrophages

At the end of the injection period (13 days for Experiment 1, 10 days for Experiment 2 and various times for Experiment 3) mice were sacrificed by cervical dislocation, the abdominal wall exposed and the peritoneal cavity injected with 6 ml of HBSS buffer. After 2 min the exudate was removed and spun at 400 g for 5 min. The cells were then washed twice with 2 ml volumes of HBSS. The cells were resuspended in RPMI with 10% fetal calf serum at a concentration of 1.5×10^6 (Expts. 1 and 3) or 0.5×10^6 (Expt. 2). After adhering cells to polystyrene flasks or microtiter wells for 2 h at 37°C in a humidified atmosphere the non-adherent cell population was removed. In Experiment 2 only, this 2 h incubation was done in the absence and presence of 100 µg/ml of azocasein. The adherent cells were washed with two further 2 ml volumes of buffer. The total non-adherent cell population which was washed off, was counted and the remaining adherent cells incubated in a further volume of RPMI with 2.5% fetal calf serum for 20 to 48 h. The supernatants were stored at -20°C for subsequent PG or TX analysis. Results were expressed as total amount of PG or TX products per unit time per 10^6 adhered cells (Expts. 1 and 3) or per unit time per ml (Expt. 2).

Kidney Slices

Kidneys were removed from azocasein injected, water injected, or untreated mice (Experiment 2 only) and freed from surrounding fat and blood vessels. Very thin slices were prepared using a Stadie Riggs micrometer. Two slices from the same kidney area of each mouse were incubated under 5% CO_2 95% O_2 for 1 h in Krebs Ringer bicarbonate buffer. The incubation medium was assayed for PG's and TX and results expressed as ng/PG or TX/100 mg wet wt/hr.

TABLE 1. Development of Amyloid in Amyloid Sensitive (CBA/J) and Resistant
(A/J) Mice Treated with Azocasein for Various Lengths of Time

DAYS	MICE	%A*
6	CBA/J	0
9	CBA/J	0
13	CBA/J	40
21	CBA/J	100
30	CBA/J	100
30	A/J	0

*A) Amyloid present as defined by characteristic green birefringence.

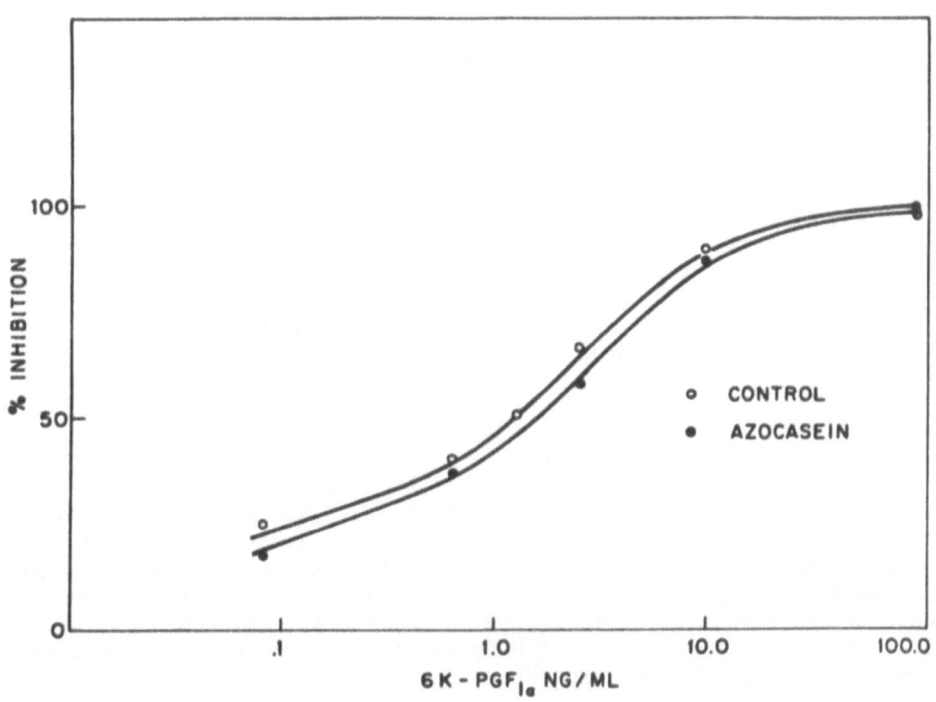

Fig. 1. The effect of azocasein on the radioimmunoassay for 6-ketoprosta-
glandin $F_{1\alpha}$ (6K-PGF$_{1\alpha}$). The percentage inhibition of binding of
labelled ligand (6-keto-PGF$_{1\alpha}$) to the antibody (specific for
6-keto-PGF$_{1\alpha}$) by a series of 6 keto PGF$_{1\alpha}$ standards in the absence and presence of 100 µg/ml of azocasein was calculated. The
presence of azocasein did not significantly alter the inhibition.
6-Keto PGF$_{1\alpha}$ is used as a measure of the unstable prostacyclin
(PGI$_2$).

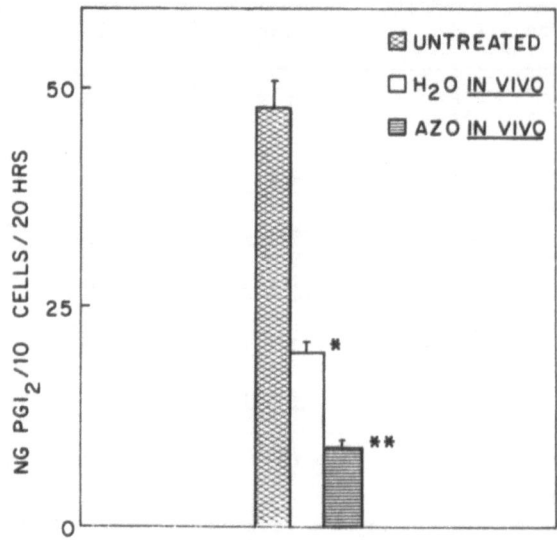

Fig. 2. Prostacyclin (PGI$_2$) levels in incubation medium from macrophages
prepared from CBA/J mice left untreated or treated in vivo with
water or azocasein (azo). CBA/J
mice were left untreated or given
13 daily injections of azocasein
or sterile water. Forty eight
hours after the last injection,
mice were sacrificed, macrophages
prepared and incubated for 20 h.
Prostaglandins in the incubation
medium were assayed radioimmunologically. *) Sterile water injections significantly (p < 0.001)
reduced PGI$_2$ production from CBA/J
macrophages. **) A further significant reduction occurred with
azocasein injections (p < .001).

Prostaglandin and Thromboxane Analysis

PGE$_2$, 6-keto-PGE$_{1\alpha}$ (as a measure of the unstable prostacylin, PGI$_2$)
and TXB$_2$ (as a measure of the unstable TXA$_2$) were assayed using a previously described radioimmunoassay [8, 9]. Although the adherent cells were
washed several times before the final incubation, the possibility does
exist that azocasein itself interfered with the radioimmunoassay. As
shown in Fig. 1 the presence of 100 µg/ml of azocasein had no effect on
the radioimmunoassay for 6-keto-PGF$_{1\alpha}$.

Cyclic Nucleotide Determinations

After 24 h incubation of macrophages 1 ml of 0.4 N ice cold perchloric
acid was added to the adherent cells and the cell layer scraped off with a
rubber policeman. Cyclic AMP was isolated by column chromatography [10]
corrected for recovery and assay radioimmunologically. Results were expressed in femtomoles per 10^6 cells.

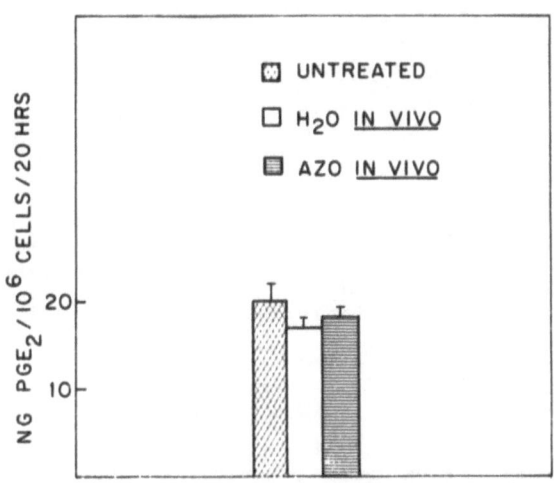

Fig. 3. Prostaglandin E₁(PGE₂) levels in incubation medium from macrophages
prepared from CBA/J mice left untreated or treated in vivo with
water or azocasein (azo). See legend
under Fig. 2. PGE₂ production from
macrophages was not altered by
sterile water or azocasein injections.

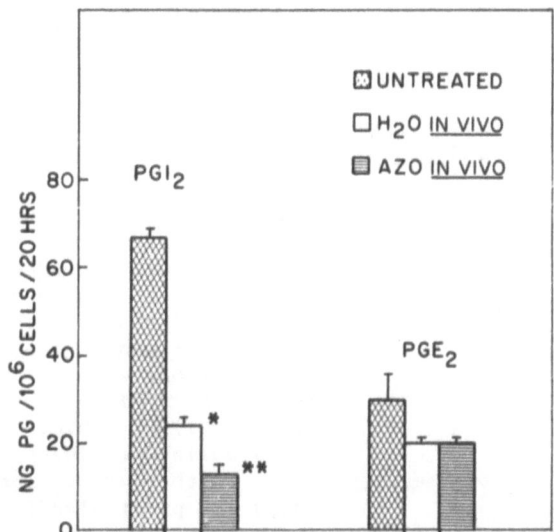

Fig. 4. Prostacyclin (PGI₂) and prostaglandin
(PGE₂) levels in incubation medium from
macrophages prepared from A/J mice left
untreated or treated in vivo with water
or azocasein (azo). A/J mice of the
same age and sex as the CBA/J mice were
treated as described in the legend under
Fig. 2. *) Sterile water injections significantly (p < .01) reduced PGI₂ production from A/J macrophages. **) A further
significant reduction occurred with azocasein injections (p < .01).

Fig. 5.
Prostacyclin (PGI$_2$) levels in incubation medium from kidney slices
prepared from CBA/J or A/J mice
left untreated or treated in vivo
with water or azocasein (azo).
Kidney slices were prepared from
the same mice treated as described
under legend Fig. 2. The slices
(approx. 80 mg wet wt.) were incubated for 1 h in a bicarbonate
buffer under 5% CO$_2$ and 95% O$_2$.
Prostaglandins were assayed radioimmunologically. PCI$_2$ and PGE$_2$
production from kidney slices was
not altered by sterile water or
azocasein injections.

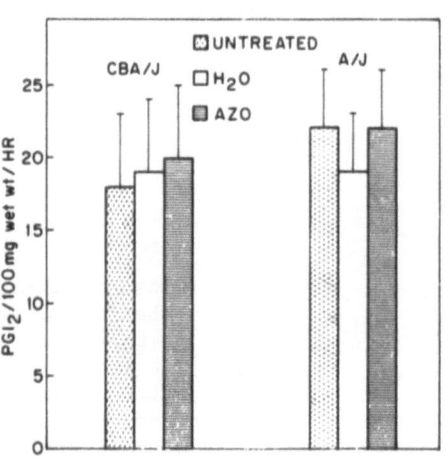

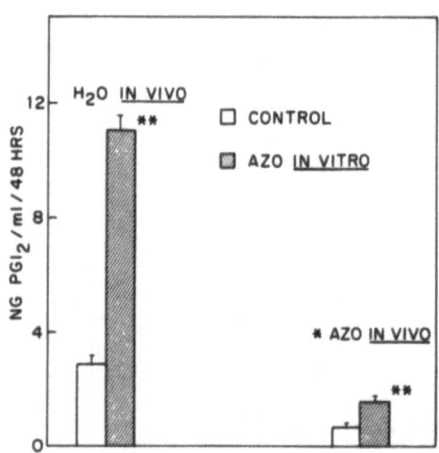

Fig. 6.

Prostacyclin (PGI$_2$) levels in incubation medium from macrophages prepared
from CBA/J mice pretreated in vivo
water or azocasein (azo) and incubated
in vitro with azocasein. Peritoneal
cells were removed from CBA/J mice after
10 injections with water or azocasein.
After 2 h in vitro exposure to azocasein
(100 µg/ml) or vehicle control, the adhered cells were incubated in fresh media
for a further 48 h. The medium was assayed for prostaglandins. *) Azocasein
pretreatment in vivo relative to water
pretreatment had significantly (p < .001)
reduced PGI$_2$. **) In vitro azocasein exposure of cells from either water or azocasein pretreated mice significantly (p<
.01) increased PGI$_2$ production.

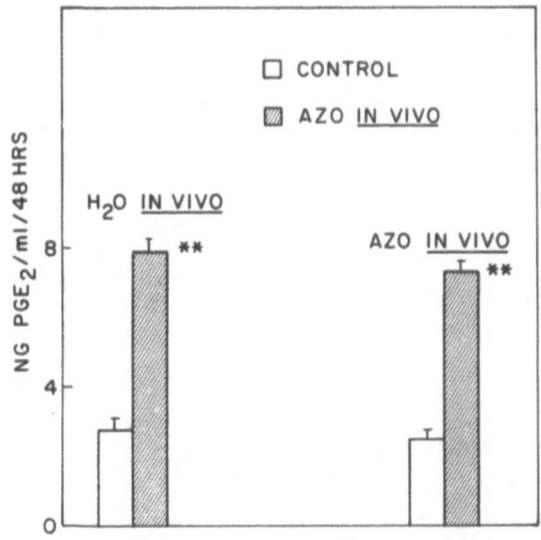

Fig. 7. Prostaglandin E_2 (PGE$_2$) levels incubation medium from macrophages
prepared from CBA/J mice pretreated
in vivo with water or azocasein
(azo) and incubated in vitro with
azocasein. See legend under Fig.
6. Azocasein pretreatment in
vivo relative to water pretreatment did not alter PGE$_2$. **)
In vitro azocasein exposure of
cells from either water or azocasein pretreated mice significantly ($p < .01$) increased PGE$_2$
production.

RESULTS

Thirteen daily injections of sterile distilled water reduced prostacyclin (PGI$_2$) production (and/or increased catabolism) from macrophages of
amyloid sensitive (CBA/J) mice (Fig. 2). A further significant reduction
($p < .001$) occurred with azocasein injections (Fig. 2). Prostaglandin
E_2 (PGE$_2$) metabolism, on the other hand, was not altered by either distilled
water or azocasein injections (Fig. 3). Identically treated, sex and age
matched amyloid resistant (A/J) mice showed this same pattern of reduced
PGI$_2$ production (Fig. 4). It was noted, however, that the macrophages prepared from untreated A/J mice produced markedly more PGE$_2$ ($p < .05$) and
PGI$_2$ ($p < .02$) than identically prepared CBA/J macrophages (Figs. 2, 3,
and 4). This reduced PGI$_2$ formation by macrophages was not found in kidney slices prepared from these same mice (Fig. 5). PGE$_2$ production in kidney slices was also unaltered.

In a second experiment in which CBA/J mice were given 10 injections of
sterile water or azocasein, it was again observed that relative to water,
azocasein given in vivo, very significantly reduced PGI$_2$ (Fig. 6) but not
PGE$_2$ (Fig. 7) production from macrophages. In contrast to this in vivo
effect of azocasein, exposure of these same macrophages to azocasein in
vitro (100 µg/ml) greatly stimulated both PCE$_2$ and PGI$_2$ production (Figs.
6 and 7).

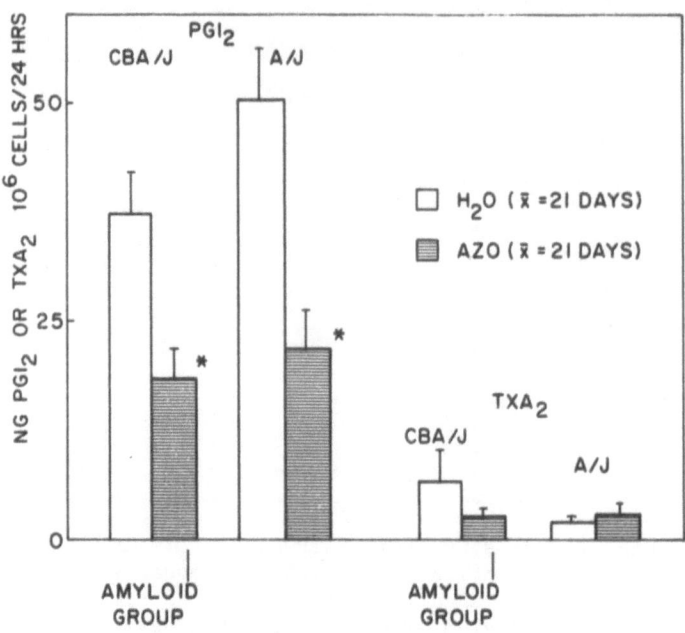

Fig. 8. Prostacyclin (PGI_2) and thromboxane (TXA_2)
levels in incubation medium from macrophages
prepared from amyloid sensitive (CBA/J) and
amyloid resistant (A/J) mice during the
amyloid period. Mice (CBA/J and A/J) were
given daily injections of azocasein or water.
After 2, 6, 9, 13, 21, or 30 days of injections, 5 mice in each group were sacrificed
and spleens removed. Spleens were examined
histologically for amyloid (Table 1). Macrophages were incubated for 24 h and prostaglandins and thromboxane assayed. PG and
TX levels of macrophages taken from mice
during the pre-amyloid period (2 to 9 injections, Table 1) and during the amyloid
period (13 to 30 injections) were meaned.
*) The group of mice with amyloid (CBA/J
mice treated with azocasein for a mean of
21 days) had a significant decrease in
PGI_2 production from macrophages ($p < .05$).
The amyloid resistant mice (azocasein
treated A/J mice) showed a similar decrease.

To determine how fast, PGI_2 was reduced in response to in vivo azocasein, mice were injected with azocasein for different lengths of time.
Table 1 shows that it took more than 9 days of azocasein injections before
any CBA/J mice developed amyloid. None of the A/J mice or any sterile water
treated mice developed amyloid even after 30 days of injections.

Often when amyloid was present in the CBA/J mice (amyloid group) there
was no difference in the amount of PGI_2 produced from CBA/J and A/J macrophages (Fig. 8). However, for 9 days prior to amyloid deposition in the
CBA/J mice (pre-amyloid group) macrophages from amyloid sensitive mice produced significantly less PGI_2 than macrophages from similarly injected A/J
mice (Fig. 8). This was because the response to azocasein occurred earlier

TABLE 2. Intracellular Cyclic Nucleotide Levels in Macrophages from Amyloid Sensitive (CBA/J) and Amyloid Resistant (A/J) Mice during the Pre-Amyloid Period

MICE	TREATMENT	FMOLES/10^6 CELLS	P
CBA/J	H_2O	465 ± 29	<.005
	AZO	656 ± 60	
A/J	H_2O	470 ± 38	>.5
	AZO	492 ± 28	

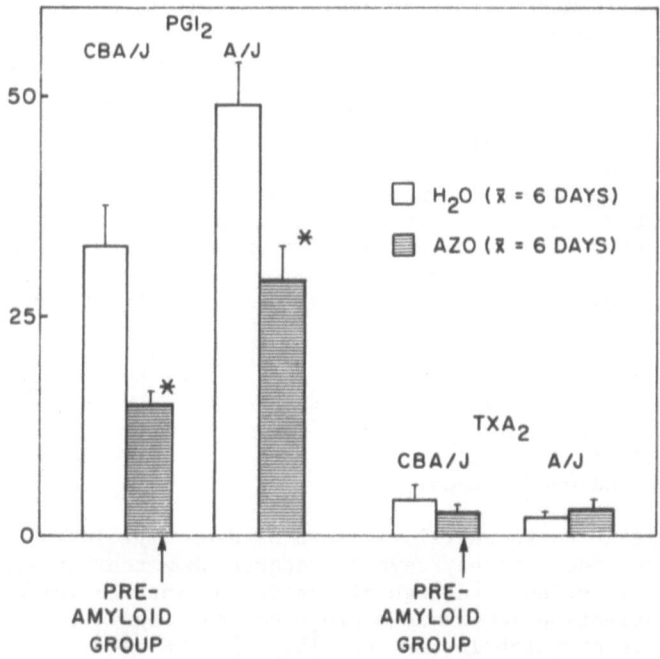

Fig. 9. Prostacyclin (PGI₂) and thromboxane (TXA₂) levels in incubation medium from macrophages prepared from amyloid sensitive (CBA/J) and amyloid resistant (A/J) mice during the pre-amyloid period. See legend under Fig. 8. *) During the pre-amyloid period (CBA/J mice treated with azocasein for a mean of 6 days) macrophages from CBA/J mice produced much less PGI₂ than A/J macrophages (p < .02).

in the CBA/J macrophage (after only 2 injections there was a 55% decrease in PGI$_2$ production relative to a 20% decrease in A/J macrophages) and because baseline PGI$_2$ production in the absence of azocasein injections was greater in the A/J mice (Figs. 4 and 9). As shown in Figs. 8 and 9, macrophages from CBA/J mice produced more TXA$_2$ than similarly prepared A/J macrophages. Azocasein injections had no significant affect on such production.

Table 2 shows that during the pre-amyloid period (7 injections of azocasein) azocasein significantly increased the cAMP content of CBA/J macrophages but not of A/J macrophages.

DISCUSSION

When amyloid susceptible CBA/J mice are injected daily with azocasein much less PGI$_2$, relative to untreated mice, is found in the medium of their subsequently incubated peritoneal macrophages. This effect can not be due to a depletion of the arachidonate precursor since PGE$_2$ and TXA$_2$ levels are not altered. Azocasein _in vivo_ (or possibly a breakdown product of azocasein or a factor released by azocasein) is either specifically inhibiting PGI$_2$ synthetase and/or augmenting the catabolism of PGI$_2$ in macrophages.

Since there was no effect on azocasein on PGI$_2$ metabolism in kidney, it would be logical to assume that accumulated azocasein by the macrophage was responsible for the altered enzyme activity. Another explanation consistent with the fact that the injection of sterile distilled water also reduced PGI$_2$ levels in incubated macrophates, would be that the stress of any injection _per se_ releases a factor which then secondarily alters the enzyme activity. The fact that _in vitro_ exposure to azocasein increased rather than decreased PGI$_2$ from incubated macrophages would also support the theory of a _in vivo_ secondary production of a factor interfering with PGI$_2$ metabolism. Ebesson [11] several years ago suggested that "stress" may have been a factor in the production of spontaneous amyloid among overcrowded male CBA/J mice. Since water or saline injections only marginally increase SAA [12], this decrease in PGI$_2$ is not altering interleukin 1 release from macrophages.

This inhibition of PGI$_2$ synthetase in macrophages by _in vivo_ azocasein injections to amyloid sensitive mice is consistent with a recent report of Scott [13]. He found that mice inoculated i.p. with C. Parvum (which may also produce amyloid in CBA/J mice) showed a reduced PGI$_2$ production from subsequently incubated macrophages.

Although there is no known relationship between amyloid and reduced PGI$_2$ production from macrophages, several reports show that prostaglandins mediate many of their effects through alteration of intracellular cAMP [4, 6, 14]. Cyclic nucleotide levels in macrophages can regulate the release of proteases capable of catabolizing SAA [15, 16]. We have found that A/J mice which are much less susceptible to experimental amyloidosis, produce more PGI$_2$ and less TXA$_2$ from their macrophages and are much slower than CBA/J macrophages to reduce their PGI$_2$ production (reflected in higher PGI$_2$/TXA$_2$ ratios) in response to _in vivo_ azocasein injections. Preliminary data (Table 2) also indicates that A/J macrophages unlike CBA/J macrophages do not alter their cAMP content in response to azocasein.

The PGI$_2$/TXA$_2$ system has been postulated to have wide biological significance in cell regulation [6]. There are several reports showing that altered PGI$_2$ production from the arterial wall may play a role in atherosclerosis. For example, species with a reduced PGI$_2$ generation in the arterial wall have a higher susceptibility to atherosclerosis [17]. We are speculating whether a susceptibility to amyloidosis may be due to similar alterations in arachidonic acid metabolism by cells of the mononuclear phagocytic system.

REFERENCES

1. K. P. W. J. McAdam and J. Sipe, Murine model for secondary amyloidosis: Genetic variability of the acute phase serum protein SAA response to endotoxins and casein, J. Exp. Med., 144, 1121-1127 (1976).
2. H. Smetana, The Relation of the reticulo-endothelial system to the formation of amyloid, J. Exp. Med., 45, 619-627 (1927).
3. G. Lavie, D. Zucker-Franklin, and E. C. Franklin, Degradation of serum amyloid protein A by surface associated enzymes of human blood monocytes, J. Exp. Med., 148, 1020-1031 (1978).
4. E. Remold-O'Donnell and H. R. Alpert, Alteration of hormone stimulated Cyclic AMP synthesis in guinea pig peritoneal macrophages, Cellular Immunol., 45, 221-229 (1979).
5. W. F. Stenson and C. W. Parker, Prostaglandins, macrophages and Immunity, J. Immunol., 125, 1-6 (1980).
6. S. Moncada and J. R. Van, Pharmacology and endogenous roles of prostaglandin endoperoxides, thrombosane A, and prostacylin, Pharmacol. Rev., 30, 293-307 (1979).
7. V. A. Ferraris, F. R. DeRobertis, R. H. Hudson, and L. Wolfe, Release of prostaglandin by mitogen and antigen stimulated leukocytes, J. Clin. Inv., 54, 378-384 (1974).
8. C. A. Leslie, Prostaglandin biosynthesis and metabolism in rat brain slices, Res. Commun. Chem. Pathol. Pharmacol., 14, 455-469 (1976).
9. C. A. Leslie, A. Pavlakis, J. Wheeler, M. Siroky, and R. J. Krane, Release of arachidonate cascase products by the rabbit bladder, Neurophysiological significance?, J. Urol., 132, 376-385 (1984).
10. C. C. Mao and A. Guidott, Anal. Biochem., 59, 64-74 (1974).
11. P. Ebbesen, Spontaneous amyloidosis in differently grouped and treated DBA/2, BALB/c, and CBA mice and thymus fibrosis in estrogen-treated BALB/c males, J. Exp. Med., 127, 387-396 (1968).
12. M. D. Bensen, M. A. Sheinberg, T. Shirahama, E. S. Cathcart, and M. Skinner, Kinetics of serum amyloid protein A in casein induced murine amyloidosis, J. Clin. Inv., 59, 412-417 (1977).
13. W. A. Scott, J. M. Zrike, A. I. Hamill, J. Kempe, and Z. A. Cohn, Activated macrophage arachidonic acid metabolism, J. Exp. Med., 155, 1148-1160 (1982).
14. I. L. Bonta, M. J. P. Adolfs, and M. W. J. A. Fieren, Cyclic AMP levels and their regulation by prostaglandins in peritoneal macrophages of rats and humans.
15. N. R. Ackerman and J. R. Beebe, Effects of Pharmacologic Agents on release of lysosomal enzymes from alveolar mononuclear cells, J. Pharmacol. Exp. Ther., 193, 603-613 (1975).
16. J. C. Khoo, E. M. Mahone, and D. Steinberg, Neutral cholesterol esterase activity in macrophages and its enhancement by cAMP dependent protein kinase, J. Biol. Chem., 256, 12659-12661 (1981).
17. H. Sinzinger, P. Clopath, K. Silberbauer, and M. Winter, Is the variation in the susceptibility of various species to atherosclerosis due to in born differences in prostacyclin (PGI_2) formation?, Experientia, 36, 321-323 (1980).

C. IN VITRO SYNTHESIS

REGULATION OF SERUM AMYLOID A SYNTHESIS IN PRIMARY

MOUSE HEPATOCYTE CULTURES*

J.D. Sipe, L.K. Chaney, E. Tatsuta,
M.F. Faber, and A.S. Cohen

Thorndike Memorial Laboratory and Division of Medicine
Boston City Hospital, The Arthritis Center
Boston University School of Medicine
Boston, Massachusetts 02118, and

Department of Internal Medicine and Clinical Toxicology
School of Medicine
University of Occupational and Environmental Health
Kitakyashbi, Japan

INTRODUCTION

Induction of serum amyloid A synthesis has been partially characterized as a sequence of cellular and molecular events involving macrophage
production of a circulating mediator Interleukin 1 (IL-1) which precedes
transcription of SAA mRNA and synthesis of SAA in liver [1]. Further
definition of these events at the molecular levels requires the use of
liver cell cultures for induction of SAA synthesis. This would permit direct analysis of the molecular chain of events that is initiated by IL-1
(or its second message) and which includes initiation and termination of
transcription and translation of SAA mRNA. In this report, we summarize
our progress toward definition of these culture conditions necessary to
mimic the in vivo situation of 1000 fold increase in SAA synthesis.

In vitro SAA synthesis has been demonstrated with hepatocytes primed
either in vivo or in vitro [2, 3, 4, 5, 6, 7, 8]. In only one case of in
vitro priming [4] with latent phase acute phase serum, rather than monokine
rich culture medium, was anything approaching the in vivo situation observed.

Our initial studies [6] were carried out with cell monolayers established for 48 h after isolation in the presence of 10% fetal calf serum.
These monolayers were then washed with serum free medium and SAA synthesis
under various culture conditions was determined. It was found that fetal
calf serum and IL-1 rich, serum free, supernatants independently stimulate
SAA production by cultured liver cells. These findings were extended to

*Supported from Grants from the U.S. Public Health Service, NIAMDD (AM 04499
and AM 07014), Multipurpose Arthritis Center, National Institutes of Health
(AM 20613), the General Clinical Research Centers Branch of the Division
of Research Resources, National Institutes of Health (RR 533), and the
Arthritis Foundation.

TABLE 1.   Effect of Normal and Acute Phase Serum on SAA Synthesis by Mouse
           Liver Cells*

Addition to Williams Medium E containing 10 mU/ml insulin	SAA ng/plate
1. None	137 ± 67
2. 10% fetal calf serum	288 ± 95
3. 10% normal human serum (SAA, 0.2 µg/ml)	240 ± 26
4. 10% acute phase human serum (SAA, 100 µg/ml)	158 ± 25
5. 10% normal mouse serum	216 ± 50
6. 10% SAA rich HDL (SAA, 250 µg/ml)	90 ± 15

*Hepatocytes were isolated [7] and established for 48 h in the presence of
10% fetal calf serum. Cells were washed and incubated with the various
sera at 10% (v/v) concentration for 24 h. Concentration of SAA (ng/35 mm
dish) was measured by radioimmunoassay [14] values expressed are the
arithemetic mean ± S.D. of the mean.

TABLE 2.   Potential Feedback Regulation of SAA Synthesis*

Source Liver Cells	SAA ng/plate		
Hours after stimulation	0-24	25-48	0-48
Normal mouse	191 ± 59	135 ± 24	228 ± 38
Acute phase mouse	210 ± 70	198 ± 42	162 ± 53

*Hepatocytes were isolated, monolayers established, and SAA measured as de-
scribed in Table 1. Culture supernatants were harvested and SAA measured
either for one 48 h period or two successive 24 h periods. Values are the
arithmetic mean ± S.D. of the mean.

TABLE 3.   Effect of Culture Conditions on SAA Synthesis by Liver Cells*

	SAA ng/µg DNA	
	Control	Stimulated
Serum present	16	80
Serum free, collagen coated	12	60
Serum free, serum pretreated	6	22

*Culture plates were either untreated, coated with native collagen [15] or
precoated with serum. SAA was determined by RIA [14] and DNA by the method
of Kissane and Robbins [16].

show that normal serum and normal mouse serum as well stimulate SAA production (Table 1). Thus there is species cross reactivity in the stimulatory
effect of serum on liver cell SAA synthesis. However, ac ute phase serum
was much less effective than normal serum and addition of SAA rich HDL resulted in less SAA synthesis than was observed for the control culture.
Further evidence for feedback inhibition of SAA synthesis is shown in Table

2. The yield of SAA from one 48 h culture was consistently less than that from two successive 24 h cultures.

It has been possible to circumvent the use of serum in the isolation of liver cells and their establishment as monolayers by using culture plates coated with collagen or fetal calf serum. After coating, the culture dishes are washed and the cells added under serum free conditions. SAA synthesis by hepatocytes cultured on collagen and serum pretreated plates was compared with liver cells cultured in the presence of fetal calf serum (Table 3). It was found that cells isolated and cultured in the absence of calf serum had reduced levels of SAA synthesis, but spontaneous SAA production could not be eliminated. Cells attached under the three conditions were able to respond to IL-1 stimulation, and those cultured in the presence of fetal calf serum exhibited the highest levels of SAA production.

Two independent studies have established that there is a major increase in the amount of translatable SAA mRNA extracted liver of acute phase stimulated as compared with unstimulated mice [9, 10]. Moreover, we have been unable, by Northern blot analysis to detect SAA mRNA in polyadenylated RNA fractions extracted from the liver of unstimulated mice.

These observations suggest that the frequently observed in vitro baseline synthesis by hepatocytes in vitro does not result from an altered regulation of translation of existing mRNA, but rather priming which occurs during the collagenase perfusion of isolation of liver cells.

The mouse model serving so well to elucidate the molecular mechanism of acute phase SAA biosynthesis is limited by the lack of a significant acute phase CRP response. This has led many laboratories to use serum amyloid P (SAP) a structurally related pentraxin as an analog for CRP in mouse. Studies of LPS treated C3H/HeJ mice suggest that the macrophage is as important to acute phase SAP elevation in mice as it is to SAA elevation. There is pronounced asynchrony in both in vivo and in vitro SAA profiles. Furthermore, synthesis of SAA and SAP has been found to differ in sensitivity to stimulation by monokines and serum in sensitivity to inhibition by cycloheximide and actinomycin D.

The recent reports of 30 fold induction of SAA mRNA transcription in the BNL cell line derived from Bab1b/C mouse embryonic liver [12] and of CRP synthesis by three human hepatoma lines [13] by supernatants of LPS-treated macrophage cultures provide an alternative to the use of primary hepatocyte cultures and promise to be particularly useful when interaction of monokines with liver cells is to be investigated.

REFERENCES

1. Sipe, J. D., Whitehead, A. S., Goldberger, G. Woo, P., Edge, M. D., Tack, B. F., Kay, R. M., Cohen, A. S., and Colten, H. R., Biochemistry (1985), in press.
2. Benditt, E. P., Hoffman, J. S., Eriksen, N., and Walsh, K. A., Ann. N.Y. Acad. Sci., 389:183 (1982).
3. Benson, M. D., and Kleiner, E., J. Immunol., 124:495-499 (1980).
4. Benson, M. D., Ann. An.Y. Acad. Sci., 389:116-120 (1982).
5. Selinger, M.J., McAdam, K. P. W. J., Kaplan, M. M., Sipe, J. D., Rosenstreich, D. L., and Vogel, S. N., Nature, 285:498-500 (1980).
6. Tatsuta, E., Shirahama, T., Sipe, J. D., Skinner, M., and Cohen, A. S., Annals N.Y. Acad. Sci., 389:467-470 (1982).
7. Tatsuta, E., Sipe, J. D., Shirahama, T., Skinner, M., and Cohen, A. S., J. Biol. Chem., 258:5414-5418 (1983).

8. Tatsuta, E., Sipe, J. D., Shirahama, T., Skinner, M., and Cohen, A. S., Arthritis and Rheumatism, 27:349-352 (1982).

9. Baumann, H., Held, W. A., and Berger, F. G., J. Biol. Chem., 259:566-573 (1984).

10. Morrow, J. F., Stearman, R. S., Peltzman, C. G., and Potter, D. A., Proc. Natl. Acad. Sci., 78:4718 (1981).

11. Sipe, J. D., in: Lymphokines, Vol. 11 (S. B. Mizel, ed.), Academic Press, New York.

12. Potter, D. A., Peltzman, C. G., and Morrow, J. F., J. Cell Biol., 99: 89a (1984).

13. Goldman, N. D., and Liu, T. Y., in: Frontiers in Biochemical and Biophysical Studies of Proteins and Membranes (T. Y. Liu, S. Sakakibara, A. N. Schecter, K. Yagi, H. Yajima, and K. T. Yasunoku, eds.), 99-107 (1983).

14. Sipe, J. D., Ignaczak, T. F., Pollack, P. S., and Glenner, G. G., J. Immunol., 116:1151-1156 (1976).

15. Obrik, B., Meth. in Enzym., 82:513-529 (1982).

16. Kissone, J. M., and Robbins, E., J. Biol. Chem., 233:184-188 (1958).

IMMUNOELECTRON MICROSCOPIC STUDY OF LIVER IN EXPERIMENTAL MURINE

AMYLOIDOSIS USING ANTI-MOUSE AA ANTISERUM

Mutsuo Takahashi, Tadaaki Yokota,
Tokuhiro Ishihara, and Fumiya Uchino

First Department of Pathology
Yamaguchi University School of Medicine
Ube, Yamaguchi, 755 Japan

ABSTRACT

With administration of amyloid-inducing agent, the synthesis of SAA
and the formation of amyloid fibrils in murine livers were examined by immunoelectron microscopy using anti-mouse AA antiserum.

The reaction products were located mainly on the microvilli of the
hepatocytes and in a few Golgi apparatus. With colchicine treatment, the
reaction products significantly increased in amount and staining intensity
in the cytoplasm of the hepatocytes. They were located within round or
oval shaped structures which were presumed to be the secretory granules derived from Golgi apparatus and some of autophagosomes.

From 24 hours to preamyloid phase (10-12 days after amyloidogenic
stimulation), Kupffer cells contained the reaction products in the phagosomes and on the surface of microvilli or pseudopods but not in the organelles concerned with protein synthesis. At 12 days, a small amount of
amyloid fibrils was detected extracellularly among the granular reaction
products in the proximity of the invaginated cytoplasm of the Kupffer cells.
At this time, amyloid fibrils surrounded by limiting membrane were seldom
detected within the cytoplasm of the Kupffer cells.

These results support the idea that SAA is synthesized by hepatocytes
and that amyloid fibrils are formed mainly extracellularly in the liver.

INTRODUCTION

Recently, synthesis of SAA by hepatocytes has been indicated by several lines of evidence obtained from hepatocyte cultures [1-3]. However,
these reports did not adequately examine how the intracytoplasmic organelles
of the hepatocytes are involved in the synthesis of SAA, and it was not
shown whether or not Kupffer cells participate in the early phase of amyloidogenesis.

This study was aimed at elucidating the precise site of SAA synthesis
and of the process of amyloid formation in murine liver at the ultrastructural level. Immunoelectron microscopy, utilizing a specific antiserum to

protein AA, has provided additional evidence to support the concept that hepatocytes are the major site of SAA synthesis. The role of Kupffer cells in the early phase of amyloidogenesis has been briefly discussed.

MATERIALS AND METHODS

Induction of SAA and Amyloidosis

Following the method of Ram et al. [4], ICR mice were given a single intraperitoneal injection of amyloid-inducing agent. Groups of ten mice were sacrificed at 6, 12, 24 h, 2, 3, 4, 5, 6, 7, 10, 12, and 14 days after the amyloidogenic stimulation. Five mice from each group were given 1 mg of colchicine in 0.2 ml saline by an intraperitoneal injection 1 or 3 h before sacrifice, and an equal volume of saline was injected intraperitoneally to the remaining five. Untreated or colchicine-treated mice were examined as controls. The liver, spleen, kidney, and lymph nodes were removed under ether anesthesia, and their fragments were fixed in a 5% buffered formalin solution. The liver specimens were also fixed in a periodate-lysine-paraformaldehyde solution or in a 2.1% glutaraldehyde solution.

Antisera

Antiserum to murine protein AA was prepared in white rabbits as previously described [5]. Normal goat serum, goat anti-rabbit immunoglobulin, and rabbit perioxidase-antiperoxidase (PAP) were obtained from DAKOPATTS (Copenhagen).

Light Microscopic Immunohistochemistry

PAP method described by Sternberger [6] was used in this study. The specificity of immunostaining was confirmed after replacing primary rabbit antiserum by non-immune rabbit serum and by antiserum absorbed with purified murine AA protein.

Ultrastructural Immunocytochemistry

Conjugation of rabbit anti-mouse AA antiserum (IgG Fab') with horseradish peroxidase was performed by the method of Wilson and Nakane [7]. Cyrostat sections of liver specimens were incubated with the peroxidase-labeled antibody for overnight at 4°C. After incubation, sections were washed and exposed to the Graham-Karnovsky solution. They were then fixed in a 1% glutaraldehyde solution for 5 min, postfixed in a 2% osmium tetroxide solution for 2 h, and embedded in Epon 812 by the inverted gelatin capsule method. Ultrathin sections stained or not stained with uranyl acetate were photographed in a Hitachi HS-8 or H-300 electron microscope.

For conventional electron microscopy, small tissue fragments from the livers were routinely processed and examined in a Hitachi H-300 electron microscope.

RESULTS

Light Microscopic Immunohistochemistry

In immunohistochemical preparations, the presence of SAA and amyloid was indicated by dark brown deposits in the livers.

At 12 h after the amyloidogenic injection, the livers showed positive

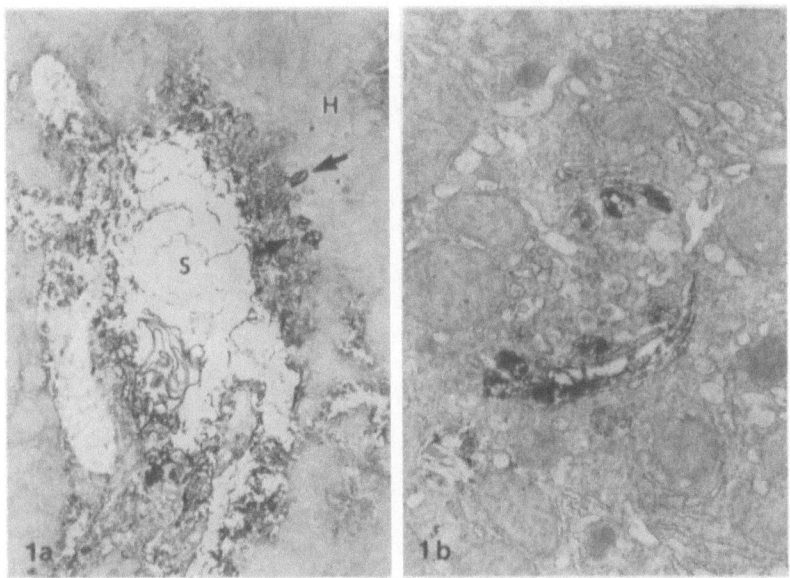

Fig. 1.   Immunoelectron micrographs of the liver at 24 h after
amyloidogenic stimulation.   a) Electron-dense precipitates of reaction products are seen on the surface
of the microvilli of hepatocytes (H) (arrows).   S -
sinusoid (×5900).   b) The reaction products are located in the cisterns and some vacuoles of the Golgi
apparatus (×18,000).

staining in the sinusoidal margins in a linear fashion.   The hepatocytes
from colchicine-treated mice were intensely stained and contained more reaction products; these products were detected as granular deposits in the
cytoplasm of the cells.   The amount and staining intensity of them in the
hepatocytes peaked between 12 and 24 h.   Thereafter, the amount of reaction
products gradually decreased.   On the 12th or 14th day, when a small amount
of amyloid deposits appeared in the liver, only small amounts of the stained
material remained in the hepatocytes.

From 24 h to preamyloid phase, the Kupffer cells occasionally contained dot-like reaction products in their cytoplasm regardless of colchicine treatment.   At 12 days, small amounts of linear or nodular accumulations of the staining were dispersely observed in the space of Disse
around the periportal areas.

No reaction product was detected in sections of the livers from untreated mice or mice treated with colchicine alone.   Sections of spleen,
kidney, and lymph nodes showed no localization of the reaction products
until amyloid deposits were detected in these organs.

Immunocytochemical Electron Microscopy

In electron microscopy, the immunoperoxidase procedure produces electron-dense precipitates which indicate the presence of SAA or amyloid
fibrils.

From 6 h to preamyloid phase, these precipitates in the liver were seen
mainly on the microvilli of the sinusoidal surface of the hepatocytes (Fig.
1a).   In contrast, very few hepatocytes contained electron-dense deposits

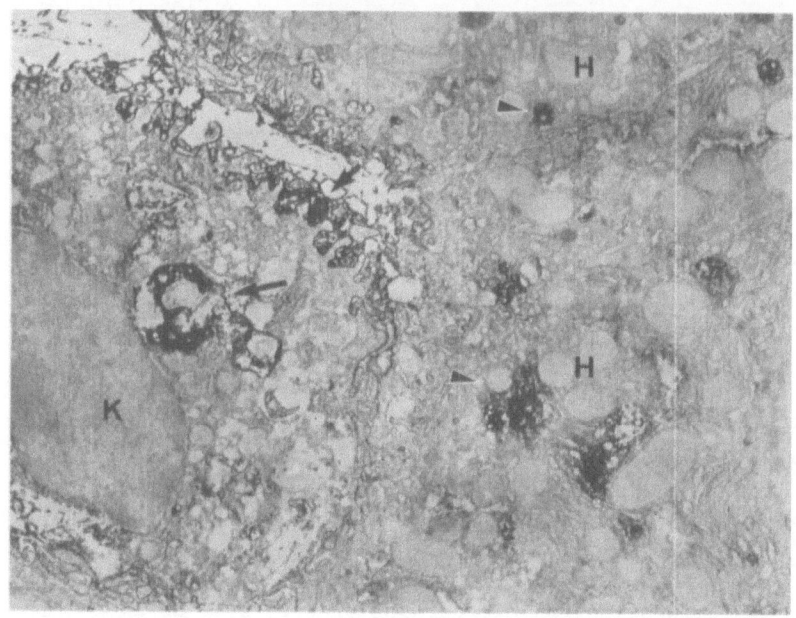

Fig. 2. Immunoelectron micrograph of the liver at 24 h after
amyloidogenic stimulation and 3 h following colchicine
treatment. The reaction products in the cytoplasm of
the hepatocyte (H) increase in amount and staining intensity (arrow heads). The Kupffer cell (K) contains
the reaction products on the invaginated cytoplasmic
membranes (short arrow) and some phagosomes (long arrow) (×8300).

in their cytoplasm; such deposits were restricted to the cisterns and some
vacuoles of the Golgi apparatus (Fig. 1b). The deposits, however, were not
clearly demonstrated in the endoplasmic reticulum of the hepatocytes.

When colchicine was administered 3 h before sacrifice, the reaction
products in the cytoplasm of the hepatocytes increased in amount and staining intensity. They were located in round or oval structures measuring
0.2–1.0 μm in diameter. By conventional electron microscopy, these structures were shown to be the secretoary granules derived from the Golgi apparatus or some autophagosomes.

In Kupffer cells, the reaction products were noted on the invaginated
cytoplasmic membranes and in some phagosomes during the observation period
of 24 h to preamyloid phase (Figs. 2, 3). At 12 days, a small amount of
amyloid fibrils was detected extracellularly among the granular reaction
products in the proximity of the invaginated cytoplasm of the Kupffer cells
(Fig. 4). At this time, amyloid fibrils, surrounded by limiting membrane
and located in close contact with lysosomal particles, were seldom detected
in the cytoplasm of the Kupffer cells. At no time was any reaction product
found in either the Golgi apparatus or the endoplasmic reticulum of the
Kupffer cells.

No reaction products were seen in control mice except for endogenous
peroxidase activity of granylocytes in the sinusoids.

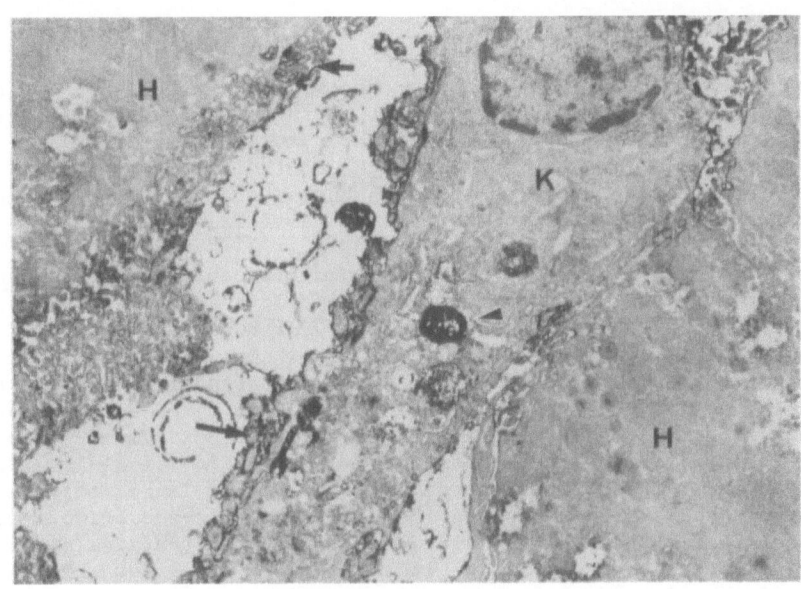

Fig. 3. At 6 days after amyloidogenic stimulation, the reaction products are located in the phagosomes (arrow
head) of the Kupffer cell (K) and on the surface microvilli of the hepatocyte (H) (short arrow) and the
Kupffer cell (long arrow) (×12,000).

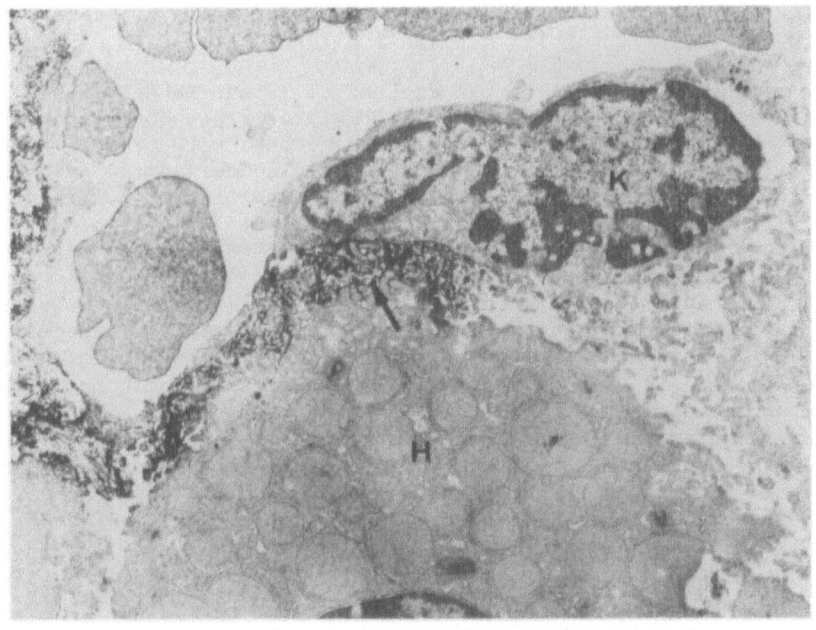

Fig. 4. At 12 days after amyloidogenic stimulation, a few amyloid fibrils (arrow) are detected extracellularly among
the granular reaction products. K) Kupffer cell, H)
hepatocyte (×12,000).

DISCUSSION

This study was aimed at determining the site of synthesis of SAA and the process of amyloid formation at the ultrastructural level. The anti-AA antiserum used in this study is specific for murine protein AA [5], and its staining specificity was confirmed in the control livers. Thus, it is reasonable to assume that the electron-dense precipitates of the immuno-labeling represent the localization of SAA and amyloid fibril.

Previous studies [1-3, 8], employing immunohistochemistry or radio-immunoassay, have demonstrated that SAA is produced in the liver by hepatocytes. The results reported here provide ultrastructural evidence to support the view that the hepatocyte is the major site of SAA synthesis. After amyloidogenic stimulation, SAA accumulated on the microvilli of hepatocytes. Although reaction products were observed in a few Golgi apparatus, they were not clearly demonstrated in the endoplasmic reticulum. Treatment of mice with colchicine induced a pronounced accumulation of SAA in the secretory granules. These findings suggest that SAA is immediately se-creted after synthesis in the hepatocytes, and that this secretion is in-hibited by colchicine. Another possible explanation is that the amount of SAA synthesized in the endoplasmic reticulum is very small, or the pre-cursor protein immediately after synthesis is antigenically different from SAA, and therefore it is not demonstrable by the method employed in our study.

It is widely accepted that the reticuloendothelial (RE) cells are in-timately involved with the genesis of amyloid [9]. Since the prime function of the RE cells are closely related to lysosomal activity, there has been speculation that lysosomes might participate in the process of amyloid for-mation [10]. This possibility was investigated by Shirahama and Cohen [11], who reported a close morphologic similarity between the lysosomal particles and the amyloid fibrils at the site of very early amyloid deposition. In this context, the localization of SAA in the Kupffer cells at an early stage of its synthesis may have significant implications.

In the present study, SAA in the Kupffer cells was largely concentrated in the phagosomes and on the surface of microvilli or pseudopods, and it was not demonstrated in the cell organelles concerned with protein synthe-sis. These findings imply that the Kupffer cells do not participate in the production of SAA. This is in agreement with the results of Selinger and co-workers [1] who, in a primary isolated cell culture system, clearly demonstrated the synthesis of SAA solely by hepatocytes. Based on the above considerations, the present findings are best interpreted as repre-senting the uptake of SAA by the Kupffer cells. It is suggested that the Kupffer cells play an important role in an early stage of amyloidogenesis in the liver. In this study, however, a small amount of amyloid fibrils was detected extracellularly among the granular reaction products in the proximity of the invaginated cytoplasm of the Kupffer cells. Furthermore, amyloid fibrils surrounded by limiting membrane were rarely detected in the cytoplasm of the Kupffer cells. Thus, although the results of our study are inconclusive, we suggest that SAA transforms to amyloid fibrils prefer-entially in the extracellular space and rarely within the cytoplasm of Kupffer cells.

ACKNOWLEDGEMENTS

We thank Dr. N. Matsumoto, Yamaguchi University, for his helpful comments on the manuscript, and Dr. K. Watanabe and his associates, Tokai University, for their pertinent advice. Supported by a Grant-in-Aid for Scientific Research of the Ministry of Education and a Research Grant for Scientific Disease from the Ministry of Health and Welfare.

REFERENCES

1. M. J. Selinger, K. P. W. J. McAdam, M. M. Kaplan, J. D., Sipe, S. N. Vogel, and D. L. Rosentreich, Nature (London), 285, 498 (1980).
2. J. S. Hoffman and E. P. Benditt, J. Biol. Chem., 257, 10518 (1982).
3. E. Tatsuta, T. Shirahama, J. D. Sipe, M. Skinner, and A. S. Cohen, Ann. N. Y. Acad. Sci., 389, 467 (1982).
4. J. S. Ram, R. A. DeLellis, and G. G. Glenner, Int. Arch. Allergy, 34, 201 (1968).
5. N. Imada, Yamaguchi Med. J., 30, 149 (1981).
6. L. A. Sternberger, P. H. Hardy, Jr., J. J. Cuculis, and H. G. Meyer, J. Histochem. Cytochem., 18, 315 (1970).
7. M. B. Wilson and P. K. Nakane, in: Immunofluorescence and Related Staining Techniques, Elsevier, Ed., North Holland Biomedical (1978), p. 107.
8. M. D. Benson and E. Kleiner, J. Immunol., 124, 495 (1980).
9. G. G. Glenner, W. D. Terry, and C. Isersky, Semin. Hematol., 10, 65 (1973).
10. F. Uchino, Acta Pathol. Jpn., 17, 49 (1967).
11. T. Shirahama and A. S. Cohen, Am. J. Pathol., 73, 97 (1973).

IMMUNOCYTOCHEMICAL STUDIES ON THE SITE OF SYNTHESIS

AND PATHWAYS OF AMYLOID PROTEIN AA*

Tsuranobu Shirahama, Martha Skinner,
Alan S. Cohen, and Orville G. Rodgers

The Arthritis Center
Boston University School of Medicine, and

The Thorndike Memorial Laboratory
and The Division of Medicine
Boston City Hospital
Boston, Massachusetts

ABSTRACT

CBA/J mice received a single subcutaneous injection of casein to provoke an acute phase response, then were sacrificed at predetermined times up to 48 h. The livers were fixed in situ with 4.0% paraformaldehyde-0.1% gluaraldehyde, and processed for immunocytochemistry against anti-mouse AA using peroxidase-antiperoxidase, avidin-biotin-peroxidase, and protein A-gold methods. The composite results of the light and electron microscopic observations revealed three major findings. 1) Primary localization of the reaction was in the hepatocyte cytoplasm and peaked at 6-8 h after the casein injection. Only certain selective hepatocyes, which were scattered over the lobule, showed this type of reaction, suggesting heterogeneity of the hepatocyte population in participation in AA synthesis. 2) In the cytoplasm, the reaction was localized on and/or in the rough endoplasmic reticulum, and the single membrane bound vesicles, vacuoles and lamellae including the Golgi complex, confirming that protein AA follows the common intracellular routes of synthesis and secretion established for other proteins. 3) The reaction was also observed on the free surface of the hepatocyte membrane including the microvilli. This reaction appeared as early as but lasted at least several hours longer than its cytoplasmic counterpart, suggesting that some retention exists before the release of AA-reactive substance from the cellular surface.

---

*Supported by grants from the United States Public Health Serve, National Institute of Arthritis, Diabetes, Digestive, and Kidney Disease (AM-04599 and AM-07014), National Institutes of Health Multipurpose Arthritis Center (AM-20613), the General Clinical Research Centers Branch of the Division of Research Resources, National Institutes of Health (RR-533) and the Arthritis Foundation.

INTRODUCTION

Recent studies have elaborated considerable details of the immunology, biochemistry, and molecular biology of the synthesis of SAA, the putative precursor of amyloid fibril protein AA and an acute phase reactant, and have established the concept that SAA is biosynthesized primarily in the liver and more specifically in the hepatocytes [1-6]. Nevertheless, credible morphologic evidence concerning this mechanism has so far been lacking.

The present report concerns our immunocytochemical studies on the loclization of the anti-AA reactive substance in the livers of mice with acute phase reactions.

MATERIALS AND METHODS

Each of 8-week old female CBA/J mice (Jackson Laboratories, Bar Harbor, Maine) was given a single subcutaneous injection of 0.5 ml of 10% casein solution. Groups of 3 mice were sacrificed at 0, 2, 4, 6, 8, 12, 16, 16, 24, or 48 h after the casein injection. Three mice were also sacrificed after receiving 30 daily casein injections [7] and then a 2-week pause period.

At sacrifice, each animal was anesthetized with an intraperitoneal injection of chloral hydrate (0.36 gm/kg), and was perfused via the adbominal vena cava with 25 ml of phosphate buffered physiological saline followed by 50 ml of 4.0% paraformaldehyde - 0.1% glutaraldehyde in 0.1 M phosphate buffer pH 7.4. Three tissue blocks not exceeding 3 mm in thickness were excised from each liver and were immersed in the same fixative for 2 h at room temperature. They were rinsed in 0.1 M phosphate buffer pH 7.4 and exposed to 1% sodium borohydrate in the same buffer for 2 h at room temperature [8].

One of the three tissue blocks was then embedded in paraffin in a routine manner. Immunohistochemical procedure was applied to a 4-micron section mounted on a microscope slide.

The second tissue block was immersed in 5% glycerol - 10% sucrose in the phosphate buffer for 2 h and then in 10% glycerol - 20% sucrose overnight for a purpose of cryoprotection. The tissue was then frozen at liquid nitrogen temperature and thawed. After rinsed in the phosphate buffer, 50 micron tissue slices were cut from the block on a Sorvall TC-2 tissue sectioner and were processed for immunocytochemistry. After the immunocytochemical staining, the tissue slices were postfixed with 2% osmium tetroxide in the same phosphate for 1 h at room temperature, and embedded in Araldite 502. Thin sections were mounted on a bare copper grid and examined in a Siemens Elmiskop I without further staining.

The last of the three tissue blocks was cut into smaller pieces. An aliquot of the small tissue pieces were postfixed in 2% osmium tetroxide in the phosphate buffer for 2 h at room temperature, and were then embedded, along with another aliquot which did not receive postfixation, in Araldite 502 through a routine procedure. The immunocytochemical reaction was carried out on the thin sections mounted on a bare nickel grid. The sections were then examined, with optional staining with 4% osmium tetroxide, in a Siemens Elmiskop I electron microscope.

The immunocytochemical reaction against anti-AA was carried out using one of the three antibody bridging methods: the peroxidase-antiperoxidase technique [9], the avidin-biotin-peroxidase complex [10], or the protein A-gold method [11].

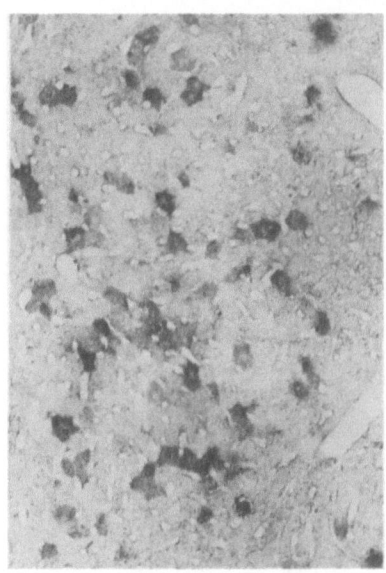

Fig. 1.   Light micrograph of a
CBA/J mouse liver, 6 h
after recieving a casein
injection. Immunohisto-
chemical preparation re-
acted against anti-mouse
AA. Positive reaction
is primarily localized
in the cytoplasm of the
selective hepatocytes
that are scattered over
the lobule. 130×.

Procedural contols were run by replacing the primary antiserum (rabbit anti-mouse AA) with normal rabbit serum or the primary antiserum absorbed with mouse serum with a high SAA level. Tissues from normal (0 h) and amyloidotic (30 daily casein injections) mouse livers were included in each processing as baseline and positive controls.

Antiserum to mouse AA was prepared in rabbits as previously described [12]. Peroxidase-antiperoxidase complex, goat anti-rabbit IgG, normal goat serum and normal rabbit serum were obtained from Cappel Laboratories, Cochranville, Pennsylvania, avidin, biotinylated horseradish peroxidase and biotinylated goat anti-rabbit IgG from Vector Labotories, Burlingame, California, and protein A-gold particles from Polysciences, Warrington, Pennsylvania.

RESULTS

The light microscopy and the electron microscopic survey of the present preparations revealed the following findings.

The control preparations where the primary antiserum had been replaced with normal rabbit serum or the primary antiserum absorbed with SAA-rich mouse serum showed no significant deposition of the reaction products.

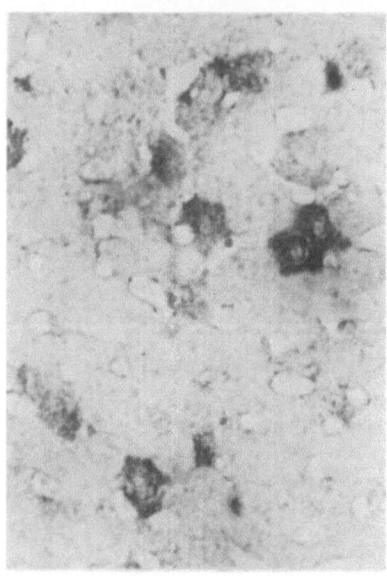

Fig. 2. A higher magnification
of an area of Fig. 1.
The cells with positive
reaction bear typical
morphologic character-
istics of the hepa-
tocyte. 330×.

In the livers from the mice that had received 30 daily casein injections and treated for immunocytochemical demonstration of anti-AA reaction,
very heavy deposition of the reaction products was localized on the amyloid
deposits.

The tissue sections from the untreated mice (at the 0 h of the casein
injection scheme) did not show any appreciable reaction against anti-AA.

In the preparations from the mice in acute phase response (2-48 h after
the casein injection), there were two major localizations of the immunocytochemical reaction against anti-AA, i.e., in the hepatocyte cytoplasm
and on the surface membrane. Only certain hepatocytes that were randomly
spread in the lobules showed the cytoplasmic reactions (Figs. 1 and 2).
The cytoplasmic reaction to the anti-AA started to be recognized at 2-4 h
after the casein injection, peaked in intensity and the number of cells involved at 6-h, and became minimal or unrecognizable at 24-48 h. The reaction on the surface membrane appeared as early as the cytoplasmic reaction,
was heaviest at 12-16 h, and still remained at 24-48 h.

Further electron microscopic analysis disclosed that the reaction products in the cytoplasm of the hepatocytes were localized on the membrane and
the attached ribosomes of the rough endoplasmic reticulum (RER), and in the
lumina of the RER, the smooth endoplasmic reticulum, the Golgi apparatus
and the single membrane bound vesicles and vacuoles. No significant reaction products were detected in and/or on other cell organelles, namely the
nucleus, mitochondria, etc. (Figs. 3-5).

About the RER, the reaction products were localized mainly on the attached ribosomes and the membrane, but also were observed on occasions in

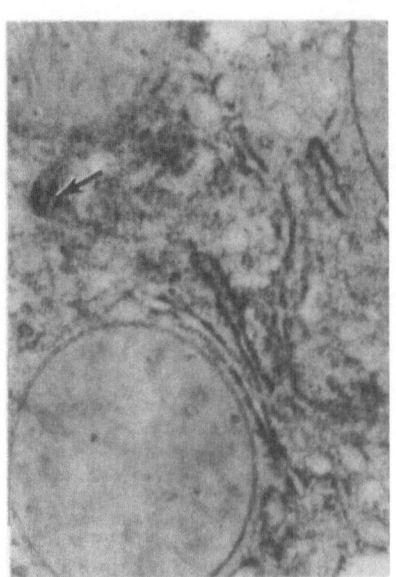 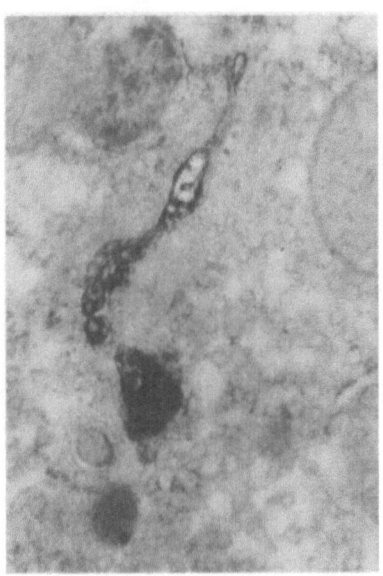

Fig. 3. Electron micrograph of
a hepatocyte of a CBA/J
mouse sacrificed 6 h
after receiving a casein
injection. Immunocyto-
chemically reacted
against anti-AA. The
reaction is localized
mainly on the attached
ribosomes and the mem-
brane of the rough
endoplasmic reticulum,
and occasionally in the
cisternae (arrow).
40,000×.

Fig. 4. Same preparation as
Fig. 3, showing an area
containing a Golgi ap-
paratus which is heavily
deposited with the reac-
tion products. 40,000×.

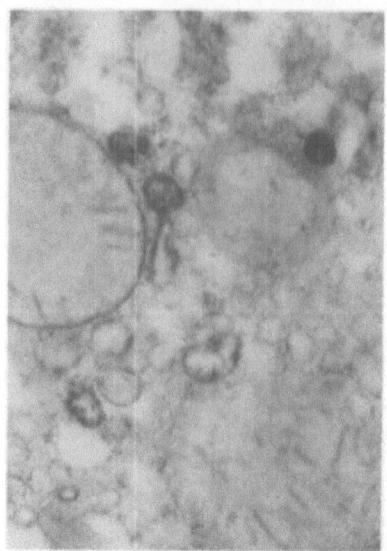 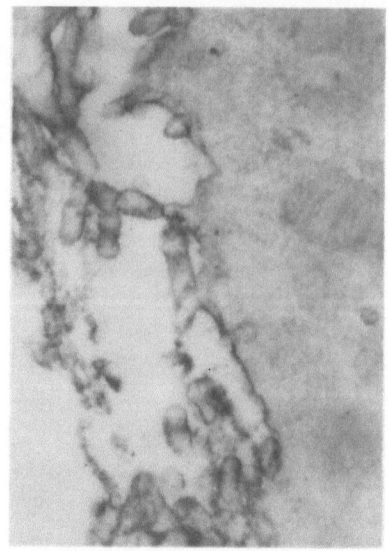

Fig. 5. Similar preparation as Figs. 3 and 4. In the peripheral cytoplasm, the contents of cytoplasmic vesicles show positive reaction. 40,000×.

Fig. 6. Electron micrograph of the sinusoidal surface of a hepatocyte of a CBA/J mouse, 16 h after a casein injection. Immunoperoxidase staining against anti-AA. The sinusoidal surface of the anti-AA reactive substance. 25,000×.

the cisternae. The cisternae of the RER were seen very rarely to be completely filled with the reaction products (Fig. 3). The SER containing the reaction products was also occasionally identified. The Golgi apparatus was often easily identifiable, for it was heavily deposited with the reaction products (Fig. 4).

Single membrane bound vesicles and vacuoles also displayed positive reaction to anti-AA. The contents with the positive reaction often filled completely the lumina of smaller vesicles, but only partially larger vesicles and vacuoles (Fig. 5).

The surface of the plasma membrane including the microvilli facing the sinusoid was often observed as if being coated with the reaction products (Fig. 6).

DISCUSSION

In the light of the current concept on the metabolism and the antigenicity of protein AA (including SAA) [13, 14], the localizations of the AA-reactive substance that were revealed in the present study in the livers from the mice in the acute phase response may reasonably be attributed to the newly synthesized AA proteins, presumably in the form of SAA. In this context, the present results can be interpreted in the following ways.

The unequivocal demonstration of the anti-AA reaction in the cytoplasm of the hepatocytes confirms, with perhaps the most direct evidence thus far, the identity of the heptatocytes as the specific cells that biosynthesize protein AA.

The localization of the anti-AA reaction only to certain hepatocytes supports the concept that participation of the hepatocyte population in the AA synthesis is not universal but a heterogeneity exists. Furthermore, because of its nature as an acute phase reactant, SAA has often been compared with another well-known, well-studied acute phase reactant, C-reactive protein (CRP) [3, 5, 15-18]. Anti-CRP reaction was observed in selective hepatocyte which were localized predominantly in the periportal and perilobular areas in rabbits being studied under experimental conditions comparable to our study [15, 16]. This distribution of the hepatocytes is different from that observed in the present study of the anti-AA reaction, and suggests that different populations of hepatocytes are involved in the synthesis of these two proteins.

The time sequential changes of the levels of biosynthetic activity of protein AA have not been directly available except from data such as fluctuation of the serum SAA levels and of the SAA content of the liver cell cultures which indicate only indirectly the levels of synthesis [3, 5, 6, 19, 20]. The time-sequential changes of the anti-AA reaction localized in the hepatocytic cytoplasm clearly demonstrated in the present study may be the first direct data and suggest that the synthesis peaks at 6-8 h after the stimulus.

The localization of the anti-AA reaction in and/or on the RER, the Golgi apparatus, the vesicles and the vacuoles confirms that amyloid protein AA follows the common routes of synthesis and intracellular pathways established for other proteins [21], including CRP (despite the fact that different hepatocyte populations may be involved in CRP and AA biosynthesis).

The accumulation of the AA-reactive substance on the free surface of the hepatocyte plasma membrane may require a different interpretation. This appeared as early as but peaked and disappeared at least several hours later than its cytoplasmic counterpart. This observation may suggest simply that the AA-related substance which had been newly synthesized and transported to the cell surface was retained there for a considerable period of time. This retention can be explained in several ways. First, apoSAA is known to be rather hydrophobic. Therefore it is possible that newly synthesized apoSAA travels the intracellular channels of secretion attaching closely to the membrane, and is brought to the cell surface still remaining to be attached to the membrane. In order to float in the plasma freely, it may need to be associated with lipoprotein [2], and therefore the several hour lapse mentioned above may represent the waiting time for the association. Other possibilities would be: 1) that the anti-AA reaction on the hepatocyte surface represents the sites of special SAA receptors, 2) that, even without special receptors, the plasma membrane has the ability (physical and/or chemical) to attract SAA, and 3) that it is an artifactual localization and simply represents the SAA concentration in the plasma.

REFERENCES

1.   M. D. Benson and E. Kleiner, J. Immunol., 124, 495 (1980).
2.   J. S. Hoffman and E. P. Benditt, J. Biol. Chem., 257, 10518 (1982).
3.   K. P. W. J. McAdam et al., Ann. N. Y. Acad. Sci., 389, 126 (1982).
4.   J. F. Morrow et al., Proc. Natl. Acad. Sci., 78, 4718 (1981).
5.   J. D. Sipe et al., Ann. N. Y. Acad. Sci., 389, 137 (1982).
6.   E. Tatsuta et al., J. Biol. Chem., 258, 5414 (1983).
7.   T. Shirahama and A. S. Cohen, Am. J. Path., 99, 539 (1980).
8.   W. D. Eldred et al., J. Histochem. Cytochem., 31, 285 (1983).

9. L. A. Sternberger, Immunocytochemistry, 2nd ed. John Wiley and Sons, New York (1979), p. 354.

10. S. M. Hsu and L. Raine, in: Advances in Immunohistochemistry (R. A. DeLellis, ed.), Masson Publishing USA, New York (1984), pp. 31-42.

11. J. Roth, in: Advances in Immunohistochemistry (R. A. DeLellis, ed.), Mason Publishing USA (1984), pp. 43-65.

12. M. Skinner et al., Lab. Invest., 36, 420 (1977).

13. A. S. Cohen et al., Lab. Invest., 48, 1 (1983).

14. T. Shirahama et al., in: Advances in Immunohistochemistry (R. A. DeLellis, ed.), Mason Publishing USA (1984), pp. 277-302.

15. I. Kishner and G. Feldman, J. Exp. Med., 148, 466 (1978).

16. S. S. Macintyre et al., Ann. N. Y. Acad. Sci., 389, 76 (1982).

17. K. P. W. J. McAdam et al., J. Clin. Invest., 61, 390 (1978).

18. P. S. Weinstein et al., Scand. J. Immunol., 19, 193 (1984).

19. E. P. Benditt et al., Ann. N. Y. Acad. Sci., 389, 183 (1982).

20. M. D. Benson et al., J. Clin. Invest., 59, 412 (1977).

21. G. Palade, Science, 189, 347 (1975).

A COMPARISON OF SERUM AMYLOID A (SAA) SYNTHESIS WITH THAT OF THE PENTRAXINS:

SERUM AMYLOID P (SAP) AND C-REACTIVE PROTEIN (CRP)*

Emiko Tatsuta†, Jean D. Sipe‡,
Tsuranobu Shirahama‡, Martha Skinner‡,
and Alan S. Cohen‡

‡Arthritis and Connective Tissue Disease Section
 Boston University School of Medicine
 Boston, Massachusetts 02118

†Department of Internal Medicine and Clinical Toxicology
 School of Medicine
 University of Occupational and Environmental Health
 Kitakyushu, Japan

ABSTRACT

Serum amyloid A (SAA) and serum amyloid P (SAP) were detected in cultures of hepatocytes which had been isolated from normal CBA/J mice by the collagenase perfusion technique. SAP production in 24 h cultures was more resistant than SAA and total protein synthesis to inhibition by actinomycin D, but was more sensitive to inhibition by 48 h. However, the production of SAP was more sensitive to cycloheximide than SAA and total protein throughout the 48 h incubation period. SAP and SAA levels in the culture media were suppressed by treatment of liver cells with 10^{-6} M of colchicine for 48 h. Inhibition of SAP production by colchicine was the same regardless of culture condition, but the effect of colchicine on SAA synthesis varied according to the presence of serum of monokine. These observations also support the concept that the two amyloid proteins are produced under different regulatory mechanisms. When C-reactive protein (CRP) was not detected in the sera of patients with severe chronic liver diseases, the SAA levels were very low. When CRP was detected, SAA values were within the normal range. Thus, in order to produce SAA, liver cells in these patients not only were viable but also maintained their specialized function.

*Supported by grants from the United States Public Health Service, National Institute of Arthritis, Diabetes, Digestive Kidney Disease (AM-04599 and AM-07014), National Institutes of Health Multipurpose Arthritis Center (AM-20613), the General Clinical Research Certers Branch of the Division of Research Resources, National Institute of Health (RR-533) and the Arthritis Foundation.

INTRODUCTION

Experimental murine amyloidosis induced by the chronic subcutaneous injection of casein, LPS, is a model of human secondary amyloidosis [1-3]. The elevation of serum amyloid A (SAA) [4] and serum amyloid P (SAP) [5] in the mouse have been studied as part of the sequence of events called the acute phase response which follows inflammatory stimulation. SAA is identified by its structural and antigenic relationship to the fibrillar protein amyloid A (AA) of the secondary amyloidosis [6, 7]. The hepatic synthesis of SAA has been confirmed in vitro by hepatocyte cultures from livers of casein and endotoxin treated mice [8, 9] and from livers of normal mice upon treatment with interleukin 1 rich macrophage supernatant and with latent period serum from LPS-treated mice [10].

Serum amyloid P (SAP) is identical to the pentraxin amyloid P that is defined as a significant constituent of all amyloid deposits [11, 12]. Histochemical studies with normal and casein treated mice suggest that liver is the major site of SAP production [13]. Our previous studies showed that SAP was produced by cultured hepatocyes from CBA/J and C3H/HeJ mice and unlike SAA was minimally stimulated with IL-1 rich macrophage supernatants [14].

The biosynthesis of SAA and SAP in vivo exhibits asynchronous acute phase profiles with respect to concentration and duration after inflammatory stimulation [15]. Our previous studies have also shown that production of SAA and SAP in vitro appear to be controlled under the different regulatory mechanism in their response to stimulation with macrophage supernatant, fetal calf serum and their susceptibility to cycloheximide [16].

In this study we sought to compare the sensitivity of in vitro SAA and SAP synthesis to actinomycin D with our earlier observations.

MATERIALS AND METHODS

Preparation of Hepatocyte Cultures

Hepatocyte cultures were prepared from livers of CBA/J mice by the perfusion technique with 50 µ/ml of collagenase type 1 (Sigman Chemical Company, St. Louis, Missouri) [17]. Two ml of cell (0.5 × 10^5/ml were incubated in 35/10 mm tissue culture plates (Falcon 3001) with a medium consisting of Williams-E medium containing 10% of fetal calf serum and 10 mU/ml of insulin. Cultures were established for 48 h and washed twice by the medium without serum just before use. After cultivation with the test media, cultures were frozen, thawed and centrifuged at 800 × g for 15 min, and suspensions were lyophilized and measured for SAP and SAA [16].

Measurement of SAA, SAP, and Protein

SAA was measured with a solid phase competitive binding assay employing mouse or human ^{125}I-AA and the respective affinity purified anti-AA antibodies [18]. Human serum was heat denatured at 60°C for one hour. SAP was measured in a similar radioimmunassay using ^{125}I-AP and affinity purified anti-AP antibodies [15]. Total protein synthesis was measured by the incorporation of [^{3}H-leucine] into TCA precipitable material [19], and exposed as dpm per plate.

Preparation of Interleukin 1 (IL-1) Rich Macrophage Supernatant

Peritoneal excudate cells from CBA/J mice activated by thioglycollate were exposed to 5 µg/ml E. coli K235 LPS in serum free RPMI 1640 for 48 h [20].

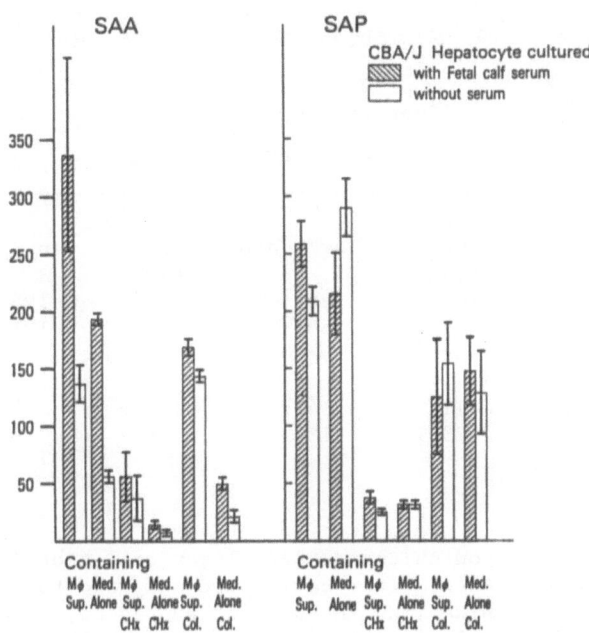

Fig. 1. Different effect of serum on serum amyloid protein synthesis. Each culture
condition was carried out with triplicate
plates of established CBA/J liver cells
and incubated for 48 h in Williams medium E plus 10 mU/ml of insulin (medium
alone, to which was added, either 10%
fetal calf serum, 10% LPS-treated CBA/J
macrophage supernatants (Msup), 30 μg/ml
of cycloheximide (CHx), or 10^{-6} colchicine.
Serum amyloid A (SAA) and serum amyloid
P (SAP) were measured for individual
plates by a solid phase radioimmunoassay and arithmetic mean − S.D. is shown.

Preparation of Human Sera and Measurement of CRP

Human sera were obtained from the patients with liver disease diagnosed
by the pathological examination, stored at −20°C prior to testing. CRP concentration were measured by a capillary precipitin test [21].

RESULTS

SAA synthesis by established cultures which were incubated for 48 h
were enhanced two fold by IL-1 rich macrophage supernatants and by 10% fetal
calf serum and was stimulated additively 5-fold by serum and monokine together. On the other hand, the serum had little effect on SAP production.
The stimulatory effect of monokine rich macrophage supernatant was minimal
(Fig. 1).

Effect of Cycloheximide on Serum Amyloid Protein Production

Protein synthesis was effectively inhibited by 30 μg/ml of cycloheximide (CHx) and the uptake of [^{3}H]-leucine for the total protein synthesis
was reduced to 92% in the presence of the inhibitor. The effect of CHx on

TABLE 1. Effect of Cycloheximide on Cultured CBA/J Liver Cell Protein
Synthesis*

	Liver cell protein					
	SAA		SAP		Total protein	
Cultured with medium	ng/plate	% production	ng/plate	% production	ng/plate	% production
alohe	156 ± 93	100	224 ± 46	100	195 ± 50	100
10% M$_\phi$ supernatant	220 ± 56	141	259 ± 91	115	191 ± 66	97.9
CHx	18 ± 7	11.5	14 ± 5	6.2	15 ± 6	7.6
CHx and 10% M$_\phi$ supernatant	36 ± 38	23.1	15 ± 12	6.7	16 ± 17	8.2

*Effect of cycloheximide on cultured CBA/J liver cell protein synthesis
Triplicate established CBA/J liver cells were cultured for 24 h with serum
free Williams medium E plus insulin to which was added, either or both 10%
M supernatants or 30 µg/ml of cycloheximide. Each value was determined
from separate experiments. SAA and SP concentration was determined for
individual plates. Total protein synthesis was measured according to
[^{3}H]-leucine uptake for individual plates.

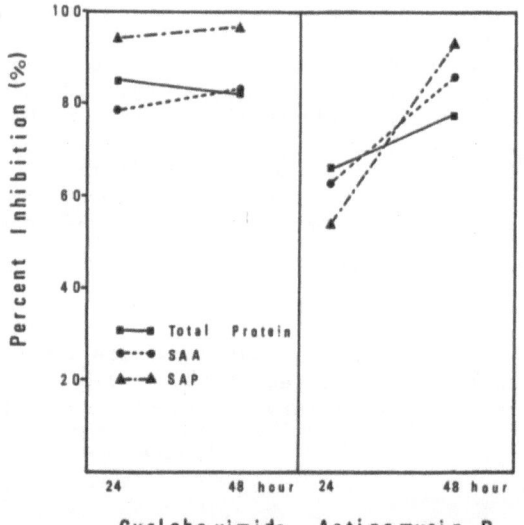

Fig. 2. Effect of actinomycin D and cycloheximide on amyloid protein synthesis.
2 µg/ml of actinomycin D or 30 µg/ml
of cycloheximide was added to the established heptatocyte cultures and
cells were incubated for the indicate
period of time. SAA, SAP, and total
protein measured by the same procedure
described other experiment. Percent
inhibition was calculated from average of two different experiments.

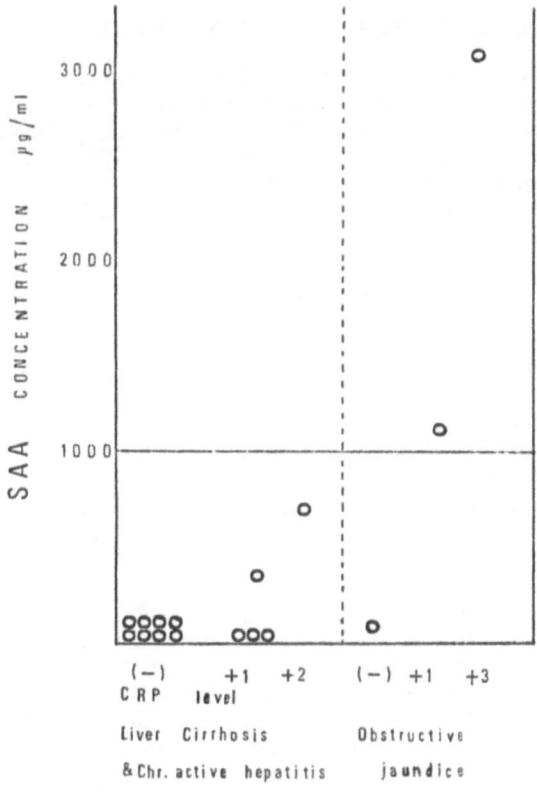

Fig. 3. Serum amyloid A levels in sera
from patients with liver dysfunction. SAA levels were measured
by radioimmunoassay. CRP concentrations were determined by
a capillary precipitin test.
+1, +2, +3 in the capillary
precipitin test indicated respectively, less than 8, 20 to
34, and 56 µg/ml. The horizontal line depicts boundaries between absence of inflammation
and mild inflammation.

SAP production was similar to that on total protein synthesis. On the contrary, the inhibition of SAA synthesis was less than that of SAP and total
protein especially in the presence of monokine (Table 1).

The Effect of Actinomycin D (AD) on Serum Amyloid Protein

The inhibition of SAP synthesis by 2 µg/ml of AD 54% at 24 h, compared
with 62% and 66% respectively for SAA and total protein synthesis. On the
other hand, the blockage of SAP synthesis by 30 µg/ml of CHx from the same
liver was 94% at 24 h and was more susceptible than SAA and total protein,
similar as previous experiment. At 48 h, the reduction of SAP by AD was
equivalent to that of CHx (Fig. 2).

The Effect of Colchicine on Amyloid Protein (Fig. 1)

Colchicine at the concentration of 10^{-6} M inhibited approximately 50% of SAA production by the cultures which were stimulated with IL-1 rich macrophage supernatant and fetal calf serum, but suppressed minimally that by the cultures with the supernatant alone. The 40% of SAP production was inhibited by the concentration of colchicine which was added to the cultures either with or without the monokine rich supernatant and fetal calf serum.

SAA and CRP Levels in Patients with Liver Dysfunction

SAA level, were measured in sera of patients with liver dysfunction and compared with the relation to the level of C-reactive protein (CRP) (Fig. 3). SAA levels in many patients with severe liver dysfunction like liver cirrhosis or chronic active hepatitis were extremely low and even when CRP was detected were minimally elevated within noninflammatory range. However, the SAA levels in sera of transitional obstructive jaundice elevated in proportion to the concentration of CRP to the inflammatory level.

DISCUSSION

The synthesis of SAA was markedly enhanced by IL-1 rich macrophage supernatant and fetal calf serum, in contrast to SAP was minimally influenced by those substances. Although previous experiments have confirmed that SAA in mouse is induced by IL-1, the stimulatory effect of fetal calf serum indicates that IL-1 may not be the only enhancer of SAA synthesisis in hepatocytes [16]. Moreover, SAA response to the IL-1 was stimulated only 200% in our in vitro system, this is quite lower than in vivo system, in which SAA has elevated 1000 fold to the normal SAA concentration [4, 15]. Previous experiments indicated that the lower SAA response in vitro results from high production following the traumatic isolation [16]. Long-term colchicine treatment has been used in the therapy of amyloidosis [24, 25]. The results of this study suggest that the mechanism of its action may not be blockage of protein secretion but rather may be reduction of protein synthesis. In this study the inhibition of SAA production by the colchicine was different in each culture condition varying presence of serum, monokines and colchicine. This might be due to each culture condition having a different effect upon the binding capacity of colchicine to cells.

This study presents another aspect of lower SAA response. In vivo SAA levels were very low in sera of CRP negative patients with severe chronic liver dysfunction and were within normal range in patients with positive CRP. In contrast, sera from patients with mild transient liver dysfunction by obstructive jaundice were elevated to mild inflammatory range in the proportion to CRP concentration. This suggests that the chronically injured livers did not sufficiently produce SAA and did not release it in spite of the inflammatory stimulation. In order to produce SAA, liver cells might be required to be viable and maintain their specialized function.

Two μg/ml of actinomycin D which is an inhibitor of mRNA synthesis blocked SAA, SAP, and total protein synthesis. The inhibitions of amyloid protein synthesis was lower than that of total protein at 24 h, and that was converted at 48 h. This might suggest that mRNA accumulated in the hepatocytes before the effect of AD on the cultures. In contrast the synthesis of SAP was more resistant to actinomycin D at 24 h than that of SAA and total protein. The differences of sensitivity between both amyloid proteins was found in the inhibition of their production to cycloheximide [16]. A recent study indicates that synthesis α_1-acid glycoprotein and other acute phase reactants in rat liver is regulated by different mechanisms [22]. This experiment also supported that the synthesis of SAP and SAA were regulated by the different productive mechanisms.

REFERENCES

1. R. Baumal, A. Acherkmann, and B. Wilson, J. Immunol., 114:1785 (1975).
2. A. S. Cohen and T. Shirahama, Am. J. Pathol., 68:441 (1972).
3. M. Skinner, T. Shirahama, M. D. Benson, and A. S. Cohen, Lab. Invest., 36:420 (1977).
4. K. P. W. J. McAdam and J. D. Sipe, J. Exp. Med., 144:1121-1127 (1976).
5. M. D. Pepys, M. Baltz, K. Gomer, A. J. S. Davis, and M. Doenhoff, Nature, 278:259-261 (1979).
6. E. P. Benditt, N. Erikson, M. A. Hermodson, and L. H. Ericcson, FEBS Letter, 16:169 (1971).
7. M. Levin, M. Pras, and E. C. Franklin, J. Exp. Med., 138:373 (1973).
8. M. D. Benson and E. Kleiner, J. Immunol., 124:495 (1980).
9. E. P. Benditt, J. S. Hoffman, N. Eriksen, and K. A. Walsh, Ann. N.Y. Acad. Sci., 389:183 (1982).
10. M. J. Selinger, K. P. W. J. McAdam, M. M. Kaplan, J. D. Sipe, S. N. Vogel, and D. L. Rosenstreich, Nature (London), 285:498 (1980).
11. E. S. Cathcart, F. R. Comerford, and A. S. Cohen, New Engl. J. Med., 273:143 (1965).
12. H. A. Bladen, M. U. Nylen, and G. G. Glenner, J. Ultrastruct. Res., 14:449 (1966).
13. M. L. Baltz, R. F. Dyck, and M. B. Pepys, Immunology, 41:59 (1980).
14. E. Tatsuta, T. Shirahama, J. D. Sipe, M. Skinner, and A. S. Cohen, Ann. N.Y. Acad. Sci., 389:467 (1982).
15. J. D. Sipe, S. N. Vogel, M. B. Sztein, M. Skinner, and A. S. Cohen, Ann. N.Y. Acad. Sci., 389:137 (1982).
16. E. Tatsuta, J. D. Sipe, T. Shirahama, M. Skinner, and A. S. Cohen, J. Biol. Chem., 285:5414 (1983).
17. P. O. Seglen, Exp. Cell Res., 82:391 (1973).
18. J. D. Sipe, T. F. Ignaczak, P. S. Pollock, and G. G. Glenner, J. Immunol., 116:1151 (1976).
19. C. E. Brinkerhoff, R. M. McMillan, J. V. Faley, and E. D. Harris, Jr., Arthritis Rheum., 22:1109 (1979).
20. J. D. Sipe, S. N. Vogel, J. L. Ryan, K. P. W. J. McAdam, and M. D. Rosenstreich, J. Exp. Med., 150:597 (1979).
21. H. C. Anderson and M. McCarty, Amer. J. Med., 8:455 (1950).
22. H. Baumann, G. L. Firestone, T. L. Burgess, K. W. Gross, K. R. Yomamoto, and W. A. Held, J. Biol. Chem., 258:573 (1983).
23. E. Tatsuta, J. D. Sipe, T. Shirahama, M. Skinner, and A. S. Cohen, Arthritis Rheum., 27:349 (1984).
24. D. Zemer, M. Pras, and E. Sohar, New Engl. J. Med., 294:170 (1976).
25. A. Rubinow, A. S. Cohen, H. Kayne, and C. A. Libbey, Arthritis Rheum. (Suppl.), 24:S124 (1981).

FURTHER STUDIES ON THE MECHANISM OF ACTION OF SURFACE ASSOCIATED PROTEOLYTIC ENZYMES ON LYMPHOCYTES AND MONOCYTES WHICH DEGRADE SAA PRECURSOR TO AA-LIKE PRODUCTS

Gad Lavie

The Division of Hematology and Center of Transfusion
Beilinson Medical Center
Tel-Aviv, Israel

ABSTRACT

AA-protein related amyloidosis is associated with prolonged chronic inflammatory reactions, which may contribute to amyloid formation by:

a) Overproduction of SAA.

b) Alteration of the amount of enzymes engaged in SAA degradation.

c) The possible introduction of changes in the biological control over the turnover of amyloid related proteins.

In this work we have examined the possibility that activation of lymphocytes and monocytes, both of which are cell types which carry surface associated elastase-type enzymes which degrade SAA, may alter the levels of these enzymes. Monocytes were activated with human α-interferon and with muramyl dipeptide, and lymphocytes were stimulated with the mitogens PHS, Con-A, and PWM. However, no marked changes in the activity of these enzymes, as determined by the kinetics of SAA degradation and the appearance of AA-like intermediate products, could be detected.

The presence of serum in the SAA degradation assays, on the other hand, was found to inhibit the catabolic pathways and sera from various clinical manifestations were found to differ in the degree of biological control over this reaction and in the patterns of degradation which were obtained. We suggest that the biological control over SAA degradation should be profoundly examined to determine its possible role in amyloid formation.

INTRODUCTION

The mechanism by which protein-AA related amyloid is formed and deposited in the tissues is commonly believed to be the result of incomplete turnover of the serum amyloid AA (SAA) precursor, resulting in the formation and accumulation of the protein AA product [1-3]. This latter protein bears a β-pleated structure which polymerizes in the tissues and sediments to form amyloid fibrils [4-6].

This process of amyloid formation seems to result from some form of imbalance in the normal cascade of turnover of SAA, and on the basis of different reports cited at [7-11] can assume the pathways shown in Fig. 1.

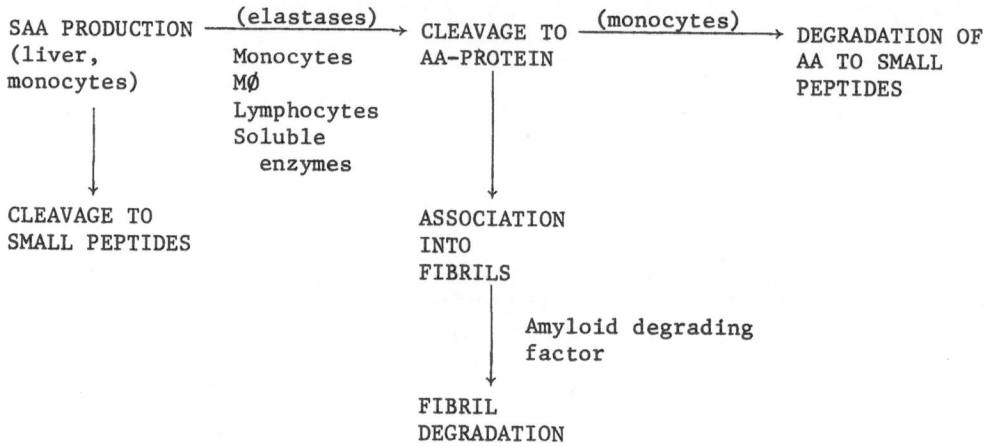

Fig. 1.   The possible pathways for the turnover and degradation of SAA.

Since AA type amyloidosis is associated with different forms of prolonged chronic inflammation, this state may contribute to the imbalance in
SAA degradation in a number of possible ways:

1. By overproduction of SAA, a protein which has been shown to behave
   as an acute phase reactant with elevated serum levels during inflammation [12-13].

2. By the possible alteration of levels of enzymes which participate
   in SAA degradation and which appear on the cell surface of monocytes as well as lymphocytes, both of which are cell types which
   are subjected to activation in response to a variety of exogenous
   stimuli. The activation processes alter the entire physiologic
   behavior and enzymatic content of the cells [14] and in mouse peritoneal macrophages activation has been shown to induce the secretion of elastase [15], collagenase [16] and other proteolytic enzymes into the extracellular environment [17].

3. The inflammatory state is also associated with alterations in the
   serum levels of inhibitors of proteolytic enzymes such as α-1 trypsin inhibitor, which may inhibit those proteolytic enzymes which
   are responsible for the breakdown of preformed AA-protein.

METHODS AND RESULTS

We have attempted to inquire whether increases in the metabolic activity of cells which produce SAA degrading enzymes affect the rates of SAA
and AA degradation and result in elevated levels of AA-like intermediate
products. First to be tested were peripheral blood monocytes. Healthy
donor mononuclear cells were isolated on ficoll-hypaque and plated in 100
mm tissue culture plates, in medium RPMI-1640 supplemented with 10% fetal
calf serum for a period of one hour for adherence. Non adherent cells were
removed by washing and the medium replaced by fresh medium, fresh medium
containing 100 units/ml of human α-interferon and a third group received
medium containing 0.1 µg/ml of N-acetyl-L-alanyl-D isoglutamine (muramyl
dipeptide - MDP) (Institute Pasteur). The monolayer of adherent cells was
incubated with the stimulants for 24 h after which time the cells were removed from the surface of the plates, washed and incubated at a concentration of 10^6 cells in 0.5 ml of medium RPMI-1640 containing 0.5 mg/ml human
SAA. The sum of 100 µl samples from the incubation medium were collected
at 0, 4, 12, and 24 h, separated on 10% SDS-polyacryl-amide gel electro-

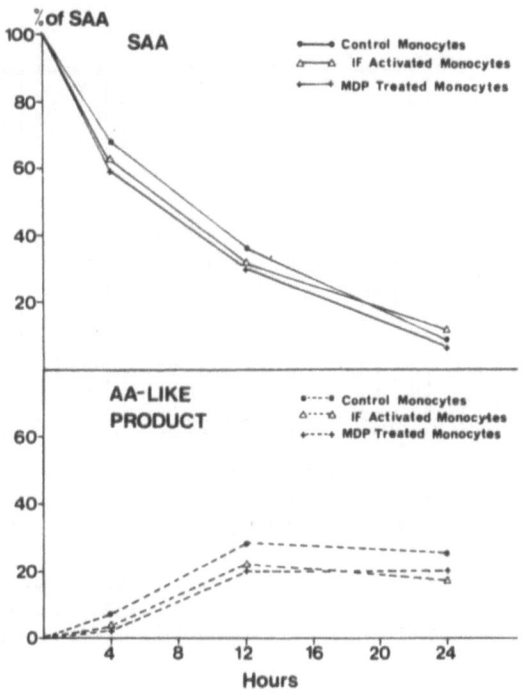

Fig. 2.   The kinetics of SAA degradation
by human peripheral blood monocytes stimulated by human α-
interferon and by muramyl dipeptide. A. (top) – rate of
elimination of SAA. B. (bottom) – rate of appearance of an
AA-like product of SAA cleavage.

phoresis (in duplicates), stained with Coomassie Brilliant Blue and the
color intensity scanned on a Gilford spectrophotometer at 540 nm. The results are shown in Fig. 2.

From part A of Fig. 2, in which the rate of elimination of the SAA
band was monitored no marked difference in the rate of SAA degradation by
monocytes pretreated with α-interferon or with muramyl dipeptide could be
observed in comparison with the rate of elimination of SAA by untreated
monocytes.

Part B of Fig. 2, in which the rate of accumulation of the AA-like degradation has been monitored shows a mild decline in the accumulation of
AA-like products following incubation with α-interferon and MDP treated
monocytes, probably due to enhanced turnover of the protein. No evidence
could be found to suggest that SAA degrading enzymes on monocytes are of
an inducible type. The surface associated elastase type enzymes on these
cells, thus, seem to be constitutive enzymes unaffected by the metabolic
activity of the cells, in contrast with the secreted type of enzyme which
has been shown to depend on the level of activation of the cell [15].

While SAA degradation by monocytes via AA-like intermediate products
is mediated by at least three different molecular weight species of cell
surface associated elastase type proteases [8], the lymphocyte is armed with
only one elastase enzyme species, and is capable of SAA degradation at a
rate substantially lower than that of monocytes. The question whether the

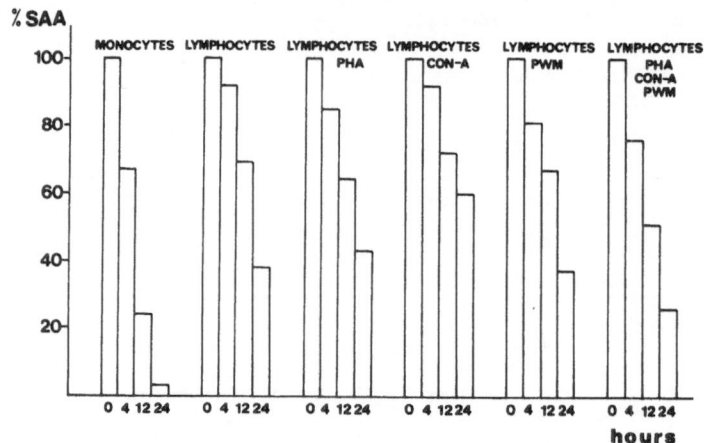

Fig. 3. The kinetics of SAA degradation by lymphocytes
stimulated by the mitogenic lectins PHA, Con-A
and Pokeweed mitogen, each applied separately
to different cell aliquots or together. Data
is presented as percent of SAA degraded after
4, 12, and 24 h of incubation with the cells.

mitogenic stimulation of lymphocytes can affect the rate of turnover of
SAA was examined by comparing the rate of SAA degradation by mitogen stimulated lymphocytes with the rate of SAA elimination by unstimulated cells.
Since only a small portion of the lymphocyte population undergoes transformation by any one lectin, a concomitant combination of three different
lectins which stimulate different subpopulations of T as well as B lymphocytes has also been studied.

PHA (Wellcome) at a concentration of 2 µg/ml, Con-A (Miles-Yeda) 20
µg/ml and Pokeweed mitogen (GIBCO) at an approximate concentration of 50
µg/ml were added to $2 \cdot 10^6$ non adherent cells purified from remaining adherent monocytes by carbonyl-iron phagocytosis followed by sedimentation
over ficoll-hypaque, and incubated for a period of three days. The cells
were washed three times with PBS containing 0.1 mM α-methyl mannoside and
incubated with SAA (0.5 mg/ml) for periods of 0, 4, 12, and 24 h. The kinetics of SAA degradation was monitored by Coomassie staining and spectrophotometric scanning of gels as described above, and the results are shown
in Fig. 3.

No significant changes in the kinetics of SAA degradation by lymphocytes seem to occur following stimulation with any one mitogen, however,
some increase in the rate of SAA turnover may be observed following lymphocyte stimulation by a combination of mitogens added concomitantly to the
cell cultures. Although it remains possible that some increase in enzyme
levels may occur on mitrogen stimulation lymphocytes and escape detection,
either because of the relatively low sensitivity of the assay, or as a result of the small percentage of cells which undergo blastogenesis, there
are no indications for marked increases in SAA degrading enzymes during
lymphocyte activation.

The constitutive nature of the enzymes engaged in the mechanism of
SAA degradation draws further attention to the biological control which
regulates this process, namely the physiologic protease inhibitors which
affect the pathways of SAA turnover.

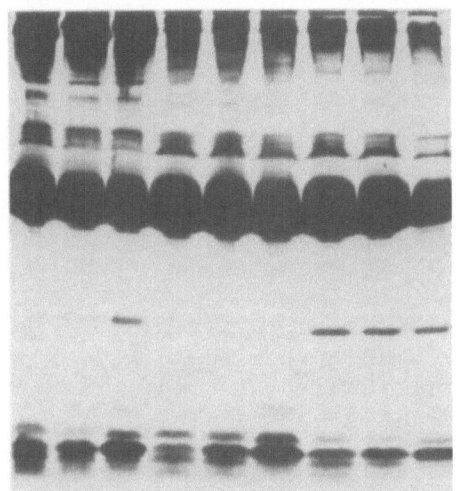

Fig. 4.   The effect of the presence of
sera from patients with a
variety of clinical conditions
on the degradation of SAA by
peripheral blood monocytes.
Assays were performed with
monocytes obtained from a
single healthy donor, cell
aliquots of which were supplemented with 10% serum: A)
from a patient with secondary
amyloidosis, B) with serum
from a patient with multiple
myeloma, C) for comparison
with degradation patterns exhibited by a healthy donor.

We have previously shown that supplementation of the incubation medium
of SAA degradation assays by monocytes with 10-15% of human serum intro-
duces a marked inhibition of the reaction [11]. This inhibition could be
demonstrated by applying supernatants of SAA degradation products onto 10-
20% SDS-polyacrylamide gradient slab gels. Degradation patterns of amyloid
related proteins can be followed because the molecular size region of both
SAA and AA proteins is relatively unmasked by other proteins. In this way
it was possible to show that purified α-1 trypsin inhibitor preparations
exhibited marked inhibition of the monocyte mediated SAA degradative activity. However, α-1 trypsin inhibitor was not the sole inhibitor of this
proteolytic activity since sera obtained from homozygous α-1 trypsin inhibitor deficient patients (ZZ-type) were found to be active in inhibiting
SAA degradation. More striking was the observation that sera from patients
who suffered from inflammatory reactions and also from AA-related amyloidosis were found to exhibit a significant diminution in the serum inhibitory
activity for SAA turnover [11], despite normal levels of serum α-1 trypsin
inhibitor. The differences in SAA degradation patterns obtained with sera
from different patients by monocytes of a single donor (run concomitantly)
are shown in Fig. 4, and seem to suggest that the cascade of SAA catabolism
is subjected to different levels of biological control in each serum sample.

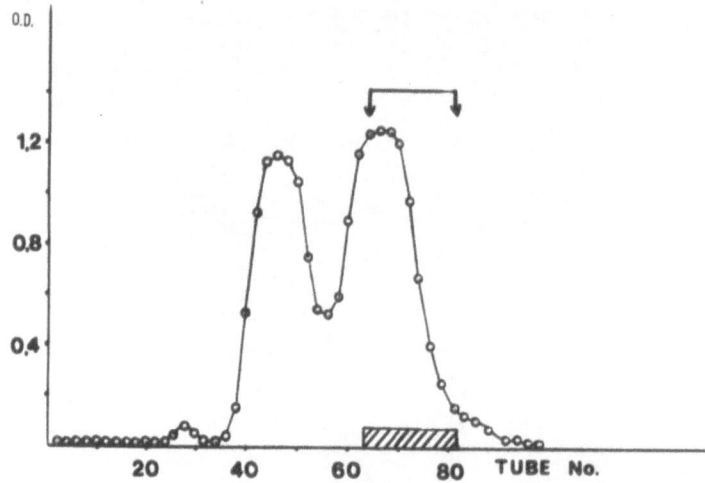

Fig. 5. Separation of serum proteins on Sephadex G-100
for the localization of the inhibitors which
regulate the monocyte mediated SAA degradation
reaction. Samples were added to the monocyte –
SAA incubation mixture at a X5 dilution of the
initial concentration found in the serum. Arrows indicate the area from which sample were
found to exhibit inhibitory activity irrespective of the strength and effectiveness of the
inhibition.

Preliminary attempts to characterize the inhibitory activity found in
normal serum consisted of separation of intact healthy donor serum on
Sephadex G-100 and determination of the inhibitory activity for SAA degradation by monocytes in each sample. The results are summarized in Fig.
5. The major inhibitory activity was found to be eluted between fractions
62-81 at the descending portion of the albumin peak. Gel analysis revealed
these fractions to contain numerous bands ranging in molecular weight from
70,000-25,000. Additional purification steps were complicated by a phenomenon of scattering of inhibitory and partial inhibitory activities and
are not available at this time. Nevertheless, the biological control over
the degradation and turnover of both SAA and AA-like cleavage products require profound evaluation because the preliminary findings suggest differences in control levels by sera of patients with various inflammatory reactions. Our attempts to measure quantitative changes in the SAA catabolic
pathways, namely the cleaving enzymes following a variety of exogenous stim-
ulations did not reveal any significant changes in enzyme levels.

REFERENCES

1. Leven, M., Pras, M., and Franklin, E. C., J. Exp. Med., 138, 373
   (1973).
2. Rosenthal, C. J., Franklin, E. C., Frangione, B., and Greenspan, J.,
   J. Immunol., 116, 1415 (1976).
3. Husby, G., and Natvig, J. B., J. Clin. Invest., 53, 1054 (1974).
4. Eanes, E. D., and Glenner, G. G., J. Histochem. Cytochem., 16, 673
   (1968).
5. Termine, J. D., Eanes, E. D., Ein, D., and Glenner, G. G., Biopolymers,
   11, 1103 (1972).
6. Cooper, J. H., Lab. Invest., 31, 232 (1974).

7. Lavie, G., Zucker-Franklin, D., and Franklin, E. C., J. Exp. Med., 148, 1020 (1978).
8. Lavie, G., Zucker-Franklin, D., and Franklin, E. C., 125, 175 (1980).
9. Skogen, B., Natvig, J. B., Borresen, A. L., and Berg, K., Scan. J. of Immunol., 11, 643 (1980).
10. Kedar, I., Ravid, M., and Sohar, E., in: Amyloid and Amyloidosis, Proc. of the III International Sympos. on Amyloidosis (G. G. Glenner, P. P. Costa, and A. F. de Freitas, eds.), Excerpta Medica, Amsterdam, (1980), p. 60.
11. Lavie, G., Franklin, E. C., and Zucker-Franklin, D., (1980), in: Amyloid and Amyloidosis, Proc. of the III International Sympos. on Amyloidosis (G. G. Glenner, P. P. Costa, and A. F. de Freitas, eds.), Excerpta Medica, Amsterdam (1980).
12. Rosenthal, J. C., and Franklin, E. C., J. Clin. Invest., 55, 746 (1975).
13. McAdam, K. P. W., and Sipe, J. D., J. Exp. Med., 144, 1121 (1976).
14. David, J. R., Fed. Proc., 34, 1730 (1975).
15. Werb, Z., and Gordon, S., J. Exp. Med., 142, 361 (1975).
16. Werb, Z., and Gordon, S., J. Exp. Med., 142, 346 (1975).
17. Unkeless, J. D., Gordon, S., and Reich, E., J. Exp. Med., 139, 834 (1974).

DOWN-REGULATION OF KUPFFER CELL ECTOENZYMES

PRECEDES DEPOSITION OF AMYLOID PROTEIN A*

Dorothea Zucker-Franklin and Alejandro Fuks

New York University Medical Center
School of Medicine
550 First Avenue
New York, N. Y. 10016

INTRODUCTION

Over the years, numerous theories have bee advanced to explain the pathogenesis of secondary amyloidosis. All theories have shared the concept that
there is an overproduction of the precursor protein. With the recognition that
the acute phase reactant serum amyloid A (SAA) is the most likely precursor of
the fibrillar AA protein deposited in tissues [1-3] it seemed not farfetched to
propose that oversprduction of SAA is responsible, at least in part, for the development of amyloidosis. A shortcoming of this theory is the observation that
the serum level of SAA does not necessarily correlate with the amount of
AA deposits, and that in some situations high levels of SAA can be maintained without any formation of fibrillar amyloid [4-6]. Therefore, additional mechanisms that have been considered are: 1) that the primary structure of the SAA molecule synthesized during stimulation is aberrant, and
2) that the cells responsible for processing SAA become impaired.

MATERIALS AND METHODS

Based on our previous work showing that peripheral blood monocytes
from patients with amyloidosis are unable to degrade SAA to completion [7-
9], we have chosen to examine the second hypothesis in greater detail. To
this end, a well established animal model for experimental amyloidosis [10,
11] was used, and isolated Kupffer cells (KC) were tested at various time
intervals during induction of amyloidosis with casein. In brief, 5 groups
of ten C57BL6/J mice received either 0, 8, 13, 18, or >30 injections of
casein. In our hands, amyloid was never detected by Congo red staining
and/or electron microscopy of the liver, spleen, or kidneys of the animals
which had received fewer than 18 injections. At the end of the injection
period, Kupffer cells (KC) were isolated by in situ perfusion of the liver
with collagenase and pronase, subsequent homogenization, Ficoll-Hypaque
centrifugation and overnight glass adhesion by a modification developed in
our laboratory for the isolation of KC from rats [12]. A concentration of
$7 \cdot 10^6$ cells per ml were plated on 35 mm petri dishes in a medium consisting
of Dulbecco's modified Eagle's (D-MEM) medium supplemented with 10% fetal
calf serum, penicillin, and streptomycin. After 48 h the Kupffer cells
were washed free of serum containing medium which was replaced with serum

*This work was supported by National Institute of Health Grants AM 012274
and AM 01431.

225

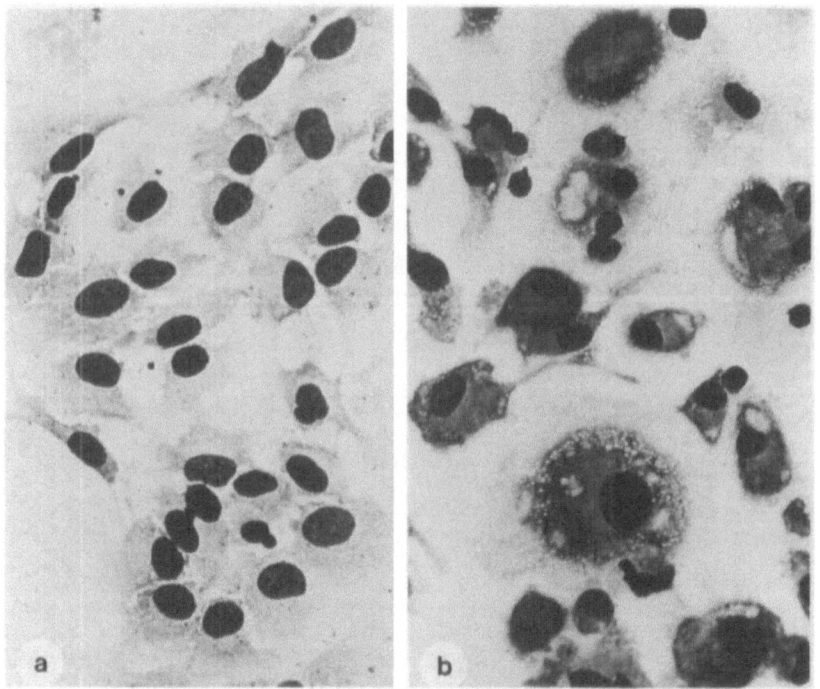

Fig. 1.   a) Kupffer cells isolated from a normal, unstimulated
          mouse. b) Kupffer cells isolated from a mouse stimu-
          lated with casein. The cells display numerous vacuoles
          and inclusions and are larger in size.

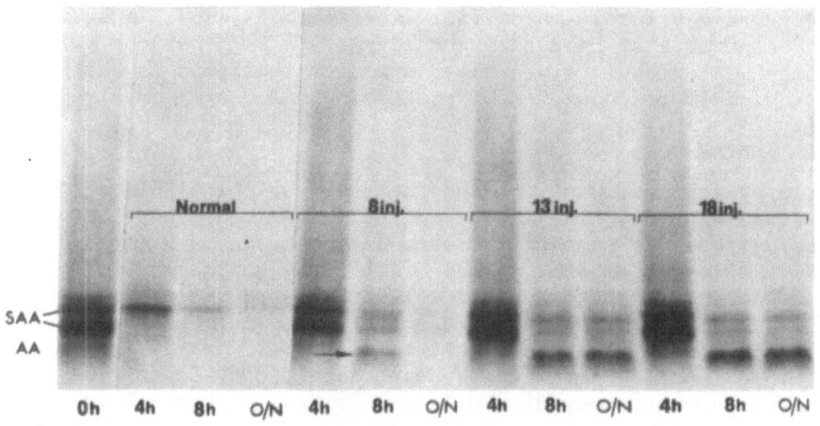

Fig. 2.   SDS – PAGE patterns obtained with supernates of
          Kupffer cells which had been incubated with SAA for
          4, 8 h, and overnight (O/N). The KC were isolated
          from normal mice and from animals which had received
          8, 13, and 18 injections of casein. KC from 8 in-
          jection mice showed an AA band after 8 h incubation
          with SAA (arrow). This band disappears on overnight
          incubation. KC from 13 and 18 injection mice also
          produce the AA cleavage product but are no longer
          able to hydrolize the peptide to completion even on
          overnight incubation.

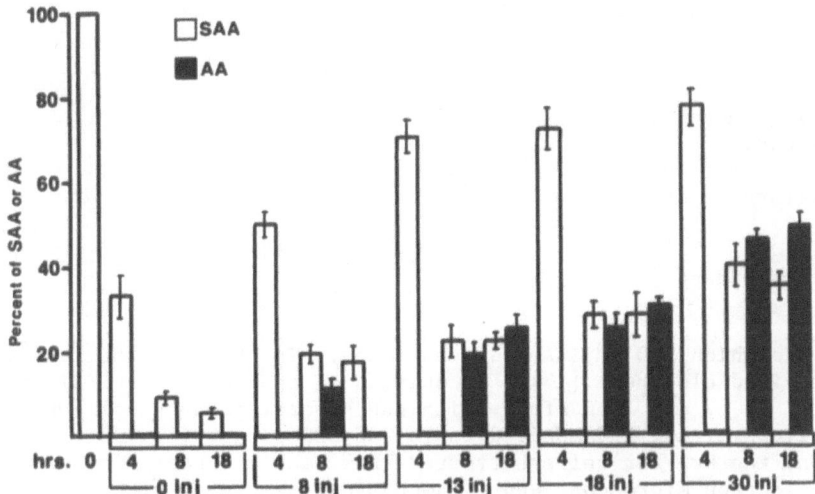

Fig. 3. Spectrophotometric quantitation of SAA and AA in the supernates of Kupffer cells which had been incubated with SAA as described in Fig. 2. Larger amounts of residual SAA and increasing quantities of AA appeared progressively as cells were isolated from animals having received an increasing number of casein injections.

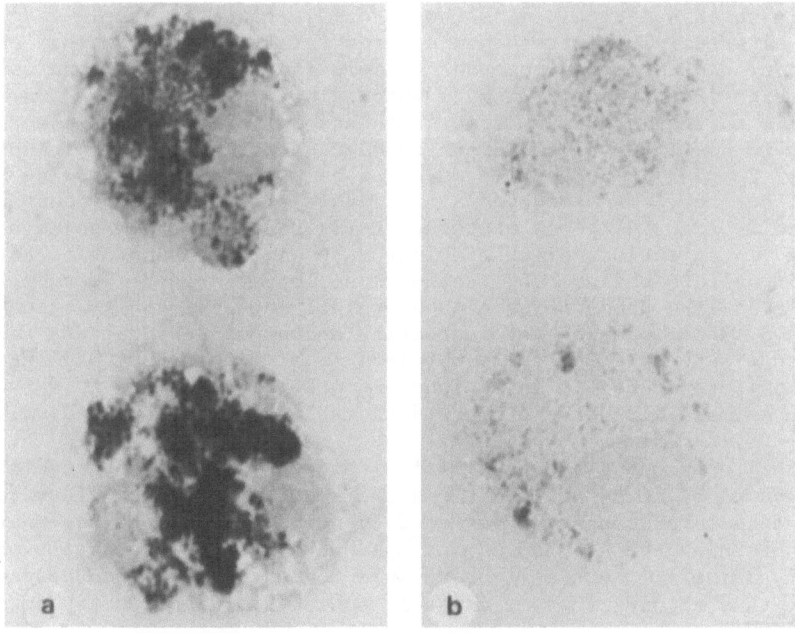

Fig. 4. a) Kupffer cells isolated from a control mouse stained for α-naphtyl butyrate esterase. The cells are strongly positive. Uneven distribution of stain is probably a preparation artifact. b) Kupffer cells isolated from a mouse having received 33 injections of casein. The cells have become virtually negative for the enzyme.

TABLE 1. Histochemistry of Kupffer cells

	Normal	Activated
Alkaline phosphase	–	–
Peroxidase	–	–
Acid phosphatase	++	++++
tartrate inhib.	+	+
ANAE	++	++
ANBE	++++	+
5'-Nucleotidase	++	+

free D-MEM to which 200 μM SAA had been added. The SAA was the same preparation described elsewhere [13]. Incubation of the cells with SAA was allowed for 0, 4, 8, and 18 h after which the supernates were collected,
dialyzed, lyophilized, and applied to 10-20% SDS polyacrylamide slab gels.
In addition, the Kupffer cells harvested from each group of mice were subjected to electron microscopy and histochemical analysis. The following
enzymes were examined: acid phosphatase, alkaline phosphatase, peroxidase,
5'-nucleotidase, lysozyme, α-naphthyl acetate esterase, and α-naphthyl
buterate esterase [14, 15].

RESULTS

The morphology of the isolated Kupffer cells obtained from unstimulated
mice are illustrated in Fig. 1a. The cells proved to be 95% viable and
phagocytic. It became immediately apparent that Kupffer cells isolated
from animals which had received as few as 8 injections of casein were morphologically altered. They spread and adhered firmly to glass within one hour
of incubation, had developed numerous vacuoles and inclusions, and more than
doubled in size (Fig. 1b). Even more surprising was the observation that
Kupffer cells harvested from animals which had only received 8 injections
of casein were no longer as efficient in degrading SAA as control Kupffer
cells (Figs. 2 and 3). Such cells were not only slower in degrading SAA to
completion, but they also produced a transient, intermediate product which
corresponded in size to the AA protein. Cells harvested from animals which
had received 13 injections of casein left an even larger amount of residual
SAA in their culture medium, and they were no longer able to degrade the
intermediate AA-like product, even on overnight incubation. As seen in
Figs. 2 and 3, there was an ever increasing amount of residual SAA and AA
in the culture supernates of cells obtained from animals that had received
increasing numbers of casein injections. Control KC isolated from frankly
amyloidotic animals did not elaborate detectable SAA into the medium.

In order to rule out the possibility that the AA-like intermediate
product produced by KC of amyloidotic animals was an aberrant cleavage
product that could no longer be degraded by normal cells, the supernate of
cultures containing the AA product was incubated with Kupffer cells obtained
from healthy animals. Such cells were able to hydrolyze the AA product to
completion, thus showing that it is still subject to digestion by normal
cells.

A few experiments were carried out to examine whether the Kupffer cell
defect was reversible. Two groups of animals, one having received 13 and

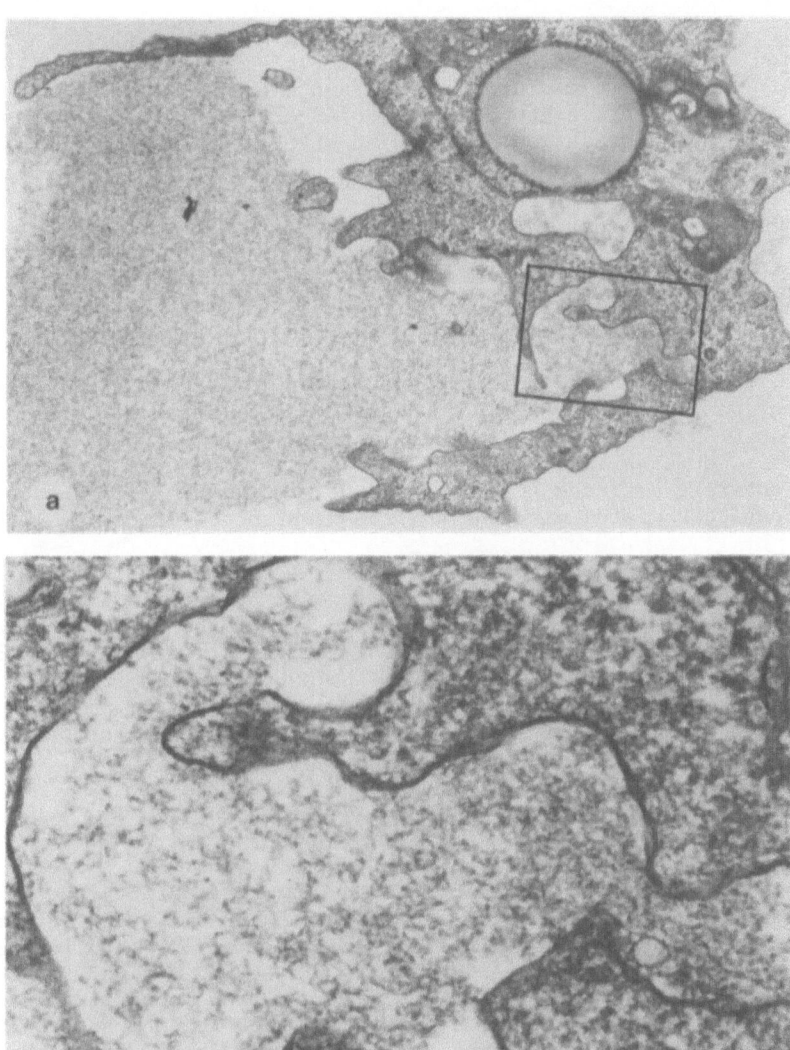

Fig. 5.   a) Detail of a Kupffer cell from a mouse which had re-
        ceived 18 injections of casein, but had not developed
        demonstable amyloid.   The cell illustrated was taken
        from a specimen of KC cultured with SAA for 18 h.
        The area in the rectangle is seen at higher resolution
        in Fig. 5b. Magnification 19,000×.   b) Higher magni-
        fication of the area delineated by the rectangle in
        Fig. 5a.   Filaments have formed in close proximity to
        the plasma membrane.   Dots represent filaments in cross
        section.   These filaments do not have the structure
        characteristic of amyloid, but may represent incom-
        pletely polymerized AA protein.   Magnification
        92,000×.

the other 20 injections of casein were chosen to determine whether Kupffer cell function could recover _in vivo_. At intervals following cessation of casein treatment, KC were isolated and the SAA assay was performed. The cells from the 13 injection group recovered after 6 weeks when they accomplished complete degradation of SAA without the appearance of the intermediate SAA product. The Kupffer cells derived from the 20 injection group required 10 weeks for complete recovery.

Because the KC impairment was likely to imply a loss of the surface-associated elastase-like enzymes responsible for processing of SAA [9], we examined whether there was evidence for down-regulation of other enzymes in KC obtained from stimulated mice. Table 1 shows a summary of the enzymes tested by histochemical means. There was a marked increase in acid phosphatase, a well studied indicator enzyme for cell activation. Most of the increment was due to the acid phosphatase moiety which is inhibitable by tartrate. Of greater interest in the context of this report was the observation of a decrease in 5'-nucleotidase and a striking diminution of α-naphthyl butyrate esterase (Figs. 4a and 5). Both the last named enzymes have been found associated with the surface membrane of monocytes [16, 17].

Lastly, we examined whether the soluble SAA cleavage product which was produced by defective KC incubated with SAA would polymerize into fibrils. For this purpose, KC of mice injected 13 times were incubated with SAA overnight and then subjected to ultrastructural analysis. Only on two occasions were fibrils seen on addition of SAA to Kupffer cells from casein injected mice whose organs were still devoid of amyloid (Fig. 5). KC from animals which had become amyloidotic could not be freed from associated amyloid fibrils and could thus not be used for these experiments.

DISCUSSION

The data recorded in this communication show that during the induction of experimental amyloidosis with casein a diminished ability of Kupffer cells to process SAA becomes evident before deposition of fibrillar amyloid can be detected. The Kupffer cell defect is manifested not only by residual SAA in the medium with which the Kupffer cell had been incubated, but also with the appearance of an intermediate product which resembles AA on SDS-PAGE. Therefore, it must be assumed that the KC had lost some of the elastase-like enzyme(s) which are believed to be involved in the hydrolysis of SAA [7, 9]. The observation is of particular interest since, after only very few injections of the stimulant, the KC resembled "activated" macrophages. They spread and adhered almost instantaneously, had numerous pinocytotic vesicles and vacuoles, and a marked increase in acid phosphatase. Although down-regulation of enzymatic activity by cells which appear otherwise activated is a novel concept, there is some precedent for the observation [16]. It has also been proposed that down-regulation of ecto-enzymes may be attributable to internalization of portions of the surface membranes [18]. This would be particularly relevant to phagocytic cells. The increase in the number of inclusions and vesicles seen in Kupffer cells from stimulated mice would support this mechanism of surface membrane modulation. The fact that stimulated KC had decreased amounts of 5'-nucleotidase and α-naphthyl butyrate esterase, enzymes which have been reported to be primarily associated with the plasma membrane, would point in the same direction. The definitive demonstration that these as well as the elastase-like enzymes are gradually lost from the surface of the cells during the amyloid induction period must await biochemical analysis of isolated plasma membranes.

Meanwhile, the data reported here and previously [7, 9], show that functional impairment of cells belonging to the monocyte/phagocytic system is, in part, responsible for the production of an intermediate cleavage product which results from incomplete processing of SAA. Whether the appearance of this presumably abnormal peptide suffices to explain fibrillogenesis or whether additional enzymatic reaction(s) are required to polymerize these molecules into the insoluble fibrillar protein recognized as amyloid A, remains to be determined.

REFERENCES

1. M. Levin, E. C. Franklin, B. Frangione, and M. Pras, J. Clin. Invest., 51:2773 (1972).
2. M. Levin, M. Pras, and E. C. Franklin, J. Exp. Med., 138:373 (1973).
3. N. Ericksen, L. H. Ericsson, N. Pearsall, D. Lagunoff, and E. P. Benditt, Proc. Natl. Acad. Sci. U.S.A., 73:964 (1976).
4. J. D. Rosenthal and E. C. Franklin, Trans. Assoc. Am. Phys., 87:159 (1974).
5. D. Zemer, M. Pras, and E. Sohar, N. Eng. J. Med., 294:170 (1976).
6. K. P. W. J. McAdam and J. D. Sipe, J. Exp. Med., 144:1121 (1976).
7. G. Lavie, D. Zucker-Franklin, and E. C. Franklin, J. Exp. Med., 148:1020 (1978).
8. G. D. Lavie, D. Zucker-Franklin, and E. C. Franklin, J. Imm., 125:175 (1980).
9. D. Zucker-Franklin, G. Lavie, and E. C. Franklin, J. Histochem. and Cytochem., 29:451 (1981).
10. H. Skinner, T. Shirahama, M. D. Benson, and S. A. Cohen, Lab. Inv., 36:420 (1977).
11. K. P. W. J. McAdam and J. D. Sipe, J. Exp. Med., 144:1121 (1976).
12. D. M. Mills and D. Zucker-Franklin, Am. J. Pathol., 54:147 (1969).
13. C. J. Rosenthal, E. C. Franklin, B. Frangione, and J. Greenspan, J. Imm., 116:1415 (1976).
14. C. Y. Li, K. W. Lam, and L. T. Yam, J. Histochem. and Cytochem., 21:1 (1973).
15. J. Lopes, D. Zucker-Franklin, and R. Silber, J. Clin. Invest., 52:1297 (1973).
16. P. J. Edelson and Z. A. Cohn, J. Exp. Med., 144:1596 (1976).
17. M. J. Bozdech and D. F. Bainton, J. Exp. Med., 153:182 (1981).
18. L. Beguinot, R. M. Lyall, M. C. Willingham, and I. Pastan, Proc. Natl. Acad. Sci., 81:2384 (1984).

SPECIFIC CHEMICAL DISSOCIATION OF FIBRILLAR
AND NON-FIBRILLAR COMPONENTS OF AMYLOID DEPOSITS

C. R. K. Hind, P. M. Collins*,
D. Caspi, M. L. Baltz,
and M. B. Pepys

MRC Acute Phase Protein Research Group
Immunological Medicine Unit
Department of Medicine
Royal Postgraduate Medical School
London W12 OHS, and

*Department of Chemistry
 Birkbeck College
 London WC1E 7HX
 United Kingdom

ABSTRACT

In systemic amyloidosis the extracellular protein deposits are composed of amyloid fibrils together with a non-fibrillar glycoprotein, amyloid P component (AP). Methyl 4,6-O-(1-carboxyethylidene)-β-D-galactopyranoside (MOβDG), a recently identified ligand for AP, was tested for its ability to produce in vitro elution of AP which had been laid down with amyloid fibrils in vivo. Millimolar concentrations of MOβDG completely dissociated AP from human and murine splenic amyloid deposits. Availability of this material thus provides for the first time the opportunity for specific molecular dissection of amyloid deposits. If MOβDG or a related substance were effective in vivo it might be of therapeutic importance.

INTRODUCTION

Amyloid P component (AP) has been detected immunochemically using antisera to AP or serum amyloid P component (SAP) in deposits or extracts of all forms of systemic amyloidosis in which it has been sought, regardless of the chemical nature of the amyloid fibril protein [1, 2]. AP is also present in deposits of all forms of localized amyloidosis [3, 4] with the possible exception of intracerebral plaques in Alzheimer's disease and senile dementia [4, 5]. Regardless of the fibril type, this non-fibrillar component is the same in all deposits and forms between 6-20% of the weight of the amyloid deposits [6]. AP is derived from circulating SAP [7], and an immunochemically cross-reactive protein (tissue AP) is also an integral constituent of normal human glomerular basement membrane and of elastic fibre microfibrils throughout the body [8, 9]. However, neither the normal physiological function of SAP or tissue AP, nor their possible role in the deposition and persistence of amyloid fibrils are known.

SAP has the capacity for calcium-dependent binding to certain specific ligands, including amyloid fibrils, fibronectin, C4-binding protein and agarose, a linear galactan hydrocolloid derived from marine algae [10-12]. The interaction with amyloid fibrils is probably a sufficient explanation for the presence of AP in amyloid deposits but it does not exclude a possible pathophysiological role for SAP or normal tissue AP in amyloidosis. The interaction with agarose is unlikely <u>per se</u> to be of any physiological importance but it has enabled us to demonstrate that the moiety recognized by SAP is the cyclic pyruvate acetal of galactose, a trace constituent of agarose [13]. We have therefore synthesized the monosaccharide, methyl 4,6-O-(1-carboxyethylidene)-β-D-galactopyranoside (MOβDG) (Fig. 1), and shown that millimolar concentrations of its R isomer inhibit and reverse <u>in vitro</u> all the known calcium-dependent binding reactions of SAP, including that with isolated AA amyloid fibrils [13].

We have now extended these observations to amyloid deposits formed <u>in vivo</u> and report here that MOβDG specifically dissociates AP from these deposits <u>in vitro</u>.

METHODS

Amyloid Deposits

Amyloid-containing human spleen was obtained at necropsy from a patient who had had rheumatoid arthritis, and murine spleen was taken from animals which had received subcutaneous injections of casein. The presence of amyloid in each case was confirmed by Congo red staining, and the presence of AP was demonstrated by immunofluorescent staining with anti-SAP antibodies [14].

Chemicals

Methyl β-D-galactopyranoside, sodium pyruvate, D-galacturonic acid, and D-galactose were obtained from Sigma London Chemical Co. Ltd. (Poole, Dorset, U.K.). The sodium salt of the R isomer of MOβDG was synthesized as described previously [13].

Antisera

Monospecific antisera to human and murine SAP were raised by immunization of sheep with the isolated pure proteins [15, 16].

Elution of AP from Amyloid Deposits

Homogenates of known weights of amyloid-containing splenic tissue were prepared and washed 10 times with 0.01 M Tris-buffered 0.138 M NaCl contain-

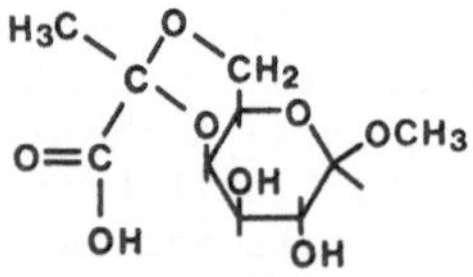

Fig. 1. Methyl 4,6-O-
        (1-carboxyethyl-
        idence)-β-D-galac-
        topyranoside
        (MOβDG).

TABLE 1. Elution of SAP from Murine Amyloid Deposits

Elution 1		Elution 2		Total eluted
Chemical	SAP (μg)	Chemical	SAP (μg)	SAP (μg)
Tris-saline-Ca	0	Tris-saline-EDTA	31	31
MOβDG	41	Tris-saline-EDTA	2	43
Tris-saline-EDTA	41	Tris-saline-EDTA	2	43

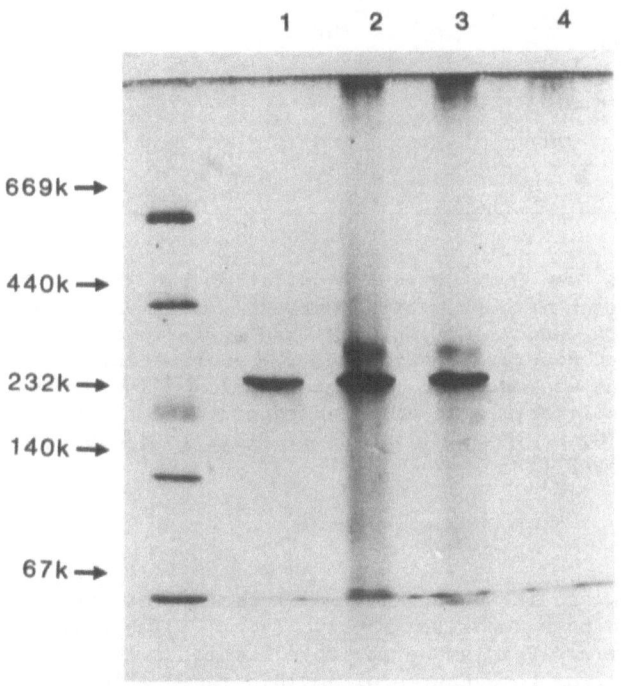

Fig. 2. 4-30% gradient PAGE showing: track 1,
isolated human SAP; trace 2, proteins
eluted from amyloid-laden spleen homogenates with 20 mM MOβDG; track 3,
proteins eluted with Tris-saline-EDTA;
proteins eluted with Tris-saline-Ca.
Positions of marker proteins of known
molecular weight are indicated by arrows.

TABLE 2. Attempted Elution of SAP from Human Amyloid-Laden Spleen

Chemical	Concentration	SAP eluted
Tris-saline-EDTA	0.01 M	100
MOβDG 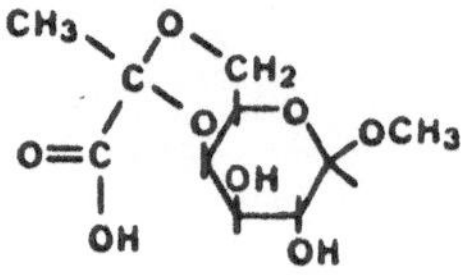	0.001 M	70
D-galacturonic acid 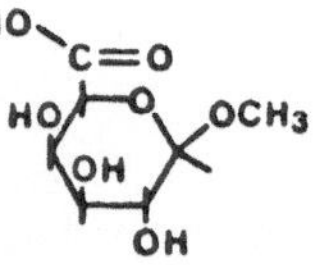	0.001–0.1 M	1–6
Methy β-D-galactopyranoside 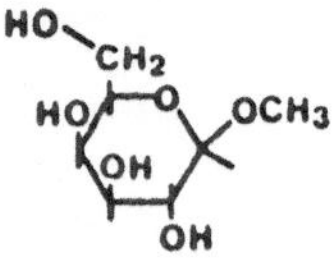	0.1 M	4
Pyruvic acid 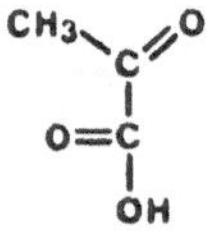	0.1 M	3

ing 0.002 M $CaCl_2$ and 0.1% wt./vol. NaN_3 at pH 8.0 (Tris-saline-Ca). Elution of AP was then attempted first with solutions of chemicals under test in Tris-saline-Ca, and then by 0.01 M Tris-buffered 0.138 M NaCl containing 0.01 M EDTA at pH 8.0 (Tris-saline-EDTA). In the control experiments Tris-saline-EDTA alone was used for complete elution. The undenatured eluates were tested by polyacrylamide gel electrophoretic analysis in 4–30% gradient gels (Pharmacia G. B. Ltd., Milton Keynes, U.K.), and by specific electro-immunoassay for SAP [12].

RESULTS

Both in man and in mouse, millimolar concentrations of MOβDG eluted the AP which had been deposited in vivo (Fig. 2, Table 1). The specificity of MOβDG in eluting AP is shown in Table 2 which summarizes the attempts to elute human SAP from homogenates of amyloid-laden spleen by chemicals with structures similar to MOβDG.

DISCUSSION

The present results show clearly that millimolar amounts of MOβDG were capable of specifically dissociating in vitro the amyloid P component from amyloid deposits which had formed in vivo, both in man and in mouse. These observations suggest that MOβDG or an analogous substance should be capable of dissociating AP from amyloid fibrils in vivo, and preliminary experiments in mice indicate that MOβDG is not acutely toxic.

Identification and availability of ligands for the calcium-dependent binding site of SAP may thus provide the first opportunity for specific molecular dissection in vivo of amyloid deposits. Such an approach may have therapeutic relevance to human amyloidosis, which remains an untreatable condition. Previous attempts at treatment have been aimed at the promotion or acceleration of amyloid fibril destruction (e.g., dimethyl sulfoxide (DMSO)), or at reducing the concentration and production of the fibril precursor (e.g., cholchicine) [17]. However, neither colchicine nor DMSO have any effect on the interaction between human SAP and isolated AA amyloid fibrils [18].

Amyloid fibrils provoke little inflammatory response in the tissues in which they are laid down, and seem not to stimulate phagocytic cells. They persist in vivo for reasons which are unclear, since isolated amyloid fibrils are sensitive to proteolysis in vitro [19]. One possibility is that AP forms a protective coating over the amyloid fibrils, thus enabling the deposits to persist. An alternative role for SAP, including its normal tissue counterpart, in amyloidosis may be as a nidus for the localization and deposition of fibril precursors. Availability of the specific ligand for SAP should help to answer these points.

ACKNOWLEDGEMENTS

This work was supported by Medical Research Council program Grant G979/51 to M. B. Pepys. C. R. K. Hind is the recipient of a MRC training research fellowship.

REFERENCES

1. M. B. Pepys, F. C. de Beer, R. F. Dyck, M. L. Baltz, S. Holdford, S. M. Breathnach, M. M. Black, C. R. Tribe, D. J. Evans, and A. Feinstein, Ann. N. Y. Acad. Sci., 389, 286 (1982).
2. C. R. K. Hind, G. A. Tennent, D. J. Evans, and M. B. Pepys, J. Pathol., 139, 159 (1983).
3. S. M. Breathnach, B. Bhogal, R. F. Dyck, F. C. de Beer, M. M. Black, and M. B. Pepys, Br. J. Dermatol., 105, 115 (1981).
4. I. F. Rowe, O. Jensson, P. D. Lewis, J. Candy, G. A. Tennent, and M. B. Pepys, Neuropath. Appl. Neurobiol., 10, 53 (1984).
5. P. Westermark, T. Shirahama, M. Skinner, A. Brun, R. Cameron, and A. S. Cohen, Lab. Invest., 46, 457 (1982).
6. M. Skinner, T. Shirahama, A. S. Cohen, and C. L. Deal, Prep. Biochem., 12, 461 (1983).
7. M. L. Baltz, D. Caspi, I. F. Rowe, C. R. K. Hind, D. J. Evans, and M. B. Pepys, this volume (1985).
8. R. F. Dyck, C. M. Lockwood, M. Kershaw, N. McHugh, V. Duance, M. L. Baltz, and M. B. Pepys, J. Exp. Med., 152, 1162 (1980).
9. S. M. Breathnach, S. M. Melrose, B. Bhogal, F. C. de Beer, R. F. Dyck, G. Tennent, M. M. Black, and M. B. Pepys, Nature, 293, 652 (1981).
10. M. B. Pepys, R. F. Dyck, F. C. de Beer, M. Skinner, and A. S. Cohen, Clin. Exp. Immunol., 38, 284 (1979).
11. F. C. de Beer, M. L. Baltz, S. Holford, A. Feinstein, and M. B. Pepys, J. Exp. Med., 154, 1134 (1981).
12. M. B. Pepys, A. C. Dash, E. A. Munn, A. Feinstein, M. Skinner, A. S. Cohen, J. Gewurz, A. P. Osmand, and R. H. Painter, Lancet i, 1029 (1977).
13. C. R. K. Hind, P. M. Collins, D. Renn, R. B. Cook, D. Caspi, M. L. Baltz, and M. B. Pepys, J. Exp. Med., 59, 1058 (1984).

14. R. F. Dyck, D. J. Evans, C. M. Lockwood, A. J. Rees, D. Turner, and M. B. Pepys, Lancet ii, 606 (1980).
15. F. C. de Beer and M. B. Pepys, J. Immunol. Methods, 50, 17 (1982).
16. M. B. Pepys, Immunology, 37, 637 (1979).
17. G. G. Glenner, N. Eng. J. Med., 302, 1283 and 1333 (1980).
18. D. Caspi and C. R. K. Hind, unpublished observations.
19. B. Skogen and J. B. Natvig, Scand. J. Immunol., 14, 389 (1981).

D. DEGRADING FACTORS

DEGRADATION OF AA-AMYLOID, CLINICAL EXPERIENCE:

AN INTRODUCTION

Otto Wegelius and Tom Törnroth

Fourth Department of Medicine
Helsinki University Central Hospital
Helsinki, Finland

The Fourth Department of Medicine in Helsinki has beside general internal medicine the responsibility for rheumatology and nephrology. Patients with rare disorders like amyloidosis and patients waiting for kidney transplantation are remitted to this department from the whole country. An accumulation of amyloid diseased patients demands efforts of both research and treatment. The frequency of amyloidosis in rheumatic patients at this university department is strikingly higher than in Rheumatism Foundation Hospital in Heinola. The prognosis of reactive amyloidosis among rheumatic patients is known to be poor. The Finnish material reported by us at the meeting in Portugal showed the same. In a cumulative survival study only a few patients survived over 15 years. These few patients with good prognosis might give a clue about the beneficial forces responsible for regression of the disease. Discovery of these mechanisms could lead us to a successful treatment.

Many reports about regression can be found in the literature. Among these are two from our department. Nine reports deal with morphological evidence of resolution of amyloid substance. Two have reports of electron microscopic findings. In reactive amyloidosis the most important target organ is the kidney. So far we have data from four patients, three of them suffering from an underlying rheumatic disease and one with bronchiectasies. During the clinical remission the amyloid deposits were still seen in either light microscopy or in electron microscopy. The latter, however, revealed a change in the ultrastructure of the amyloid substance.

This picture shows a peripheral glomerular capillary wall from an initial renal biopsy. Subepithelial amyloid deposits with clear fibrillar appearance are seen in the upper part of the picture. For comparison our pathologist Tom Törnroth has taken an subepithelial immune complex deposit to the lowest part of the picture.

These are the findings in the resolving phase. Subepithelial and intramembranous electron lucent areas containing occasional amyloid fibrils are seen in the three upper parts of the picture. For comparison similar changes in resolving immune complex glomerulonephritis are shown in the lowest part of the picture. It can be stated that the amyloid material is deposited and cleared in the same way as the immune complexes in membranous glomerulonephritis, i.e., through the basal membrane. The material in the glomeruli still stains with anti-AA (PAP method) in the resolving phase. These mesangial nodules in this semithin section are visualized with toluidine blue. The electron micrographs show their localization in the mesangium. No fibrillar structures can be seen. In higher magnification a non fibrillar, fine granular structure is obvious.

From these morphological findings we conclude: amyloid fibrils during resolution are transformed into a fine granular material; this material is still stainable with Congo red and reacts with anti AA-antiserum; staining with Congo red does not necessarily imply a fibrillar ultrastructure.

Clinical and morphological observations suggest that some enzymes are capable of resolving amyloid substance in vivo. In our efforts to find the responsible enzyme we started with serum using already reported methods, i.e., the agar diffusion method. We found that persons suffering from rheumatoid arthritis had an impaired capability to split fibrillar AA-protein compared with healthy persons. Rheumatoid arthritis with amyloidosis showed still weaker potency of degrading capacity. The enzyme belongs to the serine proteases but is not yet identified. It is not elastase. We also do not know if the serum component is active in the tissues or not. You may ask: Is the impaired degrading activity responsible for the amyloid reaction in rheumatoid arthritis? Our answer is, No. We rather believe that the overproduction of precursor protein SAA is the main reason. Our view is based on the following observations. In chronic diseases where elevated SAA levels are found for long standing, a reactive amyloidosis is a well known fact. During the course of rheumatoid arthritis the SAA, the degrading activity and its inhibitor α-antitrypsin fluctuate. When SAA during a remission decreases the degrading activity increases. This reversed balance stresses the importance of the SAA. In our studies we found a strong correlation between SAA level and progression of renal failure. As we all know CRP can equally well as SAA be used as marker of the danger for amyloid. Individual patients a good correlation between the level of these acute phase proteins and the deterioration of kidney function can be shown.

In the development and turnover of amyloid substance in AA-amyloidosis the overproduction of precursor protein is most important. Consequently, patients should be actively treated to achieve low SAA values. Special attenion should be given the rheumatic patients with initially high precursor values. SAA and CRP are good tools for evaluation in the preventive anti-amyloid treatment.

REFERENCES

1. Wegelius, O., Wafin, F., Falck, H., and Törnroth, T., Follow-up Study
    of Amyloidosis Secondary to Rheumatic Diseases, in: Amyloid and
    Amyloidosis (G. G. Glenner, P. P. Costa, and F. de Freitas, eds.),
    Amsterdam, Excerpta Medica, 183-199 (1980).
2. Wegelius, O., The Resolution of Amyloid Substance, Acta, Med. Scand.,
    212:273-275 (1982).
3. Kukhlbäck, B., and Wegelius, O., Secondary Amyloidosis, A Study of
    Clinical and Pathological Findings, Acta Med. Scand., 180:737 (1966).
4. Falck, H. Törnroth, T., Skrifvars, B., and Wegelius, O., Resolution of
    Renal Amyloidosis Secondary to Rheumatoid Arthritis, Acta Med. Scand.,
    205:651-656 (1979).
5. Törnroth, T., The Fate of Subepithelial Deposits in Acute Poststrepto-
    coccal Glomerulonephritis, Lab. Invest., 35:461 (1976).
6. Törnroth, T., Falck, H. M., and Wegelius, O., Nonfibrillar Glomerular
    Deposits in Resolving Renal Amyloidosis, in: Amyloidosis E.A.R.S.
    (C. R. Tribe and P. A. Bacon, eds.), John Wright and Sons, Ltd.,
    Bristol (1983).
7. Wegelius, O. Teppo, Anna-Maija, and Maury, C. P. J., Reduced Amyloid-
    A-Degrading Activity in Serum in Amyloidosis Associated with Rheuma-
    toid Arthritis, Br. Med. J., 287:617-619 (1982).
8. Teppo, Anna-Maija, Maury, C. P. J., and Wegelius, O., Characteristics
    of the Amyloid A Fibril-Degrading Activity of Human Serum, Scand. J.
    Immunol., 16:309-314 (1982).
9. Falck, H., Maury, C. P. J., Teppo, Anna-Maija, and Wegelius, O., Cor-
    relation of Persistently High Serum Amyloid-A-Protein and C-Reac tive
    Protein Concentrations with Rapid Progression of Secondary Amyloidosis,
    Br. Med. J., 286:1391-1393 (1983).

IN VIVO DEGRADATION OF PROTEIN SAA TO PROTEIN

AA AND INCORPORATION IN AMYLOID FIBRILS

A. Husebekk, B. Skogen,
G. Husby, and G. Marhaug

Department of Rheumatology
Institute of Clinical Medicine
University of Tomsø,
Tomsø, Norway

ABSTRACT

To groups of mice, A and B, were injected intraperitoneally with LPS
in order to induce amyloidosis. Group A got human HDL-SAA complexes intravenously in addition to LPS. The mice were sacrificed. The liver, spleen,
and kidneys from both group A and B contained moderate amounts of amyloid
examined by polarization microscopy after Congo red staining. Antiserum
to human AA/SAA was tested and showed no cross reactivity with mouse SAA or
AA.

Isolated amyloid fibrils from the mice in group A contained human protein AA. This was shown by double immunodiffusion, immunoblot, and ELISA
techniques. In contrast, mice in group B had only mouse amyloid fibrils.
The experiments provided solid evidence that SAA is the precursor for amyloid
fibril protein AA.

INTRODUCTION

Together with C-reactive protein, protein SAA is the most characteristic acute phase reactant [1]. SAA has a molecular weight of about 12,000
daltons. The protein is antigenically identical to amyloid protein AA and
the amino acid sequence is homologous in the N-terminal part. Amyloid protein AA has a molecular weight of 8600 daltons [2, 3, 4, 5, 6]. SAA is an
apoprotein to high density lipoprotein [7] and might comprise 40-50% of the
total HDL apoproteins in situations with maximal stimulation of SAA production [8]. It has been believed that SAA is the serum precursor for protein
AA in fibrillar amyloid in tissue, but the direct evidence has been lacking.
However, injections of endotoxin (LPS) in mink causes elevated concentrations of SAA and subsequent deposition of amyloid fibrils [9]. Kisilevski
noted in one of his studies that agents able to reduce the SAA levels in
mice, lead to resorption of amyloid deposits [10]. The homology in amino
acid sequence and antigenic properties between SAA and AA, indicates that
AA is derived from SAA [1, 11, 12]. It is also shown that serine proteases
in serum and on monocytes, are able to degrade SAA to a fragment with molecular weight and antigenicity identical to protein AA [11, 13, 14]. The

purpose of the present study was to investigate _in vivo_, if SAA could be converted to an AA like molecule and incorporated in amyloid fibrils.

MATERIALS AND METHODS

Preparation of Human HDL-SAA Complexes

Human HDL-SAA complexes were isolated from human acute serum by flotation in the ultracentrifuge, employing conventional technique [7, 8, 15]. LDL and VLDL was removed after centrifugation at density 1.063 g/ml, and HCL collected after centrifugation at density 1.21 g/ml, and dialyzed against 0.15 M NaCl, 2 mM EDTA.

Isolation of SAA and AA

SAA was isolated from acute phase sera by gel filtration in 10% formic acid on Bio-Gel P-60 and Sephadex G-75 (twice) as previously described [16]. Amyloid fibrils were prepared from amyloid tissues as described [3, 4]. Protein AA was isolated from dissociated fibrils by gel filtration on a Sephacryl S-200 column equilibrated with 5 M guanidine/0.1 M acetic acid, dialyzed against distilled water and lyophilized.

Induction of Amyloidosis in Mice

Amyloidosis was induced in (BALB/c × A.TH)F_1 mice by intraperitoneal injections of LPS B (Escherichia coli, B6; 026, Difco Laboratories, Michigan, USA), dissolved 1 mg/ml in PBS. Ten mice were divided in two groups, A and B, five mice in each group. Three times weekly in 4 weeks the mice were injected intraperitoneally with LPS. The last two weeks the mice in group A, was injected intravenously with human HDL-SAA complexes (0.1 ml, 10 mg/ml) in addition to LPS. The mice were sacrificed. Sections from the liver, spleen, and kidneys in each mice, were analyzed for amyloid deposits by microscopy in polarized light after Congo red staining.

Double Immunodiffusion

Double immunodiffusion was performed in 1% agarose gel in 0.025 M barbital buffer pH 8.6. The plates were developed at room temperature and examined after 24 h. Isolated SAA and AA (0.5 mg/ml) were dissolved in 0.1 M NaHCO$_3$ pH 8.3, prior to double immunodiffusion analysis.

Antisera

Antisera to human AA/SAA and mouse AA/SAA were raised in rabbits [2, 3, 16]. The antiserum to the human proteins precipitated both SAA and AA showing a reaction of antigenic identity between the two proteins. The antiserum to mouse AA/SAA precipitated only with SAA, but mouse AA clearly inhibited this reaction in double immunodiffusion. A precipitating anti-mouse AA antiserum was not available. Monoclonal mouse hybridoma antibodies reacting with human SAA, but not AA, was also used [17].

Sodium Dodecyl Sulfate-Polyacrylamide Gel Electrophoresis (SDS-PAGE)

SDS-PAGE of protein was performed as described in detail elsewhere [18].

Immunoblotting Experiments

After SDA-PAGE, the amyloid proteins were transferred to nitrocellulose filter papter (0.45 μm pore size, Schleicher and Schull, Dassel, West

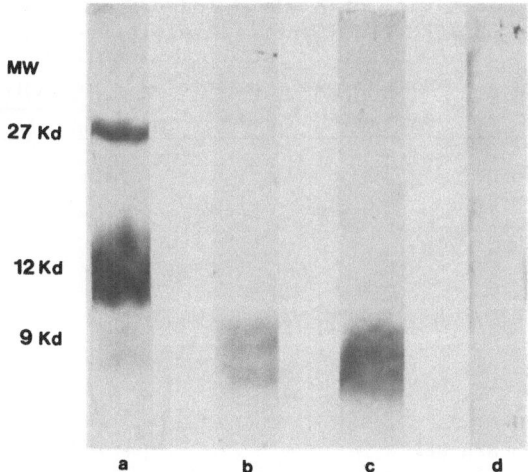

Fig. 1.   Double immunodiffusion showing anti-human AA/SAA in central well tested against amyloid protein from the mice in
group A (1), purified human AA
protein (2) and purified mouse
AA protein (3). It is seen that
amyloid from the mice in group
A contained a fibril protein
antigenically identical with
purified human AA.

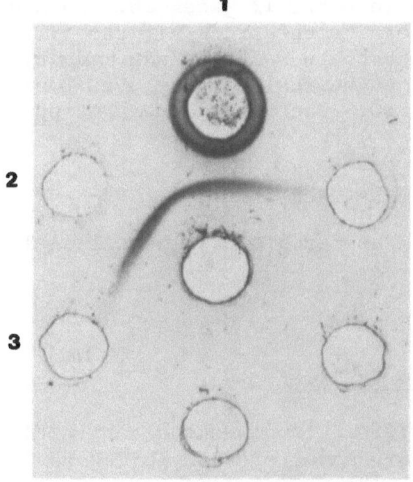

Fig. 2.   Immunoblot using anti-human AA/SAA
showing human HDL-SAA used for induction of amyloid in group A (1),
protein AA from amyloid induced with
LPS and HDL-SAA (]), purified human
AA (3), and non-reactive purified
mouse AA (4). All protein dissolved
1 mg/ml in the sample buffer. Sample size: 25 (1).

TABLE 1. Antigenic Reactivity of Amyloid Induced in Mice by LPS + Human HCL-SAA or LPS/PBS, and Control Amyloid Proteins

Antigenic materials	Mouse amyloid induced by		Human		Mouse	
	LPS+human HDL-SAA	LPS/PBS	AA	SAA	AA	SAA
Double immunodiffusion with polyclonal antisera to:						
human SAA	+	–	+	+	–	–
human AA	+	–	+	+	–	–
mouse AA/SAA	(+)*	(+)	–	–	(+)	+
Immunoblot with polyclonal anti-human AA/SAA	+	–	+	+	–	–
ELISA with:						
monoclonal anti-human SAA	–	–	–	+	–	–
polyclonal anti-human AA/SAA	+	–	+	+	–	–

* (+): Inhibition of precipitation reaction between anti-mouse SAA and mouse SAA

Germany) by overnight electrophoresis [19]. The filter paper was soaked in PBS with 3% bovine serum albumin (BSA) for 2 h to block free binding sites. Incubation was continued overnight in anti-AA diluted 1:50 in PBS/3% BSA, containing 0.1% Tween 20. After thorough washing in PBS/0.1% Tween 20 (1 h, 4–5 changes) the filter strips were incubated overnight with a protein A-horseradish peroxidase conjugate (Amersham International, Buckingamshire, England) diluted 1:1000 in PBS/0.1% Tween 20. An additional washing procedure was included before transferring all the filter strips to the substrate solution. The substrate solution was made by addition of 3 ml 0.3% 4-chloro-1-naphtol (Sigma Chemical Company, St. Louis, USA) in methanol and 1 µl 30% H_1O_2 to 50 ml PBS. The reaction was stopped after 30 min by washing the stips in H_2O.

Enzyme-Linked Immunosorbent Assay (ELISA)

ELISA was performed as described in detail earlier [20].

RESULTS

Induction of Amyloidosis in Mice

The mice were sacrificed four weeks after initiation of the amyloid induction regimen. Moderate amounts of amyloid were found in tissue section from spleen, liver, and kidneys examined after Congo red staining in polarization microscopi.

Gel Filtration of Dissociated Amyloid Fibrils

The amyloidotic organs from mice in group A and B, were pooled separately, and amyloid fibrils extracted with distilled water. The fibrils were gel filtered under dissociating conditions. Some material were excluded from the column, but a small peak was eluted corresponding to a molecular weight of 8-9000 daltons.

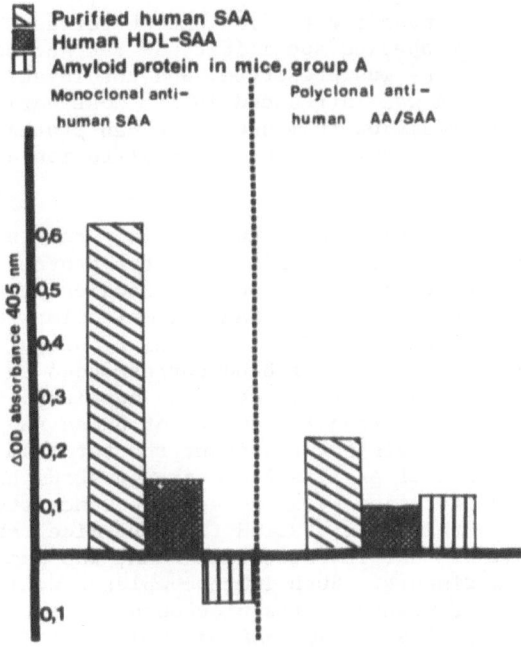

Fig. 3. Antigenic reactivity in ELISA of
human SAA, HCL-SAA and amyloid
from mice in group A, with mouse
anti-human SAA and polyclonal anti-
human AA/SAA.

Double Immuno-Diffusion Analysis of Isolated Amyloid Fibrils

The eluted 8-9000 daltons material from both group A and B mice, inhibited a reaction between mouse SAA and anti-mouse AA/SAA in double im-
muno diffusion. In addition the protein from group A precipitated with
anti human AA/SAA and gave a line of complete identity to human AA (Fig.
1). Anti human AA/SAA did not react with mouse SAA.

Immunoblot Analysis of Amyloid Fibril Proteins

The amyloid proteins from mice in both group A and B, purified human
AA and human HDL-SAA, were subjected to SDS-PAGE, transferred to nitrocellulose filter paper and exposed to antiserum to human AA/SAA. The human AA,
human HDL-SAA and the fibrils from the mice in group A, reacted with anti
human AA/SAA Fig. 2). The HDL-SAA gave two additional band in the immunoblot, one corresponding to a molecular weight of 27,000 daltons, one to
8-9000 daltons.

Enzyme-Linked Immunosorbent Assay

The ELISA experiment showed that the amyloid proteins in mice from
group A did not contain human SAA, but human AA (Table 1, Fig. 3).

DISCUSSION

Until now, the evidence that SAA is the precursor for AA, has been
lacking. Experiment with radiolabelled SAA has failed, probably because
the labelling has altered the protein (B. Skogen, unpublished observations).

In this study it was possible to distinguish between human and mouse AA, because of the strict species specificity of the antisera. The antigenicity of the injected SAA was preserved, and the injection of HDL-SAA complexes ensured that SAA was introduced in its most native form. The mice in group A had, in addition to mouse AA, human protein AA in their amyloid deposits. This was shown in the immunodiffusion and confirmed in the immunoblot and ELISA experiments.

The immunoblot showed that the immunoreacting protein had molecular weight similar to human AA, and the ELISA that the protein was lacking the C-terminal part which react with monoclonal antibodies to human SAA. Two protein bands in the immunoblot of HDL-SAA had molecular weight different from human AA. The band corresponding to the high molecular band, might represent polymers of SAA. The other band corresponded to a molecular weight of 8-9000 daltons and might represent AA complexed to HDL in serum. The amount of this AA is less than the amount of human AA protein extracted from the mice organs, and could not represent the total amount of human AA in the mice. The presence of AA like fragments in serum has been demonstrated before, but not verified by amino acid sequence studies [21]. The possibility that the protein we extracted from the mice, should represent immunocomplexes containing the injected human SAA, was excluded by the immunoblot and ELISA experiments. Such immunocomplexes would have been eluted during the initial saline washes in the procedure for extracting amyloid fibrils. The conservative nature of SAA in evolution [6, 12, 22, was probably the reason why the mice handled the human HDL-SAA complexes as their own. We conclude that the present study has demonstrated the pathway by which SAA, from its presence in HDL particles in serum, via its transformation to AA by proteolysis, is finally deposited as AA fibrils in the rissues. This has shed new light on important aspects of amyloidogenesis.

AKNOWLEDGEMENTS

This work was supported by the Norwegian Council for Science and the Humanities and the Norwegian Rheumatism Council.

REFERENCES

1. M. B. Pepys and M. L. Baltz, Adv. Immunol., 34:141 (1983).
2. G. Husby and J. B. Natvig, J. Clin. Invest., 53:1054 (1974).
3. G. Husby, K. Sletten, T. E. Michaelsen, and J. B. Natvig, Scand. J. Immunol., 1:393 (1972).
4. M. Pras, M. Schubert, D. Zucker-Franklin, A. Rimon, and E. C. Franklin, J. Clin. Invest., 47:924 (1968).
5. C. J. Rosenthal and E. C. Franklin, J. Clin. Invest., 53:1054 (1974).
6. R. F. Anders, J. B. Natvig, K. Sletten, G. Husby, and K. Nordstoga, J. Immunol., 118:229 (1977).
7. E. P. Benditt and N. Eriksen, Proc. Natl. Acad. Sci. USA, 74:4025 (1977).
8. B. Skogen, A. L. Børresen, J. B. Natvig, K. Berg, and T. Michaelsen, Scand. J. Immunol., 10:39 (1979).
9. R. F. Anders, J. B. Natvig, and G. Husby, J. Exp. Med., 143:678 (1976).
10. R. Kisilevski, L. Boudreau, and B. Foster, Lab. Invest., 48:60 (1983).
11. G. Lavie, D. Zucker-Franklin, and E. C. Franklin, J. Exp. Med., 148: 1020 (1978).
12. K. Sletten, G. Marhaug, and G. Husby, Hoppe-Seyler's Z. Physiol. Chem., 364:1039 (1983).
13. B. Skogen and J. B. Matvig, Scand. J. Immunol., 14:389 (1981).
14. B. Skogen, L. Thorsteinsson, and J. B. Natvig, Scand. J. Immunol., 11: 533 (1980).

15. R. J. Havel, H. A. Eder, and J. H. Bragdon, J. Clin. Invest., 34:1345 (1955).
16. R. F. Anders, J. B. Natvig, T. E. Michaelsen, and G. Husby, Scand. J. Immunol., 4:397 (1975).
17. G. Marhaug, G. Gaudernack, B. Bogen, and G. Husby, Clin. Exp. Immunol., 50:390 (1982).
18. R. T. Swank and K. D. Munkres, Analyt. Biochem., 39:462 (1971).
19. H. Towbin, T. Staehelin, and J. Gordon, Proc. Natl. Acad. Sci. USA, 76:4350 (1979).
20. G. Marhaug, Scand. J. Immunol., 18:329 (1983).
21. G. Marhaug, K. Sletten, and G. Husby, in: Amyloidosis E.A.R.S. (C. R. Tribe and P. A. Bacon, eds.), John Wright and Sons Limited, Bristol-London-Boston (1983), pp. 15-18.
22. K. Sletten and G. Husby, Eur. J. Biochem., 41:117 (1974).

ISOLATION AND CHARACTERIZATION OF THE INHIBITOR

OF AMYLOID DEGRADING FACTOR

Igal Kedar and Mordechai Ravid*

Cellular Immunology Section
Arthritis and Rheumatism Branch Institute
of Arthritis, Diabetes, and Digestive and Kidney Diseases
National Institutes of Health
Bethesda, Maryland 20205

*Department of Medicine
 Sackler School of Medicine
 Tel Aviv University
 Israel

ABSTRACT

The inhibitor of amyloid degrading factor is a glycoprotein of 10,000 dalton molecular weight in its inactive monomeric form. The active substance is a polymer obtained upon exposure to calcium ions. The inhibitor was isolated from serum of patients with AA amyloidosis and from amyloidotic liver tissue. The inhibitor does not block the degrading factor through a thiol groups. Restoration of amyloid degrading activity by EDTA and ascorbic acid probably takes place via their chelating effect on calcium ions thus inactivating the inhibitor.

INTRODUCTION

The vast knowledge accumulated over the last two decades about the structure and composition of amyloid did not help to elucidate the pathogenesis of this group of diseases.

We have previously shown that normal human serum contained amyloid degrading activity and that this activity was blocked by amyloidotic serum [1]. We therefore postulated the presence of an inhibitor of degradation in patients with amyloidosis and proposed that inhibition of naturally occurring amyloid degradation plays a role in amyloid deposition.

The data presented here describe the isolation of the inhibitor from amyloidotic serum and tissue, its protein nature and some of its biochemical characteristics.

253

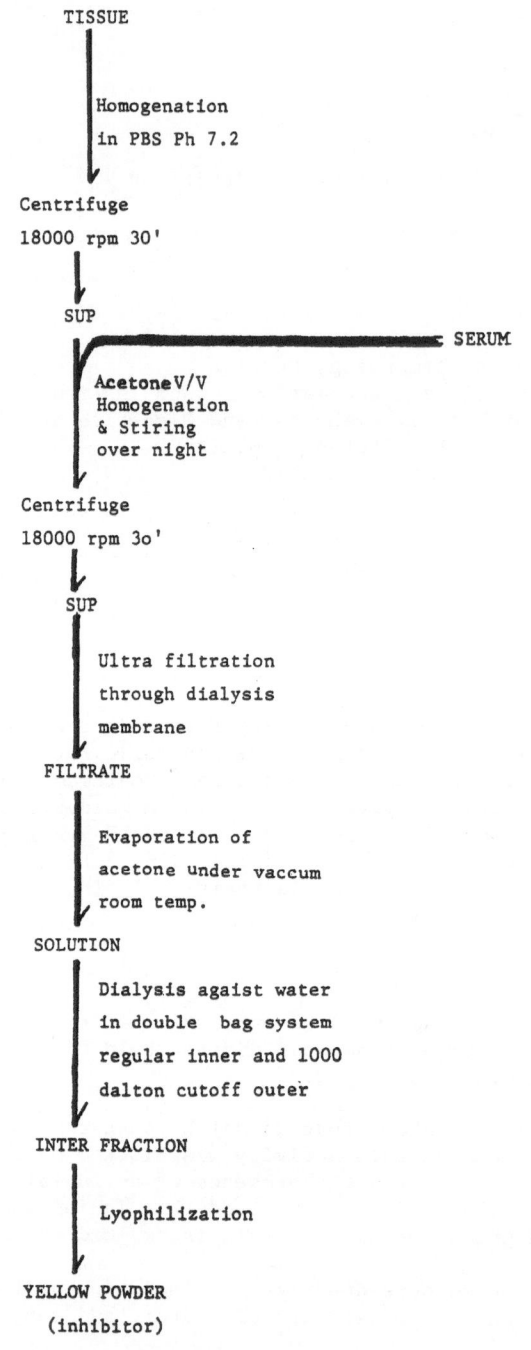

TISSUE

  Homogenation
  in PBS Ph 7.2

Centrifuge
18000 rpm 30'

  SUP ————————————————————————————— SERUM

  Acetone V/V
  Homogenation
  & Stiring
  over night

Centrifuge
18000 rpm 3o'

  SUP

  Ultra filtration
  through dialysis
  membrane

  FILTRATE

  Evaporation of
  acetone under vaccum
  room temp.

  SOLUTION

  Dialysis agaist water
  in double bag system
  regular inner and 1000
  dalton cutoff outer

INTER FRACTION

  Lyophilization

YELLOW POWDER
  (inhibitor)

Fig. 1. Procedure of inhibitor's isolation.

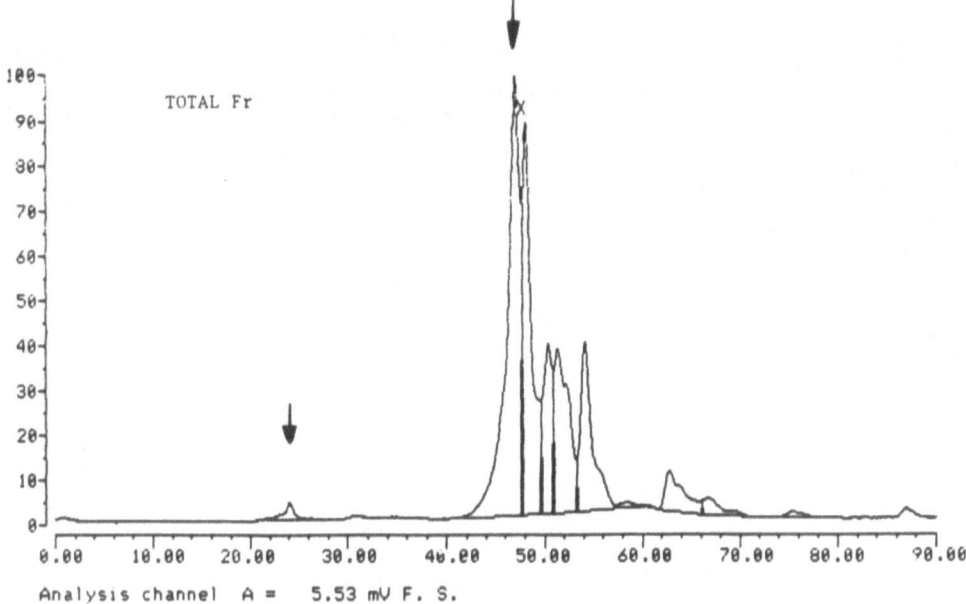

Fig. 2. HPLC profile on the interbag fraction. The arrows indicate the active fractions of the ADA inhibitor.

MATERIALS AND METHODS

Isolation of IADF (inhibitor of amyloid degrading activity)

One hundred ml of serum from a patient with AA amyloidosis or 50 gm of AA amyloidotic lives tissues served as origin. The procedure of the inhibitor isolation is described in Fig. 1. The interbag fraction was extracted by HPLC silicon column TSK-60, at a flow rate of 0.5 ml/min for 90 min. The profile of the extraction is presented in Fig. 2.

Measurement of Inhibitor Activity

The inhibitory activity of each HPLC eluted and lyophilized fraction, was determined by the measurement of its effect on amyloid degradation by the amyloid impregnated agar technique as previously described [1].

The Effect of Known Protease Inhibitors

The effect of the isolated ADA inhibitor was compared to other, known protease inhibitors. Both OH dependent and SH dependent protease inhibitors were used. The test model was the ADA of pooled normal human serum on amyloid impregnated agar. The effect of SH group donors, 2-mercaptoethanol and dithiotreitol was determined on the degrading activity of amyloidotic and normal human sera (Tables 1 and 2).

The Effect of Calcium Ions

The active HPLC fractions of the ADA inhibitor were run on 12.5% acrylamide electrophoresis at 20 mV for 6 h. Both the gel and the running buffer contained 5 mM EDTA. A parallel run was carried out without EDTA and with 2.5 mM $CaCl_2$ in the sample solution of the inhibitor. Twenty microgram of inhibitor protein were loaded in each run (Fig. 3).

TABLE 1. Inhibition of Amyloid Degrading Activity of NHS

Type of inhibitor	Amount used	% of inhibition
Native (patient's origin)	100 micgr/ml	58
N-Ethylmaleimide (NEM)	1 mM	23
p-Chloromercuribenzoic-acid (PCMB)	1 mM	25
Diethylpyrocarbonate (DEPC)	0.1%	60
$CdCl_2$	2.5 mg/ml	90
Aprotinine (trasylol)	100 units/ml	12.5
Pepstatin	1 mg/ml	Null
Leupeptin	1 mg/ml	Null
Phenylmethylsulfonyl-fluoride (PMSF)	1.5 mM	8
Sodium fluoride	0.1_s	Null
CBA/J Ø SUP	0.5 mg/ml	20

TABLE 2. S-H Influence

Serum origin	Amyloid	S-H Donor	Degradation
N.H.S.	−	2.M.E. (0.01%)	↑ (15%)
N.H.S.	−	D.T.T (1 mM)	↑ (15%)
F.M.F.	+	2.M.E. (0.01%)	⟶
F.M.F.	+	D.T.T (1 mM)	⟶
R.A.	+	2.M.E. (0.01%)	⟶
R.A.	+	D.T.T (1 mM)	⟶

Conclusions:

1. Degrading factor activity is S-H dependent.
2. Patient's Inhibitor does not block S-H groups.

     One mg of the interbag fraction (Fig. 1) was dissolved in 1 ml dis-
tilled water which contained 5 mM $CaCl_2$. A precipitate appeared. The suspension was centrifuged at 10,000 rpm for 15 min. The supernatant which
did not show ADA inhibitory activity was loaded on the same HPLC column.
The profile is shown in Fig. 4.

RESULTS

     The active fractions of ADA inhibitor are marked by arrows on the HPLC
profile in Fig. 2. The frontal peak represents 60,000 dalton molecular
weight and seems to be a polymer of the second active peak which is around
10,000 daltons. A similar pattern displaying two lines was obtained on
acrylamide gel electrophoresis (Fig. 3).

     Table 1 displays the effect of various protease inhibitors on ADA of
pooled normal human serum. The SH group inhibitors (NEM, PCMB, DEPC, and
$CalCl_2$) show a significantly higher inhibitory effect than the OH dependent
enzyme inhibitors (PMSF, trasylol, leupeptin, etc.).

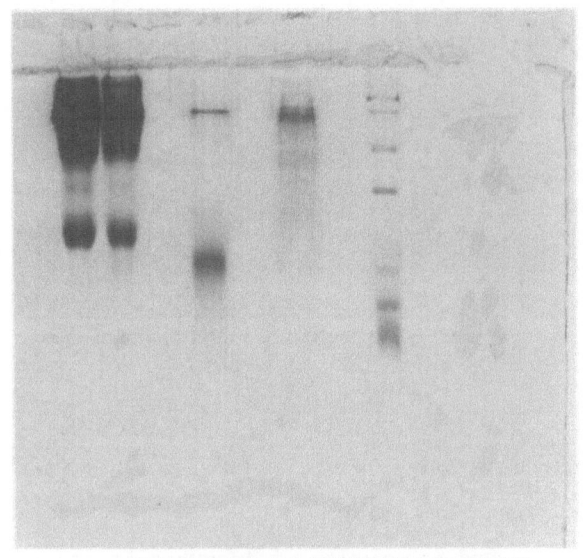

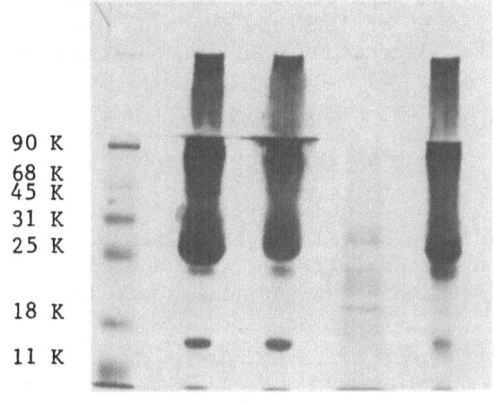

| 90 K |
| 68 K |
| 45 K |
| 31 K |
| 25 K |
| 18 K |
| 11 K |

St   N+In   N   In+Ca^{++} RA+

No   EDTA
in the system

Fig. 3. Acrylamide page electrophoresis of
the inhibitor of ADA and amyloidotic
and nonamyloidotic sera. Top) With
EDTA, mainly the 10,000 dalton mW
fraction appears. Bottom) Without
EDTA, with the addition of 2.5 mM
CaCl$_2$. Mainly the polymeric forms
appear.

The effect of supplementing the system with SH group donors is shown
in Table 2. The ADA of pooled normal human serum was increased by 15%
while there was no effect on the ADA of amyloidotic sera.

The acrylamide Page electrophoresis of the inhibitor in the presence
of EDTA (Fig. 3 - top) shows a single line corresponding to 10,000 daltons
mW. Removal of EDTA and the addition of calcium result in the appearance
of several additional lines corresponding to 20-70,000 dalton mW (Fig. 3 -

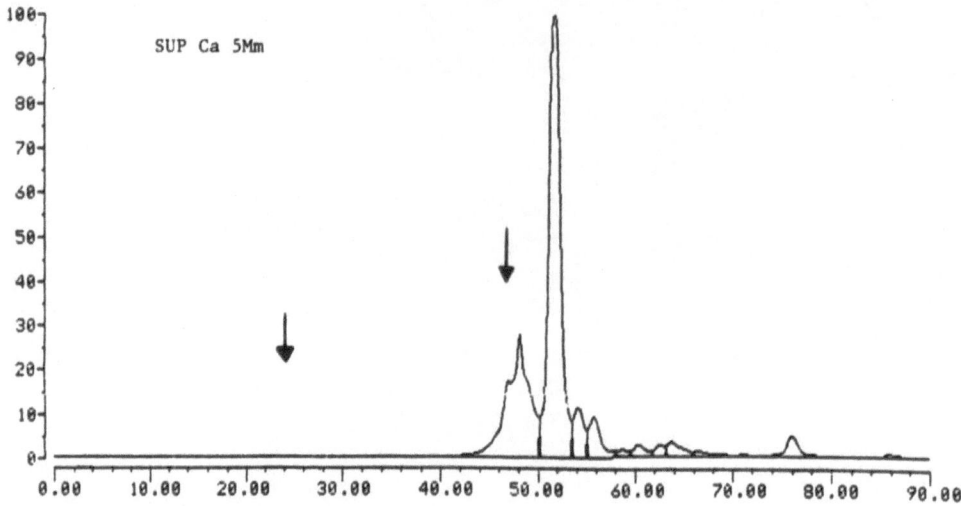

Analysis channel A = 110.61 mV F. S.

Fig. 4. HPLC analysis and separation of interbag fraction. HPLC profile
of the supernatant of interbag fraction after the addition of 5
mM $CaCl_2$. The supernatant contains no active fractions of the
inhibitor.

bottom). These lines probably represent polymers of the 10,000 dalton monomer of the inhibitor.

Following the addition of calcium the repeated HPLC profile lacks the
active peaks of the inhibitor (Fig. 4). The addition of calcium resulted
in polymerization of the inhibitor and its precipitation.

DISCUSSION

The isolation of the inhibitor of amyloid degrading activity enabled us
to define some of its characteristics.

We have been able to show that the purified inhibitor is a protein of
10,000 daltons. This is a monomer which lacks inhibitory activity. In
the presence of calcium ions, polymerization occurs. These fractions show
inhibitory activity on amyloid degrading activity of pooled normal human
serum.

It was previously shown that EDTA, ascorbic acid and citric acid could
restore the amyloid degrading activity of amyloidotic sera [1]. The effect
of these compounds is probably mediated through their chelating effect on
calcium ions. The effect of EDTA on restoration of amyloid degrading activity of amyloidotic serum was reversed by the addition of calcium ions
[2].

The amyloid degrading factor is probably an SH group dependent protease, it is readily inhibited by SH group inhibitors. However, the addition of SH group donors which increased the ADA of normal human serum had
no effect on amyloidotic serum. It therefore stands to reason that the inhibitor does not block the ADA through its SH groups, but through a different as yet unknown mechanism.

More than a decade ago we isolated a yellow powder which was able to accelerate amyloid production in the casein murine model [3]. The present experiments, in a way, close the circle by defining the nature of that yellow powder as the inhibitor of amyloid degrading factor present in human and murine serum.

REFERENCES

1. Kedar, I., Sohar, E., and Ravid, M., J. Lab. Clin. Med., 99:693-7000 (1982).
2. Scott, D. L., Bacan, and Husby, G., Arthritis Rheum., 27:Supp. 4, S77 (1984).
3. Keizman (Kedar), I., Rimon, A., Sohar, E., and Gafni, J., Acta Pathol. Microbiol. Scand., 80:Supp. 233, 172 (1972).

AMYLOID-AGAROSE PLATE TEST: ULTRASTRUCTURAL CHANGES IN THE FIBRIL

AND ITS ASSOCIATION WITH HUMAN NEUTROPHIL ELASTASE*

Martha Skinner, Tsuranobu Shirahama, Phillip Stone,
Lawreen Heller Connors, James Calore and
Alan S. Cohen

Thorndike Memorial Laboratory and Division of Medicine
Boston City Hospital
The Arthritis Center and the Biochemistry Department
Boston University School of Medicine
Boston, Massachusetts 02118

ABSTRACT

    In the amyloid agarose plate test we examined the ultrastructure of
amyloid fibrils after the clearing phenomenon caused by ethylenediamine
tetraacetic acid (EDTA) and by serum. We quantitated total fibril length
in the cleared and noncleared (control) areas by digital image analysis.
EDTA resulted in shortening of the AA fibril by 31% in 3 h and 40% in 24 h.
Serum resulted in shortening only 24% of the fibril in 3 h, but shortening
to less than one half its original length in 24 h. Further examination of
the fibrils from each of the systemic amyloid types (AL, AA, and AF) demonstrated similar clearing in agar plates. In addition, all had large amounts
of elastolytic enzyme activity in a specific assay using tritiated elastin.
The source of this fibril-bound enzyme activity was consistent with human
neutrophil elastase (HNE), since it was inhibited by an elastase specific
chloromethyl ketone inhibitor, as well as by an antibody specific for human
neutrophil elastase.

INTRODUCTION

    Kedar, et al., originally noted and others have confirmed the fact that
serum has the ability to degrade AA type amyloid fibrils in an amyloid-agar
gel preparation [1-8]. The reaction suggests that amyloid fibrils which
have been suspended in agar disappear, as a clearing zone is observed in
the agar when it is permeated by normal serum. It is not known whether this
represents enzymatic proteolysis or another form of disruption of the beta
pleated sheet amyloid fibril structure.

---

*Supported from grants from the U.S. Public Health Service, NIAMDD (AM 04499
and AM 07014), Multipurpose Arthritis Center, National Institutes of Health
(AM 20613), the General Clinical Research Centers Branch of the Division of
Research Resources, National Institutes of Health (RR 533), National Institutes of Health (HL 19717, HL 13263, HL 25229), and the Arthritis Foundation.

In all studies the fibril clearing effect is greater with serum from healthy individuals and decreased with serum from patients with an inflammatory illness. This is considered supportive evidence for the relationship of these disorders with the appearance of secondary amyloidosis. We observed the clearing phenomena to occur with EDTA alone. This prompted a series of experiments on the degrading effect of this chelating agent in comparison to the degrading effect of normal serum.

MATERIALS AND METHODS

Amyloid Plate Test

Amyloid-agarose plates were prepared using AA (secondary), AL (primary) or AF (hereditary) amyloid fibrils [9]. Top layer amyloid fibrils [10, 11] were suspended in a small volume of 0.05 M Tris (hydroxymethyl) aminomethane (Tris), buffer, pH 7.6. The suspension was added to 1% agarose which had been dissolved by heating in 0.05 M Tris, pH 7.6 and cooled to 60°C. The fibril concentration was 8 mg/10 ml agarose. Immediately after mixing, a 10 ml aliquot was poured into a flat bottom Petri dish (100 × 15 mm) and allowed to set at room temperature resulting in a hazy gel.

The amyloid-agarose plate was performed by introducing 15 μl of sample, (serum, 0.02 M EDTA or human neutrophil elastase) solution by calibrated micropipette into a 5 mm circular well cut in the agarose. A reaction was a circular zone of clearing in the hazy gel around the well. After 3 h and 24 h, specimens of the AA fibril agar plates were removed with a 2 mm punch for ultrastructural examination.

Electron Microscopy

The specimens were fixed in 1.25% glutaraldehyde–1.0% paraformaldehyde in 0.1 M phosphate buffer at pH 7.4 overnight at 4°C, and then postfixed in 1% digallic acid in 0.1 M phosphate buffer with 1.5% sucrose at pH 7.4 for 2 h at room temperature [12]. They were then dehydrated through a series of graded ethanols, and embedded in Araldite 502. Thin sections were stained with uranyl acetate and lead citrate and examined in an RCA UME-3G electron microscope.

Examination of Fibril Length

Fibril length was measured on photomicrographs (magnification 44,000 ×) taken from the cleared and control areas using a mop-3q digital image analyzer system (Zeiss, W. Germany). A template with five randomly drawn 5 cm square areas was place over each photomicrograph, insuring examination of identical areas on each totaling 12,500 mm². A writing stylus was drawn over all fibrils within each 5 cm square and total fibril length computed according to stereological measuring methods [13]. Three photomicrographs were examined from each of the 2 mm punch preparations.

Human Neutrophil Elastase Assay

AA, AL, and AF fibrils were assayed for elastin solubilizing activity. The fibrils were incubated at 37°C for 20 h in the presence of washed ^{3}H-calf ligamentum muchae elastin in 4 ml of buffer (0.05 M Tris, pH 7.6, 0.6 M NaCl, 0.05% NaN$_3$) [14, 15]. At the end of incubation the samples were mixed, centrifuged and the supernatants filtered. The amount of elastin solubilized was calculated from the level of radioactivity present corrected for the background level of radioactivity released from ^{3}H-elastin in buffer only. By comparing tubes containing ^{3}H-elastin and standard amounts of HNE, the levels of elastolytic activity were able to be expressed as HNE

TABLE 1. Human Neutrophil Elastase Activity on Amyloid Fibrils

Four mg of amyloid fibrils	ng HNE equivalents ± SE (n)		
	AA fibrils	AL fibrils	AF fibrils
Alone	1383 ± 228(2)	33 ± 2	1029
Plus elastase-specific chloromethyl ketone	33 ± 3(2)	9 ± 1(2)	62
Plus HNE antibody (rabbit IgG fraction)	49	13	N.D.
Plus alpha-1-protease inhibitor	22 ± 1(2)	7 ± 1(2)	N.D.
Plus porcine pancreatic elastase antibody	998	8	N.D.

N.D.) Not determined.

equivalents. Assays were performed on 4 mg of AA, AL, or AF fibrils either alone or including one of the following: human neutrophil elastase-specific inhibitor succinyl (L-alanyl) prolyl valyl chloromethyl ketone (CMK) [16], IgG fraction of rabbit anti-human neutrophil elastase antibody, alpha-1 protease inhibitor, or porcine pancreatic elastase antibody which was used as an unrelated control antiserum.

RESULTS

All three types of amyloid fibril (AL, AA, and AF) agarose plates showed clearing surrounding wells with serum, EDTA, or human neutrophil elastase. Clearing zones were seen within three hours and appeared to be complete after 24 h. EDTA consistently gave a clearing which was somewhat weaker in appearance than that produced by serum.

In ultrastructural studies the AA amyloid fibrils taken from a control (noncleared) area showed no significant changes at 0, 3, or 24 h. The unaltered fibrils appeared rather densely spread throughout the preparation. At 3 h both the serum and EDTA cleared areas show a significant decrease in density and in length of the fibrils compared to control preparation with little difference noted between the serum and EDTA samples. In 24 h serum and EDTA cleared areas the fibrils show a further shortening in length, which was greater in the serum cleared area. The total fibril length drawn with the digital image analyzer from a randomized 12,500 square mm area on each of the micrographs quantitated this shortening. EDTA shortened the fibril by 31% in 3 h and 40% in 24 h. Serum shortened the fibril by 24% in 3 h but to less than one half of its length in 24 h.

In the tritiated elastin assay for human neutrophil elastase, all three fibril types (AL, AA, and AF) had significant amounts of elastolytic activity (Table 1). Elastolytic activity was inhibited by the presence of a neutrophil elastase-specific synthetic inhibitor, chloromethyl ketone (CMK). The AL and AA fibrils also showed inhibition by human neutrophil elastase antibody and human alpha-1 protease inhibitor. When a control antiserum was added, no significant inhibition was noted with the AA sample. Lack of sufficient quantities of AF fibrils precluded these last three determinations.

DISCUSSIONS

The clearing phenomenon in the amyloid-agarose plate has been attributed to an effect produced by the serum on the amyloid fibril. Although the serum appears to be an important component in the reaction, the proteolytic enzyme responsible for the effect may reside on the amyloid fibril itself.

The ultrastructural studies suggest a marked disruption of the amyloid fibrils over 24 h with both EDTA and serum. This decrease in fibril length was confirmed when quantitated by digital image analysis. The ultrastructural appearance and the results of digital image analysis suggest a degradation of the amyloid fibril, perhaps by proteolysis.

In a very specific assay for an elastase we have found significant amounts of elastolytic activity to be present on isolated amyloid fibrils from all three systemic forms of amyloid disease. The dramatic inhibition of this enzyme activity by an elastase specific chloromethyl ketone inhibitor, an antibody to human neutrophil elastase and by human alpha-1-protease inhibitor strongly support the identification of this enzyme on the AA fibril, at least, as human neutrophil elastase.

In summary, we have shown that a degradation of amyloid fibrils within an agarose plate is definitely associated with a loss of total fibril length by digital image analysis. In addition, using a specific assay we have shown that fibril preparations of all systemic forms of amyloidosis contain human neutrophil elastase. These observations may be important in understanding the pathogenesis of amyloidosis with respect to the inability of variant molecular forms of precursor proteins to undergo normal proteolytic digestion.

REFERENCES

1. I. Kedar, E. Sohar, and J. Gafni, Proc. Soc. Exp. Biol. Med., 145:343 (1974).
2. I. Kedar, M. Ravid, and E. Sohar, in: Amyloid and Amyloidosis (G. G. Glenner, P. P. Costa, F. Freitas, eds.), Excerpta Medica, Amsterdam (1980), pp. 60-62.
3. I. Kedar, E. Sohar, and M. Ravid, J. Lab. Clin. Med., 99, 693 (1982).
4. C. P. J. Maury and A. M. Teppo, Lancet 2, 234 (1982).
5. M. Skinner et al., Trans. Assoc. Am. Phys., 96:437 (1983).
6. B. Skogen and J. B. Natvig, Scand. J. Immunol., 14:389 (1981).
7. A. M. Teppo, C. P. J. Maury, and O. Wegelius, Scand. J. Immunol., 16: 309 (1982).
8. O. Wegelius, A. M. Teppo, and C. P. J. Maury, Br. Med. J., 284:617 (1982).
9. E. P. Benditt et al., in: Amyloid and Amyloidosis (G. G. Glenner, P. P. Costa, F. Freitas, eds.), Excerpta Medica, Amsterdam (1980, pp. xi-xii.
10. M. Pras, M. Schubert, D. Zucker-Franklin, A. Rimon, and E. C. Franklin, J. Clin. Invest., 47:924 (1968).
11. M. Skinner, T. Shirahama, A. S. Cohen, and C. L. Deal, Prep. Biochem., 12:461 (1983).
12. O. G. Rogers, T. Shirahama, and A. S. Cohen, in: Proceedings Electron Microscopy of America 1977 (G. W. Bailey, ed.), Claitor's, Baton Rouge (1977), pp. 542-543.
13. E. R. Weibel, G. S. Kistler, and W. F. Scherle, J. Cell Biol., 30:23 (1966).
14. P. J. Stone, J. D. Calore, G. L. Snider, and C. Franzblau, J. Clin. Invest., 69:920 (1982).

15. P. J. Stone, G. Crombie, and C. Franzblau, Anal. Biochem., 80:572 (1977).
16. J. C. Powers, B. F. Gupton, A. D. Harley, N. Nishino, and R. J. Whitley, Biochem. Biophys. Acta, 485:156 (1977.

DECREASED ESTERASE ACTIVITY IN SERUM OF PATIENTS

WITH REACTIVE SYSTEMIC (AA) AMYLOIDOSIS

C. P. J. Maury, W. Junge,
and A.-M. Teppo

Fourth Department of Medicine
University of Helsinki
Helsinki, Finland, and

Laboratory Department
Kiel Hospital
West Germany

ABSTRACT

Serum esterase activities were measured in patients with AA amyloidosis and in control subjects. Patients with rheumatoid arthritis + amyloidosis had significantly reduced activities of arylesterase and paraoxonase, but not cholinesterase, as compared to healthy subjects and to disease controls including patients with rheumatoid arthritis without amyloid and patients with various nonamyloid liver and renal diseases. A significant correlation was found between serum arylesterase and amyloid degrading activity (r = 0.51, p < 0.01).

INTRODUCTION

The major constituent of the amyloid fibrils deposited in tissues of patients with inflammation-associated (reactive) amyloidosis is amyloid A (AA) protein [1, 2] which is believed to be formed from a circulating precursor, serum amyloid A protein (SAA) [3, 4]. Direct proof for this is lacking, but SAA is structurally and immunologically closely related to AA, and serine proteases of monocytic origin can cleave SAA to an AA-like fragment [5, 6]. Moreover, in conditions associated with reactive amyloidosis, elevated SAA levels are found [7, 10] and persistently high SAA levels correlate with rapid progression of amyloidosis [11]. If the underlying disease is controlled, resolution of AA amyloid may occur [12]. The molecular mechanisms involved in the resolution process are largely unknown, but they may involve serine proteases [13, 14].

We recently described an albumin-associated serine protease/hydrolase activity that is reduced in patients with reactive amyloidosis [8, 15]. Because previous studies have shown the presence of an esterase-like activity (the "albumin esterase") [16, 17] and a protease activity [18] in albumin preparations, we studied the possible relationships between various serum esterase activities and amyloid degrading activity. Significantly reduced by arylesterase and paraoxonase, but no cholinesterase, activities were found in patients with reactive amyloidosis. The arylesterase activity correlated positively with amyloid degrading activity.

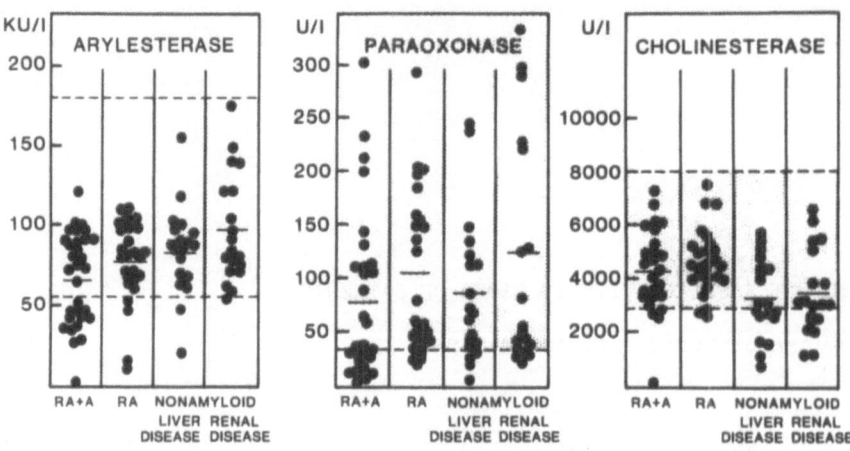

Fig. 1. Serum esterase activities in different groups of patients.
Hatched area: Reference range of activity. Details of
the patient groups are given in Methods section.

Patients and Methods

    Group RA + A consisted of 31 patients (19 women, 12 men; mean age 53
years, range 31 to 84) with rheumatoid arthritis plus amyloidosis, which
was histologically confirmed in all cases. Serum creatinine levels were
243 ± 41 µmol/L (SEM), and mean proteinuria was 4.7 ± 0.7 gm/24 h. Group
RA consisted of 26 patients (15 women, 11 men; mean age 52.2 years, range
26 to 80) with rheumatoid arthritis. None had clinical signs of amyloidosis. Their renal function was normal, and they had no proteinuria (<0.1/24
h). Because patients with liver disease may have changed esterase [19, 20]
and AA degrading activity [21], a group of patients with liver disease was
included. It consisted of 19 patients (10 women, 9 men; mean age 47.5
years, range 30 to 76) with histologically confirmed liver diseases.
Chronic active hepatitis, liver cirrhosis, fatty liver degeneration, primary biliary cirrhosis, and metastatic liver disease. Because patients
with amyloidosis had hypoalbuminemia and renal insufficiency, we included
patients with renal diseases as an additional control group. The group
consisted of 19 patients (8 women, 11 men; mean age 44.7 years, range 15
to 79) with various renal diseases, but not amyloidosis. Serum albumin
level was 20.8 ± 1.3 gm/L, creatinine 363 ± 75 µmol/L and proteinurea
3.2 ± 0.6 g/24 h.

    Serum arylesterase (EC 3.1.1.2) activity was measured with phenyl-
acetate used as substrate; details of the assay have been described elsewhere [19]. The reference values for the assay are 55 to 180 kU/L. Serum
paraoxonase activity was measured with diethyl-p-nitrophenyl phosphate as
substrate. The reference value is >35 U/L. Serum (pseudo-)cholinesterase
(EC 3.1.1.8) activity was measured with butyryl choline used as substrate
according to the recommendation of the German Society for Clinical Chemistry. The reference values are 3000 to 8000 U/L. Amyloid degrading activity was assayed as described previously [8, 15, 24].

    Previous studies have shown that the addition of inhibitors of serine
hydrolases to serum (diisopropyl fluorophosphate, methylsulfonylfluoride)
as well as physiologic inhibitors (α_1-antitrypsin or α_1-macroglobulin) inhibits the amyloid degrading activity [15]. Dialysis of sera with reduced
amyloid degrading activity against physiologic saline solution (1 h), phosphate-buffered solution (1 h), and Tris HCl buffer with 2.5 mmol/L Ca^{2+} and
1.0 mmol/L Mg^{2+} addition (2 h) did not affect the degrading activity.

TABLE 1. Number of Patients with Decreased Serum Esterase Activities
(below reference values) in the Different Patient Groups

Patient group	n	Arylesterase < 55 KU/L	Paraoxonase < 35 U/L	Cholinesterase < 3000 U/L
RA + A	31	13^x	14^{xx}	4^{xxx}
RA	26	4	4	3
Nonamyloid liver disease	19	2	4	9
Nonamyloid renal disease	19	1	5	7

The other comparisons were not significant.

^{x} $p < 0.05$ vs. Liver disease, $p < 0.02$ vs. renal disease,
$p < 0.01$ vs. all nonamyloid together.

^{xx} $p < 0.05$ vs. RA and all nonamyloid groups together.

^{xxx} $p < 0.05$ vs. liver disease.

TABLE 2. Renal Function and Degree of Proteinuria in RA + A Patients with
Reduced or Normal Arylesterase Activity

RA + A	n	Serum creatinine (μmol/L)	Proteinuria (g/24 hr)
Arylesterase < 55 kU/L	13	168 $\pm$ 21	3.1 $\pm$ 1.0
Arylesterase $\geq$ 55 kU/L	18	290 $\pm$ 64^x	5.7 $\pm$ 0.8^x

Values represent mean $\pm$ SEM.

^{x}Difference not significant.

Chi-square test and linear regression analysis were used in the statistical calculations.

RESULTS

The activities of arylesterase, paroxonase, and cholinesterase in patients in the RA + A, RA, nonamyloid liver disease and nonamyloid disease groups are shown in Fig. 1. Values in patients with systemic amyloidosis differed from those in the other patient groups with respect to arylesterase and paroxonase activities (Table 1); 13 of 31 had decreased arylesterase activity and 14 of 31 had decreased paroxonase activity. The activity of cholinesterase was similar in patients with RA with and without
amyloidosis, whereas patients with nonamyloid liver disease as well as renal

TABLE 3. Linear Regression Analysis of the Relationship between Amyloid A
Degrading Activity and Esterase Activities

	r		
Amyloid A degrading activity vs	RA + A (n = 31)	RA (n = 26)	All (n = 95)
Arylesterase	0.51[x]	0.37	0.34[xx]
Cholinesterase	0.02	0.23	0.16
Paraoxonase	0.44	0.37	0.18

[x] p < 0.01

[xx] p < 0.001

disease had decreased activity (Table 1). The combination of <55 kU/L
arylesterase plus <35 U/L paraoxonase activity was found in 32% (10/31) of
the patients with amyloidosis, but only in 4% (1/26) of the patients with
RA without any amyloidosis (p < 0.05) and in 5% (3/64) of all patients without amyloidosis (p < 0.001).

Patients with amyloidosis with decreased or normal arylesterase activity did not significantly differ from each other with respect to serum
creatinine level or degree of proteinuria (Table 2), although those with
normal activity tended to have a more severe nephropathy.

When the whole material was analyzed, significant correlations between
serum arylesterase and AA degrading activity were found (Table 3). Correlation was more evident in patients with RA and amyloidosis than in those
without amyloidosis (Table 3).

DISCUSSION

Arylesterase (aryl-esterase hydrolase, EC 3.1.1.2) are thiol enzymes
present in mammalian serum. They belong to the group of carboxylesterases
and preferentially split aromatic esters of fatty acids [25]. Their physiologic function is not known. Our results show that >40% of patients with
reactive systemic amyloidosis have a decreased arylesterase activity. The
result was the same when diethyl-p-nitrophenyl phosphate was used as substrate (paraoxonase activity). Previous studies have shown that serum
arylesterase activity is reduced in patients with liver cirrhosis and metastatic liver disease, whereas normal levels have been found in patients with
acute and chronic inflammatory liver diseases [20] corroborating the results
of this study. Because hepatic involvement in systemic reactive amyloidosis
is common, a possible explanation for the low arylesterase activity could be
liver impairment attributable to amyloid. However, with respect to liver
function, the amyloidotics with reduced arylesterase activity did not differ
from those with normal arylesterase activity. Moreover, cholinesterase activity, which is reduced in various parenchymatous liver diseases, was normal in the RA + A group. Thus systemic amyloidosis seems to represent a
disorder with reduced arylesterase activity without evidence of concomitant

significant hepatic dysfunction. The cause of the reduced activity remains unexplained, but it may be related to increased inhibitor levels.

Our previous studies have shown that the serum factor responsible for the lysing effect on AA fibrils in agar has characteristics of serine hydrolases [15]. Burlina et al. [20] have, on the other hand, shown that the behavior of serum arylesterase toward inhibitors is similar to that of serine hydrolases. This is of particular interest because our present results show a significant correlation between amyloid degrading and arylesterase activities. Moreover, the two activities seem to have other common characteristics: pH optimum stability, behavior toward inhibitors, and electrophoretic mobility [15, 19, 20, 25]. The exact molecular properties of the arylesterase measured in this study are not known, however. Arylesterase activity has been reported to be associated also with the lipoprotein fraction [22]. It is noteworthy that purified albumin preparations display both AA degrading [13], esterase [16], and serine protease [18] activities. Thus AA degrading activity in serum seems to be in many respects related to the esterase activity.

The reduced serine hydrolase activity may be directly involved in the development and progression of reactive amyloidosis. The possibility that the reduced activity is a result of the disease process should, however, also be considered.

REFERENCES

1. E. P. Benditt and N. Eriksen, Am. J. Pathol., 65:231 (1971).
2. M. Levin, E. C. Franklin, B. Frangione, and M. Pras, J. Clin. Invest., 51:2773 (1972).
3. G. Husby and J. B. Natvig, J. Clin. Invest., 53:1054 (1974).
4. R. P. Linke, J. D. Sipe, P. S. Pollock, T. F. Ignazak, and G. G. Glenner, Proc. Natl. Acad. Sci. USA, 72:1473 (1975).
5. G. Lavie, D. Zucker-Franklin, and E. C. Franklin, J. Immunol., 125: 175 (1980).
6. B. Skogen, L. Thorsteinsson, and J. B. Natvig, Scand. J. Immunol., 11: 531 (1980).
7. M. D. Benson and A. S. Cohen, Arthritis Rheum., 22:36 (1979).
8. O. Wegelius, A.-M. Teppo, and C. P. J. Maury, Br. Med. J., 284:617 (1982).
9. F. C. deBeer, R. K. Mallya, E. A. Fagan, J. G. Lanham, G. R. V. Hughes, and M. B. Pepys, Lancet, 2:231 (1982).
10. C. P. J. Maury, A.-M. Teppo, and O. Wegelius, Ann. Rheum. Dis., 41: 268 (1982).
11. H. M. Falck, C. P. J. Maury, A.-M. Teppo, and O. Wegelius, Br. Med. J., 286:1391 (1983).
12. G. G. Glenner, N. Engl. J. Med., 302:1283, 1333 (1980).
13. C. P. J. Maury and A.-M. Teppo, Lancet, 2:234 (1982).
14. A.-M. Teppo and C. P. J. Maury, Scand. J. Immunol., 18:363 (1983).
15. A.-M. Teppo, C. P. J. Maury, and O. Wegelius, Scand. J. Immunol., 16: 309 (1982).
16. S. B. Tove, Biochim. Biophys. Acta, 57:230 (1962).
17. J. Otto, A. Ronai, and O. von Demling, Eur. J. Biochem., 116:285 (1981).
18. M. Schwartz, Clin. Chim. Acta, 124:213 (1982).
19. K. Lorenz, B. Flatter, and E. Augustin, Clin. Chem., 25:1714 (1979).
20. A. Burlina, E. Michielin, and L. Galzigna, Eur. J. Clin. Invest., 7:17 (1977).
21. C. P. J. Maury, A.-M. Teppo, and M. P. Salaspuro, Clin. Chim. Acta, 131:29 (1983).
22. H. Klees, Investigations on human aryl esterase, Academic Dissertation, University of Kiel, West Germany (1983).

23. W. Junge and H. Klees, Arylesterase, in: Methods in Enzymatic Analysis (H. J. Bergmeyer, ed.), Weinheim, West Germany, Verlag Chemie
(1983).

24. I. Kedar and E. Sohar, Amyloid degrading activity of human serum, in:
Amyloid and Amyloidosis (G. G. Glenner, P. P. Costa, and A. F. Freitas,
eds.), Excerpta Medica, Amsterdam (1980).

25. K. B. Augustinsson, Ann. N. Y. Acad. Sci., 94:844 (1961).

ENHANCED DEGRADATION OF AMYLOID AA PROTEINS BY ENZYME ACTIVATION:

A POSSIBLE MODEL FOR A THERAPEUTIC APPROACH

B. Skogen and J. B. Natvig

Institute of Immunology and Rheumatology
Rikshospitalet
The National Hospital
Oslo, Norway

ABSTRACT

The capacity of plasminogen from human serum to degrade amyloid AA protein was tested using radiolabelled protein AA coupled to cyanogen bromide activated Sepharose 6 MB as substrate. Protein AA degrading activity was determined in fractions of normal human serum separated by Sephadex G 150. Each fraction was tested in the presence and absence of the plasminogen activator streptokinase. The AA degrading activity was markedly increased in fractions in which plasminogen activation had occurred. These fractions were also the same as those showing the presence of plasminogen as demonstrated by reaction with a specific anti-plasminogen antiserum. Moreover, the increase in AA degrading activity could be inhibited with antibodies to plasminogen. AA degrading activity could also be enhanced in whole human plasma by streptokinase activation.

INTRODUCTION

A variety of enzymes appear to cause a rapid degradation of the anyloid protein SAA which is the precursor of protein AA [1, 2]. Thus, enzymes of monocytic or granulocytic origin [3, 4, 5], as well as serum enzymes [6, 7] degrade amyloid AA proteins and their precursors. The purpose of the present study was to characterize the activity of plasmin as one of the proteolytic enzymes in serum which upon activation, e.g., by streptokinase, degrade protein AA.

MATERIALS AND METHODS

The details of the materials and methods are published elsewhere [8]. Briefly, the substrate was made from radioactively labelled protein AA immobilized by coupling to cyanogen bromide (CNBr) activated Sepharose 6 MB (Pharmacia AB, Uppsala, Sweden), as previously described. For control, a synthetic chromogenic substrate, S 2251 (Kabi Diagnostica, Stockholm, Sweden), was used to determine the activity of plasmin.

To determine AA degrading activity the suspended gel particles (0.2 ml) were added to the solutions to be tested for enzymatic activity, and

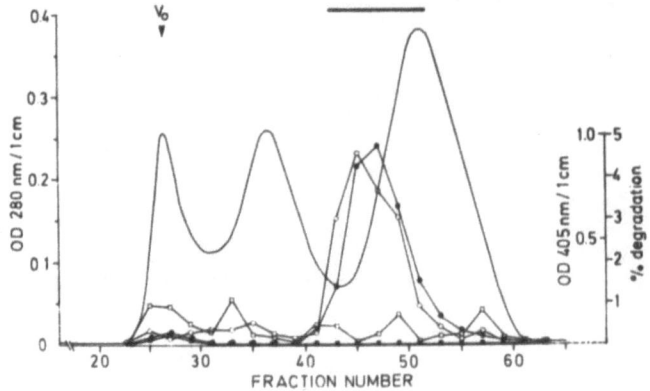

Fig. 1. Gel filtration of normal human serum on
Sephadex G 150. V_0) Void volume of the
column. The bar indicates the fractions
reacting with antiserum to human plasminogen. (■) Activity in the crude fractions
against substrate S2251. (●) Activity
against S2251 after addition of streptokinase. (□) AA-degrading activity in the
crude fractions, and (○) AA-degrading activity after addition of streptokinase.

these mixtures were incubated at 37°C. The AA degrading activity was determined by counting the radioactivity in an aliquot of the reaction solution after it had been shaken and the gel particles had sedimented. The
activity in the supernatant was calculated as a percentage of the total activity in the substrate. Elastase (E-1250, Sigma Chem. Co., St. Louis, Mo.,
USA) was dissolved in PBS at concentrations of 0.1, 0.01, and 0.001 mg/ml.
Samples (1 ml) were tested for AA degrading activity to control the applicability of the AA substrate. In parallel experiments, the serine protease
inhibitor diisopropyl fluorophosphate (DIFP, Sigma Chem. Co.) was added to
the elastase solutions to a concentration of 1 mM 30 min before addition of
the AA substrate. This showed complete inhibition. Aliquots (1 ml) of the
gel filtration fractions of normal human serum were tested for AA degrading
activity in the presence and absence of streptokinase. Streptokinase dissolved in PBS (1000 IU in 0.1 ml) was added and the samples were incubated
at 37°C for 4 h. The activity was also determined in 0.5 ml samples of normal human plasma in the presence and absence of streptokinase, which was
added as described as above.

RESULTS

     Studies on streptokinase activated gel filtration fractions of human
serum.

     The normal human serum fractions separated on a Sephadex G 150 column
under neutral conditions were tested in double immunodiffusion with an antiserum to plasminogen. The positive fractions are indicated by the bar in
Fig. 1. Then the activity against the Sepharose 6 MB-protein AA substrate
and the control plasmin substrate S 2251 was tested in each serum fraction
before and after the addition of streptokinase. As shown in Fig. 1 no or
very low enzyme activity could be encountered before activation. In contrast, upon activation a markedly increased enzyme activity occurred. This
was demonstrated both by reaction with the plasmin substrate S 2251 and by

274

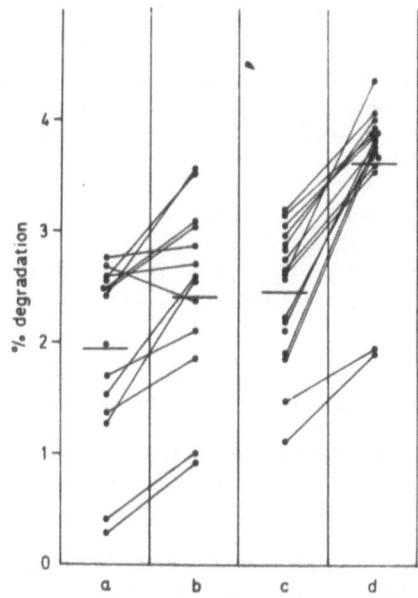

Fig. 2. Determination of AA degrading activity in human
plasma in the absence and
presence of streptokinase.
a) Plasma without streptokinase, 30 min; b) plasma
with streptokinase, 30 min;
c) plasma without streptokinase, 60 min; d) plasma
with streptokinase, 60 min.
The results from parallel
experiments are connected
by lines. The bars represent the mean values.

degradation of the protein AA substrate. The active serum fractions all
coincided with those fractions which was shown to contain plasminogen evidenced by reaction with the anti-plasminogen antiserum. In addition, the
characterization of the enzyme as being activated from plasminogen was
further demonstrated in the following inhibition studies. When the anti-
plasminogen antiserum was added (0.1 ml) to the fraction with the highest
AA degrading activity 30 min before addition of streptokinase and AA substrate, the AA degrading activity was reduced by about 85%, whereas the reduction obtained with control antibodies to sheep IgG was only about 10%.

Studies on Streptokinase Activated Human Plasma

Based on the positive experiments with serum fractions, some additional
studies were done with human plasma from healthy blood donors before and
after addition of streptokinase. In control experiments saline was used
instead of plasma. As shown in Fig. 2, a marked increase in AA degrading
enzyme activity was seen in the experiments both upon 30 min and 60 min incubation with streptokinase, as compared to untreated plasma. Saline controls with streptokinase alone did not give any degradation of protein AA,
and the background spontaneous release from the substrate was rather low.

DISCUSSION

During the last 10-15 years amyloid fibril proteins have been extensively characterized. However, we have more limited knowledge of their catabolism in normal individuals and amyloidotic patients, as well as possible therapeutic approaches to degrade or dissolve these proteins.

Enzymes of monocytic and granulocytic origin [3, 4, 5], as well as serum enzymes [6, 7] can degrade protein AA, and these enzymes appears to belong to the group of serine proteases. Thus, strong AA degrading activity was found in kallikrein-, collagenase-, and elastase preparations, and intermediate in plasmin, whereas thrombin was almost inactive [7].

There has recently been a considerable discussion on the amyloid degrading activity of serum using an agar technique developed by Kedar et al. [9]. However, accumulated evidence indicate that this is a quite difficult method with several pitfalls [10]. We have, on the other hand, developed a simple and reliable technique using protein AA coupled to Sepharose 6 MB by CNBr as substrate for measuring enzyme activity [8].

By using this method, specific enzyme activities such as that of the plasminogen/plasmin system have been clearly shown to degrade protein AA to small peptides. Similar studies of clearly defined enzyme systems which degrade protein AA or amyloid fibrils have been performed by others [11].

Some studies indicate that patients with amyloidosis may have a deficient clearing mechanism for protein AA, e.g., as demonstrated by lower activity of their monocyte associated enzymes with protein AA degrading capacity [3]. For this reason approaches to activate enzyme systems which degrade amyloid fibrils may have potential therapeutic implications. Also, the possibility for preventing the development of amyloidosis in certain exposed risk groups by enhancing their SAA/AA degrading capacity should be considered.

We have here presented the plasminogen/plasmin enzyme system which in vitro can be readily activated by streptokinase to enhance the protein AA degrading activity. Further studies along these lines are now undertaken to see whether such a system is effective to enhance degradation of protein AA upon activation in vivo. One of the problems with an activator like streptokinase when it is used in vivo is its own antigenicity. However, further access to other homologous activators such as urokinase might in the future help to get around those problems. Experiments designed to activate other enzyme systems to prevent or treat different types of amyloidosis by degrading the amyloid proteins or their precursors should have high priority.

REFERENCES

1. Anders, R. F., Nordstoga, K., Natvig, J. B., and Husby, G., J. Exp. Med., 143, 678 (1976).
2. Husebekk, A., Skogen, B., Husby, G., and Marhaug, G., Scand. J. Immunol. (in press).
3. Lavie, G., Zucker-Franklin, D., and Franklin, E. C., J. Exp. Med., 148, 1020 (1978).
4. Skogen, B., Thorsteinsson, L., and Natvig, J. B., Scand. J. Immunol., 11, 533 (1980).
5. Silverman, S. L., Cathcart, E. S., Skinner, M., Cohen, A. S., and Burnett, L., in: Amyloid and Amyloidosis (G. G. Glenner, P. P. Costa, and A. F. Freitas, eds.), Excerpta Medica, Amsterdam-Oxford-Princeton (1980), p. 420.

6. Skogen, B., Natvig, J. B., Borresen, A. L., and Berg, K., Scand. J. Immunol., 11, 643 (1980).
7. Skogen, B., and Natvig, J. B., Scand. J. Immunol., 14, 931 (1981).
8. Skogen, B., and Natvig, J. B., Scand. J. Immunol., 14, 637 (1981).
9. Kedar, I., Ravid, M., and Sohar, E., in: Amyloid and Amyloidosis (G. G. Glenner, P. P. Costa, and A. F. Freitas, eds.), Excerpta Medica, Amsterdam-Oxford-Princeton (1980), p. 60.
10. Caspi, D., Baltz, L., Feinstein, A., Munn, E. A., and Pepys, M. B., Clin. Exp. Immunol., 57, 647 (1984).
11. Skinner, M., Connors, L. H., Stone, P. J., Shirahama, T., and Cohen, A. S. (this volume) (1985).

DOES SERUM DEGRADE AMYLOID FIBRILS? FAILURE TO CONFIRM ENZYMATIC
DEGRADATION OF AMYLOID A FIBRILS AS THE BASIS OF THE SO-CALLED
"AMYLOID DEGRADING ACTIVITY" OF SERUM

D. Caspi, M. L. Baltz,
A. Feinstein*, E. A. Munn*,
and M. B. Pepys

MRC Acute Phase Protein Research Group
Immunological Medicine Unit
Department of Medicine
Royal Postgraduate Medical School
Du Cane Road
London W12 0HS, and

*AFRC Institute of Animal Physiology
 Babraham
 Cambridge, United Kingdom

ABSTRACT

Several reports from different laboratories on the capacity of serum
to degrade amyloid A fibrils have been published since the 1979 Symposium
on Amyloidosis. These are based on the observation that whole serum or isolated serum albumin causes increased translucency in turbid agarose gels
containing AA fibrils. We report here a critical study of the phenomenon
itself both in the gel and in solution.

The clearing capacity of serum samples correlated well with albumin
concentration and as previously shown by others was manifested by isolated
albumin preparations. Clearing did not involve enzymatic degradation of
amyloid fibrils. Serum albumin is known to improve the optical clarity of
agarose gels. We propose that optical clearing without degradation is the
basis of the so-called amyloid degrading activity of human serum. This
activity does not seem to be of in vivo importance in amyloidogenesis.

INTRODUCTION

Reactive systemic amyloidosis (RSA) is usually a relentless and progressive disease. Amyloid fibrils are considered to be resistant to in
vivo degradation. Instances in which the amyloid deposits have regressed
have been reported however [1]. Although rare, these cases would suggest
that degradation of amyloid is possible. The concept of an "efferent pathway" in the equilibrium of amyloid can be used hypothetically to explain
why only few of many patients at risk (those who do not degrade amyloid?)
do develop this complication. Amyloid degradation in vivo would also be
important for therapeutic prospects since recovery from amyloidosis would

279

imply clearing away of existing deposits. Against this background recent reports of the capacity of human serum to degrade amyloid A fibrils (AA-F) in vitro have attracted much attention [2-6].

All recent work on the presumed amyloid degrading activity (ADA) of human serum are based on a novel assay first reported by Kedar et al., during the 1979 Symposium on Amyloidosis [2]. The assay of ADA is based on optical clearing produced by serum of an opaque agarose gel containing AA-F. It was shown that sera from patients with RSA had a lower clearing capacity than normal sera and this fact was considered to reflect a deficiency or inhibition [4] of a serum factor capable of degrading AA-F. The assumption that clarification reflects degradation was based on electron microscopy and Congo red staining of the gels [4]. Subsequent work on ADA, either in clinical situations [3-10] or on the nature of the presumed enzyme thought to be involved [11], were based on the assumption that gel clearing reflects AA-F degradation.

We report here our study of the phenomenon designated as amyloid degrading activity and propose a non-enzymatic explanation for it.

METHOD OF ADA ASSAY

Amyloid A fibrils were extracted in water [12] from the spleen of patient with RSA. The fibril suspension was mixed with molten agarose gel at 56°C to a final concentration of 1% wt./vol. agarose and 0.65-1.25 A_{280} units/ml of AA-F. The 1.5 mm thick gel was settled in levelled Petri dishes and 4 mm diameter wells punched in it for assaying 10 µl of serum or other solutions. Pooled serum from five healthy donors served as a normal reference material. Serum concentrations of 25%, 50%, 75% in phosphate buffered isotonic saline pH 7.4 (PBS) or undiluted serum were used to construct a calibration curve. The effect of different agents on the ADA of serum or serum albumin solutions was assessed after preincubation of the serum with the specific agent as described below. Controls were incubated under identical conditions with the solvent of the agent under test and were assayed on the same gel plate.

RESULTS

A. The Clearing Phenomenon in AA-F-Agarose Gel

1. Clearing by serum and by serum albumin. After overnight incubation human serum cleared circular areas of the opaque gel around the wells. Normal sera cleared a greater area than sera from patients with RSA (219 ± 112 mm^2, n = 5 and 109 ± mm^2, n = 6, respectively). A linear correlation coefficient of 0.91 was found between the area of clearing and the concentration of albumin in the sera.

Solutions of human or bovine serum albumin at 50 g/l cleared an area similar to that cleared by normal serum.

2. Inhibition of the clearing phenomenon. Equal volumes of serum from five normal individuals were mixed with serum from five RSA patients to provide 25 different mixtures. Each serum mixed with an equal volume of normal saline served as its own control. All mixtures of sera cleared areas which were larger than those cleared by their controls, thus showing no inhibitory effect of amyloidotic serum. Other inhibitors, previously reported to inhibit ADA [4, 11], were assayed and compared to similarly diluted sera. None of the agents had any influence on the ADA (Table 1).

TABLE 1. Materials Which Did Not Affect the Clearing Phenomenon

Inhibitor	Final concentration	Preincubation
Alpha 1 anti-trypsin	2–3.2 μM	30 min/37°C
Aprotinin	10^2–10^5 U/ml	6 h/37°C
PMSF	0.5–5.0 mM	Overnight 23/°C
NaF	0.1–5.0 mg/ml	30 min/23°C
NaN$_3$	0.0.–0.1 mg/ml	30 min/23°C

PMSF) Phenylmethylsulfonylfluoride.

TABLE 2. Enhancement by Isolated Albumin of the Clearing Capacity of Amyloid Patients' Sera

Exp.	Serum	Final dilution	Additive	Final albumin concentration (g/l)	Area of clearing (mm^2)
1	NHS	2/3	PBS	33.3	119
	Pt serum	2/3	PBS	12.7	54
	Pt serum	2/3	HSA	55.7	133
	Pt serum	2/3	BSA	55.7	123
2	NHS	1/2	PBS	25.0	80
	Pt serum	1/2	PBS	9.5	52
	Pt serum	1/2	HSA	34.5	99
	Pt serum	1/2	BSA	34.5	113

NHS) Normal human serum; Pt) patient; PBS) phosphate buffered saline; HSA) human serum albumin; BSA) bovine serum albumin.

3. Enhancement of the clearing phenomenon. The clearing capacity of amyloidotic serum increased in a dose dependent fashion when human or bovine serum albumin was added to it (Table 2). Sodium citrate (10 mg/ml) and ascorbic acid (0.004–50 mg/ml), previously reported [4] to enhance ADA of sera from patients with RSA, did not affect the clearing capacity in our hands. EDTA (0.1 mg/ml), another enhancing factor reported previously [4], cleared AA-F-agarose gel even in the absence of serum. The clearing produced by EDTA was prevented by CaCl$_2$ in molar excess.

The effect of temperature on the rate of clearing was studied at 4°C and 37°C. A 40% increase in the rate of clearing was noticed after 8 h at 37°C. This modest increase is compatible with better diffusion of the serum at high temperature but definitely not with temperature effect on an enzymatic reaction.

4. Effect of proteolytic enzymes on the AA-F gel. Both pronase and trypsin (10 μg/ml-1 mg/ml) are capable of degrading amyloid fibrils (see below). These same enzymes produced no clearing effect in the AA-F agarose during up to 48 h of incubation.

5. Electron microscopy of AA-F agarose. The AA-F agarose gels of the assay were stained with uranyl acetate and lead citrate after fixation with osmium tetroxide, dehydration and embedding in araldite. The appearance of gels containing AA-F was not significantly different from plain agarose gel

since the latter had a dispersed fibrillar ultrastructure. Similarly, the appearance of cleared zones of the AA-F agarose did not differ from that of uncleared, untreated zones in the gel.

6. Congo red staining. Using 0.05%-0.01% wt./vol. Congo red or 0.05% Sirius red in water we could show no lack of staining in the cleared zones of the gel, though these did have a more translucent orange-red appearance than the rest of the turbid gel. Cryostat tissue sections of amyloidotic kidney incubated in normal serum, amyloid patients' serum or PBS, stained identically with alkaline Congo red. Similarly, a homogenate of amyloidotic tissues was incubated for 24 h in excess of normal serum, amyloidotic serum or PBS. The pellets were washed, smeared on glass and stained with alkaline Congo red. Again, no difference in the Congophilia was shown.

B. The Effects of Albumin and Proteinases on AA-F in Solution

1. Immediate clearing. When serum albumin solution was added at a final concentration of 5-10 g/l to a turbid suspension of AA-F an immediate clearing was noticed. This observation was not possible with whole serum due to the intrinsic mild turbidity and color of the serum.

2. Low molecular weight degradation products. ^{125}I labelled AA-F were incubated with normal serum, albumin solution, pronase (1% wt./wt.), trypsin (10% wt./wt.) or PBS. After overnight incubation the mixtures were separately dialyzed against an identical volume of water and the dialyzable radioactivity was counted. While pronase and trypsin increased the radioactivity of the dialyzate by 50% as compared to PBS, no increase was noted after treatment with serum or serum albumin.

When AA-F were run in SDS polyacrylamide gel electrophoresis (SDS-PAGE) under reducing conditions a group of bands with apparent molecular weights between 8 K and 18 K was observed. The same pattern persisted after treatment of the AA-F with albumin. In contrast, pronase and trypsin caused complete disappearance of all these bands (Fig. 1). As mentioned above, these same enzymes did not have any clearing effect in the AA-F-agarose gel.

3. Electron microscopy. AA-F in water were treated with either PBS, albumin (10 mg/l), normal sera or pronase (10 μg/ml). After incubation the suspensions absorbed to carbon films were negatively stained with sodium silicotungstate. Pronase degraded almost all fibrils but serum, albumin or PBS had no effect on their appearance and dimensions.

DISCUSSIONS

Several reports [1-11] including our own [13] confirm the observation that serum clears agarose gel containing AA-F. The phenomenon has been ascribed to amyloid degrading activity but no direct evidence for degradation has been published. Kedar et al. [4] described electron microscopic disappearance of fibrils from the cleared area while Schneller et al., mentioned a "structural change" of the fibrils [3]. We could not achieve satisfactory electron microscopy of the fibrils in agarose gel due to the fibrillar background of the gel itself. In solution, however, the morphology of the AA-F remained unchanged following incubation with serum or serum albumin. Loss of Congophilia in the cleared zones in the AA-F gel was considered to be further evidence for degradation of AA-fibrils. We cannot confirm this observation and consider the change in the staining at the cleared area solely as a result of loss of turbidity.

The interpretation of the optical clearing as an expression of degradation was perpetuated in further experiments using enzyme inhibitors, thus

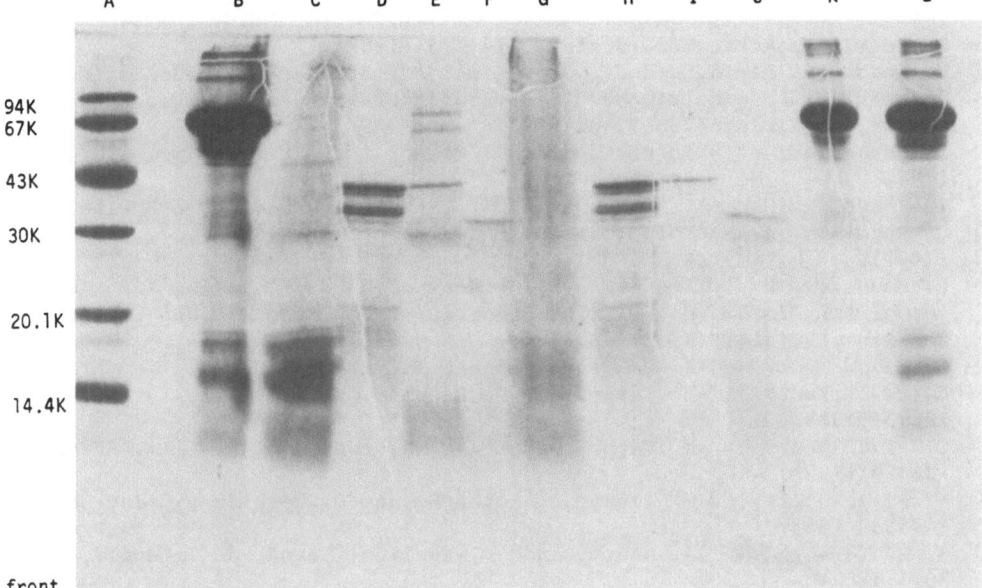

Fig. 1. Analysis by SDS-PAGE (15%) of AA fibrils after incubation with albumin or proteinases. Lane A, marker proteins of known molecular weight; lanes B and L, AA-F plus HSA; lane C, AA-F plus PBS; land D, AA-F plus pronase; lane F, AA-F plus trypsin; lane H, pronase alone; lane J, trypsin alone; lane K, HSA alone.

leading to the attribution of the activity to a serine esterase [11]. We could not confirm an inhibitory effect of PMSF and other reported agents. Moreover, we wonder whether the reported 50% inhibition of ADA [11] by PMSF, which was gradual and dose dependent, justifies an interpretation of enzymatic blockade. The same considerations are true for other reported inhibitors, e.g., 53% inhibition with diisopropyl fluorophosphate and 30% inhibition with aprotinin [11].

We suggest that the nature of the so-called amyloid degrading activity is a non-enzymatic optical clearing. The phenomenon depends upon the albumin level; it occurs instantaneously and does not involve degradation of amyloid fibrils. Serum albumin also has optical effects in other instances. It is used commercially to improve the transparency of agarose gel [14, 15] and is also capable of clearing agarose gels impregnated with totally different fibrils such as non-collagenous reticulin [16]. The mechanism of the optical phenomenon is still unknown. However, the inter-relationships between calcium and albumin on the one hand, and the clearing produced by EDTA and prevented by $CaCl_2$ on the other, might be of interest.

It is difficult to see an _in vivo_ role for amyloid clearing activity of serum in the pathogenesis of amyloidosis. Decreased clearing activity apparently reflects hypoalbuminemia, an effect of RSA or its causative condition, rather than a pathogenetic mechanism in amyloidosis.

ACKNOWLEDGEMENT

This work was supported by Medical Research Council programme Grant G979/51 to M. B. Pepys.

283

REFERENCES

1. O. Wegelius, Acta, Med. Scand., 214:273 (1982).
2. I. Kedar, M. Ravid, and E. Sohar, in: Amyloid and Amyloidosis (G. G. Glenner, P. P. e Costa, and A. Falcao de Freitas, eds.), Excerpta Medica, Amsterdam (1980), p. 60.
3. S. Schneller, M. Skinner, and A. S. Cohen, Arthritis Rheum., 23:743 (1980).
4. I. Kedar, E. Sohar, and M. Ravid, J. Lab. Clin. Med., 99:693 (1982).
5. O. Wegelius, A.-M. Teppo, and C. P. J. Maury, Brit. Med. J., 284:617 (1982).
6. P. Maddison, P. A. Bacon, A. F. Strachan, and C. R. Tribe, in: Amyloidosis E.A.R.S. (C. R. Tribe and P. A. Bacon, eds.), John Wright and Sons, Bristol (1983), p. 124.
7. C. P. J. Maury and A.-M. Teppo, Lancet ii, 234 (1982).
8. C. P. J. Maury, A.-M. Teppo, and P. Rannio, Eur. J. Clin. Invest., 13:73 (1983).
9. C. P. J. Maury, A.-M. Teppo, and M. P. Salaspuro, Clin. Chim. Acta, 131:29 (1983).
10. C. P. J. Maury, A.-M. Teppo, B. Forseth, and O. Wegelius, Clin. Sci., 64:453 (1983).
11. A.-M. Teppo, C. P. J. Maury, and O. Wegelius, Scand. J. Immunol., 16:309 (1982).
12. M. Pras, M. Schubert, D. Zucker-Franklin, A. Rimon, and E. C. Franklin, J. Clin. Invest., 47:924 (1968).
13. D. Caspi, M. L. Baltz, A. Feinstein, E. A. Munn, and M. B. Pepys, Clin. Exp. Immunol., 57:647 (1984).
14. K. B. Guiseley and D. W. Renn, in: Agarose Information Booklet, Marine Colloids Division, FMC Corporation, U.S.A. (1977).
15. D. W. Renn, personal communication.
16. D. L. Scott, R. Stone, P. Bracken, and P. A. Bacon, Presented at the British Society for Rheumatology, Bristol (April 4, 1984).

E. HEREDITARY AND FAMILIAL (AF) AMYLOIDOSIS

STATEMENT REGARDING NOMENCLATURE FOR THE PROTEIN KNOWN AS PREALBUMIN,

WHICH IS ALSO (RECENTLY) CALLED TRANSTHYRETIN

DeWitt S. Goodman

Professor of Medicine
Columbia University
New York, New York 10032

Recent studies on the heredofamilial amyloidoses have demonstrated that the amyloid deposits in tissues in patients with familial amyloidotic polyneuropathy (FAP) are derived from a variant (mutant) form of the plasma protein previously known as prealbumin. This protein, prealbumin, has been extensively studied in several laboratories throughout the world during the past two decades. Its primary structure was reported in 1974, and its full three-dimensional structure has been determined by high resolution x-ray crystallography. Its biological/physiological roles include a role in retinol (vitamin A) transport, through forming a complex with retinol-binding protein, and a role in thyroid hormone transport.

The term "prealbumin" is an unsatisfactory one. At the present time, the prefix "pre" in the name of a protein refers to a biosynthetic precursor, containing a signal/leader sequence (a "pre" piece that is usually cleaved cotranslationally as part of the protein's processing in the cell). The term "prealbumin" hence suggests that this protein is a precursor of albumin. In fact, this protein is neither a precursor form, nor is it related to serum albumin in any way. Accordingly, a more appropriate name is needed.

Because of these considerations, the Nomenclature Committee of the International Union of Biochemistry (NC-IUB), and the IUB-International Union of Pure and Applied Chemistry Joint Commission on Biochemical Nomenclature (JCBN), have recommended that this protein be called "transthyretin." This name is an apt, descriptive one, since the protein is a transport protein for both thyroid hormone and retinol-binding protein. The name is consistent with accepted modern usage for other transport proteins (e.g., transferrin). The recommendation that the name transthyretin should be used was published in the 1981 Newsletter of the above committees, that appeared in Arch. Biochem. Biophys., 206:458-462 (1981); Eur. J. Biochem., 114:1-4 (1981); Hoppe-Seyler's Z. Physiol. Chem., 362:IV (1981); and J. Biol. Chem., 256:12-14 (1981).

Accordingly, I wish to recommend that investigators in the amyloid field adopt the recommended term "transthyretin" as the name for this protein. Since research concerning variant transthyretins and FAP is likely to expand in the near future, it would be advisable that this nomenclature adoption be made as soon as possible, so that the future scientific literature will have the same name used in the biochemical literature and the amyloid field. I recognize that it is sometimes difficult for investigators to give up a name that has been used for a number of years, and with which they are fully familiar. Many workers found it very difficult in the 1960s to give up the familiar and established terms DPN and TPN, for the terms NAD and NADP. The change was, however, recognized as highly desirable and has been of value for the teaching and practice of science concerning these compounds. Similarly, the adoption of the term transthyretin for the protein known as prealbumin would clearly be of value with regard to future teaching and research concerning this protein.

FAMILY STUDIES OF TRANSTHYRETIN (PREALBUMIN) AND ITS METHIONINE 30 VARIANT

IN PORTUGUESE PATIENTS WITH FAMILIAL AMYLOIDOTIC POLYNEUROPATHY

Maria Joao Mascarenhas Saraiva‡,
Pedro Pinho Costa†, Steven Birken*,
and DeWitt S. Goodman*

*Department of Medicine
 Columbia University College of Physicans and Surgeons
 New York, New York,

†Centro de Estudos de Paramiloidose
 Hospital de Santo Antonio
 Porto, Portugal

‡Department of Biochemistry
 Instituto de Ciencias Biomedicas
 Universidade do Porto
 Porto, Portugal

INTRODUCTION

The association of human plasma transthyretin (TTR, a protein usually referred to as prealbumin) with amyloid deposits in familial amyloidosis of autosomal inheritance is now well established. Thus, in 1978, Costa et al., reported that a protein component of the amyloid fibrils that accumulate in tissues of patients with familial amyloidotic polyneuropathy (FAP), Portuguese type, is closely related to TTR [1]. Subsequently, investigators using both chemical and immunohistochemical methods found that a TTR-related protein constitutes the major protein component of amyloid deposits of FAP patients from Japan [2], the United States (from various ancestral origins [3-5], and other countries [3, 6] as well. It was postulated that in FAP a genetic mutation may have occurred, leading to the production of an abnormal TTR molecule, which is abnormally degraded, bound, or precipitated in the tissues as amyloid fibrils.

Within the past two years, the presence of an abnormal TTR in FAP patients has been reported by several groups. Thus, the major protein of amyloid in a Jewish patient was reported to be a TTR variant with a glycine for threonine substitution at position 49 [7]. This was followed by descriptions of a TTR variant with a methionine for valine substitution at position 30 as the major constituent of amyloid. This variant TTR (which we shall refer to a TTR(Met^{30})) was described by us in Portuguese patients with FAP, where we demonstrated its presence in blood plasma and in amyloid deposits [8-10]. The same variant TTR has also been demonstrated in patients of Swedish ancestry [11], and in Japanese patients with FAP [12, 13].

Detailed studies of the properties of the purified amyloid protein AF$_p$ from Portuguese patients with FAP showed that the protein resembled plasma

TTR in forming a stable tetrameric structure, and in its binding affinities for both thyroxine and retinol-binding protein (RBP) [10]. Studies on the purified plasma TTR from the same FAP patients showed no differences from normal TTR with regard to a wide range of physical-chemical properties [14].

The finding of a biochemical marker for a disease that usually becomes manifest relatively late in life raises the question of the detection of carriers of the abnormal protein in the preclinical phase. Accordingly, studies were undertaken in families with FAP in order to address the following questions:

a) Does TTS(Met^{30}) circulate in plasma of affected individuals before clinical symptoms appear? If so, what are the relative levels of the variant TTR compared to normal TTR in younger asymptomatic subjects as compared to FAP patients?

b) Does TTR(Met^{30}) circulate in those FAP patients with late onset of clinical symptoms [13]? If so, does it circulate in a pre-clinical phase?

TTR(MET^{30}) IN ASYMPTOTOMATIC FAP OFFSPRING

Presence of TTR(Met^{30}) in Asymptomatic FAP Offspring

In order to address the question of whether TTR(Met^{30}) circulates in the plasma of asymptomatic FAP children, we isolated TTR from individual serum samples by an efficient small scale procedure involving: i) chromatography on Blue Sepharose [16]; and ii) affinity chromatography on human plasma RBP linked to Sepharose [17]. Portions of the purified TTR samples were then subjected to CNBr cleavage. Detection of "abnormal" peptides (as compared to those obtained with normal TTR) was effected by both HPLC and SDS-PAGE analysis using methods similar to those employed previously with samples of AFp [10]. These methods are based on the fact that normal TTR possesses only one methionine residue at position 13 [18]; CNBr treatment cleaves the protein into two peptide fragments: a small peptide, residues 1-13 (called peptide C_1, and labeled CNBr1 in Fig. 1), and a large peptide, residues 14-127 (called peptide C_2, and labeled CNBr2 in Fig. 1; with AFp samples and TTR from the plasma of FAP patients, CNBr treatment produces extra peptide fragments (as compared to TTR): an intermediate peptide (called peptide C_a and labeled CNBr a in Fig. 1) and a larger fragment (called peptide C_b and labeled CNBr b in Fig. 1). The aberrant peptide C_a is readily observed on HPLC analysis of CNBr digests [10]. Peptide C_b can be visualized as a single peptide band, of apparent molecular weight of approximately 12,000 on SDS-PAGE analysis [10]. Both fragments have never been detected on analysis of CNBr digests of normal TTR.

Our first investigation of the possible presence of TTR(Met^{30}) in FAP children involved in one family with five offspring, none of whom had clinical evidence of FAP. The abnormal CNBr fragments C_a and C_b were observed, respectively, on HPLC and on SDS-PAGE analysis, in two of the five offspring, but not in the other three subjects. Thus, these analyses demonstrated that TTR(Met^{30}) can be detected in plasma in asymptomatic at-risk offspring of FAP patients.

Family Studies

The previous observation that TTR(Met^{30}) circulates in FAP in a pre-clinical phase led us to extend our family analysis and screen for the variant TTR in several other FAP kindreds. The results obtained with the first six families studies are summarized in Fig. 2. The variant TTR was found in 12 of the 21 offspring examined in this particular study. Within

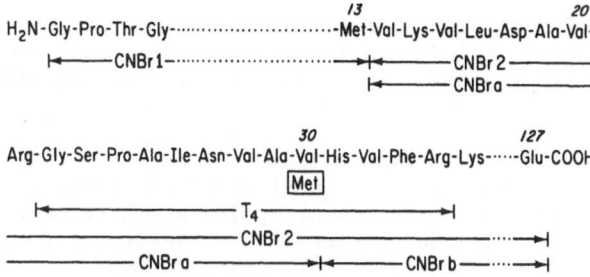

H₂N-Gly-Pro-Thr-Gly·············Met-Val-Lys-Val-Leu-Asp-Ala-Val-

Arg-Gly-Ser-Pro-Ala-Ile-Asn-Val-Ala-Val-His-Val-Phe-Arg-Lys-·····-Glu-COOH

Fig. 1.   Partial amino acid sequence of the
           human TTR subunit taken from Kanda
           et al. [16].   The nomenclature of the
           peptides is as follows: T4, tryptic
           peptide 4; CNBr 1 and 2, CNBr frag-
           ments of normal transthyretin; CNBr a
           and b, additional CNBr fragments of
           the amyloid fibril protein.   The Met
           residue (enclosed in a box) below Val
           30 indicates the difference found
           between AFp and TTR.

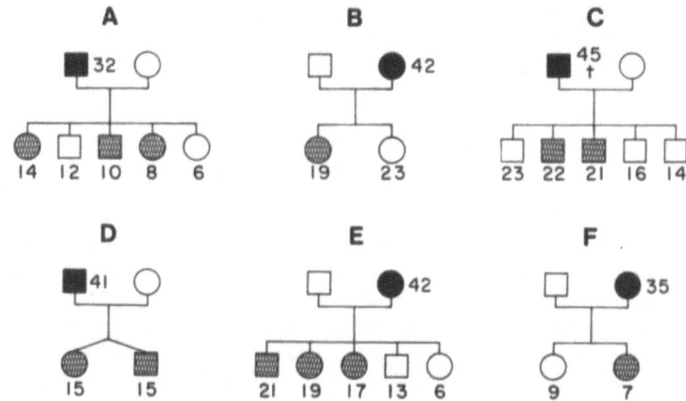

Fig. 2.   A composite diagram showing the partial pedi-
           grees of six families with FAP, and the dis-
           tribution of the variant "abnormal" TTR found
           among their asymptotomatic children.   Symbols:
           □) male; ○) female; ■), ●) FAP patients □),
           ○) healthy persons not carrying the biochem-
           ical marker (the variant TTR) for FAP; ▦),
           ▦) asymptomatic carriers of the biochemical
           marker for FAP.   The numers indicate the ages
           of the patients and their offspring at the
           time the sera were collected.

the ages of 6 to 23 years, TTR(Met³⁰) was detected as early as 7 years, with
no predilection for either sex.

    An important observation emerging from this study was that the fre-
quency and distribution of the variant TTR in the FAP offspring are consistent with the autosomal dominant manner of inheritance typical of the
Portuguese form of FAP [19].   This distribution was also evident on analysis

of plasma TTR of offspring of affected members of a large kindred with FAP. In this large kindred (including 3 generations of normal and affected persons) the variant TTR was never found in offspring of non-affected family members.

A mixture of both normal TTR and the variant TTR(Met^{30}) was found in the circulation of the asymptomatic carriers of the variant TTR. Thus, both FAP patients [10], and affected offspring are heterozygous for the variant TTR, a feature also consistent with an autosomal dominant trait.

The 2 TTR genes apparently present in affected persons (one for normal TTR and one for the variant TTR) are likely to represent co-dominant alleles at a single locus. Both genes are expressed in affected subjects. We do not know the reasons that account for the reduced amounts of the mutant TTR relative to normal TTR observed in the plasma of FAP patients [10]. One explanation might be a reduced rate of synthesis of the variant as compared with the normal TTR subunit. Alternatively, both TTR subunits might be produced at similar rates, but a particular species containing the variant TTR might be removed more rapidly than normal TTR from plasma, either because of more rapid degradation and/or its deposition in tissues.

Relative Levels of TTR(Met^{30}) in Asymptomatic FAP Offspring

The reduced levels of TTR(Met^{30}) relative to normal TTR usually found in FAP patients prompted us to investigate the relative levels of TTR(Met^{30}) compared to normal TTR, in asymptomatic offspring. For this study, following the identification of the carriers of the variant TTR by the methods described above, portions of TTR isolated from plasma of TTR(Met^{30}) carriers were digested with trypsin under highly controlled conditions. The resulting tryptic peptides were separated by HPLC using the same conditions as those previously described with samples of plasma TTR from FAP patients [10]. FAP-TTR tryptic peptide maps have been found to be identical to those of normal TTR with one distinct difference. This difference consists of the presence of a peak in the FAP-TTR peptide map that is not present with normal, and that elutes after tryptic peptide T4 (residues 22 to 34 in Fig. 1). This "abnormal" peak represents tryptic peptide T4*, consisting of peptide 4 but with a methionine residue replacing valine at position 30 [8-10]. Thus the ratio of the amount of peptide T4* to peptide T4 can give us an estimate of the relative amounts of TTR(Met^{30}) as compared to normal TTR in a given sample.

The ratios of the variant TTR to normal TTR in asymptomatic carriers varied from individual to individual and ranged from 0.2 to 0.6 in a study of 7 subjects. These ratios were not different from the ratios we have found in FAP patients when assayed individually. We observed no correlation between the relative levels of the abnormal TTR and either age or total TTR serum levels. Furthermore, total TTR serum levels were not significantly different in non-carriers and asymptomatic carriers of the mutant TTR. This is in contrast with the reduced TTR plasma levels generally found in FAP patients with clinical disease [14]. Thus TTR levels cannot be used in asymptomatic FAP children in a predictive way.

TTR(MET^{30}) IN A FAP KINSHIP WITH LATE ONSET OF CLINICAL SYMPTOMS

Although slightly different phenotypic clinical expressions exist among the different ethnic and geographic varieties of FAP, these syndromes all exhibit prominent peripheral neuropathy. Future studies are needed to determine whether or not these different clinical forms of FAP represent mutations in the TTR molecule other than the mutations reported at position 49 (Thr → Gly) and at position 30 (Val → Met).

We have examined a large kinship in which the Portuguese variety of FAP manifests a late onset, usually appearing clinically in the sixth decade of life as described by Andrade [15]. Using the methodology described above (CNBr cleavage and tryptic peptide mapping) we investigated whether TTR(Met^{30}) is present in the sera of these patients. TTR(Met^{30}) was detected in the sera of these late onset FAP patients and was also present in the sera of some of their asymptomatic offspring. The distribution of the variant TTR among the offspring was also consistent with the autosomal mode of inheritance of FAP. Thus, in view of these results, it appears that some other unknown factor must be responsible for the differences in the clinical expression in these particular patients as compared to the usual form of FAP.

SUMMARY

In summary, these studies have demonstrated the following: 1) The variant TTR(Met^{30}) can be detected in asymptomatic children of FAP patients. 2) The distribution of the mutant TTR within families with FAP is consistent with the autosomal dominant mode of inheritance of FAP. 3) TTR levels are not reduced in asymptomatic FAP offspring who are carriers of the mutant TTR. This contrasts with the reduced TTR levels found in FAP patients, and indicates that TTR levels cannot be used as a predictive marker in the preclinical phase of the disease. 4) TTR(Met^{30}) also circulates in the late onset forms of FAP. The factor or factors that might be responsible for the late onset of FAP require further study.

Although the detailed mechanisms that lead to amyloid formation are unknown the presence of the variant TTR(Met^{30}) appears to constitute a direct and true genetic marker of the disease. We believe that the presence of the mutant TTR constitutes an important parameter that can be used in genetic counseling in asymptomatic at-risk offspring and as a future guide to newer approaches to prevention and therapy.

ACKNOWLEDGEMENTS

This work was supported by National Institutes of Health grants HL-21006, AM-05968, and HD-15454.

REFERENCES

1. P. P. Costa, A. S. Figuerira, and F. R. Bravo, Proc. Natl. Acad. Sci., 75:4499 (1978).
2. S. Tawara, S. Araki, K. Toshimori, H. Nakagowa, and S. Ohtaki, J. Lab. Clin. Med., 98:811 (1981).
3. M. C. Dalakis and W. K. Engel, Arch. Neurol., 38:420 (1981).
4. M. D. Benson, J. Clin. Invest., 67:1035 (1981).
5. M. Skinner and A. Cohen, Biochem. Biochem. Res. Commun., 99:1326 (1981).
6. M. Pras, E. C. Franklin, F. Prelli, and B. Frangiona, J. Exp. Med., 154:989 (1981).
7. M. Pras, F. Prelli, E. C. Franklin, and B. Frangione, Proc. Natl. Acad. Sci. USA, 80:539 (1983).
8. M. J. M. Saraiva, D. S. Goodman, P. P. Costa, R. E. Canfield, and S. Birken, 31:533A (1983).

9. M. J. M. Saraiva, P. P. Costa, S. Birken, and D. S. Goodman, Trans. Assoc. Amer. Phys., 96:261 (1983).
10. M. J. M. Saraiva, S. Birken, P. P. Costa, and D. S. Goodman, J. Clin. Invest., 74:104 (1984).
11. F. E. Dwulet and M. D. Benson, Proc. Natl. Acad. Sci. USA, 81:694 (1984).
12. S. Tawara, M. Nakazato, K. Kangawa, H. Matsuo, and S. Araki, Biochem. Biophys. Res. Comm., 116:880 (1983).
13. M. Nakazato, K. Kangawa, N. Minamino, S. Tawara, H. Matsuo, and S. Araki, Biochem. Biophys. Res. Commun., 122:712 (1984).
14. M. J. M. Saraiva, P. P. Costa, and D. S. Goodman, J. Lab. Clin. Med., 102:590 (1983).
15. C. Andrade, in: Handbook of Clinical Neurology, 21:119 (1975).
16. E. Giannazza and P. Arnaud, Biochem. J., 201:129 (1982).
17. M. Navab, A. K. Malia, Y. Kanda, and D. S. Goodman, J. Biol. Chem., 252:5100 (1977).
18. Y. Kanda, D. S. Goodman, R. E. Canfield, and F. J. Morgan, J. Biol. Chem., 249:6796 (1974).
19. C. Andrade, M. Canijo, and D. Klein, Humangenetik, 7:163 (1969).

SERUM CONCENTRATIONS OF PREALBUMIN AND RETINOL BINDING

PROTEIN IN FAMILIAL AMYLOID PATIENTS FROM 15 KINSHIPS*

Lawreen Heller Connors, Martha Skinner,
and Alan S. Cohen

Thorndike Memorial Laboratory and Division of Medicine
Boston City Hospital,

Arthritis Center
Boston City Hospital School of Medicine
Boston, Massachusetts 02118

ABSTRACT

We have quantitated the levels of serum prealbumin (PA) by rate nephelometry in 33 individuals with AF from 15 unrelated kinships. PA concentrations in the AF group were significantly depressed as compared to normal
individuals and patients with primary amyloidosis (AL). Serum levels of
retinol binding protein (RBP), the linker molecule complexing PA to Vitamin
A, were near normal in the AF patients. In 54 unaffected "at risk" relatives from 2 AF kinships, serum PA and RBP levels were not significantly
different from normal values. PA concentrations were compared to serum
levels of the acute phase reactants, C-reactive protein (CRP) and serum
amyloid A (SAA). Abnormally depressed amounts of PA corresponded to higher
than normal concentrations of CRP and SAA in the AL and AA sera. However,
in the AF group, lower than normal serum PA levels were not accompanied by
abnormally elevated amounts of CRP and SAA. These data suggest that abnormal serum PA concentrations in patients with AF are a true manifestation
of the disease, not simply a reflection of a negative acute phase response.
Depressed plasma PA levels in AF may represent the expression of the genetic
abnormality.

INTRODUCTION

Familial amyloidosis (AF), an autosomal dominant disorder, is one of
three systemic forms of amyloid disease. Biochemical characterization of
AF amyloid fibrils has identified monomeric prealbumin (PA) as the major
protein constituent [1-5]. Normally, prealbumin is a stable, soluble

---

*Supported by grants from the U.S. Public Health Service, NIAMDD (AM 04599
 and AM 07014), Multipurpose Arthritis Center, National Institutes of
 Health (AM 206013), from the General Clinical Research Centers Branch of
 the Division of Research Resources, National Institutes of Health (RR 533),
 and the Arthritis Foundation.

tetramer (M_r = 54,980 daltons) which functions as a carrier protein for retinol and thyroxine [6]. Plasma transport of retinol occurs via the complex formed between PA and retinol binding protein (RBP). All four sub-units of PA are identical (M_r = 13,745 daltons) and contain no attached sugar or lipid groups. The secondary structure of the monomer is ordered significantly in an anti-parallel β-conformation with little α-helix [7, 9]. Serum concentrations of PA are usually 200-300 μg/ml [9] although in cases of liver disease, malnutrition and trauma, plasma levels are depressed [10-12]. In addition, PA is a recognized negative acute phase reactant and lowered concentrations manifest in response to inflammatory stimuli [13].

The circulating concentrations of PA and RBP in patients with AF and their "at risk" relatives were examined to determine any abnormalities consistent throughout all kinships. Previous studies have reported lower than normal serum PA levels in AF affected individuals [14-16]. One kinship of AF patients in Indiana and their "at risk" relatives have been found to have depressed PA, as well as depressed RBP serum concentrations [14]. Separate rate nephelometric assays were developed to quantitate accurately the levels of serum PA and RBP in AF patients and their relatives. In addition, concentrations of PA were measured in sera from individuals with one of the other two systemic amyloid types, primary (AL) or secondary (AA) amyloidosis. PA levels in the three forms of systemic amyloidosis were compared to concentrations of the acute phase reactants, serum amyloid A (SAA) and C-reactive protein (CRP) in corresponding sera.

MATERIALS AND METHODS

Patients with AL, AA, or AF amyloidosis were seen at the Clinical Research Center of the Thorndike Memorial Laboratory. Sera were collected from 33 patients with AF from 15 different kinships, 55 unaffected relatives "at risk" for AF from 2 kinships, 28 patients with AL, 25 patients with AA and 20 normal individuals. The samples were stored in glass tubes at -20°C until evaluated.

Rate nephelometric analyses were all performed using the Beckman Immunochemistry System II (Beckman Instruments, Inc., Fullerton, California). Separate assays for PA and RBP were developed and run manually using commercial antibodies raised in rabbits to human PA and RBP, respectively (Calbiochem-Behring Corp., La Jolla, California). In both systems, calibration curves were constructed with commercial normal serum (Calbiochem-Behring Corp.) as the reference serum. In the PA assay, the optimal dilution of the antiserum was 1:6. The standard curve obtained using the diluted antibodies was linear in the PA concentration range between 140-558 mg/ml [18]. Serum RBP was quantitated nephelometrically using a 1:4 dilution of the antiserum to RBP. A calibration curve was constructed and displayed linearity between 0.02-1.9 mg/dl RBP. CRP was measured immuno-nephelometrically in the automated mode using the Beckman ICS commercial CRP kit. Serum concentrations of SAA were quantitated by RIA, using a solid phase, competitive binding technique on microtitration plates according to the method of Sipe and coworkers [19].

RESULTS

The nephelometrically determined plasma PA levels were evaluated in logarithmic terms to obtain a more Gaussian distribution of data points. Mean values are expressed both in logarithmic and geometric forms (Table 1). The variations of the geometric means are expressed as 95% confidence intervals (C.I.).

TABLE 1. Serum PA Concentrations (μg/ml) Determined
by Rate Nephelometry in Patients with AF
and At Risk Relatives Compared to Normal
Individuals and Other Amyloid Types

Group	N	Mean (S.D.)§	Geometric Mean (95% C.I.)
Normal	20	2.42 (0.099)	263 (163,424)
AF	33	2.15 (0.236)*†	141 (48,410)
AF "at risk"	55	2.36 (0.098)	229 (147,357)
AL	28	2.30 (0.207)	200 (75,531)
AA	25	2.27 (0.253)	186 (56,620)

§ $\log_{10}$ transformed data

* differs from normals, "at risk" (p < .01)
† differs from AL (p < .05)

TABLE 2. Serum RBP Concentrations Determined by
Rate Nephelometry

Group	No.	Mean mg/dl (S.D.)
Normal	20	4.9 (1.1)
AF	25	4.4 (0.8)
AF "at risk"	54	5.7 (2.5)

Markedly lower PA concentrations were noted in serum samples from 33
individuals with AF. In this group, which was comprised of patients' sera
from 15 unrelated kinships, the geometric mean was 141 μg/ml. A geometric
mean of 263 μg/ml was calculated from the quantitative data obtained on 20
normal individuals. PA levels in unaffected relatives considered "at risk"
for AF were near normal (geometric mean = 229 μg/ml). Twenty-eight AL amyloid samples rendered a geometric mean PA value of 200 μg/ml, which was
also near normal. Lower levels of PA were noted in the sera of 25 AA amyloid patients (geometric mean = 186 μg/ml). Serum PA amounts in individuals
with AF were significantly depressed when compared to normal levels (p <
0.01). In addition, this group differed significantly from the "at risk"
relatives (p < 0.01) and AL amyloid patients (p < 0.05). None of the other
three groups, including the "at risk" relatives, were significantly different from each other or normal values.

The mean concentrations of RBP in 25 patients with AF (4.4 mg/dl) and
54 "at risk" relatives (5.7 mg/dl) were both within the accepted normal
range of 3.0-7.0 mg/dl (Table 2). Nephelometrically determined RBP levels

TABLE 3.   Serum PA and RBP Concentrations in AF Kinships

Patient Kinship	No.	PA ug/ml Mean (S.D.)	No.	RBP mg/dl Mean (S.D.)
A	5	108 (42)	5	4.2 (.88)
B	4	67 (22)	4	3.6 (.19)
C	3	142 (27)	2	3.8 (.35)
D	2	171 (54)	2	4.8 (.40)
E	2	182 (43)	2	4.7 (.40)
F	2	260 (67)	1	5.5
G	1	211	1	5.1
H	1	239	1	4.1
I	1	138	1	4.2
J	1	170	1	5.5
K	1	248	1	4.3
L	1	167	1	4.8
M	1	209	1	5.0
N	1	197	1	4.8
O	1	103	1	4.8

in sera from 20 normal individuals yielded an average value of 4.9 mg/dl.
PA and RBP mean concentrations for each of the fifteen kinships studied
were evaluated (Table 3). The distribution of serum PA and RBP levels in
the AF patients and their unaffected "at risk" relatives from 2 kinships
were schematized with respect to normal ranges (Fig. 1).

Serum levels of PA in patients with AF, AL, and AA amyloidosis were
compared to corresponding concentrations of the acute phase proteins, SAA,
and CRP (Table 4). Acute inflammation is indicated by levels of SAA > 1000
ng/ml, CRP > 10 µg/ml and PA < 200 µg/ml. Lower than normal PA levels occurred in 76% of the AF patients, while only 41% had abnormal amounts of
SAA and 6% showed increased concentrations of CRP. In the AL and AA groups,
about one-third and two-thirds, respectively, of the patients had abnormal
values.

DISCUSSION

Nephelometric quantitation of serum PA showed significantly lower
levels in AF patients when compared to concentrations in the other two systemic forms of amyloidosis and normal values. The lowered concentration
did not represent a negative acute phase response in the AF group as all

TABLE 4. Comparison of Acute Phase Proteins SAA, CRP, and PA on Patients with AF, AL, and AA

Median (Range) Concentrations and % abnormal *

Group (n)	SAA ng/ml	% elevated	CRP ug/ml	% elevated	PA ug/ml	% depressed
AF (17)	861 (168–3,675)	41%	<6 (<6– 17.9)	6%	148 (50.4–326)	76%
AL(18)	945 (273–2,625)	39%	<6 (<6– 33.2)	17%	219 (72.8–591)	39%
AA (17)	10,500 (105->20,000)	82%	15.7 (<6– 162)	65%	190 (65.1–461)	65%

* abnormal values
SAA > 1000 ng/ml
CRP > 10 ug/ml
PA < 200 ug/ml

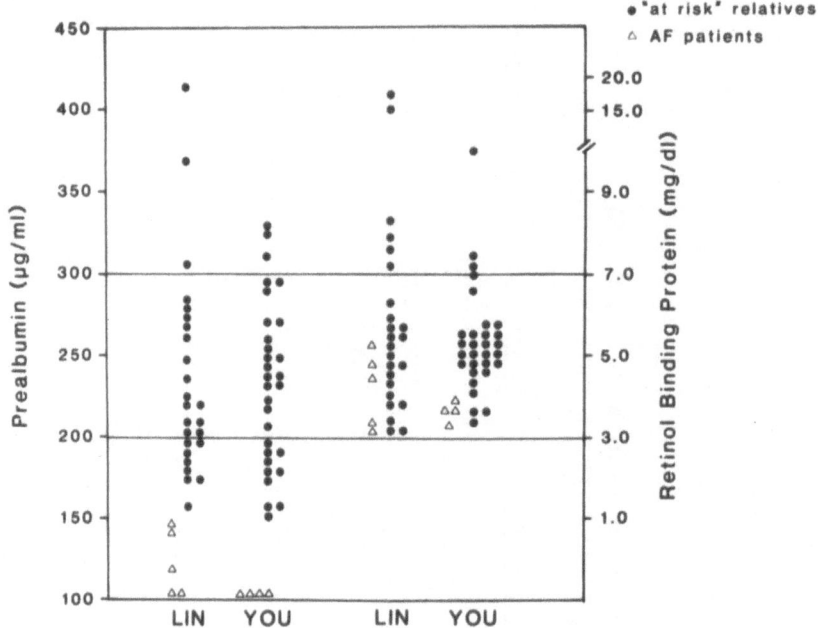

Fig. 1. Relative distribution of serum prealbumin and retinol
binding protein concentrations in two unrelated kinships of familial amyloid patients and their "at risk"
relatives. The area displayed within the horizontal
lines represents accepted normal concentrations range.

serum albumin levels were normal and none had malnutrition or a protein
losing enteropathy. The relatives from two of these AF afflicted kinships,
who did not have amyloidosis, but were "at risk" to develop the disease,
had normal concentrations of serum PA. Presently, it is thought that a
variant prealbumin which has been found in the serum of AF patients may be
the precursor protein for the amyloid fibrils in these individuals. It is
not yet known at what stage of development the aberrant prealbumin occurs
in affected individuals. Whether or not AF patients with lowered levels of
prealbumin once exhibited normal concentrations has never been determined.
The absence of this abnormal prealbumin concentration state in the "at
risk" relatives suggests that the onset of the disease may result from an
age-dependent triggering of a genetically predetermined metabolic abnormality.

     In our studies the concentrations of RBP were examined in AF and "at
risk" sera and found to be normal. One study on an AF kinship from Indiana
has reported depressed levels of PA and RBP in the patients and some of
their "at risk" relatives [14]. This suggests certain laboratory abnormalities may precede by years the disease onset, at least in thier kinship.

     CRP and SAA concentrations, which are routinely analyzed in our lab-
oratory, were compared to PA levels in corresponding sera (Table 4). This
comparison allowed us to correlate two well recognized positive acute phase
proteins with a negative acute phase protein in determining the inflammatory response of the three systemic forms of amyloidosis. Depressed amounts
of PA in patients with AF did not show corresponding elevations in CRP or
SAA within this group, suggesting that the lower than normal PA concentrations in individuals with familial amyloidosis are not a reflection of inflammation. Rather, they are a true manifestation of the disease. In con-

trast, AL amyloid results were consistent with a mild to moderate inflammatory response, and AA amyloid results with a moderate to severe inflammatory response as might be anticipated.

REFERENCES

1. M. Pras, E. C. Franklin, F. Prelli, and B. Frangione, J. Exp. Med., 154:989 (1981).
2. M. Skinner and A. S. Cohen, Biochem. Biophys. Res. Comm., 99:1326 (1981).
3. M. D. Benson, J. Clin. Invest., 67:1035 (1981).
4. S. Shoji and A. Okano, Neur., 31:186 (1981).
5. S. Tawara, S. Araki, K. Toshimori, H. Nakagawa, and S. Ohtaki, J. Lab. Clin. Med., 98:811 (1981).
6. F. W. Putnam, The Plasma Proteins, Academic Press, New York, pp. 57 (1975).
7. C. C. F. Blake, M. J. Geisow, I. D. A. Swan, C. Rerat, and B. Rerat, J. Mol. Biol., 88:1 (1974).
8. C. C. F. Blake, M. J. Geisow, S. J. Oatley, B. Rerat, and C. Rerat, J. Mol. Biol., 121:339 (1978).
9. F. R. Smith and D. S. Goodman, J. Clin. Invest., 20L2426 (1971).
10. S. Skrede, J. P. Blomhoff, K. Elgjo, and E. Gjone, Scand. J. Clin. Lab. Invest., 35:399 (1975).
11. P. Douville, J. Talbot, R. Lapoint, and L. Belanger, Clin. Chem., 28: 1706 (1982).
12. M. J. Solomon, M. F. Smith, J. B. Dowd, B. R. Bistrian, and G. L. Blackburn, J. Urology, 119:350 (1978).
13. P. S. Shetty, K. E. Watrasiewica, R. T. Jung, and W. P. T. James, Lancet ii, 230 (1979).
14. M. D. Benson and F. E. Dwulet, Arth. Rheum., 26:1493 (1983).
15. M. J. M. Saraiva, P. P. Costa, and D. S. Goodman, J. Lab. Clin. Med., 102:590 (1983).
16. M. Skinner, L. H. Connors, A. Rubinow, C. A. Libbey, J. D. Sipe, and A. S. Cohen, Am. J. Med. Sci. (in press).
17. L. H. Connors, M. A. Gertz, M. Skinner, and A. S. Cohen, J. Lab. Clin. Med., 104:538 (1984).
18. J. S. Sipe, T. F. Ignaczak, P. S. Pollack, and G. G. Glenner, J. Immunol., 116:1151 (1976).

PRE-ALBUMIN AND RETINOL BINDING PROTEIN SERUM CONCENTRATIONS IN THE

BRAZILIAN TYPE (PORTUGUESE) OF FAMILIAL POLYNEUROPATHY*

Ana Paula Nunes, Levy Waisbach,
and Morton A. Scheinberg

Division of Immunology
Instituto do Câncer
"Arnaldo Vieira de Carvalho"
(Santa Casa de São Paulo)

INTRODUCTION

Familial amyloid polyneuropathy (FAP) is an inherited disorder, character-ized by the extracellular deposition of fibrillary amyloid protein in various organs.

The major manifestations are dissociated sensory disturbance and auto-nomic dysfunction in the early phase followed by motor neuropathy. Family trees carrying this disorder have been reported from various countries in-cluding Portugal, Finland, Germany, Japan, and Brazil [1].

Several researchers have reported by chemical analysis or immunochemi-cal techniques that these amyloid deposits in these hereditary types of amyloidosis contain pre-albumin [2, 3]. In addition, it has been reported that alterations of serum pre-albumin and retinol binding protein concen-trations occur at least in one of the familial forms described, e.g., the Indiana type raising the possibility that the diagnosis of these abnormali-ties can occur prior to expression of the disease [4].

In the present study we have looked at the serum levels of PA and RBP in patients with the Brazilian form of FAP (identical to the Portuguese) in an attempt to determine whether serum abnormalities could be detected in un-affected relatives prior to disease manifestations as well as in patients with polyneuropathy.

MATERIALS AND METHODS

Serum samples from 37 members were studied and compared to twenty nor-mal controls. The ages are 16 to 40 with a mean age of 28 years.

Concentrations of pre-albumin and retinol were measured by radial immunodiffusion using commercially available assay plates from Calbiochem Behring (La Jolla, California).

---

*This is publication No. 42 from the Division of Immunology-IAVC. Grants for these investigations were provided by the CNPq and FAPESP.

TABLE 1. Pre-Albumin and Retinol Binding Protein Levels in Amyloid
Patients Siblings of Amyloid Patients and Controls

Group Tested	PA (mg/dl ± S.D)	RBP (mg/dl ± S.D)
Patients (17)	27.9 ± 6.0	3.6 ± 1.1
Siblings of Patients (20)	28.7 ± 6.2	3.5 ± 1.1
Normal Controls (20)	29.9 ± 6.0	3.9 ± 0.5

RESULTS AND DISCUSSION

Serum PA and RBP levels are presented in Table 1. No significant differences were observed in the men concentration of RBP and PA levels of
amyloid patients, unaffected relatives and normal controls.

The present data show that both pre-albumin and retinol binding protein serum concentrations are not different in patients with FAP and unaffected, and do not differ from the values observed on a control population.

The reason or reasons for the discrepant results here observed from
those reported in the Indiana type are not clear at the present time since
similar reagents were used on both studies and several investigations including our own point to the presence of a pre-albumin variant in the
serum that may be related to amyloid fibril formation [5].

The commercial antiserum employed in our study is directed against
the whole molecule of the pre-albumin and would probably not differentiate
the variant from the normal pre-albumin. We are now in the process of
raising anti-sera against the variant PA and hope to further extend the
current observations.

SUMMARY

Serum pre-albumin (PA) and retinol binding protein (RBP) concentrations
were determined in patients with familial polineuropathy and non-affected
relatives using commercial radial immunodiffusion plates.

No significant differences were observed in the serum levels in PA and
RBP in any of the groups studied. In spite of the fact that the amyloid
deposits in this disease contain pre-albumin serum PA and RBP levels are
normal in patients with this disease and normal relatives precluding the
possibility that they may be identified prior to clinical expression.

REFERENCES

1.   Andrade, C., Areki, S., Block, W. D., Cohen, A. S., Jackson, C. E.,
     Juroway, Y., McKusick, V. A. Nisson, J. Sohar, E., Van Allen, M. W.,
     Arthritis and Rheumatism, 13:902-915 (1970).
2.   Costa, P. P., Figueira, A. S. Bravo, F. R., Proc. Nat. Acad. Sci.
     (U.S.A.), 75:4449-4503 (1978).
3.   Benson, M. D., J. Clin. Invest., 67:1035-41 (1981).
4.   Bensen, M. D., Dwulet, F. E., Arthritis and Rheumatisms, 26:1493-8
     (1983).
5.   Benson, M. D., Dwulet, F. E., Greipp, P. R., Scheinberg, M. A., Clin.
     Research (in press).

CLINICAL INVESTIGATIONS OF AUTONOMIC HEART REGULATION

AND RENAL FUNCTION OF FAMILIAL AMYLOIDOTIC POLYNEUROPATHY

Shukuro Araki*, Shinichi Ikegawa*,
Jinro Nagata*, Yoshihiro Kimura*,
and Yutaka Horio†

*The First Department of Internal Medicine
 Kumamoto University Medical School

†Division of Cardiology
 Kumamoto University Medical School Hospital
 1-1-1 Honjo
 Kumamoto, Japan 860

ABSTRACT

    Familial amyloidotic polyneuropathy (FAP) is a systemic disease and
its main symptoms are polyneuropathy and autonomic dysfunction. Stokes-
Adams syndrome and renal involvements can be the cause of death.

    The effects of atropine and isoproterenol on the cardiac conduction
sytem in FAP were studied using surface ECG and His bundle electrograms.
Intravenous administration of 1 mg atropine sulfate induced prolongation of
the sinus cycle length and sinus node recovery time, but isoproterenol shortened the conduction system. The therapeutic doses of atropine may be potentially detrimental for conduction blocks in FAP, but isoproterenol may
have beneficial effects.

    For the quantitative and non-invasive measurements of the autonomic
dysfunction in FAP, a coefficient of variation (CV) of R-R intervals in
ECG was investigated, and compared to the age-matched normal controls. The
mean of CV was significantly decreased in FAP in their 30's and 40's. This
examination is a valuable method for detecting early involvement of the
autonomic dysfunction of the heart.

    The renal function was investigated in 23 cases of FAP. Patients were
classified into four stages according to the degree of their ADL and the
degree of sensory impairment. Proteinuria was noted in the early stage,
and creatinine clearance was most closely related to the disease progress.

INTRODUCTION

    In 1968, a large focus of familial amyloidotic polyneuropathy (FAP),
in the Arao area of Kumamoto, Japan, was reported by Araki et al. [1]. In
October 1984, they summarized the clinical and genetic manifestations in
90 individuals from 8 pedigrees to conclude that FAP is transmitted in an

autosomal dominant manner of inheritance with a high penetrance rate, and is fatal within about 8 years after the onset of the disease [2]. The disease is characterized by autonomic dysfunctions and sensory dominant mixed-type polyneuropathy affecting the lower extremities more severely than the upper [3]. The postmortem findings disclosed that amyloid deposits were found not only in peripheral and autonomic nerves, but also in the heart, kidney, spleen, thyroid, and gastrointestinal tract [4].

The present paper describes the results of our latest studies on FAP patients: 1) the electrophysiological effects of atropine and isoproterenol on the cardiac conduction system, 2) the quantitative analysis of the impaired autonomic nervous control of the heart, and 3) the renal involvement.

1. Adverse Effects of Atropine on the Cardiac Conduction System

The abnormality of cardiac rhythm, conduction disturbances, and orthostatic hypotension have been frequently reported in FAP. Stokes-Adams attack due to disturbances of cardiac impulse formation or conduction is an especially important clinical problem in the management of FAP patients [5, 6].

Therapeutic doses of atropine in the human heart usually induce shortening of the sinus cycle length, sinus node recovery time, sinoatrial conduction time, atrial refractory periods, atrioventricular (A-V) nodal conduction time, and A-V nodal refractory periods [7, 8]. In general, therefore, atropine is accepted to be a first-choice drug for prophylaxis or for treatment of bradyarrhythmias and cardiac conduction disturbances. However, we have recently observed that atropine has a detrimental effect on sinus node automaticity in FAP [9, 10].

1) Patients and methods: Ten patients with FAP had specific symptoms and signs, and amyloid deposits were confirmed by biopsy. All medications were discontinued 72 h before the study. Surface electrocardiogram (ECG) was recorded in 10 patients before and after intravenous administration of 1 mg atropine sulfate. On another day, detailed electrophysiologic studies of the cardiac conduction system were performed on 8 patients using a His bundle electrogram (HBE).

Electrocariographic leads I, II, V_1 and intracardiac electrograms were simultaneously displayed on a multichannel oscilloscope (CS-800, Fukuda-Denshi) and recorded on a photocorder (Type 2901, Yokogawa Electric Work) at a paper speed of 100 mm/sec. Intracardiac electrograms were recorded at a filter frequency setting of 1000 Hz and a time constant of 0.003 sec.

After completing the control studies, 1 mg atropine sulfate was administered intravenously to 8 patients, and the same studies done on the control were repeated 5-10 min after injection. Refractory periods of the atrium and A-V node were measured at the driven cycle length identical with that in the control state. Sixty min after atropine, isoproterenol was administered in 6 patients by continuous drip infusion at a rate of 0.5 µg/min, and the same studies done on the control were performed 10 min after the infusion was stabilized. Refractory periods of the atrium and A-V node were measured at the basic cycle length of 600 msec.

2) Results: Intravenous administration of atropine sulfate induced prolongation of the sinus cycle length (SNCL) in 6 of 8 (75%), the sinus node recovery time (SNRT) in 4 of 6 (66%), the A-V nodal conduction time in 4 of 7 (57%), the effective refractory periods of the atrium (AT-ERP) and A-V node (AVN-ERP) in 4 of 6 (67%) and in 3 of 7 patients (43%), respectively.

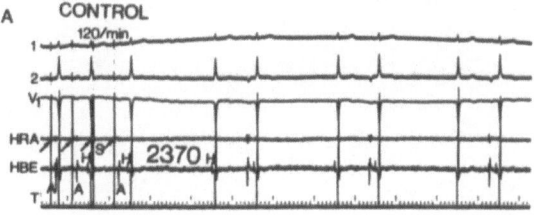

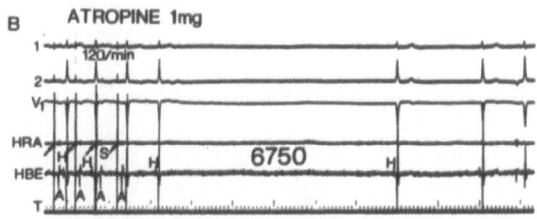

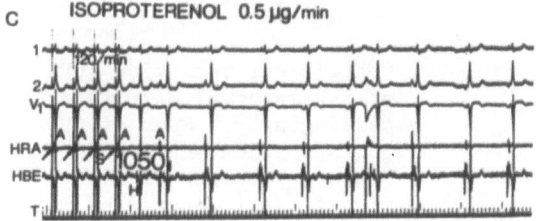

Fig. 1.   Effects of atropine and isoproterenol
          on the sinus node of A-V nodal recov-
          ery time.   Atrial pacing was carried
          out at a paced rate of 120/min.   Con-
          trol state (panel A):   the automa-
          ticity of the sinus node was mark-
          edly suppressed and the A-V junc-
          tion beat occurred 2370 msec after
          the stop of atrial pacing.   After
          atropine (panel B):   the automaticity
          of the A-V node was suppressed more
          than in the control state.   The A-V
          junctional beat occurred 6750 msec
          after the stop of atrial pacing.
          After isoproterenol (panel C):   the
          automaticity of the sinus node en-
          hanced and the sinus node recovery
          time was shortened to 1050 msec.
          Each panel shows, from top to bot-
          tom, the standard electrocario-
          graphic leads I, II, V_1 and high
          right atrial electrogram (HRA), His
          bundle electrogram (HBE) and time
          lines (T) at 100 mm/sec.   S or
          black arrow mark = stimulation
          artifact.

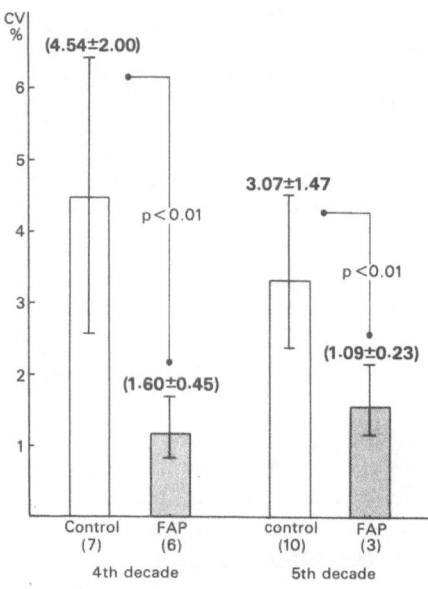

Fig. 2. Coefficient variation (CV)
of R-R interval of electrocardiography. Mean of CV
in FAP patients and con-
trols. The mean of CV was
significantly decreased in
FAP patients in their 30's
and 40's, as compared to
the age-matched controls.

Continuous intravenous administration of isoproterenol shortened the
SNCL, SNRT, A-V interval and refractory periods of the atrium and A-V node
in all patients [8, 9, 10] (Fig. 1).

Comments

Cardiac arrhythmias, including sinus arrest, sinoatrial block, A-V
block, and bundle branch block are frequently therapeutic problems in FAP.

Atropine is widely used for treatment of sinus bradycardia, sinoatrial
block, first degree and second A-V blocks, and so on. However, the above
results show that therapeutic or higher doses of atropine might be useless,
or potentially detrimental, for cardiac arrhythmias in some patients with
FPA, and that isoproterenol might be useful for the treatment of brady-
arrhymias or conduction blocks in FAP. In FAP patients with Stokes-Adams
attacks due to conduction blocks or impulse formation, a cardiac pacemaker
should be implanted early, since the cardiac contractile function was relatively well preserved in FAP.

2. A Quantitative Investigation of Autonomic Dysfunction
of the Heart in FAP Patients

The function of the autonomic nervous system in FAP patients was investigated by a quantitative and non-invasive technique using the coefficient of variation (CV) of the R-R interval of an electrocardiogram (ECG).
This was thought to reflect the vagal control of sinoatrial node [11].

While the patients were lying on a bed quietly for 15 min, a continuous ECG was recorded. R-R intervals were measured during 100 beats. Mean and standard deviation and coefficient of variation (CV) were calculated by Autonomic R-100 (MEC) [12].

The subjects were 11 FAP patients, 7 males and 4 females, age 27 to 63 years (mean of 38.6). The duration of illness varied from 3 to 16 years (mean 6.5). The control group comprised 43 healthy individuals, 23 males and 20 females, age 21 to 66 years (mean of 39.2).

In normal controls, the correlation coefficient between CV and age was -0.73 ($p < 0.01$). CV reduced in parallel to the age. The mean of CV in 6 FAP patients in their 30's (the 4th decade) was 1.60 ± 0.45 (mean $\pm$ SD), as compared to the age-matched normal control (4.54 ± 2.00). The mean of CV in 3 FAP patients in their 40's (the 5th decade) was 1.09 ± 0.23 (mean $\pm$ SD), as compared to the age-matched normal controls (3.07 ± 1.47) (Fig. 2).

The mean of CV was significantly decreased in FAP patients. But the difference in the mean of CV in the 50's and beyond was statistically insignificant.

Comments

Pathological studies of the autonomic nervous system and conduction system of the heart in the autopsy cases have disclosed severe amyloid deposition in the sympathetic ganglia, trunk, and vagus nerves [13, 14]. Recently, Kimura found that nerve fascicles in the epicardium showed amyloid deposition and marked loss of myelinated nerve fibers. In the sinoatrial node, the unmyelinated nerve fibers were markedly depleted and cardiac muscle fibers were degenerated. Degeneration of specialized muscle fibers was rather conspicuous in the bundle branches running in the subendocardial regions [14].

According to our study by the quantitative and non-invasive technique of using CV of the R-R interval of an ECG, and by pathological study, it appears that the autonomic control of the heart in FAP is impaired in both the sympathetic and parasympathetic nervous system. Measurements of R-R interval variation in the ECG is a valuable quantitative method for the evaluation of an autonomic dysfunction in FAP of the 4th to 5th decades.

3. Renal Involvement in FAP

In pathological studies, heavy amyloid deposits have been observed in the kidneys of both Japanese and Portuguese FAP patients [4]. Most FAP patients developed dysuria during the progress of the illness, and cystometry showed neurogenic bladder [15]. Since there have been few reports available on renal involvement in FAP, we studied in relation to the clinical stage of daily activity (ADL) and to clinical symptomatology.

We classified the clinical stage of FAP into 4: Stage I - sensory symptoms slight in feet and no restriction in ADL, Stage II - sensory impairment in lower extremities and slight ADL restriction with difficulty in working, Stage III - sensory impairment in 4 extremities and moderate ADL restriction with home stay, and Stage IV - generalized sensory impairment and severe ADL restriction with bed ridden state.

The subjects were 23 FAP patients, 13 males and 10 females, ages 24 to 47 years. The duration of illness varied from 1 to 10 years. Five FAP patients belonged to stage I, 2 to stage II, 12 to stage III, and 4 to stage IV. The tests performed in the series included urinary protein, serum total protein, BUN, PSP (15 min), Ccr, and Fishberg tests.

Proteinuria was noted in the early stage, but urinary protein contents showed a relation to the clinical stage. Serum protein, especially albumin, showed a decrease correlatively to each stage. BUN and serum creatinine were elevated at the end stage. Among the renal function tests, creatinine clearance was most closely related to the clinical stage.

Comments

A 38 year old male had developed polyneuropathy and autonomic neuropathy at age 33. He was at clinicial stage II at age 38, and at the same time renal function studies, before suicide, showed proteinuria and decrease in PSP. BUN (25 mg/dl) and serum creatinine (1.5 mg/dl) were unremarkable. Pathological studies disclosed hyalinization of the glomerulus with marked amyloid deposition [14].

The above study and pathological observation suggest that the renal lesion of FAP is caused mainly by involvement of the glomerulus. Moreover, it seems likely that dysuria and infections of the urinary tract are also factors of renal dysfunction.

SUMMARY

Our recent studies on FAP treated electrophysiological aspects of autonomic heart regulation and pathophysiological aspects of renal involvement.

1. Therapeutic doses of atropine may be useless or potentially detrimental for bradyarrhythmias or conduction blocks in some patients with FAP, but isoproterenol may have beneficial effects on those arrhythmias in FAP.

2. Examination for coefficient variation (CV) of the R-R interval in the ECG is a valuable quantitative and non-invasive method for detecting early involvement of the autonomic dysfunction of the heart in FAP.

3. FAP patients were classified into 4 stages according to the degree of their activity in daily life and the degree of sensory impairment. The renal involvements was examined in each stage. Proteinuria was noted in the early stage, and creatinine clearance was most closely related to the disease progress.

REFERENCES

1. S. Araki, S. Mawatari, M. Ohta, A. Nakajima, and Y. Kuroiwa, Arch. Neurol., 18:593 (1968).
2. S. Araki, S. Ikegawa, and J. Nagata, (Abst.), The 17th International Congress of Internal Medicine, Kyoto, 121 (1984).
3. S. Araki, Brain and Development, 6:128 (1984).
4. T. Shirabe, M. Hashimoto, S. Araki, S. Mawatari, and Y. Kuroiwa, in: Progress in Neuropathology (H. M. Zimmerman, ed.), Vol. II, Grune and Stratton, Inc., New York, pp. 409-420 (1973).
5. T. Sawayama, T. Kurihara, and S. Araki, Br. Heart. J., 40:1288 (1978).
6. B. O. Olofsson, R. Andersson, and B. Furberg, Acta. Med. Scand., 208: 77 (1980).
7. M. Akhtar, A. N. Damato, A. R. Caracta, et al., Am. J. Cardiol., 33: 333 (1974.
8. J. K. Bissett, N. D. B. DeSoyza, J. J. Kane, et al., Cardiovasc. Res., 9:73 (1975).
9. Y. Horio, T. Okajima, T. Ono, et al., Chest, 82:190 (1982).

10. Y. Horio, K. Matsuyama, M. Rokutanda, et al., Jap. Circul. J., 48:474 (1984).
11. T. Wheeler and P. J. Watkins, Br. Med. J., 4:584 (1973).
12. S. Kageyama, S. Mochio, and M. Abe, Neurol. Med., Japan, 9:594 (1978).
13. S. Kito, Y. Yamamura, H. Tokinobu, et al., Annual Report of the Ministry of Health and Welfare (ARMHW). Primary Amyloidosis Research Committee, Japan, p. 167 (1982).
14. Y. Kimura, Unpublished data.
15. N. Yanagisawa and S. Ikeda, ARMHW, Primary Amyloidosis Research Committee, Japan, 261 (1984).

IDENTIFICATION OF AMYLOID PREALBUMIN VARIANT IN FAMILIAL AMYLOIDOTIC POLY-

NEUROPATHY OF JAPANESE ORIGIN;   THREE PATIENTS OF DIFFERENT PEDIGREES

Satoru Tawara*, Masamitsu Nakazato†, Kenji Kanagawa‡,
Yoshio Takaba**, Hisayuki Matsuo‡, and
Sukuro Araki††

*The Department of Internal Medicine
 Yamaga City Hospital,

†The Third Department of Internal Medicine

‡The Second Department of Biochemistry

**Miyazaki Medical College
 Arao City Hospital, and

††The First Department of Internal Medicine
 Kumamoto University Medical School

ABSTRACT

The primary structure of four amyloid fibril proteins [AFj(INOK), AFj(INOT), AFj(TAMK), and AFj(SHIK)] isolated from different organs of three patients of type 1 FAP with different pedigrees was identified by comparing with that of normal human serum prealbumin using peptide mapping on a reverse phase column by high performance liquid chromatography. After cyanogen bromide cleavage, all amyloid fibril proteins demonstrated a unique peptide (CB-II) and four N-terminal peptides with successively accumulated deletion of N-terminal three amino acids (Gly, Pro, Thr). Tryptic digestion also revealed a unique peptide (T 4' or T 4") and twenty one peptides normally composing prealbumin.

Amino acid analyses and microsequence analyses of the peptides significantly proved that a valine residue at position 30 in normal prealbumin was replaced by a methionine residue. This change requires only one base change (GUG to AUG) in the nucleotide. Type 1 FAP in Japanese is an autosomal dominant metabolic disorder of a variant prealbumin.

INTRODUCTION

The dominantly inherited amyloidotic polyneuropathy (FAP) described by Andrade in 1952 [1] is characterized by a slowly progressive sensorimotor polyneuropathy initially affecting the lower extremities and later the hands. Autonomic dysfunction and loss of pain and temperature perception occur in early phase. Type 1 FAP patients in Japan [2] show basically similar clinical features as those in Portugese patients; autosomal dominant inheritance, begin late in the third decade or early in the fourth decade with death within several years to 25 years. In a previous paper, we reported the amyloid substance from type 1 FAP patients in Japan was a fibrillar component which was immunologically and biochemically related to prealbumin [3]. Recently neuropathic amyloidosis of "Jewish" origin was reported to be characterized clinically by impairment of vision and had the deposition of variant amyloid prealbumin (Thr-49 to Gly) [4]. This study reports the difference between the peptide mappings from amyloid proteins of type 1 FAP patients in Japan and that from normal human serum pre-albumin by high performance liquid chromatography (HPLC) and amino acid microsequence analyses of unique peptides and discusses the pathogenesis of this disease.

MATERIALS AND METHODS

Amyloid fibrils were obtained from the autopsied kidney and thyroid tissues from three FAP patients according to the published methods. Case 1, a 49 year old woman (SHI) and case 2, a 56 year old man (INO) had lived in Arao city, Japan. The diagnosis in case 1 and 2 was made by the clinical features, the pedigrees and amyloid deposits in the peripheral nerves, as described by Tawara et al. [3]. Case 3 is a 55 year old woman (TAM) who began to notice tingling sensation in the lower extremities and also diarrhea and constipation alternatively at the age of 38 followed by weakness and arrhythmia and finally died with complete AV block seventeen years after the onset.

Normal human serum prealbumin (PreA) (No. 101169) was purchased from Behringwerke, A. G., Marburg-Lahn, West Germany. The amyloid fibrils were denatured in 6 M guanidine HCl buffered at pH 8.5 with 0.5 M Tris containing 2 mM EDTA and 0.17 M dithiothreitol and were fractionated on a Sephadex G-100 column (2.6 × 67 cm) previously equilibrated with 5 M guanidine HCl in 1 M acetic acid [5, 6]. The molecular weight and the purity of each protein fractionated through Sephadex G-100 were determined in 17% poly-acrylamide gels containing 0.1% NaDoSO$_4$ according to Laemmli [7]. The purity of the protein was further confirmed by high performance liquid chromatography (HPLC) on a reverse phase C 18 column (0.4 × 25 cm, TSK ODS SIL: Toyo Soda, Tokyo, Japan) or on a C 18 μ-Bondapak (0.4 × 25 cm, Waters Associates, USA). The isolated amyloid fibril proteins (AFjs) and PreA were reduced and S-carboxymethylated (RCM) according to the published methods [8]. RCM samples were cleaved by a 200 fold excess (w/w) of cyanogen bromide (CNBr) (Nakarai Chemical Ltd., Kyoto, Japan) in a shielded state for 24 h. After lyophilization, homoserine lactone was changed to homoserine in 0.2 M ammonium bicarbonate. RCM samples were digested by trypsin treated with N-tosyl-phenyl alanine chloromethyl ketone (purchased from Worthington Biochemical Co.) in 50 mM Tris HCl, pH 8.0, for 2 h at 37°C (1:40-50 ratio of enzyme/substrate) after denaturation with 70% formic acid. The enzymatic digestion was terminated by the addition of 1 M acetic acid and boiled for 3 min. The CNBr or tryptic peptides were isolated by HPLC on a reverse phase column (TSK ODS SIL, 0.4 × 25 cm, Toyo Soda Co.), using two Hitachi model 635 pumps with a linear gradient of 0-60% acetonitrile (Katayama Chemicals, Osaka, Japan) in 0.1% trifluoroacetate and distilled water (pH 2.5) for 80 min. The solvents were HPLC grade and degassed prior to use. The peptides were detected by absorbance at 210 nm and 280 nm by using a variable wavelength detector from Hitachi. Poorly separated tryptic peptides using the TSK ODS SIL column were rechromatographed on a C 18 μ-Bondapak column (0.4 × 25 cm, Waters Associates) with a gradient of 0-50% acetonitrile in 10 mM ammonium folate (pH 4.0). The isolated peptides were pooled, lyophilized, and used for amino acid sequence analyses.

Amino acid analyses of peptides and proteins were carried out on a Hitachi 835-50 automatic amino acid analyzer using ninhydrin system after hydrolysis in 5.7 M HCl in evacuated sealed tubes at 100° for 24 h. Half

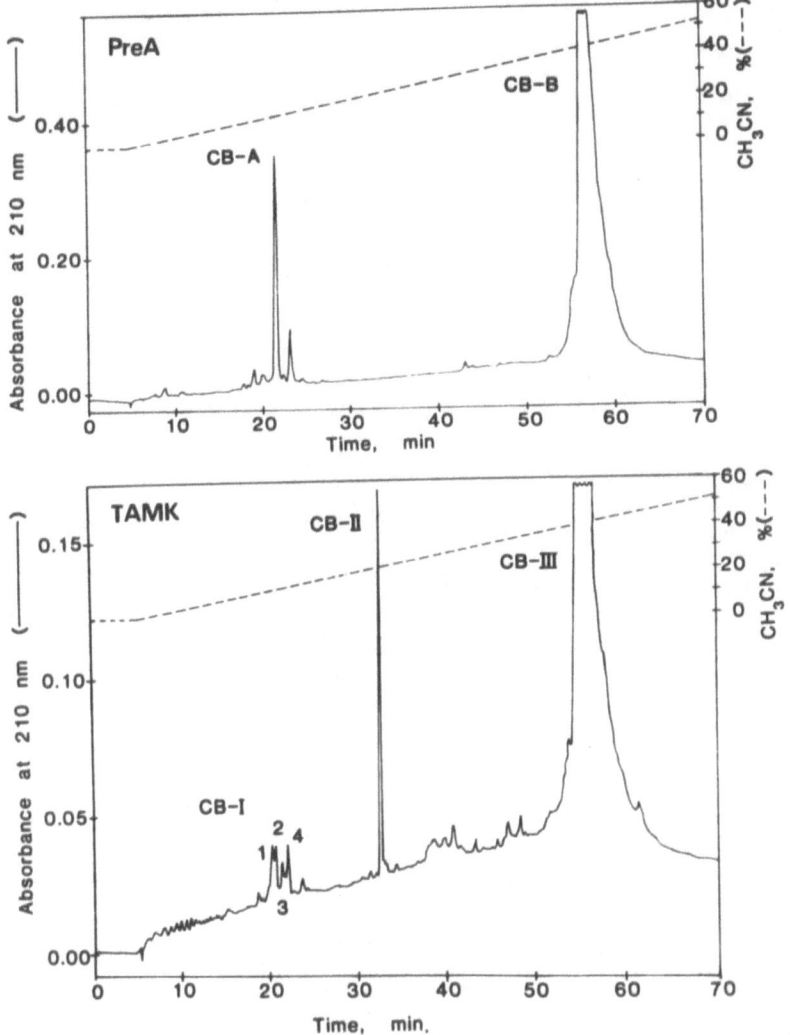

Fig. 1. Separation of CNBr cleaved peptides by reverse phase
column. Samples were reduced and carboxymethylated.
Flow rate: 2 ml/min. Conditions: see the text.

cystine was analyzed as cysteic acid after performic acid oxidation of the
samples, which was not reduced nor S-carboxymethylated, as described by
Simpson [9]. The microsequences of the abnormal peptides were determined
by amino acid analyzer (Waters Associates) after digestion by carboxypeptidase A or B for 15-75 min. The microsequence (22-30) of the CNBr cleaved
peptide in amyloid protein was identified by comparing the latent time in
HPLC with that of the peptide synthesized in our laboratory [10].

RESULTS

The gel filtrated pattern of amyloid fibrils on a Sephadex G-100 column
yielded three peaks as described before. The void (peak I) contained several materials of higher molecular weights and a protein of MW about 14,000.
Peak II contained two components MW 14,000 and 34,000. Peak III was composed of only a protein of MW 14,000. After CNBr treatment, HPLC or RCM

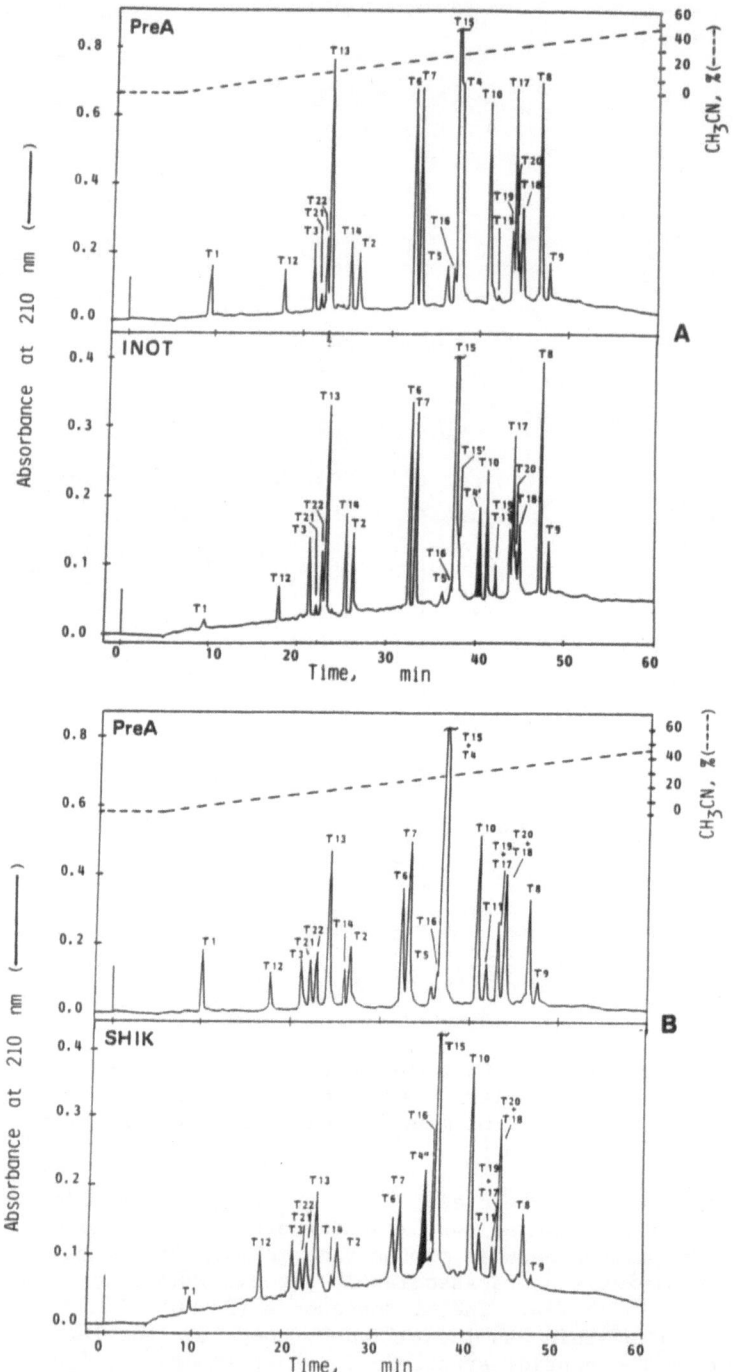

Fig. 2. Separation of tryptic peptides by reverse phase
column. A) A peak containing T4 and T15 or T15
and T15' was further separated as described in
the text. T15' was the peptide containing amino
acids of position from 81 to 102 of normal prealbumin. B) Conditions: Same as described in
Figs 1 or 2A.

316

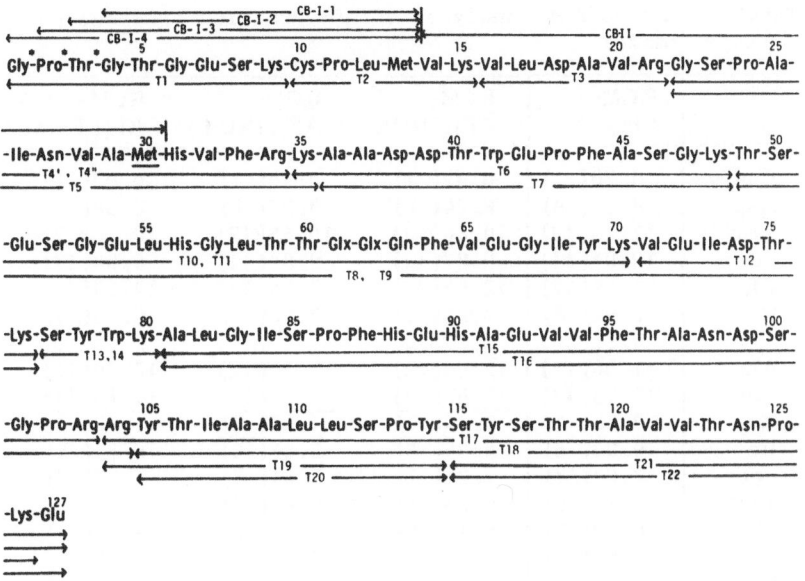

Fig. 3.   The amino acid sequence of AFj proteins (INOK, INOT,
          TAMK, and SHIK). T) Tryptic peptides; CB) CNBr com-
          ponents. N-Terminal Gly, Pro and Thr were found to
          be partially deleted.

peak III proteins from the kidney and thyroid tissues revealed three components. HPLC of peak II proteins showed a similar pattern. RCM-PreA
showed a different pattern on the same TSK ODS SIL column after CNBr treatment (Fig. 1).

The entire components of RCM-PreA and amyloid peak III protein from
the kidney and thyroid were digested by TPCK treated trypsin and revealed
twenty two peaks respectively by HPLC on a TSK ODS SIL column (Fig. 2A and
2B). Tryptic peptides T4' and T4" were not obtained from normal human serum
prealbumin. No normal T4 was observed in the mappings of trypsin digestion
of RCM-AFjs. T4" was oxidized form of T4'.

Amino acid analysis of RCM-AFj(INOK), RCM-AFj(INOT), RCM-AFj(TAMK) revealed that this protein had one more methionine and one less valine residue and less threonine, proline, and glycine residues than normal human
prealbumin (Table 1). Amino acid sequence analyses of the second component
(Fig. 1, CB II) isolated by HPLC after CNBr cleavage of AFj(INOK), AFj(TAMK)
disclosed that this component exactly agreed with the amino acids of normal
prealbumin from the 14th to the 30th with only one amino acid substitution,
methionine for valine at position 30 (Table 2, Fig. 3). Amino acid analyses
of the four minor peaks of the first component (Fig. 1, CB-I-1,2,3,4) obtained after CNBr cleavage of AFj(INOK) indicated that CB-I-1 was devoid of
three N-terminal amino acids (Gly-Pro-Thr), CB-I-2 lacked two N-terminal
amino acids (Gly-Pro) and only Gly was missed in CB-I-3 (Table 3). The
raio of CB-I-1:CB-I-2:CB-I-3:CB-I-4 was 39:19:18:24. HPLC analyses of the
tryptic peptides from RCM-AFjs and PreA indicated two points of differences
(Fig. 2, Table 4): one was that the new tryptic peptide T4' was found in
AFj instead of the peptide T4 of normal prealbumin. This T4' and T4" contained one methionine instead of valine. The other was that the amount of
the peptide T1 (amino acid position 1 to 9) was smaller than that of normal
prealbumin.

TABLE 1.   Amino Acid Analyses of AFj Proteins (residue per mole)

	RCM-PreA	RCM-AFj(INOK)	RCM-AFj(INOT)	RCM-AFj(TAMK)
CmCys	0.70(1)	0.92(1)	0.90(1)	0.92(1)
Asp	8.07(8)	8.24(8)	8.27(8)	8.38(8)
Thr	11.24(12)	10.66(12)	10.65(12)	10.20(12)
Ser	10.01(11)	9.87(11)	9.84(11)	9.84(11)
Glu	11.99(12)	12.06(12)	12.25(12)	12.64(12)
Pro	7.94(8)	7.23(8)	7.00(8)	6.86(8)
Gly	9.98(10)	9.28(10)	9.30(10)	9.67(10)
Ala	11.96(12)	12.04(12)	12.00(12)	12.00(12)
Val	11.13(12)	10.46(11)	10.27(11)	10.13(11)
Met	0.82(1)	1.65(2)	1.51(2)	1.90(2)
Ile	4.94(5)	4.98(5)	5.07(5)	5.31(5)
Leu	7.03(7)	7.21(7)	7.51(7)	7.77(7)
Tyr	4.98(5)	4.93(5)	4.89(5)	4.87(5)
Phe	4.93(5)	5.18(5)	5.10(5)	4.80(5)
Lys	7.83(8)	8.00(8)	8.10(8)	8.95(8)
His	3.85(4)	3.97(4)	3.84(4)	3.89(4)
Trp	1.04(2)	1.28(2)	1.32(2)	1.24(2)
Arg	4.00(4)	4.20(4)	4.35(4)	5.34(4)
Total	127	127	127	127

TABLE 2.   Amino Acid Compositions (residue per mole) of CNBr Peptides (CB-II)

	AFj(INOK) CB-II	AFj(TAMK) CB-II		AFj(INOK) CB-II	AFj(TAMK) CB-II
CmCys					
Asp	2.10(2)	2.14(2)	Ile	1.02(1)	1.00(1)
Thr			Leu	1.03(1)	0.98(1)
Ser	1.03(1)	1.57(1)	Tyr		
Glu			Phe		
Pro	1.11(1)	1.06(1)	Lys	1.00(1)	1.00(1)
Gly	1.15(1)	1.19(1)	His		
Ala	3.01(3)	3.07(3)	Trp		
Val	4.03(4)	3.69(4)	Arg	1.00(1)	1.00(1)
Met	0.74(1)	0.85(1)			
Position				14--30	14--30

The second component (CB II) obtained by HPLC after CNBr cleavage of AFjs was further digested by TPCK treated trypsin. One of two tryptic peptides was composed of amino acids of normal prealbumin position 22 to 30 except Met-30. The latent time of this peptide in HPLC was exactly the same as that of the synthesized peptide of Met-30 from position 30 to 22 in our laboratory.

TABLE 3.   Amino Acid Compositions (residue per mole)
           of CNBr Peptides (N-terminals)

	PreA CB-A	AFj(INOK)			
		CB-I-1	CB-I-2	CB-I-3	CB-I-4
CmCys	0.82(1)	0.83	0.83	0.85	0.84(1)
Asp					
Thr	1.85(2)	0.83	1.44	1.56	1.64(2)
Ser	0.95(1)	0.92	0.91	0.94	0.88(1)
Glu	1.00(1)	0.96	0.96	1.00	0.92(1)
Pro	2.18(2)	1.05	1.12	1.53	1.95(2)
Gly	2.79(3)	1.79	1.94	1.92	2.49(3)
Ala					
Val					
Met	0.69(1)	0.77	0.74	0.73	0.73(1)
Ile					
Leu	0.99(1)	0.96	0.98	0.97	0.97(1)
Tyr					
Phe					
Lys	1.00(1)	1.00	1.00	1.00	1.00(1)
His					
Trp					
Arg					
Position	1--13	4--13	3--13	2--13	1--13

TABLE 4.   Amino Acid Compositions (residue per mole)
           of Tryptic Peptides from AFj Proteins and
           Prealbumin

	PreA T 4	AFj(INOK) T 4'	AFj(INOT) T 4'	AFj(SHIK) T 4"
CmCys				
Asp	1.12(1)	1.16(1)	1.04(1)	1.10(1)
Thr				
Ser	1.04(1)	1.16(1)	0.95(1)	0.98(1)
Glu				
Pro	1.14(1)	1.19(1)	0.98(1)	1.08(1)
Gly	1.13(1)	1.19(1)	1.02(1)	1.08(1)
Ala	2.07(2)	2.00(2)	1.86(2)	1.99(2)
Val	2.83(3)	1.85(2)	1.72(2)	1.96(2)
Met	0 (0)	0.90(1)	0.81(1)	0.93(1)
Ile	1.00(1)	1.00(1)	0.89(1)	1.00(1)
Leu				
Tyr				
Phe	1.03(1)	1.05(1)	1.00(1)	1.01(1)
Lys				
His	0.90(1)	0.94(1)	0.91(1)	0.95(1)
Trp				
Arg	1.05(1)	0.94(1)	1.00(1)	1.00(1)
Position	22--34	22-34	22-34	22-34

DISCUSSION

Inherited systemic amyloidosis of a neuropathic form (familial amyloidotic polyneuropathy, FAP) was classified into four clinical types according to the distinctive clinical features. The primary structures of amyloid fibril proteins isolated from type 1 FAP patients of "Jewish" [4], Japanese [10], Swedish [11], and Portuguese [12] origins were recently reported to be variant prealbumins. We had previously elucidated the novel primary structure of AFj(INO) protein isolated from kidney of case 2. Here we report the primary structure of amyloid fibril protein from the tissues of three other Japanese patients of different backgrounds, in comparison with that of normal human serum prealbumin. Our studies reveal three main characteristics of AFj(INOT), AFj(TAMK), and AFj(SHIK) proteins, which are all variant forms of prealbumin. The first finding was that the variant prealbumin significantly had only one amino acid substitution at position 30, methionine for valine. The second finding was that each AFj protein is composed of four different proteins; a variant prealbumin and three related proteins which successively and accumulatedly deleted the N-terminal three amino acids (Gly, Pro, Thr). Amino acid analyses of the whole component of AFj proteins also revealed these two findings (Table 1). The third finding was that these AFj proteins contained no peptide T4 of normal prealbumin structure.

Regarding the primary structure of amyloid fibril protein of type 1 FAP, AF proteins from Swedish origin [AFs(GRO)] [11] and Portuguese origin [Afp] [12] were confirmed to have the same amino acid substitution (30 Met for Val) as our AFj proteins had. But SKO neuropathic amyloidosis of "Jewish" origin [4] was reported to have amyloid fibril protein [AFje(SKO)] of a different amino acid substitution at position 49. About SKO 3 protein, the position of amino acid substitution is still controversial. Since our recent study [13] revealed that SKO 3 protein has only one amino acid replacement at position 33, the amino acids of position from 30 to 33, namely β-strand B could be the major factor in the structural perturbation of variant amyloid prealbumin.

Regarding the complexity of the N-terminal amino acids of amyloid fibril protein (AF), there are two data. AFp was reported to have a normal N-terminal peptide in the map of tryptic digestion, but no C1 peptide in the map of CNBr cleaved samples. N-Terminal heterogeneity has been suggested in AFs reported by Skinner et al. [14]. Since our recent study [15] confirmed that the patient KURO has serum variant prealbumin of normal N-terminal, soluble serum variant prealbumin could be transformed into insoluble amyloid fibrils after proteolysis of its N-terminals. The possibility is still present that this N-terminal heterogeneity could arise only from destruction of the protein during isolation and purification.

Although our AFj proteins and AFp respectively revealed no T4 peptides, AFs(GRO) [11] and AFje(SKO) [4] were reported to have partially normal peptides (30 Val) or (49 Thr). The presence of normal structure of prealbumin may be related to clinical features such as the onset of the disease or the presence of visual impairment.

From these three characteristic findings and our recent report [16] that FAP patients have serum variant prealbumin, we can conclude that type 1 FAP in Japanese patients is a metabolic disease of a variant prealbumin (30 Met).

REFERENCES

1. C. Andrade, Brain, 75:408 (1952).
2. S. Araki, S. Mawatari, M. Ohta, A. Nakajima, and Y. Kuroiwa, Arch. Neurol., 18:593 (1968).
3. S. Tawara, S. Araki, K. Toshimori, H. Nakagawa, and S. Ohtaki, J. Lab. Clin. Med., 98:811 (1981).
4. M. Pras, F. Prelli, E. C. Franklin, and B. Frangione, Proc. Natl. Acad. Sci. USA, 80:539 (1983).
5. M. Pras, M. Schubert, D. Z. Franklin, A. Rimon, and E. C. Franklin, J. Clin. Invest., 47:924 (1968).
6. G. G. Glenner, M. Harada, and C. Isersky, Preparative Biochem., 2:39 (1970).
7. U. K. Laemmli, Nature, 227:680 (1970).
8. A. M. Crestfield, S. Moore, and W. H. Stein, J. Biol. Chem., 238:662 (1963).
9. R. J. Simpson, M. P. Neuberger, and T. Y. Liu, J. Biol. Chem., 241:1936 (1976).
10. S. Tawara, M. Nakazato, K. Kangawa, H. Matsuo, and S. Araki, Biochem. Biophys. Res. Commun., 116:880 (1983).
11. F. E. Dwulet and M. D. Benson, Proc. Natl. Acad. Sci. USA, 81:694 (1984).
12. M. J. M. Saraiva, S. Birkin, P. P. Costa, and D. S. Goodman, J. Clin. Invest., 74:104 (1984).
13. Submitted by Dr. Nakazato.
14. M. Skinner and A. S. Cohen, Biochem. Biophys. Res. Commun., 99:1326 (1981).
15. M. Nakazato, K. Kangawa, N. Minamino, S. Tawara, H. Matsuo, and S. Araki, Biochem. Biophys. Res. Commun., 122:712 (1984).
16. M. Nakazato, K. Kangawa, N. Minamino, S. Tawara, H. Matsuo, and S. Araki, Biochem. Biophys. Res. Commun., 122:719 (1984).

MONOCLONAL ANTIBODIES TO SERUM PREALBUMIN OF A PATIENT

WITH FAMILIAL AMYLOIDOTIC POLYNEUROPATHY

C. J. Rosenthal, M. E. Martin,
and A. Huq

Department of Medicine
Downstate Medical Center-SUNY
450 Clarkson Avenue
Brooklyn, New York 11203

ABSTRACT

In the present study we prepared a monoclonal antibody (m. ab.) to the abnormal serum prealbumin previously found (Tawara, et al.) in the amyloid fibrils of patients with Familial Amyloidotic Polyneuropathy (FAP). Prealbumin (PA) was isolated from the plasma of a 34 year old male of Ashkenazi Jewish extraction with FAP (accompanied by typical clinical presentation and course) and injected into three BALB/c mice whose spleens were removed after appropriate boosting. Splenic lymphocytes (1×10^8) were fused with 2×10^7 nonsecretory P3 × U1 myeloma cells according to a modification of Kohler and Milstein's technique using HAT selection medium. Clones, obtained through the limiting dilution method, were tested for the production of m. ab. to PA on dishes with U bottom wells into which the following proteins were absorbed: pur PA, PA_{FAP}, Albumin, BSA, Ovalbumin, IgG, SAA, AA, and serum from two patients with FAP and 5 normal individuals. The amount of m. ab. binding to these respective proteins was determined using ^{125}I labelled goat antimouse serum.

Based on their pattern of reactivity with PA and PA_{FAP} three m. abs. were selected. Two of them, 1C8-4 and 3C10-2, appeared to have different binding affinity for PA (three times stronger for the 1C8-4 m. ab.) but reacted equally well with normal PA and PA_{FAP}. The third m. ab., 2D12-7 consistently showed stronger affinity for PA_{FAP} than for normal PA. None of the m. abs. to PA reacted with any of the other proteins. When the 3 m. abs. to PA were used to recognize amyloid fibrils in liver and nerve biopsies obtained from the FAP proband and his father (using the PAP immunoenzymatic method) the bioptic materials were stained reddish brown when all m. abs. to prealbumin were used (somewhat more intensely with the 2D12-7 m. ab.) but did not stain when an antibody to Kappa light chain was used. Thus, it appears that the amino acid substitution in the PA_{FAP} can be recognized as an antigenic variant by a sensitive hybridoma.

INTRODUCTION

The chemical structure of amyloid fibrils in patients with familial amyloidotic neuropathy type I of Portuguese and Japanese origin started to be elucidated when Costa et al. [1] found that a protein with MW of 14,000 daltons extracted from fibril concentrates of kidneys, thyroid and peripheral nerves of patients with FAP appeared to be antigenically identical to normal prealbumin as recognized by a polyclonal antibody to human prealbumin, a protein that has over 50% of its native form as a β pleated sheet structure [2].

It was later found [2] that half of the amino acids comprising this protein, designated AF_p [2] have the same number of residues as prealbumin while the other half varies from the normal prealbumin structure by only one to three residues [2]. However, Saravia, Costa, and Goodman were unable to find physical, chemical, nor antigenic differences between the prealbumin extracted from the sera of 24 patients with FAP and that of 18 normal controls [3]. Finally, Tawara, et al., [4] recently reported the purification of an abnormal prealbumin from a Japanese patient with FAP. This protein differs from the normal tetrameric structure of prealbumin by a single amino acid substitution at position 30 (valine residue replaced by the fact that the three of the repetitive components of the abnormal prealbumin have deletions of the N terminal amino acid residues [4].

It is the existence of this microheterogeneity of the prealbumin structure of AF_p that led us to postulate that the production of monoclonal antibodies to the serum prealbumin of a patient with FAP may lead to an antibody capable of differentiating the FAP prealbumin from the normal prealbumin.

This became possible when, during the last 5 years, we had cared for a patient with characteristic clinical manifestations seen in FAP but with an ancestry not usually seen in this disease, i.e., an Ashkenazi Jewish family from Poland.

METHODS

Patient on Study

A 34 year old W/M of Ashkenazi Jewish extraction presented to us 5 years ago with a few months history of paresthesias (numbness) in his lower extremities, intermittent diarrhea, difficulties in having or maintaining an erection and an early goiter. His father, born in Poland, died at age 51 of systemic amyloidosis established at autopsy performed at our institution. His physical examination initially was remarkable for slight global thyroid enlargement, borderline liver enlargement (vertical span of 14 cm.) and peripheral neuropathy of the lower extremities with decrease of the deep tendon reflexes. EEG confirmed his significant peripheral neuropathy while a sural nerve biopsy and a rectal valve biopsy revealed amyloidosis. 99m-Technetium diphosphonate body scanning indicated increased uptake by patients's heart and muscles. During the following two years, despite therapy with DMSO patient developed bilateral footdrop (requiring special supporting devices), complete impotence (requiring a penile prosthesis), further enlargement of his thyroid, vitreous deposition of amyloid bilaterally and slight cardiomegaly. Since his enrollment in the plasma exchange program [5] $1^1/_2$ years ago, implemented by us for patients with systemic amyloidosis, his disease had first a stationary course with subjective improvement and decrease of the densitometry of 99m-Tc-diphosphonate radioactivity over patient's heart. However, more recently, he showed further slight deterioration of his lower extremity neuropathy with muscle atrophy and inability to walk. The plasma exchange therapy made available a significant source of prealbumin.

Prealbumin purification was performed following Rask's technique [6]. In brief, concentrated supernatant resulting from plasma precipitation with 40% ammonium sulfate was applied to a DEAE-Sephadex A50 column in 0.02 M Tris/HCl, 0.2 M NaCl, pH 7.4 and eluted with a linear gradient of 0.2 to 0.6 M NaCl. The peak enriched in prealbumin was detected by Ouchterlony immunodiffusion [7] then concentrated and dialyzed against 0.02 M Tris/HCl, 0.25 M NaCl, pH 7.2 and applied to a second DEAE-Sephadex A-50 column. It was then eluted with a linear gradient of 0.25 to 0.4 M NaCl. The peak containing prealbumin was dialyzed against 2 mM Tris/HCl pH 8.0 and then applied to a Sephadex G-200 column from which it was eluted with the same buffer. Finally, it was dialyzed vs. distilled water, lyophilized and tested for purity by SDS-PAGE.

Monoclonal antibodies to prealbumin were produced applying Kohler and Milstein's technique [8] with some modifications [9]. Three BALB/c female mice were immunized with 200 µg pure prealbumin subcutaneously followed by two intramuscular boosts at three week intervals and finally by an intraperitoneal boost. Three days later the animals were sacrificed. 1×10^8 spleen cells obtained from the immunized mice were fused with 2×10^7 nonsecretory murine myeloma cells of the P3 × U1 line. The fusion was performed in the presence of 30% PEG 4000 solution which was kept in contact with the cells for 8 min including a 3 min centrifugation period. Following washing and resuspension in HAT selective medium the cells were then dispersed into 96 well plastic trays. The production of antibody by the fused cells was tested within 2-3 weeks by a solid phase RIA using ^{125}I goat antimouse antibody to detect the binding of the m. ab. with the antigens absorbed in the wells of a 96 well U bottom plastic plate. The chosen hybridomas were cloned by limiting dilution, re-assayed and m. abs. were then produced in large scale in the supernatant of established hybridoma cell lines as well as in mouse ascitic fluid following injection of hybridoma cells in the peritoneal cavity of BALB/c mice primed with pristane.

Immunoenzymatic staining was performed with some of the selected m. abs. which reacted with the amyloid deposited in the bioptic material obtained from the proband on study and from his father's organs.

The peroxidase-antiperoxidase method [10] was applied. In brief, formalin fixed paraffin embedded tissues were deparaffinized and then incubated successively with 1% rabbit serum at 22°C and then 1% anti PA_{FAP} m. ab. (to be tested) in 1% rabbit serum for 48 h at 4°C. Finally, sections were treated with 1:20 rabbit antimouse IgG in Tris buffer. The reaction was then developed with the peroxidase-antiperoxidase soluble complex (1:50 dilution in Tris buffer with 1% rabbit serum) followed by treatment with 0.01% H_2O_2 and 0.05% diaminobenzidine tetrahydrochloride.

RESULTS

Among the hybridoma clones resulting from cell fusion of P3 × U1 murine myeloma cells with the spleen cells of the mice immunized with pure prealbumin from the patient with FAP, five of them secreted antibodies in satisfactory titers. They were immunologically defined as belonging to the IgG class when tested with a panel of class specific goat antimouse immunoglobulin antibodies.

None of the antiprealbumin monoclonal antibodies gave precipitin reactions in Ouchterlony immunodiffusion gels. Their reaction with prealbumin was easily detectable in a solid phase radioimmunassay which was also used for their selection (see Methods). These m. abs. were stable when kept at low temperatures up to -70°C but their reaction with prealbumin did not occur if kept at temperatures higher than 60°C for more than 10 min.

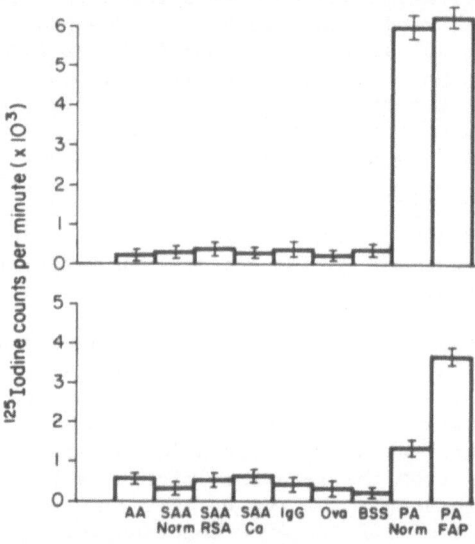

Fig. 1. Monoclonal antibodies to PA_FAP; their binding affinity to various antigens (upper graph: reactions of m. ab. 1C8-4; bottom graph: reactions of m. ab. 2D12-7). SAA Norm) SAA extracted from normal persons; SAA RSA) SAA extracted from patients with reactive systemic amyloidosis; SAA Ca) SAA extracted from patients with metastatic cancer; IgG) human immunoglobulin G; Ova) ovalbumin; BSA) bovine serum albumin; PA Norm) prealbumin purified from normal serum, PA FAP) prealbumin purified from the FAP patient's serum.

These m. abs. were produced in relatively large amounts in continuous cell cultures maintained for more than 6 months as well as in ascitic fluid in BALB/c mice innoculated with the hybridoma cells. Monoclonality was demonstrated in the ascitic fluid by the presence of an IgG band with restricted heterogeneity on electrophoresis. When tested by RIA against a panel of antigens including normal prealbumin, FAP prealbumin, bovine serum albumin, ovalbumin, human immunoglobulin G, SAA extracted from a patient with reactive systemic amyloidosis, SAA from normal donor and finall AA (see Fig. 1), the m. abs. showed no reaction above the background radioactivity with any of the proteins tested with the exception of prealbumin.

Two patterns of reactivity with normal and FAP prealbumin were noted: one characteristic of the 2D12-7 m. ab. which binds approximately three times stronger with FAP prealbumin than with normal prealbumin. The other pattern was similar for all the remaining monoclonal antibodies which showed equal affinity for both normal and FAP prealbumin. Two of them, exemplified by the 1C8-4 m. ab., appear to give stronger reaction with prealbumin than the other two exemplified by the 3C10-2 m. ab. (Table 1). The m. abs. 2D12-7 and 1C8-4 were selected for production in large amounts in mouse ascitic fluid.

TABLE 1. Monoclonal Antibodies to PA$_{FAP}$ Binding Affinity for Various Antigens (1 μg/ml)*

m. ab.†	AA	SAA$_{RSA}$‡	SAA$_N$**	BSA	Ova	PA$_N$	PA$_{FAP}$
IC$_{8-4}$	238 (0.6)	322 (0.8)	285 (0.7)	344 (0.9)	274 (0.6)	6038 (15)	6189 (154)
3C$_{10-2}$	224 (0.6)	330 (0.8)	281 (0.7)	320 (0.8)	295 (0.7)	2012 (5.1)	2070 (52)
2D$_{12-7}$	551 (1.3)	561 (1.4)	319 (0.8)	301 (0.7)	224 (0.6)	1318 (3.3)	3925 (98)

*The results are expressed as mean counts per minute of ^{125}Iodine in three wells with identical experimental conditions and (in parenthesis) as a percentage of the total ^{125}I c.p.m. detected in control wells in which no antigen antibody reaction occurred.
†m. ab.) Monoclonal antibody.
‡RSA) Reactive systemic amyloidosis donor.
**N) Normal donor.

TABLE 2. Reaction of the Two Different m. abs. to PA$_{FAP}$ Against Undiluted and 1000 Times Diluted Sera*

Serum donors	Undiluted serum		1:1000 diluted serum	
	2D12-7 m. ab.	C8-4 m. ab.	2D12-7 m. ab.	1C8-4 m. ab.
D$_1$	5820	8820	220	35
D$_2$	5540	8540	285	35
D$_3$	5980	8980	290	40
D$_4$	5430	9800	330	85
D$_5$	5700	8925	280	35
D$_{FAP}$	5350	7550	185	35

*The reaction is expressed in counts per minute of radioactive ^{125}Iodine contained by the goat antimouse antibody representing the second antibody of the "sandwich reaction."

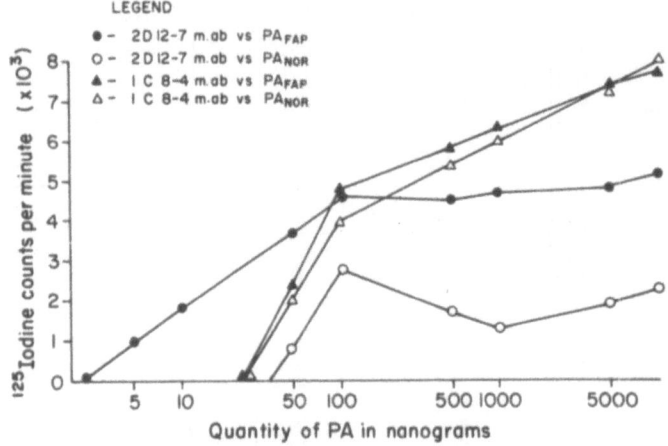

Fig. 2. Binding reaction curves of monoclonal antibodies to FAP prealbumin for prealbumin purified from normal serum (PA HDR) and for that
from the serum of the FAP patient (PA$_{FAP}$).
●) Reaction of 2D12-7 m. ab. against PA$_{FAP}$;
○) reaction of 2D12-7 m. ab. against PA NOR;
▲) reaction of 1C8-4 m. ab. against PA$_{FAP}$;
△) reaction of 1C8-4 m. ab. against PA NOR.

Their affinity for normal prealbumin and FAP prealbumin was further
tested by the solid phase RIA using a large range of dilutions of the antigens. As seen on Fig. 2 the steepest part of the reaction curve of 2D12-7
m. ab. with prealbumin was within nanogram amounts of antigen. At a concentration of 5-25 ng/0.1 ml 2D11-7 m. ab. was able to detect only FAP prealbumin while at a concentration of 50 ng/.1 ml the affinity of 2D11-7 m.
ab. for PA$_{FAP}$ was four times stronger than for normal PA (Fig. 2). This
m. ab. was not useful in RIA when microgram amounts of antigens were used.
Instead 1C8-4 m. ab. reacted equally well with normal and FAP prealbumin
over a larger range of antigen concentrations for 50 ng to 50 µg. When
microgram amounts of PA are detectable, the reaction of normal PA with
1C8-4 m. ab. is 50-100% stronger than that of 2D12-7 m. ab. with FAP prealbumin and 300% stronger than the reaction of 2D12-7 m. ab. with normal
prealbumin (Fig. 2).

It is only when 5 to 50 nanograms of prealbumin are used in the reaction that the affinity of 2D12-7 m. ab. for FAP prealbumin is 50-100%
stronger than that of 1C8-4 m. ab. for FAP (Fig. 2).

When the quantity of prealbumin in the sera of five normal donors and
of the patient with FAP from which the apparently abnormal prealbumin was
extracted was measured by the same solid phase RIA using the two m. abs.
previously characterized it was found that both m. abs. gave similar results (Table 2) for the quantity of prealbumin found in normal sera and in
the serum of the patient with FAP; they indicated the presence of approximately 30% less prealbumin in the latter. It is only at a very low dilution of the sera tested (Table 2) that a difference was noted between the
FAP patient's serum and normal serum and between various m. abs. The
2D12-7 m. ab. detected nanogram amounts of prealbumin while at that dilution level the 1C8-4 m. ab. was unable to detect any prealbumin-specific
radioactivity (above the radioactive background) (Table 2).

When the 2D12-7 and 1C8-4 m. abs. were used in the previously described immunoperoxidase (PAP) method for detecting amyloid deposits in bioptic sections of the sural nerve of the patient from whom the FAP prealbumin was extracted as well as in those obtained from the brain and liver of his father and from the liver of two cases of reactive systemic (secondary) amyloidosis, reddish brown staining of amyloid deposits, primarily surrounding vessels, was seen only in the sections obtained from the FAP patient and his father. When the same method of staining was performed using an antibody to a Kappa light chain as a control no reddish-brown stain was seen. The PAP staining was somewhat more intense when the 2D12-7 m. ab. was used than when the 1C8-4 m. ab. was tested.

DISCUSSION

Since their discovery in 1975 [8] it was realized that monoclonal antibodies have some unusual serological properties and that they are capable of recognizing only small portions of the amino acid sequence of a molecule [11]. This led us to produce a monoclonal antibody to serum prealbumin extracted from a patient with FAP which could differentiate the FAP prealbumin from normal prealbumin. Previous data generated by Costa et al. [1] and Saravia et al. [3] appeared to suggest that the normal and FAP prealbumin may have an identical structure in view of their identical physicochemical properties and identical antigenic characteristics demonstrated by the use of polyclonal antibodies. However, other structural studies suggested that the FAP prealbumin molecule [2] has a microheterogeneous composition which was clearly confirmed by the recent work of Tawara et al. [4].

Our current study which led to the production of a m. ab. (2D11-7) with much greater affinity for the FAP prealbumin than for the normal prealbumin and of 4 other m. abs. with equal affinity for the two molecules confirmed the existence of minor structural differences in the FAP prealbumin isolated from the FAP patient on study. The fact that 2D12-7 m. ab. reacts to a lesser degree with normal prealbumin indicated that it likely recognizes only a small fragment of the amino acid chain of the prealbumin molecule of which only a few residues are specific for the FAP prealbumin, while the others are shared with the normal prealbumin.

This cross reactivity of a monoclonal antibody with two different molecules was previously reported for other m. abs. [11] and is due to the recognition by the m. abs. of identical structural components in the two molecules. Because of this cross reactivity as well as because the abnormal prealbumin is mixed in the serum of FAP patients with normal prealbumin, the 2D12-7 m. ab. was unable to differentiate, in a standard sandwich RIA, the serum of FAP patients from that of normal patients. However, as indicated in Fig. 2 this distinction may be possible when patients serum tested this solid phase RIA were significantly diluted (1:1000 and more). Due to a higher affinity of the 2D12-7 m. ab. for the FAP prealbumin than for the normal prealbumin this m. ab. was able to detect nanogram amounts of prealbumin while the other m. abs. (1C8-4, etc.) were unable to recognize any prealbumin. Thus, the parallel use of 2D12-7 and 1C8-4 m. abs. in the solid phase RIA could help recognize the presence of abnormal FAP prealbumin in the 1:1000 diluted serum of patients with FAP; this assumption might be confirmed only if the heterogeneity of the prealbumin molecule of the patient herein presented (of Ashkenazi Jewish extraction) is found similar to that of FAP patients of Portuguese or Japanese origin. This may be the case in view of the fact that phenotypic manifestations of our patient have been almost identical with those of other patients with type I neuropathic familial amyloidosis and his disease had an autosomal dominant hereditary transmission as in all other cases of type I neuropathic familial amyloidosis.

This form of hereditary amyloidosis was previously recognized in patients who did not have a Portuguese or Japanese ancestry. Libbey et al. [12] reported similar clinical manifestations in a family of English and German ancestry whose members developed the disease in their seventh decade of life while Frangione and Pras (unpublished observation) recognized the disease in a young patient of Ashkenazi Jewish extraction born in Poland like the patient we studied. In some of these cases, using immunoperoxidase techniques, prealbumin was demonstrated in the amyloid deposits [12]; likewise it was found in the amyloid deposits recognized in the bioptic materials of the case herein reported.

The production in large amounts of this monoclonal antibody to the abnormal FAP prealbumin of a patient with type I neuropathic heredity amyloidosis could have further application in the early diagnosis of this disease before the appearance of clinical manifestations as well as a possible therapeutic agent through the formation of immune complexes with the circulating abnormal prealbumin present in these patients, followed by the rapid clearance of these complexes by the kidney. The latter application would likely be successful without unwanted side effects if further attempts to produce monoclonal antibodies to FAP prealbumin may generate an antibody devoid of cross reactivity with normal prealbumin.

ACKNOWLEDGEMENT

We gratefully acknowledge the excellent assiatance of Ms. S. Amrani in preparing this manuscript. This study was supported, in part, by NIH Grant No. 5R01AM2008006.

REFERENCES

1. P. P. Costa, A. S. Figueira, and F. R. Bravo, Proc. Natl. Acad. Sci. USA, 75:4499 (1978).
2. G. G. Glenner, New Engl. J. Med., 302:1283 (1980).
3. M. J. M. Saravia, P. P. Costa, and D. S. Goodman, J. Lab. Clin. Med., 102:590 (1983).
4. S. Tawara, M. Nakazato, K. Kangawa, et al., Biochem. Biophys. Res. Commun., 116:880 (1983).
5. C. J. Rosenthal, R. W. Kula, N. Solomon, and R. DeVita, Proceed. IV. Int. Symp. Amyloidosis.
6. L. Rask, P. A. Peterson, and S. F. Nilsson, J. Biol. Chem., 246:6087 (1971).
7. O. Ouchterlony, Progr. Allergy, 5:1 (1958).
8. G. Kohler and C. Milstein, Nature 256:495 (1975).
9. S. Fazekas de St. Groth and Schedeger, J. Immunol. Meth., 35:1 (1980).
10. L. A. Sternberger and S. A. J. Joseph, Histoch. Cytochem., 27:1424 (1979).
11. C. Milstein, in: Monoclonal Antibodies in Clinical Medicine (A. J. McMichael and J. W. Fabre, eds.), Academic Press, London-New York-Paris, etc. (1982), p. 3.
12. C. A. Libbey, A. Rubinow, T. Shirahama, C. Deal, and A. S. Cohen, Amer. J. Med., 76:18 (1984).

SALIENT STRUCTURAL FEATURES OF LOW MOLECULAR WEIGHT AMYLOID FIBRIL PROTEINS

IN FAMILIAL AMYLOID POLYNEUROPATHY OF JAPANESE ORIGIN

Tomotaka Shinoda, Fuyuki Kametani,
Hiroshi Tonoike, and Shozo Kito

Department of Chemistry
Tokyo Metropolitan University
Setagaya-ku Tokyo 158, and

Department of Medicine
Hiroshima University
Hiroshima, Japan 734

ABSTRACT

A unique amyloid fibril protein with a molecular weight of 8 K daltons, in addition to one with 14 Kd, has been isolated from an autopsy specimen of a patient with familial amyloid polyneuropathy of Japanese origin. It consisted of 73 amino acid residues and had cross reactivity with an anti-serum against normal plasma prealbumin. Following the extensive purification by reverse phase high performance liquid chromatography, it was digested with trypsin and the resulting peptides, after the purification by HPLC, were completely sequenced. The results disclosed that it had a unique sequence which corresponded with that of the residues from Gly-6 to Tyr-78 of normal prealbumin, except for a single amino acid replacement of methionine for valine at position 30 (normal prealbumin numbering). Besides the component, we also isolated from the affected tissues of patients with this disease an additional protein with similar molecular weight, but it was immunochemically distinct from Am43 (8 Kd) and normal prealbumin. A partial characterization was also made on this amyloid-related non-pre-albumin protein.

INTRODUCTION

Familial amyloid polyneuropathy (FAP) is a pathological condition having an autosomal dominant mode of inheritance, characterized by systemic depositions of amyloid fibrils and progressive disorder of the peripheral nerves [1]. In 1978, Costa et al. [2] described evidence that protein from amyloid deposits from an individual with Portuguese type FAP was antigenically related to plasma prealbumin. Subsequently, it was structurally identified as a variant form of the plasma prealbumin with a single amino acid replacement of methionine for valine at position 30 [3].

In Japan, two large foci of FAP (designated FAPj) have been reported [4]. Recent biochemical analyses have demonstrated that a variant prealbumin with the valine-methionine replacement at position 30 was also involved in these cases [5]. More recently, we have confirmed by recombinant DNA techniques that this replacement involved a single base substitution of G for A in a valine codon [6]. In the course of studies on FAPj, we have isolated a unique protein with a molecular weight of 8 K daltons, and have identified as a fragment corresponding to the residues from 6 to 78 of the variant prealbumin with the Val-Met interchange at position 30. Besides the component, we have also isolated from the affected tissues an additional protein with simimilar molecular weight, but it was immunochemically distinct from the plasma prealbumin. A partial characterization was also made on this unique component.

MATERIALS AND METHODS

    Amyloid fibril proteins Am43 and Am46. In each case, amyloid fibrils were extracted from amyloid-laden kidney according to the reported procedures [2, 5]. The materials were further purified by reverse phase HPLC using a column of Hitachi 3013-O macroreticular resin (0.4 × 25 cm) equilibrated with 20% CH_3CN-0.1% trifluoroacetic acid (TFA), pH 2.5. The column was eluted at a flow rate of 0.5 ml/min with a linear gradient of increasing CH_3CN concentration (20-70% in 0.1% TFA) [7].

    Trypsin digestion and the peptides separation. Rechromatographed AE-Am43 (8 Kd) (2, 5 mg) was suspended in 1.0 ml of 0.1 M NH_4HCO_3, pH 8.1 and was digested with 0.05 mg of TPCK treated trypsin (2× crystllized, Worthington). Aliquots of the digest were purified by reverse phase HPLC on a column of Hitachi 3013-O resin (0.4 × 25 cm) using a linear gradient of increasing CH_3CN concentration (10-15%) in 0.1% TFA, pH 2.5 [7]. AE-Am46 (8 Kd) component was treated in the same way as described.

    Amino acid analyses and sequence determination. Peptides (1.5-2 N mole) were hydrolyzed with 0.5 ml of 6 N HCl at 110°C for 24 h, and amino acids were analyzed on a Hitachi KLA-5 analyzer. The sequence of each peptide (20-60 N mole) was determined by manual Edman degradation method and PTH-amino acids were identified by HPLC as reported [7].

RESULTS AND DISCUSSION

    As shown in Fig. 1A, typical amyloid fibrils can be seen in the crude extracts from which Am43 (8 Kd) component has been purified. After the fractionation with Sephadex followed by repeated purifications by reverse phase HPLC, the material gave a single band on SDS-disc electrophoresis. The electron micrograms of desalted and lyophilized component is given in Fig. 1B. In contrast to amyloid fibrils in the crude extract, it became less sharp, and the striped patterns disappeared.

    Table 1 summarizes the amino acid compositions of the purified amyloid proteins of different molecular weights which have been isolated from three different cases from Ogawa-Village focus. For comparison, Afj(INO) from Aro focus [5] and of normal plasma prealbumin are also shown. As a whole, the compositions of the 14 Kd AFjs are very similar to each other, and seem to be in good agreement with that of the normal plasma prealbumin, except for higher contents in glutamic acid and methionine for AFjs. On N-terminal analysis, PTH-glycine was obtained from each case as the major product, suggesting that they were homogeneous by this criterion.

    As for the low molecular weight component Am43 (8 Kd), since it has been isolated from FAP tissues and has given a positive reaction with anti-plasma prealbumin antiserum, and since a similar protein has not been iso-

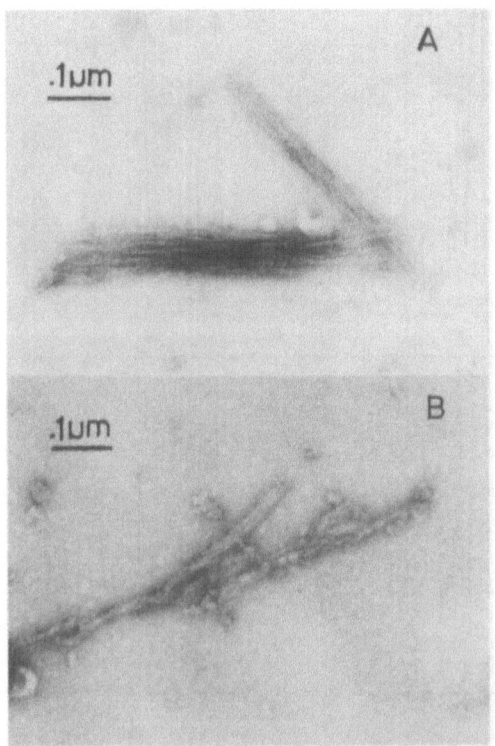

Fig. 1. Electron micrograms of amyloid fibril
proteins. Top: Crude fibrils in
water extract (precipitated with 0.15
M NaCl). Bottom: Lyophilized fibrils
after the degradation with 8 M urea.

TABLE 1. Amino Acid Compositions (mole %) of AFj Proteins in
Comparison with Normal Plasma Prealbumin

	Am14 14000	Am16 14000	Am16 30000	Am43 8000	INO(5) 14000	prealbumin
Lys	6.0	6.0	6.6	8.4	6.5	6.3
His	2.9	2.7	3.8	2.7	3.2	3.1
Arg	3.7	4.4	2.5	4.3	3.4	3.1
Asp	8.6	8.5	8.3	10.0	6.7	6.3
Thr	7.6	7.2	6.5	5.1	8.7	9.4
Ser	9.1	7.3	8.9	8.1	8.1	8.7
Glu	12.1	14.4	13.8	13.4	9.9	9.4
Pro	5.4	6.0	5.6	5.5	5.9	6.3
Gly	8.6	6.0	11.9	7.9	7.6	7.9
Ala	8.4	9.3	8.1	6.7	9.9	9.4
Cys	trace	trace	trace	trace	1.4	0.8
Val	7.3	7.1	5.3	7.7	8.6	9.4
Met	1.2	1.3	1.1	1.6	0.8	0.8
Ile	4.7	3.4	4.3	4.3	4.0	3.9
Leu	7.3	6.2	6.4	9.1	5.9	5.5
Tyr	3.2	3.6	2.8	1.9	4.0	3.9
Phe	3.9	4.4	3.9	4.2	4.2	3.9
Trp	(+)	(+)	(+)	(+)	1.0	1.6

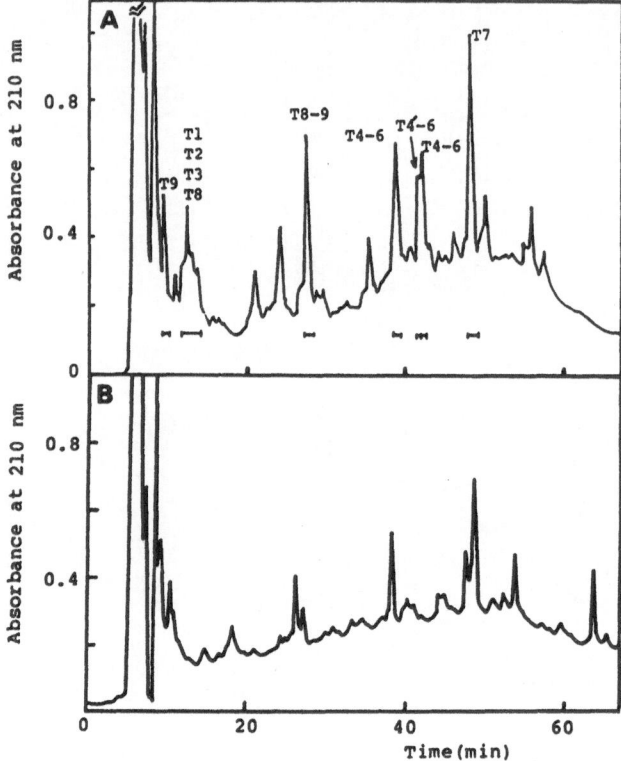

Fig. 2. Separation of tryptic peptides by reverse phase HPLC. A) AE-Am43 (8 KD); B) AE-Am46 (8 Kd). The digests were separated with a column of Hitachi 3013-0 macroreticular resin (0.4 × 25 cm) using a linear gradient of an increasing CH_3CN concentration (10-50%) in 0.1% TFA, pH 2.5. Flow rate, 0.5 ml/min.

lated from the normal control autopsy tissues, it is regarded as one of the constituents of the amyloid fibrils. In this context, we have undertaken a sequence analysis to see if there is any sequence homology with plasma prealbumin. Using a manual Edman degradation technique, the N-terminus sequence of the component was shown to be Gly-Glu-Ser-Lys- as its major sequence, by contamination with a minor sequence of Cys-Pro-Leu-. The major sequence was identical with that of the residues from Gly-6 to Lys-9 of normal plasma prealbumin, suggesting that it initiated with Gly-6 in the sequence of normal plasma prealbumin.

Figure 2A shows elution profiles in reverse phase HPLC of the tryptic peptides obtained from AE-Am43 (8 Kd). Following the rechromatography by HPLC, altogether 10 distinct peptides were isolated. The overall yields were between 7 and 30%. Among these peptides, T4-6 and T4'-6 had the same sequences except that a valine residue for T4'-6, while a methionine for T4-6, was respectively identified at the 9th position in each peptide. The sequence of T4'-6 was essentially identical with that of the residues from Glt-22 to Lys-48 of the normal plasma prealbumin, whose sequence has been reported by Kanda, et al. [8]. Thus, it was assumed to occupy the corresponding region in the sequence of AE-Am43 (8 Kd). Likewise, peptide T4-6

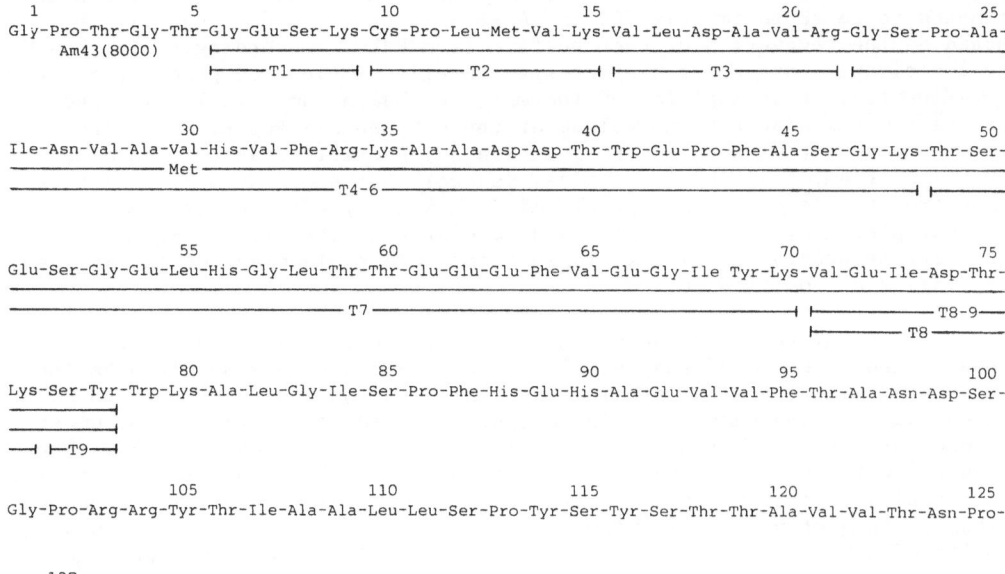

```
    1                 5                    10                     15                     20                      25
Gly-Pro-Thr-Gly-Thr-Gly-Glu-Ser-Lys-Cys-Pro-Leu-Met-Val-Lys-Val-Leu-Asp-Ala-Val-Arg-Gly-Ser-Pro-Ala-
      Am43(8000)    ├─────────────────────────────────────────────────────────────────────────────────
                    ├──────T1──────┤ ├─────T2─────────┤ ├──────T3──────┤ ├─

          30                   35                  40                     45                      50
Ile-Asn-Val-Ala-Val-His-Val-Phe-Arg-Lys-Ala-Ala-Asp-Asp-Thr-Trp-Glu-Pro-Phe-Ala-Ser-Gly-Lys-Thr-Ser-
────────────── Met ─────────────────────────────────────────────────────────────────────────────┤ ├─
                              ├──────────T4-6──────────┤

          55                  60                    65                     70                      75
Glu-Ser-Gly-Glu-Leu-His-Gly-Leu-Thr-Thr-Glu-Glu-Glu-Phe-Val-Glu-Gly-Ile Tyr-Lys-Val-Glu-Ile-Asp-Thr-
─────────────────────────────────────────T7──────────────────────────────┤ ├───────── T8-9───┤
                                                                            ├──────────T8────────┤

          80                  85                    90                     95                      100
Lys-Ser-Tyr-Trp-Lys-Ala-Leu-Gly-Ile-Ser-Pro-Phe-His-Glu-His-Ala-Glu-Val-Val-Phe-Thr-Ala-Asn-Asp-Ser-
──────────────────┤
──────────────────┤
──┤ ├─T9─┤

          105                  110                   115                    120                     125
Gly-Pro-Arg-Arg-Tyr-Thr-Ile-Ala-Ala-Leu-Leu-Ser-Pro-Tyr-Ser-Tyr-Ser-Thr-Thr-Ala-Val-Val-Thr-Asn-Pro-

    127
Lys-Glu
```

Fig. 3. Amino acid sequence of a low molecular weight amyloid fibril pro-
         tein (Am43 (8 Kd)). For convenience, the sequence is shown in
         line with that of normal prealbumin. Tryptic peptides are given
         the prefix T and are numbered consecutively in their order in the
         sequence.

TABLE 2. Amino Acid Compositions (mole %) of Non-Prealbumin
          AFj-Related Proteins and of a Variant Prealbumin-
          Related AFj Am14(14000)

	Am 7 10000	Am14 8000	Am46 8000	Am14 14000
Lys	4.0	4.6	6.5	6.0
His	2.7	2.3	2.7	2.9
Arg	3.8	4.0	5.3	3.7
Asp	8.5	10.7	9.7	8.6
Thr	7.7	5.2	5.5	7.6
Ser	7.5	7.5	4.9	9.1
Glu	13.1	12.9	11.9	12.1
Pro	3.0	6.5	5.9	5.4
Gly	8.4	8.6	7.9	8.6
Ala	8.9	7.8	9.2	8.4
Cys	trace	trace	trace	trace
Val	8.5	7.2	6.3	7.3
Met	0.8	1.1	1.8	1.2
Ile	5.2	5.0	5.8	4.7
Leu	7.6	9.3	9.3	7.3
Tyr	5.3	3.3	3.4	3.2
Phe	4.9	4.1	3.7	3.9
Trp	(+)	(+)	(+)	(+)

could be located at the same position as peptide T4'-6. The ratio was estimated to be approximately 30% of T4'-6 and 70% of T4-6, respectively, based on the recoveries of each peptide from HPLC. Accordingly, it should be conceivable that there are two structurally distinct components, one has a valine residue at position 30 (normal prealbumin numbering) while another having a methionine for the valine at the corresponding position. The former component with valine at position 30, possibly existed as a minor fraction of amyloid fibril proteins, is best understood as a catabolic fragment from the normal plasma prealbumin. Likewise, the one with a methionine at that position, is also regarded as one of the catabolic intermediates of an aberrant prealbumin with a single amino acid replacement of methionine for valine at position 30.

In Fig. 3, the amino acid sequence of the entire AE-Am43 (8 Kd) is shown. The sequence of the normal plasma prealbumin is also given as the reference. There are two prealbumin-related components in AFjAm43 (8 Kd) which exist in the same molecular weights of 8 Kd, and have the common sequences except for the valine-methionine replacement at position 30. The sequence with the valine-type, existing as a minor fraction, is essentially identical with that of residues from Cys-10 to Tyr-78 of normal plasma prealbumin, suggesting that it might have been derived from the corresponding region of normal plasma prealbumin. The methionine-type component, the major fraction, could therefore be considered to have been derived from the corresponding region of the variant prealbumin. The above findings, strongly suggests that a variant prealbumin with the valine-methionine replacement at position 30 or its catabolic fragment is also in close association with the amyloid fibril protein in Ogawa-Village type FAP.

During a search for AFj proteins, we have recently isolated an additional unique protein component from the autopsy specimens of patients with FAPj. This component, designated Am46 (8 Kd), showed an apparent molecular weight of 8 K daltons on SDS-disc electrophoresis. It did not react with either of the antisera against normal plasma proteins, or ones against amyloid-related proteins, such as AA, AF, and AL. The manual Edman degradation yielded PTH-Ser as its major product, suggesting that its N-terminus was serine. Table 2 summarizes the amino acid compositions of Am46 (8 Kd) together with those of variant prealbumin-related AFjAm14 (14 Kd). It has higher contents in aspartic and glutamic acids and leucine as compared with those of the normal plasma prealbumin, but has somewhat decreased amounts in threonine and serine. In Fig. 2B, an elution profile of the tryptic peptides from AE-Am46 (8 Kd) is shown in comparison with that of the AE-Am43 (8 Kd). The difference in the patterns is apparent, in comparison with the data on immunochemical examinations, as well as in amino acid composition. Although these peptides are only partially characterized at present, we would suggest that the unique protein component may also participate in the formation of the amyloid fibrils in the affected tissues of patients with this disease.

AKNOWLEDGEMENTS

This work was supported in part by a grant-in-aid from the Ministry of Health and Welfare Primary Amyloidosis Research Committe and the Ministry of Education, Science, and Culture of Japan.

REFERENCES

1. C. Anddrade, Brain, 75:408 (1952).
2. P. P. Costa, A. S. Figueria, and F. R. Bravo, Proc. Natl. Acad. Sci., USA, 75:4499 (1978).

3. F. E. Dwulet and M. D. Benson, Biochem. Biophys. Res. Comm., 114:657 (1983).
4. S. Araki, S. Mawatari, M. Ohta, A. Nakajima, and Y. Kuroiwa, Arch. Neurol., 18:593 (1968).
5. S. Tawara, M. Nakazato, K. Kangawa, H. Matsuo, and S. Araki, Biochem. Biophys. Res. Comm., 116:880 (1983); T. Shinoda, F. Kametani, H. Tonoike, H. Miyachi, S. Kito, and M. Inokawa, Ann. Rep. Minist. Health Welfare Prim. Amyloid. Res. Committ., 331 (1984); F. Kametani, H. Tonoike, A. Hoshi, T. Shinoda, and S. Kitto, submitted (1984).
6. H. Sasaki, Y. Sakaki, H. Matsuo, I. Goto, Y. Kuroiwa, I. Sahashi, A. Takahashi, T. Shinoda, and T. Isobe, submitted (1984).
7. T. Shinoda, N. Takahashi, T. Takayasu, T. Okuyame, and A. Shimizu, Proc. Natl. Acad. Sci. USA, 78:785 (1981); F. Kametani, T. Takayasu, S. Suzuki, T. Shinoda, T. Okuyama, and A. Shimizu, J. Biochem., 93: 421 (1983); T. Shinoda, K. Yoshimura, F. Kametani, and T. Isobe, Biochem. Biophys. Res. Comm., 117:587 (1983); H. Tonoike, F. Kametani, A. Hoshi, T. Shinoda, and T. Isobe, submitted (1984).
8. Y. Kanda, D. S. Goodman, R. E. Canfield, and F. J. Morgan, J. Biol. Chem., 249:6796 (1974).

IMMUNOHISTOCHEMICAL STUDIES ON AUTOPSIED ORGANS OF FAMILIAL AMYLOID POLYNEUROPATHY IN RELATION WITH AMYLOID PROTEIN

Rie Miyoshi, Shozo Kito,
Yasuhiro Yamamura, Masae Inokawa,
Eiko Itoga, and Takenobu Kishida

Third Department of Internal Medicine
Hiroshima University School of Medicine
1-2-3, Kasumi Minami-Ku
Hiroshima, 734, Japan

ABSTRACT

These days, much progress has been achieved on biochemical studies of amyloidogenesis and the relationship between clinical types and amyloid-proteins has been well documented.

It has been suggested that prealbumin is likely to be a candidate as the precursor protein of familial amyloidosis (FA). In our previous studies, the authors confirmed that DMSO administration to FA patients resulted in increased urinary excretion of retinol binding protein. In this study immunohistochemical examinations on 6 autopsy cases of FA were done with use of antibodies against prealbumin, retinal binding protein and protein AA.

In the results, positive immunoreactivities against prealbumin and retinol binding protein were obtained corresponding with deposits of Congo red-philic substances. Moreover, distributions of immunoreactivities against these two substances showed the almost same patterns within a particular organ of each individual case. It was especially noteworthy that protein AA-positive substances were confirmed in the thyroid gland of one FA case together with prealbumin- and retinol binding protein-positiveness, since protein AA has been considered specific for secondary amyloidosis.

All these results strongly supported the idea that several proteins were involved in amyloidgenesis of which exact mechanism has not yet clarified.

INTRODUCTION

Recently, biochemical studies on amyloid fibril protein have achieved much progress and it is advocated that clinical type of amyloidosis should be reclassified according to the major component of amyloid protein. The fact that in primary amyloidosis and amyloidosis with myeloma, Bence Jones protein is excreted in urine has been well documented, whereas high concentration of serum protein SAA has been pointed out in cases of secondary

TABLE 1. Clinical Manifestations of Familial Amyloidosis Cases Studied

Case	S.M.	S.A.	K.S.	N.S.	K.M.	H.M.
Age at onset	29	23	32	35	36	25
Age at death	41	36	36	41	54	34
Duration of illness	12	13	4	6	18	9
Symptoms at onset	paresthesia in the first toe	paresthesia	nausea	burning sensation in the ankle	paresthesia in the toes	nausea anorexia abdominal pain
Cause of death	brain abscess general infection	malnutrition	unidentified	malnutrition pneumonia	cardiac insufficiency respiratory insufficiency chronic renal failure	unidentified

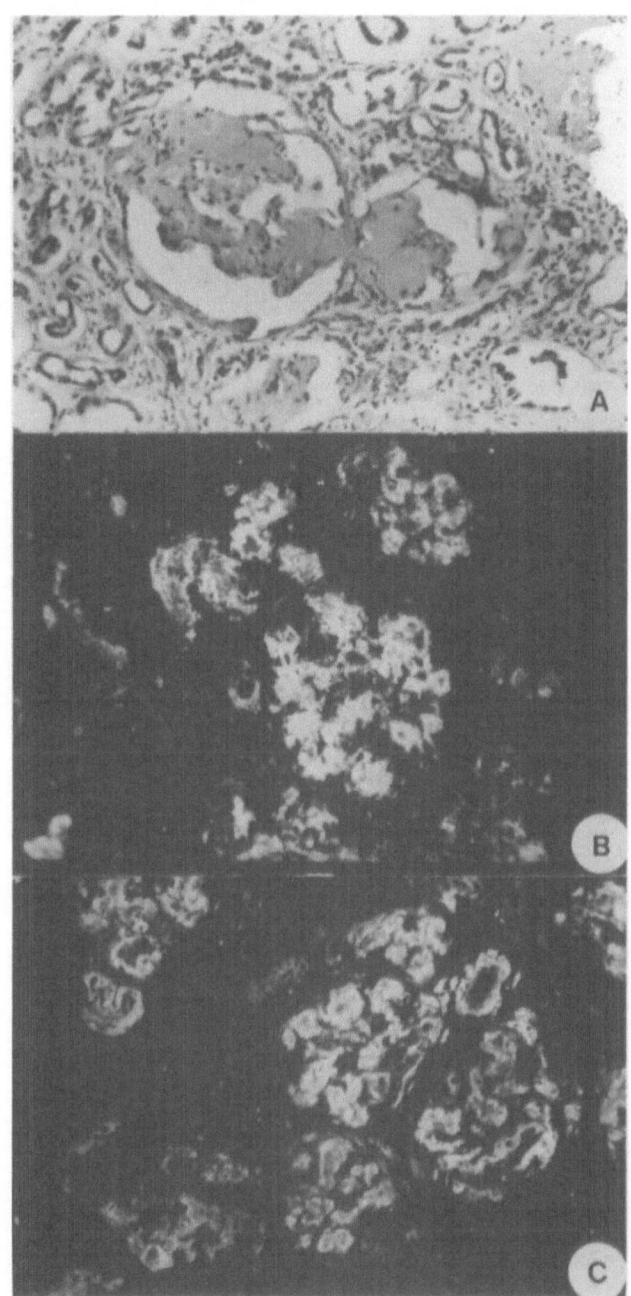

Fig. 1.   Microphotographs of the kidney of K.M. case. 1-a. Congo red
stain (×400). The Congo red-philic substance are deposited largely
in the glomerulus. 1-b. Immunohistochemical stain with use of a
human prealbumin-specific antibody (×400). There is prealbumin-
like-immunoreactivity of which the distribution pattern is consistent with that of the Congo red-philic substances. 1-c. Immunohistochemical stain with use of a human retinol binding pro-
tein-specific antibody (×400). Positive immunoreactivity is observed in the same pattern to that of plate 1-b.

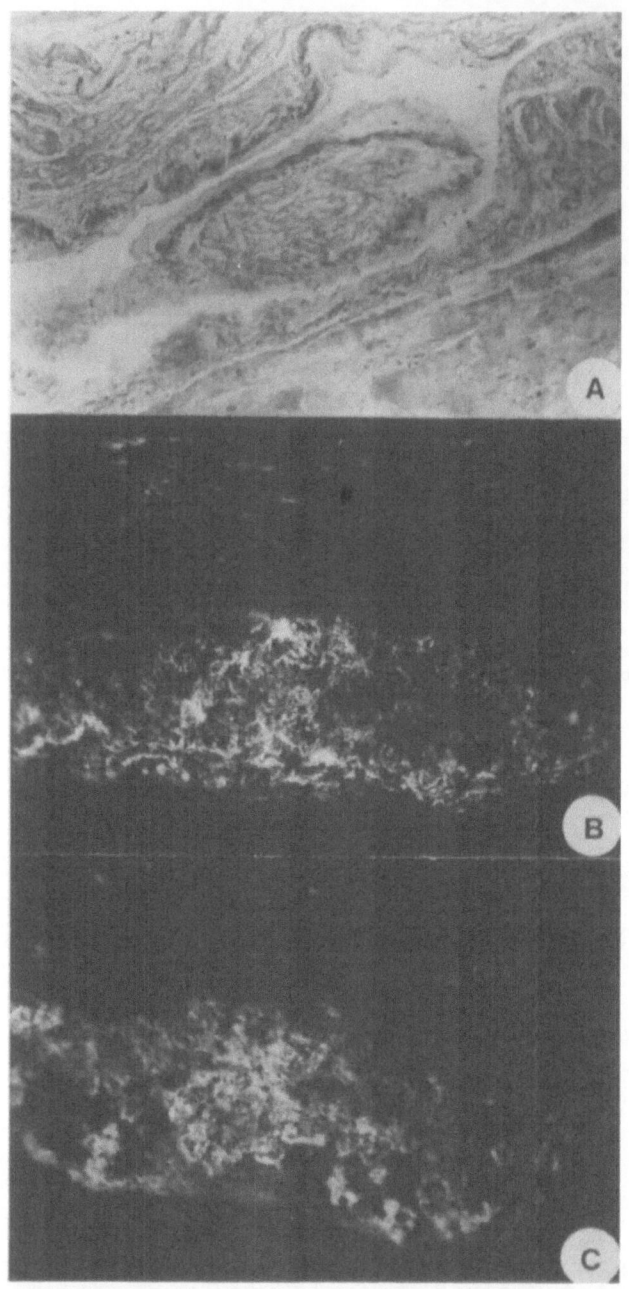

Fig. 2.   Microphotographs of the heart of S.A. case. 2-a. Congo red stain
(×400). Deposits of Congo red-philic substance are noticed in the
subendcardial region. 2-b. An immunohistochemical picture
against human prealbumin (×400). Prealbumin positive substances
are deposited also in the subendcardial region. 2-c. Human
retinol binding protein immunohistochemistry in the same region
(×400). Deposition of retinol binding protein is evidently observed in the similar way to prealbumin immunohistochemistry.

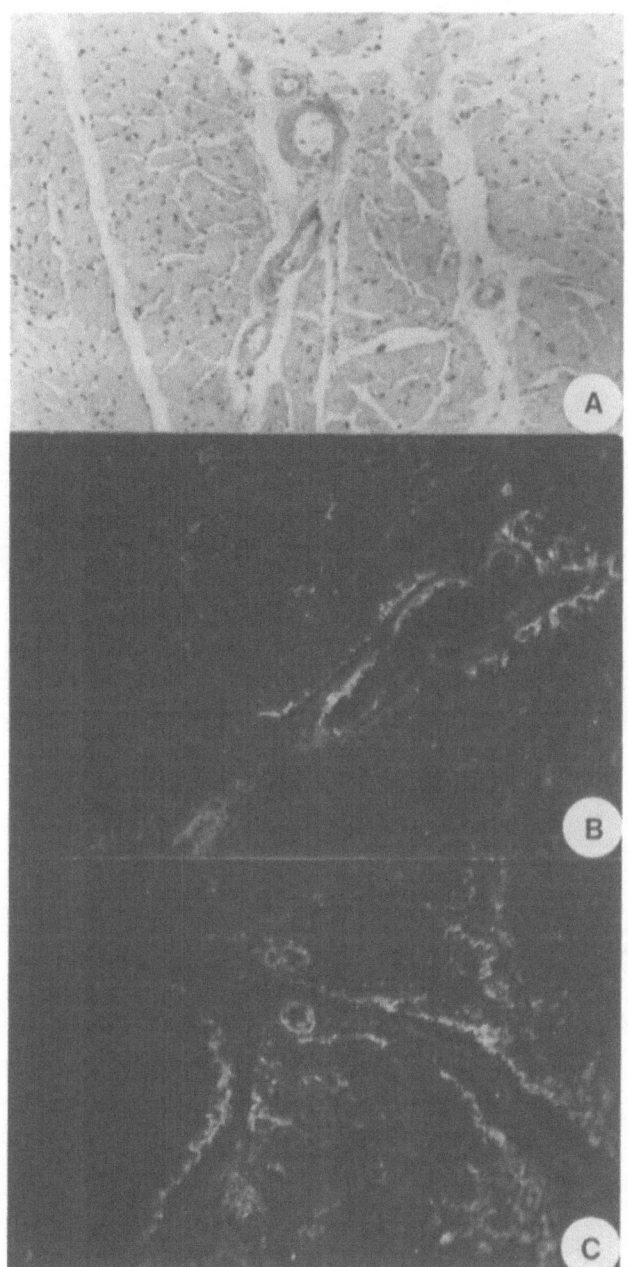

Fig. 3. Microphotographs of the heart of K.S. case. 3-a. Congo red stain
         (×400). Congo red-philic substances are deposited surrounding
         the interstitial blood vessels within the myocardium, while cardiac
         muscle fibers are atrophic. 3-b. Immunohistochemistry with use
         of human prealbumin antibody (×400). There are prealbumin-like-
         immunoreactive substances in the perivascular regions. 3-c. Im-
         munohistochemistry with use of human retinol binding protein anti-
         body (×400). Retinol binding protein is also accumulated within
         the myocardium.

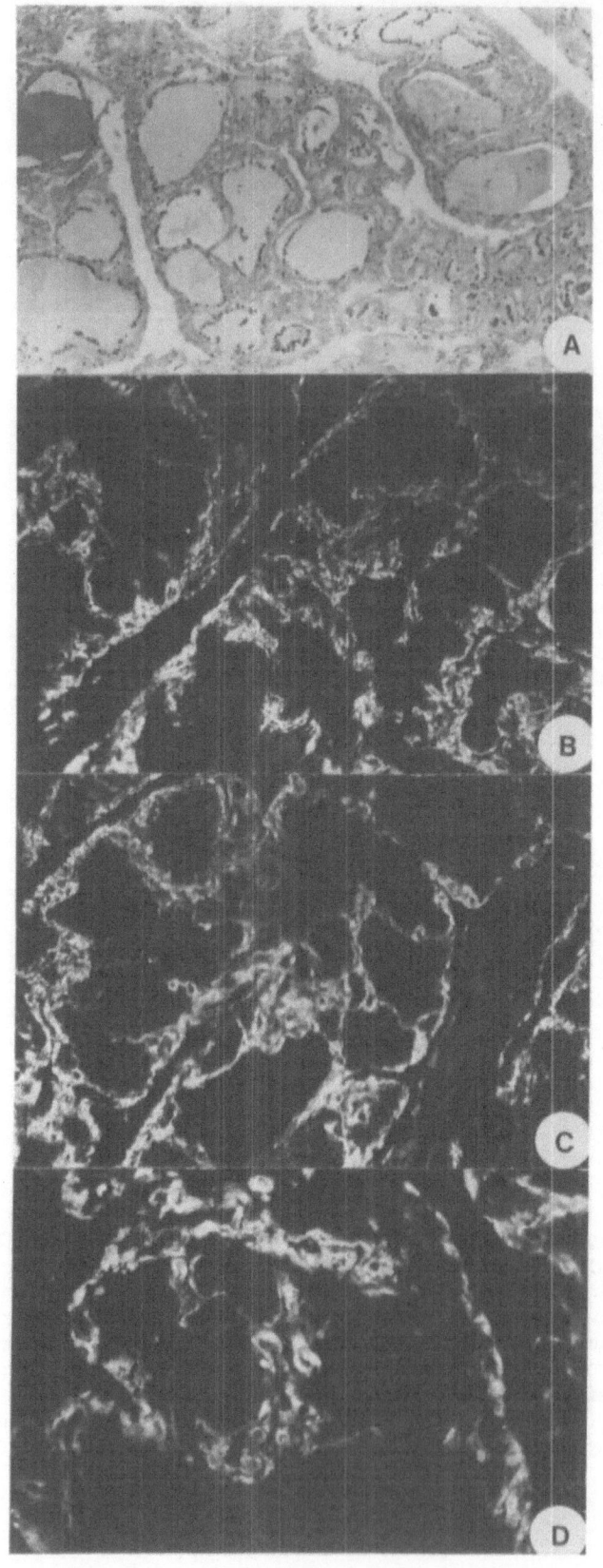

344

amyloidosis [1]. Recently, Costa, Pras and other research workers showed good evidences to support the hypothesis which regards prealbumin as a candidate for precursor protein of amyloid fibrils in Portuguese type of familial amyloid polyneuropathy (FAP) [2]. In our previous papers, the authors confirmed that urinary excretion of retinol binding protein was much increased by therapeutic administration of DMSO to FAP patients [3]. This result is significant since retinol binding protein combines easily with prealbumin in blood plasma.

In this paper, the authors performed immunohistochemical studies on autopsy organs of FAP cases originating from Magano prefecture, Japan using antibodies against various amyloid related proteins.

METHODS

Examined objects were six cases of FAP of which clinico-pathological summaries were shown in Table 1. Of six cases, four were males. All the cases had characteristics typical of FAP. Hematoxilin eosin and Congo red stains were performed on the kideny, heart and thyroid gland of these cases. Antibodies used for immunohistochemical studies were those against human prealbumin, human retinol binding protein and protein AA. Antibodies against prealbumin and retinol binding protein were purchased from commercial sources. The antiserum against protein AA was prepared by injecting protein AA extracted from the spleen of a secondary amyloidosis case into rabbits.

As for immunohistochemical techniques, fluorescent antibody technique was applied. Formalin fixed tissues were embedded in paraffin and cut in 6 μm thickness sections. These sections were incubated with antibodies for 30 min at 37°C, which was followed by another 30 min incubation with FITC-labeled anti-rabbit IgG goat IgG. Careful comparison between Congo red-philic sites and immunohistochemical positive regions was done.

RESULTS

Figure 1 shows histological pictures of the kidney of K. M. case as stained by Congo red (Fig. 1-a), prealbumin antibody (1-b) and retinal binding protein (1-c). Congo red stains revealed that there were amyloid deposits mainly in the glomerulus and partly in the Henle's loop of the urinary tubules. Distributions of both prealbumin- and retinol binding protein-like-immunoreactivity were consistent with the sites of Congo red-philic substance. In Fig. 2 of the heart of S.A. case, amyloid deposits were most prominent in the subendcardial regions (Fig. 2-a), where substances with positive prealbumin and retinol binding protein immunoreactivities were also most remarkably observed (Fig. 2-b, c). Prealbumin-

---

Fig. 4. Microphotographs of the thyroid gland of N.S. case. 4-a. Congo red stain (×400). Congo red positive substances are diffusely distributed in the interstitial tissue, whereas the follicules are atrophic. 4-b. An immunohistochemical picture with use of human prealbumin antibody (×400). Profuse prealbumin deposition in the interstitium is seen. 4-c. An immunohistochemical picture with use of human retinol binding protein (×400). Retinol binding protein is accumulated as much as Congo red positive substance and prealbumin. 4-d. Protein AA-like-immunoreactivity in the thyroid gland of a familial amyloidosis case (×400). This finding is noteworthy since protein AA has been considered specific to the amyloid substance in secondary amyloidosis.

and retinol binding protein-like-immunoreactivities were also observed
within the myocardium with lesser degrees. In the heart of K.S. case,
amyloid deposits were observed surrounding the interstitial blood vessels
within the myocardium (Fig. 3-a). Similar distribution patterns were observed by immunohistochemical stains for prealbumin and retinol binding
protein (Fig. 3-b, c). Histological examination of the thyroid gland of
case N.S. showed prominent deposits of amyloid substances in the interstitium with resultant atrophy of the parenchymal gland (Fig. 4-a). As in
the above-mentioned cases, localization of prealbumin and retinol binding
protein positiveness were consistent with amyloid deposits, with preponderance in the interstitium (Fig. 4-b, c). It was especially noteworthy that
protein AA-like-immunoreactivity was observed in the interstitium of the
thyroid gland of this case (Fig. 4-c), since protein AA has been considered
essentially specific to secondary amyloidosis.

DISCUSSION

     Histological and immunohistochemical examinations were done on 10
organs, 6 cases of FAP. In the results, immunoreactive positiveness against
prealbumin and retinol binding protein corresponded to Congo red-philic
sites in all the examined materials. In addition, immunoreactive sites
against prealbumin were almost identical to those against retinol binding
protein within the same organ. This suggested that within the amyloid-
laden organs, retinol binding protein was binding with prealbumin as in
blood plasma and thus contributing to aggregation to form amyloid
fibril protein. This hypothesis is partly supported by our previously experiments of urinary protein analysis after DMSO administration in which
excretion of retinol binding protein was confirmed [3]. Recently, Ishii
reported that DMSO administration to one patient of Alzheimer's disease
with amyloid deposits in the brain resulted in excretion of retinol binding protein [4]. On the other hand, Shinoda extracted and purified not only
a variant prealbumin with one amino acid deplacement but also normal prealbumin from an organ of FAP cases [5]. From these results, it should be
concluded that further studies are needed before one asserts amyloid precursor protein of FAP is exclusively a prealbumin variant. We proved
existence of protein AA-like-immunoreactivity in the thyroid gland of an FAP
case together with prealbumin and retinol binding protein positiveness.
This means that protein AA is not necessarily the specific to secondary
amyloidosis and relationship between clinical types of amyloidosis and biochemical characteristics of deposited protein is more complex than has
been considered so far.

     Amyloid fibril protein was considered a complex protein aggregated
into anti parallel β-pleated structure. Authors have paid attention to
retinol binding protein, urinary acid glycoprotein (UAGP extracted and purified from urine of an FAP patient) and α_1-microglobulin which shoed immunological cross reactivity with UAGP [3, 6]. In our experiments,
DMSO administration to FAP patients resulted in not only excretion of retinol binding protein but also that of IgA. It is a well known fact that
IgA is easy to make a complex with α_1-microglobulin which may be related with
amyloidogenesis in FAP according to our previous study [5-9]. All these results show that amyloidognesis is not as simple as only one precursor protein
playing a major role. Probably all these above-mentioned proteins, especially retinol binding protein, are contributing to amyloidogenesis as prealbumin is doing.

REFERENCES AND NOTES

1. M. Levin, M. Pras, and E. C. Franklin, J. Exp. Med., 138:373 (1973).
2. P. P. Costa, A. A. Figueira, and F. R. Bravo, Proc. Natl. Acad. Sci. USA, 75:4499-4503 (1978).
3. S. Kito, E. Itoga, Y. Ito, T. Kishida, Y. Yamamura, T. Shinoda, and Y. Yaguchi (G. Glenner, P. Costa, F. Freitas, eds.), 153-165 (1979).
4. T. Ishii, S. Haga, K. Kosaka, and K. Kato, Annual Report of the Ministry of Health and Welfare Primary Amyloidosis Research Committe, Japan, 1983 (in press) (1984).
5. T. Shinoda, F. Kametani, K. Sotoike, H. Miyachi, S. Kito, and M. Inokawa, Annual Report of the Ministry of Health and Welfare Primary Amyloidosis Research Committee, Japan, 1983 (in press) (1984).
6. E. Itoga and S. Kito, Jpn. J. Human Genet., 27:319-334 (1982).
7. S. Kito, K. Kamiya, E. Itoga, T. Kishida, M. Yamamoto, K. Nagano, and I. Iwasaki, Annual Report of the Ministry of Health and Welfare Amyloidosis Research Committee, Japan, 1977, 26-27 (1978).
8. S. Kito, K. Kamiya, and T. Shinoda, Annual Report of the Ministry of Health and Welfare Amyloidotic Neuropathy Research Committee, Japan, 1978, 21-22 (1979).
9. S. Kito, K. Kamiya, E. Itoga, T. Kishida, Y. Yamamura, S. Takegawa, and M. Usui, Annual Report of the Ministry of Health and Welfare Amyloidotic Neuropathy Research Committee, Japan, 1978, 27-28 (1979).
10. S. Kito, E. Itoga, K. Kamiya, T. Kishida, and Y. Yamamura, European Neurology, 19:141-151 (1980).
11. S. Kito, E. Itoga, Y. Ito, T. Kishida, Y. Yamamura, and M. Usui, Annual Report of the Ministry of Health and Welfare Amyloidotic Neuropathy Research Committee, Japan, 1979, 9-10 (1980).
12. Table 1. All these cases were derived from Ogawa village, Nagano prefecture of Japan, where second largest conglomeration of familial amyloidosis had been discovered by the authors. The authors observed clinical pictures of these cases throughout the entire course of the disease.

STUDIES ON BLOOD MARKERS AND AMYLOID FIBRIL

IN THE ARAO FOCUS OF FAMILIAL AMYLOID POLYNEUROPATHY

S. Sakoda*, T. Suzuki*, S. Higa*,
M. Ueji*, S. Kishimoto*, K. Titani†,
A. Hayashi‡, H. Matsumoto**,
T. Sasazuki††, K. Omoto‡‡,
Y. Takaba***, and A. Nakajima†††

*The third Department of Internal Medicine, Osaka
 University Hospital, Fukushima-ku, Osaka 553, Japan

†Department of Biochemistry, University of Washington
 Seattle, Washington, USA

‡Osaka Medical Center and Research Institute for Maternal
 and Child Health, Osaka, Japan

**Department of Legal Medicine, Osaka Medical College, Japan

††Department of Human Genetics, Medical Research Institute
 Medical Research Institute, Tokyo Medical and Dental
 University, Tokyo, Japan

‡‡Department of Anthropology, Faculty of Science, The
 Univeristy of Tokyo, Tokyo, Japan

***The Arao City Hospital, Japan

†††The Nakajima Medical Clinic, Japan

ABSTRACT

To investigate the genetic origin of familiar amyloid polyneuropathy
(FAP) in the Arao district of Japan, the amyloid-laden kidneys of 4 patients
from 3 affected families were examined for the primary structure of amyloid
fibril protein and blood samples from 21 patients with FAP and 81 normal
family members among 7 affected families were tested for 30 blood markers.
The amyloid fibril protein isolated was identified as a prealbumin variant,
in which an amino acid substitution of a methionine for a valine occurred
at position 30, irrespective of the patient or the family. The relatively
rare variants, group sepecific component Gc*1A2 and phosphoglucomutase
PGM1*7, were distributed over 3 affected families. No phenotype attributable to Caucasians was found. The results of the study on the amyloid
fibril protein suggests that patients with FAP in Arao might have the same
mutation and the existence of Gc*1A2 and PGM1*7 in 3 of 7 families suggests
the possibility that the FAP mutation occurred once and subsequently spread
to 7 families.

INTRODUCTION

Type 1 familial amyloid polyneuropathy(FAP) has a curious geographic distribution: there are large foci in Portugal [1], Sweden [2], and Japan [3] but the disease is rare elsewhere. The Arao district, one of two large foci in Japan, is located in Kyushu where Portuguese first came in the middle of the 16th century and remained for about a hundred years. Whether FAP in Japan has a Portuguese ancestry or not is an interesting enigma [4]. Our previous genealogical survey [5] revealed that FAP in the Arao district of Japan affects nearly one hundred patients among 9 families but did not provide any information about the origin of the disease. To elucidate the origin of the FAP gene in Arao, we analysed the primary structure of the amyloid fibril and examined 30 polymorphic genetic markers in blood in members of several affected families.

MATERIALS AND METHODS

I. Analysis of Amyloid Fibril Protein

Materials: Amyloid laden kidneys were obtained at the autopsies of 4 patients with FAP in the Arao district. Case 1, a 47-year-old man, is a member of the U family; case 2, a 41-year-old women is a member of the S family; case 3, a 51-year-old man is a member of the H family; and case 4, a 46-year-old woman, is a sister of case 3. These family names are those used in our previous report [5]. Control analyses were performed on a kidney obtained from a 52-year-old woman who died from a myocardial infarction.

Isolation and Fractionation of Amyloid Fibril. Amyloid fibrils were extracted from the kidneys by the method of Pras et al. and applied to a Sephadex G-100 column [7]. The third peak (P3) material was reduced with dithiothreitol and SO-carboxymethylated by the method of Crestfield et al. [8]. The mixture was then loaded on a column of UltroPac TSK-G2000 SW with a precolumn [9]. Subsequent purification of the major fraction from the gel filtration column was achieved by reversed phase high performance liquid chromatography (HPLC) performed with a Varian 5000 liquid Chromatograph on a column of Synchropak RP-P (Synchrom) using a trifluoroacetic acid (Pierce)-acetonitrile (Burdick & Jackson) system [10]. The major peak was further purified by rechromatography.

Amino Acid Sequence Analyses. After SO-carboxymethylation, the amyloid protein was digested with TPCK-trypsin (Worthington). The digest was injected into a reversed phase HPLC column, Synchropak RP-P [9]. Automated sequence analysis was performed with an Applied Biosystems 470A Protein Sequencer using a program adapted from Hunkapiller et al. [11].

For comparative studies, normal human prealbumin (kindly provided by Dr. Y. Kanda, Nippon Medical School) was also treated by the same procedure as the P3 material.

II. Analysis of Genetic Markers in Blood

21 patients with FAP and 81 normal family members from 7 affected families (Table 1) in Arao donated blood for examination. Each subject was typed for 9 blood groups, 8 serum protein markers, 12 red cell enzymes, and HLA [12]. The nine blood groups included ABO, MN, P, Rh, Kell, Kidd, Duffy, Lutheran and Diego; the eight serum protein markers included haptoglobin, transferrin, group specific component (Gc), protease inhibitor, second component of complement, factor B, Gm, and Km; and the 12 red cell enzymes in-

TABLE 1. Distribution of Gc*1A2 and PGM1*7
Phenotype among 7 Families

Family	Gc*1A2	PGM1*7
U	+	+
Sa	+	+
S	−	−
Tn	−	−
Tu	+	−
Ni	−	−
H	−	−

included acid phosphatase, 6-phosphogluconate dehydrogenase, esterase D, glutamic-pyruvic transaminase, glutamic-oxaloacetic transaminase, phospho-hexose isomerase, lactate dehydrogenase, adenosine deaminase, uridine-5-monophosphate Kinase, glyoxalase 1, abnormal hemoglobin, and phosphogluco-mutase-1 (PGM1).

RESULTS

I. Analysis of Amyloid Fibril Protein

The Sephadex G-100 gel-filtration of amyloid fibrils from FAP kidneys gave a void volume peak (P1) with a shoulder (P2) on the descending limbs and a retarded peak (P3) [9]. Neither P2 nor P3 was obtained from the control kidney.

Tryptic peptides of each P3 predominant protein were compared with those of prealbumin of known primary structure [13] by reversed phase HPLC. Although only the HPLC chromatogram of case 1 is shown in Fig. 1, identical chromatograms were obtained in the 3 other cases, indicating that the primary structure of the P3 predominant protein from each of the 4 cases is essentially identical. However, T1', with slightly shorter retention time than T1, was isolated from P3. Sequence analysis of the peptide T1' yielded the major sequence of Thr-Gly-Thr-Gly-Glu-Ser-Lys ———————, which appears to be from the amino terminus of the protein (Fig. 2). T3 and T4 of prealbumin appear to be replaced by T3' and T4' in P3. Amino acid analysis showed that T3 and T4 of prealbumin are derived from residues 22-34 and 22-35, respectively, and T3' and T4' only differ by containing one less valine and one methionine. Sequence analysis of T3' from P3 of each of the 4 cases identified the Val-Met replacement at residue 30.

Further differences between prealbumin and P3 predominant protein were not explored in the present study, except for peptide T7 containing residues 61 and 62 which had been identified as Glx and Glx in a study of human prealbumin by Kanda et al. [13]. Sequence analysis of the peptide identified residues 61 through 63 as Glu-Glu-Glu, the last one of which differs from Gln-63 in prealbumin.

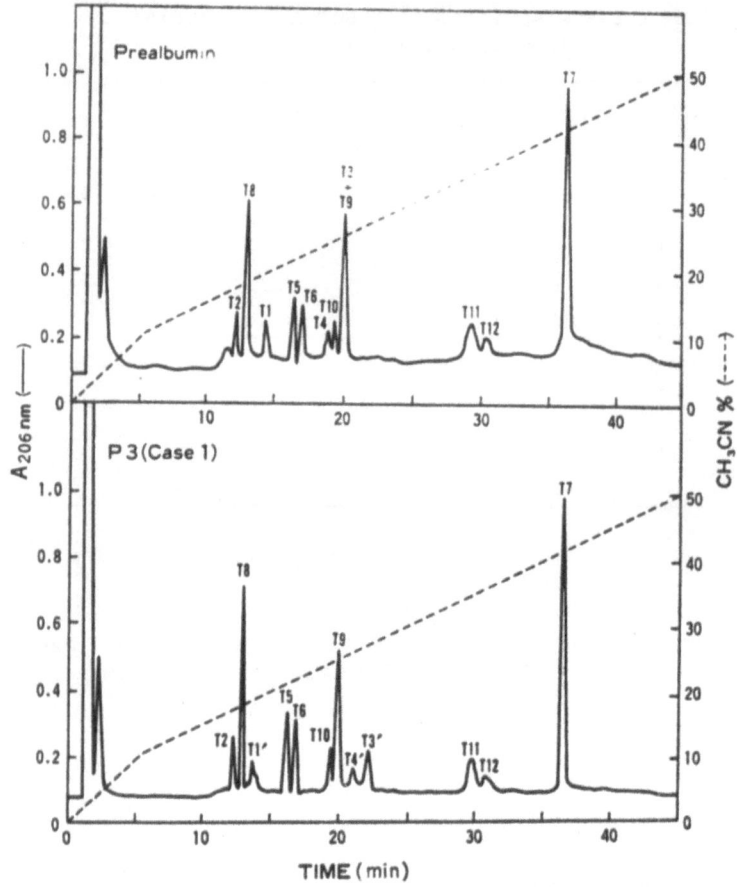

Fig. 1.   Separation of tryptic peptides of prealbumin and
the P3 predominant protein (case 1) by reversed
phase HPLC.

II.   Analysis of Genetic Markers in Blood

Relatively rare variants of Gc*1A2 and PGM1*7 were found in 3 of 7
families affected with FAP (Table 1). Phenotypes attributable to Caucasians, for example K+ in the Kell group, were not found in this study.

DISCUSSION

The present study on the primary structure of the amyloid fibril from
4 patients with FAP in Arao confirmed the finding of Tawara et al. [14] that
this protein has valine-methionine replacement at residue 30 in prealbumin,
and, moreover, suggested that FAP in Arao might result from a single mutation. The existence of the relatively rare variants, Gc*1A2 and PGM1*7 in
3 of 7 families suggested the possibility that the FAP mutation might have
occurred once and subsequently spread to 7 families.

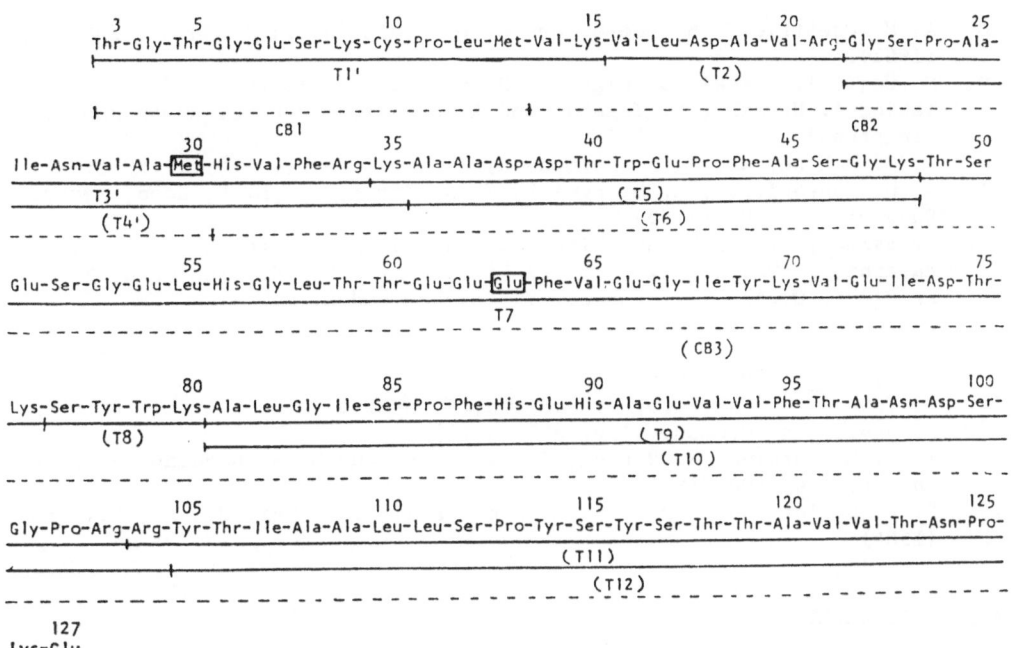

Fig. 2. Amino acid sequence of the P3 predominant protein (4 cases). The sequence shown herein was derived by sequence analysis of T1', T3', and T7, and by comparison of the tryptic peptides with those of human prealbumin of known primary sequence [13]. Peptides, of which the sequences were assumed to be identical to those of pre- albumin, are shown in parentheses. Met and Glu (residues 30 and 63), which differ from Val and Gln in human prealbumin, are en- closed. The human prealbumin numbering system is used [13].

Recently it has been demonstrated that the structure of the amyloid fibril protein in three large FAP foci, i.e., Portugal [15], Sweden [16], and Japan is identified as a prealbumin variant which has the Val-Met re- placement at residue 30. Although phenotypes peculiar to Caucasian were not found in this study, extended analysis of genetic markers in blood might elucidate whether the FAP mutation occurred independently in each focus.

REFERENCES

1. C. Andrade, M. Canijo, D. Klein, and A. Kaelin, Humangenetik, 7, 163 (1969).
2. R. Andersson, Acta Med. Scand. Suppl., 590, 1 (1976).
3. S. Araki, S. Mawatari, M. Ohta, A. Nakajima, and Y. Kuroiwa, Arch. Neurol., 18, 593 (1968); S. Kito, N. Fujimoti, M. Yamamoto, E. Itoga, Y. Toyoizumi, T. Kakizaki, Z. Mitsui, H. Ichikawa, T. Morinaga, K. Wakatsuki, S. Satoh, and I. Iwasaki, Nippon Rinsho, 31, 2326 (1973).
4. C. Andrade, S. Araki, W. D. Block, A. S. Cohen, C. E. Jackson, Y. Kuroiwa, V. A. Mckusick, J. Nissim, E. Sohar, and M. W. Van Allen, Arthr. Rheum., 13, 902 (1970).
5. S. Sakoda, T. Suzuki, S. Higa, M. Ueji, S. Kishimoto, A. Hayashi, N. Yasuda, T. Takaba, and A. Nakajima, Clin. Genet., 24, 334 (1983).
6. M. Pras, M. Shubert, D. Zucker-Franklin, A. Rimon, and E. C. Franklin, J. Clin. Invest., 47, 924 (1968).
7. G. G. Glenner, M. Harada, and C. Isersky, Prep. Biochem., 2, 39 (1972).

8. A. M. Crestfield, S. Moore, and W. H. Stein, J. Biol. Chem., 238, 622 (1963).

9. M. Ueji, T. Suzuki, S. Higa, S. Sakoda, S. Kishimoto, K. Titani, K. Takio, A. Hayashi, Y. Takaba, and A. Nakajima, Jpn. J. Human Jenet. (in press).

10. W. C. Mahoney and M. A. Hermodson, J. Biol. Chem., 255, 11199 (1980).

11. M. W. Hunkapiller, R. M. Hewick, W. J. Dryer, and L. E. Hood, Methods Enzymol., 91, 399 (1983).

12. S. Sakoda, T. Suzuki, S. Higa, M. Ueji, S. Kishimoto, Y. Wada, A. Hayashi, H. Matsumoto, T. Miyazaki, T. Sasazuki, K. Nishimura, M. Egami, K. Omoto, K. Tokunaga, Y. Takaba, and A. Nakajima, Jpn. J. Human Genet., 29, 51 (1984).

13. Y. Kanda, D. S. Goodman, R. E. Canfield, and F. J. Morgan, J. Biol. Chem., 249, 6796 (1974).

14. S. Tawara, M. Nakazato, K. Kanzawa, H. Matsuo, and S. Araki, Biochem. Biophys. Res. Commun., 116, 880 (1983).

15. M. J. M. Saraiva, S. Birken, P. P. Costa, and D. S. Goodman, J. Clin. Invest., 74, 104 (1984).

16. F. E. Dwulet and M. D. Benson, Pro. Natl. Acad. Sci. U.S.A., 81, 694 (1984).

ACKNOWLEDGEMENT

We thank Dr. Y. Wada, Dr. K. Nishimura, Miss T. Miyazaki, Miss M. Egami, Mr. K. Tokunaga, Dr. T. Tsuru, Dr. K. Shida, and Mr. H. Kido for their cooperation, and thank Dr. K. A. Walsh for this encouragement and valuable discussions, and thank Mr. R. D. Wade and Mrs. S. Kumar for their skillful technical assistance. Thanks are due to Prof. J. Miller, University of British Columbia, for looking over the manuscript. This work was supported by grants for Specific Diseases and for Monitoring Study of Congenital Disorders from the Ministry of Health and Welfare, Japan, and by grants from the National Institute of Health (GN 15731).

FAMILIAL AMYLOIDOTIC POLYNEUROPATHY TYPE I AND TYPE II: CHARACTERIZATION OF TWO DISTINCT GENETIC DEFECTS AND IDENTIFICATION OF CARRIERS OF EACH GENE

Merrill D. Benson and Francis E. Dwulet

Indiana University School of Medicine
Richard L. Roudenbush Veterans
Administration Medical Center
Indianapolis, Indiana

ABSTRACT

Familial amyloidotic polyneuropathy (FAP) Type I and FAP Type II have previously been classified on the basis of clinical presentation. Amyloid fibrils have been isolated from the tissues of patients with FAP Type I (Swedish) and FAP Tyep II (Indiana-Swiss) and the subunit protein of each type of amyloid structurally characterized as a variant of prealbumin. The FAP Type I prealbumin has a methionine for valine amino acid substitution at position 30 of the 127 residue molecule. FAP Tyep II subunit has a glycine for threonine substitution at position 49 as has been reported previously for amyloid from a Jewish patient in Israel. Carriers of the FAP Type I genetic defect have been identified by cleavage of their plasma prealbumin with cyanogen bromide. This generates two extra peptides because CNBr cleaves the variant prealbumin at both methionine residues. This difference from normal is readily seen by HPLC analysis of the cleaved prealbumins. Carriers of FAP Type II prealbumin have been shown to have significantly depressed plasma retinol binding protein concentrations. These two separate methods allow identification of carriers of the aberrant prealbumin genes before expression of the disease and may be useful in genetic counseling.

INTRODUCTION

A number of kindreds from around the world have been described with familial amyloidotic polyneuropathy (FAP) [1]. In all cases where amyloid tissue deposits from patients with FAP have been chemically characterized the amyloid has been found to contain prealbumin. This is true for the Portuguese, Japanese, and Swedish-American kindreds with this disease [2, 3, 4, 5]. We have previously described a prealbumin variant which was isolated from amyloid fibrils and plasma of patients with hereditary amyloidosis of Swedish origin [6, 7]. This variant has a single amino acid change, a methionine for valine at position 30 from the amino terminus. Similar findings have now been reported for the subunit protein of hereditary amyloid in Japan and also for hereditary amyloid in Portugal [2, 3]. The only other structural abnormality of prealbumin that has been confirmed in hereditary amyloidosis is the finding of a glycine for threonine interchange at position 40 of the prealbumin subunit protein isolated from a patient with hereditary amyloidosis in Israel [8].

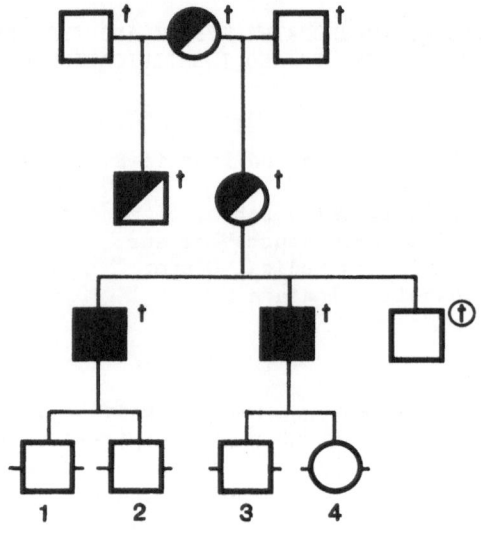

KEY

■ Affected

◐ Presumed Affected

† Deceased

-□- Before Usual Age of Onset

① Died Before Usual Age of Onset

Fig. 1.   Abbreviated Swedish kindred
          to show four children ages
          22-32 without clinical
          disease.

Clinically the hereditary amyloidoses have been classified by the clinical presentation of the neuropathy and associated organ system involvement [1]. FAP Type I is associated with initial lower extremity sensorimotor neuropathy progressing to symmetrical polyneuropathy. Impotence and bowel dysfunction are common. Death is often from renal insufficiency. Kindreds in Portugal, Japan and the United States have been described. FAP Type II usually presents with a compressive neuropathy of the wrist giving the carpal tunnel syndrome and only later is associated with symmetrical polyneuropathy. Vitreous opacities from amyloid deposits are common. Death frequently is due to restrictive cardiomyopathy. Kindreds in Indiana and Maryland that are of German or German-Swiss origins have been described with this syndrome. FAP Type III is associated with symmetrical peripheral neuropathy with prominent renal involvement giving the nephrotic syndrome. FAP Type IV is the designation given to those familial amyloids with cranial involvement.

Our studies have centered on describing the structural abnormalities of prealbumin which are associated with FAP Type I and Type II. We have used different chemical methods to identify the carriers of the variant prealbumin genes.

MATERIALS AND METHOD

Subjects

Four offspring from 2 patients with FAP Type I of Swedish variety were studied (Fig. 1). We originally described this kindred in 1975 and subsequently have shown the variant prealbumin with methionine for valine at position 30 in amyloid fibril deposits of 2 patients who died with this disease.

Serum samples from 68 members of the Indiana kindred with FAP Type II originally described by Rukavina et al. in 1956 were studied (Fig. 2). These sera included 9 members who have proven systemic amyloid, 21 children of these 9 amyloid patients, 6 siblings of the amyloid patients, and 32 other nonaffected kin. Amyloid fibrils were isolated from cardiac tissue of one member of this kindred who died with restrictive cardiomyopathy.

Amyloid Subunit Protein Isolation

Amyloid fibrils were isolated as described previously. Isolated fibrils were reduced and alkylated and the solubilized proteins fractionated by size exclusion chromatography. Structural analysis was done by amino acid sequencing of tryptic digests of subunit proteins.

Prealbumin Isolation

Prealbumin was isolated from plasma by a combination of ion exchange, affinity chromatography and size exclusion chromatography. Cyanogen bromide cleavage of prealbumin was accomplished by dissolving 3 mg of prealbumin in 1 ml of deoxygenated 70% formic acid. An equal weight of cyanogen bromide was added and the mixture allowed to stir at room temperature in the dark for 24 h. Samples were diluted with distilled water and lyophil-

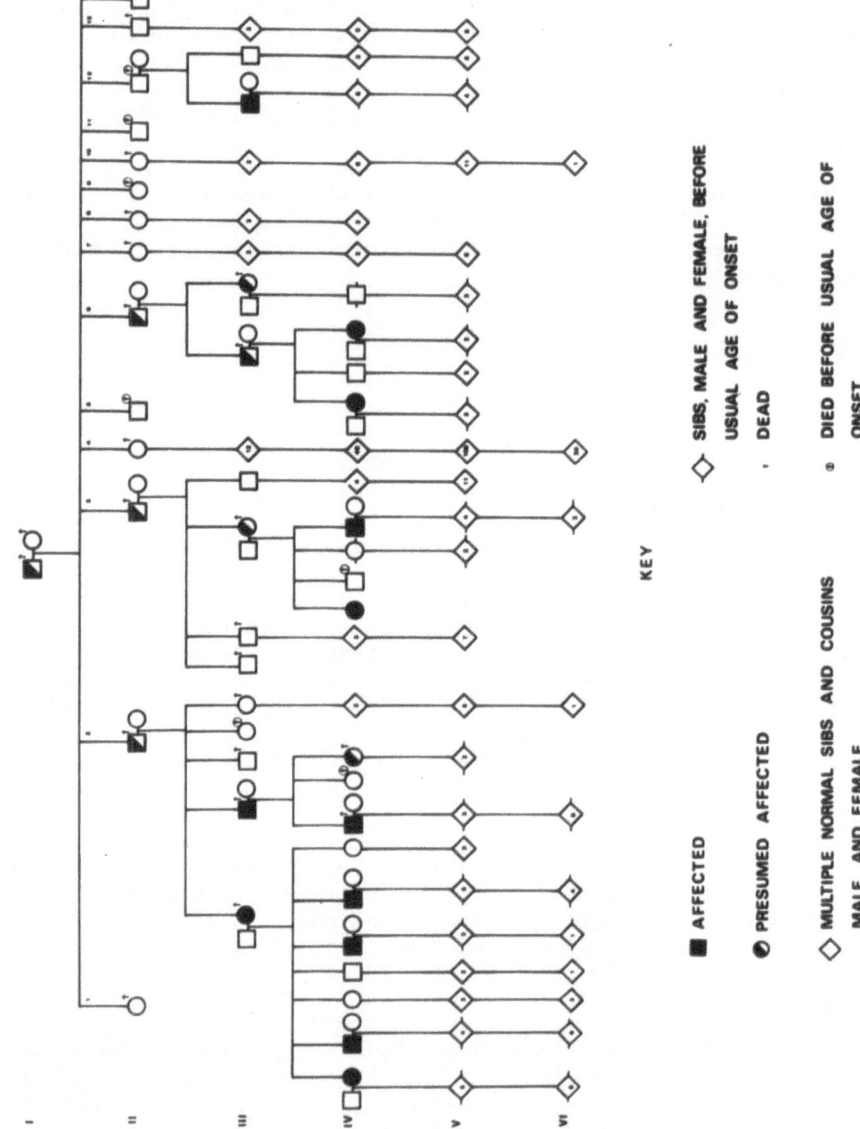

KEY

AFFECTED

PRESUMED AFFECTED

MULTIPLE NORMAL SIBS AND COUSINS
MALE AND FEMALE

SIBS, MALE AND FEMALE, BEFORE
USUAL AGE OF ONSET

DEAD

DIED BEFORE USUAL AGE OF
ONSET

Fig. 2. Indiana–Swiss kindred with FAP Type II.

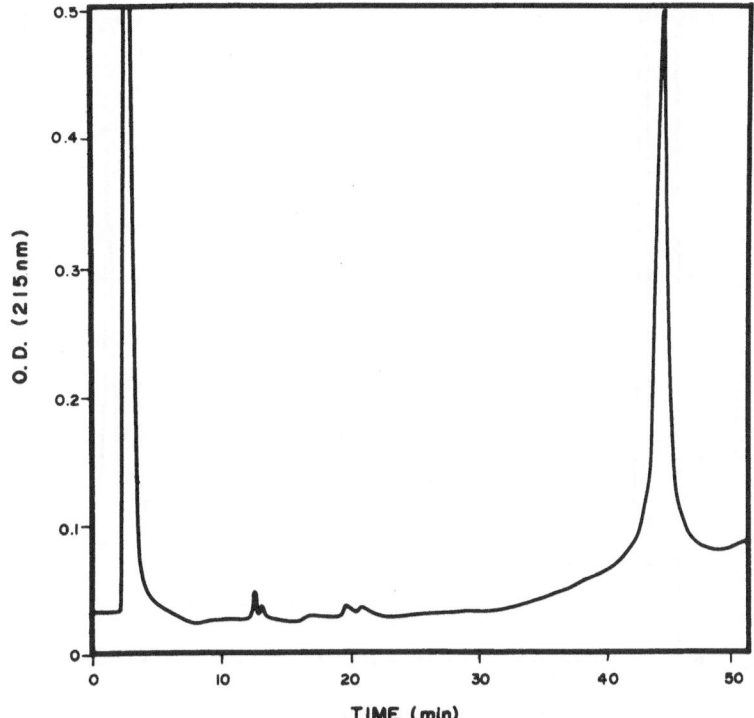

Fig. 3. HPLC separation of CNBr peptides of normal prealbumin on a reverse phase C-18 column. Peptide
1-13 elutes at 12 min. Peptide 14-127 elutes at
44 min.

ized. Cleaved peptides were fractionated by HPLC on a Synchrom RPP column
using a gradient of 2-propanol.

Amino Acid Sequence

Sequence analyses were carried out on a Beckman 890C automatic se-
quentor. For peptides, 3 mg of polybrene was added with each sample. All
samples were converted to the phenylthiohydantoin derivative by heating at
80°C in 1M HCl for 10 min and the phenylthiohydantoin amino acids were
identified by chromatography on a Waters gradient HPLC system.

Concentrations of prealbumin and retinol binding protein were determined
by radial immunodiffusion using assay plates from Calbiochem-Behring (La
Jolla, California). Means ± standard errors of the means were determined
for prealbumin and retinol binding protein levels in all groups. Analysis
of variance and multiple contrasts were used to compare groups.

RESULTS

Isolation of plasma prealbumin from 4 children of 2 brothers who died
with FAP Type I yielded between 8 and 13 mg per 100 ml of plasma. This
yield was 35-50% of theoretical. Separation of cyanogen bromide peptides
of the isolated prealbumin preparations gave two patterns. The first pattern was seen with normal prealbumin from an individual without amyloidosis
and 2 of the offspring of FAP Type I patients. This pattern showed two

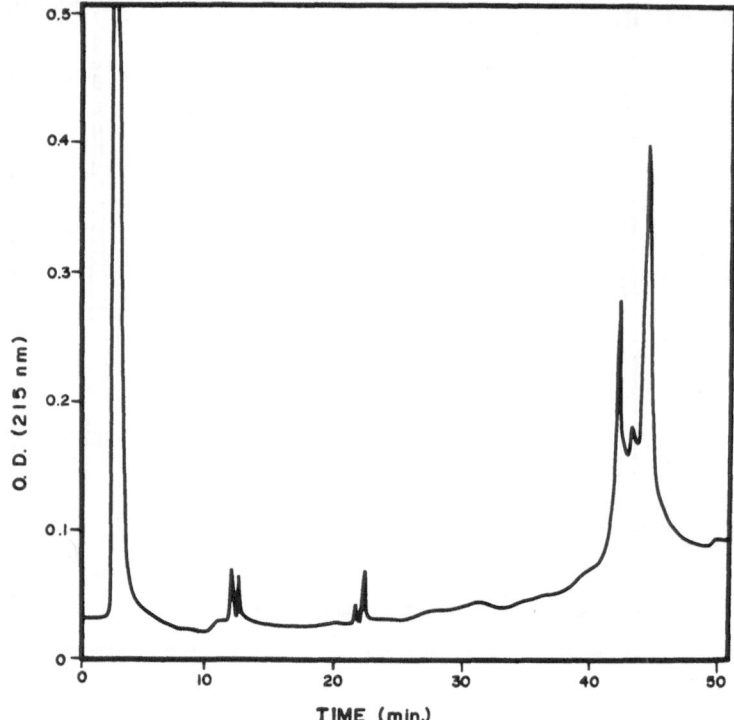

Fig. 4.　HPLC separation of CNBr peptides of prealbumin
from individuals who are carriers of the variant
prealbumin gene.　Peptide 14-30 elutes at 22 min.
Peptide 31-127 elutes at 42 min.

major peaks (Fig. 3).　A second pattern was seen for the cyanogen bromide
cleaved prealbumin of the 2 other offspring of FAP Type I patients (Fig.
4).　This pattern showed 4 peptides and was consistent with the prealbumin
being a mixture of normal prealbumin and the variant prealbumin which had
2 methionines.　Amino terminal sequence analysis of these 4 peaks revealed
that CBI was the amino terminal peptide.　CB2 is the peptide representing
positions 14-127, CBV1 represents 14-30 of the aberrant prealbumin protein.
CBV2 is the variant peptide from position 30-127.

Chromatography of FAP Type II amyloid fibrils which had been reduced
and alkylated on CL6B gave several retarded peaks (Fig. 5).　The smallest
molecular weight peak was shown to be homogeneous by SDS-PAGE and had a
molecular mass of approximately 14,000 daltons.　This protein did not react
with commercial antihuman prealbumin and when subjected to sequence analysis gave no amino acid sequence.　This was interpreted as being consistent
with a blocked amino terminus.　Cleavage of this protein with cyanogen
bromide gave 2 peptides.　The smaller peptide was blocked and therefore
assumed to be the amino terminal peptide, the second peptide gave a normal
prealbumin sequence starting with position 14.　Separation analysis of each
isolated tryptic peptide was completely homologous to the tryptic peptides
of normal plasma prealbumin except for one peak.　This peptide was homologous with the normal prealbumin sequence from position 49-70 except that
the amino terminus showed both threonine and glycine.

Serum prealbumin concentrations in patients with the Indiana kindred
with FAP Type II are seen in Fig. 7.　The concentrations for patients with

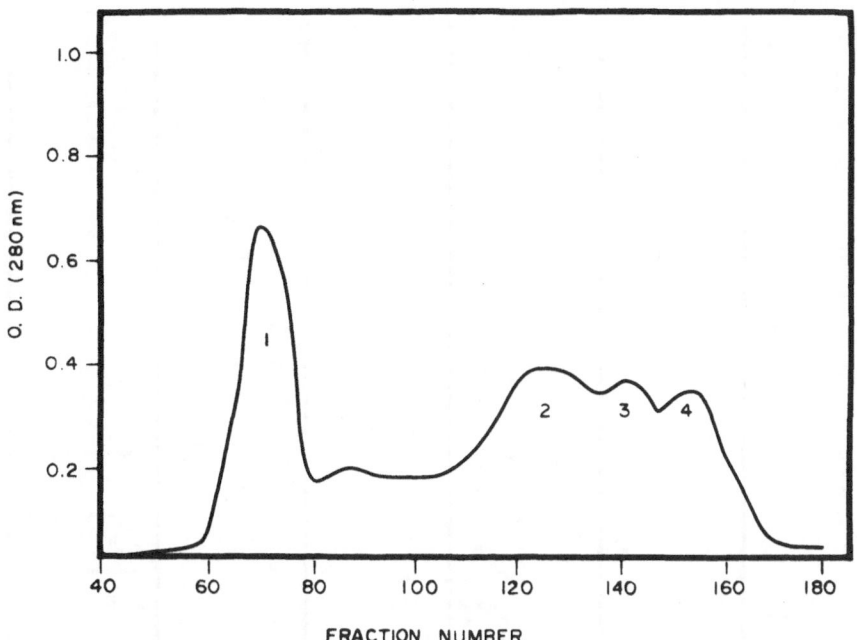

Fig. 5. Separation of FAP Type II amyloid on CL6B. Peak 4 has a molecular weight of approximately 14,000.

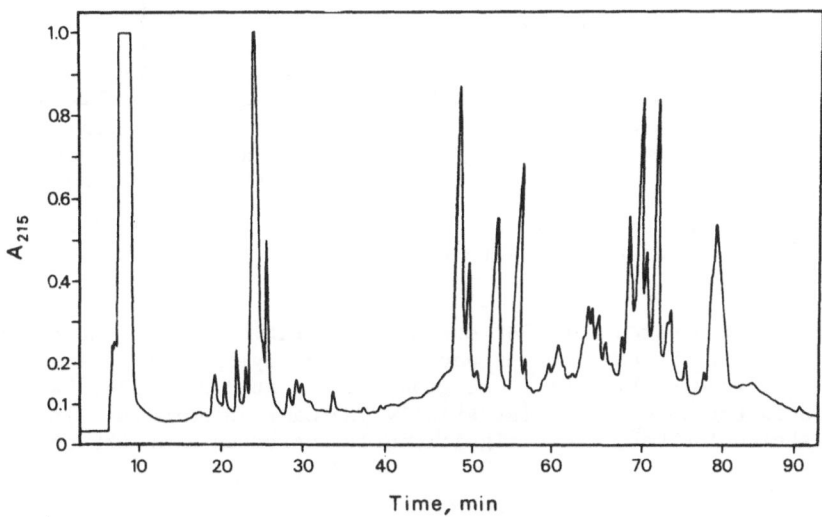

Fig. 6. Separation of tryptic peptides of peak 4 material on HPLC. The peak at 80 min was shown to have both threonine and glycine residues at the amino terminus.

amyloidosis was significantly lower than normal (p < .001). The mean pre-albumin concentration for the children of patients with clinical amyloidosis was not significnatly lower than normal. Serum retinol binding protein levels for the amyloidosis patients was significantly lower than normals (p < .001) (Fig. 8). In addition, the children of amyloid patients had a

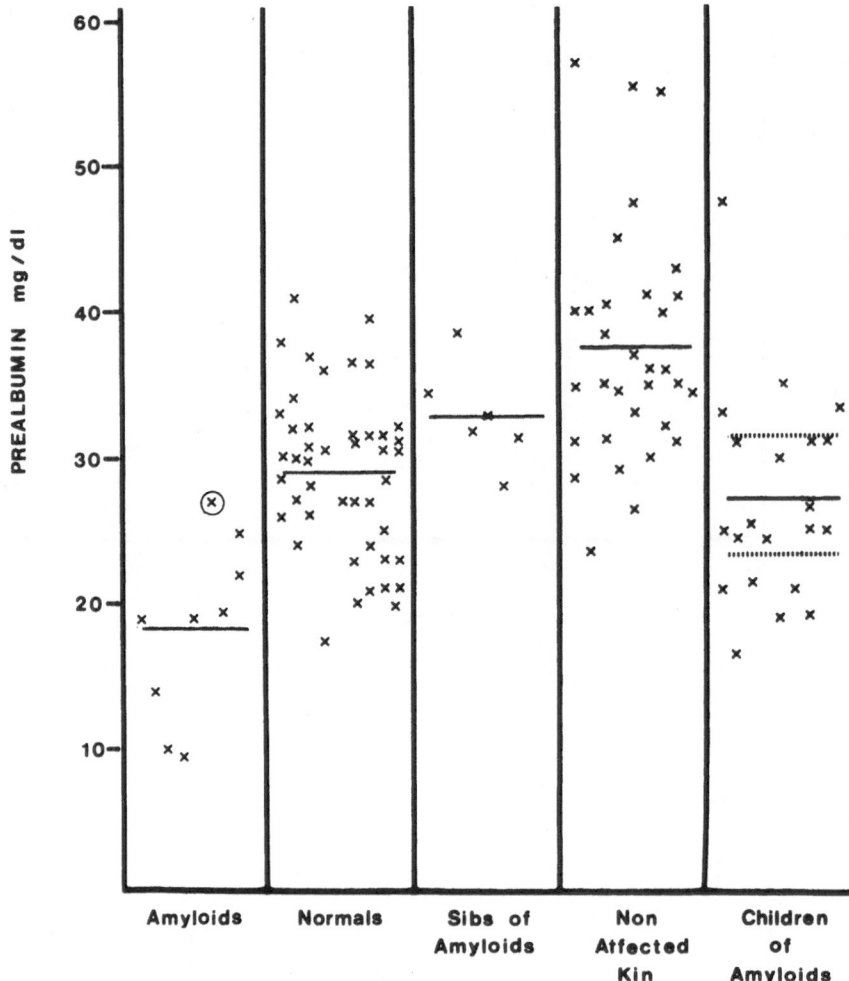

Fig. 7. Serum prealbumin concentrations in individuals from the
         Indiana kindred with FAP Type II.

significantly depressed mean RBP serum concentration. More interestingly
the RBP data for the children of patients with amyloidosis separated into
two distinct groups (Fig. 9). One group, designated high RBP, had a mean
serum concentration wich was essentially the same as normals. The second
group, labeled low RBP, had a significantly depressed mean RBP concentration.

DISCUSSION

     We have now been able to identify distinct structural abnormalities
in plasma prealbumin which are associated with both FAP Type I and FAP Type
II. In FAP Type I there is a methionine for valine interchange at position
30 of the prealbumin molecule. This is present in the circulating prealbumin and is found in the amyloid fibrils along with normal prealbumin.
The simplest explanation of these findings is that there is one gene for
plasma prealbumin and that the patients with FAP Type I are heterozygous,
having a variant prealbumin allele that codes for a methionine instead of
a valine at position 30. This represents a one base change.

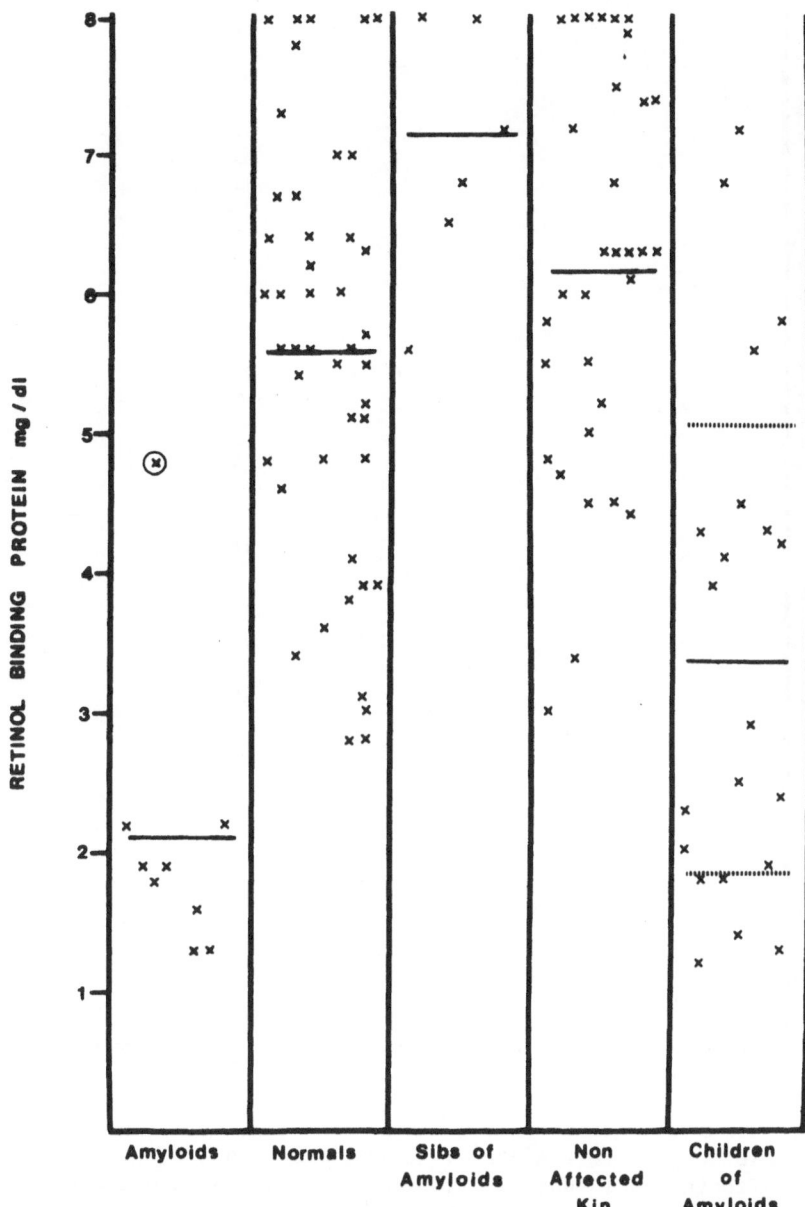

Fig. 8. Serum RBP concentrations in the same individuals as in Fig. 7.

In FAP Type II (Indiana-Swiss) the structural variation in prealbumin is a glycine for threonine substitution at position 49 from the amino terminus. This also represents a one base change in the gene coding for prealbumin. This amino acid substitution has been previously described by Pras et al. in a Jewish patient of European extraction. It should appear that this genetic abnormality is shared by other ethnic groups.

Of prime interest is the ability to identify carriers of the variant prealbumin genes before the onset of the clinical syndrome of FAP. Both

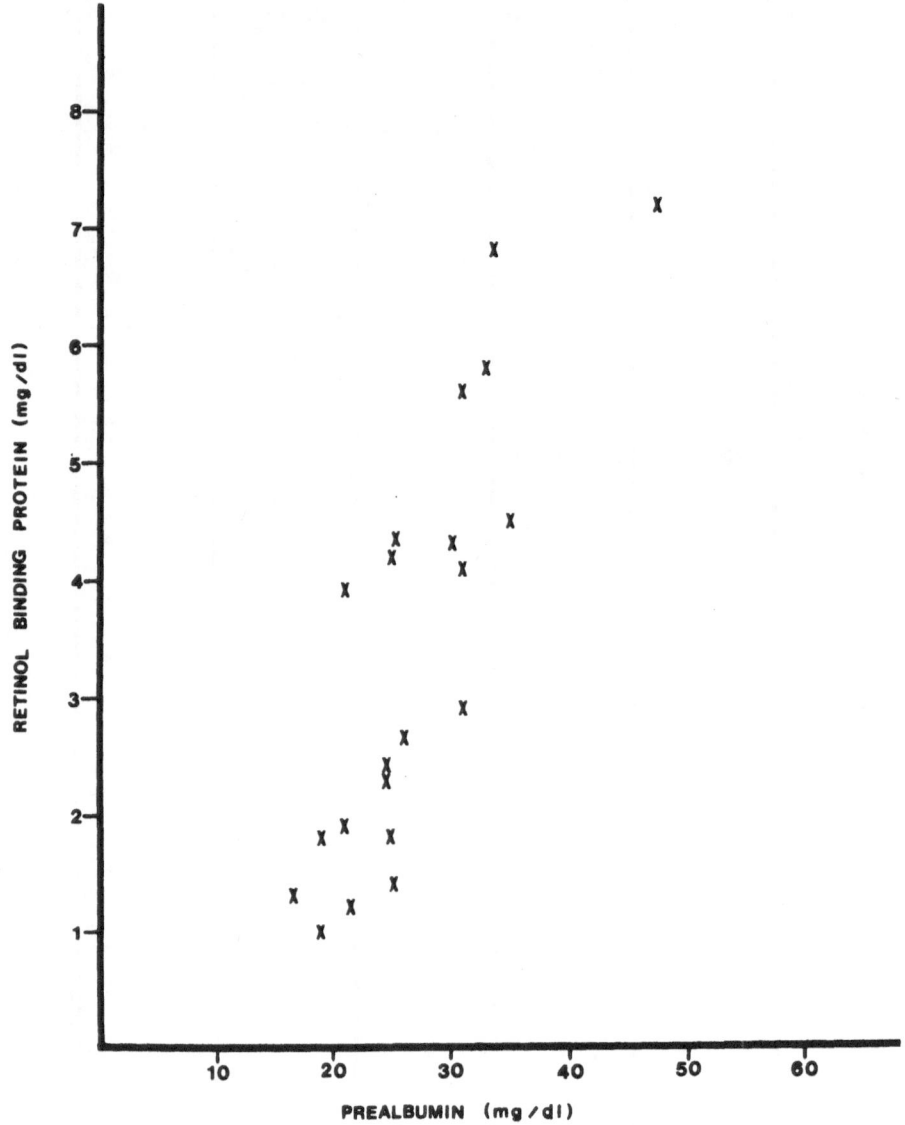

Fig. 9. Plot of PRE versus RBP serum concentrations for children of
affected individuals. Obvious segregation into two groups is
seen.

the Swedish patients with FAP Type I and the Indiana-Swiss patients with
FAP Type II tend to develop neuropathy after they have had their children
and, therefore, have passed the variant prealbumin gene onto one-half of
their children. While DNA analysis would obviously give the most versa-
tility in screening patients for these aberrant genes, we do have methodologies to identify carriers of the Type I and Type II genes prior to child-
bearing years.

The FAP Type I carriers are easily identified by subjecting their
plasma prealbumin to cyanogen bromide cleavage. Normal plasma prealbumin
gives 2 peptides because the molecule contains only one methionine and
cyanogen bromide cleaves only at methionines. Carriers of the aberrant

Type I gene have a mixture of normal and variant prealbumin in their plasma. Cyanogen bromide cleavage of this prealbumin mixture results in 4 peptides. These differences are easily determined by HPLC on a reverse phase C-18 column. We have done mixing experiments and shown that the sensitivity of this method is at a level where as little as 1% variant prealbumin can be detected. Recently a radioimmunoassay using polyclonal antiserum that identifies the cyanogen bromide cleaved aberrant peptide has been described [9]. This affords a second method of identifying the carriers of the FAP Type I gene.

We have not yet identified the variant prealbumin for FAP Type II in circulating plasma. The fact that both normal and variant prealbumin are found in the amyloid fibril subunit protein, however, indicates that FAP Type II amyloid fibril formation is analogous to FAP Type I fibril formation. Therefore, we would expect to find the aberrant prealbumin in the plasma when we have had the opportunity to search for it. Pras et al. did not report analysis of plasma prealbumin from the Jewish patient that they reported [8]. The chemical analysis for the variant prealbumin with the glycine for threonine interchange is not as easily accomplished as the cyanogen bromide cleavage of the FAP Type I prealbumin. Chemical analysis of the FAP Type II prealbumin requires tryptic digestion, and the plasma prealbumin is relatively resistant to proteolysis. Even so, under proper denaturing conditions such as we have used for the fibril subunit protein, the protein is cleaved between position 48 and 49 and identification of the aberrant peptide requires only amino terminal determination of the isolated peptide. Alternatively determination of serum RBP levels promises to be a quick method to screen for carriers of the abnormal prealbumin gene [10]. In the future it should be possible to develop antisera which will identify this amino acid substitution, since as with the methionine for valine interchange in FAP Type I prealbumin, the glycine for threonine is in a position where the surface of the undenatured molecule would be distorted. Indeed the valine at position 30 and the threonine at position 49, while on different beta strands, are adjacent to each other in the x-ray crystallographic pattern.

In conclusion we have described the structural abnormalities associated with both FAP Type I of Swedish origin and FAP Type II (Indiana-Swiss). Each prealbumin variant can be identified by the proper chemical analysis and these methods can be used to generate data for genetic counseling. In the future, since we know the protein abnormalities, we will be able to define the DNA abnormalities and develop faster more versatile genetic analyses.

ACKNOWLEDGEMENTS

This work was supported by VA Medical Research (MRIS 583-0888), and grants from RR-00750 (GCRC), United States Public Health Service, National Institute of Arthritis, Metabolism and Digestive Diseases (AM 20582 and AM 7448), The Arthritis Foundation, and The Grace M. Showalter Foundation.

REFERENCES

1. Andrade, C., Araki, S., Block, W. D., Cohen, A. S., Jackson, C. E., Kuroiwa, Y., McKusick, V. A. Nissim, J., Sohar, E., and Van Allen, M. W., Arthritis Rheum. 13:902-915, 1970.
2. Saraiva, M. J. M., Birken, S., Costa, P. P., and Goodman, D. S., J. Clin. Invest. 74:104-119, 1984.
3. Tawara, S., Nakazato, M., Kangawa, K., Matsuo, H., and Araki, S., Biochem. Biophys. Res. Commun. 116:880-888, 1983.

4. Benson, M. D., J. Clin. Invest. 67:1035–1041, 1981.
5. Skinner, M. and Cohen, A. S., Biochem. Biophys. Res. Commun. 99:1326–1332, 1981.
6. Dwulet, F. E. and Benson, M. D., Biochem. Biophys. Res. Commun. 114:657–662, 1983.
7. Dwulet, F. E. and Benson, M. D., Proc. Natl. Acad. Sci. USA 81:694–698, 1984.
8. Pras, M., Prelli, F., Franklin, E. C., and Frangione, B., Proc. Natl. Acad. Sci. USA 80:539–542, 1983.
9. Nakazato, M., Kangawa, K., Minamino, N., Tawara, S., Matsuo, H., and Araki, S., Biochem. Biophys. Res. Commun. 122:719–725, 1984.
10. Benson, M. D. and Dwulet, F. E., Arthritis Rheum. 26:1493–1498, 1983.

FAMILIAL AMYLOIDOTIC POLYNEUROPATHY TYPE I: CHARACTERIZATION OF THE
PREALBUMIN AMYLOID SUBUNIT AND PRECURSOR PROTEIN

Merrill D. Benson and Francis E. Dwulet

Indiana University School of Medicine and
Richard L. Roudbush Veterans Administration Medical Center
Indianapolis, Indiana

ABSTRACT

The prealbumin amyloid subunit protein from individuals with hereditary
amyloid of Swedish origin has been isolated and characterized by amino acid
sequencing of the entire molecule. Comparison with normal prealbumin peptides showed that an amino acid substitution of methionine for valine had
occurred at position 30. This variant prealbumin was also found in the
plasma of patients with FAP Type I where it accounted for approximately
one-third of the circulating prealbumin. In the amyloid fibril the variant
prealbumin represented approximately two-thirds of the subunit protein with
the other one-third being normal prealbumin. From this structural information and the known three dimensional structure of prealbumin a mechanism
for amyloid formation is proposed. It involves formation of the amyloid
fibrils by aggregation of prealbumin dimers or tetramers. Each dimer must
contain at least one variant peptide chain while the tetramer must contain
at least two abnormal chains. Either of these models could explain the observed amount of normal prealbumin in amyloid fibrils. No proteolytic
processing of this molecule is required because the entire undegraded prealbumin molecule is found in the fibrils.

INTRODUCTION

In 1977 we first described an American family of Swedish origin with
autosomal dominant hereditary amyloidosis which presented as a familial amyloidotic polyneuropathy Type I [1]. This kindred had three generations
afflicted with FAP Type I since the original family immigrated to the United
States from Sweden. The disease is characterized by symmetrical ascending
polyneuropathy. Death is usually from renal failure, although significant
cardiac amyloid has also been noted. One individual in this kindred had
the classic scalloped pupil of FAP Type I. Since our last report on this
kindred, another individual has died of renal insufficiency and another has
presented with severe sensorimotor neuropathy at age 37. Affected members
in this kindred usually have presentation of neuropathy in the lower extremities between ages 35 and 45 and most individuals die by age 50. We
have now been able to define the molecular abnormality associated with this
disease and, therefore, can formulate hypotheses on the pathogenetic mechanisms involved in amyloid deposition.

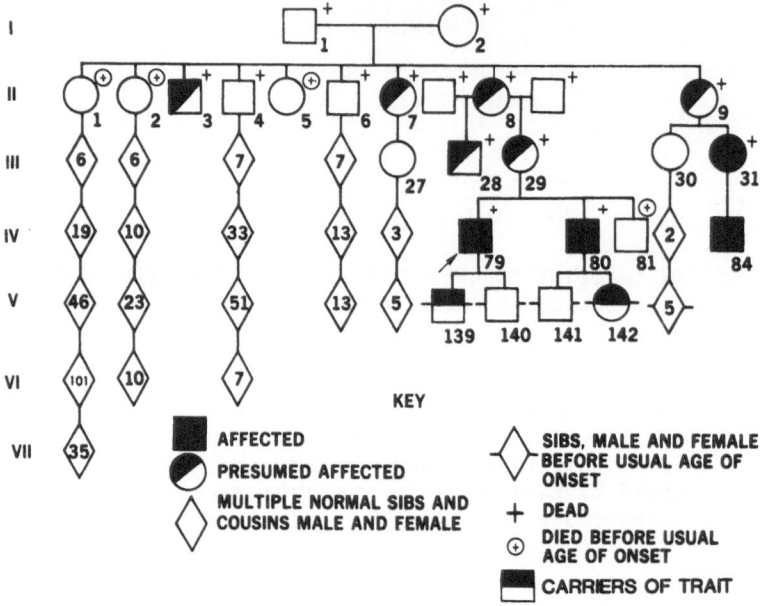

Fig. 1. Updated genealogic tree of Swedish kindred.

MATERIALS AND METHODS

The updated genealogic tree can be seen in Fig. 1. Individuals IV 79 and IV 80 have died and their tissues were made available for these studies. Individual IV 84 whose mother died of systemic amyloidosis is now 39. He has had peripheral neuropathy and bladder dysfunction for approximately 2 years. Individuals V 139, V 140, V 141, and V 142 range in age from 22 to 32 and none has symptoms of FAP.

Isolation of Amyloid Fibril and Plasma Prealbumin Proteins

Amyloid fibrils were isolated from the kidneys of patients IV 79 and IV 80 as previously described [2]. After reduction and alkylation the amyloid subunit protein was isolated by gel filtration on Sephadex G-100. Prealbumin was isolated from plasma as previously described using a combination of ion exchange, affinity, and size exclusion chromatography [3].

Alkylated amyloid subunit protein and plasma prealbumin isolated from patient IV 80 were each suspended in 1.5 ml of water and enough 1 M ammonium hydroxide was added to solubilize the proteins. The solutions were deoxygenated with nitrogen gas and the pH adjusted to pH 8.2 with 0.2 M NH_4HCO_3. The proteins were denatured in a boiling water bath for 5 min and then cooled. Diphenylcarbamoyl chloride-treated trypsin was added to an enzyme substrate ratio of 2:100 (wt/wt) and the mixture was kept at 37° for 8 h. The reaction was terminated by lyophilization. Tryptic peptides were isolated by HPLC on an Ultrasphere C-18 column and impure pools were rechromatographed on an alkylphenyl μ-Bondapak column. The amyloid and plasma prealbumin proteins were also cleaved with cyanogen bromide. Five mg of each protein were dissolved in 1 ml of deoxygenated 70% formic acid to which was added an equal weight of cyanogen bromide. The mixture was kept in the dark at room temperature for 24 h and the reaction terminated by dilution and lyophilization.

Amino Acid Sequencing

Amino acid sequence analysis was carried out on Beckman 890C automatic sequenator using the 0.1 M quadrol program (121078). For peptides, 3 mg of polybrene was added and one cycle in which phenyl isothiocyanate was not added was carried out to remove impurities. The anilinothiazolinone derivatives were converted to the phenylthiohydantoins by heating at 80°C in 1 M HCl for 10 min. The phenylthiohydantoin amino acids were identified on a Waters gradient HPLC system equipped with an Altex Ultrasphere C-18 column. Peaks were identified by their absolute and relative retention times. Amino acid derivatives not clearly identified were reconverted to the free amino acid by hydrolysis at reduced pressure in 5.7 M HCl/0.1% $SnCl_2$ at 150°C for 12 h and identified on a Beckman 119C amino acid analyzer.

RESULTS

The yield of prealbumin from plasma ranged between 35 and 55% of theoretical. The use of Affi-gel Blue in the isolation of plasma prealbumin afforded a means of separating retinol binding protein from the prealbumin under nondenaturing conditions. A final step of sieve chromatography on AcA-34 resulted in pure prealbumin as judged by immunodiffusion and SDS-PAGE. The isolation of amyloid fibrils has been described previously and resulted in a homogeneous subunit protein of molecular mass 14,000 daltons.

Elution profiles of the tryptic digests of the amyloid protein and the plasma prealbumin from normal and amyloid patients can be seen in Fig. 2. The only difference between the profiles was the appearance of a new peak (12B) in the prealbumin from the amyloid subunit protein. Amino acid analysis of these fractions showed that peaks 12 and 12A have the same composition and peak 12B was identical except for the replacement of a methionine for a valine. All of the structure of the prealbumin protein was determined by sequence analysis as can be seen in Fig. 3 except for the blocked amino terminal peptide which was placed by composition analysis. Peptide 12B of both the plasma prealbumin of the amyloid patient and the amyloid subunit fibril protein showed the methionine at position 30.

A number of chymotrypsin-like cleavages were observed and may be the result of the long digestion time that was required for these proteins.

DISCUSSION

There are several significant findings from these studies which help us understand amyloid fibril formation. 1) There is only one amino acid substitution in the variant prealbumin associated with FAP Type I (Swedish). The entire molecule has been sequenced and no other substitutions have been found [2]. This is consistent with the methionine substitution being the determining factor in amyloid formation. 2) The variant prealbumin is present in circulating plasma in an amount of suggest that there is one gene with codominant alleles determining the expression of prealbumin. The affected individuals with amyloidosis are obviously heterozygous because they have both normal and the variant prealbumin. This is entirely consistent with the autosomal dominant nature of FAP Type I. 3) Both variant and normal prealbumin are found in the amyloid fibrils. This is consistent with either the prealbumin dimer or tetramer having one or more variant monomers being the basic building block of the fibril. This is not consistent with the prealbumin tetramer being reduced to monomeric form prior to amyloid fibril formation. If the dimer, which is the more stable unit, is the building block of the fibril, this is consistent with both intra-dimer association and external surface structure being important factors

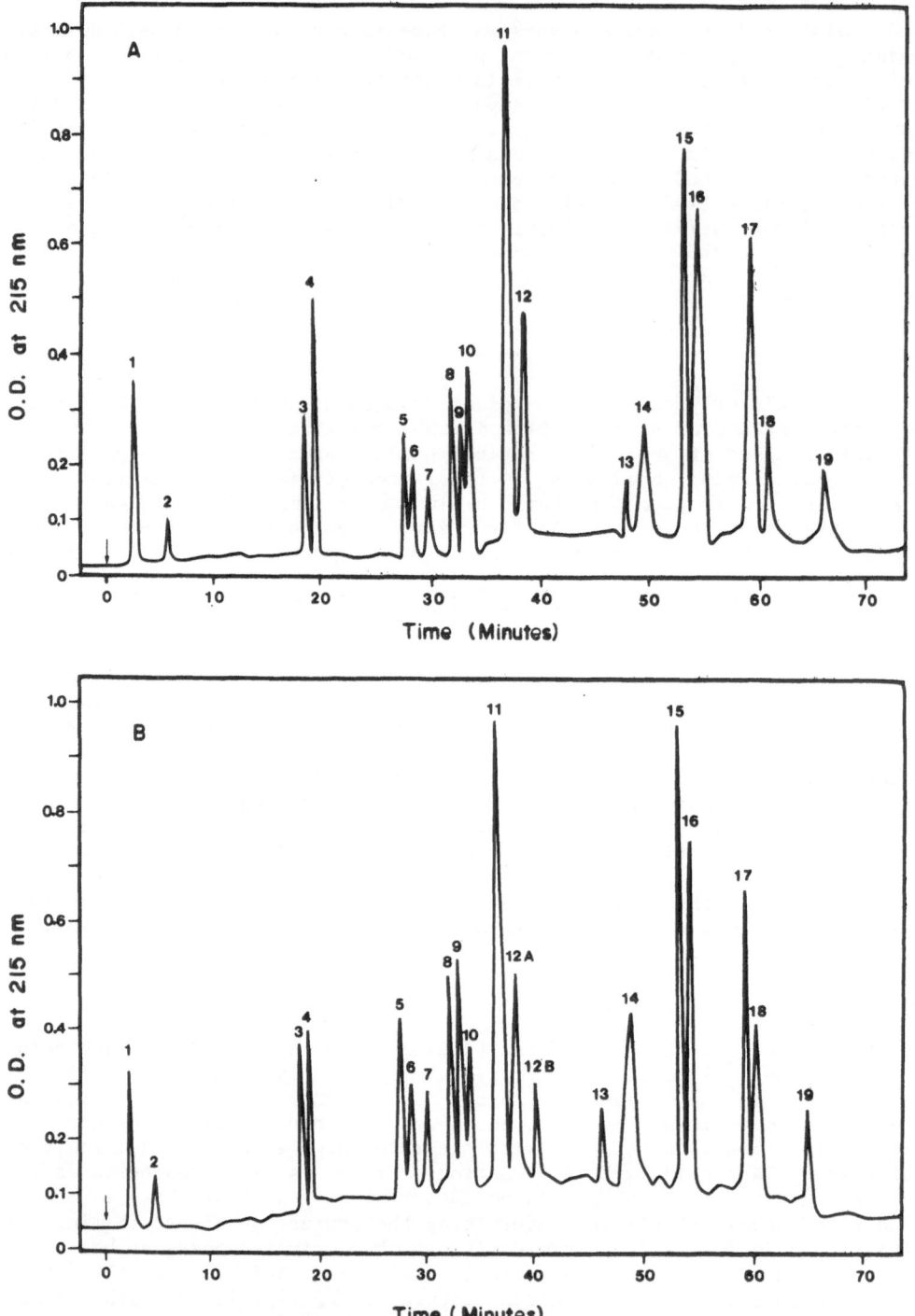

Fig. 2. HPLC separation of tryptic peptides (A) of normal prealbumin, (B) of plasma prealbumin from patient IV 79, and (C) of amyloid sub-unit protein from patient IV 79. Peak 12B is the peptide from 22-31 having Met at position 30. Peak 12A is the normal peptide 22-31 with Val at position 30.

370

in the aggregation that would cause fibril formation. A similar finding may be present in the dimeric Bence-Jones proteins which give immunoglobulin type amyloidosis. 4) While less than 50% of circulating prealbumin is the variant form in the FAP Type I patients, greater than 50% of the fibril subunit protein is represented by the variant. This enrichment of the variant protein in the fibrils is consistent with the prealbumin dimer being the building block of the amyloid fibril. In this model any prealbumin dimer which is made of two normal monomers would be excluded from the fibril. 5) While both the variant and normal prealbumin proteins isolated from the amyloid fibrils have a blocked amino terminus, both of the precursor proteins in the serum have the normal unblocked glycine residue at the amino terminus. This suggests that there is modification perhaps by acetylation of the amino terminus of the proteins at the time of or after incorporation into the amyloid fibrils.

All of the above factors are in agreement with the hypothesis that plasma prealbumin is the reservoir from which the amyloid fibrils form. A single amino acid substitution was also noted by Pras et al., for patient SKO who had hereditary amyloidosis [4]. Those investigators did not show an abnormal prealbumin in the plasma, however, so it is not known at this time whether a situation similar to the FAP Type I Swedish patients exists. Evaluation of the two known amino acid substitutions associated with pre-albumin type amyloidosis namely, the Swedish variety with methionine at position 30 and the amyloid reported for SKO and the FAP Type II (Indiana-Swiss) with glycine at position 49 reveals an interesting pattern. The x-ray crystallographic structure of human prealbumin is well known [5].

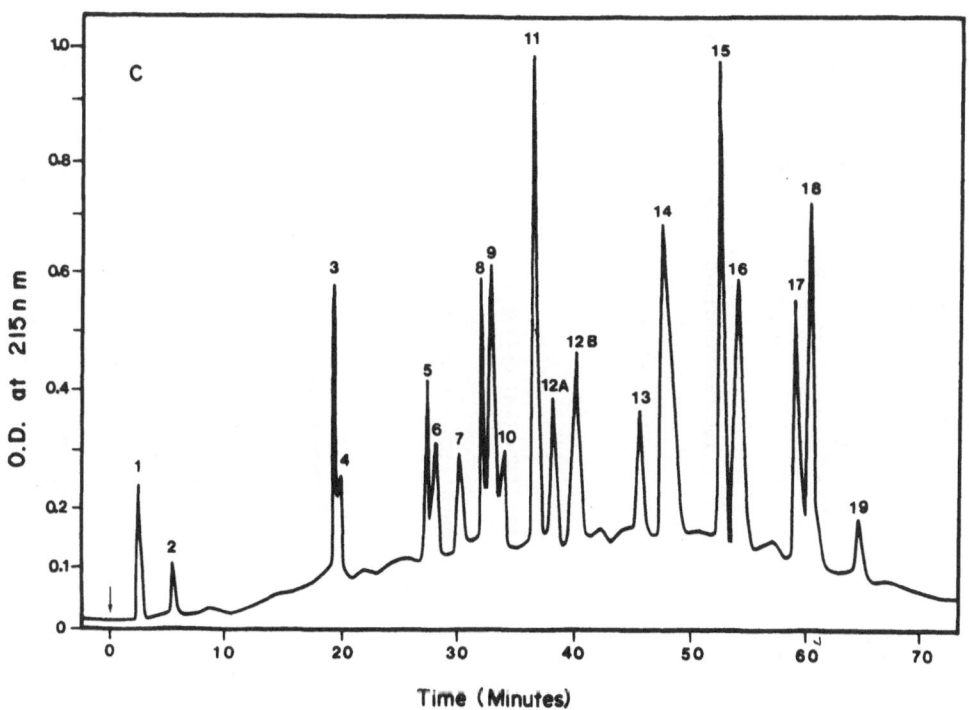

(A) TBPA Sequence

Gly-Pro-Thr-Gly-Glu-Ser-Lys-Cys-Pro-Leu-[Met]-Val-Lys-Val-Leu-Asp-Ala-Val-Arg-Gly-Ser-Pro-Ala-
                    10   20

Ile-Asn-Val-Ala-Val-His-Val-Phe-Arg-Lys-Ala-Ala-Asp-Asp-Thr-Trp-Glu-Pro-Phe-Ala-Ser-Gly-Lys-Thr-Ser-
          30 [Met]   40   50

Glu-Ser-Gly-Glu-Leu-His-Gly-Leu-Thr-Glu-Glu-Glu-Phe-Val-Glu-Gly-Ile-Tyr-Lys-Val-Glu-Ile-Asp-Thr-
                    60   70

Lys-Ser-Tyr-Trp-Lys-Ala-Leu-Gly-Ile-Ser-Pro-Phe-His-Glu-His-Ala-Glu-Val-Val-Phe-Thr-Ala-Asn-Asp-Ser-
                    80   90   100

Gly-Pro-Arg-Arg-Tyr-Thr-Ile-Ala-Ala-Leu-Leu-Ser-Pro-Tyr-Ser-Tyr-Ser-Thr-Thr-Ala-Val-Val-Thr-Asn-Pro-
                    110   120

Lys-Glu

(B) CNBr Peptides of Normal TBPA

CB1   1   Gly-Pro-Thr-Gly —————————— 13

CB2   14   Val-Lys-Val-Leu —————————————————————— 127

CNBr Peptides of Variant TBPA

CB1   1   Gly-Pro-Thr-Gly —————————— 13

CBV1   14   Val-Lys-Val-Leu ———— 30

CBV2   31   His-Val-Phe-Arg —————— 127

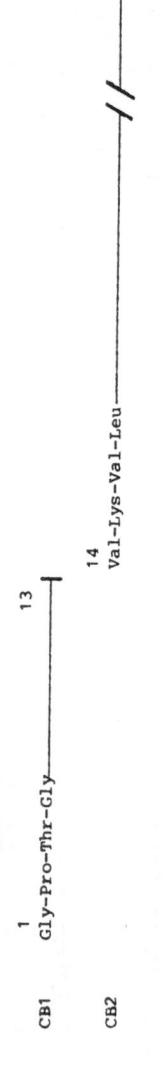
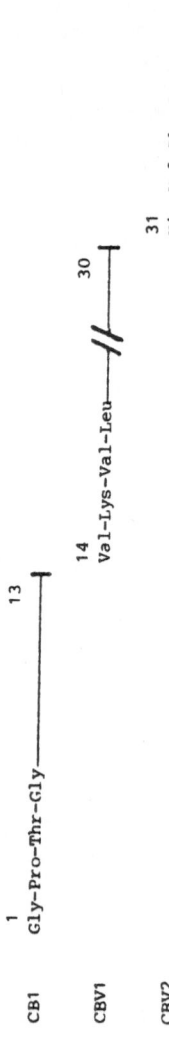

Fig. 3.   A) Amino acid sequence of normal and FAP Type I prealbumin showing the extra methionine at position 30. B) Schematic representation of peptides of FAP Type I prealbumin cleaved with CNBr.

Both the Val-Met interchange at position 30 and the Thr-Gly interchange at position 49 are in close proximity. Position 30 is the second residue on the amino terminus of beta strand B while position 49 is the carboxyl terminal residue of beta strand C. For FAP Type II the change from threonine to glycine would cause a major change in secondary structure. Threonine has a high beta sheet forming potential while glycine has a low one and it is hypothesized that such a change would distort the surface of the prealbumin molecule in this area. For the FAP Type I protein the valine has a high beta forming potential while methionine has a much lower one. Methionine also would occupy a greater volume and thus distort this area of the molecule. If the fibril building block is the stable dimer, the interaction of dimers with distorted surfaces could lead to fibril formation. At this stage it is only an hypothesis but this is an hypothesis that lends itself to being tested.

ACKNOWLEDGEMENTS

This work was supported by Veterans Association Medical Research (MRIS 583-0888), and grants from RR-00750 (GCRC), United States Public Health Service, National Institute of Arthritis, Metabolism and Digestive Diseases (AM 20582 and AM 7448), The Arthritis Foundation, and The Grace M. Showalter Foundation.

REFERENCES

1.   Benson, M. D., and Cohen, A. S., Ann. Intern. Med., 86:419-424 (1977).
2.   Dwulet, F.E., and Benson, M. D., Proc. Natl. Acad. Sci. USA, 81:694-698 (1984).
3.   Dwulet, F. E., and Benson, M. D., Biochem. Biophys. Res. Commun., 114:657-662 (1983).
4.   Pras. M., Prelli, F., Franklin, E. C., and Frangione, B., Proc. Natl. Acad. Sci. USA, 80:539-542 (1983).
5.   Blake, C. C. F., Geisow, M. J., Oatley, S. J., Rerat, B., and Rerat, C., J. Mol. Biol., 121:339-356 (1978).

IMMUNOHISTOCHEMICAL STUDIES ON HEREDITARY AMYLOIDOSIS

OF THE FINNISH TYPE

H. M. Falck and P. Westermark

Fourth Department of Medicine
Helsinki University Central Hospital
Helsinki, Finland

Department of Pathology
University Hospital
Uppsala, Sweden

ABSTRACT

The amyloid fibril protein of the Finnish familial amyloidosis (AF_F) has been only partially characterized, i.e. it is only known to differ from protein AA immunologically and by its amino acid composition. Six tissue specimens from five patients with this disease and five known control tissues were stained by the peroxidase-antiperoxidase (PAP) method using 10 antisera against known fibril proteins and serum prealbumin. These proteins were AP, AA, four ALs, AS_{C1} (prealbumin-related), AF_D (Danish familial cardiomyopathy, prealbumin-related) and gamma trace (related to the fibril protein in Icelandic hereditary cerebral hemorrhage with amyloidosis). The tissues of AF_F strained negatively with all antisera except anti-AP suggesting that the fibril protein of AF_F is none of the proteins known so far.

INTRODUCTION

The Finnish type hereditary amyloidosis (AF_F), first described by Meretoja in 1969 [1], is a systemic form of amyloidosis with a relatively mild course in most cases. Its main clinical signs are corneal lattice dystrophy and cranial neuropathy [2]. So far, the amyloid fibril protein of this amyloidosis has been only partially characterized. The overall amino acid composition of this protein differs from that of protein AA and the protein does not react with anti-AA [3]. Most other forms of familial amyloidosis have been found to be composed of prealbumin-related proteins [4, 5, 6], or, in the case of the Icelandic hereditary cerebral hemorrhage with amyloidosis, of a protein related to gamma trace protein [7]. It has also been possible to identify these proteins in tissue sections by immunohistochemical methods [7, 8, 9]. In this study an attempt was made to identify the amyloid fibril protein of AF_F by the peroxidase- anti-peroxidase (PAP) method.

TABLE 1. Immunohistochemical Staining by the PAP Method of Amyloid in Finnish Familial Amyloidosis (AF_F) and Some Controls

Amyloid Type	Tissue	Autopsy/ Biopsy	Antisera Against									
			AP	AA	AL κI	AL κIII	AL λII	AL λIV	ASC1	AF_D*	pre- alb.	gamma trace†
AF_F	kidney	a	+	-	-	-	-	-	-	-	-	-
AF_F	salivary gland	a	+	-	-	-	-	-	-	-	-	-
AF_F	kidney	b	+	-	-	-	-	-	-	-	-	-
AF_F	kidney	b	+	-	-	-	-	-	-	-	-	-
AF_F	nerve	b	+	-	-	-	-	-	-	-	-	-
AF_F	skeletal muscle	b	+	-	-	-	-	-	-	-	-	-
Controls												
AA	kidney	a	+	+	-	-	-	-	-	-	-	-
AL_{κ}I	kidney	a	+	-	+	±	-	-	-	-	-	-
AL_{κ}III	kidney	a	+	-	-	+	-	-	-	-	-	-
AL_{λ}II	kidney	a	+	-	-	-	+	-	-	-	-	-
AL_{λ}IV	kidney	a	+	-	-	-	-	+	-	-	-	-
AS_{C1}	heart	a	+	-	-	-	-	-	+	±	+	-

*Danish familial cardiomyopathy, prealbumin-related, antiserum provided by G. Husby, Tromsø, Norway.
†Antiserum provided by A. Grubb, Malmö, Sweden.

MATERIALS AND METHODS

The tissue specimens studied were four biopsies from four patients and two autopsy samples from one patient (Table 1). The tissue sections were stained by the PAP method [10] using a variety of antisera covering most known amyloid fibril proteins. These included antisera against the proteins AP, AA, four ALs (κ_I, κ_{III}, λ_{II}, λ_{IV}), AS_{C1} (prealbumin-related), AF_D (Danish familial cardiomyopathy, prealbumin-related), gamma trace (related to the fibril protein in Icelandic hereditary cerebral hemorrhage with amyloidosis), and commercially available anti-prealbumin (DAKO, Copenhagen, Denmark). Known positive controls were used for all antisera except that against gamma trace protein.

RESULTS

The results are summarized in Table 1. All tissue specimens from patients with the Finnish familial amyloidosis stained negatively with all antisera except anti-AP. The control staining showed that the antisera were specific for the same type of amyloid with some cross reactivity between two κ-type amyloids. No reactions were seen when the antisera were replaced by normal rabbit serum.

DISCUSSION

These results suggest that the amyloid fibril protein of Finnish familial amyloidosis is none of the proteins known, so far, to be amyloid proteins of systemic amyloidosis. Interestingly, the protein seems not to be prealbumin-related as it is in most other neuropathic familial amyloidoses. This exclusion is not completely certain but its reliability is increased by the negative results with three different antisera against prealbumin-related proteins. Furthermore, immunohistochemical methods seem to be reliable according to several other studies [8, 9]. The final identification of the protein must await further studies.

ACKNOWLEDGEMENTS

This study was supported by the Swedish Medical Research Council, the research Fund of King Gustaf V and Finska Lakaresällskapet.

REFERENCES

1. J. Meretoja, Ann. Clin. Res., 1, 314 (1969).
2. J. Meretoja, In Amyloidosis, O. Wegelius, A. Pasternack, Eds. (Academic Press, London, 1976).
3. J. Meretoja, T. Holmén, T. Meretoja, R. Penttinen, Med. Biol., 56, 17 (1978).
4. P. P. Costa, A. S. Figueira, F. R. Bravo, Proc. Natl. Acad. Sci. USA, 75, 4499 (1978).
5. M. D. Benson, J. Clin. Invest., 31, 190 (1981).
6. S. Tawara, M. Nakazato, K. Kangawa, H. Matsuo, S. Araki, Biochem. Biophys. Res. Commun., 116, 880 (1983).
7. R. P. Linke, Clin. Neuropathol., 1, 172 (1982).
8. D. H. Cohen, H. Feiner, O. Jensson, B. Frangione, J. Exp. Med., 158, 623 (1982).
9. G. G. Cornwell III, W. L. Murdoch, R. A. Kyle, P. Estermark, P. Pitkänen, Am. J. Med., 75, 618 (1983).
10. L. A. Sternberger, Immunocytochemistry, 2nd ed., (John Wiley & Sons, New York, 1979).

LATE ONSET HEREDITARY AMYLOIDOSIS IN A FAMILY

FROM TEXAS*

Caryn A. Libbey, Alan Rubinow, Tsuranobu Shirahama,
Chad Deal, and Alan S. Cohen

The Thorndike Memorial Laboratory
and Department of Medicine
Boston City Hospital, and

The Arthritis Center
Boston University School of Medicine
Boston, Massachusetts 02118

ABSTRACT

    A new kinship of German-English ancestry with familial amyloid poly-
neuropathy (FAP) is described. Four siblings of a large Texan family have
been studied with what appears to be an autosomal dominant transmission.
The onset is very similar to the Andrade (Portuguese) type I FAP in that
autonomic dysfunction and sensory findings precede motor involvement. This
particular family however is unique in that the age of onset is the seventh
decade in all members affected to date. Renal involvement appears to be
less prominent and has occurred several years after onset of polyneuropathy
symptoms. In contrast to other types of familial amyloid, scalloped pupils
have not been seen. The clinical symptoms of cardiac and gastrointestinal
involvement became manifest more slowly (10 or more years after first neuropathic symptoms) in this elderly onset Texan family. The pattern of disease, however, was similar to that of typical FAP type I. Immunohistochemical staining techniques have shown that the amyloid is prealbumin.
These data indicate characteristics of FAP may be a broader continuum of
disease processes rather than a single definite entity.

    Since Andrade first described familial amyloidosis in Portugal in 1952
[1], several other types of familial amyloidosis have been described [2].
The Portuguese form is manifest as a predominantly sensory peripheral neuropathy with autonomic nervous system involvement. This is transmitted as
an autosomal dominant pattern. The age of onset is usually between 25 and
35 years and generally the course is probresive leading to death in 10 to

---

*This study was supported by grants from U.S. Public Health Service NIAMDD
 (AM-04599 and AM-7014), Multipurpose Arthritis Center, National Institutes
 of Health (AM-20613), the General Clinical Research Centers Branch of the
 Division of Research Resources, National Institutes of Health (RR-533),
 and the Arthritis Foundation.

12 years. Similar clinical patterns have been described in Swedish [3, 4, 5], Japanese [6], and other [7] kindred. Other familial amyloid syndromes have been described with prominent upper extremity neuropathy but without the marked renal and autonomic involvement of the Portugese type patterns [2]. More prolonged survival characterizes these latter types.

We describe here a family of German-English ancestry with familial amyloid polyneuropathy. The affected family members have resembled more clinically the findings in the Andrade (Portuguese) type I with familial amyloid polyneuropathy [8], but this family appears unique in that the age of onset has been in the seventh decade in affected family members. Renal and ocular findings also have not been a prominent part of the disease. Immunocytochemical studies have shown prealbumin in biopsied amyloid tissue.

SUBJECTS

The family is a large one, with 12 siblings in the first generation. Three of the older brothers died of cardiac disease in their fifties. Two sisters were found to have familial amyloid polyneuropathy and were referred to the Thorndike Memorial Laboratory at Boston City Hospital for evaluation. Further investigation revealed amyloidosis in two younger brothers (patients I-9 and I-10).

CASE REPORTS

Patient I-6

This 74 year old woman was in good health until the age of 59 when she noted the recurrence of stress incontinence that persisted despite a Marshal-Marchetti procedure. In 1973, biopsy showed amyloid infiltration of the bladder wall. Fecal incontinence was also noted at this time. Ten years after the onset of sensory and motor symptoms she walked with a wide based gait and required the use of a cane for ambulation. In 1978 she was referred to the Thorndike Clinical Research Center for evaluation.

Physical examination at that time revealed no postural hypotension, no scalloping of the pupils, or no vitreous opacities. Findings on cardiovascular, pulmonary and abdominal examinations were normal. Neurologic evaluation revealed marked motor weakness in her legs, the distal muscles being more severely affected. Deep tendon reflexes (ankles and brachioradialis) were absent and weak reflex responses of the triceps, biceps, and the knees were obtained. Senstations of pin prick and temperature were absent to the knees and the wrists in a stocking-glove distribution. Perception of vibration was decreased in the toes and ankles but the position sense and graphesthesia were normal. Sphincter tone was hypotonic.

Pertinent laboratory data revealed normal liver and kidney function. There was no proteinuria, and immunoelectrophoreses of serum and urine showed no light chains. A 24 h fecal fat excretion was 33.3 grams. Electrocardiography was normal but a 24 h Holter monitor showed frequent multifocal premature ventricular contractions. Echocardiography gave results consistent with a hypertrophic nonobstructive cardiomyopathy and an ejection fraction of 51%.

Nerve conduction velocity studies showed decreased nerve conduction in all extremities, especially in legs, consistent with a diffuse peripheral neuropathy. Amyloid deposition was confirmed in the bladder, skin, and rectal biopsy specimens and in an abdominal fat aspirate [9, 10]. During the following 3 years the patient continued to have steatorrhea and loss of weight. She finally died from acute renal failure after an episode of pyelonephritis. Autopsy was not performed.

Patient I-7

A 71 year old woman, had a very similar clinical presentation. She was in good health until the age of 61 when she noted the vague onset of anorexia, early satiety and slowly progressive weakness and numbness in her legs. Five years later she had a 60 pound weight loss, difficulty digesting her food, nocturnal diarrhea alternating with constipation and urinary urgency and incontinence. Radiologic studies revealed slightly dilated esophagus. Rectal biopsy specimen revealed amyloid.

Physical examination demonstrated a frail cachectic woman with postural hypotension. No scalloping of the pupils or vitreous opacities were seen. The heart, lungs, and the abdominal examination were unremarkable. Neurologic exmination showed decreased pin prick and temperature sensation in the arms and legs reaching to the elbows and groin area respectively. Vibration, light tough, and position sense were impaired but to a lesser extent. Deep tendon reflexes were absent in the legs and decreased in the biceps and the triceps. The patient's gait was unsteady but cerebellar function was normal.

Laboratory investigations revealed normal serum and urine immunoelectrophoreses. Renal and liver functions were normal. Steatorrhea with 11.1 grams of fecal fat per 24 h was present. Nerve conduction velocities were unobtainable along the tibial and peroneal nerves consistent with a long standing peripheral neuropathy. A hypoflexic neurogenic bladder unresponsive to urecholine was also observed. Cardiac evaluation showed a PR interval of 0.24 seconds on electrocardiography. Rectal, skin, and abdominal fat biopsy specimens were found to contain amyloid. Reexamination two years later showed progression of neuropathy with decreased sensation to upper arm and groin. At this time she was able to ambulate only with a walker. She died at the age of 74 with acute renal failure. An autopsy was not performed.

Patient I-9

The brother of the above patients, a 65 year old male was well until the age of 62 when he first noted hoarseness and dysphagia with solid food intake. Shortly afterwards diarrhea 2 or 3 times per week was noted. Endoscopy revealed distal esophagitis and a superficial esophageal biopsy specimen did not show amyloid. A rectal biopsy did show amyloid. Additional problems included impotence, difficulty with urination, anorexia, weight loss and open angle glaucoma.

Physical examination was remarkable for orthostatic changes in blood pressure. No abnormalities were noted in the patient's skin, eye, heart, or abdomen. Tone of the anal sphincter was normal. Neurological examination revealed decreased sensation in the distribution of the fourth lumbar dermatome thought to be consistent with a radiculopathy secondary to lumbar spinal stenosis. There was no evidence for a peripheral neuropathy. Laboratory studies showed normal liver and kidney functions. Immunoelectrophoreses of serum and urine demonstrated no M component or free light chains. Electrocardiography showed a PR interval of 0.20 seconds and a prolonged QT interval of 40 seconds. Premature ventricular contractions and occasional runs of slow ventricular tachycardia was seen on a Holter monitor. Evaluation of the patient's impotence revealed nocturnal penile tumescence and no spontaneous erections. Doppler studies showed a normal penile blood supply and a biopsy showed amyloid in the corpus cavernosum. Skin and abdominal fat specimen showed amyloid.

Patient I-10

A 63 year above patients was well with the exception of occasional episodes of diarrhea. Rectal biopsy showed nonspecific colitis and no amyloid. The patient denied any neurologic symptoms, weight loss, or impotence. An abdominal fat aspirate performed as part of the first family screening contained amyloid.

Physical examination showed no postural hypotension. There was no scalloping of the pupils and vitreous opacities were not observed. Findings on examination of the heart, abdomen, peripheral nerves and skin were normal. Laboratory data showed normal renal and gastrointestinal function. Electromyography and nerve conduction velocities had normal findings. In the year after his initial evaluation, the patient noted the onset of occasional clumsiness and stumbling, dysphagia with solid food intake and easy bruisability of the skin. Reevaluation revealed a mild generalized peripheral neuropathy, abnormal cine-esophagographic result and amyloid in the rectal, abdominal fat and skin biopsy specimens.

Family Studies

At four family gatherings in the past five years, sixty two members at risk from ages 21 to 68, were evaluated for the development of familial amyloid polyneuropathy. A detailed history and physical examination has been performed as well as a biopsy of the abdominal fat aspirate. Other than patient I-10, no other new members have been found to be affected by amyloid polyneuropathy.

Prealbumin Testing

Tissue from the penile biopsy specimen of patient I-9 was formalin-fixed and embedded in paraffin blocks. Sections of tissue were tested by an immunocytochemical technique [11] for the presence of prealbumin.

RESULTS AND COMMENTS

Tissue sections from the penile biopsy stained with Congo red demonstrated the characteristic green birefringence of amyloid when viewed under polarized light. There was prominent uptake of the anti-prealbumin and anti-AF_S anti-serums and a weaker uptake with the anti-AP areas corresponding to amyloid deposition. There was no reaction with anti-AA or control anti-serum.

The onset of clinical disease in the seventh decade in all affected family members is a unique feature in this family. The usual ages at which the symptoms begin are 25 to 35 years in the Portuguese [1] and 25 to 50 in the Swedish and Japanese kinships [4, 7].

Analysis of 46 Portuguese kinships in which affected persons had an age of onset of over 40 years of age, revealed 6 families in which there was a tendency for an earlier age of onset in successive generations [12]. Consequently, we are unable to predict with any certainty that younger unaffected family members in our family will be free of the disease until the seventh decade. We plan, therefore, to obtain abdominal fat specimens at regular intervals in the hope of establishing the diagnosis in its preclinical stages. The annual family reunions of this kindred provide a unique opportunity to closely monitor the entire family.

Other kindreds of German ancestry with heredofamilial amyloidosis have been described. Erbsloh [13] described a German kinship orginating from

382

Portugal with type I familial amyloid polyneuropathy; an additional family was reported on by Delank et al. [14] but there were no older identifiable ancestors. The Rukavina form of amyloid neuropathy (type II familial polyneuropathy) was described in a large Maryland family of German ancestry [15, 16]. In contrast to type I familial amyloid polyneuropathy the onset is later in life, primarily involves the upper limbs and is often associated with the development of vitreous opacities.

Recent biochemical studies have established that prealbumin is the amyloid fibril protein in type I familial amyloid polyneuropathy in families of Portuguese [17], Swedish [18, 19], and Polish-Jewish [20] origin. The demonstration of the prealbumin in the amyloid deposit in patient I-9 suggests that this family has biochemical as well as clinical characteristics consistent with similar kinships with type I familial amyloid polyneuropathy of diverse geographic origin.

REFERENCES

1. C. Andrade, Brain, 75:408 (1952).
2. C. Andrade et al., Arth. Rheum., 13:902 (1970).
3. R. Anderson, Acta Med. Scand., Suppl. 590, 1 (1976).
4. M. D. Benson and A. S. Cohen, Ann. Intern. Med., 86:419 (1977).
5. A. S. Cohen, A. Rubinow, D. Ginter, and F. Wilsonn, in: Amyloid and Amyloidosis (G. G. Glenner, P. P. Costa, and F. Freitas, eds.), Excerpta Medica, Amsterdam (1979), pp. 78-85.
6. S. Araki et al, Arch. Neurol., 18:593 (1968).
7. M. W. Van Allen, J. A. Frolich, and J. R. Davis, Neurology, 19:10 (1969).
8. A. S. Cohen, in: The Metabolic Basis of Inherited Disease (J. B. Stanbury, J. B. Wyngaarden, and D. S. Fredrickson, eds.), McGraw-Hill, New York (1979), pp. 1273-1294.
9. C. A. Libbey, M. Skinner, and A. S. Cohen, Arch. Int. Med., 143:1549 (1983).
10. P. Westermark and B. Stenkvist, Arch. Int. Med., 132:522 (1973).
11. T. Shirahama, M. Skinner, and A. S. Cohen, Histochemistry, 72:161 (1981).
12. A. Bastos Lima and A. Martins da Silva, in: Amyloid and Amyloidosis (G. G. Glenner, P. Costa, and A. Freitas, eds.), Excerpta Medica, Amsterdam (1980), pp. 99-105.
13. F. L. Erbsloh, Mater. Med. Nordmark, 13:157 (1961).
14. H. W. Delank et al., Artzl. Forschung., 19:401 (1965).
15. J. G. Rukavina et al., Medicine, Baltimore, 35:239 (1956).
16. M. Mahloud et al., Medicine, Baltimore, 48:1 (1969).
17. P. Costa, A. S. Figueria, and F. R. Brava, Proc. Natl. Acad. Sci. USA, 75:4499 (1978).
18. M. Skinner and A. S. Cohen, Biochem. Biophys. Res. Commun., 99:1326 (1981).
19. M. D. Benson, J. Clin. Invest., 67:1035 (1981).
20. M. Pras, E. C. Franklin, P. Prelli, and B. Frangione, J. Exp. Med., 154:989 (1981).

GENETIC HETEROGENEITY OF FAMILIAL AMYLOID

POLYNEUROPATHIES OF JEWISH TYPE

Mordechai Pras*, Frances Prelli†
Joseph Gafni*, and Blas Frangione†

*Heller Institute
 Sheba Medical Center
 Tel-Hashomer, Israel

†New York University Medical Center
 Department of Pathology
 550 First Avenue
 New York, N. Y. 10016

ABSTRACT

The Jewish SKO amyloid protein is a prealbumin monomer with two amino acid substitutions. Glycine is substituted for Threonine at position 49 and Isoleucine for Phenylalanine at position 33. The distribution of these components is different in thyroid and spleen suggesting tissue specificify in amyloid disposition. The SKO variant differs from the prealbumin proteins found in the Portuguese, Japanese and Swedish Familial Amyloid Polyneuropathies. Additional prealbumin variants will be expected when the amyloid proteins of the facial and upper limb amyloid neuropathies as well as the Van Allen kinship can be studied.

INTRODUCTION

In May, 1980 our only patient with Jewish familial amyloid polyneuropathy died at the age of 29. He shot himself in the abdomen to insure hospitalization and the utilization of his body for a better understanding of his disease.

The patient's death occurred after a relatively short illness of four years. Until the age of 25 he was a healthy young man who served in the Israeli army as a paratrooper, married and had a son. His earliest complaints were of visual disturbances and impotence. Vitreous opacities were noted, and progressed to cause blindness that required vitrectomy two years later. Frequency and incontinence of the urine appeared at the age of 26 and parasthesias and weakness of the lower limbs at the same time.

Deterioration was progressive accompanied by muscle wasting diarrhea and fecal incontinence.

The father, an Ashkenazi Jew born in Poland, had suffered virtually from the same clinical picture and died of bleeding gastric erosions at the age of 36.

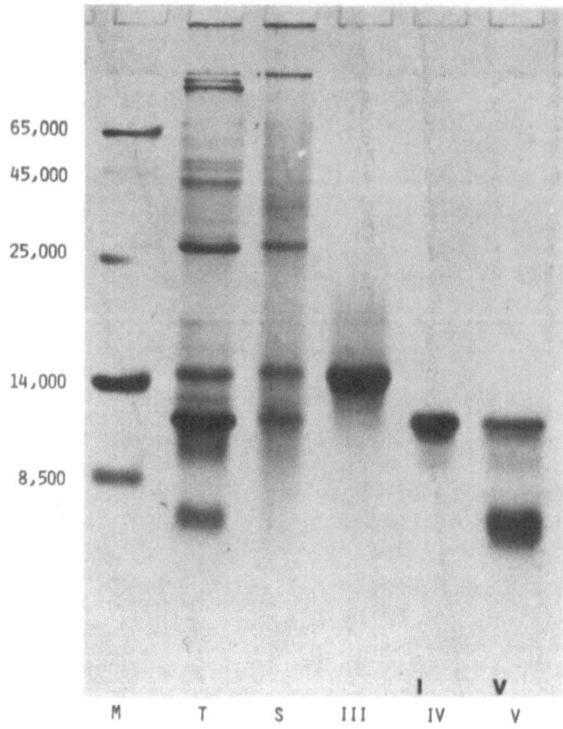

Fig. 1.   SDS-PAGE 17% slab gel of impure
amyloid fibrils extracted from thyroid
(T) and spleen (S). Peaks III, IV,
and V are purified components. M,
markers; bovine serum albumin, 67,000
mol. wt.; ovalbumin, 45,000 mol. wt.;
chymotrypsinogen A, 25,000 mol. wt.;
ribonuclease A, 13,700 mol. wt.; and
AA protein, 8,000 mol. wt.

Autopsies in both father and son confirmed systemic amyloidosis:
spinal nerves and autonomic nerves as well as striated muscles, thyroid,
spleen and adrenals showed massive amyloid deposits.

The thyroid was the source for extraction of the amyloid fibrils.
SDS gel electrophoresis of the isolated fibrils demonstrated a unique pattern: in addition to P component three major protein bands could be distinguished. The first protein of 14K, the second of about 10K and the last
one of 5K (Fig. 1).

After complete reduction in guanidine these three proteins were isolated on Sephadex and ACA Ultrogel columns. The proteins were studied by
amino acid sequencing and showed them to have the same amino terminal. The
next step was to cleave the 14K dalton protein by cyanogen bromide and the
10K protein was subjected to trypsin digestion.

The amino acid sequence of all the proteins obtained from SKO amyloid
fibrils demonstrated that they were homologous to serum prealbumin: the
14K protein was the intact prealbumin monomer; the 10K protein, its carboxy
terminal fragment from residues 49 to 127, and the 5K protein its 48 amino
terminal residues (Fig. 2). However in position 49 we detected mainly

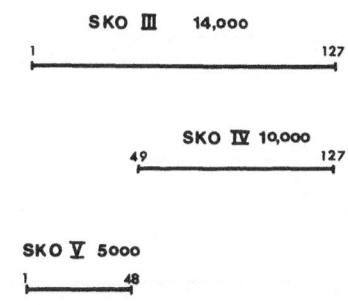

Fig. 2. Diagram of the three proteins obtained from the SKO amyloid fibrils.

glycine [1]. Small amounts of threonine which is the residue reported to be present in normal prealbumin was present [2]. These findings indicated that a normal and a variant prealbumin were present in the tissue of this patient and presumably in the serum. The antibodies developed in rabbits against the 10K protein (positions 49-127) with mainly glycine as its amino terminal amino acid [3], reacted against the 14K, and 10K isolated proteins as well as the patient's serum. The antibodies raised showed specificity since they did not react against normal sera, isolated normal prealbunin and against the Portuguese isolated prealbumin provided to us kindly by Dr. Saraiva. Because of differences in the yield of Thr/Gly at position 49 detected in amyloid fibrils extracted from thyroid and spleen and a search for further heterogeneity we decided to analyze the intact prealbumin (14K) by isolating their tryptic peptides. Very recently our Japanese friends Dr. Nakazato and Dr. Araki and associates wrote us about another substitution in position 33 of our 14K protein. We repeated the study according to their modification of pretreating the protein with 70% formic acid and found beside the glycine substituting for threonine at position 49 that isoleucine substituted for phenylalanine at position 33. In this instance the amyloid fibrils were extracted from the spleen instead of the thyroid. On the other hand when similar studies were conducted in our laboratory with the 14K protein obtained from thyroid Phe was obtained at position 33 instead of Ile (Phe is the residue present in normal prealbumin) [2]. These findings clearly show that at least two amino acid substitutions are present in prealbumin variant SKO and that the composition of amyloid fibrils present in different organs is not the same, indicating tissue specificity in amyloid deposition. Work is in progress to demonstrate whether both substitutions, namely Ile and Gly are present in one, two or more distinct molecules.

Since Andrades' classical description of familial amyloid polyneuropathy among Portuguese in 1952 [4], it has been described in numerous families of various ethnic origins. They can be divided into three prototype entities by gross differences in the clinical symptoms that initiate and dominate their disease [5].

The fact that familial amyloid polyneuropathies are restricted various ous ethnic origins, often separated geographically, and that clinical variations can be detected even in the various forms of the lower limb familial amyloid polyneuropathy suggests that different FAPs could be due to genetic polymorphism. The clinical picture of the Japanese and Swedish polyneuropathy is virtually identical to the Portuguese type although among the Swedes average age of the onset is 20 years later than in the Portuguese-Japanese patients.

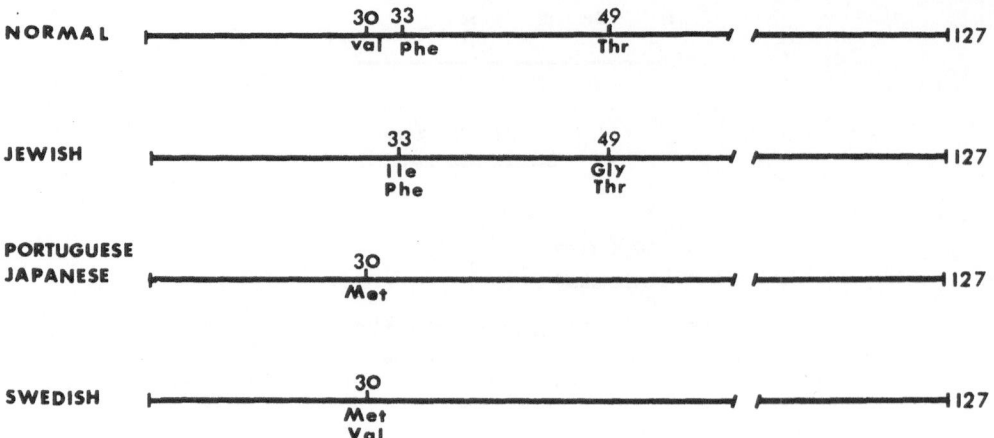

Fig. 3. Genetic heterogeneity of FAP of different types. Numbers indicate the position of amino acid substitutions.

The family of Irish-English-Scottish origin described by Van Allen is of special interest because its members suffered also from clinical symptoms that cannot be attributed to systemic amyloidosis [6]. The fact that 11 out of 12 affected members are male raises the question of sex influence that does not occur in other forms of familial amyloid polyneuropathies. Out of the 12 affected members that suffered from neuropathy, nine suffered from aggression form of peptic ulcer with numerous performations and bleeding. Nine manifested renal failure without nephrotic syndrome and at autopsy the amyloid deposits in the kidneys were too minute to account for renal insufficiency. Therefore, nonamyloidotic renal disease, peptic ulceration as well as cataract and deafness that occurred each in five members must be considered as independent phenotypic expression of a pleiotropic gene. Unfortunately, the amyloid fibrils of this Iowa family were never studied and characterized.

In our Jewish family, visual disturbances due to amyloid vitreous deposits were the first symptoms in the father and son [3]. Amyloid vitreous deposits although striking in our patients occur in other forms of FAP in some Japanese, Swede, and Portuguese patients. But we can hardly recall in the literature another family in which amyloid deposits in the eyes were so striking and occur so early in the course of the disease.

In summary: presently we recognize two prealbumin variants characterized by amino acid substitutions which appear to be related to the development of familial amyloid polyneuropathy (Fig. 3). In the Portuguese [7], Japanese [8], and Swedish [9] types methionine replaces valine at position 30, in the Jewish type glycine substitutes threonine at position 49 and isoleucine-phenylalanine at position 33. In two instances both the variant and the normal prealbumin molecules were present in tissue and/or serum. Our findings seem to indicate that different phenotypic expression in patients with familial amyloidosis polyneuropathy, are due to different gene types. Since other clinical forms of FAP has been described [6, 10, 11] further heterogeneity can be expected.

ACKNOWLEDGEMENTS

The work was supported by USPHS Grant #AM 01431.

ADDENDUM

Nakazato et al. (Biochem. Biophys. Res. Comm. 123:921, 1984) have reported the sequence analysis by tryptic peptide mapping of the 14,000 dalton component of a 0.5 mg sample of SKO splenic amyloid that we have provided. They found an isoleucine replacement for a phenylalanine at position 33. However, they failed to identify the previously reported amino acid substitution glycine for threonine at position 49.

We have reexamined the 14,000, 10,000, and 5,000 dalton components of amyloid derived from both the thyroid and spleen using the methods originally applied by us and those of Nakazato et al.

Both methods confirm the glycine for threonine substitution at position 49 regardless of organ source. 10%-40% of threonine was also detected at this position, reaffirming the heterogeneity previously reported. The isoleucine for phenylalanine substitution at position 33 was present only in fibrils obtained from the spleen.

REFERENCES

1. M. Pras et al., Proc. Natl. Acad. Sci., 80, 539 (1983).
2. Y. Kanda et al., J. Biol. Chem. 249, 6796 (1974).
3. M. Pras et al., J. Exp. Med. 154, 989 (1981).
4. C. Andrade, Brain 75, 408 (1952).
5. G. Glenner et al., in "The Metabolic Basis of Inherited Diseases," McGraw-Hill, New York, pp. 1468 (1983).
6. M. W. Van Allen et al., Neurology 19, 10 (1969).
7. M. J. M. Saraiva et al., J. Clin. Invest., 74, 104 (1984).
8. S. Tawara et al., Biochem. Biophys. Res. Commun. 116, 880 (1983).
9. F. E. Swelet and M. D. Benson, Proc. Natl. Acad. Sci., 81, 594 (1984).
10. J. Meretoja, Ann. Clin. Res., 1, 314 (1969).
11. J. G. Rukavina et al., Medicine, 35, 239 (1956).

PREALBUMIN NATURE OF THE AMYLOID IN FAMILIAL

AMYLOID CARDIOMYOPATHY OF DANISH ORIGIN

G. Husby*, P. J. Ranløv†,
K. Sletten‡, and G. Marhaug**

*Department of Rheumatology
 The University Hospital of Tromsø, Tromsø, Norway

†Department of Medicine B
 Central Hospital, Hillerød, Denmark

‡Institute of Biochemistry
 University of Oslo, Oslo, Norway

**Department of Rheumatology
  The University Hospital of Tromsø, Tromsø, Norway

ABSTRACT

Amyloid obtained from the myocardium of a patient (Han) with familial amyloid cariomyopathy of Danish origin was studied. Gel filtration and electrophoresis of purified and denatured amyloid fibrils Han revealed various fractions ranging in molecular weight from 40,000 to 8000 daltons. Amyloid Han and fractions reacted with an antiserum against amyloid Han showing a reaction of identity with each other; partial identity between Han and humn prealbumin was observed, while no reaction was seen with AA or AL proteins. Cardiac tissue sections from Han showed reactivity with antisera to amyloid Han, prealbumin and protein AP, but not with anti-AA or anti-AL in indirect immunofluorescence. Amino acid composition and sequences studies of a protein fraction of amyloid Han with molecular weight 15,000 daltons confirmed the structural relationship with prealbumin.

INTRODUCTION

Frederiksen and co-workers [1] described in 1962 a Danish family with amyloid cardiomyopathy verified in five out of twelve siblings in one generation, probably inherited autosomal dominant. The affected siblings died from heart failure between 40 and 50 years of age, and cardiac symptoms and signs were the only ones which could be related to amyloid deposits. In all cases examined at autopsy, the myocardium was heavily infiltrated, while only microdeposits of amyloid were found in other organs or tissues including peripheral nerves, striated muscle and the intestines.

Some family members of the next generation have now reached the age of 40 years or more, and two of them have died from heart failure 43 and 44 years old, respectively. We have had access to autopsy material from the latter patient. Because the affected members of the family suffered a very distinct clinical form of dominantly inherited amyloidosis, we found it of interest to study the structural properties of amyloid isolated from this patient. Detailed clinical, pathologic and genetic data will be reported later.

MATERIALS AND METHODS

Source of Amyloid

Amyloid fibrils were prepared from the myocardium obtained at autopsy from patient Han who died from cardiac failure at the age of 44 years. He was the son of sibling No. 11 in the generation with familial amyloid cardiomyopathy described by Frederiksen et al. [1] and was given No. 11.1 in the pedigree reported by these authors.

Extraction and Purification of Amyloid Fibril Proteins

Myocardial tissue was cut into small pieces and subjected to extraction of amyloid fibrils with water after repeated washings of homogenized tissue with physiological saline [2]. The fibril-containing water supernatants were lyophilized, treated with 6 M guanidine and a reducing agent, 0.05 M dithiothreitol (DDT), plus 1.0 mM EDTA, and thereafter subjected to gel filtration on Sephadex G-100 under dissociating conditions as described [3, 4]. In some experiments the reduced fibril preparation was also alkylated with 0.3 M iodoacetamide [4] before application to the column. Selected protein fractions eluted from the Sephadex G-100 column were subjected to polyyacrylamide gel electrophoresis (PAGE) as described [5] and were also used for amino acid composition and sequence studies after gel filtration on a Sephadex G-25 fine column [4].

Immunologic Studies

Double diffusion and immunoelectrophoresis in 1% agarose gel was used for immunologic characterization of crude alkali-degraded amyloid fibrils (DAM) and purified amyloid protein fractions obtained by gel filtration [4]. In addition, the following human amyloid proteins were used as controls: Protein AA [6], various AL proteins [7] and the amyloid P-component (AP) [8]. Prealbumin was purchased from Behringwerke AG, Germany. Antiserum to amyloid Han was produced in rabbits by immunization with amyloid fibrils denatured with 0.1 M NaOH [4]. Antisera to AA and various AL proteins have been described before [7] while anti-AP was purchased from Atlantic Antibodies, Westbrook, Maine, USA and anti-prealbumin and anti-retinol binding protein (RBP) from Behringwerke AG, Germany.

Immunohistochemical Studies

Indirect immunofluorescence (IIF) was used to characterize amyloid deposits directly in frozen tissue sections from Han. Frozen sections from various tissues with amyloid deposits of known chemical composition [9] was used for control in addition to tissue specimens from corresponding normal organs. Rabbit or goat antisera to the various antigens mentioned above was used as first layer, and fluorescein isothiocyanate (FITC) labelled swine anti-rabbit or -goat IgG (DAKO Immunoglobulins A/S, Copenhagen, Denmark) as second layer in the IIF technique. Serially cut sections stained with Congo red were examined by polarization microscopy.

Structural Studies

The amino acid composition was determined from 24 hrs acid hydrolyzates and was analyzed on a BIOTRONIK LC 5000 Amino Acid Analyzer. Edman degrada-

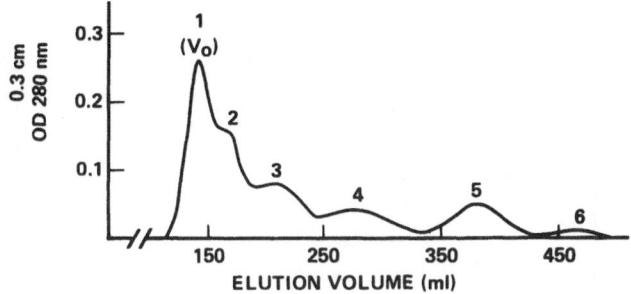

Fig. 1. Gel filtration of amyloid fibrils Han
treated with 6 M guanidine, 0.05 M DTT
on a 1.5 × 87 cm Sephadex G-100 column
with 5 M guanidine in 0.1 M acetic acid
as eluent.

tion was performed using a JEOL 47K Sequence Analyzer and the PTH-amino
acid derivatives analyzed as described [10]. The protein was cleaved with
cyanogen bromide in 70% formic acid and the lyophilized material was taken
up in 10% acetic acid for gel filtration [6]. Some undissolved material
was centrifuged down and used for Edman degradation.

RESULTS

Polarization microscopy of sections stained with Congo red showed that
the myocardial tissue from Han was heavily infiltrated with amyloid. Up to
75% of the area of the view fields exhibited the typical green birefringence
when sections from different parts of the myocardium were stained with Congo
red and examined by polarization microscopy. The yield of water-extracted
cardiac amyloid Han was 1200 mg of lyophilized fibrils per 20 g of fresh
tissue. Also the fibril preparation stained specifically with Congo red
and showed green birefringence under polarized light.

Gel Filtration and Electrophoresis

The elution profile obtained when dissociated and reduced amyloid Han
was gel filtered on Sephadex G-100 is shown in Fig. 1. Five retarded protein fractions (peak 2-6) were eluted in addition to the void volume (Vo,
peak 1) material excluded by the column. Molecular weights of the proteins
eluted in the various peaks were estimated [4] to be approximately 40,000
(peak 2), 30,000 (peak 3), 20,000 (peak 4), 15,000 (peak 5) and 8000 (peak
6). Relative protein yield of the fractions was 27% (Vo, peak 1), 18%
(peak 2), 19% (peak 3), 15% (peak 4), 15% (peak 5) and 6% (peak 6). Alkylation of the reduced protein material before gel filtration did not alter the
elution profile of amyloid Han. Material from the protein peak 5 was selected for further structural studies.

Immunologic Studies

The immunodiffusion studies of amyloid Han and its fractions are summarized in Table 1. Both DMA Han and the protein fractions 1-5 separated
by gel filtration (Fig. 1) reacted with anti-Han, all showing a reaction of
antigenic identity with each other, while no reaction was obtained with the
8000 molecular weight material in peak 6. However, the protein fraction 1
(Vo) showed a much weaker reaction than the other fractions. Anti-Han reacted with prealbumin, the precipitation lines of amyloid Han spurring over

393

TABLE 1. Antigenic Reactivity of Crude and Fractionated Amyloid Han, Control Amyloid Preparations, and Serum Proteins

		Protein fractions of amyloid Han											
	DAM Han	1(Vo)	2	3	4	5	6	AA	AL	AP	Pre-alb.	Whole serum	Retinol binding protein
Mol wt		>50,000	40,000	30,000	20,000	15,000	8,000						
Reaction with antisera to:													
DAM Han	+*	+/-	+	+	+	+	-	-	-	-	+*	+	-
AA	-	-	-	-	-	-	-	+	-	-	-	-	-
AL	-	-	-	-	-	-	-	-	+	-	-	-	-
AP	-	-	-	-	-	-	-	-	-	+	-	+	-
Prealbumin	+**	-	-	+	+	+	-	-	-	-	+**	+	-
Retinol binding protein	-	-	-	-	-	-	-	-	-	-	-	+	+

*The precipitation line of amyloid Arv spurred over that of prealbumin, i.e., a reaction of partial antigenic identity.
**The precipitation line of prealbumin spurred over that of amyloid Han.

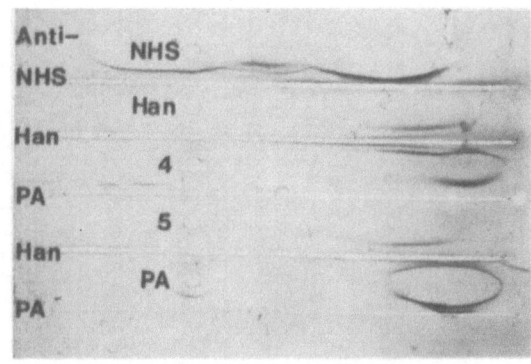

Fig. 2. Immunoelectrophoresis of normal
human serum (NHS), crude amyloid
Han and its protein fractions 4
and 5 (Fig. 1) and prealbumin (PA)
against anti-NHS, anti-amyloid Han
and anti-prealbumin.

that of prealbumin, thus showing a reaction of partial antigenic identity.
Also anti-prealbumin reacted with amyloid Han and its protein fractions 3,
4, and 5, showing a reaction of partial identity with prealbumin (the precipitation line of prealbumin spurring over that of amyloid Han) while no
reaction was obtained with the fractions 1 (Vo), 2 and 6. This clearly
showed that amyloid Han and its subfractions 3, 4, and 5 shared antigenic
determinants with normal prealbumin. No reaction between amyloid Han and
antisera to the amyloid proteins AL, AA, AP or retinol binding protein was
obtained with the immunodiffusion technique used (Table 1). Both anti-
amyloid Han and anti-prealbumin precipitated with a component in normal
human serum which was antigenically identical with prealbumin.

To summarize the immunologic findings: It was clear that degraded
amyloid Han and its fractions (except fraction 6) were antigenically identical when tested against anti-amyloid Han. In addition, amyloid Han and
its fractins 3-5 also showed antigenic relationship with prealbumin, but
not with the other amyloid proteins, retinol binding protein or other serum
proteins detected by anti-whole human serum. The partial antigenic identity
observed between prealbumin and amyloid Han showed that both shared antigenic
determinants, but also that both had determinants not shared by the other.

Immunoelectrophoresis using antisera to amyloid Han and prealbumin
(Fig. 2) revealed the same pattern of reactivity as the double diffusion experiments. Crude amyloid Han and its gel filtration fraction 4 reacted with
both antisera showing an electrophoretic mobility similar to that of prealbumin (slightly anodic to albumin), while fraction 5 and 1, 2, and 3 (not
shown) migrated somewhat slower. It was also seen that fraction 4 showed
two precipitation lines reflecting the rather asymmetric shape of the protein peak on Sephadex G-100 (Fig. 1).

The IIF studies demonstrated bright staining of amyloid deposits in the
myocardium of Han when the frozen sections were incubated with anti-amyloid
Han (Fig. 3), anti-prealbumin or anti-AP. With all three antisera the
fluorescent areas corresponded to the birefringent material revealed by polarization microscopy of adjacent sections stained with Congo red. Preabsorption of each of the three antisera with their respective antigens
abolished the immunofluorescence staining. No specific IIF reaction was
obtained when cardiac sections were treated with antisera to AA, AL, or RBP.

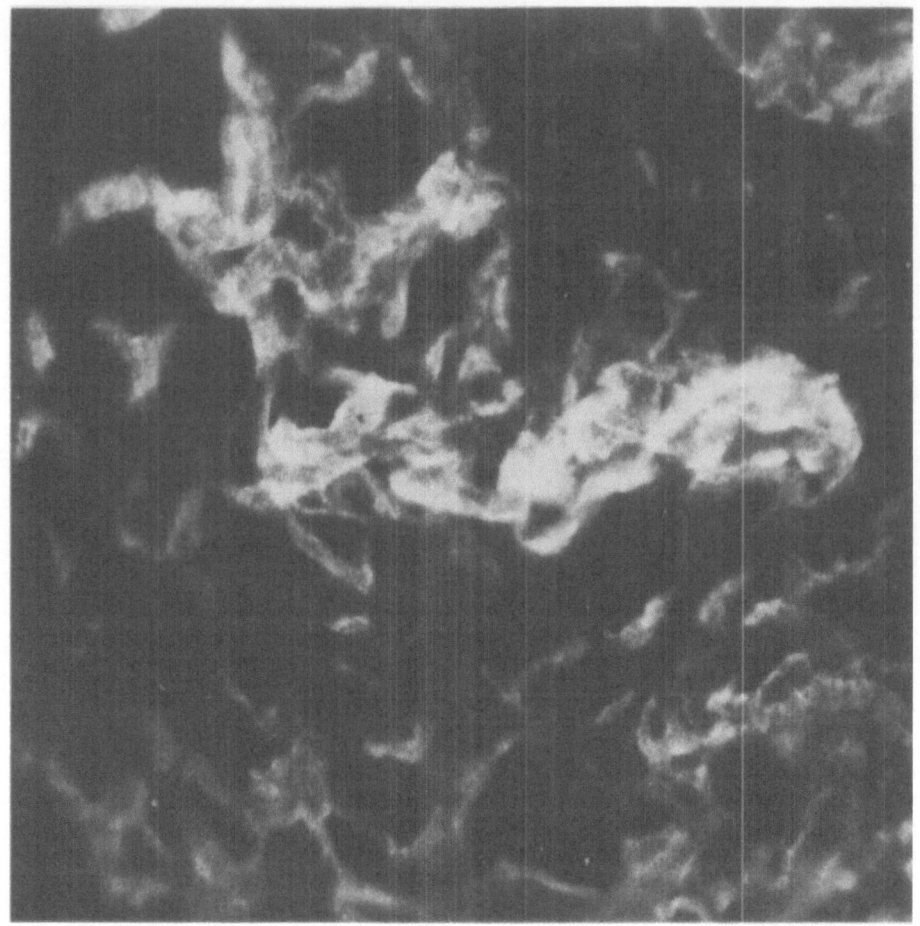

Fig. 3. Immunofluorescence micrograph. Cardiac tissue section from Han
         stained with anti-amyloid Han showing bright fluorescence of
         amyloid infiltrating the myocardium. (Orig. magnification ×400).

Renal, splenic or hepatic tissue sections from Han did not stain with any
of the antisera used, nor did staining with Congo red reveal amyloid material in these tissues; the same was also seen with the normal myocardium
used for control.

Amino Acid Studies

     The amino acid composition of the protein in fraction 5 showed clearly
that the composition was similar to that of prealbumin (Table 2). N-terminal analysis revealed several amino acid residues in each step. However,
in step 2 and 5, glycine was found to be the main derivative, and the yield
was about 40% and 10% of the material applied. The N-terminal sequence of
prealbumin has glycine in positions 1, 4, and 6 (Kanda et al., 1974). The
results indicated that the protein has a ragged N-terminal with a different
amino acid sequence. Edman degradation of an undissolved fraction from the
bromide cleaved material revealed the following sequence:

                    Val-Lys-Val-Leu-Asp-Ala

TABLE 2. Amino Acid Composition of Amyloid Protein Fraction
5 Determined after 24 hrs Acid Hydrolyses

	Residues per molecule	
Aspartic acid	8.1	(8)*
Threonine	11.2	(12)
Serine	12.0	(11)
Glutamic acid	14.3	(12)
Proline	8.1	(8)
Glycine	10.6	(10)
Alanine	10.4	(12)
$^1/_2$ Cystine	Trace	(1)
Valine	8.1	(12)
Methionine	1.5	(1)
Isoleucine	5.6	(5)
Leucine	7.3	(7)
Tyrosine	5.3	(5)
Phenylalanine	5.1	(5)
Histidine	5.3	(4)
Lysine	7.4	(8)
Arginine	4.2	(4)
Tryptophan	N.D.	(2)

*Numbers in brackets are from the amino acid composition
of prealbumin (Kanda et al., 1974).

this amino acid sequence corresponds to positions 14 to 19 in prealbumin
and is thus the cyanogen bromide fragment 2 [11]. We also suspect that
Leucine in position 110 of normal PA is replaced by methionine in fraction
V of amyloid Han.

DISCUSSION

Familial amyloidosis includes a variety of disease syndromes caused by
the deposition of amyloid fibrils in different tissues and organs. Except
for familial Mediterranean fever (autosomal, recessive), all syndromes appear to be inherited as an autosomal dominant trait [12]. Many forms of
systemic, familial amyloidosis are characterized by polyneuropathy (FAP),
which is distributed in a characteristic fashion in the different families
reported [12].

The present case Han represent familial amyloid cardiomyopathy occurring in a Danish family [1], characterized by gross infiltration of amyloid
in the myocardium, but only nonsymptomatic, minor depositions of amyloid in
peripheral nerves or other organs, a syndrome which has not been described
in any other family, and is thus clinically distinct from FAP. Fredriksen
et al. [1] reported on only one sibship and could thus not establish the
mode of inheritance of the amyloid cardiomyopathy, although it was suggested to be autosomal dominant. Genetic studies of the following generations
will clarify this question.

The amyloid fibrils isolated from patients with FAP have been shown to
be related to prealbumin or variants of this protein in families of Portuguese [13], Swedish [14, 15], Jewish [16, 17], Japanese and German/English
[19] origin. Amyloid fibrils related to prealbumin therefore appear to have
a high tendency to localize to peripheral nerves. The present data of the

cardiac amyloid Han proved that it was also related to prealbumin, showing that prealbumin-related amyloid may severely affect cardiac tissues as well. Amyloid of prealbumin nature has also been found in cases of non-familial senile cardiac amyloid [20].

An example of dominantly inherited amyloid which is not of prealbumin nature is hereditary cerebral hemorrhage with amyloidosis, which very recently has been shown to be related to gamma trace protein [21].

The immunologic studies revealed a marked antigenic cross-reactivity between amyloid Han and normal human prealbumin, but both protein materials also exhibited antigenic specificities. The specificities could represent conformational changes in the amyloid fibril protein, but could also be due to substitutions among its amino acid residues, i.e., a change in the primary structure of the protein. Thus the prealbumin-like amyloid protein from FAP of Jewish origin described by Pras et al. [17] was mutant, the threonine in position 49 in normal serum prealbumin being substituted by glycine in the amyloid protein, showing that the Jewish form of FAP can be regarded as an inborn error of metabolism. Whether mutation has taken place in the prealbumin-like amyloid protein Han described here, will eventually be confirmed by the further amino acid sequence studies presently in progress. Preliminary studies, however, have indicated a replacement of leucine in position 110 of normal PA by methionine in amyloid protein Han.

The IIF studies confirmed the immunoreactivity of cardiac amyloid Han in situ, and bright IIF staining was obtained with both anti-Han and anti-prealbumin. Protein AP was also demonstrated in the cardiac amyloid deposits. Although not being an amyloid fibril protein, AP thus appears to be almost invariably present in amyloid deposits, regardless of their chemical composition and clinical relationship [22], the only known exception being some intracerebral amyloids [23]. However, the significance of protein AP in the formation of amyloid is not known.

Pras et al. [16, 17] showed that both intact prealbumin-like protein and differently sized fragments were co-isolated from their Jewish FAP amyloid preparation. The molecular weight (approximately 15,000 daltons) and the amino acid composition and partial sequence suggested the protein fraction 5 of amyloid Han to be monomeric prealbumin (molecular weight 14,000) or a variant of this protein, while fraction 6 may represent a fragment of the protein in fraction 5. The small size of the protein fraction 6 may be responsible for its lack of antigenic reactivity. Amino acid studies presently in progress will elucidate this question. Interestingly the presence of intact protein and fragments of the same protein has also been observed in amyloid of AA [24, 25] and AL [7] type. Furthermore, the protein fractions 2, 3, and 4 may represent polymers or aggregates of intact or fragmented protein Han, while a normal tissue component [26] also present in amyloids of AA and AL types [27] seemed to make up most of the proteins in fraction 1 (results not shown). All the protein fractions of amyloid Han are presently subjected to further structural studies to be reported later.

ACKNOWLEDGEMENTS

The autopsy of the patient (Han) was performed at the Insitute of Pathology, Svendborg Hospital, Svendborg, Denmark. We are grateful for the help and cooperation provided by Drs. W. Kiaer and A. Thamsen of that Institute.

This work was supported by the Norwegian Council of Science and the Humanities, The Norwegian Rheumatism Research Council and by Kaptajnløytnant

Jensen and Hustrus Foundation. The authors thank Ms. Kirsti Rønne and Ms. Jessie Juul for technical assistance and Ms. Anita Skoge Hoel for typing the manuscript.

1. T. Frederiksen, H. Gøtzsche, N. Harboe, W. Kiaer, and K. Mellemgaard, Am. J. Med., 33, 328 (1962).
2. M. Pras, D. Zucker-Franklin, A. Rimon, and E. C. Franklin, J. Exp. Med., 130, 777 (1969).
3. M. Harada, C. Isersky, P. Cuatrecasas, D. Page, H. A. Bladen, E. D. Eanes, H. R. Keiser, and G. G. Glenner, J. Histochem. Cytochem., 19, 1 (1971).
4. G. Husby, K. Sletten, T. E. Michaelsen, and J. B. Natvig, Scand. J. Immunol., 1, 393 (1972).
5. G. Marhaug and G. Husby, Clin. Exp. Immunol., 45, 97 (1981).
6. K. Sletten and G. Husby, Eur. J. Biochem., 41, 117 (1974).
7. G. Husby, K. Sletten, N. Blumenkrantz, and L. Danielsen, Clin. Exp. Immunol., 45, 90 (1981).
8. K. Holck, G. Husby, K. Sletten, and J. B. Natvig, J. Immunol., 10, 55 (1979).
9. G. G. Cornwell, III, G. Husby, P. Westermark, J. B. Natvig, T. E. Michaelsen, and B. Skogen, Scand. J. Immunol., 6, 1071 (1977).
10. K. Sletten, J. B. Natvig, G. Husby, and J. Jull., Biochem. J., 195, 561 (1981).
11. Y. Kanda, D. S. Goodman, R. E. Canfield, and F. J. Horgan, J. Biol. Chem., 249, 6796 (1971).
12. G. G. Glenner, T. F. Ignaczak, and D. L. Page, in: Metabolic Basis of Inherited Disease, Ed. 4, NewYork, McGraw-Hill Book Co., Inc., p. 1308 (1978).
13. P. P. Costa, A. S. Figueira, and F. R. Bravo, Proc. Natl. Acad. Sci. USA, 75, 4499 (1978).
14. M. D. Benson, J. Clin. Invest., 67, 1035 (1981).
15. M. Skinner, A. S. Cohen, Biochem. Biophys. Res. Commun., 99, 1326 (1981).
16. M. Pras, E. C. Franklin, F. Prelli, and B. Frangione, J. Exp. Med., 154, 989 (1981).
17. M. Pras, F. Prelli, E. C. Franklin, and B. Frangione, Proc. Natl. Acad. Sci. USA, 80, 539 (1983).
18. S. Tawara, S. Araki, K. Toshimori, H. Nakagawa, and S. Ohtaki, J. Lab. Clin. Med., 98, 811 (1981).
19. C. A. Libbey, A. Rubinow, T. Shirahama, C. Deal, and A. S. Cohen, Am. J. Med., 76, 18 (1984).
20. K. Sletten, P. Westermark, J. B. Natvig, Scand. J. Immunol., 12, 503 (1980).
21. D. H. Cohen, H. Feiner, O. Jensson, and B. Frangione, J. Exp. Med., 158, 623 (1983).
22. M. B. Pepys, M. L. Baltz, Adv. Immunol., 34, 141 (1983).
23. P. Westermark, T. Shirahama, M. Skinner, A. Brun, R. Cameron, and A. S. Cohen, Lab. Invest., 46, 457 (1982).
24. K. Møyner, K. Sletten, G. Husby, and J. B. Natvig, Scand. J. Immunol., 11, 549 (1980).
25. K. Waalen, K. Sletten, G. Husby, K. Nordstoga, Eur. U. Biochem., 104, 407 (1980).
26. G. Husby and K. Sletten, Acta. Pathol. Microbiol. Scand. (C), 85, 153 (1977).

399

DIAGNOSIS OF FAMILIAL AMYLOIDOTIC POLYNEUROPATHY

BY RECOMBINANT DNA TECHNIQUES

H. Sasaki*, Y. Sakaki*, H. Matsuo†,
I. Goto*, Y. Kuroiwa*, I. Sahashi‡,
A. Takahashi‡, T. Shinoda**,
T. Isobe††, and Y. Takagi*

*Kyushu University
 Faculty of Medicine Fukuoka 812

†Miyazaki Medical College
 Kiyotake 889-16

‡Aichi Medical College
 Nagakute 480-11

**Tokyo Metropolitan University
  Tokyo 158, and

††Kobe University
  Kobe 650, Japan

ABSTRACT

An amino acid substitution of Met for Val at position 30 or plasma prealbumin is closely related to familial amyloidotic polyneuropathy. The cDNA for normal human prealbumin was cloned and its nucleotide sequence was determined. The results showed that the nucleotide substitution responsible for the Val → Met change results in formation of new restriction sites for BalI and NsiI. Based on the results, a method was developed for diagnosis of the disease presymptomatically and prenatally.

INTRODUCTION

Recent biochemical studies revealed a close relationship between familial amyloidotic polyneuropathy (FAP) and human plasma prealbumin [1-6]. In the Japanese type of FAP, a prealbumin variant with a single amino acid replacement of methionine for valine at position 30 is thought to lead to amyloid fibril formation [3, 6]. This paper describes cloning and sequence analysis of the cDNA for normal human prealbumin, and presents a simple method for detection of the mutation based on our findings. This method should be useful for diagnosis of FAP presymptomatically and prenatally.

MATERIAL AND METHODS

Construction and Screening of a Human Liver cDNA: Poly(A)$^+$RNA was prepared from normal human liver by use of guanidine hydrochloride and oligo(dT)cellulose chromatography [7, 8]. Double-stranded cDNA was synthesized from 2 μg of liver mRNA as described by Okayama and Berg [9] and approximately 30,000 independent recombinant colonies were obtained.

These colonies were screened on nitrocellulose filters with oligo-nucleotide probes. Hybridization were carried out as described by Cohn et al. [10].

Subcloning and Nucleotide Sequence Analysis: Restriction endonuclease fragments of the cDNA subcloned into pUC 13 at appropriate restriction sites. The recombinant plasmids were isolated by alkaline lysis [11], pre-cipitated with polyethylene glycol [12], and used as templates for sequence determination by the dideoxy method [13]. DNA sequencing was carried out bidirectionally with both obverse and reverse primers.

Preparation of DNA from Human Blood: Peripheral blood samples (10-20 ml) were obtained from two normal healthy adults and three patients with FAP from the Arao area, Kumamoto prefecture, Japan. DNA was isolated from collected leukocytes by the procedures described by Ryan et al. [14] with some modifications.

Preparation of Probes and Southern Blot Hybridization Analysis: The prealbumin cDNA was subcloned into plasmid pSP64 [15] and transformed into Escherichia coli stain HB101. The resulting recombinant plasmid was linear-ized and subjected to the transcription reaction with SP6 polymerase for generating hybridization probes [16].

Samples of 5-10 μg human DNA were completely digested with restriction endonuclease NsiI or BalI under the conditions recommended by the manufac-turers. After electrophoresis through 0.7% agarose gel, the DNAs were de-natured in situ and transferred to nylon membrane filters (Bio-Rad, Zeta-Probe) by the procedure of Southern [17]. Prehybridization, hybridization and washing of the filters were performed as described by Zinn et al. [16].

Materials: Sequencing primers were obtained from Pharmacia P-L Bio-chemicals. Enzymes were purchased from Promega Biotec (USA), New England Biolabs (USA), Takara Shuzo Co., Ltd. (Kyoto, Japan), and Nippon Gene Co., Ltd. (Toyama, Japan) and radio-isotopes were from Amersham (England).

RESULTS AND DISCUSSION

Isolation and Characterization of Prealbumin cDNA

We employed the colony hybridization technique with synthetic oligonu-cleotide probes to pick up prealbumin cDNA clones from a human liver cDNA library. As a result, three of the four possible clones (pHPA15, 21, 27) were found to contain at least part of cDNA for human prealbumin. Since clone HPA27 had the longest insert (about 600 bp) and was expected to in-clude a full-length cDNA for prealbumin, its complete nucleotide sequence was determined. The results of DNA sequence analysis and the deduced amino acid sequence are shown in Fig. 1. The sequence appears to include the entire region coding for the precursor for prealbumin, and a hydrophobic N-terminal peptide of 20 amino acid residues, predicted from our data, seems to have the expected characteristics of a signal peptide [18].

Detection of the Mutation in FAP Patients

In the Japanese type of FAP, a prealbumin variant with a single amino acid replacement of methionine for valine at position 30 was reported [3, 6]. The most remarkable feature of the cDNA sequence is that the genetic change, which could case the Val → Met change, (GTG → ATG), leads to for-mation of new restriction sites for BalI(TGGCCG → TGGCCA) and NsiI(GTGCAT →

ATGCAT). This indicates that the mutation in the prealbumin gene of FAP patients could be easily detected by the sensitivity of the gene to <u>Bal</u>I and/or <u>Nsi</u>I.

```
                                          -20
                                         Met Ala Ser His Arg Leu Leu Leu Leu Cys
                     ACAGAAGTCCACTCATTCTTGGCAGG ATG GCT TCT CAT CGT CTG CTC CTC CTC TGC
                     ˙                                                           ˙
                     1                                                          50
                     -10                                      -1  1
                     Leu Ala Gly Leu Val Phe Val Ser Glu Ala Gly Pro Thr Gly Thr Gly Glu
                     CTT GCT GGA CTG GTA TTT GTG TCT GAG GCT GGC CCT ACG GGC ACC GGT GAA
                                                                   ˙
                                                                  100
                              10                                      20
                     Ser Lys Cys Pro Leu Met Val Lys Val Leu Asp Ala Val Arg Gly Ser Pro
                     TCC AAG TGT CCT CTG ATG GTC AAA GTT CTA GAT GCT GTC CGA GGC AGT CCT
                                                                          ˙
                                                                         150
                                     30                                      40
                     Ala Ile Asn Val Ala Val His Val Phe Arg Lys Ala Ala Asp Asp Thr Trp
                     GCC ATC AAT GTG GCC GTG CAT GTG TTC AGA AAG GCT GCT GAT GAC ACC TGG
                                  ‾‾‾‾‾‾‾‾̣‾‾‾‾‾‾                            ˙
                                                                          200
                                          50
                     Glu Pro Phe Ala Ser Gly Lys Thr Ser Glu Ser Gly Glu Leu His Gly Leu
                     GAG CCA TTT GCC TCT GGG AAA ACC AGT GAG TCT GGA GAG CTG CAT GGG CTC
                                                                      ˙
                                                                     250
                              60                                      70
                     Thr Thr Glu Glu Glu Phe Val Glu Gly Ile Tyr Lys Val Glu Ile Asp Thr
                     ACA ACT GAG GAG GAA TTT GTA GAA GGG ATA TAC AAA GTG GAA ATA GAC ACC
                                                                          ˙
                                                                         300
                                     80                                      90
                     Lys Ser Tyr Trp Lys Ala Leu Gly Ile Ser Pro Phe His Glu His Ala Glu
                     AAA TCT TAC TGG AAG GCA CTT GGC ATC TCC CCA TTC CAT GAG CAT GCA GAG
                                                                  ˙
                                                                 350
                                          100
                     Val Val Phe Thr Ala Asn Asp Ser Gly Pro Arg Arg Tyr Thr Ile Ala Ala
                     GTG GTA TTC ACA GCC AAC GAC TCC GGC CCC CGC CGC TAC ACC ATT GCC GCC
                                                                      ˙
                                                                     400
                     110                                      120
                     Leu Leu Ser Pro Tyr Ser Tyr Ser Thr Thr Ala Val Val Thr Asn Pro Lys
                     CTG CTG AGC CCC TAC TCC TAT TCC ACC ACG GCT GTC GTC ACC AAT CCC AAG
                                                                      ˙
                                                                     450
                     127
                     Glu ***
                     GAA TGAGGGACTTCTCCTCCAGTGGACCTGAAGGACGAGGGATGGGATTTCATGTAACCAAGAGTA
                                                       ˙
                                                      500
                     TTCCATTTTTACTAAAGCAGTGTTTTAACTCATATGCTATGTTAGAAGTCAGGAGAGACAATAAAAC
                               ˙                                              ‾‾‾‾‾‾‾‾
                              550
                     ATTCCTGTGAAAAAAAAAAA...
                     ˙
                     600
```

Fig. 1. Nucleotide sequence of prealbumin cDNA. Amino acids deduced from the nucleotide sequence are also shown. The presumed signal peptide is shown in italics. Asterisks show the stop codon at the C-terminus. A putative poly A signal is indicated by a wavy line. A dot at position 30 shows the presumed mutation site which causes Val → Met change in FAP patients. Regions in which new restriction sites could be formed by the Val → Met change are underlined.

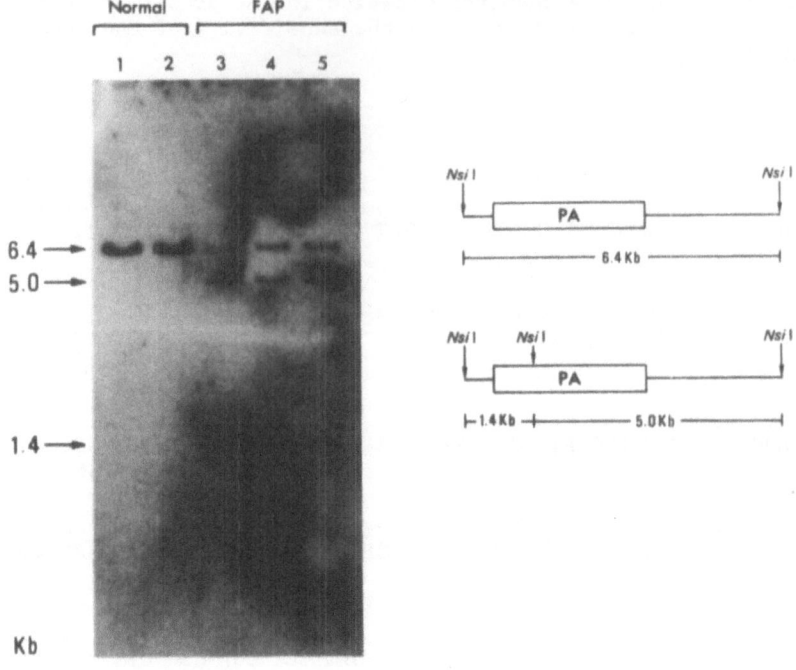

Fig. 2. Detection of a new restriction site for NsiI in the
mutated prealbumin gene. Lanes 1 and 2 represent
DNA samples from two normal individuals and lanes
3-5 those from three FAP patients. The box designated PA in the schematic drawing represents the
chromosomal prealbumin gene.

To test whether the DNA of patients has the new restriction sites expected, DNAs were prepared from two healthy normal subjects and three patients with FAP, and the prealbumin genes were analyzed by Southern hybridization as described in MATERIALS AND METHODS.

The hybridization patterns with restriction endonuclease NsiI are
shown in Fig. 2. The DNAs of the two normal individuals gave only a single
hybridization band of 6.4 Kb (lanes 1 and 2), whereas those of the FAP patients gave two additional bands of 5.0 Kb and 1.4 Kb (lanes 3-5). As illustrated schematic on the right, this can be explained by the presence of
a new restriction site for NsiI in the prealbumin locus. Similar results
were also obtained for BalI.

These results indicate that a mutation in the prealbumin gene can
easily be detected by use of restriction endonuclease BalI and/or NsiI.
The normal bands given by these FAP patients indicate that the patients are
all heterozygous for the mutant gene. Since the Val → Met change at position 30 in prealbumin was also observed in Swedish and Portuguese types of
FAP [4, 5], we believe that this method provides a method for diagnosis of
these three types of FAP presymptomatically and prenatally.

REFERENCES

1. Costa, P. P., Figueira, A. S., and Bravo, F. R., Proc. Natl. Acad.
    Sci. USA, 75:4499-4503 (1978).
2. Pras, M., Prelli, F., Franklin, E. C., and Frangione, B., Proc. Natl.
    Acad. Sci. USA, 80:539-542 (1983).

3. Tawara, S., Nakazato, M., Kangawa, K., Matsuo, H., and Araki, S., Biochem. Biophys. Res. Commun., 116:880-888 (1983).
4. Dwulet, F. E., and Benson, M. D., Proc. Natl. Acad. Sci. USA, 81:694-698 (1984).
5. Saraiva, M. J. M., Birken, S., Costa, P. P., and Goodman, D. S., J. Clin. Invest., 74:104-119 (1984).
6. Kametani, F., Tonoike, H., Hoshi, A., Shinoda, T., and Kito, S., Biochem. Biophys. Res. Commun. (1984) (in press).
7. Deeley, R. G., Gordon, J. I., Burns, A. T. H., Mullinix, K. P., Binastein, M., and Goldberger, R. F., J. Biol. Chem., 252:8310-8319 (1977).
8. Aviv, H., and Leder, P., Proc. Natl. Acad. Sci. USA, 69:1408-1412 (1972).
9. Okayama, H., and Berg, P., Mol. Cell. Biol., 2:161-170 (1982).
10. Cohn, D. H., Ogden, R. C., Abelson, J. N., Baldwin, T. O., Nealson, K. H., Simon, M. I., and Mileham, A. J., Proc. Natl. Acad. Sci. USA, 80:120-123 (1983).
11. Birnboim, H. C., and Doly, J., Nucleic Acids Res., 7:1513-1523 (1979).
12. Lis, J. T., and Schleif, R., Nucleic Acids Res., 2:383-389 (1975).
13. Sanger, F., Nicklen, S., and Coulson, A. R., Proc. Natl. Acad. Sci. USA, 74:5463-5467 (1977).
14. Ryan, J., Barker, P. E., Shimizu, K., Wigler, M., and Ruddle, F. H., Proc. Natl. Acad. Sci. USA, 80:4460-4463 (1983).
15. Krainer, A. R., Maniatis, T., Ruskin, B., and Green, M. R., Cell, 36:993-1005 (1984).
16. Zinn, K., DiMaio, D., and Maniatis, T., Cell, 34:865-879 (1983).
17. Southern, E. M., J. Mol. Biol., 98:503-517 (1975).
18. Perlman, D., and Halvorson, H. O., J. Mol. Biol., 167:391-409 (1983).

BIOCHEMICAL NATURE OF FAMILIAL AMYLOIDOTIC POLYNEUROPATHY

AND A NEW DIAGNOSTIC METHOD BY RADIOIMMUNOASSAY

M. Nakazato*, T. Kurihara*,
K. Kangawa†, N. Minamino‡,
S. Tawara**, and H. Matsuo†

*The Third Department of Internal Medicine
†Department of Biochemistry and
‡Department of Anesthesiology
 Miyazaki Medical College
 Kiyotake, Miyazaki 889-16, Japan

**Division of Medicine
  Yamaga City Hospital
  Yamaga

Familial amyloidotic polyneuropathy (FAP) in Japan is clinically similar to that of Portugal. We have reported that amyloid fibril protein isolated from Japanese FAP cases is composed of a prealbumin variant in which
a valine residue at position 30 is replaced by a methionine (Tawara
et al., 1983). Furthermore, we have clarified that this prealbumin
variant is present in the sera of Japanese FAP patients. There has been no
definite method to detect this progressive illness before clinical manifestations appear. For the purpose of developing a new, noninvasive diagnostic method, we have established a radioimmunoassay (RIA) using a nonapeptide corresponding to the subsequence [22-30] of the prealbumin variant.
The serum levels of the prealbumin variant in normal individuals, FAP patients, asymptomatic members of FAP families, primary and secondary amyloidosis cases are studied. The present RIA serves as a simple and definite
method for an early detection of this disease and an appropriate genetic
advice can be given to FAP patients and their families.

METHODS

Identification of a Prealbumin Variant in the Sera
of Japanese FAP Patients

Serum prealbumin was isolated from Japanese FAP patients by loading on
columns of Affi-Gel Blue and then Mono Q (Nakazato et al., 1984). Purified serum prealbumin was treated with cyanogen bromide, incubated in
0.2 M ammonium bicarbonate and then trypsinized. The resulting fragments
were loaded on a column of reverse phase high performance liquid chromatography (HPLC). Then, amino acid and sequence analyses of tryptic pep-

```
              5              10              15             20             25
Gly-Pro-Thr-Gly-Thr-Gly-Glu-Ser-Lys-Cys-Pro-Leu-Met-Val-Lys-Val-Leu-Asp-Ala-Val-Arg-Gly-Ser-Pro-Ala-
                                    ↓
              30             35              40             45             50
-Ile-Asn-Val-Ala-Met-His-Val-Phe-Arg-Lys-Ala-Ala-Asp-Asp-Thr-Trp-Glu-Pro-Phe-Ala-Ser-Gly-Lys-Thr-Ser-

              55             60              65             70             75
-Glu-Ser-Gly-Glu-Leu-His-Gly-Leu-Thr-Thr-Glu-Glu-Glu-Phe-Val-Glu-Gly-Ile-Tyr-Lys-Val-Glu-Ile-Asp-Thr-

              80             85              90             95             100
-Lys-Ser-Tyr-Trp-Lys-Ala-Leu-Gly-Ile-Ser-Pro-Phe-His-Glu-His-Ala-Glu-Val-Val-Phe-Thr-Ala-Asn-Asp-Ser-

              105            110             115            120            125
-Gly-Pro-Arg-Arg-Tyr-Thr-Ile-Ala-Ala-Leu-Leu-Ser-Pro-Tyr-Ser-Tyr-Ser-Thr-Thr-Ala-Val-Val-Thr-Asn-Pro-

     127
-Lys-Glu
```

Fig. 1. Amino acid sequence of the serum prealbumin variant, where Val at
         position 30 in normal prealbumin is replaced by Met.

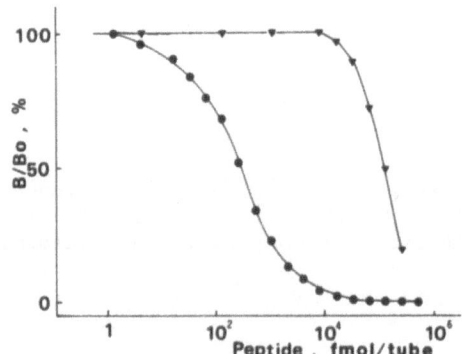

Fig. 2. Inhibition of binding of
         ^{125}I-labeled FAP nonapeptide
         to the antiserum raised
         against FAP nonapeptide by
         serial dilution of unlabeled
         ligands, i.e., FAP nonapep-
         tide (●), a tridecapeptide
         corresponding to the sub-
         sequence [22-34] in normal
         prealbumin (▼). Antiserum
         was used at a final dilution
         of 1:50,000.

tides were performed. The results revealed that there was a prealbumin
variant containing a single amino acid substitution of a methionine for
valine at position 30 in the patients' sera along with normal prealbumin.
This prealbumin variant was identical to the prealbumin variant derived
from amyloid fibrils of Japanese FAP patients. Amino acid sequence of the
prealbumin variant was demonstrated in Fig. 1.

408

Radioimmunoassay for the Prealbumin Variant

The nonapeptide amide (Gly-Ser-Pro-Ala-Ile-Asn-Val-Ala-Met-NH$_2$) corresponding to the subsequence [22-30] of the prealbumin variant was synthesized by solid phase techniques, conducted on a p-methylbenzhydrylamine resin. The nonapeptide amide was treated with cyanogen bromide in 70% formic acid. The resulting COOH-terminal homoserine lactone was converted into homoserine by incubating in 0.2 M ammonium bicarbonate (pH 8.0) at 40°C for 24 h. Conversion to homoserine was confirmed by HPLC. We designated a nonapeptide with a homoserine at the COOH-terminus as FAP nonapeptide.

FAP nonapeptide was conjugated with bovine thyroglobulin by the glutaraldehyde method. The resulting antigenic conjugate was used for immunizing New Zealand White rabbits. [Tyr^0]-FAP nonapeptide was radioiodinated by the lactoperoxidase method. The ^{125}I-labeled peptide was purified by loading on a reverse phase HPLC column. RIA procedure was described in our previous report (Nakazato et al., 1984). The antiserum raised against FAP nonapeptide recognized this peptide with high affinity at a final dilution of 1:50,000. Mean binding of ^{125}I-labeled FAP nonapeptide to the antiserum was 300 fmole/tube and the measurable range of the assay was 4-10^4 fmole, as demonstrated in Fig. 2. Cross-reactivity of a tridecapeptide corresponding to the subsequence [22-34] of normal prealbumin was markedly low (0.4%) in comparison to that of FAP nonapeptide and other tryptic peptides did not appreciably cross-react with the antiserum. Therefore, this RIA specifically detected the prealbumin variant with a Met^{30} substitution. Moreover, the RIA was reproducible with the intra-assay variability of ±7.5%, and the coefficient of variation of the interassay variability was 6.8%.

Prior to examining the serum level of the prealbumin variant, this RIA was checked to preclude assay of any cross-reactive substances in the serum as described previously (Nakazato et al., 1984). This RIA was specific for detecting the subsequence in the prealbumin variant with Val → Met replacement at position 30.

Serum Concentration of the Prealbumin Variant

The subjects studied here consisted of 60 normal individuals aged from 2 to 60 years with a mean age of 32.4 ± 9.8 (SD) years; 14 Japanese FAP cases (7 males and 7 females) aged from 25 to 49 years with a mean of 36.6 ± 7.7 years; 22 asymptomatic members of FAP families aged from 6 to 64 years with a mean of 28.8 ± 18.7 years; 3 cases of primary amyloidosis aged 43, 55, and 56 years; and 4 cases of secondary amyloidosis associated with rheumatoid arthritis or polymyositis aged 36, 46, 59, and 59 years. All the amyloidotic patients were definitely diagnosed by biopsy studies.

The sera (5 µl) of FAP patients, normal individuals, members of families with FAP, and primary or secondary amyloidosis cases were lyophilized. The sera were treated with cyanogen bromide in 70% formic acid for 48 h and then re-lyophilized. Afterwards, the resulting fragments were incubated in 0.2 M ammonium bicarbonate (pH 8.0) at 40°C for 24 h. They were then digested with TPCK-treated trypsin at 37°C for 2 h. Thereafter, soy trypsin inhibitor was added to the buffer to stop the reaction. The recovery rate of the RIA was 61%. Samples were assayed by the procedure previously reported and the serum level of the prealbumin variant was determined (Nakazato et al., 1984). In addition to the prealbumin variant, the serum level of total prealbumin was determined by using a single radial immunodiffusion plate for prealbumin (Behringwerke).

The serum levels of the prealbumin variant in 60 normal individuals ranged from 0.08 to 0.16 mg/dl with a mean of 0.12 ± 0.02 mg/dl. However,

TABLE 1. The Serum Levels of the Prealbumin Variant and
Total Prealbumin in 14 Japanese FAP Patients

Case Number	Age Sex	Age of Onset (yrs)	Duration of Illness (yrs)	Prealbumin Variant (mg/dl)	Total Prealbumin (mg/dl)
No. 1	25/M	23	2	9.59	16.6
No. 2	29/M	27	2	7.60	17.2
No. 3	30/F	25	5	11.80	20.0
No. 4	30/M	27	3	9.93	23.9
No. 5	31/M	26	5	11.36	23.6
No. 6	31/F	27	4	7.59	15.8
No. 7	33/M	32	1	11.67	22.4
No. 8	37/F	30	7	7.41	25.0
No. 9	39/F	32	7	9.36	18.4
No.10	42/M	32	10	8.34	20.6
No.11	44/F	37	7	9.52	19.8
No.12	45/M	38	7	13.23	21.7
No.13	47/F	44	3	8.18	13.3
No.14	49/F	39	10	6.46	16.9
Mean	36.6	31.4	5.2	9.43	19.7

TABLE 2.   The Serum Levels of the Prealbumin
           Variant and Total Prealbumin in 10
           Non-Inheriting FAP Families

Subject	Age Sex (yrs)	Prealbumin Variant (mg/dl)	Total Prealbumin (mg/dl)
1	30/M	0	36.7
2	31/M	0	26.8
3	33/F	0	26.8
4	39/F	0	30.7
5	43/F	0	28.0
6	50/F	0	29.6
7	53/M	0	41.5
8	58/F	0	24.8
9	62/M	0	35.8
10	64/M	0	25.9
Mean	46.3	0	30.7

these results did not indicate that the prealbumin variant was present at this concentration in normal human serum based on the findings described below. Prealbumin was isolated from normal human serum by Affi-Gel Blue affinity chromatography and anion exchange chromatography. Purified serum prealbumin was cleaved by cyanogen bromide and trypsinized, then applied to reverse phase HPLC. Each fraction was submitted to the RIA for FAP nonapeptide. Immunoreactivity was not observed at the elution position of FAP nonapeptide derived from the prealbumin variant. A small amount of immunoreactivity was noted at the elution position of a tridecapeptide corresponding to the subsequence [22-34] of normal prealbumin. It had been already clarified that the tridecapeptide cross-reacted up to 0.4% with the antiserum. Therefore, the value of the prealbumin variant in normal human serum was verified to originate from the cross-reactivity to the tridecapeptide derived from normal serum prealbumin and the prealbumin variant was not present in normal human serum. With respect to total serum prealbumin in normal individuals, the value ranged from 24.0 to 35.8 mg/dl with a mean of 30.6 ± 4.4 (SD) mg/dl.

Table 1 summarized the serum levels of the prealbumin variant and total prealbumin in 14 Japanese FAP patients. The serum levels of the prealbumin variant ranged from 6.46 to 13.23 mg/dl with a mean of 9.43 ± 1.99 mg/dl. The serum levels of the prealbumin variant were not related to the age of onset, sex, nor the duration of the illness of FAP patients. Not only the case whose duration of illness was 10 years (Case 10, 14), but also the case with a duration of illness for less than a year (Case 7) had high serum levels of the prealbumin variant. The serum levels of the total prealbumin ranged from 13.3 to 25.0 mg/dl with a mean of 19.7 ± 3.4 mg/dl, which were about 2/3 of the control values.
mg/dl with a mean of 19.7 ± 3.4 mg/dl, which were about 2/3 of the control values.

Table 2 summarized the serum levels of the prealbumin variant and total prealbumin in 10 unaffected members of FAP families, whose ages were above 30 years. It should be noted that the value of the serum prealbumin variant in these family members ranged from 0.10 to 0.15 mg/dl, which was within normal limits. By the same token as in normal individuals, the prealbumin variant was not actually present in the sera of non-inheriting family members and the data obtained by the RIA resulted from the cross-reactivity to normal serum prealbumin.

The serum levels of the prealbumin variant and total prealbumin of 12 children of FAP patients were studied. Six children had the same levels of the prealbumin variant and total prealbumin as controls. On the other hand, the other six had high serum levels of the prealbumin variant, which ranged from 7.38 to 14.21 mg/dl with a mean of 11.80 ± 1.68 mg/dl. These high values were not significantly related to their ages, nor sex. No difference was noted in the serum level of total prealbumin between the two groups of children.

DISCUSSION

FAP results from the systemic deposition of amyloid fibrils which are most likely formed by the serum prealbumin variant and a small amount of other constituents. Quantitative analysis of the serum prealbumin variant could become an important clue to the definite diagnosis of this disorder and it could help to elucidate the pathophysiological mechanism of amyloid deposition.

Normal prealbumin is composed of four identical subunits of 127 amino acid residues. The structural difference between normal prealbumin and the prealbumin variant is only one amino acid replacement. Thus, it is difficult to differentiate the two by the direct immunological method using an antiserum against a whole molecule of the prealbumin variant. Since the prealbumin variant has a methionine for valine substitution at position 30, cyanogen bromide cleavage occurs at position 30. However, in normal prealbumin cyanogen bromide cleavage does not occur at the position. A nonapeptide corresponding to the subsequence [22-30] is specifically derived from the prealbumin variant by cyanogen bromide cleavage followed by tryptic digestion. The prealbumin variant is now measured quantitatively by the RIA using FAP nonapeptide.

Japanese FAP patients have high serum levels of the prealbumin variant from the early stage of this illness. The serum prealbumin variant is not present in normal individuals, nor in primary or secondary amyloidosis cases, nor in non-inheriting family members. The serum prealbumin variant is required to develop this disorder. Measurement of the serum prealbumin variant is a promising, new, and noninvasive diagnostic method for the disease. The present study also shows that serum prealbumin of FAP patients consists of normal prealbumin and the prealbumin variant in an approximately equal ratio. The ratio probably indicates that normal prealbumin and the prealbumin variant are the products of a nearly co-dominant expression of two allelic genes in the heterogeneous state. Very recently it has been clarified that one of the patients' prealbumin alleles has undergone mutation resulting in G to A transition in the 5' terminal position of the valine codon and this transition is reponsible for a methioine for valine substitution.

We have clarified that the serum prealbumin variant forming amyloid fibrils exists in subclinical stages in the sera of children of FAP patients. Children having high serum levels of the prealbumin variant will most likely develop this illness; therefore, they have to be observed closely. An early genetic advice to asymptomatic family members and a wide screening test among relatives of diseased families can be performed by studying the serum prealbumin variant. Furthermore, quantitative analysis of the serum prealbumin variant can be used as an objective index in the process of developing an effective treatment in the future. The prealbumin variant with a methionine for valine substitution at position 30 is present in the sera of FAP patients originating in Sweden (Dwulet and Benson, 1983) and Portugal (Saraiva et al., 1984) as well as Japan. Therefore, this RIA is widely applicable to this intractable familial disorder in the world for the purpose of an early diagnosis and constructive genetic advice.

Sasaki, Sakaki, Takagi, their colleague and Matsuo have recently developed another method for diagnosis of FAP based on the recombinant DNA techniques. cDNA for human prealbumin was cloned and its nucleotide sequence was determined. The results showed that the nucleotide substitution responsible for the Val → Met change resulted in formation of new restriction sites for BalI and NsiI. By Southern blot hybridization analysis, the expected restriction sites were actually detected in the prealbumin locus of FAP patients. Thus, FAP can also be diagnosed by this method prenatally and in early subclinical stages.

REFERENCES

Dwulet, F. E., and Benson, M. D., Biochem. Biophys. Res. Commun., 114:657 (1983).

Nakazato, M., Kangawa, K., Minamino, N., Tawara, S., Matsuo, H., and Araki, S., Biochem. Biophys. Res. Commun., 122:712 (1984).

Nakazato, M., Kangawa, K., Minamino, N., Tawara, S., Matsuo, H., and Araki, S., Biochem. Biophys. Res. Commun., 122:719 (1984).

Saraiva, M. J., Birken, S., Costa, P. P., and Goodman, D. S., J. Clin. Invest., 74:104 (1984).

Tawara, S., Nakazato, M., Kangawa, K., Matsuo, H., and Araki, S., Biochem. Biophys. Res. Commun., 116:880 (1983).

CLINICAL AND PATHOLOGICAL STUDIES OF FAMILIAL AMYLOID POLYNEUROPATHY (FAP),

WITH SPECIAL REFERENCE TO NEPHROPATHY AND CARDIOPATHY

Shu-ichi Ikeda*, Norinao Hanyu*,
Nobuo Yanagisawa*, Minoru Hongo*,
Hisao Oguchi*, and Nobuo Ito†

*Department of Medicine
 Shinshu University School of Medicine
 Matsumoto 390, Japan

†Department of Pathology
 Shinshu University School of Medicine
 Matsumoto 390, Japan

ABSTRACT

We made a clinicopathological study of 48 cases with FAP in Nagano Prefecture, Japan. The age of onset ranged widely from 16 to 62 years. The main neurological manifestations were polyneuropathy which started in the legs and progressed in an ascending fashion, and various autonomic dysfunctions. Cranial nerves were also affected in the advanced stage, producing facial palsy and bulbar signs. Clinically apparent renal dysfunction was infrequent, but some cases showed a remarkable nephropathy with heavy proteinuria from an early stage. Cardiac involvement was frequent. Electrocardiographic abnormalities with conduction disturbances appeared at first and cardiac biopsy revealed positive amyloid deposition, and congestive heart failure due to severe amyloid heart disease occurred in the terminal stage. We propose that Japanese FAP provide a broad clinical spectrum affecting more systemic organs than previously known.

INTRODUCTION

Familial amyloid polyneuropathy (FAP) is the most common form of heredofamilial amyloidosis. The disease was first described by Andrade in Portugal in 1952 [1] and since then a large number of afflicted kinships have been reported from several other countries; at present four clinical phenotypes are recognized on the basis of neuropathic patterns and different systemic organ involvement [2, 3].

The clinical pictures of Japanese FAP have already been reported to be similar to those of Portuguese FAP (type I FAP) [4, 5]. However, as many kinships with this disease have recently been found in our country, Japanese FAP seems to provide a broad clinical spectrum. In this paper, we deal with the clinicopathological study of Japanese FAP with special attention to nephropathy and cardiopathy, both of which have been thought to be rare in type I FAP.

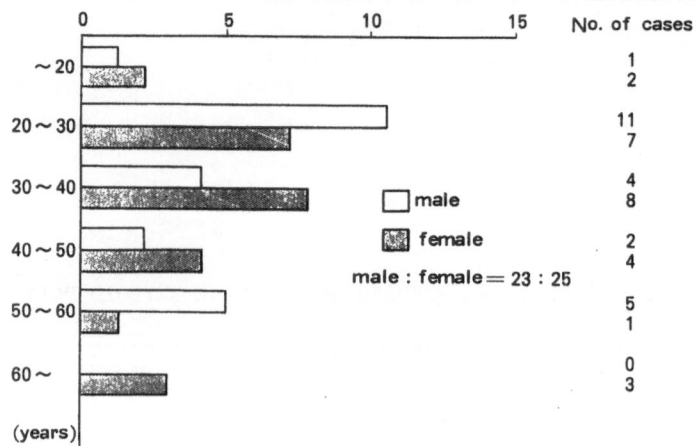

Fig. 1

TABLE 1

Symptoms	Number of cases
Dysesthesia in the lower limbs	21
Weakness of the lower limbs	3
Anorexia	2
Severe constipation	9
Uncontrollable diarrhea	2
Impotence	4
Orthostatic fainting	3
Bullous formations	1
Hematuria	1
Decreased visual acuity	2

TABLE 2

Signs and symptoms	No.	Signs and symptoms	No.
Neuropathic signs		Urinary and fecal incontinence	21
Distal sensory dullness		Trophic changes of the skin	
with dissociation	46	and anhidrosis	31
Distal amyotrophy and weakness	38	Others	
Sensory dullness of the anterior		Arrhythmia	17
thoracoabdominal wall	24	Congestive heart failure	2
Facial weakness	7	Goiter	4
Facial sensory dullness	3	Macroglossia	12
Bulbar signs	6	Edema	8
Decrease or loss of taste	7	Bullous formations	12
Autonomic symptoms		Charcot's joint	3
Anorexia, nausea and vomiting	28	Stokes—Adams attack	8
Alternating constipation		Implantation of	
and diarrhea	38	artificial pacemaker	8
Hypotension	14	Pupillary abnormalities	12
Orthostatic hypotension	27	Glaucoma	2
Impotence	18	Vitreous opacity	2
Dysuria	30	Hyperreflexia in the extremities	9

416

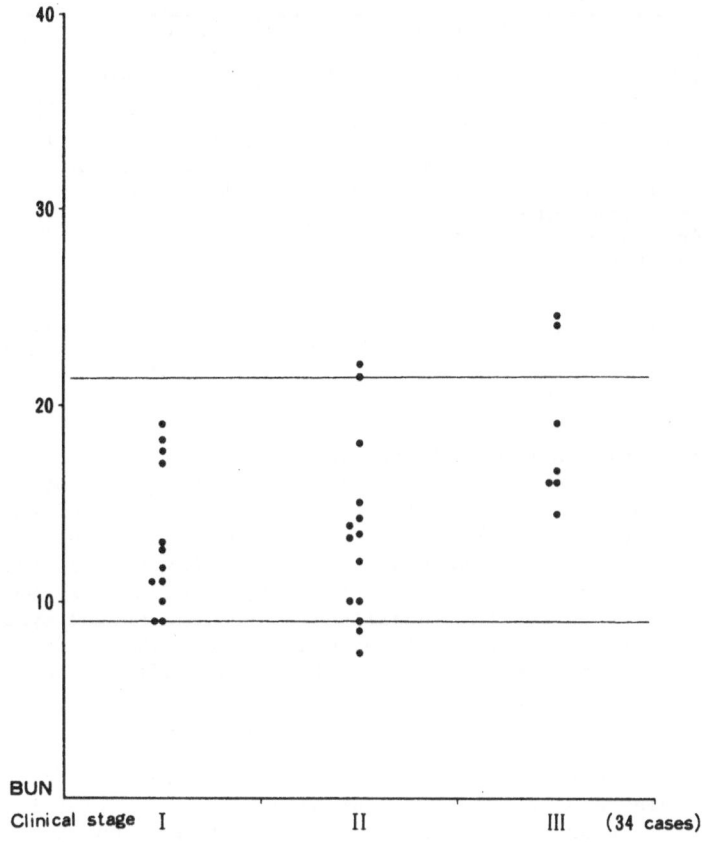

Fig. 2. The clinical stages of FAP are divided into
three groups according to Coutinho et al. [8].
Stage I: The patients can walk unaided, Stage
II: Patient can move with help, Stage III: Patient is bedridden.

Clinical Pictures

During the past ten years we have found 48 cases with FAP from 31
families (45 cases from 30 families in Ogawa village and neighboring area
[6], and 3 cases from 1 family in Miyata village without any genealogical
relation to the families in the former) in Nagano Prefecture, Japan. All
cases were shown to have amyloid deposition by one or more biopsies of the
stomach, rectum, myocardium, skin and sural nerve.

The age of onset ranged widely from 16 to 62 years (Fig. 1), but in
about half of the cases it was between 25 and 35 years. The most frequent
initial symptom was dysesthesia in the lower limbs, sometimes associated
with an intolerable burning or shooting pain in the legs. Next came digestive symptoms including severe constipation, uncontrollable diarrhea or
anorexia. Severe constipation frequently preceded other symptoms by
several years. Impotence in males was also an important initial complaint
(Table 1).

The clinical manifestations frequently observed are listed in Table
2. Two of the main ones were polyneuropathy and autonomic dysfunction.

TABLE 3

	Family M		Family S		
Case	1	2	3	4	
Age & Sex	52, F	51, F	44, F	43, F	37, F
Nephropathy					
Age at detection	48	45	40	35	
Edema	−	+	+++	+	(−)
Proteinuria	1–3g/day	100–300mg/dl	5–6g/day	2–3g/day	
BUN (mg/dl)	35	25	60	20	
Neurological manifestations					
Age at onset	51	45	36	38	26
Neuropathic signs					
Upper extremities	−	+	++	−	+
Lower extremities	+	+++	+++	+	++
Autonomic disorders	+	++	+++	+	++

Severity of symptoms :+: slight, ++: moderate, +++: remarkable

Sensory dullness with dysesthesia started in the legs and progressed in an ascending fashion. Although at an early stage disturbance of thermal and pain senses predominated, later all senses were lost with diffuse amyotrophy and weakness in the limbs, and about half of these cases showed sensory dullness of the anterior thoracoabdominal wall. Cases in an advanced stage revealed diminished or absent tendon reflexes, especially in the lower limbs; 8 cases with neuropathy localized in the legs showed symmetrically increased tendon reflexes in all limbs without Babinski's sign at our first examination, but several years later their tendon reflexes were diminished or absent. At a later stage lower cranial nerves were also affected, presenting as facial weakness with lagophthalmos, facial sensory dullness, decrease or loss of tastes and bulbar signs. Several autonomic symptoms invariably appeared in the course of the disease and in particular, digestive symptoms including severe anorexia, periodic nausea and vomiting and alternating constipation and diarrhea with incontinence continually distressed and exhausted patients. Cardiac involvement often revealed various patterns of arrhythmia, and 8 cases with illness for more than 7 years experienced Stokes–Adams syndrome due to sinus arrest or complete atrioventricular block and had pacemakers implanted. Moreover, congestive heart failure was seen in 2 cases at the terminal stage. Goiter, macroglossia, Charcot's joint and ocular lesions also occurred.

Nephropathy in FAP

To investigate renal function in FAP we examined blood urea nitrogen (BUN) in 34 cases in different clinical stages (Fig. 2). One bedridden case was in a state of renal failure (BUN: 73); other revealed almost normal values, while slight proteinuria was observed in 6. However, in addition to these 34 cases, we had another 4 who showed severe nephropathy from an early stage. Clinical pictures of these 4 cases and one case without nephropathy in the same family are summarized in Table 3.

Case 1, as a representative case, was a 52 year-old thin female who had been suffering from bilateral glaucoma caused by amyloid deposition since the age of 44. At 48 proteinurea was detected and by the age of 51 coldness of the legs, constipation and orthostatic fainting had appeared. Physical examination revealed only hypotension, slight muscular weakness and dissociated sensory loss of the legs. Motor and sensory nerve conduction velocities were normal in both upper and lower limbs. Laboratory studies revealed albuminurea, increased BUN and creatinine, and moderately delayed excretion of phenolsulfonaphthalein. Needle biopsy of the right kidney showed prominent amyloid deposition in the glomeruli and vessels in

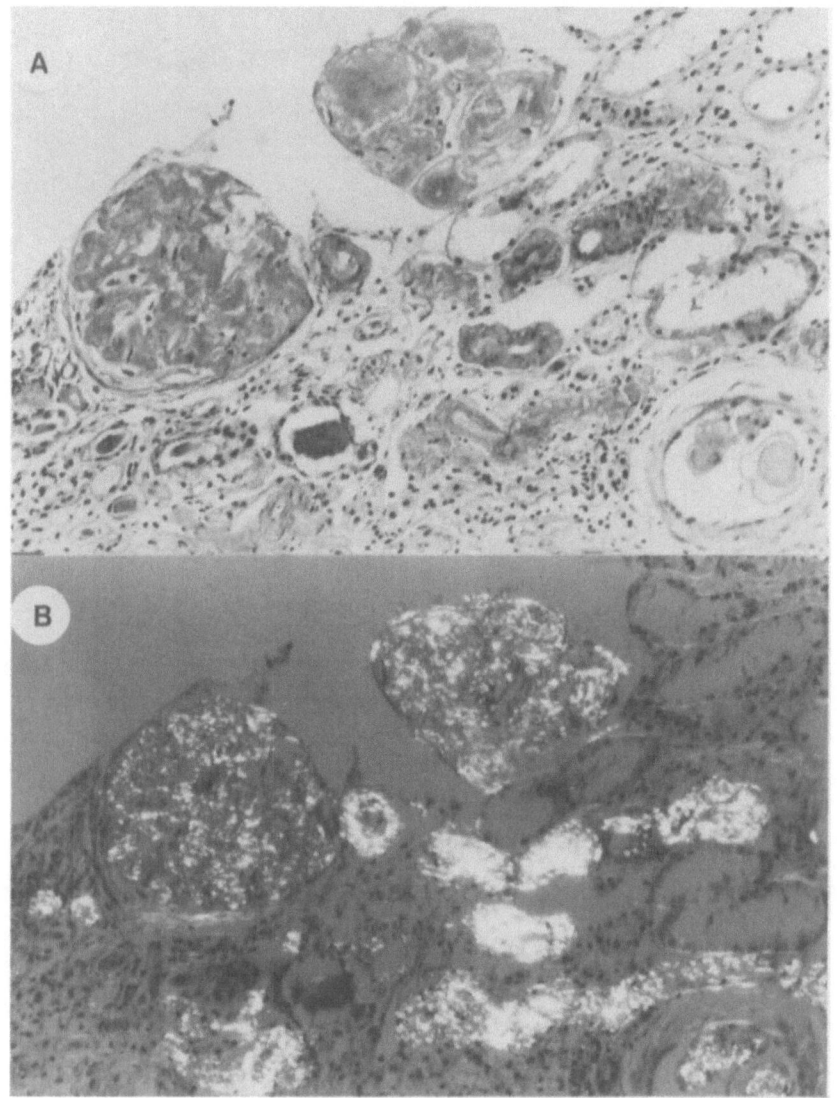

Fig. 3. Renal biopsy finding from case 1. A: Congo red stain,
B: Same section viewed through crossed polars. There
are severe amyloid depositions in the glomeruli and
vessel walls. Original magnification ×150.

the preparation with Congo red stain (Fig. 3-A, B). Later her neuropathy
slowly progressed and several autonomic dysfunctions appeared.

Cardiopathy in FAP

To determine cardiac involvement in FAP, we examined the electrocardiogram (ECG), endomyocardial biopsy and cardiothoracic ratio (CTR) on the
thoracid roentogenogram. ECG was recorded from 22 cases and 20 cases
showed abnormalities (Table 4), which included various patterns of conduction disturbances, low voltage in the standard limb leads and QS configuration in the right precordial leads (Fig. 4). Four cases lacked these find-

TABLE 4

1) QRS changes	No. of cases
Low voltage in the standard limb leads	1
QS in the right precordial leads	7
Decreased voltage of R waves and deep S waves in the right precordial leads	6
Small R waves in leads V_5 and V_6	14
2) Abnormal left axis deviation	5
3) Ischemic ST–T changes	6
4) Rhythm and conduction disturbances	
Sinus arrest	2
Ectopic atrial rhythm	1
Atrial fibrillation	1
1st atrioventricular block	9
2nd atrioventricular block	1
Complete atrioventricular block	2
Right bundle branch block alone	2
Right bundle branch block with anterior hemiblock	3
Left bundle branch block	1

TABLE 5

ECG changes	No. of cases			
	Total	Clinical stage		
		I	II	III
Low voltage in the standard limb leads	1			1
QS in the right precordial leads				
Decreased voltage of R waves and deep S waves in the right precordial leads	6		2	4
Small R waves in leads V_5 and V_6	4	3	1	

TABLE 6

Patient	Age	Sex	Duration of symptoms(yr)	Clinical stage	Cardiac symptoms	CTR(%)	Amyloid deposition
1	40	M	2	I	no	50	moderate
2	38	F	3	I	no	44	severe
3	46	F	6	I	no	38	severe
4	59	M	4	II	no	47	moderate
5	59	M	6	II	no	41	severe
6	49	F	9	II	S–A	49	severe
7	49	F	28	III	S–A	50	severe

Abbreviations: M = male, F = female, S–A = Stokes–Adams syndrome

ings, but disclosed a characteristic pattern of decreased voltage of R waves and deep S waves in the right precordial leads and small R waves in leads V_5 and V_6 (Fig. 5). Cases with low voltage in the standard limb leads and QS configuration in the right precordial leads showed more advanced neurological signs than these 4 (Table 5).

We performed transvenous right ventricular endomyocardial biopsy in 7 cases. Paraffin-embedded samples were cut and were stained with H & E and 1% Congo red. Some were used for electron-microscopic examination. Moderate or severe amyloid deposition was observed in all, including 5 cases without any cardiac symptoms (Table 6). In the subendocardium patchy deposits of amyloid were seen, and in other regions myocardial cells

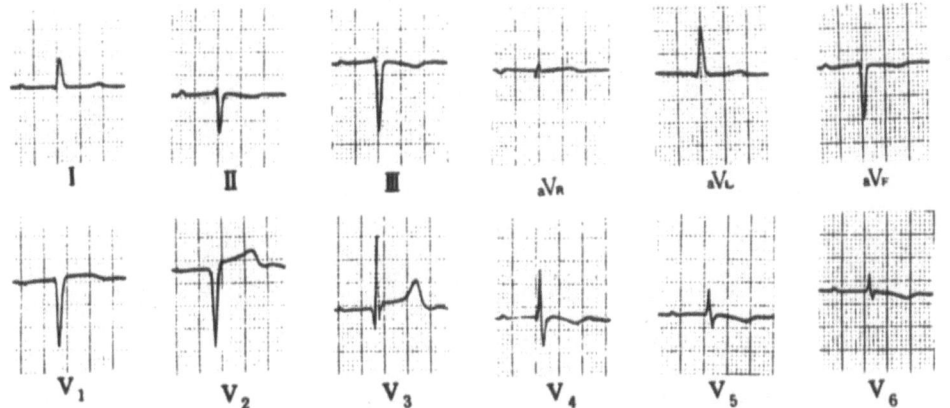

Fig. 4. ECG from a case in the advanced stage showing prolongation of P-Q interval, left axis deviation, QS configuration in V₁ and V₂ and small R waves in V₅ and V₆.

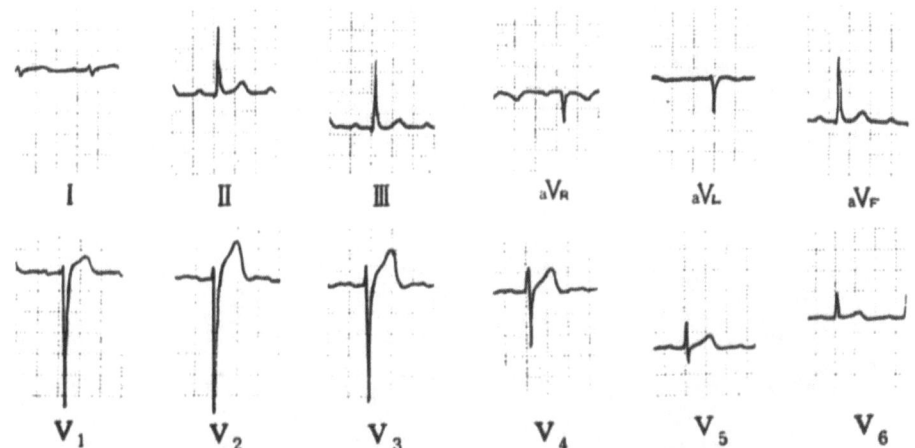

Fig. 5. ECG from a case in the early stage showing decreased R waves and deep S waves in V₁ and V₃ and small R waves in V₅ and V₆.

were surrounded by rings of amyloid, resulting in degeneration (Fig. 6-A, B and C). In severely affected regions only amyloid rings were observed. There were deposits also in the vascular walls and connective tissues.

CTR was measured in 33 cases in different clinical stages (Fig. 7). Most showed neither cardiac enlargement nor clinically overt heart failure, but three cases in stage III had an enlarged heart and 2 of them suffered from congestive heart failure. The following case is representative of severe amyloid heart disease.

A 61-year-old man was first admitted to our hospital because of muscular weakness and dysesthesia in the lower limbs. His neurological symptoms had been present for three years and his younger sister and cousin had similar neurological disabilities. On examination, neuropathic signs including muscular atrophy and weakness, sensory dullness with dissociation, and diminished or absent tendon reflexes were prominent in the lower extremities and were moderate in the hands and forearms. ECG showed first

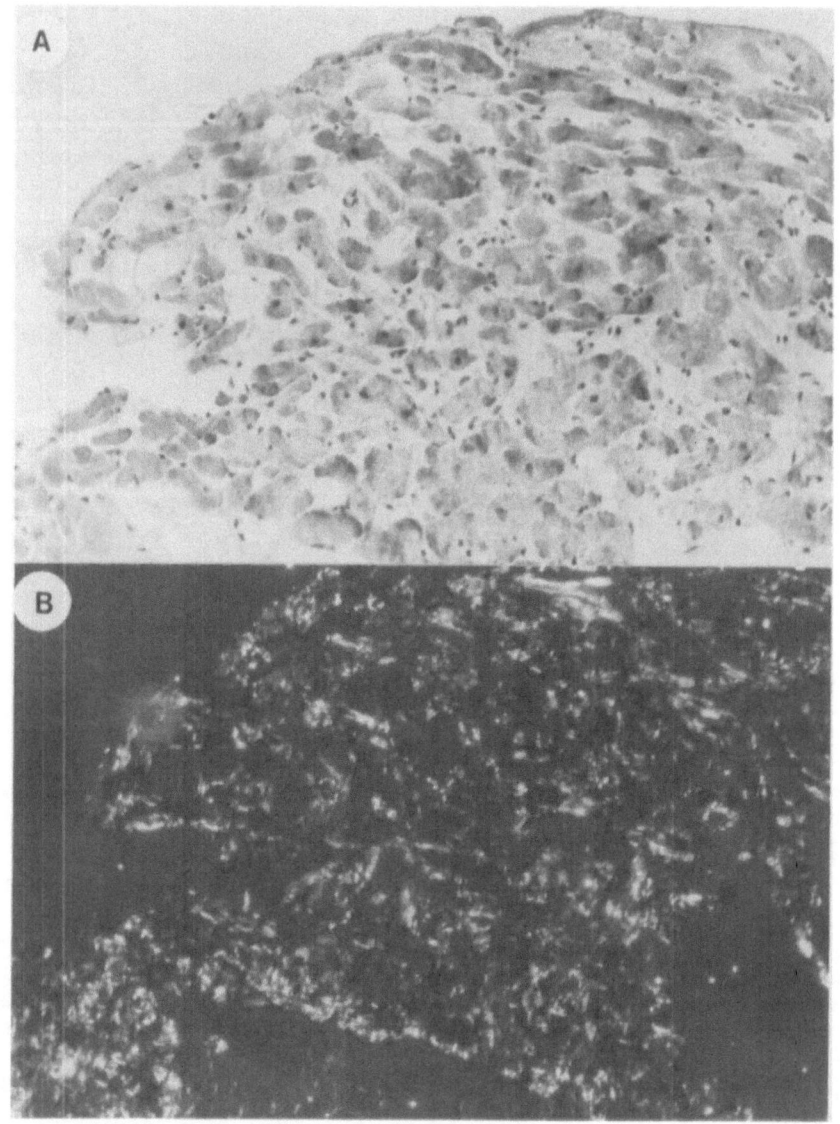

Fig. 6A, B.

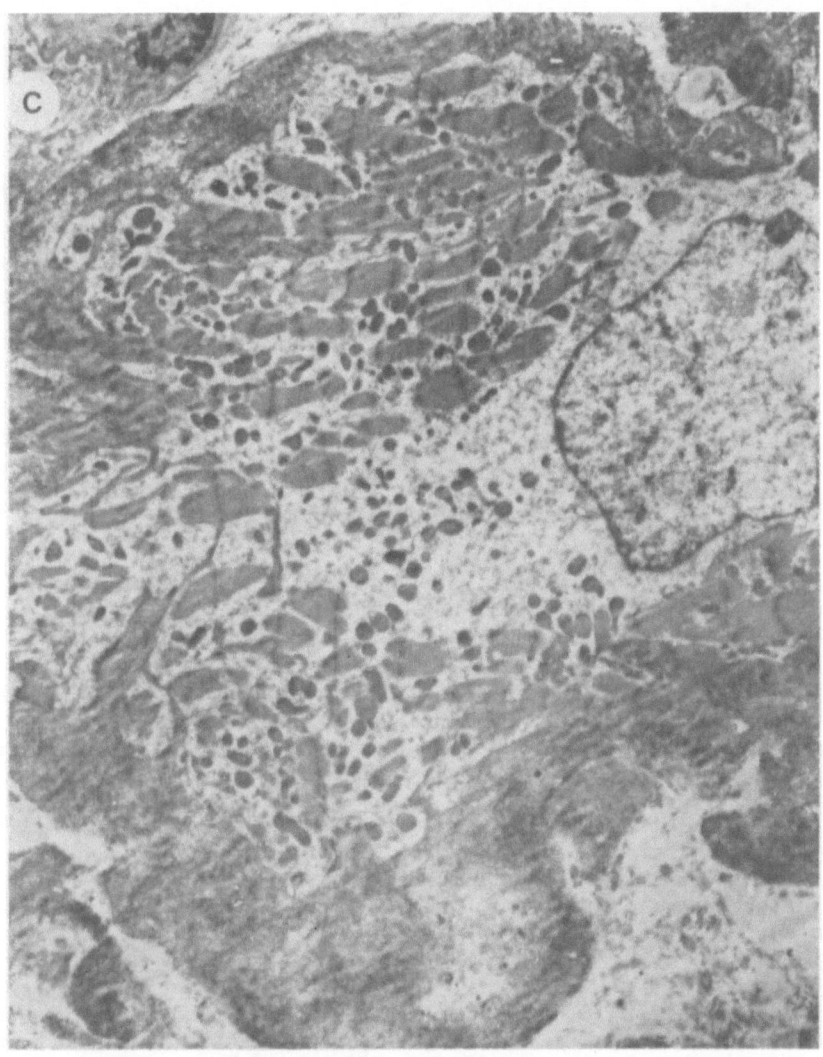

Fig. 6. Cardiac biopsy findings from case 3. A: The section
stained with Congo red. There are remarkable deposits of
amyloid in the myocardium. Original magnification ×150.
C: Electron photomicrograph at low magnification. Degenerated myocardial cell is surrounded by dense layer of
amyloid fibril. Original magnification ×4500.

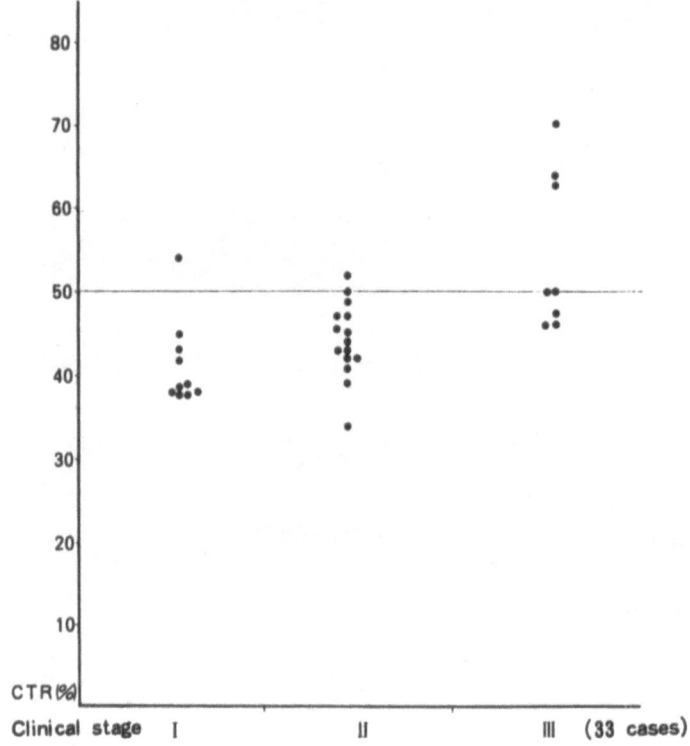

Fig. 7.   The clinical stages of FAP are the same as in
          Fig. 2.

degree atrioventricular block and right bundle branch block with anterior
hemiblock, but there were no cardiac symptoms and the cardiac shadow on
the thoracic roentogenogram was normal (Fig. 8-A).   Amyloid deposition was
found in both gastric and sural nerve biopsies.   Impotence and gastrointestinal disorders subsequently appeared.   At age 63 he had a pacemaker implanted because of complete atrioventricular block and at age 65 he was
hospitalized complaining of precordial discomfort.   Examination showed
cardiac enlargement with bilateral pleural effusion and edema in the legs.
Echocardiography disclosed increased thickness of the ventricular septum
and left ventricular wall with diminished motion and pericardial effusion.
He was diagnosed as having congestive heart failure due to amyloid heart
disease.   Administration of furosemide relieved his cardiac symptoms and
right heart catheterization performed just before discharge showed normal
pressure pulses, but his cardiac output was reduced (3.0 1/min).   Figure
8-B is his thoracic roentogenogram at this time.   The cardiac shadow is
considerably enlarged over that at first admission.   Four months later he
was readmitted because of orthopnea and remarkable general edema.   His condition again improved with the administration of furosemide, but he died
suddenly from subarachnoid hemorrhage 20 days after admission.   Necropsy
findings showed that he had an arteriovenous malformation of the spinal
cord which produced the fatal subarachnoid hemorrhage.   Amyloid had accumulated extensively in the peripheral nerves, vagal nerve and sympathetic
ganglia (Fig. 9-A, B).   Cardiac weight was increased (600 g) and there was
marked hypertrophy of the left ventricular wall and ventricular septum
(Fig. 10).   Microscopic examination showed remarkable deposition of amyloid
in the myocardium, especially in the subendocardial region.

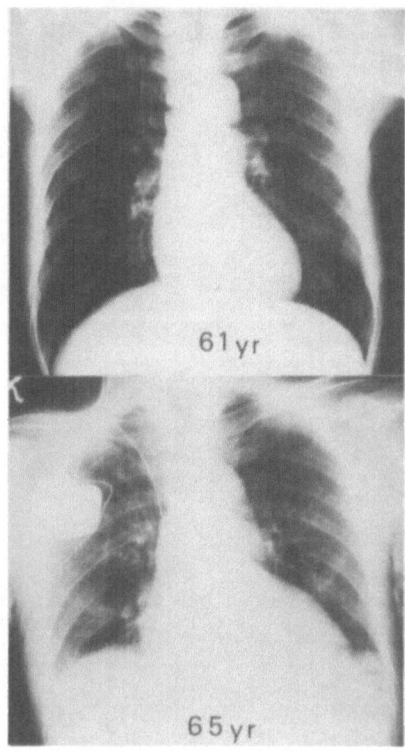

Fig. 8. The change of cardiac
shadow on the thoracic
roentogenogram.

DISCUSSION

Neurological Manifestations

Araki et al. [4] reported the first Japanese cases of FAP from Arao city in Kumamoto Prefecture, in the southern part of the country; their clinical pictures were said to be similar to those of Portuguese FAP (type I FAP) [5], and Kito et al. [6] came to much the same conclusion from a clinical study of cases with FAP from Ogawa village in Nagano Prefecture, in the central part of Japan. In our cases, the age of onset showed a wider range than previously described in Japan and corresponded closely with the reports from Swedish [7] and Portuguese [8] families with FAP. The neurological manifestations of progressive polyneuropathy starting in the legs and various autonomic dysfunctions satisfied the criteria for type I FAP [2] except for the cranial nerve involvement, but this cranial neuropathy was only seen in the cases at an advanced stage and was easily distinguishable from that of type IV FAP [9].

Nephropathy

The absence of remarkable nephropathy was used to differentiate type I FAP from type III (Van Allen's form) [10]. In fact Andrade mentioned in his original report that kidney was severely affected by amyloid deposition [1], but later reports [8, 11] stated that there was no nephrotic syndrome nor uremia in the cases of Portuguese origin, and in Swedish FAP amyloid deposition in the kidney was found to be insignificant on necropsy [12].

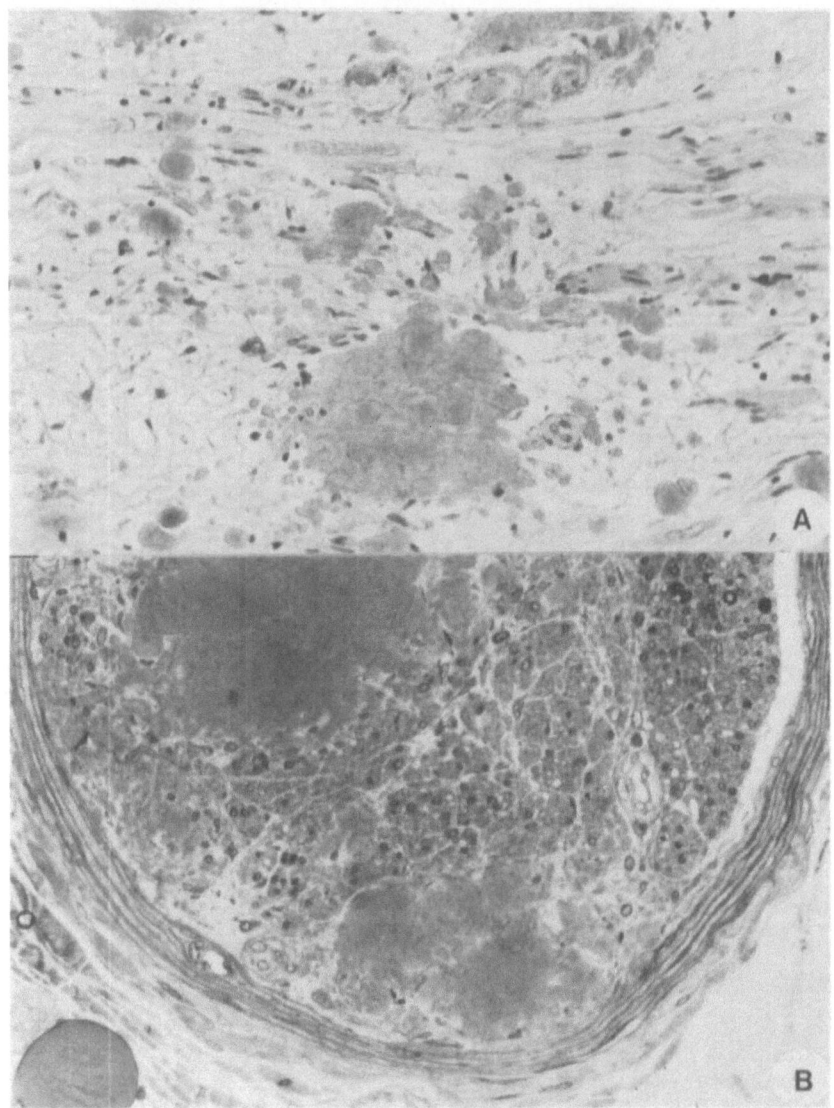

Fig. 9. A: Sciatic nerve stained with Klüver Barrera. Heavy
deposits of amyloid are present and remaining myelinated
nerves are few. Original magnification ×300. B: Toluidine blue stain of vagus nerve embedded in an epoxy-resin
mixture. The conglomerate deposits of amyloid are visible. Original magnification ×300.

In most of our cases renal function was relatively preserved even at the
more advanced stage. However, some cases from the same area showed severe
nephropathy with marked proteinuria from the start, although their neurological manifestations were identical with those of cases without nephropathy, and renal biopsy from one of them disclosed prominent deposition of
amyloid in the glomeruli and vessels. Clinical pictures similar to these
cases were reported as a familial generalized amyloidosis characterized by
initial involvement of peripheral nerves in the lower extremities by Benson
et al. [13].

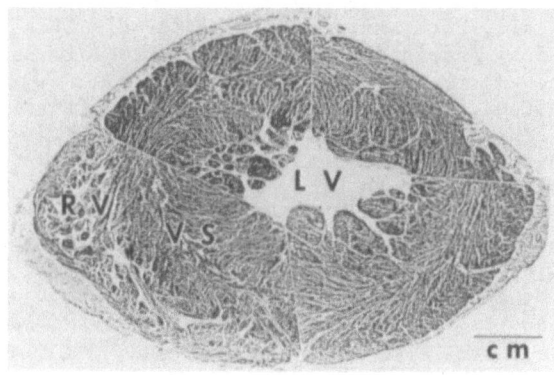

Fig. 10. Transverse plane of the heart showing thickened ventricular septum
and left ventricular wall.

Cardiopathy

It was reported that cardiac involvement frequently showed various
electrocardiographic abnormalities with conduction disturbances but did not
cause cardiac insufficiency in Portuguese [14, 15] and Japanese FAP [16].
On the other hand, in Swedish [17] and English FAP [18] some cases suffered
from severe amyloid heart disease with congestive heart failure. In the
present study the incidence of prominent cardiopathy was indeed low, but
cardiac biopsy disclosed that the myocardium was involved from the early
stage; this finding was supported by the electrocardiographic changes which
frequently preceded cardiac symptoms. Moreover, it is notable that amyloid
deposition heavy enough to cause cardiac hypertrophy with congestive heart
failure occurred in some cases in the terminal stage, and the appearance
of these enlarged hearts closely resembled that of amyloid hearts seen in
other forms of systemic amyloidosis [19].

In conclusion, it is clear from our study that the clinical pictures
of Japanese FAP are variable and that the significant nephropathy and cardiopathy which were very often seen in the nonhereditary generalized amyloidosis [20, 21] may occur in addition to the predominant polyneuropathy and
autonomic dysfunction. There are, therefore, some differences between
Japanese FAP and Portuguese FAP, and the former seems to provide a broader
clinical spectrum of systemic disease.

REFERENCES

1. C. Andrade, Brain, 75:408 (1952).
2. M. Mahloudji et al., Medicine, 48:1 (1969).
3. A. S. Cohen and M. D. Benson, in: Peripheral Neuropathy, P. J. Dick,
    P. K. Thoma, and E. H. Lambert, Ed. (Philadelphia, 1975), Chapter 53.
4. S. Araki et al., Arch. Neurol., 18:593 (1968).
5. C. Andrade et al., Arthritis Rheum., 13:902 (1970).
6. S. Kito et al., Eur. Neurol., 18:141 (1980).
7. R. Andersson, Acta Med. Scand., Suppl., 590:1 (1976).
8. R. Coutinho et al., in: Amyloid and Amyloidosis, G. G. Glenner,
    P. P. Costa, A. F. Freitas, Ed. (Excerpta Medica, 1980), p. 88.
9. J. Meretoja, Ann. Clin. Res., 1:314 (1969).
10. M. W. Van Allen et al., Neurology, 19:10 (1969).

11. J. S. Hota et al., Path. Microbiol., 27:809 (1964).
12. P. A. Hoer and R. Andersoon, Acta Path. Microbiol. Scand. Sect. A, 83:309 (1975).
13. M. D. Benson et al., Ann. Intern. Med., 86:419 (1977).
14. E. Coelho et al., Amer. J. Cardiol., 8:624 (1961).
15. A. F. Freitas and A. Barbedo, Adv. Cardiol., 21;206 (1978).
16. T. Okajima et al., Kumamoto Med. J., 35:11 (1982).
17. R. Andersson, Acta Med. Scand., 188:85 (1970).
18. A. Zalin et al., Br. Med. J., 12:65 (1974).
19. L. M. Buja et al., Amer. J. Cardiol., 29:394 (1970).
20. A. S. Cohen, N. Engl. J. Med., 277:628 (1967).
21. J. R. Wright and E. Calkins, Medicine, 60:429 (1980).

CARDIAC DISORDERS AND AUTONOMIC NERVOUS SYSTEM
INVOLVEMENT IN FAMILIAL AMYLOIDOSIS

Yasuhiro Yamamura, Shozo Kito, Masanori Shimoyama,
Akio Abe, Hiroaki Matsubayashi, Nobuyuki Anzai*,
and Tomoki Nakano†

Third Department of Internal Medicine
Hiroshima University School of Medicine
Hiroshima, Japan

*Higashi Nagano National Hospital
 Nagano, Japan

†Nagano Chuo Hospital
 Nagano, Japan

ABSTRACT

To clarify the pathogenesis of cardiac involvement in familial amyloidosis, the authors studied histological changes of the autonomic nervous system and conduction system of the heart in seven cases with this disease. Postmortem examination revealed that the autonomic innervation of the heart was impaired in both sympathetic and parasympathetic nervous system. The specialized conduction system was involved most severely and regularly in the sinus node, and to a lesser extent, in the atrioventricular node, His bundle and its periphery. Dual damage to the sinus node through autonomic denervation and degeneration of the specialized conduction system accounts for arrhythmias and conduction disturbances frequently associated with this disease.

INTRODUCTION

Although familial amyloidosis of Andrade (Portuguese-Japanese) type is clinically manifested by peripheral neuropathy, the disease often accompanies uncontrollable cardiac involvement with various forms of arrhythmias and conduction disturbances on electrocardiogram [1]. The morphological background for these electrocardiographic abnormalities has been attributed to direct amyloid infiltration of the specialized conduction system of the heart, but it has also been pointed out that in cardiac amyloidosis involvement of the specialized conduction system is not fully correlated with rhythm and conduction disturbances. In this paper we studied cardiac disorders from the view point of the autonomic nervous system control of the heart.

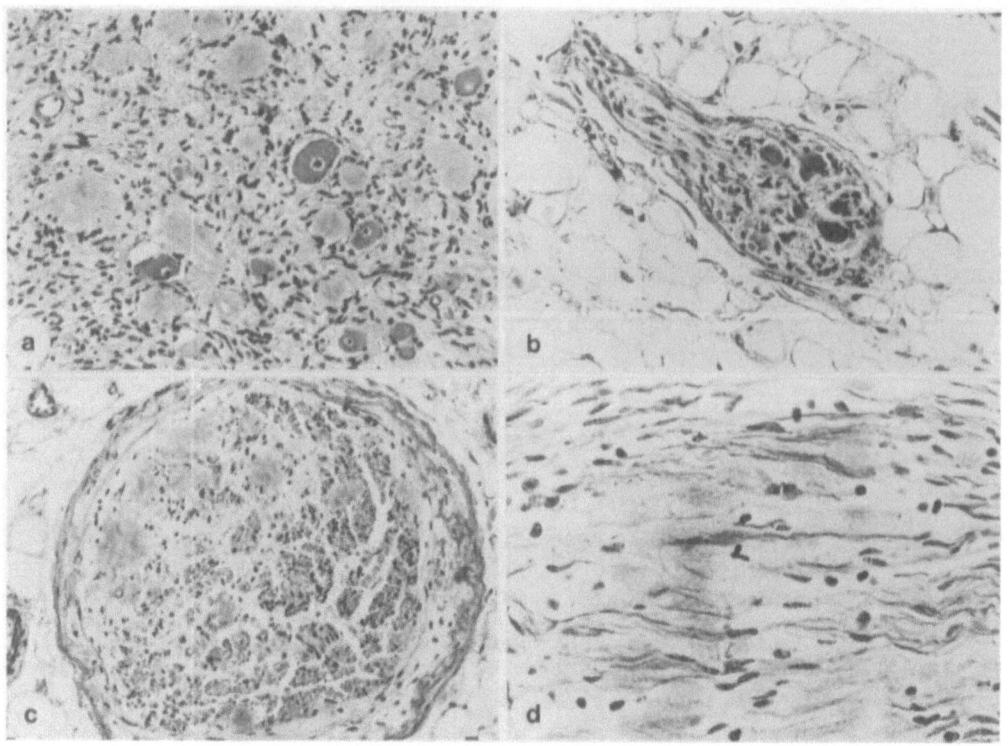

Fig. 1. Autonomic nerves and ganglia. (a) Amyloid deposit and atrophy of
nerve cells in a cervical sympathetic ganglion. H.E., ×180. (b)
A small ganglion in the epicardial connective tissue at the junction of the superior vena cava and right atrium showing amyloid deposit. H.E., ×150. (c) A nerve fascicle in the epicardial connective tissue near the sinus node showing amyloid deposit and fibrosis. Masson trichrome, ×150. (d) Degeneration and loss of unmyelinated fibers in a nerve fascicle in the epicardial connective
tissue near the sinus node. Bodian, ×180.

MATERIALS AND METHODS

     The materials are seven autopsy cases of familial amyloidosis from
Ogawa village, Nagano Prefecture, Japan. The seven cases belonged to six
pedigrees, consisting of three males and four females. The age at death
ranged from 35 to 54 (average 43) years-old, the age at onset ranged from
24-50 (average 34) years-old, and the duration of affection from 4 to 18
(average 10) years. All the cases had sensorimotor polyneuropathy of glove-
stocking type of distribution with autonomic symptoms and signs of a variable combination. In addition all the cases had anemia, malnutritional
state and emaciation. Two had struma, and two had hepatosplenomegaly.
Four cases had cardiomegaly on chest X-ray films, of which two were diagnosed clinically to have heart failure. Electrocardiographs showed low
voltage pattern on limb leads and QS pattern on right chest leads in all
cases. Sinus arrhythmia was found in 2 cases, sinus tachycardia in 1,
sinus bradycardia in 3, transcient sinus arrest in 2, sinoatrial block in
3, atrioventricular block in 6 and bundle branch block in 3. Six cases had
Stokes-Adams syndrome, and four had artificial pace-maker transplanted.

     Autopsy materials were fixed in 10% formalin solution. For the study
of the autonomic nervous system and conduction system of the heart the

430

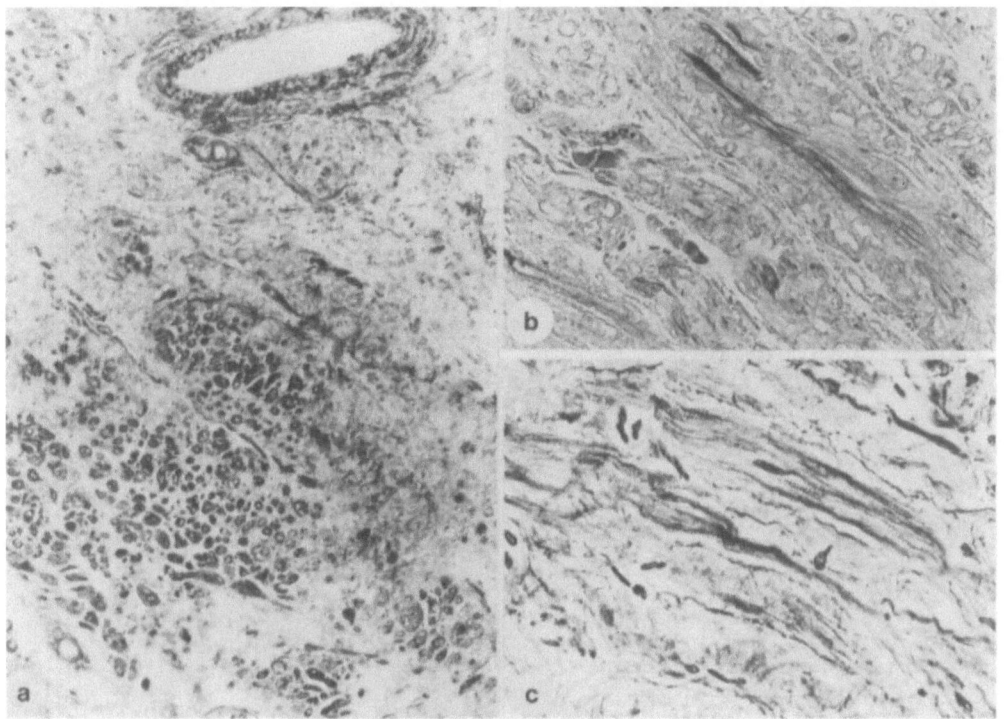

Fig. 2.   Sinus node.   (a) A section of the node after Hudson's method.
Severe atrophy of specialized cardiac muscle fibers and fibrosis
but slight amyloid deposit are noted. H.E., ×76. (b) A transverse
section of the right wall of the superior vena cava at its junction
with the right atrium, cutting through the sinus node. Loss of
specialized cardiac muscle fibers and ring-formed amyloid deposit
are observed. Masson trichrome, ×150. (c) A silber impregnation
preparation of the sinus node showing few remaining nerve fibers.
Bodian, ×380.

cervical sympathetic ganglia and vagal nerves, multiple blocks of the heart
including the sinus node, atrioventricular node. His bundle and intra-
septal bundle branches were cut off en block. The sinus node was removed
in a single block and subdivided after the method of Hudson in five hearts,
and in another two the blocks were subdivided horizontally. Paraffin embedded sections were stained with hematoxylin-eosin, Congo red, Masson
trichrome, Klüver-Barrera and Bodian's silver impregnation.

RESULT

    In the cervical sympathetic ganglia amyloid deposition was conspicuous.
Ganglion cells were strophic and slightly to moderately reduced in number
(Fig. 1a). In the vagal nerve marked loss of both myelinated and unmyelinated fiber along with deposition of amyloid substance were observed. Small
autonomic ganglia in the epicardial connective tissue at the junction of
the superior vena cava and the right auricle had atrophic nerve cells and
amyloid deposit (Fig. 1b). Small nerve fascicles in and around the sinus
node had extensive amyloid deposit (Fig. 1c) and contained only a few nerve
fibers (Fig. 1d).

431

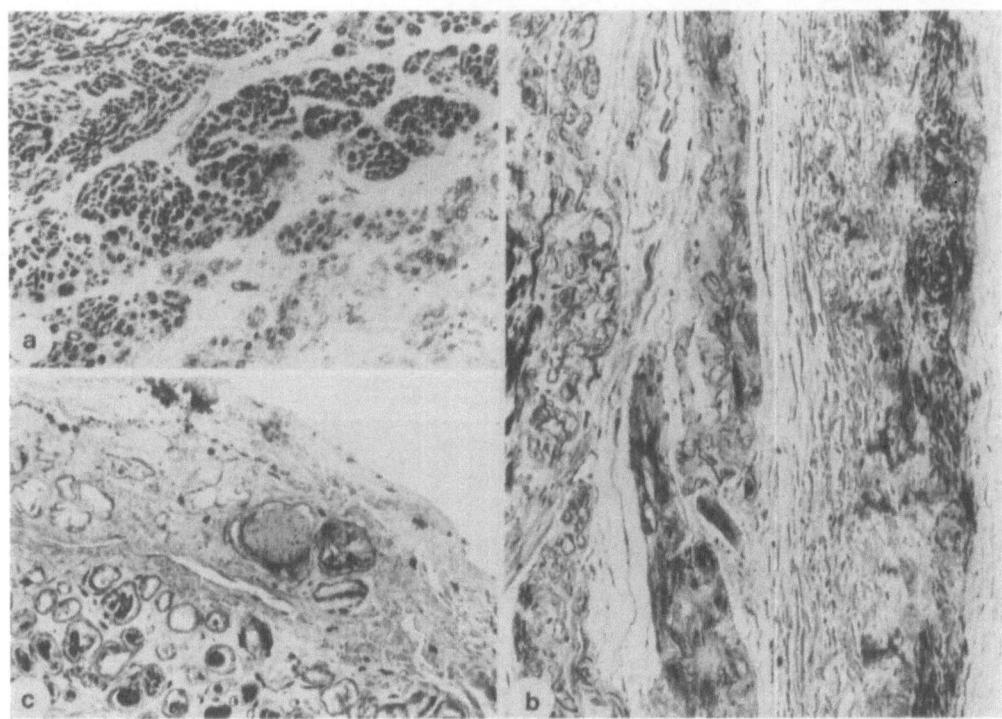

Fig. 3. Atrioventricular node and peripheral conduction system. (a) Degeneration and atrophy of specialized cardiac muscle fibers in portion of the atrioventricular node with moderate amyloid deposition, as seen in the right lower of the picture. H.E., ×56. (b)
Heavy deposition of amyloid in the subendocardial regions and degeneration of cardiac muscle and right bundle branches. Masson
trichrome, ×180. (c) Degeneration of specialized cardiac muscle
fibers of the right bundle branch. Around atrophic fibers or
surrounding empty lumina amyloid deposit in ring form is seen.
Masson trichrome, ×250.

Histological examination of specimens including the sinus node revealed
that there was marked deposition of amyloid in the subintimal region of the
superior vena cava and subendocardial tissue of the right atrium and valvu-
lar leaflets, and specialized cardiac muscle fibers of the sinus node were
largely reduced with residual amyloid rings and were partially replaced by
scar (Fig. 2a, 2b). Remaining specialized cardiac muscle fibers of the
sinus node were small in number and atrophic, and Bodian preparations disclosed that unmyelinated nerve fibers, which were to be observed abundant in
this region in normal subjects, were almost completely lost (Fig. 2c). In
the atrioventricular node degeneration, atrophy and decrease in number of
specialized cardiac muscle fibers were observed (Fig. 3a), but the histological alteration was rather mild in degree and variable from case to case.
The bundle of His had relatively well integrated structure. In the septal
walls amyloid deposition was marked along the endocarium, and the bundle
branches as well as ordinary cardiac muscle fibers showed degeneration and
atrophy with amyloid deposit, and there were numerous empty ring form structures of amyloid deposit in the region abutting the subendocarcial tissue
(Fig. 3b, 3c). Observation of serial sections showed these changes of

bundle branches were often focally accentuated and not continuous along their course.

DISCUSSION

Most long standing cases with familial amyloidosis show various types of arrhythmias and conduction disturbances on electrocardiographs [1]. Abnormal rhythms include sinus tachycardia, sinus bradycardia, atrial fibrillation and flutter and other types of arrhythmias. In advanced stages of sick sinus syndrome, atrioventricular junctional escape rhythm, junctional bradycardia are occasionally encountered. Conduction disturbances include sinoatrial block, atrioventricular block, bundle branch block and so on. These electrocardiographic abnormalities often occur admixed or changing from time to time in the individual. In cases with familial amyloidosis from Portugal it was reported that they rarely developed chronic congestive heart failure and their main cardiac manifestations were arrhythmias and conduction disorders [1]. It is also the case in familial amyloidosis in Japan, although our experience suggested heart failure could not absolutely be excluded in late stages of the disease. To clarify the pathological backgrounds of these electrocardiographic changes in familial amyloidosis a systematic investigation is necessary not only of the specialized conduction system but also of the autonomic nervous system which supplies a reciprocal, i.e., sympathetic and parasympathetic, innervation to the sinus node of the heart.

In the previous paper [2], we reported that in cases with familial amyloidosis coefficient variation of R-R intervals of electrocardiographs, which is considered to be a parameter of the vagal control of the sinus node, are markedly reduced, suggesting impaired vagal control. The present morphological study provided more concrete evidence for the importance of autonomic nervous system involvement. In all the seven cases of familial amyloidosis with typical clinical and electrocardiographic abnormalities during life the autonomic nerves and ganglia concerned with the cardiac control showed atrophy, degeneration and a decrease in number of nerve cells and fibers. Of special importance is the pathology of the sinus node, where, in addition to marked reduction in number and degeneration of specialized cardiac muscle fibers, unmyelinated nerve fibers to innervate the sinus node were massively depleted. This observation indicates that innervation of the sinus node, of both sympathetic and parasympathetic nervous system, is impaired, and, furthermore, the sinus node is incapacitated through conduction system involvement by amyloid.

In amyloid heart disease it has been a subject of controversy whether or not the frequently associated electrocardiographic abnormalities can be explained by amyloid infiltration within the specialized conduction system. James [3] found extensive amyloid deposit in the specialized conduction system correlating with associated electrocardiographic disturbances in five cases of amyloidosis (four cases of primary, one case of secondary). Ridolfi et al. [4], examining 23 patients with senile cardiac amyloidosis, concluded that direct amyloid infiltation did not account for the majority of electrocardiographic disturbances. James suggested that electrocardiographic disorders might be due to neurogenic influence on the heart. The authors of the present paper consider that, with different extents of nerve lesion between familial amyloidosis and other types of amyloidosis, involvement of autonomic innervation as well as of the specialized conduction system, especially of the sinus node, are the common and main pathogenesis of arrhythmia and conduction disturbances in amyloid heart.

REFERENCES

1. A. F. DèFreitas, A. Barbedo, Adv. Cardiol., 21, 206 (1978). S. Araki,
    T. Sawayama, Annual Report Ministry Health Welfare on Amyloidosis,
    167 (1978). S. Kito, N. Anzai, M. Yamada, S. Miyazawa, Y. Hayashibe,
    E. Itoga, Annual Report Ministry Health Welfare on Amyloid Neuropathy,
    105 (1980). S. Kito, E. Itoga, K. Kamiya, T. Kishida, Y. Yamamura,
    Eur. Neurol., 19, 141 (1980). S. Kito, E. Itoga, Y. Ito, T. Kishida,
    Y. Yamamura, T. Shinoda, Y. Yaguchi, Amyloid and Amyloidosis, Proceed.
    111 Internat. Symp. on Amyloidosis, ed. G. G. Glenner, P. P. Costa,
    F. de Freitas, Excerpta Medica, Amsterdam, 153 (1980). S. Ikeda,
    M. Shindo, N. Yanagisawa, S. Harta, Jap. J. Med., 71, 787 (1982).
2. Y. Yamamura, S. Kito, H. Tokinobu, E. Itoga, T. Kishida, M. Shimoyama,
    M. Hironaka, M. Togo, T. Mochizuki, T. Nakano, Y. Hirohashi, N. Anzai,
    Autonom. Nerv., 21, 8 (1984).
3. T. M. James, Ann. Intern. Med., 65, 29 (1966).
4. R. L. Ridolfi, B. H. Burkley, G. M. Hutchins, Am. J. Med., 62, 677
    (1977).

TREATMENT OF ORTHOSTATIC HYPOTENSION IN FAMILIAL AMYLOID POLYNEUROPATHY

WITH L-THREO-3,4-DIHYDROXYPHENYLSERINE

T. Suzuki, S. Sakoda, S. Higa,
M. Ueji, S. Kishimoto,
A. Hayashi*, Y. Takaba†
and A. Nakajima‡

Third Department of Internal Medicine, Osaka University
Hospital Osaka, Japan

*Osaka Perinatal Center and Research Institute for Maternal
 and Child Health

†Arao City Hospital

‡Nakajima Medical Clinic

ABSTRACT

To investigate the use of L-threo-3,4-dihydroxyphenylserine (L-threo-DOPS), a precursor of (-)-norepinephrine, as a therapeutic agent for orthostatic hypotension in familial amyloid polyneuropathy (FAP), we studied the metabolism of stable isotope-labelled L-threo-DOPS, and then administered DL-threo-DOPS to FAP patients for a long term. $[^{13}C, ^{2}H]$-L-threo-DOPS was synthesized, and 100 mg was infused into two normal subjects and two FAP patients. During the infusion, plasma and urine specimens were obtained. To determine endogenous and labelled norepinephrine in biological fluids, a novel method was developed using gas chromatography/mass spectrometry. The results revealed that the increase in norepinephrine in biological fluids after L-threo-DOPS was attributable to the increase in L-threo-DOPS-derived norepinephrine. Subsequently, a long term therapeutic trial of the effect of DL-threo-DOPS on orthostatic hypotension was carried out in four FAP patients. The administration of DL-threo-DOPS for four to eight months was effective in two patients, but its clinical efficacy was difficult to evaluate accurately in the remaining two.

INTRODUCTION

Orthostatic hypotension is one of the most embarrassing manifestations in amyloidosis, particularly in type 1 familial amyloid polyneuropathy (FAP). Based on biological findings, which suggest peripheral norepinephrine depletion [1], and an exaggerated cardiovascular response to infused norepinephrine [2], we adopted L-threo-3,4-dihydroxyphenylserine(L-threo-DOPS), an unphysiologic precursor of (-)-norepinephrine, to treat orthostatic hypotension in FAP. Racemic DL-threo-DOPS orally administered for 4 weeks improved postural dizziness and syncope, and enhanced daily activity [3]. We also demonstrated that L-threo-DOPS substantially elevates plasma norepinephrine levels and enormously increases urinary excretion of norepinephrine [4]. However, there is no evidence that the increase in nore-

TABLE 1. Urinary Excretion of Free Endogenous and Labelled Norepine-phrine (NE) after Infusion 100 mg [^{13}C,D]-L-threo-DOPS over 2 h into a Normal Subject and an FAP Patient

Time(h)	Endogenous NE(μg)		Labelled NE(μg)	
	Normal	FAP	Normal	FAP
0- 3	17.3	3.2	184.8	98.0
3- 6	9.9	6.5	40.7	217.3
6- 9	6.2	0	13.9	25.0
9-12	3.9	0.8	5.8	10.3
12-24	11.3	0	4.2	4.9
0-24	48.6	10.4	249.3	355.5

pinephrine in biological fluids is attributable to L-threo-DOPS-derived norepinephrine, rather than to preformed endogenous norepinephrine released by L-threo-DOPS.

In the present study, we examined the metabolism of stable isotope-labelled L-threo-DOPS and carried out long-term thrapeutic trials of the effects of DL-threo-DOPS on orthostatic hypotension in patients with FAP.

Metabolism of Stable Isotope-Labelled L-threo-DOPS

L-threo-DOPS with a deuterium and a ^{13}C atom in the β position ([^{13}C,^{2}H]-L-threo-DOPS) was synthesized, and 100 mg was infused for 2 h into two normal subjects and two FAP patients. After the influsion, plasma and urine samples were obtained at various intervals for determining endogenous and labelled (-)-norepinephrine. Standard [^{13}C,^{2}H]-(-)-norepine-phrine was prepared *in vitro* from [^{13}C,^{2}H]-L-threo-DOPS by crude aromatic L-amino acid decarboxylase obtained from rat kidney. Endogenous and labelled norepinephrine in biological fluids was isolated by boric acid gel and assayed by gas chromatography/mass spectrometry using (±)-isoproterenol as an internal standard, as described elsewhere [5].

Table 1 gives the urinary output of free endogenous and labelled norepinephrine after infusion of labelled L-threo-DOPS into a normal sub-jects and an FAP patient. Urinary excretion of endogenous norepinephrine by the FAP patient who had orthostatic hypotension remained low, as re-ported previously [1]. In contrast, large amounts of free labelled norepi-nephrine are excreted in both subjects. Although the initial excretion of labelled norepinephrine was delayed in the FAP patient, the 24-h excretion was rather higher than in the normal subject.

Infusion of labelled L-threo-DOPS into normal subjects and a FAP pa-tient in whom orthostatic hypotension was not developed induced only a slight, if any, increase in plasma levels of endogenous norepinephrine and produced only small amounts of labelled norepinephrine in the plasma. In another FAP patient who had orthostatic hypotension, however, the plasma levels of total norepinephrine was elevated from 36 pg/ml to 156 pg/ml

TABLE 2. Long-Term Therapeutic Trial of Orthostatic Hypotension with DL-threo-DOPS in Four FAP Patients

Case#	Age(years) and sex	Duration of illness(years)	Clinical stage	Duration of therapy(months)	Clinical efficacy
1	34 M	7	2	8.5	+
2	37 M	8	3	3	±
3	29 M	9	3	8	±
4	35 F	10	2	4.5	+

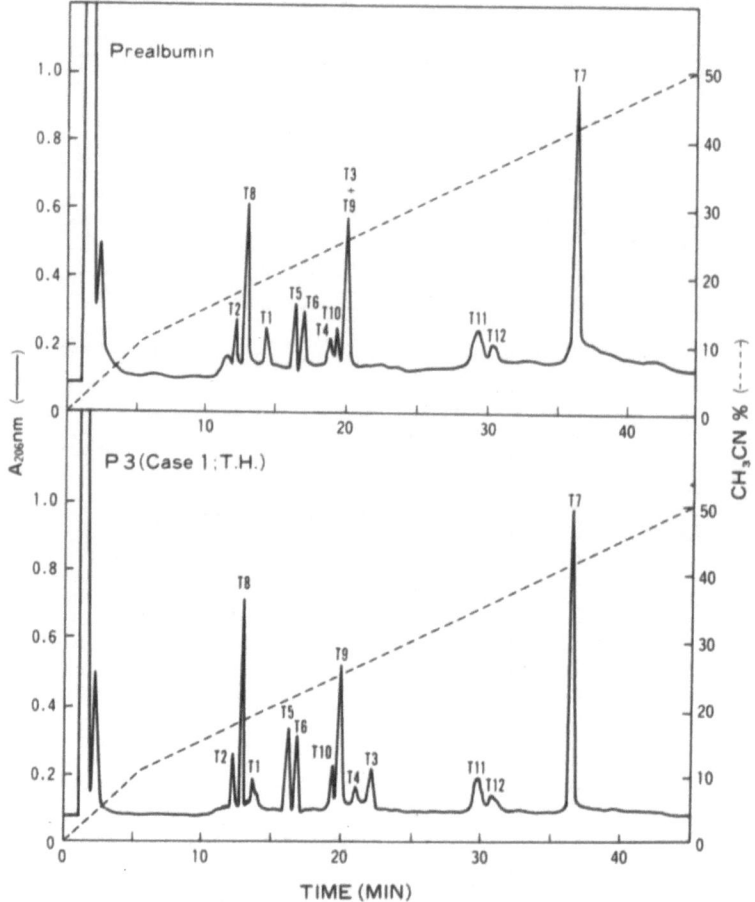

Fig. 1. Separation of tryptic peptides of prealbumin and
the P3 predominant protein (case 1) by reversed
phase HPLC.

during infusion. This elevation was clearly due to labelled norepinephrine.
When the patient stood at the end of infusion, both endogenous and labelled
norepinephrine increased slightly.

The results obtained give evidence that the increase in norepinephrine
in biological fluids after the administration of L-threo-DOPS is attributable to L-threo-DOPS-derived norepinephrine. Much higher enrichment of
urine with labelled norepinephrine suggests that most of it might be
synthesized in the kidney and excreted immediately.

Long Term Therapeutic Trial of Orthostatic Hypotention

with DL-threo-DOPS

A long-term therapeutic trial of orthostatic hypotension with DL-threo-
DOPS was carried out in four FAP patients (Table 2).

During the course of the chronic administration of DL-threo-DOPS to
Cases 1 and 4, plasma L-threo-DOPS and norepinephrine concentrations, and
adrenergic function were measured: various stimuli, such as Valsalva's
maneuver, Schellong's test, and the norepinephrine infusion test were given
while blood pressure was monitored continuously from a fine catheter, con-

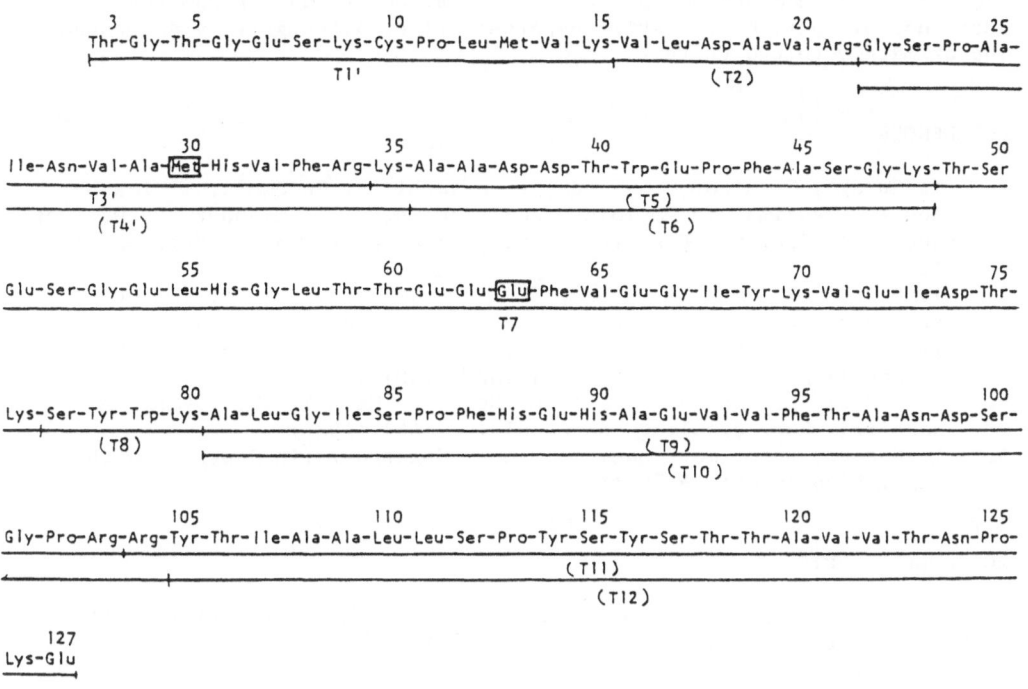

Fig. 2. Amino acid sequence of the P3 predominant protein (4 cases). The
sequence shown herein was derived by sequence analysis of T1', T3',
and T7, and by comparison of the tryptic peptides with those of
human prealbumin of known primary sequence [13]. Peptides, of
which the sequences were assumed to be identical to those of prealbumin, are shown in parentheses. Met and Glu (residues 30 and
63), which differ from Val and Gln in human prealbumin, are enclosed. The human prealbumin numbering system is used [13].

nected with a transducer, in a radial artery and was displayed on a Gilson
unigraph. The concentrations of DL-threo-DOPS and norepinephrine in plasma
were determined as described previously [4].

DL-threo-DOPS, 1200 mg to 1600 mg, administered for 8 months to Case
1, who had suffered from orthostatic hypotension and bradycardia attack,
elevated blood pressure in both the supine and standing position, and reduced the fall in blood pressure on standing, consequently improving the
postural dizziness and syncope. The effect of DL-threo-DOPS on preventing
a bradycardia attack was transient. No side effect was observed during
treatment. DL-threo-DOPS, 800 mg to 1200 mg, administered for 4.5 months
to Case 4 improved the orthostatic dizziness, but the trial was discontinued because of the patient's vague uneasiness, headache, and insomnia.
In Cases 2 and 3, who were far advanced and almost confined to bed, the
clinical efficacy of the drug was difficult to evaluate accurately although
the patients reported subjective improvement.

The results of Schellong's test before and 2 months after treatment
began in Case 4 revealed that the fall in systolic and diastolic blood
pressure was reduced by treatment. Plasma norepinephrine concentration
when the patient was in supine position was elevated to normal range by
treatment, but the response to standing was still defective. The patient
did not show a blood pressure "overshoot" response to the Valsalva's

maneuver even when she was on treatment. Blood pressure responses to infused norepinephrine were still hypersensitive, although they decreased approximately to two thirds.

REFERENCES

1. T. Suzuki, S. Higa, S. Sakoda, A. Hayashi, Y. Yamamura, Y. Takaba, and A. Nakajima, in Amyloid & Amyloidosis, G. G. Glenner, P. P. Costa, and A. A. Freitas, Eds. (Excerpta Medica, Amsterdam, 1980), pp. 113-119.
2. T. Suzuki, S. Higa, I. Tsuge, S. Sakoda, A. Hayashi, Y. Yamamura, Y. Takaba, A. Nakajima, Eur. J. Clin. Pharmacol., 17:429 (1980).
3. T. Suzuki, S. Higa, S. Sakoda, A. Hayashi, Y. Yamamura, Y. Takaba, A. Nakajima, Neurology (Ny), 31:1323 (1981).
4. T. Suzuki, S. Hia, S. Sakoda, M. Ueji, A. Hayashi, Y. Takaba, A. Nakajima, Eur. J. Clin. Pharmacol., 23:463 (1982).
5. T. Suzuki, Proc. Jap. Soc. Med. Mass Spectrom. (in Japanese with English abstract), 9:89 (1984).

ACKNOWLEDGEMENTS

We thank the Sumitomo Pharmaceuticals Co. Ltd., for synthesizing stable isotope-labelled L-threo-DOPS. We are grateful to Dr. J. Yoshida for considerable assistance, Drs. S. Higa, K. Kimura, and T. Doi for the valuable suggestions, Drs. S. Kurinami, K. Tsuru, and H. Kawashima for cooperation, Mrs. M. Okada for technical assistance, and Prof. J. Miller for reviewing the manuscript. The work was supported by grants for Specific Disease from the Ministry of Health and Welfare.

REVIEW OF CLINICAL RECORDS AND THERAPEUTIC TRIALS IN FAMILIAL

ANYLOIDOTIC POLYNEUROPATHY (TYPE 1) IN JAPAN

Sinichi Ikegawa, Shukuro Araki,
and Jinro Nagata

The First Department of Internal Medicine
Kumamoto University Medical School
Kumamoto 860, Japan

ABSTRACT

Since 1967, when a large focus of familial amyloidotic polyneuropathy (FAP) in Kumamoto, Japan, was reported by Araki, considerable experience has been accumulated at Kumamoto University. We reviewed all the clinical data of FAP from 1967 to 1984. Subjects were 734 members of 303 families in 8 pedigrees. There were 90 FAP patients, and 50 cases were examined. Average of onset was 33.2 years old, and duration of illness was 8.8 years. The initial symptoms and the clinical manifestations were evaluated, and it was perfectly uniform and virtually identical to the Portuguese. The penetrance rate was as high as 100%.

DMSO was applied to 18 FAP patients. Subjective improvements were observed in 8 cases. But the disease progressed under the DMSO treatment and it was discontinued. We tried other symptomatic treatment such as MAO-I and tyramine for orthostatic hypotension, opthalmologic operation for keratoconjunctivitis sicca, and isoproterenol for bradyarrhythmias. These treatments were effective for some cases, but other new drugs are greatly needed.

INTRODUCTION

In 1967, a large focus of familial amyloidotic polyneuropathy (FAP) in Kumamoto prefecture, Japan, was reported by Araki [1, 2]. Since then, many identical FAP patients were found and considerable experiences have been accumulating at Kumamoto University. In the north district of Kumamoto prefecture, there is the second largest focus of FAP in Japan, and clinical pathological, biochemical, and genetic approaches have been carried out. In this paper, we reviewed all the clinical data from 1967 to 1984, and report about the present status of the therapy for FAP.

EPIDEMIOLOGY AND CLINICAL FEATURES

1. Epidemiology

To confirm the clinical data, we inquired into census registers of 734 members who were related to FAP families (1820-1984). We reviewed all the

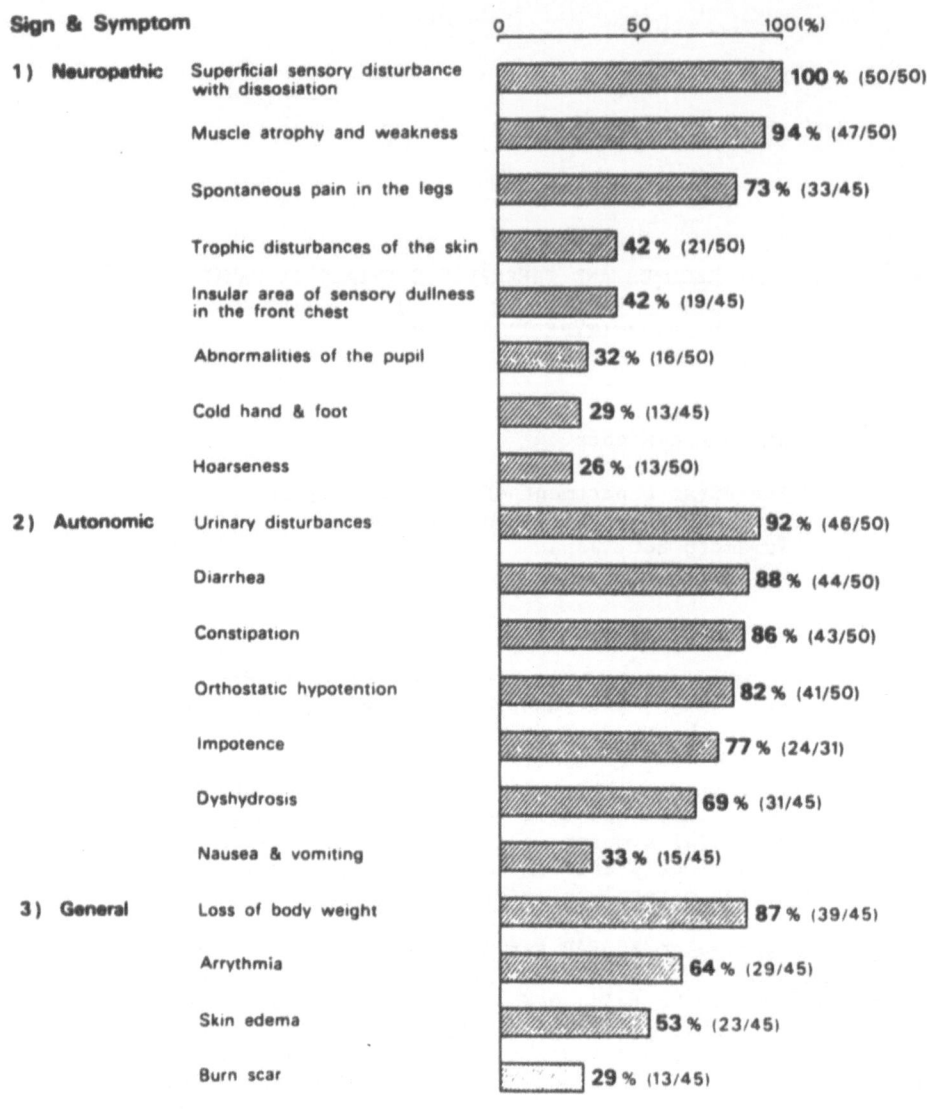

Sign & Symptom

1) **Neuropathic**
   - Superficial sensory disturbance with dissosiation — 100 % (50/50)
   - Muscle atrophy and weakness — 94 % (47/50)
   - Spontaneous pain in the legs — 73 % (33/45)
   - Trophic disturbances of the skin — 42 % (21/50)
   - Insular area of sensory dullness in the front chest — 42 % (19/45)
   - Abnormalities of the pupil — 32 % (16/50)
   - Cold hand & foot — 29 % (13/45)
   - Hoarseness — 26 % (13/50)

2) **Autonomic**
   - Urinary disturbances — 92 % (46/50)
   - Diarrhea — 88 % (44/50)
   - Constipation — 86 % (43/50)
   - Orthostatic hypotention — 82 % (41/50)
   - Impotence — 77 % (24/31)
   - Dyshydrosis — 69 % (31/45)
   - Nausea & vomiting — 33 % (15/45)

3) **General**
   - Loss of body weight — 87 % (39/45)
   - Arrythmia — 64 % (29/45)
   - Skin edema — 53 % (23/45)
   - Burn scar — 29 % (13/45)

Fig. 1. Clinical manifestations of FAP in Kumamoto (1967–1984).

available records from 1967 to 1984 in order to investigate whether they
have clinical features of FAP or not. They consisted of 303 families and
they were classified into 8 pedigrees. We found 90 individuals who had a
clinical history of FAP, and we confirmed diagnoses in 50 patients by typical clinical pictures and positive nerve or rectal biopsies. General information, common symptoms and signs and some laboratory data were inserted
in the IBM 5550 computer and the results were evaluated. There were 31
males, and 19 females. Twenty six of them were biopsied, and 9 were autopsied. Most of them (89%) were dwellers in Arao area of Kumamoto, Japan.

2. Clinical Features

Initial Symptoms. The age of initial symptoms represented was from
16 to 58 years old, and the mean of onset was 33.2 years old. Initial
symptoms of the 44 examined cases were as follows.

Alternating diarrhea and constipation was the most common initial symptoms (39%) and decrease of superficial sensation in the feet came next (20%). In 15% of male, sexual impotency was first recognized. In 11% of the cases, the disease began by distal dominant paresthesia in the feet. Nausea (7%) and light headedness (5%) were initial complaints in some cases.

Clinical Symptoms. Clinical manifestations of FAP in Kumamoto are listed in Fig. 1. Major symptoms and signs consisted of: 1) polyneuro-pathy, 2) autonomic neuropathy, and 3) generalized emaciation. The symptoms of sensory dominant type of peripheral neuropathy started in the lower limbs. Dissociation of sensory impairment was common, with pain and temperature sensation most severely affected in the early stage of the illness. An insular area of sensory dullness in the front chest was frequently observed. Abnormalities of the pupils and hoarseness were found in some cases.

Autonomic nervous system involvements, such as urinary incontinence, disturbances of gastrointestinal motility, orthostatic hypotension, sexual impotency and dyshydrosis were also common.

General manifestations, as loss of body weight, cardiac arrhythmic, and skin edema were frequently observed.

The clinical manifestations of Japanese FAP in Kumamoto were perfectly uniform, and virtually identical to those of the Portuguese [3].

Prognosis. The prognosis of this disease was invariably fatal. The average age of death was 44.2 years old (33–67 y.o.), after the duration of illness of 8.8 years (4–18 y). The common cause of death was urinary tract infection, arrhythmia, uremia, and bronchopneumonia.

Genetics. From the viewpoint of genetics, the inheritant pattern of this disease was autosomal dominant. There were 39 patients in 71 siblings who had a FAP parent. Appearance rate of these cases was 54.9% (39/71 × 100). Ideal apperance rate was 50%, so "penetrance rate" was about 100% (54.9/50 × 100). There have been no cases of so-called mild syndrome in the affected families.

THERAPEUTIC TRIALS

Although there were no specific therapy for amyloidosis, dimethyl sulf-oxide (DMSO) and other symptomatic treatment were tried to decrease the symptoms.

1. DMSO

DMSO was given to 18 FPA patients by method of skin, oral, and anal applications. Six patients continued the therapy and 12 patients discon-tinued at the time of evaluation in July 1983. Six patients showed some improvement in sensory disturbance, gait disturbance, diarrhea, and pol-lakisuria. But the effectiveness was subjective, and no objective improve-ment was observed, and course of the illness was progressive under treat-ment of DMSO. Side effects of DMSO therapy were seen in 8 cases. There were dermatitis in 7 cases, nausea in 2 cases when the skin application was given. In oral administration, there were nausea, and vomiting in 5 cases, liver dysfunction in 2 cases and hematemesis in one. Anal application caused diarrhea in one. The DMSO therapy was discontinued.

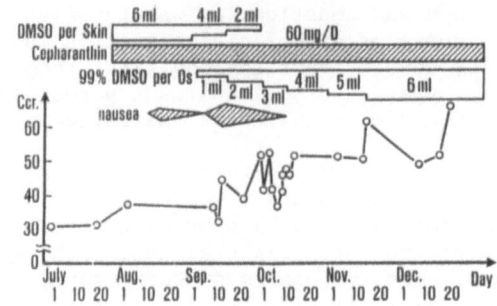

Fig. 2.   Combined therapy of FAP with
DMSO and cepharanthin. Creatinine clearance was gradually improved by the therapy.

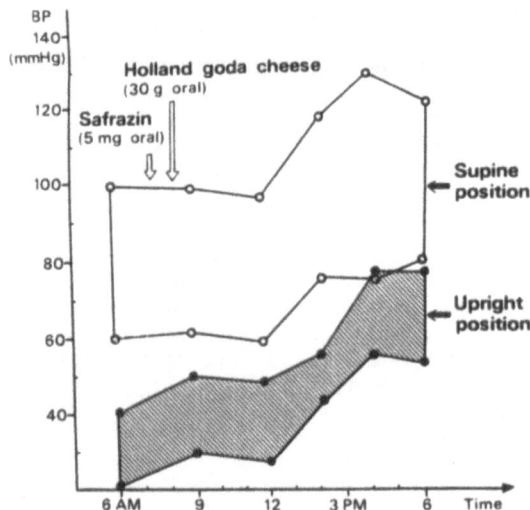

Fig. 3.   Combined therapy of MAO-I and
tyramine. A 36-year-old, male
FAP patient. Orthostatic hypotension was improved by the
therapy.

2.   Other Symptomatic Therapy

We tried some symptomatic treatment for a 36-year-old male FAP patient
(I.U.), who had severe orthostatic hypotension, dissociated sensory disturbances, muscle wasting, renal dysfunction, and diarrhea.

DMSO 6 ml/day and cepharanthin 60 mg/day were prescribed. The clinical symptoms of FAP were not improved after 4 month therapy, however,
creatinine clearance was gradually increased from 30 ml/min to 50-60 ml/min
(Fig. 2). The pacemaker was implanted for his sick sinus syndrome, but
syncope attacks still remained. On supine position, his blood pressure was
138/42 mm Hg, and on upright position, his blood pressure fell down to 60/42
mm Hg, we prescribed monoamine oxidase inhibitor (Safra) 5 mg/day at 8:30
AM. This cheese was rich in tyramine (20 r/g) [4]. From 3 to 4 hours

later, his blood pressure increased and syncope attacks stopped during the day time (Fig. 3). In his hospital stay, he developed keratoconjunctivitis sicca due to corneal sensory disturbances and decrease of lacrimation. An operation was performed to block the lacrimal pathway, and visual disturbances improved remarkably. Other symptomatic treatments such as L-threo DOPS for orthostatic hypotension [5], loperamide hydrochloride for diarrhea, domperidone for nausea, and maprotiline for depressive state, isoproterenol and pacemaker for bradyarrhythmia [6], were effective for FAP symptoms.

CONCLUSIONS

We reviewed clinical data of FAP from 1967 to 1984, in Kumamoto prefecture, Japan.

Subjects were 734 members from 8 pedigrees. There were 90 FAP patients, and 50 cases were examined. Average of onset was 33.2 years old, and duration of illness was 8.8 years. The initial symptoms and the clinical picture of FAP was perfectly uniform and almost similar to those of the Portuguese. The penetrace rate was as high as 100%.

DMSO was applied to 18 FAP patients. Subjective improvements were observed in 6 cases. Side effects were seen in 8 cases. The disease was progressive under the treatment of DMSO. Other symptomatic treatments such as MAO-I and tyramine for orthostatic hypotension, opthalmologic operation for keratoconjunctivitis sicca, were effective for some cases, but other new drugs are greatly required.

REFERENCES

1. S. Araki, S. Mawatari, Y. Murai, and A. Nakajima, Jap. J. Clin. Med., 25, 1570 (1967).
2. S. Araki, S. Mawatari, M. Ohta, A. Nakajima, and Y. Kuroiwa, Arch. Neurol., 18, 593 (1968).
3. C. Andrade, Brain, 75, 408 (1952).
4. R. N. Nanda, et al., Lancet, 27, 1164 (1976).
5. T. Suzuki, S. Higa, S. Sakoda, et al., Neurology, 31, 1323 (1981).
6. Y. Horio, T. Okajima, T. Ono, et al., Chest., 82, 190 (1982).

F.   IMMUNOGLOBULIN (AL) AMYLOIDOSIS

LIGHT CHAIN VARIABLE REGION SUBGROUPS OF MONOCLONAL

IMMUNOGLOBULINS IN AMYLOIDOSIS AL

Alan Solomon,* Robert A. Kyle,†
and Blas Frangione‡

*Department of Medicine, Knoxville Unit, University of
 Tennessee College of Medicine, Knoxville, Tennessee

†Division of Hematology and Internal Medicine, Mayo Clinic
 and Mayo Foundation, Rochester, Minnesota

‡Department of Pathology, New York University Medical
 Center, New York, New York

ABSTRACT

We have reported previously that λ light chains of the VλVI subgroup
are preferentially associated with amyloidosis AL(λ) - based on the finding
that 5 of 20 λ Bence Jones proteins from such patients were classified
serologically and chemically as members of this uncommon V region isotypic
subgroup representing $\sim$10 percent of normal λ chains. Subsequently, using
specific anti-λVI antisera, we have identified 6 additional λVI Bence Jones
proteins and 1 IgGλVI protein, all of which were obtained from patients
with histologically proven amyloidosis. We have determined the complete
amino acid sequence of 3 λVI light chains and found that each protein contains a 2-residue V region insertion between positions 68 and 69 - a finding unique to proteins of this λ chain subgroup. The non-λVI chains were
classified immunochemically as members of either the λI, λII, λIII, or λIV
subgroup. Although monoclonal non-λVI proteins are found in patients with
amyloidosis AL(λ), the striking association of a particular V region isotype with amyloidosis AL appears to be limited to λVI proteins. No such
association has been evident in patients with amyloidosis AL(κ). Serological analyses with specific anti-κI, anti-κII, anti-κIII, and anti-κIV antisera of monoclonal Igκ from 34 such patients revealed that the frequence
of distribution of the 4 κ chain V region subgroups approximates that found
among non-amyloid associated κ-type proteins. Whether amyloid-associated
light chains, especially λVI chains, possess distinct structural features
that render them "amyloidogenic" or, alternatively, the light chain degradative process is abnormal in patients with amyloidosis AL remains to be
established.

INTRODUCTION

Amyloidosis AL is characterized by the tissue deposition of fibrillar
protein constituted of monoclonal light chains corresponding to the variable (V) domain or to the V domain plus a portion of the constant (C) domain [1]. The counterparts of these proteins are usually found in the
monoclonal serum Ig or urinary Bence Jones proteins (i.e., M-proteins)

TABLE 1. Prototype Sequences for the First 23 Amino Acids (framework region 1) of the Four κ and Six κ Human Light Chain Subgroups*

Subgroup	1	2	3	4	5	6	7	8	9	10	11	12	13	14	15	16	17	18	19	20	21	22	23
κ Chain Subgroup																							
κI	Asp	Ile	Gln	Met	Thr	Gln	Ser	Pro	Ser	Ser thr	Leu val	Ser	Ala val	Ser	Val	Gly	Asp	Arg	Val	Thr	Ile	Thr	Cys
κII	Asp	Ile val	Val	Met leu	Thr	Gln	Ser	Pro	Leu	Ser	Leu	Pro	Val	Thr	Pro	Gly	Glu	Pro	Ala	Ser thr	Ile	Ser	Cys
κIII	Glu	Ile	Val	Leu met	Thr	Gln	Ser	Pro	Gly ala	Thr	Leu	Ser	Leu val	Ser	Pro	Gly	Glu asp	Arg	Ala val	Thr ala	Leu	Ser	Cys
κIV	Asp	Ile	Val	Met leu	Thr	Gln	Ser	Pro	Asn asp	Ser thr	Leu	Ala	Val	Ser	Leu	Gly	Glu	Arg	Ala	Thr	Ile	Ser asn	Cys
λ Chain Subgroup†																							
λI	PCA‡	Ser	Val	Leu	Thr	Gln	Pro	Pro	Ser		Val ala	Ser	Gly ala	Ala thr	Pro	Gly	Gln	Arg	Val	Thr	Ile	Ser	Cys
λII	PCA	Ser	Ala	Leu	Thr	Gln	Pro	Ala arg/pro	Ser		Val ala	Ser	Gly	Ser	Pro	Gly	Gln	Ser	Ile val	Thr	Ile	Ser	Cys
λIII	Ser§	Tyr	Glu val	Leu	Thr	Gln	Pro asp	Pro	Ser		Val	Ser	Val	Ser ala	Pro	Gly	Gln	Thr	Ala	Arg ser	Ile	Thr	Cys
λIV		Ser	Glu	Leu	Thr	Gln	Pro asp	Pro	Ser		Val	Ser	Val	Ala ser	Pro leu	Gly	Gln	Thr	Val ala	Arg	Ile	Thr	Cys
λV	PCA	Ser	Ala	Leu	Thr	Gln	Pro	Pro	Ser		Ala	Ser	Gly	Ser	Pro	Gly	Gln	Ser	Val	Thr	Ile	Ser	Cys
λVI	Asn asp	Phe	Met	Leu	Thr	Gln	Pro	His	Ser		Val	Ser	Glu	Ser	Pro	Gly	Lys	Thr	Val	Thr	Ile	Ser	Cys

*The amino acid residue occurring exclusively or most often at a designated position is shown *capitalized*; the next most common residue is indicated in *lower case* (sequence data from Ref. 8).

†For comparison of κ and λ chain FR1 sequences, a gap is introduced between positions 9 and 11 (Ref. 8).

‡PCA represents pyrrolidone-carboxylic acid.

§This residue is deleted in some λIII chains.

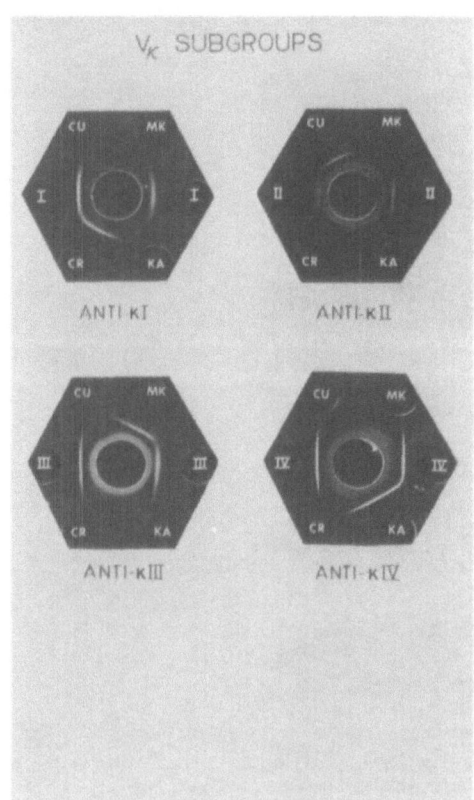

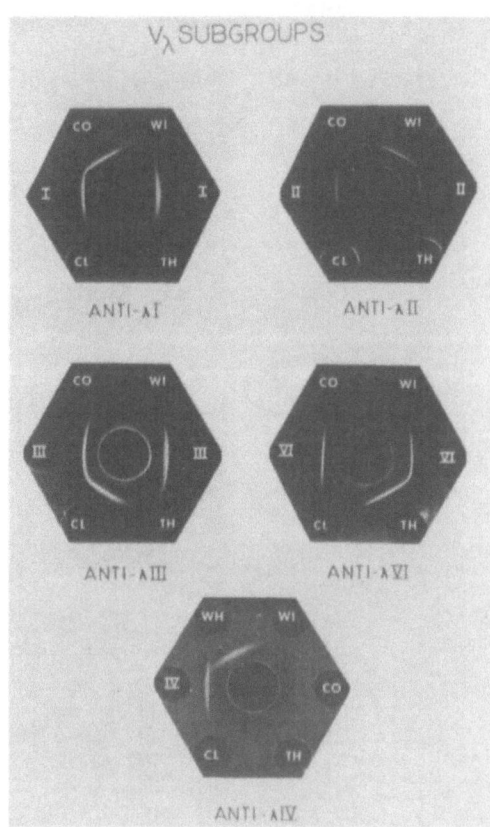

Fig. 1. Serologic detection of human light chain V-region subgroups.
Immunodiffusion analyses of κ and λ Bence Jones proteins (0.2 mg/
ml) representative of the chemically-defined [8] V_κ subgroups I,
II, III, and IV and of the V_λ subgroups I, II, III, IV, and VI.
The center wells contain V_κ and V_λ subgroup-specific antisera as
indicated. The V region subgroup of the reference κ and λ light
chains in the outer antigen wells are indicated by the Roman nu-
merals. (Left). Proteins CR, CU, MK, and KA are classified as
κI, κII, κIII, and κIV, respectively. (Right). Proteins CO, WI,
CL, WH, and TH are classified as λI, λII, λIII, λIV, and VI, respectively. From Ref. 7, with permission of the publisher.

which are manifestations of a benign or malignant B cell-related disorder
in patients with amyloidosis AL [2, 3]. The pathogenesis of this disease
remains unknown but several observations imply that certain types of light
chains are more "amyloidogenic" than others. First, λ-type light chains are
found more frequently among the M-proteins of patients with amyloidosis AL
in contrast to the predominance of κ chains among normal Igs and non-amyloid
associated M-proteins [3]. More striking is the preferential association
of λ chains of a particular V region subgroup, $V_\lambda VI$, with the amyloid process. Proteins of this subgroup were first recognized through chemical
analyses of amyloid fibril protein [4, 5]. Subsequently we found that
λVI-type monoclonal serum and urinary Igs were invariably obtained from patients with amyloidosis AL [6]. Our initial report described the detection
with a specific anti-λVI antiserum of 5 λ Bence Jones proteins and 1 IgGλ
protein which, by sequence analysis, had the primary structural properties
characteristic for the chemically-defined V_λ subgroup $V_\lambda VI$. All 6 proteins
were obtained from patients with histologically proven amyloidosis. The
frequency of occurrence of λVI light chains in patients with amyloidosis

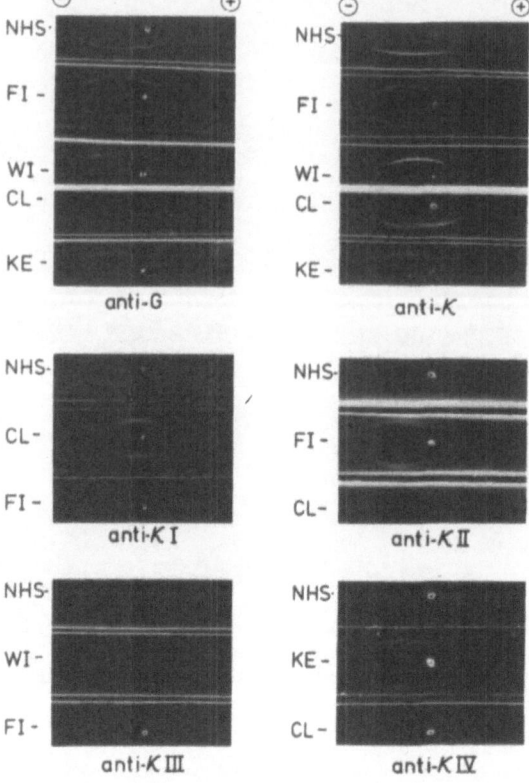

Fig. 2. Identification with specific anti-
         light chain antisera of the V_κ
         subgroup of intact monoclonal κ-type
         immunoglobulins. Immunoelectrophoretic
         analyses in 1 percent agar-3 percent
         PEG gels of serum specimens containing
         IgGκI (CL), IgGκII (FI), IgGκIII (WI),
         and IgGκIV (KE) monoclonal proteins.
         The antisera employed are rendered
         specific for κ light chains (anti-κ)
         and γ heavy chains (anti-G), and for
         κI (anti-κI), κII (anti-κII), κIII
         (anti-κIII), and κIV (anti-κIV) light
         chains.

ALλ was found to be 3- to 5-fold higher than expected based on the ∿10 percent incidence of λVI light chains in the normal Igλ population and on our analyses of monoclonal serum and urinary λ type M-proteins in patients with this disorde

MATERIALS AND METHODS

     The availability of antisera to the chemically defined V region sub-
groups of human κ and λ chains has made possible the continued investigation of serological and chemical features of light chain components found
in patients with amyloidosis AL. The methods used for the isolation and
purification of Bence Jones proteins and for immunochemical analyses are
described in detail elsewhere [7]. Briefly, monoclonal M-components were
isolated by zone electrophoresis on a polyvinyl resin (Pevikon-980, Mercer
Chemical Corp., N. Y.) and purified by gel filtration through agarose gel
columns (Ultrogel, LKB). Rabbits were immunized with Bence Jones proteins

or V region fragments and, by appropriate absorption, the antisera were rendered specific for the 4 chemically-defined [8] V region subgroups of human κ chains, $V_{\kappa}I$, $V_{\kappa}II$, $V_{\kappa}III$, and $V_{\kappa}IV$, and for 5 of the 6 chemically-defined V region subgroups of λ chains, $V_{\lambda}I$, $V_{\lambda}II$, $V_{\lambda}III$, and $V_{\lambda}VI$ (the proteins classified λV react with our specific anti-λII antisera). The prototype subgroup sequences of the first (amino-terminal) 23 amino acids that constitute the first framework region (FR) of the light polypeptide chain V region are shown in Table 1.

The V region subgroups of Bence Jones proteins and isolated light chains were established cy comparative immunodi-fusion analyses in which an appropriate reference light chain of known amino acid sequence was used with each V region-specific antiserum (Fig. 1). Similarly, these antisera were also used to determine the light chain V region subgroup of isolated and purified intact monoclonal Ig molecules. While it has been possible to determine by immunoelectrophoresis the light chain subgroup of non-isolated monoclonal Igs (as shown in Fig. 2 for κ-type Igs), the presence of heavy chains decreases the expression of light chain V region subgroup antigens, making the serological classification of light chains on intact monoclonal Igs more difficult as compared to that of free light chains. To circumvent this problem, we developed a microtechnique [9] using relatively small amounts of isolated monoclonal Igs that have been mildly reduced, alkylated, and treated to ensure that their presence in the reaction mixture of free light chains is sufficient to react in double immunodiffusion analyses with our anti-V region specific light chain antisera (Fig. 3).

Through our determination of V region subgroup of light chains from monoclonal Igs, we have obtained additional data confirming the preferential association of λVI proteins with the amyloid process. Serological analyses of the V region subgroup of 97 λ-type Bence Jones proteins revealed the percent of λI, λII + λV, λIII, λIV, and λVI proteins to be 26, 38, 22, 3, and 11, respectively. Among 20 amyloid-associated λ chains, 11 were classified as λVI, 7 as λII + λV, and 2 as λIII (Table 2). Since our earlier report [6], we have identified 7 additional λVI light chains (6 Bence Jones proteins and 1 IgGλ protein) all of which were obtained from patients with histologically proven amyloidosis. The λVI nature of the Bence Jones protein was established in 5 of 6 patients after the diagnosis of amyloidosis had been substantiated. For the 2 others, the discovery that the Bence Jones protein of one patient and the light chain of the IgG protein of the second were λVI led to retrospective review of tissue specimens that showed, in both cases, the presence of amyloid.

Among our patients with renal amyloidosis and the nephrotic syndrome, the electrophoretic and immunochemical detection of λVI Bence Jones proteinuria was made difficult by the presence of large amounts of non-Ig urinary proteins (especially transferrin and albumin) relative to the amount of Bence Jones protein. The electrophoretic analysis of urine specimens from patients with and without renal amyloidosis is shown in Fig. 4. The marked albuminuria is evident in specimens from the amyloidosis AL(λVI) nephrotic patients GIO, THOM, and CUR in contrast to non-nephrotic patients MOR and SUT in whom the amyloid process did not involve the kidneys. For patients MOR and SUT, the presence of an aberrant (monoclonal) urinary protein is unambiguous (Fig. 4); this component was readily identified immunoelectrophoretically with anti-λ and anti-λVI antisera as a λVI light chain. For the 3 other patients, the Bence Jones component was obscured by transferrin and the immunoelectrophoretic analysis of unconcentrated urine specimens failed to disclose the M-component. The detection of the λVI Bence Jones protein in urine specimens from patients GIO, THOM, and CUR was made possible by immunofixation in which specific anti-κ, anti-λ, and anti-λVI antisera were employed as shown in Fig. 5 for patients GIO and THOM. By

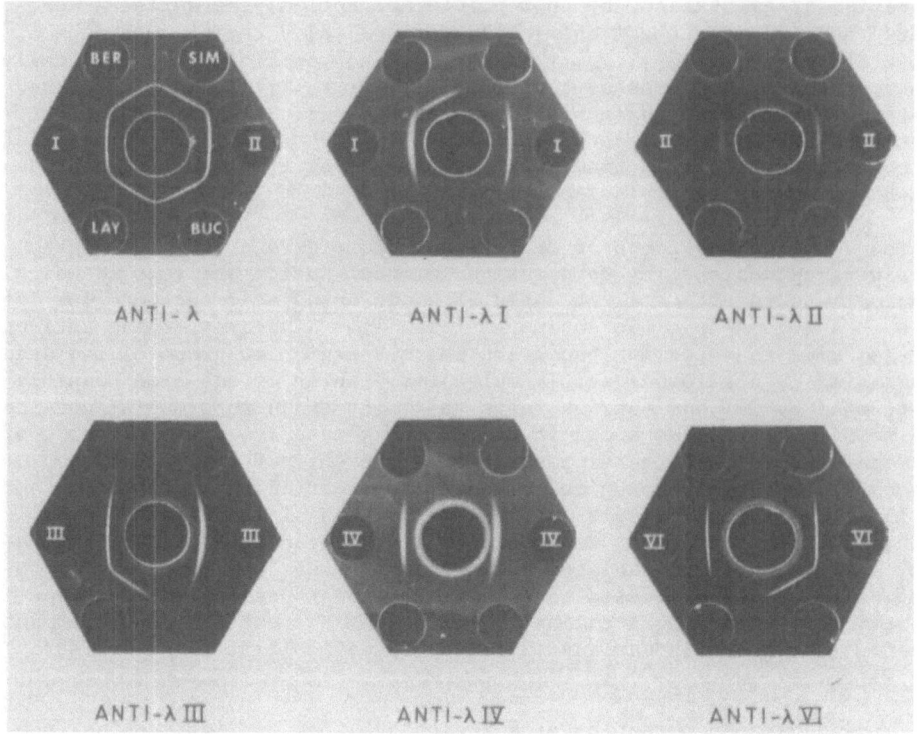

Fig. 3.   Identification with specific anti-light chain antisera of
          the V$_\lambda$ region subgroup of light chains dissociated from re-
          duced-alkylated monoclonal λ-type immunoglobulins.   The
          outer antigen wells in each pattern contained, at a concen-
          tration of 10 mg/ml, the treated IgD protein BER (BER), IgG
          proteins LAY (LAY) and BUC (BUC), and reference λI, λII,
          λIII, λVI Bence Jones proteins (0.2 mg/ml) as indicated by
          the Roman numerals. The central wells contained (as indi-
          cated) anti-λ chain and specific anti-λI, anti-λII, anti-
          λIII, anti-λIV, and anti-λVI antisera. Based on their re-
          activity the λ light chains of proteins BER, SIM, LAY, and
          BUC were classified as λI, λII, λIII, and λVI, respectively.

immunoelectrophoretic analyses, λVI protein was readily detected in patients
GIO and THOM's lyophilized urin specimens reconstituted to a total concentration of ∿20 mg/ml.   In the case of patient CUR, a higher concentration
of urinary protein (60 mg/ml) was necessary for the detection of this component (Fig. 6).

     We have determined the complete V region sequence of 3 λVI Bence Jones
proteins - protein SUT (10) and proteins MOR and THOM (B. Frangione, to
be published). Although the structural basis for the striking association
of λVI light chains with amyloidosis AL(λ) is not as yet known, two observations are of note: first, sequence analyses of λVI proteins have
shown that members of this subgroup uniquely contain a 2-residue insertion
at positions 68 and 69 in the V region (FR3) preceded by a hydrophobic
residue at position 67, as found in protein AR [11], NIG-48 [12], SUT [10],
and in the two other λVI amyloid-associated proteins that we have sequenced (Fig. 7). Second, the susceptibility of λVI light chains to a
specific site of proteolytic cleavage is also evidenced by the molecular
weight, chemical, and serological analyses of λVI-related amyloid fibril

454

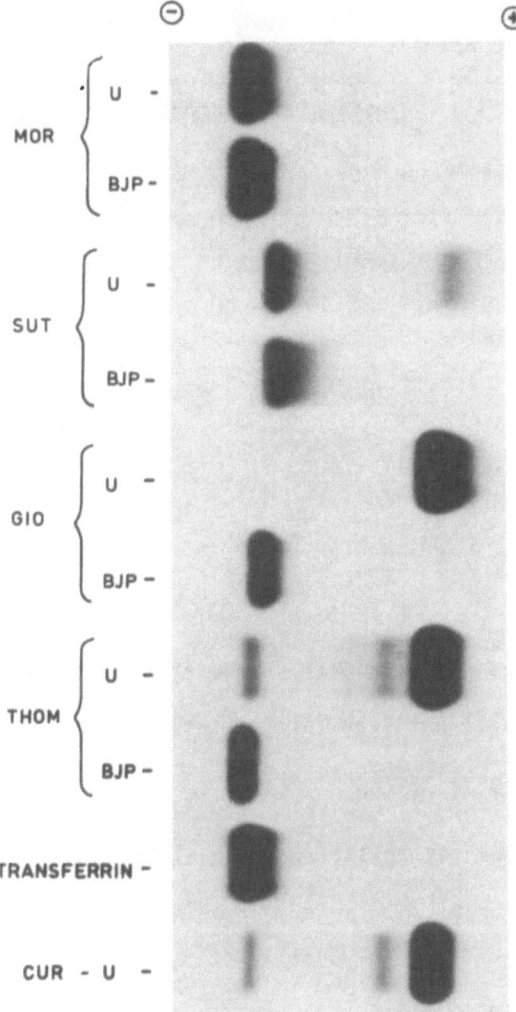

Fig. 4.   Agarose gel electropherogram (Paragon™
Electrophoresis System, Beckman) of
urine (U) specimens and isolated Bence
Jones proteins (BJP) from patients with
λVI-associated amyloidosis AL.   The
samples were at a protein concentration
of ∿10 mg/ml.

proteins AR [11], MUL [13], and GIO [6].   All 3 proteins have a molecular
weight of ∿17-18,000 and lack the ∿60 carboxyl-terminal residues of the
light chain C region.   Although the 3 amyloid components express $V_{\lambda VI}$-re-
lated antigenic determinants, they are deficient in C region determinants.
The lower molecular weight of these λVI amyloid fibril proteins (AR and
GIO), as compared to that of the intact λVI Bence Jones protein GIO, is
evident in the SDS-polyacrylamide gel electropherogram depicted in Fig. 8.
In the case of patient GIO, we have found that aminoterminal sequence of
the Bence Jones protein and of the amyloid extracted from spleen [14] to
be identical (Fig. 9).   The lack of C region sequence of the amyloid fibrils
is also reflected in their expression of λ chain determinants.   The 3 amy-

TABLE 2. Relation of V Region Subgroups of λ-Type Bence Jones Proteins and Amyloidosis AL(λ)

Patient classification	Number	$V_{\lambda I}$	$V_{\lambda II,V}$	$V_{\lambda III}$	$V_{\lambda IV}$	$V_{\lambda VI}$
		\multicolumn{5}{c}{V_λ region subgroups[*]}				
Amyloid	20	0	7	2	0	11
Nonamyloid[†]						
N	26	11	7	7	1	0
or						
U	51	14	23	12	2	0
Total	97	25 (26%)	37 (38%)	21 (22%)	3 (3%)	11 (11%)

[*]Based on serological analyses with specific anti-λI, anti-λII, anti-λIII, anti-λIV, and anti-λVI antisera (proteins classified chemically as λV react with specific anti-λII antisera).

[†]N, no amyloid evident clinically and/or histologically; U, unknown.

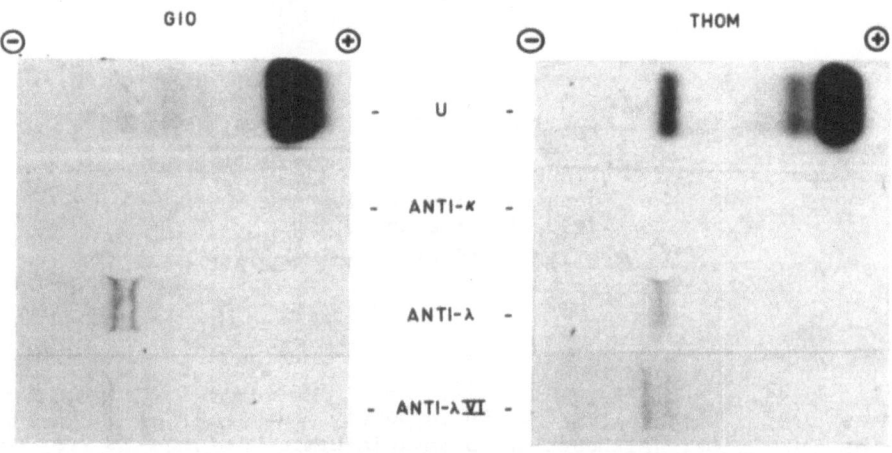

Fig. 5. Identification by immunofixation electrophoresis of λVI Bence Jones protein in urine (U) specimens of amyloidosis AL patients GIO and THOM. After electrophoresis on agarose gel, the membranes were stained with specific antisera as indicated. Depending on the antiserum employed, the specimens were diluted appropriately to obtain optimum precipitin reactions.

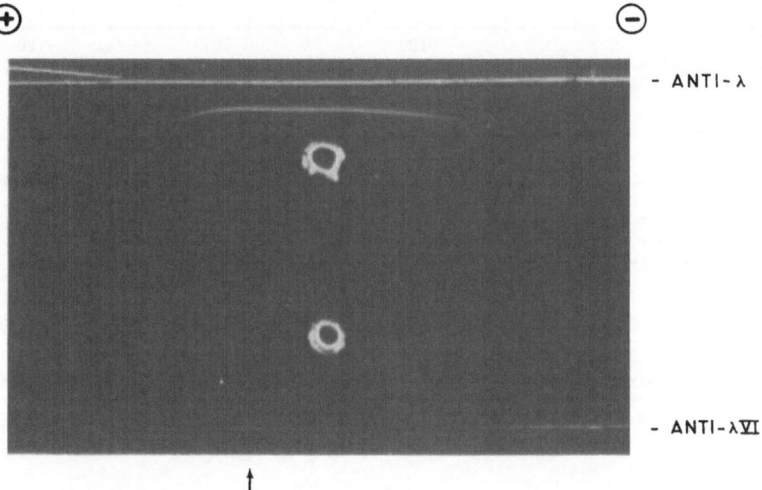

Fig. 6. Detection by immunoelectrophoresis of λVI Bence Jones
         protein in a urine specimen (60 mg/ml) from a patient
         (CUR) with renal amyloidosis and nephrosis. The lo-
         cation of the monoclonal λ chain is shown by the arrow.
         The antiserum troughs contained anti-λ light chain
         (anti-λ), and specific anti-λVI light chain (anti-λVI)
         antisera.

loid components (GIO, AR, and MUL) were recognized by our anti-λVI antisera but not with anti-λ chain antisera having specificity for intact λ
light chains (Fig. 10).

Whether λVI light chains are unusually susceptible to proteolysis in
the C region at position ∿154 and whether such ∿154-residue fragments are
amyloidogenic is not known. Likewise, the signifcance of the 2-residue
insertion in the V region of λVI proteins is not apparent. From the X-ray
crystallographic data on the λ Bence Jones dimer McG [15], the Lys^{154} residue is located on an outside loop at the carboxyl-terminal end of the 3-1
strand and thus is potentially susceptible to endopeptidase cleavage. The
V region conformation of λVI proteins would also differ from that of non-
λVI light chains because of the 2-residue insertion at positions 68 and
69 plus the hydrophobic residue at position 67. This insertion enlarges
the loop formed between the 4-3 and 4-4 strands with the hydrophobic residue serving to stabilize the polar charged loop. The importance of the
residue at position 67 is evidenced in the structure of protein McG where
Lys^{67} interacts with the first complementarity determining region [16].
Further, the potential for V domain interaction would be enhanced by the
aspartyl residue insertion at position 68 which can form a salt bridge with
the histidyl residue at position 8 that has been found in all λVI proteins
except for NIG-48 [12]. In collaboration with Dr. M. Schiffer, we are
currently attempting to crystallize our λVI proteins in order to determine
how these λVI-associated V region sequence differences affect the antigen
binding site.

Our analyses of non-λVI-type monoclonal Igs found in serum specimens
from patients with primary or myeloma-associated amyloidosis has demonstrated that such components contain either λI, λII, λIII, or λIV light
chains. We have not found a predominance of a particular V region subgroup

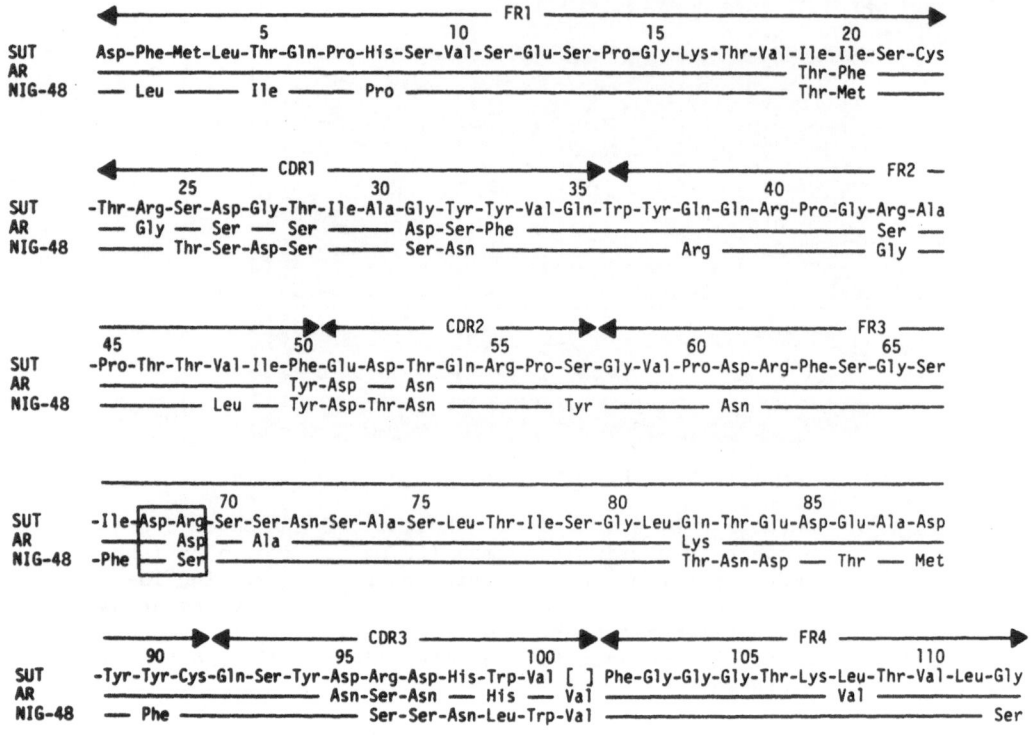

Fig. 7. The amino acid sequence of the first 112 residues constituting the
V region of the λVI Bence Jones protein SUT in comparison with
that of the λVI amyloid protein AR [11] and the λVI Bence Jones
NIG-48 [12]. Sequences of proteins AR and NIG-48 that are
homologous to protein SUT are indicated by a solid line. The
unique 2-residue insertion at positions 68 and 69 is indicated by
an enclosed box. [ ], deletion of the residue at position 101 in
protein SUT; FR, and CDR, framework and complementarity determining
regions, respectively.

among these proteins. Because of limited structural data, no common feature
is as yet evident among non-λVI amyloid-associated light chains or amyloid
fibrils.

     To ascertain if there is a preferential association of a particular
V region subgroup of κ chains with amyloidosis, AL, we analyzed serologically κ Bence Jones proteins and monoclonal Igκ proteins from patients with
histologically proven amyloidosis. Based on our serological analyses with
specific anti-V$_\kappa$ antisera, we found that among 121 unselected κ-type Bence
Jones proteins the percent of κI, κII, κIII, and κIV light chains was 56,
10, 30, and 4 percent, respectively (Table 3). Among 13 of the amyloid-
associated κ Bence Jones proteins, 8 were classified as members of the V$_{\kappa I}$
subgroup, 4 as V$_{\kappa II}$, and 1 as V$_{\kappa IV}$. The frequency of κI amyloid-related
proteins is comparable to that of κI light chains among normal Igκ, that of
κII proteins 3-fold higher, and that of κIII (and κIV) proteins less than
expected. Our analyses of the V region light chain subgroup of 34 monoclonal serum IgG, IgA, and IgM κ-type Igs from patients with amyloidosis
showed that the distribution of κI, κII, κIII, and κIV light chains approximates that found among non-amyloid associated Igκ.

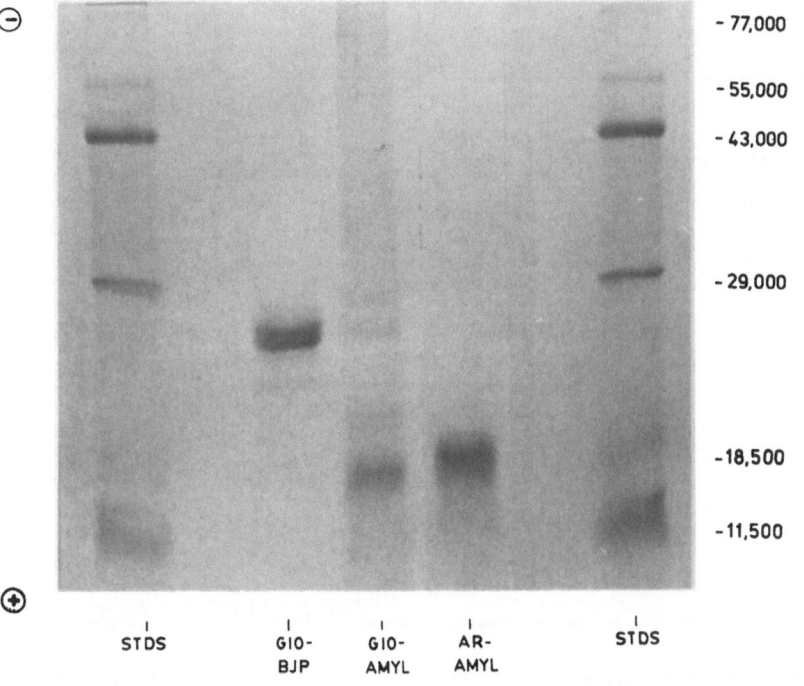

Fig. 8.   SDS-polyacrylamide gel electropherogram of λVI Bence Jones protein
and amyloid fibril proteins. Before electrophoresis, 50 μg of
the Bence Jones protein and the amyloid fibrils, and 75 μg of a
mixture of reference standard proteins (3 mg/ml) were reduced and
denatured by heating them for 5 min at 82°C in 0.1 ml of a 0.125
M Tris HCl buffer, pH 6.8, containing 2.3 percent SDS and 10 percent 2-mercaptoethanol. The treated proteins were applied (25
μl) to a 12 percent gel (4.5 percent stacking gel) prepared in a
0.375 M HCl buffer, pH 8.8, and electrophoresed for 1 h at 20 mA,
1 h at 30 mA, and 3 h at 40 mA. The gel was stained with 0.2
percent Coomassie brilliant blue R-250 in 100 percent methanol:
10 percent acetic acid (v:v) and decolorized in 10 percent meth-
anol:5 percent acetic acid (v:v). The molecular weights of the
reference standard proteins are as indicated. GIO-BJP, Bence
Jones protein GIO; GIO-AMYL and AR-AMYL, proteins extracted from
splenic amyloid fibrils of patients GIO [6] and AR [11], respectively. STDS, reference standard proteins (molecular weight):
cytochrome C (11,500); β-lactoglobulin (18,500); carbonic anhy-
drase (29,000); ovalbumin (43,000); catalase (55,000); and transferrin (77,000).

These results do not as yet indicate a preferential association of a
V_K subgroup with amyloidosis AL(κ). Of potential interest, however, is the
finding that all 8 our our κI amyloid-associated Bence Jones proteins are
members of a $V_{κI}$ sub-subgroup as defined by their reactivity with several
of our anti-κI antisera [17]. These proteins as well as other κI chains
for which the complete V region sequence is known [8] but no clinical or
pathological data are available (e.g., Bence Jones proteins HAU, BI, SCW,
KUE), can be distinguished immunochemically from other κI chains (e.g.,
Bence Jones proteins ROY, AU, AG). Similarly, certain of our anti-κII
antisera recognize antigenic differences among κII chains [17] and also
distinguish the κII amyloid-associated proteins (e.g., Bence Jones protein
TEW) from other (presumably non-amyloid) κII proteins (e.g., Bence Jones

TABLE 3. Relation of V Region Subgroups of κ-Type Bence Jones Proteins and Amyloidosis AL(κ)

Patient classification	Number	V_κ region subgroups[*]			
		$V_{\kappa I}$	$V_{\kappa II}$	$V_{\kappa III}$	$V_{\kappa IV}$
Amyloid	13	8	4	1	0
Nonamyloid[†]					
N	16	9	0	6	1
or					
U	92	51	9	28	4
Total	121	68 (56%)	13 (10%)	35 (30%)	5 (4%)

[*]Based on serological analyses with specific anti-κI, anti-κII, anti-κIII, and anti-κIV antisera.

[†]N, no amyloid evident clinically and/or histologically; U, unknown.

POSITION	1	2	3	4	5	6	7	8	9	10	11	12	13	14	15	16	17
GIO (BJP)	Asp	Phe	Met	Leu	Thr	Gln	Pro	His	Ser	Val	Ser	Glu	Ser	Pro	Gly	Lys	Thr
GIO (AMYL)											(?)						

	18	19	20	21	22	23	24	25	26	27	28	29	30	31	32	33	34
GIO (BJP)	Val	Thr	Ile	Ser	Cys	Thr	Gly	Ser	(Ser)	Gly	(Ser)	Ile	Ala	(?)	Asn	Phe	Val
GIO (AMYL)														(Ser)			

Fig. 9. The amino acid sequence of the first 34 residues of the λVI Bence Jones protein (BJP) GIO in comparison with that of the amyloid fibril protein (AMYL) GIO. Sequences of amyloid GIO that are homologous to Bence Jones protein GIO are indicated by a solid line. (Ser), residue tentatively identified; (?), residue not identified.

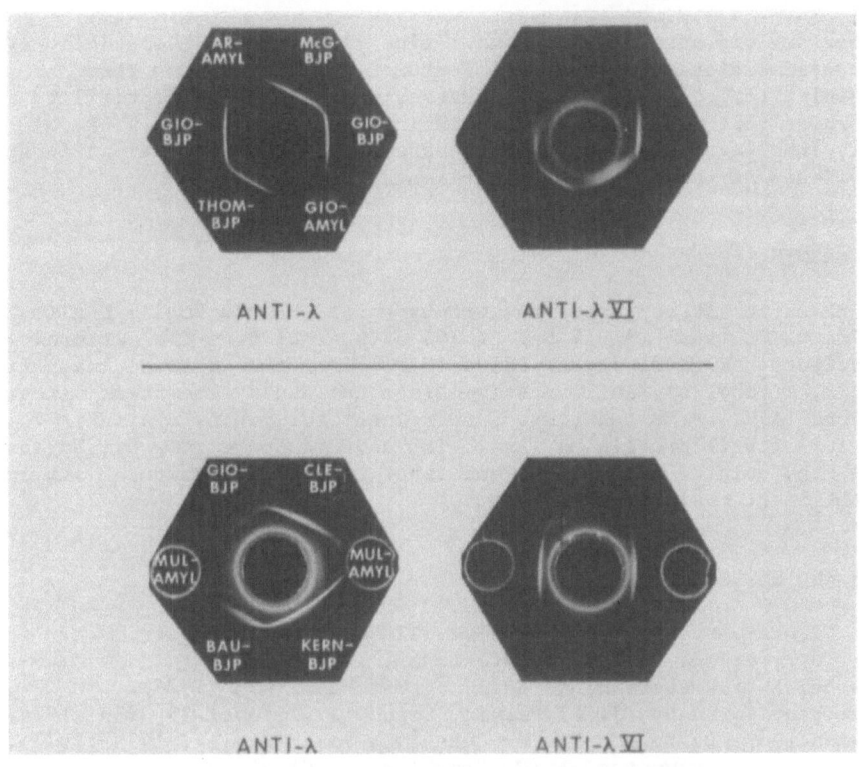

Fig. 10.   Immunodiffusion analysis of amyloid
fibril proteins and Bence Jones proteins. (Upper) The outer antigen
wells contained the λVI Bence Jones
proteins GIO (GIO-BJP) and THOM (THOM-
BJP), the λV Bence Jones protein McG,
(McG-BJP), and the amyloid fibril proteins GIO (BIO-AMYL) and AR (AR-AMYL).
The center wells in the patterns on
the left contained an anti-λ chain
antiserum and on the right an anti-λVI
antiserum. (Lower) The outer antigen
wells contained the amyloid fibril
protein MUL (MUL-AMYL) and the λVI
Bence Jones protein GIO (GIO-BJP) and
the λIII Bence Jones proteins CLE (CLE-
BJP), KERN (KERN-BJP), and BAU (BAU-
BJP). The center wells contained anti-λ
and anti-λVI antisera as indicated. The
concentration of the Bence Jones proteins dissolved in 0.15 M NaCl and the
amyloid fibril protein in 6 M guanadine·
HCl were 0.2 mg/ml and 5 mg/ml, respectively.

461

Jones proteins CUM and NIM). In two cases, limited sequence analyses of κIII chain-related amyloid fibril proteins have shown uncommon substitutions [18, 19] but whether such proteins are characteristically associated with amyloidosis is unknown.

Whether amyloid-associated κ- and λ-type light chains, especially λVI proteins, possess distinct structural features [3] that render them "amyloidogenic" (e.g., conformation, charge, solubility, susceptibility to specific proteolytic cleavage, tissue binding specificity, etc.) or, alternatively, the light chain degradative process is abnormal in patients with amyloidosis AL remains to be established.

ACKNOWLEDGEMENTS

This research was supported in part by United States Public Health Research Grants CA 10056 (A.S.) and CA 16835 (R.A.K.) from the National Cencer Institute; AM 01431 and AM 02594 (B.F.) from the National Institute of Arthritis, Metabolism, and Digestive Diseases; and by the Stein Cancer Research Fund (A.S.). We thank Dr. Gunnar Husby for making available to us the amyloid fibril protein AR [11]. The authors appreciate Dr. Marianne Schiffer's many helpful discussions and input regarding structural implications of the light chain sequence data.

REFERENCES AND NOTES

1. G. G. Glenner, N. Engl. J. Med. 302, 1283, 1333 (1980).
2. W. D. Terry et al., J. Clin. Invest. 52, 1276 (1973).
3. T. Isobe, E. F. Osserman, N. Engl. J. Med. 290, 473 (1974).
4. K. Sletten, G. Husby, J. B. Natvig, Scand. J. Immunol. 3, 833 (1974).
5. M. Skinner, M. D. Benson, A. S. Cohen, J. Immunol. 114, 1433 (1975).
6. A. Solomon, B. Frangione, E. C. Franklin, J. Clin. Invest. 70, 453 (1982).
7. A. Solomon, Methods Enzymol. (in press).
8. E. A. Kabat, T. T. Wu, H. Bilofsky, M. Reid-Miller, H. Perry, "Sequences of Proteins of Immunological Interest," U.S. Dept. of Health and Human Services (1983).
9. C. L. McLaughlin, A. Solomon, J. Immunol. 113, 1369 (1974).
10. B. Frangione, T. Moloshok, A. Solomon, J. Immunol. 131, 2490 (1983).
11. K. Sletten, J. B. Natvig, G. Husby, J. Juul, Biochem. J. 195, 561 (1981).
12. N. Takahashi et al., J. Biochem. 86, 1523 (1979).
13. D. Cohen, M. Pras, E. C. Franklin, B. Frangione, Am. J. Med. 74, 513 (1983).
14. M. Pras, M. Schubert, D. Zucker-Franklin, A. Rimon, E. C. Franklin, J. Clin. Invest. 47, 924 (1968).
15. A. B. Edmundson, K. R. Ely, E. E. Abola, M. Schiffer, N. Pangiotopoulos, Biochemistry 14, 3953 (1975).
16. M. Schiffer, personal communication.
17. A. Solomon, C. L. McLaughlin, J. Immunol. 106, 120 (1971).
18. K. Sletten, P. Westermark, P. Pitkänen, N. Thyresson, O. K. Olstad, Scand. J. Immunol. 18, 557 (1983).
19. We have determined the sequence of the first 29 residues of an amyloid-associated Bence Jones protein INU classified serologically as κIIIa [17] and found them to be identical to that of the κIII protein TI [8] with the exception that the residues at positions 1, 9, 11, and 13 were aspartyl, alanyl, valyl, and valyl, respectively (A. Osmand, A. Solomon, M. Kosaka, unpublished studies).

STRUCTURAL STUDIES OF THE VARIABLE REGION OF IMMUNOGLOBULIN LIGHT-CHAIN-TYPE

AMYLOID FIBRIL PROTEINS

Knut Sletten*, Per Westermark†
and Gunnar Husby‡

*Department of Biochemistry
 University of Oslo, Oslo, Norway

†Institute of Pathology
 University of Uppsala, Uppsala, Sweden

‡Department of Rheumatology
 The University Hospital of Tromsø, Norway

ABSTRACT

AL proteins, six of the k-type and ten of the λ-type, were isolated from amyloid fibrils obtained from amyloid-laden organs of patients with plasma cell dyscrasias. The AL proteins were subgroups in VkI, VkIII, VλI, VλII, VλIII, VλIV and VλVI. The molecular weight ranged from 12 to 22 kD. At least 4 of the k-type and 5 of the λ-type AL proteins contained carbohydrate. Elucidation of the primary structure of three AL-chains subgrouped in VλI, VλII and VλIII, revealed several positions where some unique amino acid interchanges had occurred. A comparison of AL-chains and Bence Jones proteins from patients without amyloidosis, indicated that the homology between two AL-chains of the same subgroup was less than that between an AL-chain and a Bence Jones protein. Location of oligosaccharide chains were established by amino acid sequence analyses of glycopeptides. The glycosylation sites were located in the CDR 1, CDR 3 and the FR 4.

INTRODUCTION

Tissue deposition of amyloid material is a pathological process resulting in functional disturbances of various organs [1]. The major component of the amyloid material is the fibrils which vary in composition. Thus in primary systemic and in myeloma-associated amyloidosis, the fibrils consist of immunoglobulin light-chains or fragments thereof. These proteins of immunoglobulin light-chain origin are being designated AL-chains [2]. The lower molecular weight found for these AL-chains is mainly attributed to the absence of a C-terminal part which contribute so that the antigenic determinants in the C-terminal region are being lost [3].

Structural studies of AL-chains have revealed that they are derived from homogeneous light chains of both the k- and the λ-type. The AL-chains could, with one exception, be classified in the already established subchains subgroups in VλVI [5] have a special interest since they more frequently appear in patients with primary or myeloma-associated amyloidosis than in patients without amyloidosis. The results so far, have also regroups delineated through sequence analyses of Bence Jones proteins and light chains isolated from monoclonal immunoglobulins [4]. However, AL-chains subgroups in VλVI [5] have a spe _al interest since they more frequently appear in patients with primary or myeloma-associated amyloidosis than in patients without amyloidosis. The results so far, have also revealed that AL λ-chains are found more often than the k-chains, which is in contrast to that observed from patients without amyloidosis [1]. The reason why only some immunoglobulin light chains are involved in the amyloidogenesis is still unknown, but unusual amino acid sequences and substitutions have been reported in several AL-chains [5, 6]. In the present paper, structural studies of AL-chains containing carbohydrate is described.

MATERIALS AND METHODS

Amyloid fibrils were extracted with distilled water [7]. Lyophilized fibrils were defatted with chloroform-methanol (2:1), dissolved in 6 M dithiothreitol and gelfiltered on a 2.6 × 90 cm Sepharose 6 B column, equilibrated with 5M guanidine HCl in distilled water and eluted with the same solution under continuous registration of the absorbancy at 280 nm. The fractions containing the main retarded peak were pooled, dialysed exhaustively against distilled water and lyophilized, redissolved in 5 M guanidine HCl in distilled water 0.1 M dithiothreitol and applied to a 1.6 × 90 cm Sephacryl S300 column, other conditions being the same as above. Pooled fractions were dialyzed exhaustively against distilled water and lyophilized. SDS gel-electrophoresis was performed as described [8].

Amino Acid Analyses

Amino acid composition on acid hydrolysed polypeptides was determined as described [9]. Approximately 10 nmol was applied to the BIO CAL BC-200 automatic amino acid analyser, and from a 1/2 to 5 nmol was applied to a Biotronik LC 5000 amino acid analyser. A special program was used for analyses of polypeptides containing carbohydrates.

Carbohydrate Analyses

A complete composition of carbohydrates in glycopeptides was determined after hydrolysis in 2 M HCl-methanol for 18 h at 85°C and derivatized in trifluoroacetic acid - acetonitrile (1:1) [10]. Samples were analysed by gas chromatography with a fused silica capillary column (0.2 mm × 25 ml). Values from double or triple analyses were used.

Proteolytic Digestion

Tryptic digestion of carboxymethylated protein was performed in 0.2 M NH₄HCO₃, pH 8.5, containing 2 M urea [9]. The urea solution was prior to use chromatographed on a mixed bed resin (AG 501-X8). Digestions with thermolysin, chymotrypsin and Staphylococcus aureus were as described [11].

Chemical Cleavage

The protein was cleaved by cyanogen bromide and by BNPS-skatole as described [11, 13].

Purification of Peptides

Peptides were purified by gel-filtration, by ion-exchange chromatography, high performance liquid chromatography and thin-layer chromatography as described [6, 9, 11, 14].

TABLE 1. Characteristics of Amyloid Fibril Proteins of Immunoglobulin-κ Light Chain Origin

Patient	Clinical classification	Organ studied	Molecular weight	Subgroup	Carbohydrate	Reference
Es305	Primary amyloidosis	Tongue	12,000	VκI	?	Westermark et al.,1981
547/74	Myelomatosis	Spleen	22,000	VκI	+	Westermark et al.,1981
594/79	Primary amyloidosis	Heart	15,000	VκI	?	Westermark et al.,1981
Wr	Localized amyloidosis	Larynx	13,000	VκI or VκIII	+	Westermark et al.,1981
KSA	Localized amyloidosis	Skin	14,000	VκIII	+	Sletten et al.,1983
Sol24	Primary amyloidosis	Spleen	17,000	VκIII	+	Sletten et al.,1983

TABLE 2. Characteristics of Amyloid Fibril Proteins of Immunoglobulin-λ Light Chain Origin

Patient	Clinical classification	Organ studied	Molecular weight	Subgroup	Carbohydrate	Reference
EPS	Waldenström's macroglobulinaemia	Liver	20,000	VλI	+	This paper
Es492	Primary amyloidosis	Spleen	18,000	VλII	+	This paper
612/80	Primary amyloidosis	Spleen	?	VλII or VλI	Trace	This paper
MOL	Primary amyloidosis	Spleen	22,000	VλIII	+	This paper
808	Primary amyloidosis	Spleen	18,000	VλIII	+	Natvig et al.,1981
758	Myelomatosis	Tongue	17,000	VλIII	Not tested	Natvig et al.,1981
GIL	Multiple myeloma	Spleen	16,500	VλIV	Trace	This paper
AR	Primary amyloidosis	Spleen	16,000	VλVI	−	Sletten et al.,1981
RS	Primary amyloidosis	Spleen	16,000	VλVI	Not tested	Natvig et al.,1981
145/84	Primary amyloidosis	Spleen	14,000	VλVI	+	This paper

TABLE 3. Amino Acid Sequence Data on Human VλI Light Chains

```
                    5              10             15             20
AL EPS      Glp-Ser-Val-Leu-Thr-Gln-Pro-Pro-Ser-Leu-Ser-Ala-Ala-Pro-Gly-Gln-Arg-Val-Ser-Ile-Ser-Cys-Ser-
AL NIG-51   ──────────Ala──────Gly-Val────────Ser──────Ile──
B.J. NEW    ──────────Val──────────────Lys──────Thr──


                   27E            30             35             40             45
AL EPS      Gly-Ser-Ser-Ser-Asn-Ile-Gly-Lys-Asn-Tyr-Val-Asp-Trp-Tyr-Gln-Gln-Leu-Pro-Gly-Thr-Ala-Pro-Lys-
AL NIG-51   ──────────Arg──────Thr──Asn──────────Val──Ala──
B.J. NEW    ──────Gly──────Thr──Asn──────Ser──His──His──


                    50             55             60             65
AL EPS      Leu-Leu-Ile-Phe-Asn-Asn-Asn-Lys-Arg-Pro-Ser-Gly-Ile-Pro-Asp-Arg-Phe-Ser-Gly-Ser-Lys-Ser-Gly-
AL NIG-51   ──────Val-Tyr-Ser────────Gln-Trp──────Val──
B.J. NEW    ──────Tyr-Glu-Asp────────────Ile──Ala──


                    70             75             80             85             90
AL EPS      Thr-Ser-Ala-Thr-Leu-Gly-Ile-Thr-Gly-Leu-Gln-Thr-Gly-Asp-Glu-Ala-Ile-Tyr-Tyr-Cys-Gly-Thr-Trp-
AL NIG-51   ──────Ser──────Ala──────Ser──────His-Ser-Glu──────Asp──────Phe──────Ala──
B.J. NEW    ──────Ala──────────────Arg──────────Asp──────────Asp──────Ala──


                    95    96                           100*                    105
AL EPS      Asp-Asn-Arg-Arg- D - D -Ser-Val-Phe-Gly-Gly-Gly-Thr-Asn-Val-Thr-Val-Val-Gly-Gln-Pro-Lys
AL NIG-51   ──────Asp-Ser-Leu-Asp-Gly-Pro────────────────────Lys-Leu──────Leu
B.J. NEW    ──────Ser-Ser-Leu-Asn-Ala-Val────────────────────Lys──────Leu
```

467

Amino acid sequence determination and analyses of the resulting PTH-derivatives were performed as described [9]. Samples of 20 to 100 nmol were used.

RESULTS

A large number of sequence data on immunoglobulin light chains have by now been studied, but only limited and incomplete data are available for AL-chains. In order to elucidate a relationship between the structure and the pathogenic function of AL proteins a more detailed investigation was undertaken. The amyloid fibril proteins were purified by sequential gel-filtration under dissociating conditions. The purity of the AL-proteins were tested by SDS polyacrylamide gel electrophoreses and N-terminal analyses. Table 1 shows some characteristical features of six amyloid fibril proteins of immunoglobulin-k-light-chain origin, isolated from patients with primary or myeloma associated amyloidosis. All AL k-chains could according to results obtained by N-terminal analyses be placed in either the VkI or the VkIII subgroup. Correspondingly, ten AL λ-chains were tested and found to belong to the VλI, VλII, VλIII, VλIV and VλVI subgroup (Table 2). The molecular weight of the isolated AL-chains vary in size from about 12 to 22 kDalton, which is in accordance with what others also have reported [4].

Determination of the amino acid composition of the different AL-chains revealed that at least nine of the fifteen proteins analysed contained hexosamine. In order to investigate this further, structural studies of AL-chains from different subgroups were started. The amino acid sequence determination involved automatic Edman degradation of polypeptides obtained after cleaving the protein with trypsin, thermolysin, BNPS-skatole and cyanogen bromide. The entire V-region structure of AL-chain EPS is presented in Table 3, and compared with that of another AL-chain, AL NIG-51 [15] and the VλI Bence Jones protein NEW [16]. A comparison of the two AL proteins shows that there are 34 amino acid residues which differ. Only three of these may be attributed to more than one-base mutations (positions 10, 32, and 85) and two residues come from the additional positions; 95A and 95B, found in AL NIG-51. A comparison of the AL protein EPS and the Bence Jones protein NEW reveals 26 differences, of which only 4 may be attributed to more than one base mutations, namely positions 34, 50, 85 and 96, and 2 residues from positions 95A and 95B in protein NEW. These results show that the AL protein EPS belongs to subgroup VλI, and that there is a greater homology between AL protein EPS and Bence Jones protein NEW than between the 2 AL proteins. The differences observed, are in both cases mainly distributed in the complementarity-determining region, CDR3.

Structural studies of another AL-chain, ES492, resulted in the amino acid sequence of the V-region, shown in Table 4, together with the sequence of the Bence Jones protein VIL [17]. A comparison of these 2 proteins reveals 24 differences, of which 7 may be attributed to more than one-base mutations, namely positions 26, 28, 29, 30, 32, 93 and 95B. It is interesting to note that 5 of these positions are distributed in the complementarity-determining region, CDR1, which is different from what was observed when the AL protein EPS was compared with a Bence Jones protein. The amino acid sequence showed that the AL protein ES492 belongs to subgroup VλII.

Structural studies of a third AL protein of the λtype, AL MOL, revealed an amino acid sequence shown in Table 5. For comparison, the Bence Jones protein BAU [18] of the VλIII subgroup is added. The numbering sys-

TABLE 4. Amino Acid Sequence Data on Human VλII Light Chains

```
                    5              10             15             20
AL Es 492 Glp-Ser-Ala-Leu-Thr-Gln-Pro-Ala-Ser-Val-Ser-Gly-Ser-Pro-Gly-Gln-Ser-Ile-Thr-Ser-Cys-Ala
B.J.  VIL His——————————————————————————————————————————Leu————————————————————————————Thr

              25      27 27a 27b      30             35             40
                              *
AL Es 492 Gly-Thr-His-Ser-Asp-Val-Asn-Phe-Thr-Asx-Ala-(Glx-Ser)Trp-Tyr-Gln-Leu-His-Pro-Gly-Ile-Ala-Pro
B.J.  VIL Ser——————Gly-Gly-Tyr-Asn-Tyr-Val——————Phe————————Gln————————Thr

              45             50             55             60             65
AL Es 492 Lys-Leu-Met-Ile-Phe-Asp-Val-Ser-Asn-Arg-Pro-Ser-Gly-Val-Ser-Asn-Arg-Phe-Ser-Gly-Ser-Lys-Ser
B.J.  VIL ——————Ile——————Ser-Glu——————Arg——————————Asp

              70             75             80             85      *    90
AL Es 492 Gly-Asn-Thr-Ala-Ser-Leu-Thr-Ile-Ser-Gly-Leu-Gln-Ala-Glu-Asp-Glu-Ala-Asp-Tyr-Tyr-Cys-Ser-Ser
B.J.  VIL Ala————————

              95 95A 95B     100            105
AL Es 492 Phe-Thr-Asp-Thr-Thr-Gln-Leu-Val-Val-Phe-Gly-Gly-Gly-Thr-Lys-Leu-Thr-Val-Leu-Gly-Gln-Pro
B.J.  VIL Tyr-Thr-Ser-Ser-Asn-Ser- D————————
```

TABLE 5. Amino Acid Sequence Data on Human VλIII Light Chain

```
                5              10             15              20
AL   MOL ──Tyr-Glu-Leu-Thr-Gln-Pro-Pro-Ser-Val-Ser-Val-Ser-Pro-Gly-Gln-Thr-Ala-Thr-Ile-Thr-Cys-Ser
B.J. BAU ──────────Gly──────────────Leu──────────────────────────────────────────────────Ser

                25             30             35              40             45
AL   MOL Gly-Asp-Lys-(─────Leu-Gly-Glu-Ser-Tyr)-Tyr-Asp-Trp-Tyr-Gln-Gln-Ser-Pro-Gly-Gln-Ser-Pro-Leu-Leu
B.J. BAU ────────────Gln──────────Val-Cys──────────────Lys──────────────────────────────Val

                50             55             60              65
AL   MOL Val-Ile-Tyr-Glu-Gly-Asp-Lys-Arg-Pro-Ser-Gly-Ile-Pro-Glu-Arg-Phe-Ser-Gly-Ser-Asn-Ser-Gly-Asn
B.J. BAU ────────────His-Asp-Ser──────────────────────────────────────────────────────Thr

                70             75             80              85         90*
AL   MOL Thr-Ala-Thr-Leu-Thr-Ile-Ser-Gly-Thr-Glu-Ser-Met-Asp-Glu-Ala-Asp-Tyr-Tyr-Cys-Gln-Ala-Trp-Asn
B.J. BAU ────────────────────Gln-Ala──────────────────────────────────────────────Asp

                95             100            105
AL   MOL Ser-Ser-Val-Leu-Phe-Gly-Gly-Gly-Thr- Lys-Leu-Thr-Val-Leu-Gly-Gln-Pro
B.J. BAU ────────────Tyr──Thr──────Ile
```

tem used is that adapted by Kabat et al., [19]. The amino acid residues in positions 27-32 are tentatively identified because of no overlapping peptide. These two proteins differ in 17 positions and 6 of these are differences in terms of more than one-base mutations, namely positions 31, 33, 34, 39, 50 and 52. Positions 92 could be a result of deamidation. The homology seen in this case shows clearly that the AL proton MOL belongs to the VλIII subgroup. And further more, the observation shows that there is a greater homology between the AL protein and the Bence Jones protein than the homology between the two AL proteins, EPS and NIG-51, in subgroup VλI.

Initially, amino acid analyses revealed that these three AL proteins contained hexosamine (Table 2) and a complete carbohydrate composition was made on two of them. The results, together with the composition of an N-glycosidically linked oligosaccharide derived from a Bence Jones protein SM of the λ-type [20] is shown in Table 6. The content of glucosamine is in AL-chains very similar to that in the glycopeptide derived from protein SM, while there is small variations in the content of mannose and galactose. The content of glucose is most probably due to contamination from the Sephadex columns being used for purification.

From AL protein EPS, a tryptic peptide T-10 and a thermolytic peptide Th-19 was isolated and characterized, and both was shown to contain glucosamine. Edman degradation revealed that they were derived from the same region of the protein, they namely contained a -Phe-Gly-Gly-Gly- sequence which is so typical for positions 98-101 in light chains (Table 3). The carbohydrate was established to be covalently attached to the asparagine residue in position 103, which together with residues 104 and 105 (Table 3) forms a part of an appropriate acceptor sequence for N-glycosylation. The composition of the carbohydrate linked to peptide Th-19 is in good agreement with that found for the protein, except for the content of fucose. However, they may in part be explained by the results obtained from thin-layer chromatography and high performance liquid chromatography of peptides T-10 and Th-19, which established a heterogeneity in the oligosaccharide.

From the AL protein Es492 a cyanogen bromide fragment, CB-1, containing residues 1-47 (Table 4) was found to contain only one residue each of glucosamine and sialic acid. Thermolytic digestion yielded a peptide containing one of the two residues of histidine in the protein, in addition to approximately one residue of glucosamine. Edman degradation of the peptide revealed that the disaccharide was covalently linked to the asparagine residue in position 28 of the protein (Table 4). Other structural studies established the sequence of -Phe-Thr- in position 29 and 30, which again would form an acceptor sequence for N-glycosylation. Evidence for a second glycosylation site was obtained from a tryptic peptide T-5, contained residues 67-103 (Table 4), and which revealed a carbohydrate composition shown in Table 6. The content of sialic acid and glucosamine deviates from that found totally in the protein. The tryptic peptide was digested with protease aureus which yielded a peptide, Pa-2, containing 2.5 residues of glucosamine. Edman degradation of the peptide established the position of residues 84-98, except for position 89, where a very low yield of serine derivative was detected. However, as the yield in the other cycles were normal, and the peptide contained only two residues of aspartic acid which were taken care of in positions 85 and 93, we suggest that the carbohydrate is O-glycosidically linked to a serine residue in position 89.

From the third AL protein MOL, of subgroup VλIII, a tryptic peptide, T-4, containing glucosamine was purified, and a complete carbohydrate composition was determined (Table 6). Except for a lower content of sialic acid and glucosamine the carbohydrate content is very similar to that

TABLE 6. Carbohydrate Composition of AL Proteins, of Glycopeptides Derived from Them and of an N-Glycosidically Linked Oligosaccharide Derived from a Human Bence Jones Protein SM

	Residues per polypeptide molecule					
	Fucose	Mannose	Galactose	Glucosamine	Sialic acid	Glucose
B.J. SM VλII (20)	0.8	3.0	1.7	4.2	1.3	
AL EPS VλI	0.6	3.5	1.9	3.7	0.8	2.5
AL EPS T-10 (Pos. 96-111)*				3.0		
AL EPS Th-19(Pos. 97-105)		3.1	2.0	3.5	1.8	
AL Es492 VλII		1.6	1.3	2.0	0.6	1.9
AL Es492 CB-1(Pos. 1-47)				1.0	1.0	15.0
AL Es492 Th-7(Pos. 23-28)*				0.6		
AL Es492 T-5 (Pos. 67-103)	0.3	2.0	1.2	3.0	3.6	
AL Es492 Pa-2(Pos. 84-103)*				2.5		
AL MOL VλIII*				4.		
AL MOL T-4 (pos. 62-103)	0.6	2.6	1.8	2.2	trace	trace

N-glycosidically linked in the Bence Jones protein SM [20]. The tryptic peptide T-4, contained one residue of methionine, the only one in the protein, which established the location to position 62-103. The exact position of the glycosylation site could not be elucidated, but as T-4 and the cyanogen bromide fragment CB-2 contained carbohydrate, the site has to be between position 82 and 103 (Table 6). From the amino acid sequence, the residues in position 92, 93 and 94 would fulfill an appropriate acceptor sequence for N-glycosylation.

DISCUSSION

The reason why some immunoglobulin light chains give rise to amyloid fibrils is still obscure. Several groups have, however, suggested that certain regions of the AL-chains could be amyloidogenic [4, 5, 6, 9]. The theory for this assumption was that some rather uncommon interchanges of amino acids, and as in the case of the VλVI, an insertion of two amino acids in the FR3, had occurred. In order to test this theory, more extensive structural studies have to be performed. The amino acid sequence of the three AL-chains here presented revealed some rather unique amino acid replacements. In AL EPS of the VλI subgroup, an isoleucine residue in position 85 was found, and this residue has previously not been observed in this position in human λ-light chains. In AL Es492 of the VλII subgroup, a histidine in position 26, an asparagine in 28, a phenylalanine in 29 and a threonine in 30 in addition to a -Phe-Thr- sequence in positions 91 and 92 have not been observed in these positions in human λ-light chains. The same is also true for the serine residue in position 39 in AL MOL of the VλIII subgroup. A comparison of the two AL-chains, EPS and NIG-51, and the Bence Jones protein NEW, showed that there is a greater homology between an AL-chain (EPS) and a Bence Jones protein (NEW) than that between two AL-chains of the same subgroup. This interesting observation is also being supported by the homology seen when the AL Es492 and AL MOL was compared with a Bence Jones protein (Tables 4 and 5) of the same subgroup.

Another interesting feature seen with these AL-chains, was the content of carbohydrate. Among the 14 AL-chains analyzed, at lease 9 of them contained hexosamine. This is more than 4 times higher than that reported for light chains isolated from patients with multiple myeloma, and supposedly without amyloidosis [21]. For those light chains where the glycosylation site has been determined, the carbohydrate was found to occur between positions 25 and 34, and between 65 and 94 [22]. And recently a glycosylation site at position 107 in a VkI protein obtained from a monoclonal IgG1 was elucidated [22]. The amino acid sequence data for AL EPS showed clearly that the carbohydrate was linked to an asparagine residue in position 103, which is in the framework region 4 (FR4) and is thus among the J-mini-genes for λ-light chains. It is interesting to note that this glycosylation site is the first case where carbohydrate has been reported in this region of a λ-chain, however, it is in the same region as that observed in the k-chain [22].

In the other AL-chain, Es492, the elucidated amino acid sequence has evidence for two glycosylation sites. One of them was at the asparagine residue in position 28, which is in the CDR1 and where carbohydrate has been reported to occur [22]. The second site is most probably located at the serine residue in position 89, which is in the CDR3. In this region carbohydrate has been detected earlier [22]. In the third AL-chain, MOL, the elucidated primary structure gave evidence for an attachment of carbohydrate between positions 82 and 103. The protein has an appropriate sequence for N-glycosylation in positions 92, 93 and 94, which would be the most likely site.

The carbohydrate composition obtained for the two glycopeptides from AL EPS and AL MOL, is with a few exceptions similar to what have been reported [20]. The differences could be explained by a heterogeneity observed during purification of the glycopeptides. The carbohydrate composition found for the glycopeptides in AL Es492, is very peculiar, for which we have no explanation. Very little is, however, known about the oligosaccharide chains in light chains of myeloma proteins, and especially from these partially degraded AL-chains.

The presence of oligosaccharides in proteins have been shown to play important biological functions [23]. This includes the stabilization of protein conformation and thereby prevent its degradation by proteases. The glycosylations could also interfere with the folding of a domain or with the association of heavy and light chains.

REFERENCES

1. G. G. Glenner, W. D. Terry, and C. Isersky, Semin. Hematol. 10, 65 (1973). G. Husby, Ann. Clin. Res. 7, 154 (1975).
2. E. P. Benditt, A. S. Cohen, P. P. Costa, E. C. Franklin, G. G. Glenner, G. Husby, E. Mandema, J. B. Natvig, E. F. Osserman, E. Sohar, O. Wegelius and P. Westermark, Amyloid and Amyloidosis. G. G. Glenner, P. P. Costa, A. F. Freitas, Eds. (Excerpta Medica, Amsterdam 1980) p. XI.
3. J. B. Natvig, P. Westermark, K. Sletten, G. Husby, and T. Michaelsen. Scand. J. Immunol. 14, 89 (1981).
4. G. G. Glenner, New Eng. J. Med. 302, 1283 and 1333 (1980).
5. K. Sletten, G. Husby, and J. B. Natvig, Scand. J. Immunol. 3, 833 (1974); M. M. Skinner, D. Benson and A. S. Cohen, J. Immunol. 114, 1433 (1975), N. Takahashi, T. Takaysu, T. Isobe, T. Shinoda, T. Okuyama, and A. Shimizu, J. Biochem. 86, 1523 (1979), B. Frangione, T. Moloshok, and A. Solomon, J. Immunol. 131, 2490 (1983).
6. P. Westermark, K. Sletten, P. Pitkänen, J. B. Natvig, and C. E. Lindholm, Molec. Immunol. 19, 447 (1982), K. Sletten, P. Westermark, P. Pitkänen, N. Thyresson, O. K. Olstad, Scand. J. Immunol. 18, 557 (1983).
7. M. Pras, M. Schubert, D. Zucker-Franklin, A. Rimon, and E. C. Franklin, J. Clin. Invest. 47, 924 (1968).
8. R. T. Swank and K. D. Mundres, Anal. Biochem. 39, 462 (1971).
9. K. Sletten, J. B. Natvig, G. Husby, and J. Juul, Biochem. J. 195, 561 (1981).
10. C. H. Bolton, J. R. Clamyr and L. Hough, Biochem. J. 96, 5c (1965).
11. K. Sletten and G. Husby, Eur. J. Biochem. 41, 117 (1974), B. Austen and E. Smith, Biochem. Biophys. Res. Commun. 72, 411 (1976).
12. I. Kawasaki and H. A. Itano, Anal. Biochem. 48, 546 (1972).
13. A. Fontana, Methods Enzymol. 25, 419 (1972).
14. K. Sletten, G. Marhaug, and G. Husby, Hoppe-Seyler's Z. Physiol. Chem. 364, 1039 (1983).
15. N. Takahashi, T. Takayasu, T. Shinoda, S. Ito, T. Okuyama, and A. Shimizu, Biomed. Res. 1, 321 (1980).
16. B. Langer, M. Steinmetz-Kayne, and N. Hilschmann, Hoppe-Seyler's Z. Physiol. Chem. 349, 945 (1968).
17. H. Ponstingl and N. Hilschmann, Hoppe-Seyler's Z. Physiol. Chem., 352, 859 (1971).
18. K. Baczko, D. G. Braun, and N. Hilschmann, Hoppe-Seyler's Z. Physiol. Chem. 355, 131 (1974).
19. E. A. Kabat, T. T. Wu, H. Bilofsky, M. Reid-Miller, and H. Perry, Sequences of Proteins of Immunological Interest. U.S. Department of Health and Human Services (1983).

20. F. A. Garver, L. S. Chang, C. R. Kiefer, J. Mendicino, E. W.
    Chandrasekaran, T. Isobe, and E. F. Ossermand, Eur. J. Biochem.,
    115, 643 (1981).
21. H. C. Sox and L. Hood, Proc. Natl. Acad. Sci., U.S.A. 66, 975 (1970).
22. G. Savvidou, M. Klein, C. Horne, T. Hofmann, and K. F. Dorrington,
    Molec. Immunol. 18, 793 (1981).
23. H. Schachter, Clin. Biochem. 17, 3 (1984).

AMYLOIDOGENICITY AND SUBGROUPS OF HUMAN LAMBDA

BENCE JONES PROTEINS

Takashi Isobi,* Hiroshi Tonoike,†
Fuyuki Kametani,† and Tomotaka Shinoda*

*Department of Medicine
 Kobe University School of Medicine, Kobe, Japan

†Department of Biochemistry
 Tokyo Metropolitan University, Tokyo, Japan

ABSTRACT

The nature of Bence Jones protein (BJP) NIG-77 (Kor) has been biochemically characterized. This BJP λ easily forms white and viscous precipitates in the cold in more than 8 mg/ml. This insolubility property is
ascribed to one tryptic peptide involving residues 23-46, which corresponds
with the first complementarity-determining regions (CDR) of the V-domain of
BJP.

Complete sequence analysis has been carried out to see if there is
any correlation between the primary structure and amyloidogenicity. On the
basis of sequence homology of CDR as well as whole variable region, BJP
NIG-77 has been classified in subsubgroup Vλ I-2 closely related to
amyloidosis, in contrast to presumably non-amyloidogenic subsubgroup Vλ
I-1 (1).

INTRODUCTION

By amino acid sequence analysis, amyloid fibril proteins from primary
and myeloma-associated amyloidosis have been found to be homologous to the
variable domain of immunoglobulin light chains [2]. However, only limited
and rather incomplete sequence data are available on AL, which seem to be
insufficient to elucidate between primary structure and amyloidogenicity
[3]. In this context, an attempt has been made to determine full amino
acid sequence of one Bence Jones protein with special interest as to whether
the BJP has any particular characteristic in primary structure compared
with other BJPs, since the case producing this BJP demonstrated clinically
dramatic changes from myeloma to systemic amyloidosis in the clinical
course.

MATERIALS AND METHODS

The detailed case report (Kor) is described separately in this pro-
ceeding of the symposium [4]. BJP NIG-77 (according to numbering in our

laboratory, also designated as Kor) was isolated from the urine in the following procesures: (1) fractionation with 60% saturation of ammonium sulfate, (2) DEAE-Sephadex A-50 column chromatography (2.6 × 40 cm, in 10 mM phosphate, pH 8.1, with a linear gradient in NaCl (0-0.3 M). (3) Column chromatography with CM-Sepharose CL-6B (2.6 × 40 cm, in 10 mM Na-acetate, pH 4.5 with linear gradient in NaCl (0-0.3 M).

The methods of further purification, and characterization with immuno-electrophoresis, disc-and SDS-disc electrophoresis, amino acid analysis of protein and peptides, complete reduction and aminoethylation, N- and C-terminal analyses have been described [4]. The purified and amino-ethylated BJP (25 mg in 20 mM NH_4HCO_3) was digested with 1,25 mg of TPCK-trypsin (2 × crystallized, Worthington) at 37°C for 4 h at pH 8.1. The digest was chromatographed first by HPLC with Hitachi 3013-C resin, (0.4 × 25 cm with an increasing concentration of the equilibrium buffer, 0.5 to 50% CH_3CN-0.25% to 25% isopropanol-4 mM to 0.4 M $NH_4CH_3SO_3$, pH 6.4) and peptides were further purified by reverse phase HPLC with a column of Hitachi 3013-0 (0.4 × 25 cm with an increasing concentration of buffer, 5 to 40% CH_3CN = 0.1% trifluoroacetic acid, pH 2.5). Fractions containing peptides were pooled and lyophilized.

Sequence analysis of the peptides (20-60 n mole) was carried out by manual Edman degradation method and PTH-amino acids were identified by HPLC under the reported conditions [1]. The nomenclature of the peptides of the protein, given the prefix T for the trypsin peptides and V for the V region, is followed as described [1]. Sequence of tryptic peptides are numbered consecutively in their order in the sequence.

RESULTS AND DISCUSSION

Crude material of BJP NIG-77 (Kor) was obtained by ammonium sulfate precipitation and was dialyzed against distilled water. Figure 1 shows a primary separation profile of the crude material through DEAE-Sephadex A-50, resulting in 4 peaks. Peak III in Fig. 1, reacted immunologically with anti λ antiserium, was further applied on CM Sepharose CL-6B column, yielding one major peak together with 3 minor peaks. This purified speci-men was lambda chain type, and the majority was existed in covalent dimers with an apparent molecular weight of 47 K daltons estimated by SDS-Disc electrophoresis. The N-terminus of the protein was not detected by Edman degradation, suggesting that it was blocked. None of the other N-terminal amino acids was detected in a significant amount. Therefore, the final preparation was considered to be homogeneous and was used for the subse-quent study.

Figure 2 shows an elution profile in the separation by HPLC of the tryptic peptides obtained from aminoethylated BJP NIG-77. Following the re-chromatography of several peaks, a total of 19 distinct peptides cover-ing the entire region of the protein were obtained. Of these, 8 peptides (TVI-TV7) were belonged to the V region. Yield of these peptides ranged between 15 and 80%. The amino acid compositions and sequences of the whole peptides were determined. The alignment of these peptides were conducted by homology with the other BJP λ chains reported previously. Figure 3 shows the amino acid sequence of the entire light chain of BJP NIG-77. It has 216 amino acid residues in total without any appreciable contamination with carbohydrates. The constant region occupying 105 residues has a rare amino acid replacement with the OZ (+) marker. It has the isotypes Is (-), Mcg (-), Kern (-) and Mz (-), respectively.

The variable region initiated with a blocked terminus and consisted of 111 amino acid residues including two additional ones at positions 27b and

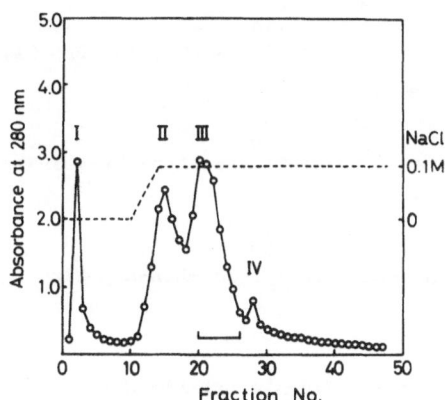

Fig. 1. Primary separation profile
of the crude material of
BJP NIG-77 (Kor) through
DEAE-Sephadex A-50.

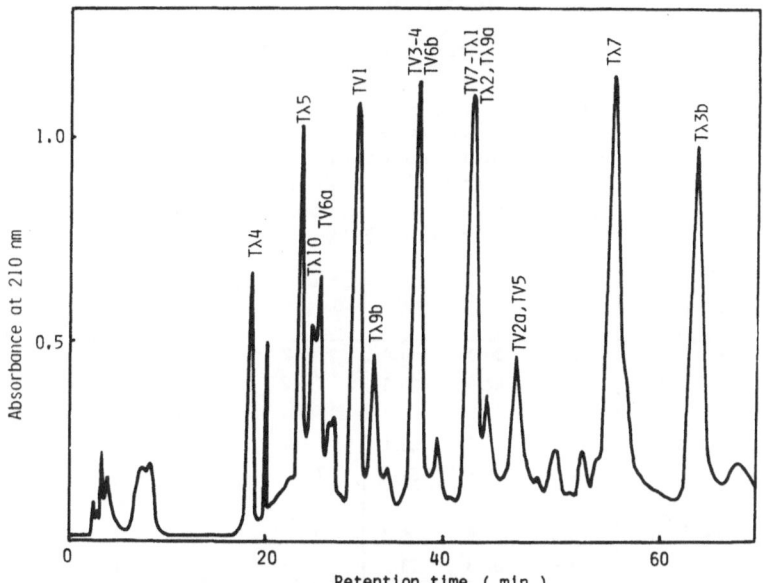

Fig. 2. Elution profile by HPLC of the tryptic peptides obtained from aminoethylated BJP, of which TVI to TV7
belongs to V region.

27c. The sequence is characteristic of the Vλ I light chains. There are
two tryptophan residues, one at position 36 and the other at 92, which is
consistently present in all the Vλ I light chains thus for sequenced.
Table 1 shows a comparison of the V region sequence of BJP NIG-77 and other
5 BJPs. Since the V region of light chains is made up of four frame work
regions separated by three complementary-determining regions (CDR), the
sequence homologies are demonstrated in Table 1 in three different ways,
(1) the entire V region, (2) four frame work regions and (3) three CDR.
The additional data on the presence or absence of clinical amyloidosis and

```
  1                              10                         TV1        20
Glp-Ser-Val-Leu-Thr-Gln-Pro-Pro-Ser-Ala-Ser-Gly-Thr-Pro-Gly-Gln-Arg-Val-Thr-Ile-


      TV2a                       30                                    40
Ser-Cys-Ser-Gly-Ser-Thr-Ser-Asn-Ile-Gly-Ser-Asn-Thr-Val-Thr-Trp-Tyr-Gln-His-Leu-


          TV2b                50                                        60
Pro-Gly-Thr-Ala-Pro-Lys-Leu-Leu-Ile-Tyr-Ser-Asn-Asp-Gln-Arg-Pro-Ser-Gly-Val-Pro-


      TV3-4            TV5       70                                     80
His-Arg-Phe-Ser-Gly-Ser-Lys-Ser-Gly-Ala-Ser-Ala-Ser-Leu-Ala-Ile-Ser-Gly-Leu-Gln-


                           TV6a 90                                     100
Ser-Glu-Asp-Glu-Thr-Asp-Tyr-Tyr-Cys-Ala-Thr-Trp-Asp-Asp-Ser-Leu-Asn-Gly-Pro-Val-


            TV6b            110        TV7-Tλ1        190
Phe-Gly-Gly-Gly-Thr-Lys-Val-Thr-Val-Gln-Gly-Gln-Pro-Lys--------Lys-----Ser-COOH
```

Fig. 3. Amino acid sequence of the entire light chain of BJP NIG-77 (Kor).

TABLE 1. Sequence Homology (%) of Vλ of BJP
NIG-77 (Kor) to Other 5 BJPs, Together
with the Data of the Presence or Absence of Clinical Amyloidosis and
in vitro Insolubility

BJP	No. of residues	V-region	Frame work	CDR	Vλ Subgroup Subsubgroup	Clinical Amyloid	In Vitro Insolubility
Kor	111	100.0	100.0	100.0	I − 2	+	+
51	111	82.0	82.5	80.6	I − 2	+	+
64	111	73.9	80.0	58.1	I − 1	−	−
New	111	72.0	77.5	58.1	I − 1	−	?
AR	110	60.0	68.8	36.7	VI	+	+
48	110	53.6	61.3	33.3	VI	+ ?	+

in vitro insolubility property of BJPs are also indicated. When the entire
V regions are compared, NIG-77 and NIG-51 has a close similarity (82.0%)
and only moderate degrees of homology (72.0 to 73.9%) are seen between
NIG-77 and two other BJPs (64, New), which are other members of Vλ I sub-
group. There are low degrees of homology (53.6 to 60.0%) of NIG-77 with
BJPs AR and NIG-48 belonging to subgroup Vλ VI. When the total framework
regions are compared, there are no remarkable differences of homology
among BJPs of subgroup I, although differences are seen between subgroups
I and VI. On the other hand, when the total CDR are compared, proteins
NIG-77 and -51 share the highest homology, in contrast to 2 other BJPs
NIG-64 and New of Vλ I subgroup, and also markedly contrasted to subgroup
VI proteins. On the basis of these data, the assignment of a subgroup Vλ
I is further divided into two distinct subsets of the structure, designated

subsubgroups Vλ I-1 and Vλ I-2, respectively [1]. If we look at the biological and physio-chemical aspects of these proteins in connection with
primary structure, two proteins belonging to subsubgroup I-2 have definite
association with systemic amyloidosis, with positive for insoluble property
in vitro. In contrast, two proteins classified in subsubgroup I-1 have
neither association with amyloidosis nor insolubility property as shown in
Table 1. As far as two proteins of subgroup VI are concerned, they are
associated with amyloidosis and also with insolubility property.

Insolubility property is one of the characteristics of physicochemical
nature in BJP NIG-77. During the course of the purification, BJP NIG-77
tended to precipitate in more than 8 mg/ml in protein concentration and in
low temperature. Moreover, it was noted that the tryptic peptide TV 2b
(residues 23-46), consisting of 24 residues including the first CDR (hyper-
variable region 1, HV 1), had also a characteristic property in solubility.
When a solution of the peptide, over 50 μg/ml in buffers such as 10 mM
NH_4HCO_3, pH 8.1, was allowed to stand at 4°C for few days, white and
viscous precipitates appeared. Thus, the peptide is presumably responsible
for the insolubility property of the whole chain. It may be conceivable
that insolubility of the proteins seems to be in some ways correlated to
the intrinsic property to produce β-pleated sheet conformation, typical
of amyloid fibril proteins [1, 5].

REFERENCES

1.   T. Shinoda, K. Tinani, F. W. Putnum, J. Biol. Chem., 245, 4463
     (1970); T. Shinoda, T. Takahashi, T. Takayasu, T. Okuyama, A.
     Shimizu, Proc. Natl. Acad. Sci. USA, 78, 785 (1980); F. Kametani,
     T. Takayasu, S. Suzuki, T. Shinoda, T. Okuyama, A. Shimizu, J. Bio-
     chem., 93, 421 (1983).
2.   G. G. Glenner, D. Ein, E. D. Eines, H. A. Bladen, W. Terry, D. L.
     Page, Science, 174, 712 (1971); G. G. Glenner, W. Terry, J. Harada,
     C. Isersky, D. Page, Science, 172, 1150 (1971); G. G. Glenner, New
     Engl. J. Med., 302, 1283 (1980).
3.   F. W. Putnum, E. J. Whitley, C. Paul, J. N. Davidson, Biochemistry,
     12, 3763 (1973); J. W. Fett and H. F. Deutsch, Biochemistry, 13, 4102
     (1974); N. Takahashi, T. Takayasu, T. Shinoda, S. Iot, T. Okutani,
     A. Shimizu, Biochem. Res., 1, 321 (1980); K. Sletten, J. B. Natvig,
     G. Husby, J. Juel, Biochem. J., 195, 561 (1981).
4.   T. Isobe, S. Hata, Y. Imai, S. Shiozawa, T. Fujita, T. Shinoda, in
     Proceedings of 4th International Symposium (1985).
5.   A. Solomon and C. L. McLaughlin, J. Biol. Chem., 244, 3393 (1969);
     T. Isobe, K. Takatsuki, F. W. Tishendorf, S. Birken, E. F. Osserman,
     Clin. Immunol. Immunol., 19, 15 (1981).

APPEARANCE OF SYSTEMIC AMYLOIDOSIS IN MYELOMA

WITH AMYLOIDOGENIC BENCE JONES PROTEIN

Takashi Isobe, Sachiko Hata,
Yasuo Imai, Shunichi Shiozawa,
Takuo Fujita, and Tomotaka Shinida*

Third Division
Department of Medicine
Kobe University School of Medicine
Kobe, Japan

*Department of Chemistry
 Tokyo Metropolitan University
 Tokyo, Japan

ABSTRACT

The patient (K. Kor), 55 year old female, had two phases of clinical manifestations in the course. The first one year is characterized by myeloma giving rise to osteolytic lesions, plasma cell proliferations in the bone marrow and urinary BJP of lambda type. Subsequent 8 months manifested amyloidosis with another variety of manifestations, including low voltage with sick sinus syndrome in ECG, progressive fall of blood pressure and macroglossia with amyloid deposits demonstrated by biopsy. It is noteworthy that the urinary excretion of BJP has decreased in amount along with the appearance of amyloidosis, suggestive of different catabolism of BJP in amyloidosis. The BJP, easily formed viscous precipitated in vitro, belong to V I-2 (sub-subgroup) washih is presumably amyloidogenic in character.

INTRODUCTION

The purpose of this report is to describe clinical and pathologic observations which have been made in the course of less than 2 years of a patient with systemic AL amyloidosis. This case is considered to lend support to the presence of amyloidogenic Bence Jones protein (BJP). The biochemical analysis of the amyloidogenic nature of the BJP in the present case will be described separately in this proceedings of the symposium [1]. In this regard, comparison before and after the appearance of amyloidosis will provide some clues to the pathologic processes of amyloidosis [2].

CASE PRESENTATION

K. Kor, 55 year old female, visited the orthopedic clinic because of pain of the right hip joint on walking. She transfered to the Third Division

sion, Department of Medicine after the histological diagnosis of plasmacytoma was made by a iliac-bond biopsy. She was found to be obese. Her
body weight was 62 kg and height 152 cm. Her blood pressure was 144/86
mmHg. There was no evidence of macroglossia, cardiomegaly or hepatosplenomegaly. Neurological examination was negative. Laboratory data included a red blood cell count of $456 \times 10^4/mm^3$, hemoglobin 13.6 g/dl,
platelet $32.3 \times 10^4/mm^3$, white cell count 8,800/mm^3 with a normal deffer-
ential, serum cholesterol 188 mg/dl, blood urea nitrogen 13 mg/dl, uric acid
5.0 mg/dl, serum creatinine 0.8 mg/dl, serum calcium 9.2 mg/dl, phosphorus
3.3 mg/dl, CRP +3 and ESR 77 mm/hour. There were normal values of function
tests for the thyroid, lever and kidneys. Serum total protein was 6.7
g/dl consisting of albumin 3.6, α_1-globulin 0.3, α_2-0.7, β-1.0 and γ-globu-
lin 1.1 g/dl without any monoclonal spike. Serum immunoglobulin measure-
ment revealed IgG 1,740 mg/dl, IgA 590 mg/dl, IgM 92 mg/dl, IgE 16 μ/ml and
IgD undetectable.

Urinary protein excretion ranged between 0.2 to 1.0 g/24 h. Cellulose
acetate electrophoresis disclosed a monoclonal spike in the urine, which
was identified as BJP of lambda type. X-ray survey showed multiple punched-
out lesions in the skull, the right pelvis and the femur, together with com-
pression fracture of the 1st and 3rd lumbar spines. Bone scintography
showed an abnormal accumulation of 99 m Technetium at the lumbar spines,
right pelvis and bilateral ribs. Although the diagnosis of plasmacytoma
was made based on the biopsied material from the iliac bone, plasma cells
occupied only 2.4% of the nucleated cells in the specimen from the sternum
and 1.2% from the iliac crest bone marrow cespiation. Chemotherapy was
instituted by continuous administration 2 mg/day melphalan with 10 mg/day
prednisolone, which induced a good response of subsidence of subjective
complaints in 2 months in spite of no remarkable changes of daily excretion
of urinary BJP.

She had been doing well for the subsequent 6 months, when she started
to notice weakness, dyspnea, light headedness and body weight loss of 16
kg within 6 months. At that time she was found to have macroglossia,
lowered blood pressure 94/78 mmHg and low voltage of the limb leads in ECG.

Because these clinical manifestations were suggestive of amyloidosis,
a biopsy of the tongue was performed, confirming this histological diagnosis of amyloidosis. On re-admission, she was emaciated and poorly nourished.
Her body weight was then 48 kg and blood pressure was 66/52 mmHg. Laboratory data included red blood cell $388 \times 10^4/mm^3$, hemoglobin 12.4 g/dl,
platelet $15.6 \times 10^4/mm^3$, white cell count 4,200 with a normal differential,
serum cholesterol 221 mg/dl, blood urea nitrogen 13 mg/dl, uric acid 5.3
mg/dl, serum creatinine 0.9 mfg/dl, serum calcium 10.4 mg/dl, phosphorus
3.7 mg/dl, CRP (-) and ESR mm/hour. A serum total protein was 4.9 g/dl
consisting of albumin 2.3, α_1-globulin 0.2, α_2-0.7, β-0.7, γ-globulin 1.0
g/dl, without monoclonal spike. Serum immunoglobulin concentration was IgG
795 mg/dl, IgA 350 and IgM 52 mg/dl. Daily protein excretion into the
urine ranged between 0.5 to 1.0 g. It is noteworthy that the monoclonal
peak of BJP in the urine decreased in size on cellulose acetate electrophoresis compared with the size of albumin, together with the diminution
of daily excretion of BJP in the urine (Fig. 1).

The patient exhibited the clinical manifestations of cardiac failure
probably due to cardiac amyloidosis, since there were suggestive changes
in ECG's within a year from normal to abnormal findings including low
voltage, junctional rhythm and sick sinus syndrome as shown in Fig. 2.
Another supportive evidence of cardiac amyloidosis was an abnormal echogram
of the heart, which demonstrated hypertrophic intraventricular septum towards the apex with thickness of 12 to 21 mm in association with partially
akinetic and echogenic area. Comparison of routine chest X-rays also

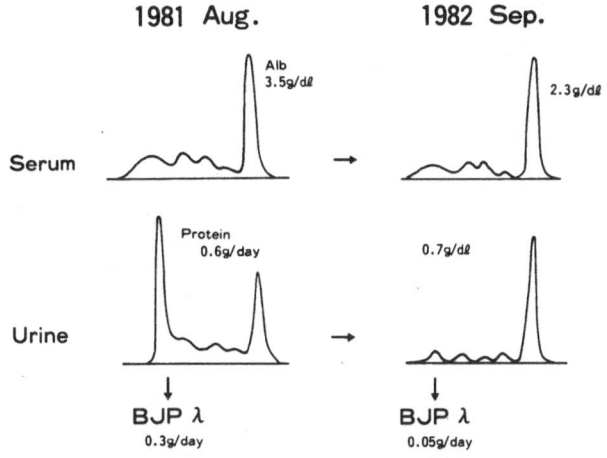

1981 Aug.   1982 Sep.

Serum

Alb
3.5g/dl

2.3g/dl

Urine

Protein
0.6g/day

0.7g/dl

BJP λ
0.3g/day

BJP λ
0.05g/day

Fig. 1.   Monoclonal peak of BJP of the urine de-
          creased in size on cellulose acetate
          electrophoresis compared with the size
          of albumin, together with the diminu-
          tion of daily excretion of BJP in the
          urine.

showed the enlargement in cardiac silhouette within a year. Her clinical
condition deteriorated with cardiac failure and edema. She died 8 months
after the appearance of signs of amyloidosis and 16 months after the diagnosis of myeloma.

     Autopsy diagnosis was systemic amyloidosis associated with multiple
myeloma. As to myeloma, multiple punched out lesions of bones were found
in the sternum and the vertibral bodies of thoratic 12th to lumbar 3rd
spines. There were nodular and diffuse infiltration of lambda chain positive plasmacytes. Amyloid depositions were mainly on vessel wall and in
the parenchyma, in varied organs, especially in the tongue and in the
heart including the conductive system. Other organs are involved by amyloid
markedly in kidneys, adrenals, and spleen, and moderately in liver pancreas, lung, thyroid, parathyroid, submucosal lesions of gastrointestinal
tracts, ovaries and several lymph nodes. Associated and other findings
were tuberculous lymphadenitis in peripancreatic node, pseudomembranous
gastorcolitis, nephrolithiosis of the left renal pelvis and submucosal
bleedings.

     In summary, this patient exhibited two phases of clinical manifesta-
tions in her course. The first phase of one year is characterized by myeloma of osteolytic lesions, plasma cell proliferations in the bone marrow
and urinary BJP of lambda type. Another variety of manifestations lasting a
subsequent 8 months represented systemic AL amyloidosis including macro-
glosia, progressively lowered blood pressure and ECG abnormalities. Table
1 showed the major differences of signs and symptoms between myeloma-phase
and amyloidosis-phase. Particular noteworthy is that urinary excretion of
BJP tended to decrease in amount along the appearance of amyloidosis.

THE NATURE OF BJP KOR

     BJP of this patient was isolated, purified and then characterized.
Insolubility property is one of the characteristics of physicochemical na-

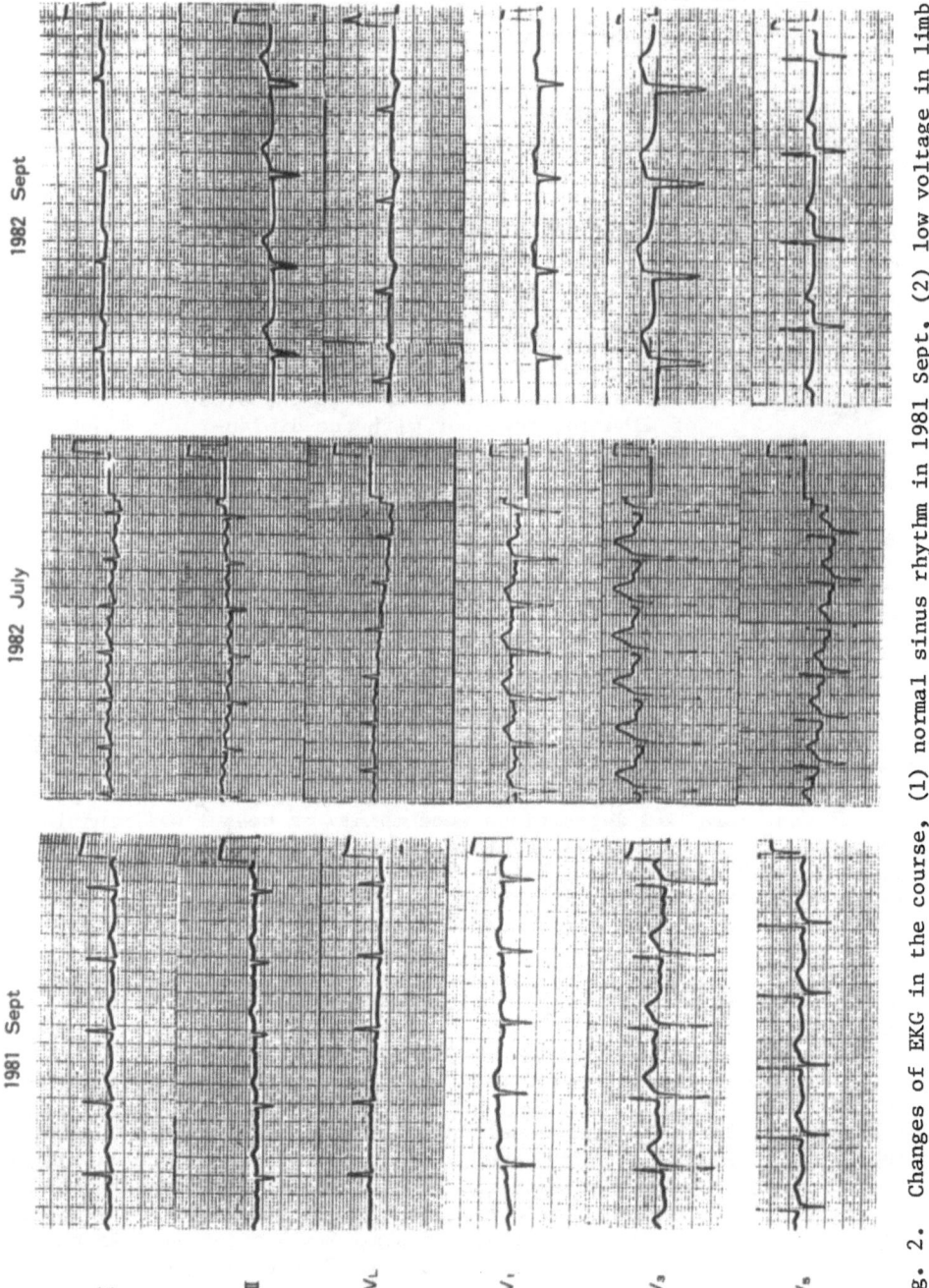

Fig. 2. Changes of EKG in the course, (1) normal sinus rhythm in 1981 Sept, (2) low voltage in limb leads and poor progression of R waves in the right precordial leads in 1981 July and (3) sick sinus syndrome with intraventricular conduction delay in 1982 Sept.

TABLE 1. Two Phases of Clinical Features of Case Kor from Multiple Myeloma to Systemic Amyloidosis

		1981 Aug.	1982 Sep.
		Plasmacytoma Pelvis	Amyloidosis
Serum MP		(−)	(−)
Tp	(g/dℓ)	6.7	4.9
Alb	(g/dℓ)	3.5	2.3
γ-gl	(g/dℓ)	1.1	1.0
Urine		BJP λ	BJP λ
Protein	(g/day)	0.6	0.7
Alb	(g/day)	0.2	0.6
BJP	(g/day)	0.3	0.05
Marrow			
Plasma cells (%)		1.2~2.4	5.6
Bone X-P		Osteolytic	Osteolytic
ECG		Normal	→ Low voltage in limb leads
			→ Sick sinus syndrome
BP	(mmHg)	134/96	→ 94/78 → 66/52
Tongue		Normal	Macroglossia
Body weight	(kg)	64	→ 48 → 45

ture in BJP Kor. During the processes of purification, BJP Kor tended to precipitate in more than 8 mg/ml in protein concentration and in low temperature, which considerably hindered the isolation of the protein.

As to its biochemical nature, this BJP was classified into subgroup Vλ I and further sub-subgroup Vλ I-2 on the basis of homology of the data of amino acid sequence in the variable region. So far, sub-subgroup Vλ I-2 is found in BJPs only from the patients with amyloidosis [1]. Table 2 summerizes the nature of BJP Kor. The detailed data will be reported separately in this proceedings [1].

DISCUSSION

It is rather unusual to see a change of the clinical course from one disease to the other. The present case exhibited two phases of clinical features, starting with those of myeloma, followed by appearance of amyloidisis. Thus, the case may provide the subject of extensive consideration and investigation. Manifestations of myeloma were based on bone destructive lesions, whereas appearance of new symptoms was related to amyloid deposi-

TABLE 2. Physico-Chemical and
Biochemical Nature of
BJP Kor

Kor BJP

λ

Dimer in the urine

C-region isotype

OZ$^+$, IS$^-$, Kern$^-$, McG$^-$

V-region

Subgroup VλI, VλI − 2

Insoluble property

Whole chain, more than 8 mg/mℓ

Tryptic peptides (23−46) in Vregion

tion in the tongue which demonstrated macroglossia and in the heart suggested by low voltage and conduction disturbance of ECG as well as abnormal thickenings on cardiac echogram as shown in Figs. 1 and 2. It may be worthy to evaluate echograms of the heart to detect some abnormal findings related to amyloid, because of recently increasing application to practical medicine and its simplicity.

AL amyloidosis consists of primary amyloidosis and myeloma-associated amyloidosis. These two groups constitute different aspect of the same disease process [2]. The most frequent initial symptoms are weakness or fatigue, loss of weight, ankle edema, dyspnea, paresthesia and light headedness and signs of purpura, enlargement of the liver and tongue, orthostatic hypotension and congestive heart failure, all of which just occurred in the course of the present case except purpura [2, 3]. Although not seen in this case, nephrotic syndrome, malabsorption, peripheral neuropathy, and the carpal tunnel syndrome are found in some cases of AL amyloidosis. The electrocardiogram shows various changes including low voltage, junctional escape beats and sick sinus syndrome due to amyloid infiltration, all of which again occurred in the present case [4].

As to protein abnormalities in AL amyloidosis, Isobe and Osserman summarized 100 cases of amyloidosis, 46% of the patients with amyloidosis had BJP only without a serum M-protein, as compared with 21% of cases of myeloma without associated amyloidosis [2]. There was also a higher proportion of λ type BJP in the amyloidosis group. Similar studies by Kyle in USA and Isobe in Japan also supported the BJP predominance in amyloidosis [3]. The most interesting feature in the present case is the changes of protein electrophoresis in the serum and urine. Serum albumin decreased, corresponding to the increased albuminuria. Especially noteworthy is that the diminution of BJP in proportion as well as in daily-amount of excretion, which is suggestive of an unusual catabolism of amyloidogenic BJP not in the urine but into specific tissues. This speculation may be valid in cases of AL amyloidosis due to a different catabolism of M-protein operative in the pathogenesis of amyloidosis. In this regard, it may be conceivable that insolubility of the proteins seems to be in some ways correlated to the intrinsic property to produce β-pleated sheet conformation, typical of amyloid fibril proteins [2, 5]. Further experiments on the production and catabolism of BJP in amyloidotic and non-amyloidotic patients is worthy of pursuit.

REFERENCES

1. T. Isobe, H. Tonoike, F. Kametani, T. Shinoda, in: Proceedings of 4th International Amyloidosis Symposium (1985).
2. E. F. Osserman, K. Takatsuki, N. Talal, Seminars in Haematology 1, 3 (1964); T. Isobe and E. F. Osserman, New Engl. J. Med., 290:473 (1974); G. G. Glenner, New Engl. J. Med., 302:1283 (1980).
3. R. A. Kyle and E. D. Bayrd, Medicine, 54:271 (1975); T. Isobe, M. Tomita, J. Matsumoto, T. Fujita, Jap. J. Med., 22:117 (1983).
4. R. L. Ridolfi, B. H. Bulkley, G. M. Hutchins, Am. J. Med., 62:677 (1977).
5. A. Solomon and C. L. McLaughlin, S. Biol. Chem., 244:3393 (1969); T. Isobe, K. Takatsuki, F. W. Tishchendorf, S. Birken, E. F. Osserman, Clin. Immunol. Immunopath., 19:15 (1981).

COMPLETE PRIMARY STRUCTURE OF AN IMMUNOGLOBULIN λII-

CHAIN DERIVED AMYLOID FIBRIL PROTEIN (HAR)

M. Eulitz and R. P. Linke*

Institut f. Hämatologie der GSF
Abt. Immunologie
Landwehrstr. 61
D-8000 München 2, West Germany

*Institut f. Immunologie der Ludwig
 Maximilians Universität
 München, West Germany

ABSTRACT

An amyloid fibril protein was isolated from the spleen of a patient
(HAR) suffering from an IgD, λ myeloma. The isolated fibril protein has
a molecular weight of 5000 dalton. Its amino acid sequence was established
by automatic degradation of the whole fragment and by studies on tryptic
and thermosinolytic peptides. The fragment showed maximal homology to
human λII-immunoglobulin light chains. It commences at two positions, 8
and 9 and extends to the position 67 of a prototype sequence. The missing
N-terminal hepta- or octopeptide most probably had been cleaved off from
the N-terminus of the parent L-chain during amyloidogenesis. This is
strikingly similar to results obtained by limited in vitro digestion of
some human λ-Bence Jones proteins with formation of amyloid-like material.
In addition two peptides, not covalently bound to the V-region fragment and obviously derived from the connection between variable and constant part have been
isolated from the tryptic digest of the amyloid fibrils and sequenced.

INTRODUCTION

Since the work of Glenner and associates [6, 7] it is generally accepted,
that amyloid fibril proteins identified in patients with B-cell tumors or plasma
cell dyscrasias have their origin in monoclonal immunoglobulin light chains.
Amyloid fibril proteins are rarely deposited as uncleaved immunoglobulin light
chains [19]. However, in most cases the major amyloid fibril proteins consist
of fragments of monoclonal immunoglobulin light chains (abbreviated AL) [3, 5,
10, 20]. As amino acid sequence studies on isolated amyloid fibril proteins have
shown, most of the AL-fibril proteins comprise the whole V-region of immunoglobulin L-chains and to a varying extent parts of the constant region. As reviewed
by Glenner [8] the average molecular weight of all reported fibril proteins is
approximately 14,000 daltons.

A special finding was the description of a subgroup of human λ-chains
(λVI), which was found to be associated in many cases with amyloidosis

[14, 16, 17]. This association occurs more frequently, than would be expected from the concentration of this subgroup in normal serum immunoglobulins [17].

Despite intensive efforts to identify structural or antigenic peculiarities among "amyloidogenic" immunoglobulin L-chains, so far no such general applicable principles could be defined [8].

Based on chemical evidence and in vitro studies Al-amyloid fibril proteins are identified as proteolytic degradation products of monoclonal L-chains, as for instance Bence Jones proteins. The enzymes responsible for this pathogenetic mechanism are not defined yet. Also the complete primary structure of AL-amyloid fibril proteins is known only in a few cases.

In extending the studies on AL-type amyloid fibrils, we describe here the complete amino acid sequence of an amyloid fibril protein (HAR), isolated from the spleen of a patient with IgD, λ myeloma, which showed some unusual features.

MATERIALS AND METHODS

Amyloid fibrils were isolated from the spleen (65 gr) of a patient who died with IgD, λ-myeloma and generalized amyloidosis. After extraction according to Pras [12], the amyloid fibril protein was purified by gel filtration on Sephadex G-100 (Pharmacia, Uppsala, Sweden) as already described [3]. After reduction with dithiothreitol and alkylation of the sulfhydryl groups with iodoacetamide, the fibril protein was subjected to stepwise automatic degradation in a Beckman 890 C sequenator (Beckman Instr., Fullerton, Cal.) equipped with a cold trap accessory.

Tryptic peptides were generated from the amyloid fibril protein by incubation with TPCK-Trypsin for 4 h at 37°C in 0.1 M methylmorpholine-acetate buffer pH 8.0. An insoluble precipitate was formed during the incubation. This precipitate was spun down by centrifugation at 12,000 rpm in a table top centrifuge and cleaved further by incubation with thermolysin (ratio 1:100) for 16 h at 37°C also in the methyl-morpholine buffer pH 8.0. Tryptic and thermosinolytic peptides were purified separately by high performance liquid chromatography on a column (4.6 × 250 mm) of Lichrospher RP$_{18}$, 5μ particle diameter, (Merck AG, Darmstadt) employing a linear gradient from 0.1% trifluoroacetic acid to the same solution with 70% acetonitrile within 55 min at 50°C column temperature. The separated peptides were checked for purity by thin layer chromatography on silica gel 60 coated glass plates (20 × 20 cm) (Merck AG, Darmstadt) in a solvent system of methanol:chloroform:ammonia 2:2:1 (v/v/v). The peptides were detected after spraying with fluorescamine according to Schiltz et al. [18].

The amino acid composition of the tryptic or thermosinolytic peptides was estimated in an automatic amino acid analyzer model 5000 (Biotronik Instr./Frankfurt) after hydrolysis in contant boiling hydrochloric acid at 105°C for 24 h.

The amino acid sequence of the tryptic or thermosinolytic peptides was evaluated either by automatic degradation in the Beckman Sequenator with polybrene (Pierce, Rockford, Ill.) as carrier or in some cases by manual degradation with 4-N,N-dimethylaminoazobenzene 4'-isothiocyanate (DABITC) (Fluka AG, Buchs, Switzerland) essentially as described by Chang et al. [1].

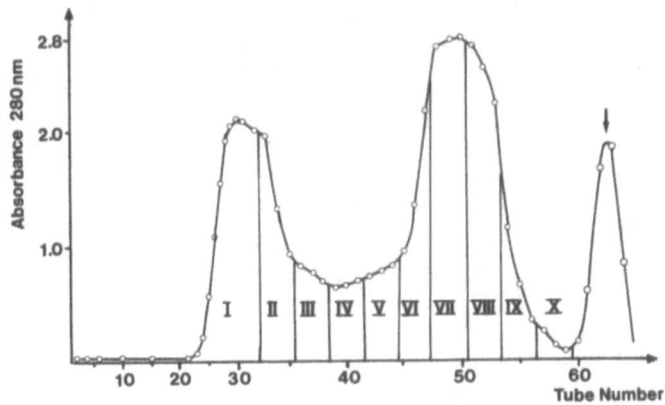

Fig. 1.   Gel filtration of amyloid fibril protein Har
          on Sephadex G_{100}. The water extracted fibril
          protein was dissolved in 5m guanidine-hydro-
          chloride in 0.1 m Tris-HCl buffer pH 8.0.
          Undissolved material was centrifuged off. About
          450 mg material in a volume of 10 ml was
          applied to a column (2 × 100 cm) filled with
          Sephadex G_{100}. Elution was performed with 5
          m guanidine hydrochloride in 0.1 m Tris-HCl
          buffer pH 8.0. Flow rate 12 ml/h. Volume/
          tube = 6 ml. The absorbancy was measured at
          280 nm against the elution buffer. Fractions
          were taken as indicated by roman figures. The
          arrow marks the position were ε-DNP-lysine
          elutes from the column.

RESULTS

    Water extracted, lyophilized amyloid fibrils were dissolved in 5 M
guanidine-hydrochloride 0,1 M Tris, pH 8.0. Undissolved material was removed by centrifugation. The clear solution was separated in a Sephadex
G-100 column (2 × 100 cm) and eluted in the same solvent with a flow rate
of 12 ml/h. Volumes of 6 ml were collected per tube. The absorption profile at 280 nm is shown in Fig. 1. Fractions were collected as indicated
in Fig. 1. Fraction VI of Fig. 1 containing a polypeptide chain of about
5000 daltons by SDS-polyacrylamide-electrophoresis was reduced, carboxymethylated and subjected to automatic degradation. The amino acid sequence
of this peptide could be determined up to position 41, histidine, shown in
Fig. 2. About 70% of the chain commences with alanine and about 30% with
serine. Also the following degradation cycles gave two amino acids in about
the same ratio. The amino acid sequences deduced from the different yields
of PTH-amino acids are in accordance with a displacement of one residue at
the N-terminus of the polypeptide chain. We concluded from this finding,
that an intact λII-light chain must have been cleaved at the positions 8 and
9 of the variable region. From the supernatant after tryptic digestion of
protein HAR all peptides spanning the positions 44 to 67 of the variable
region could be isolated by HPLC, characterized by amino acid analysis and
sequenced, either by automatic degradation or by the manual DBITC-method
[1].

    The precipitate, which has been formed during the digestion with tryp-
sin was cleaved further with thermolysin and the resulting peptides were
isolated likewise by the HPLC-method and sequenced. The complete primary

```
                     10              20                    30
PROTEIN NEI  PCA S A L T Q P A S V S G S P G Q S I T I S C T G T T S D V G S Y N F V S W Y
PROTEIN HAR              A S V S G S P G Q S V T I S C T G T S S D V G G Y N Y V S W Y

            40            50              60            68
PROTEIN NEI  Q Q N P G K A P K L M I Y E G N K R P S G V S N R F S G S K . . . . . .
PROTEIN HAR  Q Q H P G K A P R L I I Y D V N K R P S G A P D R F S G S
```

ALIGNMENT OF THE SECOND FRAGMENT OF PROTEIN HAR TO THE CONNECTION BETWEEN V_L- AND C_L- REGION

```
            100              110                120               130
PROTEIN NEI  G T R V T V L S Q P K A A P S V T L F P P S S E E L Q A N K A T V L . . . . . .
PROTEIN HAR      L T V L S Q P K A A P S V T L F P P S S E E L Q A N K
```

Fig. 2. Comparison of the amino acid sequence of the amyloid fibril
protein Har with the human V II protein Nei. Protein Har
was aligned to protein Nei [4] for maximal homology. Stretches
which show the same amino acid are boxed. The one letter code
for amino acids according to Dayhoff [2] was choosen. The
symbols mean: A = alanine, C = cysteine, D = Aspartic acid,
E = glutamic acid, F = Phenylalanine, G = glycine, I = isoleucine, K = lysine, L = leucine, M = methionine, N = asparagine, P = proline, Q = glutamine, R = arginine, S = serine,
T = threonine, V = valine, W = tryptophan, Y = tyrosine, PCA =
pyrrolidone carboxylic acid.

structure of the amyloid fibril protein HAR could be deduced from the sequence data of the degradation of the amyloid fibril protein and from the
studies of the tryptic and thermosinolytic peptides as given in Fig. 2.

Comparison with already known sequences of human immunoglobulin
L-chains showed maximal homology of protein HAR to proteins of the subgroup
λII. As mentioned before, the amyloid fibril protein commences with two
different amino acids, i.e. 8 and 9 of the variable region and extents up
to position 67.

In an attempt to confirm the results we digested also fraction VII of
Fig. 1 with trypsin. Beside the peptides already known from the digestion
of fraction VI we found unexpectedly two additional tryptic peptides, which
also have been sequenced. The peptides could be aligned to the positions
103-110 of the V-region and 111-129 of the adjacent C-region. Obviously
both peptides originate from a fragment not covalently bound but associated
to the amyloid fibril protein.

DISCUSSION

In the AL forms of amyloidosis the amyloid fibril proteins deposited
in tissues and organs consist mainly of fragments of immunoglobulin
L-chains [3, 5, 10, 20]. This is also true here for the reported sequence
of the fibril protein HAR. In contrast to many other amyloid fibril pro-

teins, protein HAR does not represent the complete V-region. It commences
with alanine, respectively serine at positions 8 and 9 of the λII-light
chains. As the N-terminus of proteins in this subgroup is normally blocked,
it can be concluded that the amyloid fibril protein HAR represents only a
fragment of the parent protein. The possibility that the main fragment may
also be blocked can be ruled out, because the starting yield in the automatic degradation was about 80 percent of the expected value. This yield
is only possible, if the N-terminal amino group is practically fully acces-
sible to the phenylisothiocyanate. Furthermore, all thermosinolytic peptides could be aligned to the sequence. Especially no peptide with a
blocked N-terminus was found. For these reasons it is very likely that the
amyloid fibril protein HAR is produced by limited proteolysis from a blocked
λII-chain. In addition the inhomogeneous N-terminus can be taken as evidence for proteolytic cleavage.

Whether the related L-chain is really blocked could not be tested, because the patient did not excrete significant amounts of Bence Jones proteins. Experiments to isolate the λ-chain from the IgD myeloma protein are
under way.

Protein HAR shows a striking chemical similarity to amyloid like material produced in vitro be digestion of λI-Bence Jones proteins by incubation with proteolytic enzymes. Glenner and associates [7] found that
pepsin could cleave off a tripeptide from the λI bence Jones protein NIC,
whereas Linke et al. [11] reported the removal of a tetrapeptide from Bence
Jones protein CAR, also by pepsin. In protein HAR a hepta- or octopeptide
must have been cleaved off in vivo. Another clear similarity exists in respect to the length of fibril protein HAR and the in vitro produced amyloid-
like fragments. The NIC-fragment had a molecular weight of 4600 dalton and
the CAR-fragment one of 6000 daltons. Protein HAR being of similar size,
however is a typical in vivo produced amyloid fibril protein. Thus, at
least in this case, the proteolytic process which lead to the formation of
amyloid protein HAR may more closely resemble the in vitro process.

There is only one other amyloid fibril protein, whose amino acid sequence is known in full length, i.e. protein AR [16]. Protein HAR in contrast to protein AR is a rather small fragment not extending to the constant region. The C-terminus of protein HAR is (in contrast to protein AR)
homogeneous.

In another case the isolation of two light chain fragments with a molecular weight of 11300 and 14500 daltons from an IgG₃ λ plasmocytoma was
reported by Isobe et al. [9]. Both fragments showed a blocked N-terminus
and originated from the same precursor protein. Although the amino acid
sequence of an isolated peptide from one of the fragments shows close
homology to the positions 67-90 of λII-immunoglobulin light chains, there
are great differences in respect to the amino acid regions, from which the
amyloid protein HAR was derived.

A quite unexpected finding was the isolation of two adjacent peptides
from the connection of the variable and the constant region of protein
HAR. We conlude, that this second fragment is not covalently bound to the
V-region derived fragment of protein HAR, because both peptides do not contain cysteine and no peptides alignable to the positions 68-103 could be
found. As x-ray crystallographic studies on protein NEW [13] with a resolution of 2 Å have shown, there exist a close connection between residues
8-13 of the variable region and residues 102-108 at the beginning of the
constant region, confirmed by hydrogen bridges. It is suspected, that this
connection has been maintained also after the proteolytic disintegration
of the monoclonal immunoglobulin L-chain.

ACKNOWLEDGEMENT

This work was supported in part by the Sonderforschungsbereich 0207 (Projects Lp 12 and Lp 13) of the University of München.

REFERENCES

1. Chang, J. Y., Brauer, D., and Wittman-Liebold, B, FEBS-Letters, 93: 205 (1978).
2. Dayhoff, M. O. (Ed.), Vol. 4, "Atlas of Protein Sequence and Structure," National Biomedical Research Foundation, Silver Spring, Md. (1969).
3. Eulitz, M. and Lonke, R. P., Hoppe Seylers Z. Physiol. Chem., 363:1374 (1982).
4. Garver, F. A. and Hilschmann, N., Eur. J. Biochem., 26:10 (1972).
5. Glenner, G. G., Harbaugh, J., Ohms, J. J., Harada, M., and Cuatrecasas, P., Biochem. Biophys. Res. Comm., 41:1287 (1970).
6. Glenner, G. G., Terry, W. D., Harada, M., Isersky, C., and Page, D. L., Science, 172:1150 (1971).
7. Glenner, G. G., Ein, D., Eanes, E. D., Bladen, H. A., Terry, W. D., and Page, D. L., Science, 174:712 (1971).
8. Glenner, G. G., New Engl. J. Med., 302:1283 and 1333 (1980).
9. Isobe, T., Takatsuki, K., Tischendorf, F. W., Birken, S., and Osserman, E. F., Clin. Immunol. Immunopathol., 19:55 (1981).
10. Kimura, S., Guyer, R., Terry, W. D., and Glenner, G. G., J. Immunol., 109:891 (1972).
11. Linke, R. P., Zucker-Franklin, D., and Franklin, E. C., J. Immunol., 110:21 (1973).
12. Pras, M., Schubert, M., Zucker-Franklin, D., Rimon, A., and Franklin, E. D., J. Clin. Invest., 47:924 (1968).
13. Poljack, R. J., Amzel, L. M., Chen, B. L., Phizackerley, R. P., and Saul, F., Proc. Natl. Acad. Sci. USA, 71:3440 (1974).
14. Skinner, M., Benson, M. D., and Cohen, A. S., J. Immunol., 114:1433 (1975).
15. Sletten, K., Husby, G., and Natvig, J. B., Scand. J. Immunol., 3:833 (1974).
16. Sletten, K., Natvig, J. B., Husby, G., and Juul, J., Biochem. J., 195:561 (1981).
17. Solomon, A., Frangione, B., and Franklin, E. C., J. Clin. Invest., 70:453 (1982).
18. Schiltz, E., Schnackerz, K. D., and Gracy, R. W., Anal. Biochem., 79:33 (1977).
19. Terry, W. D., Page, D. L., Kimura, S., Isobe, T., Osserman, E. F., and Glenner, G. G., J. Clin. Invest., 52, 1276 (1973).
20. Westermark, P., Sletten, K., and Natvig, J. B., Acta. Pathol. Microbiol. Scand., C89:199 (1981).

SOME STRUCTURAL FACTORS INVOLVED IN AMYLOID FIBRIL

FORMATION BY LAMBDA VI LIGHT CHAIN PROTEINS*

Francis E. Dwulet, Kandice Strako,
and Merrill D. Benson

Indiana University School of Medicine and
Richard L. Roudebush Veterans
Administration Medical Center
Indianapolis, Indiana

ABSTRACT

Recent studies on the structures of lambda VI proteins have revealed
that these molecules have a high propensity to form amyloid deposits. Of
the 13 lambda VI proteins reported in the literature 12 have been shown to
be incorporated into AL amyloid. Of these proteins only the myeloma protein NIG48 and the amyloid proteins AR and SUT have been subjected to complete sequence analysis. To improve this data base we report the complete
structure of the amyloid protein WLT. This molecule has 134 amino acid
residues and consists of the entire variable region, joining segment and
first tryptic peptide of the constant region. Phylogenetic analysis of
these proteins reveals that the 3 amyloid proteins (WLT, AR and SUT) are
more closely related to each other than to protein NIG48. Separating the
variable regions into framework and complementarity determining regions
and recalculating the phylogenetic comparisons identifies substitutions
in the framework regions of protein NIG48. These findings support the
hypothesis that the formation of AL amyloid is a result of the structure of
the FR regions of the precursor molecule.

INTRODUCTION

During the last several years there has been increased interest in the
structures of immunoglobulin (AL) amyloid proteins. This has been most
dramatic in the study of the labmda VI proteins which have been found to
have a high propensity for amyloid formation. Of the 13 proteins in this

---

*This work was supported by VA Medical Research (MRIS 583-0888), and grants
 from RR-00750 (GCRC), United States Public Health Service, National Institute of Arthritis, Metabolism and Digestive Diseases (AM 20582 and
 AM 7448), The Arthritis Foundation, and The Grace M. Showalter Foundation.

subgroup which have been reported [1, 2] 12 have been shown to form AL amyloid. Unfortunately, only 3 of these proteins have been subjected to complete sequence analysis. Proteins AR and SUT were isolated from individuals with AL amyloid while protein NIG48 was obtained from a myeloma patient. Because of this characteristic property to form amyloid fibrils it is tempting to say that this molecule has some feature which predisposes it to form these deposits. However, no analysis of the structures of these proteins have successfully identified unique structural elements. This is partly due to the limited number of structures which are currently available. To increase this structural data we report here the complete sequence of lambda VI amyloid protein WLT and an analysis of the structural relatedness of all complete lambda VI proteins.

MATERIALS AND METHODS

Amyloid Isolation

Amyloid-laden tissue was obtained post mortem from patient WLT, a 43 year old male with rapidly progressing systemic amyloidosis, who died of renal failure. Amyloid fibrils were isolated from 30 g of spleen by standard procedures [3]. The fibrils were denatured in 6M guanidine and the disulfide bonds reduced with dithiothreitol and alkylated with iodoacetic acid. The subunit protein was isolated by chromatography on a column of Sepharose CL6B equilibrated in 4M guanidine. Pooled fractions were dialyzed against distilled water and lyophilized.

Enzymatic Digestions

Amyloid subunit protein WLT (6 mg) was dissolved in 2 ml of 0.1M ammonium bicarbonate buffer to which was added 0.12 mg (2% by weight) of TPCK-trypsin (Worthington). The digest was allowed to progress for 12 hours at 37° when it was terminated by freezing and lyophilization. The staph protease digest was done in a similar manner except 0.3 mg (5% by weight) of enzyme (Miles) was used and the digest maintained at 37° for 24 hours before lyophilization.

Peptide Separation

The digests were dissolved in 40% acetic acid and the peptides separated by reverse phase high pressure liquid chromatography. Teh tryptic digest was separated on an Altex Ultrasphere C-18 column (1 × 25 cm) using a 0.025M ammonium acetate pH 5.0 buffer and a 0-50% gradient of acetonitrile. The staph protease digest was separated on a Synchrom RPP column (1 × 25 cm) equilibrated in 0.1% trifluoroacetic acid and eluted with 0-45% 2-propanol gradient.

Sequence Analysis

All protein and peptide samples were degraded in a Beckman 890C sequenator using the Edman procedure. All technical aspects of the degradation and PTH identification have been described previously [4].

Phylogenetic Analysis

The phylogenetic relationships of the 4 lambda VI proteins was accomplished using the method of Bogardt et al. [5]. This procedure uses nearest neighbor analysis to identify the minimum number of DNA mutations to account for the observed amino acid differentes. This analysis was performed on the entire variable regions as well as on the framework and complementarity determining regions.

```
                          5                   10                  15              20              25
          |------------------------------------ FR1 -----------------------------------------------|
WLT     Asn-Phe-Met-Leu-Thr-Gln-Pro-Leu-Ser-Val-Ser-Gly-Ser-Pro-Glu-Lys-Thr-Val-Thr-Ile-Ser-Cys-Thr-Gly-Ser-
SUT                       Asp                             His  Glu                Ile                 Arg
AR                        Asp                             His  Glu                Phe
NIG48                     Leu        Ile             Pro  Glu  Gly                Met                 Arg-Thr


          |--------- CDR1 ----------|            30                  35       |----- FR2 ----|  40          45                  50
WLT     Ser-Gly-Ser-Ile-Gly-Ser-Asn-Tyr-Val-Gln-Trp-Tyr-Gln-Gln-Arg-Pro-Gly-Ser-Ala-Pro-Thr-Asn-Val-Ile-Tyr-
SUT                      Asp   Thr   Ala-Gly-Tyr                                           Thr              Phe
                                                                                          Thr
AR                       Asp   Gly   Ala-Asp-Ser-Phe
NIG48                    Asp         Ala                    Arg              Gly                       Thr-Leu


          |-------- CDR2 --------|           55                  60          65                  70       |--- FR3 ---|  75
WLT     Glu-Asn-Asn-Gln-Arg-Pro-Ser-Glu-Val-Asp-Arg-Phe-Ser-Gly-Ser-Ile-Asp-Ser-Ser-Ser-Asn-Ser-Ala-Ser-
SUT                      Asp-Thr                   Gly              Arg
                                                                   Asp   Ala
AR                       Asp-Asp                   Gly                    Ala
NIG48                    Asp-Thr                   Tyr-Gly         Asn          Phe


                        80                  85                  90                  95         |------ CDR3 ------|  100
WLT     Leu-Thr-Ile-Ser-Gly-Leu-Lys-Thr-Glu-Asp-Glu-Ala-Asp-Tyr-Tyr-Cys-Gln-Ser-Tyr-Asp-Asn-Asn-Asn-His-Val-
SUT                               Gln                                              Arg-Asp-His  -  Trp
AR                    Thr-Asn-Asp                                            Thr                 Ser  His-His
NIG48                                        Phe                        Met                      Ser-Ser  Leu-Trp


          |---- FR4 ----|      105                 110
WLT     Val-Phe-Gly-Gly-Gly-Thr-Arg-Leu-Thr-Val-Leu-Gly-
SUT                                 Lys
AR                                  Lys-Val
NIG48                               Lys                              Ser          Constant Region
```

Fig. 1. The complete amino acid sequence of the variable region of protein WLT. The structures of amyloid protein AR and SUT and myeloma protein NIG48 are also shown. Only residues which are different from the WLT sequence are noted and all blank residues are the same as for the WLT protein. The framework (FR) and complementarity determining residues (CDR) regions are marked above the sequences.

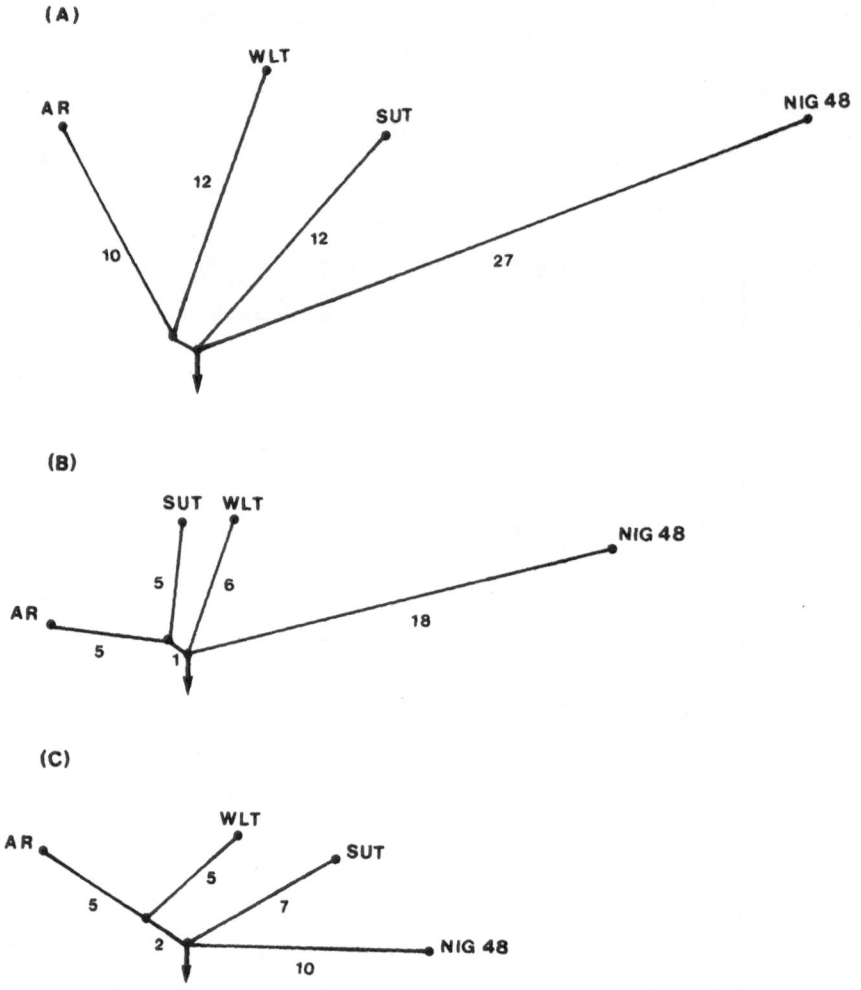

Fig. 2. (A) The phylogenetic comparisons of the complete lambda VI
variable regions. All numbers represent the minimum number of DNA substitutions needed to change one protein sequence to the adjacent structure. (B) Phylogenetic analysis of the lambda VI FR regions. (C) The phylogenetic
analysis of the CDR regions.

RESULTS

The WLT amyloid sample gave a standard profile on the CL6B column.
There was a void volume peak followed by a large included peak with small
amounts of protein on the leading and tailing edges. The major included
peak accounted for 65% of the recovered protein and from sequence analysis
was found to be at least 95% pure. SDS-PAGE confirmed this purity and gave
a molecular mass of 15,000 daltons. The entire sequence of this protein
was determined by the overlapping of sequence data from the whole protein
sequenator run, the tryptic peptide, staph protease peptides and the chymotrypsin subdigestion of tryptic peptides. Only one amino acid was found
at each position and every residue was identified from at least 2 peptides.
The protein was found to contain 134 amino acid residues which included the
entire variable region, joining segment and first complete tryptic peptide

of the constant region. The complete sequence of the variable region of the WLT protein along with the other complete lambda VI proteins can be seen in Fig. 1.

The protein was fragmented readily by both the trypsin and staph protease and only one unexpected cleavage was seen for both proteases. For trypsin the usually resistant Arg-Pro bond at residues 40-41 was cleaved in high yield and for staph protease a low yield of cleavage at the Trp-Tyr bond at residues 36-37 was also seen. All other cleavages were at arginine and lysine for trypsin and at glutamic acid for the staph protease. All peptides from both digests were isolated in a high state of purity from the reverse phase high performance liquid chromatography and no further purifications were necessary.

DISCUSSION

This is the fourth lambda VI protein whose structure has been determined. The protein was isolated from amyloid fibrils in very high yield and was found to be homogeneous at its amino and carboxyl terminals. The unique sequence of the first framework region as well as the 2 residue insert at residues 68 and 69 clearly identify this protein as belonging to the lambda VI subgroup. From Fig. 1 it can be seen that the WLT protein has 9 unique substitutions which are found at positions 8, 12, 15, 30, 47, 52, 58, 96, and 107. Of these changes the leucine at position 8 and the glutamic acid at position 58 have the largest changes in side chain characteristics.

The phylogenetic comparisons of the lambda VI proteins are shown on Fig. 2. The comparisons of the 4 variable regions can be seen on Fig. 2a. From this it appears that the 3 amyloid proteins are more closely related to the ancestral sequence (about 12 differences apiece) than the NIG48 sequence (27 differences). In Fig. 2B the same analysis was performed on the substitutions in the framework residues. These results are even more dramatic. Again the 3 amyloid proteins form a cluster of limited variability (6 changes) while the NIG48 protein has three times the number of substitutions (18 changes). Finally in Fig. 2C the phylogenetic relationships of the complementarity determining regions are presented. From this profile it can be seen that all the proteins have from 7 to 10 differences from the proposed ancestral sequence. A residue by residue comparison of the substitutions reveals no systematic pattern to the amino acid replacements. These findings indicate that the unique differences between the lambda VI amyloid and myeloma proteins appear to reside in the framework residues. Also, these sequence changes do not appear to be completely random but instead show some clustering in FR2 (residues 38-48) and FR3 (residues 82-90) regions. Since these residues form part of the interchain binding region and the outside surface of the molecule, it is expected that such molecules would have very different physical properties.

From these observations we are led to propose a possible mechanism for lambda VI AL amyloid formation. It would appear that the structure of lambda VI amyloid proteins are consistently different from the myeloma protein and that these differences are of major importance for the formation of the deposits. In addition the changes also occur in 2 specific locations in the molecule. First, there appear to be major differences in the interchain binding regions. These changes would be expected to alter the association constant for the formation of light chain dimers and thus indicates the potential importance of aggregation state in fibril formation. Second, the amyloid proteins seem to have additional hydrophobic residues on their outside surface (WLT, Leu 8; SUT, Ile 20; and AR, Phe 33). These residues may act as nucleation sites for subunit aggregation and resultant amyloid formation.

REFERENCES

1.   Solomon, A., Frangione, B., and Franklin, E. C., J. Clin. Invest., 70:453-460 (1982).
2.   Cohen, D., Pras, M., Franklin, E. C., and Frangione, B., Am. J. Med., 74:513-518 (1983).
3.   Dwulet, F. E. and Benson, M. D., Biochem. Biophys. Res. Commun., 114:657-662 (1983).
4.   Dwulet, F. E. and Benson, M. D., Proc. Natl. Acad. Sci. USA, 81:694-698 (1984).
5.   Bogardt, R. A., Jones, B. N. Dwulet, F. E., Garner, W. H., Lahman, L. D., and Gurd, F. R. N., J. Mol. Evol., 15:197-218 (1980).

POLYMORPHISM IN A KAPPA I PRIMARY (AL) AMYLOID

PROTEIN (BAN)*

Francis E. Dwulet, Timothy P. O'Conner
and Merrill D. Benson

Indiana University School of Medicine and
Richard L. Roudebuch Veterans
Administration Medical Center
Indianapolis, Indiana

ABSTRACT

To identify any potential relationships between protein structure and
primary (AL) amyloid formation it is best to study amyloid proteins from
subgroups for which there is a large sequence data base and for which x-ray
crystallographic data are available. The kappa I subgroup is ideal for
these studies. A large number of kappa I myeloma proteins have undergone
complete sequence analysis and high resolution x-ray crystallographic data
are available for protein REI. In addition the complete structure of
kappa I AL amyloid protein MEV has been reported. With such a data base
we began the study of kappa I amyloid protein BAN. This molecule was
found to contain 126 amino acid residues and consists of the entire variable region, joining segment and the first complete tryptic peptide of the
variable region. There are two unique features of this protein. First,
it is glycosylated. The normal arginine at position 61 has been replaced
with an asparagine to which is attached a glucosamine-containing carbohydrate chain. Second, the protein is not monoclonal but instead contains
2 different residues at positions 104 and 105. Analysis of the amyloid
proteins reveal that each contains specific mutations where threonine is
replaced by isoleucine and tyrosine by phenylalanine. From the x-ray
structure these substitutions are located in positions to cause self-aggregation and amyloid fibril formation.

INTRODUCTION

Attempts to identify the causes of immunoglobulin (AL) amyloid has
been thwarted because of a number of factors. These include the large number of subgroups in the kappa [4] and lambda [6] families. The high muta-
bility of the complementarity determining residue (CDR) regions and the

---

*This work was supported by VA Medical Research (MRIS 583-0888), and
grants from RR-00750 (GCRC), United States Public Health Service, National
Institute of Arthritis, Metabolism and Digestive Diseases (AM 20582 and
AM 7448), The Arthritis Foundation, and the Grace M. Showalter Foundation.

random accumulation of substitutions in the framework (FR) regions which make the identification of potential structure altering amino acid changes difficult. Finally, the very limited number of complete AL amyloid sequences in the literature reduces the probability of identifying any substitution patterns. To alter this situation we have begun the study of kappa I amyloid proteins. This subgroup was chosen because of several characteristics. First the subgroup accounts for about 20% of all AL amyloid deposits. Second there are a large number of sequenced myeloma kappa I proteins in the literature to provide nonamyloid controls for the evaluation of amino acid substitution patterns. Third the subgroup has a restricted mutation pattern which will simplify substitution comparisons' and lastly there is x-ray structure data for a kappa I variable region which will help in the evaluation of the effects of amino acid substitutions. With these factors in mind we began the structural studies of kappa I amyloid protein BAN.

MATERIALS AND METHOD

Amyloid Isolation

Amyloid-laden tissue was obtained post mortem from patient BAN, a 43 year old man who died from renal insufficiency. Amyloid fibrils were isolated from spleen tissue by previously reported procedures [1]. One hundred fifty milligrams of fibril preparation was dissolved in 8 ml of 6M guanidine hydrochloride, 0.5M TRIS pH 8.5 and reduced with 80 mg of dithiothreitol. The sample was then alkylated with 193 mg of iodoacetic acid and the soluble proteins separated by chromatography on a column of Sepharose CL6B.

Enzymatic Digestion

BAN amyloid subunit protein (6–8 mg) was dissolved in 2 ml of 0.1M ammonium bicarbonate buffer before the addition of the desired enzyme. For the tryptic digest 0.12 mg (2% by weight) of Worthington TPCK-trypsin dissolved in pH 3.0 water was added to the sample. The digest was maintained at 37°C for 12 h. The chymotrypsin digest was performed using the same conditions as for the trypsin digest. Finally the protein was fragmented with 0.3 mg (5% by weight) staph protease (Miles). The reaction was maintained at 37° for 24 h. All digests were stopped by freezing and lyophilization.

Peptide Separation

The tryptic digest was dissolved in 0.5 ml of 50% acetic acid and applied to a Synchrom RPP column (1 × 25 cm) in 0.1% trifluoroacetic acid and the peptides eluted with a gradient of 0–50% acetonitrile. The chymotrypsin digest was applied to an Altex Ultrasphere C-18 column (1 × 25 cm) and eluted with the same buffer system as used for the tryptic digest. Finally the staph protease digest was separated on a Synchrom RP-8 column (1 × 25 cm) and the peptides eluted with a 0–50% gradient of 2-propanol in 0.1% trifluoroacetic acid. When necessary pools were repurified on a Waters microbondapakphenyl column (4.1 × 300 mm).

Sequence Analysis

All protein and peptide samples were degraded in a Beckman 890C sequenator using the Edman degradation. All technical aspects of the degradation and identification of the phenylthiohydantoins have been described previously [2].

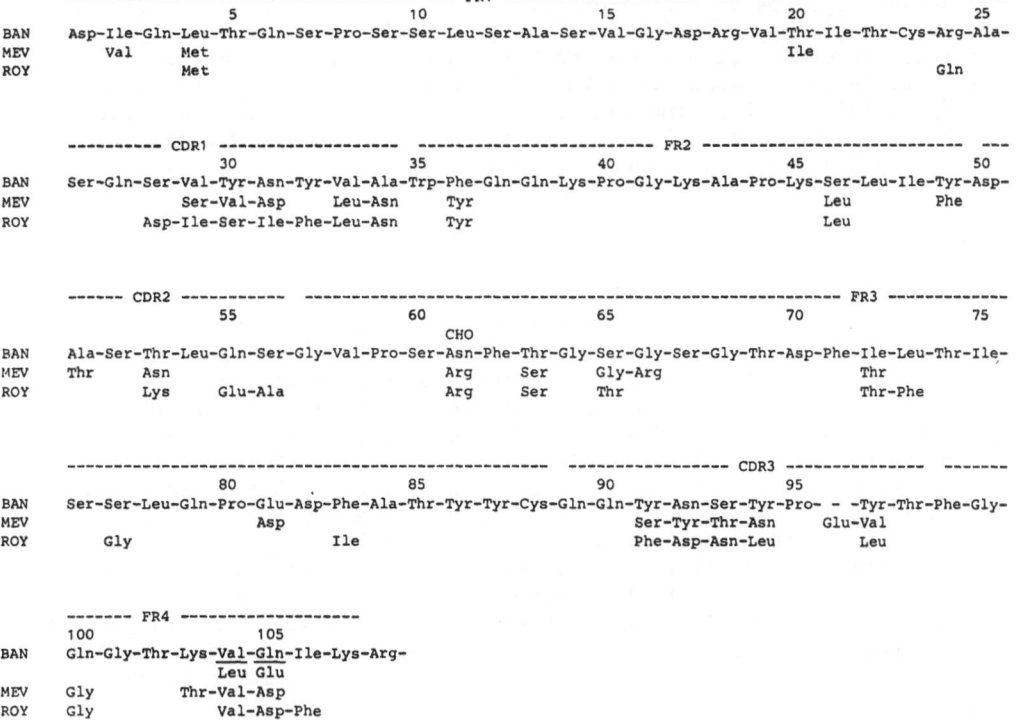

Fig. 1. The complete amino acid sequence of the variable region of protein
BAN is presented. Also, the complete variable region sequence of
kappa I amyloid protein MEV is shown but only those residues which
are different from the BAN protein are shown while the constant
residues are not printed. The kappa I myeloma protein ROY is shown
for comparison.

Analysis of Amino Acid Substitutions

Using the x-ray crystallographic structure of protein REI [3] the effect of the BAN substitutions were evaluated. This was accompalished using
a computer graphic modeling program (FRODO) [4] on an Evans and Sutherland
instrument. The effect of substitutions on surface topography, side chain
packing and inter light chain interactions were evaluated.

RESULTS

The BAN amyloid material gave a standard separation profile on the
CL6B column. The major included peak accounted for greater than 60% of
the recovered material and showed amino terminal homogeneity of greater
than 95% by sequence analysis. SDS-PAGE confirmed this purity and gave a
molecular mass of 14,000 daltons. The entire structure was determined from
the whole protein and tryptic peptide sequences. The chymotrypsin and
staph protease digests were used to confirm substitutions and overlap peptides.

The molecule was found to contain 126 residues encompassing the entire
variable region, joining segment and first tryptic peptide of the constant
region. The sequence of the BAN variable region as well as that of kappa
I amyloid protein MEV and myeloma protein ROY are shown on Fig. 1. There are

two unique features to this protein. First the molecule is glycosylated. The usual arginine at position 61 has been replaced by an asparagine to which is attached a glucosamine carbohydrate chain. The second is that the molecule is not monoclonal but instead has 2 amino acid residues at positions 104 and 105. The computer graphics program found that all of the BAN substitutions could fit into the REI protein without changing significantly the basic beta sheet structure.

DISCUSSION

This is the second kappa I amyloid protein to have its structure completely determined. The subunit protein was isolated in high yield from the fibril preparation and was found to be size homogeneous. This protein contains a number of unique substitutions located in both complementarity determining regions (CDR) and framework regions (FR). In the CDR regions only the tyrosine at position 30 is a unique residue never before reported. In the FR regions the phenylalanine at positions 36 (FR2) as well as the asparagine-linked carbohydrate as position 61 (FR3) and the isoleucine at 72 (FR3) have all never been observed in previous kappa I protein structures. Finally the serine at position 46 (FR2) has been reported in a DNA sequence [5] but this is the first protein found to contain these substitutions. A comparison of the BAN amino acid changes to those found in the MEV sequence [6] reveals unique substitutions in these 2 amyloid proteins. Both molecules have 2 unique amino acid replacements where isoleucine replaces threonine (BAN 72, MEV 20) and phenylalanine replaces tyrosine (BAN 36, MEV 49).

The presence of 2 sequences in the joining segment at positions 104 and 105 could be explained by a number of mechanisms:

1) The precursor proteins are derived from 2 clones of cells with the same variable region but different joining segments.

2) Both proteins are derived from a single cell, but during DMA rearrangement 2 J-segments were attached to the V-region and upon subsequent divisions one or the other J-segment was deleted.

3) Early in the cellular growth of this cell line 2 somatic mutations were incorporated into the J-segment sequences to account for the differences.

Whatever the mechanism the event had to occur early in the process to account for the nearly 1:1 ratio of the 2 sequences.

An evaluation of how the BAN substitutions fit into the known three dimensional structure of protein REI was accomplished using a computer graphics system. The asparagine linked carbohydrate at position 61 is on a beta turn in FR3. It is located on the surface which points away from the antigen binding site and into the space between the variable and constant regions. There appears to be plenty of room for this moiety without distortion of spatial relationships. The most important effect will be the loss of the salt bridge to the arginine side chain but this might be replaced by linkage to one of the glucosamine sugars. The isoleucine replacement at position 72 is in the middle of a beta strand facing out into the solvent. From the computer graphics it was determined that this isoleucine would fit easily into the available space. The surrounding residues are all small (serine and threonine) and form a nearly uniform flat surface. Thus, the isoleucine will form a hydrophobic site which will project from the smooth hydrophilic surface. The substitution of phenylalanine for tyrosine at position 36 occurs in the middle of a beta strand which is part of the variable domain interaction region. This side chain is one of the contact residues between the 2 variable domains. Since the phenylalanine is smaller than the tyrosine it fits easily into the available space, however, the phenylalanine is much more hydrophobic than the tyrosine and will greatly increase the hydrophobicity of the interior surface of the variable domain. All other FR substitutions fit easily into the available spaces and would appear to cause little change in structure. The substitutions in the CDR regions, because of their inherent flexibility, would seem to fit easily into the binding site. The 2 tyrosine residues at positions 94 and 96 (CDR3) do seem to be of structural importance because the presence of aromatic or hydrophobic amino acids at these locations increases the association constants for these light chains [7].

From these findings a mechanism for the formation of AL amyloid can be suggested. Two structural features are necessary for monoclonal light chains to form amyloid deposits. First the light chain dimer must have a high association constant (K_D about 10^4 M^{-1} or greater) and second a specific substitution must be present on the outside beta sheet layer which positions a hydrophobic amino acid (usually isoleucine) on the aqueous surface. The primed light chain dimers are then proteolytically cleaved by specific proteases into dimeric variable domain size fragments. The microenvironment then induced these dimeric fragments to self-aggregate and form fibril complexes.

This hypothesis is supported by a number of experimental observations. A second kappa I amyloid protein (NIE) whose structure we are presently determining (data not shown) has been found to be a partial hybrid of the BAN and MEV substitutions. The NIE protein has the isoleucine at position 20 (like MEV) and the phenylalanine at position 36 (like BAN). This sharing of substitutions unique to amyloid proteins gives strong support for the importance of these residues for amyloid formations. The importance of the high association constant of the variable region dimers in amyloidogenesis is probably responsible for preponderance of lambda chains in amyloid deposits. This is because lambda chains in general have a higher association constant than do kappa chains [7] and thus fewer substitutions would be needed to make lambda chains form amyloid deposits.

REFERENCES

1. Dwulet, F. E. and Benson, M. D., Biochem. Biophys. Res. Commun., 114:657-662, 1983.
2. Dwulet, F. E. and Benson, M. D., Proc. Natl. Acad. Sci. USA, 81:694-698, 1984.
3. Epp, O., Lattman, E. E., Schiffer, M., Huber, R., and Palm, W., Biochemistry, 14:4943-4952, 1975.
4. Jones, T. A., J. Appl. Cryst., 11:268-272, 1978.
5. Bentley, D. L. and Rabbitts, T. H., Nature 288:730-733, 1980.
6. Eulitz, M. and Linke, R. P., Hoppe-Seyler's Z. Physiol. Chem., 363: 1347-1358, 1982.
7. Stevens, F. J., Westholm, F. A., Solomon, A., and Schiffer, M., Proc. Natl. Acad. Sci. USA, 77:1144-1148, 1980.

ANALYSIS OF THE MONOCLONAL COMPONENTS IN SYSTEMIC

AL-AMYLOIDOSIS

Jan Marrink, Theo Ockhuizen,
Sven Janssen, Martin van Rijswijk,
and Enno Mandema

Department of Internal Medicine
University Hospital
Groningen, The Netherlands

SUMMARY

The amyloid fibril protein in systemic AL-amyloidosis has been shown
to be derived from monoclonal immunoglobulin components (MC). In this study
the MC were analyzed in patients with systemic AL-amyloidosis and compared
to patients with a M-component who were not suffering from amyloidosis.
Typing of the monoclonal components revealed a pronounced shift to the Bence
Jones (BJ) type of the M-component in patients with AL-amyloidosis (41%
versus 6% in the general M-component associated disease group). Moreover
a shift in favor of the lambda type of the MC in patients with systemic
AL-amyloidosis was noticeable (kappa/lambda-ratio in AL-amyloidosis 0.55
versus 1.63 in the non-amyloidosis group). The application of the sensitive and specific immunofixation technique for the detection of M-components
in serum and/or urine is highly recommended. In this way the number of
idiopathic systemic AL-amyloidoses will decrease in favor of the number of
monoclonal gammopathy-associated AL-amyloidosis.

INTRODUCTION

In general systemic amyloidosis can be subdivided into two categories
depending on the nature of the main constituent of the amyloid fibril.
Whereas in primary and myeloma-associated amyloidosis (AL-amyloidosis) the
fibrils are derived from monoclonal immunoglobulins and/or their fragments,
in secondary amyloidosis (AA-amyloidosis, associated with chronic inflammatory diseases) the main constituent of the fibrils is supposed to be derived from an acute phase reactant (serum amyloid A protein, SAA). Though
the application of the potassium permangante method enables to distinguish
between AA and AL-amyloidosis (Van Rijswijk et al. [1]) - since AA amyloid
looses its affinity for Congo red after incubation with potassium permanganate - in practice it became apparent that within the AL-amyloid group a
further subdividion could be made on the basis of the actual finding of the
immunoglobulin precursor. In myeloma-associated systemic amyloidosis (MM-
AL) the monoclonal component is an associated finding. In a second group
a monoclonal component (M-component) can be identified in the serum and/or
urine of AL-amyloid patients with plasmacell dyscrasia other than multiple
myeloma (designated as monoclonal gammopathy-associated amyloidosis (MG-AL).

As a third group within AL-amyloidosis should be considered those patients with idiopathic systemic amyloidosis in whom no M-component can be detected. A proper classification of idiopathic versus MG/MM-associated AL-amyloidosis is important in relation to the identification of the precursor of amyloid in the individual patient. This in turn might have implications for further treatment.

The finding of the immunoglobulin constituent, being a complete immunoglobulin molecule (or a fragment, which will be readily excreted into the urine) will depend on the specificity and the sensitivity of the immuno-chemical methods applied.

In this study the M-components were analyzed in 34 patients with AL-amyloidosis and compared to those found in 621 patients without systemic amyloidosis.

METHODS

The presence of M-components in serum and/or urine was established by menas of immuno-electrophoresis according to Scheidegger [2]. Specific antisera were obtained from Behringwerke A.G. (Marburg, West-Germany) and from Dakopatte (Copenhagen, Denmark). Urine was concentrated about 100 times using Minocon-B 15 concentration units (Amicon Corp., Lexington, Mass., USA). Total protein in the urine was established by means of the Bio Rad system (Rio Rad Chem. Div., Richmond, Ca., USA). Protein-electro-phoresis of serum and urine was done on agarose sheets with the Panagel electrophoresis system (Milliport Biomedica). Immunofixation was performed using the commercial Universal Electrophoresis kit from Corning (Palo Alto, Ca., USA), following the manufacturers recommendations. The potassium per-manganate method - to distinguish the AA and AL amyloid populations - was applied as described earlier [1].

PATIENTS

96 amyloid patients entered the study. Of these 40 could be typed as having AL-amyloidosis.

As a control population those patients not suffering from amyloidosis in whom a M-component was found in serum and/or urine were used. Between the years 1965 and 1984 in 621 patients with some form of plasmacell dys-crasia, and not associated with amyloidosis, attending our clinic, a M-com-ponent was demonstrated by immunochemical techniques.

RESULTS

AL-Amyloidosis/M-Components/Associated Disease

Of the 96 amyloid patients 40 were of the AL-type, thus 41%. Of these 40 AL-amyloid patients, 6 (15%) belonged to the group in whom no M-component was detected (designated as idiopathic systemic AL-amyloidosis), 14 (35%) could be classified as systemic AL-amyloidosis associated with a (apparent bening) monoclonal gammopathy (MG-AL), whereas in 20 (50%) multiple myeloma was associated with the systemic AL-amyloidosis (MM-AL).

Thus 34 out of 96 (35%) of all amyloid patients have a monoclonal com-ponent in their serum and/or urine. Moreover 34 out of 40 (85%) of the AL-group show this monoclonal spike.

TABLE 1.   Type of M-Component in Patients Without and With AL-Amyloidosis (n, %)

	IgG	IgA	IgM	IgD	BJ	Total
MC	364 (58)	92 (15)	124 (20)	5 (1)	35 (6)	621 (100%)
MC-AL	15 (44)	4 (12)	1 (3)	0 (0)	14 (41)	34 (100%)

TABLE 2.   Type of MC in AL-Amyloidosis with Respect to the Association MG/MM (n, %)

	IgG	IgA	IgM	BJ	Total
MG-AL	5 (36)	1 (7)	1 (7)	7 (50)	14 (100%)
MM-AL	10 (50)	3 (15)	0 (0)	7 (35)	20 (100%)

TABLE 3.   Light Chain Type of M-Components in MC and AL-Amyloidosis

	kappa-type	lambda-type	K/L-ratio
MC	385	236	1.63
MG-AL	4 ⟍	10 ⟍	0.40 ⟍
	12	22	0.55
MM-AL	8 ⟋	12 ⟋	0.67 ⟋

Furthermore this finding illustrates that of a total of 655 patients with a M-component this is associated with amyloidosis in about 5% of the cases (34 patients having AL-amyloidosis).

AL-Amyloidosis/M-component Type

Table 1 comprises the results of the comparison of the type of M-components in the AL-amyloid patients and those in the general MC-population. Compared to the MC-group the patients with AL-amyloidosis show a pronounced shift to the MJ-type of the monoclonal component (6% versus 41%).

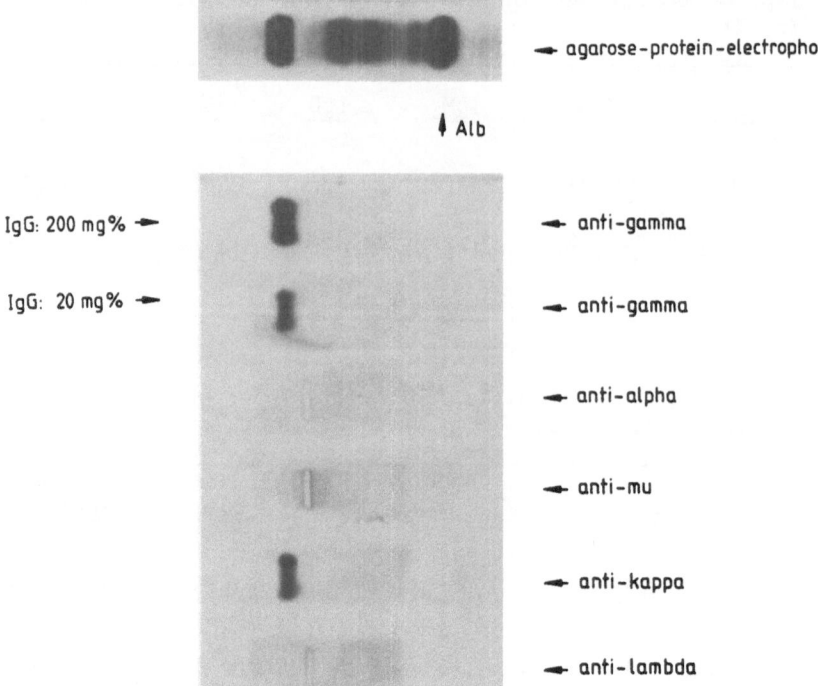

Fig. 1. Protein-electrophoresis and immunofixation of serum. After
agarose protein-electrophoresis specific antisera are
spread on the surface of the gel. In this way the band in
the gamma region can be types as a IgG(K) M-component.

AL-Amyloidosis/M-Component Type/Associated Disease

Table 2 analyses the type of the monoclonal component in AL-amyloidosis
with respect to the associated monoclonal gammopathy (MG-AL) or multiple
myeloma (MM-AL).

From this table it is obvious that the shift toward the BJ-type of the
M-component in AL-amyloidosis is more pronounced in MG-AL than in MM-AL
(50% versus 35%).

Light-Chain Type in AL-Amyloidosis

Table 3 gives the results of typing the M-components according to the
light-chain (kappa/lambda ratio).

Thus patients with AL-amyloidosis show a shift in the kappa/lambda ratio in favor of the lambda type of the monoclonal component (0.55 versus
1.63). Moreover these results illustrate that the increase of the lambda
type of the M-component in systemic AL-amyloidosis is more pronounced in
MG-AL than in MM-AL (0.40 versus 0.67).

Methodology of Typing M-Components

In general by immuno-electrophoresis we were able to detect the majority of the M-components in serum and urine of the patients. Immunofixation however showed to be more sensitive and specific for the detection
of M-components present in low concentrations, in particular for the detec-

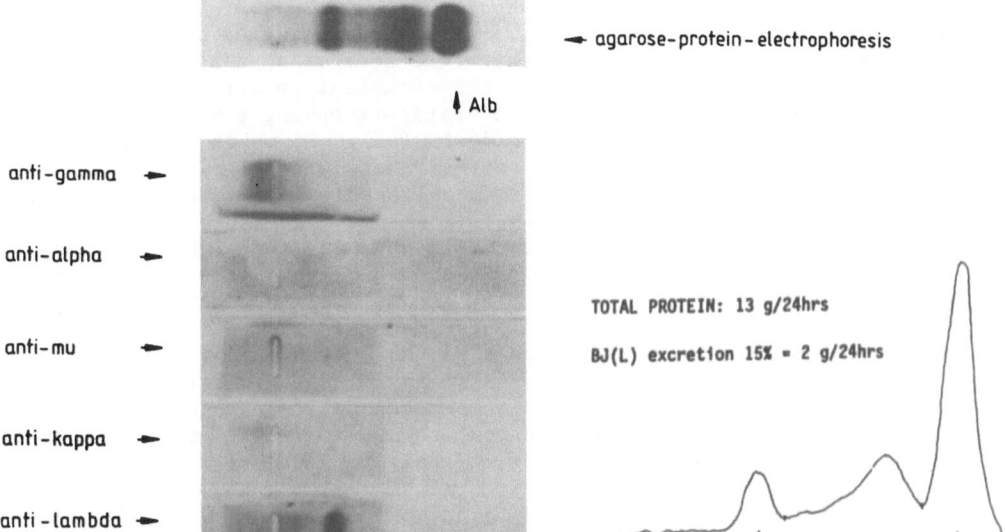

Fig. 2.   Protein-electrophoresis and immunofixation of urine.   Immunofixation detected a MJ(L) M-component in the unconcentrated urine at
a concentration of around 2 grams per 24 h.

tion of MJ-proteins in the urine.   Immunofixation not only enables the detection of the M-component, but also provides the means to establish its
concentration using the percentage of the M-component on the electropherogram and the total protein content.

Figure 1 gives a typical example of the detection of a M-component in
the serum of a patient.   By means of immunofixation the band in the gamma
region of the protein profile could easily be typed as a IgG(k) M-component.
In our hands a concentration of 20 mg per 100 ml is easily detectable.   In
34 patients having AL-amyloid a M-component was demonstrated.   In 18 of
them the monoclonal protein in the serum was found to be associated with
the presence of light-chains in the urine.   In 6 other patients the presence
of a monoclonal spike could be based solely on the findings in the concentrated urine, in 4 cases a kappa and in 2 cases a lambda light-chain was
involved.   Figure 2 shows how by means of the immunofixation technique,
applied on unconcentrated urine, the band in the protein profile is typed
as a BJ(L) M-component.   The total protein excretion in this patient (13
grams per 24 h) revealed a BJ-excretion of about 2 grams.   In our hands a
concentration of 200 mg BJ per liter can be easily detected in this way.
Moreover by a 100-fold concentration of the urine prior to immunofixation
a BJ concentration down to 2 mg per liter can be measured (which is at the
excretion level of a normal individual).

DISCUSSION

The existence of a spike in the beta/gamma-region on cellulose-ace-
tate/agarose serum electrophoresis is a hallmark of a monoclonal proliferation of B lymphocytes.   This monoclonal gammopathy can be associated with
a variety of diseases, the main being multiple myeloma (around 50%).
Others being macroglobulinaemia, lymphoma, leukemia, connective tissue
diseases, amyloidosis and miscellaneous (Ameis et al. [3]).   The associated
finding M-component/AL-amyloidosis therefore depends on two phenomena: the

finding of an M-component and the diagnosis of amyloidosis. Thus it is of utmost importance that an adequate laboratory investigation on M-components is undertaken in those patients; moreover the reverse approach of looking for amyloid positivity in those having a M-component in serum and/or urine should be considered. Of a total of 655 patients having a M-component we found 34 patients suffering from amyloidosis (5%). Of these AL-amyloid patients 20 were multiple myeloma associated whereas in 14 patients a monoclonal gammopathy association could be established. In 6 other AL-amyloid patients, designated as idiopathic systemic AL-amyloidosis, a M-component could not be detected. We think that due to an inadequate laboratory investigation (plus the reverse approach as outlined above) the percentage of idiopathic amyloid patients within the AL-amyloid group generally observed is overestimated (too many patients are classified as idiopathic 'in sensa strictu' because a M-component has not been found). Even in our study the percentage of idiopathic systemic amyloidosis is still 15%. It should be mentioned however that this number relates to patients analyzed at a time the technique of immunofixation was not available yet and of whom no serum/urine samples were stored for re-analysis.

Analysis for M-components should be performed on serum and urine (100 times concentrated) using protein electrophoresis (screening), immuno-electrophoresis and/or immunofixation. One should however be aware of some pitfalls:

- the so-called 'dip-stick' screening on proteinuria is negative for Bence Jones proteins,
- classical 'heat-test' for BJ is too insensitive. In our hands a positive reaction was only found at concentrations over 600 mg/L,
- no general proteinuria does not imply no BJ-proteinurea (matter of detection level). Normal proteinuria is defined as being below 100 mg/L whereas normal BJ-proteinuria should not exceed 5 mg/L.

Taking these recommendations into account one can detect a M-component in serum at a concentration of 20 mg/100 ml using the immunofixation technique. The latter technique should be the method of choice since particularly at low concentrations one might easily miss the presence of a M-component by application of the conventional immuno-electrophoresis due to masking by the polyclonal determinants. The same holds true for the analysis of the urine. By immunofixation we were able to detect properly the presence of monoclonal light chains at concentrations above 200 mg/L. Therefore concentration of the urin prior to immunofixation enables one to measure BJ-proteinuria at levels down to 2 mg/L.

In this way we analyzed the monoclonal components in 34 patients with amyloidosis and compared them to the M-components found in patients not suffering from this disease. Three main conclusions can be drawn from our observations. 1°: compared to the MC-group the patients with AL-amyloidosis show a shift to the BJ-type of the monoclonal component. 2°: patients with AL-amyloidosis show a shift in the kappa/lambda ratio in favor of the lambda type of the monoclonal component. 3°: with the introduction of more sensitive immunochemical techniques (immunofixation) the number of idiopathic systemic AL-amyloidosis has decreased in favor of the number of MG-AL.

Our observations as summarized in the first and second conclusion fit with those reported by Ameis et al. [3] who in a large survey of M-components found a 50% prevalence of BJ protein in 'primary generalized amyloidosis' and a K/L-ratio of 0.48. Out of 1242 cases in 2.5% the diagnosis of amyloidosis was made. Our higher percentage (5%) probably can be attributed to our third conclusion. The advantages of immunofixation over immunoelectrophoresis for the detection of monoclonal immunoglobulins have been recently advocated by others as well [4, 5].

REFERENCES

1. M. H. van Rijswijk and C. W. G. J. van Heusden, Am. J. Pathol., 97:43 (1979).
2. J. J. Scheidegger, Int. Arch. Allergy Appl. Immunol., 7:103 (1955).
4. A. Ameis, H. S. Ko, W. Pruzanski, Can. Med. Ass. J., 114:889 (1976).
4. E. Pascali, A. Pezzoli, A. Chiarandini, Cln. Chem., 28:1404 (1982).
5. J. T. Whicher, Clin. Chem., 29:402 (1983).

STRUCTURAL AND IMMUNOLOGIC STUDIES OF A KAPPA AMYLOID

FIBRIL PROTEIN*

Morie A. Gertz, Martha Skinner, Alan S. Cohen,
Lawreen Heller Conners, and
Robert A. Kyle

Thorndike Memorial Laboratory and
Division of Medicine
Boston City Hospital, and the
Arthritis Center
Boston University School of Medicine
Boston, Massachussets 02118

Mayo Foundation
Rochester, Minnesota 55905

ABSTRACT

In primary amyloidosis (AL) the fibril is composed of a monoclonal
immunoglobulin light chain and portions thereof. No specific alterations
in the proteins' primary structure have been identified that predispose
certain light chains to preferentially form amyloid fibrils. The classification of all forms of amyloidosis is based on the structure of the amyloid
fibril. We determined the N-terminal sequence of an amyloid fibril (PAG)
and found it to be of the kappa I immunoglobulin subclass. No specific
structural alterations were identified in this partial sequence that
account for its formation of amyloid fibrils. The ability to develop light-
chain subclass-specific antisera to amyloid fibril proteins could permit
immunochemical identification of amyloid deposits of light-chain origin.
Antiserum produced to the fibril protein did not react in immunodiffusion
with two other purified kappa I proteins. This antiserum may be directed
to unique antigenic sites present on the immunizing protein and would therefore be unable to recognize homologous proteins.

INTRODUCTION

Systemic amyloidosis is generally classified based on the chemical
composition of the fibril protein [1]. In primary amyloidosis or myeloma-

---

*Supported by grants from the U.S. Public Health Service, National Institute
of Arthritis Metabolism and Digestive Disease (AM 04599 and AM 07014), from
the General Clinical Research Centers Branch of the Division of Research
Resources, National Institute of Health (RR 533), Multipurpose Arthritis
Center, National Institute of Health (AM 20613 and CA-16835) and the
Arthritis Foundation.

associated amyloidosis, the fibril consists of a monoclonal immunoglobulin light chain or portions thereof and is designated AL [2]. It has been suggested that certain immunoglobulin light chains have a unique primary structure that makes them amyloidogenic. Nonetheless, no unique primary sequence alterations have been recognized that specify an "amyloidogenic" property in immunoglobulin light chains. To determine whether such a structure exists requires compilation of detailed sequence data on many amyloid fibrils.

The AL protein may often be composed of only the N-terminus (variable portion) of an immunoglobulin light chain, and antisera to intact kappa or lambda light chains will frequently fail to recognize antigenic determinants on the amyloid fibril [3]. In contrast to the situation with AA or AF, the cross-reactivity of anti-AL may be limited to the AL protein of the same or a few individuals [4-9], and a great difficulty could be encountered in developing a subclass-specific AL antisera. The ability to develop a panel of subclass-specific antisera to various amyloid fibril proteins could permit immunocytochemical or immunofluorescent identification of amyloid deposits of light-chain origin.

In this study, we determined the N-terminal sequence of an amyloid fibril that belongs to the kappa I immunoglobulin subclass. Attention was given to any structural alterations that could lead to amyloid fibril formation. Antiserum was produced to this protein and characterized as to its ability to identify other amyloid fibril proteins.

MATERIALS AND METHODS

Source of Material

At postmortem examination, a 58-year-old woman (patient PAG) was diagnosed as having primary amyloidosis (AL). Two months previously, she had been hospitalized and was found to have an enlarged tongue and a serum creatinine level of 1.8 mg/dl. Three days before her death, she was rehospitalized with hepatomegaly, a 4.5 kg loss of weight, and orthopnea. Serum protein electrophoresis and immunoelectrophoresis showed a monoclonal IgA kappa protein. Her hospitalization was complicated by an episode of cardiac standstill. She could not be resuscitated after a second cardiac arrest the following day.

Purification of Amyloid Fibril Protein

All tissues were stored frozen at $-20°C$ until used. Twenty grams of amyloid-rich liver were repeatedly homogenized in saline and citrate, followed by water [10]. Fibrils used for analysis were taken from the first three water washes, exhaustively dialyzed, and lyophilized. Eight milligrams of fibrils were solubized in 6 M guanidine, 0.1 M Tris, 0.01 M EDTA at pH 7.6, and then reduced with 40 mg of dithiothreitol. After centrifugation, the supernatant was fractionated by gel filtration on a 90 × 2.5 cm Sepharose 6 B column eluted with 4 M guanidine, 0.1 M Tris, 0.01 M EDTA.

Polyacrylamide Gel Electrophoresis

Sodium dodecylsulfate (SDS) disc gel electrophoresis was performed in 15% acrylamide on the four retarded column fractions and compared with molecular weight standards" immunoglobulin heavy chain (mol. wt. 53,000), immunoglobulin light chain (mol. wt. 23,000), lysozyme (mol. wt. 14,300), and insulin (mol. wt. 6,000) [11]. Gels were stained with Coomassie blue and destained in 7.5% acetic acid/10% methanol.

Amino Acid and Sequence Analysis

Amino acid analyses were performed on a JEOL-5-AH analyzer. Samples were hydrolyzed in 6 N HCl under nitrogen in sealed glass tubes at 110°C for 18 h [12]. Sequence analysis was performed on the peak 4 protein using a Beckman Sequencer Model 890C, utilizing the Edman and Begg procedure [13]. The aminothiazolinones were converted to the phenylthiohydantoin (PTH) derivatives by incubation in 1 N HCl at 80°C for 10 minutes. The PTH-amino acids were extracted in ethyl acetate or ecovered in the aqueous phase. PTH-amino acid derivatives were identified by high-performance liquid chromatography (Varian 5000) using a reverse-phase MCH 5 column [14]. Results were confirmed by back hydrolysis of the PTH derivatives to their free amino acids, followed by amino acid analysis.

Preparation of Antisera

Antiserum was produced in New Zealand white rabbits by injection of PAG peak 4 in phosphate-buffered saline/Freunds' adjuvant. After 4 weekly injections, a monthly booster dose of guanidine-denatured PAG amyloid fibrils in complete Freunds' adjuvant was administered. Serum was obtained one week after each injection.

Immunodiffusion Analysis

Immunodiffusion was performed in 0.6% agarose gels. Unadsorbed antisera to various amyloid proteins was placed in central wells 6 mm in diameter. Antigens consisted of purified AL proteins at a concentration of 1 mg/ml in phosphate-buffered saline. Plates were incubated for 30 min at 37°C and then placed in a humidified chamber at room temperature overnight.

RESULTS

Fractionation of the fibrils of Sepharose 6B gave a void volume and three retarded peaks. SDS polyacrylamide gel electrophoresis showed multiple faint bands corresponding to molecular weights in excess of 30,000 for peaks 2 and 3. Analysis of peak 4 showed a single dominant band with a molecular weight of 14,500 and a second band of lesser intensity of molecular weight 23,000.

Amino acid analysis revealed large amounts of serine and glutamic acid with little histidine and methionine (Table 1). There results are similar to previously reported amino acid analyses of amyloid. N-terminal amino acid sequencing was carried out to 40 residues. The N-terminus Asp-Ile-Gln-Met identifies PAG as kappa I subclass (Table 2 [16]. The kappa I amyloid fibril proteins sequenced in our laboratory to 20 and 25 residues, respectively, are LEP and MAG [17, 18]. PAG differed in residue 14 from the former and had no differences from the latter.

Anti-PAG was tested for reactivity against each of the purified PAG peaks. A precipitin line of identity was detected with peaks 3 and 4. No reaction was obtained with peaks 1 and 2. No reaction was obtained with any peak tested against commercial anti-kappa antisera. When anti-PAG was tested against LEP and MAG antigens, both kappa I amyloid proteins, no reaction was obtained (Table 3). No reaction was obtained when anti-PAG was tested for reactivity with normal serum or purified fibrils of kappa$_3$ or lambda origin. To serve as a control each purified fibril preparation was tested in immunodiffusion with antisera prepared to its respective fibril, and in each case a precipitin line of identity was obtained.

TABLE 1. Amino Acid Analysis of Amyloid PAG, Peak 4

Amino Acid	Residues/1000
Lysine	44
Histidine	15
Arginine	45
Aspartic Acid	81
Threonine	73
Serine	118
Glutamic Acid	129
Proline	64
Glycine	91
Alanine	75
Valine	56
Valine	56
Methionine	22
Isoleucine	34
Leucine	73
Tyrosine	34
Phenylaline	47

DISCUSSION

PAG amyloid protein represents the 10th reported variable kappa I
fibril protein partially sequenced. Analysis revealed a major protein of
14,500 daltons and a second quantitatively minor protein of 23,000 suggesting the presence of both an intact immunoglobulin light chain and a fragment thereof in the amyloid deposits. Sequence analysis revealed no ambi-
guity suggesting that the two proteins are identical for the N-terminal 40
residues and that the major protein with molecular weight 14,500 is the
N-terminal fragment of the quantitatively minor 23,000 protein.

This patient had a monoclonal IgA kappa immunoglobulin in the serum.
Since 23,000 is the molecular weight of an intact immunoglobulin light
chain, we postulate that the patient's fibril was composed predominantly
of the N-terminal fragment from an intact light chain but also contained
the intact light chain. It has been suggested previously that the formation
of amyloid fibrils containing light chains and their variable region as a

TABLE 2. Sequence of PAG (A kappa_I) Amyloid Fibril Protein

1	2	3	4	5	6	7	8	9	10	11	12	13	14	15	16	17	18	19	20
asp	ile	gln	met	thr	gln	ser	pro	ser	ser	leu	ser	ala	(ser)	val	gly	asp	arg	val	thr

21	22	23	24	25	26	27	28	29	30	31	32	33	34	35	36	37	38	39	40
(ile)	thr	(cys)	gln	ala	(ser)	gln	ala	(ser)	(thr)	tyr	tyr	(gly)	asn	trp	tyr	gln	gln	lys	pro

( ) indicates residue identification was equivocal

TABLE 3. Immunodiffusion of Amyloid Fibril Proteins Against
Subclass-Specific Antisera

Amyloid protein	Anti-PAG	Anti-MAG	Anti-kappa III	Anti-lambda
PAG	+	−	−	−
MAG	−	+	−	−
LEP	−	+	−	−
BRAITH(kappa III)	−	−	+	−
BURT(lambda)	−	−	−	+
Human Serum	−	−	−	−

major protein component can occur as a result of copolymerization of the light chain with its N-terminal fragment [19].

Antisera produced from purified PAG did not cross react with two other fibril proteins of the same immunoglobulin light-chain subtype (Table 3). It should be useful in the classification of amyloid if the various subtypes of AL fibrils could be identified immunochemically. Reports have shown varying results [6-8, 20, 21].

One report described specific antibodies against AL protein that could identify primary amyloid deposits by immunohistochemistry. This antibody was used to successfully classify 3 patients with myeloma-associated amyloidosis, all of whom had a lambda Bence Jones protein [22]. That report concluded that the antiserum produced against one amyloid protein could be used for detection and typing of other AL proteins. As stated, our results could not confirm this, at least in the kappa I subclass. Anti-PAG did not cross-react with purified fibrils of LEP and MAG, despite their common kappa I origin. Presumably, antiserum produced in the former group of experiments was to an idiotypic determinant common to all members of that light-chain subclass [22, 23]. In our experiments, the antiserum produced may only be capable of recognizing idiotypes unique to the immunizing protein and therefore incapable of recognizing homologous proteins. The lack of cross-reactivity between commercial antiserum against intact light chains recognizes determinants located in the constant region of the light-chain molecule. Since the C-terminus is presumed deleted in the production of the 14,500 fragment, no antigenic sites remain to react with commercial antisera. The absence of cross-reactivity also suggests that only trace amounts of the intact light chain are present in the intact fibril, amounts below the limit of detection by immunodiffusion.

We are aware of 86 kappa proteins that have been partially sequenced. Ten of these proteins are of amyloid fibril origin (12%). This incidence of amyloid proteins among all sequenced kappa I immunoglobulin light chains exceeds the incidence of amyloid proteins found in other subclasses that have been sequenced. This finding supports the hypothesis that kappa I light chains may be more amyloidogenic than other kappa subclasses. In a similar vein, Cohen et al. [24] reported that 16 or 19 lambda VI proteins identified were derived from cases of amyloidosis. However, immunologic studies of 49 cases of primary amyloidosis all derived from lambda light chains revealed only 7 belonging to the lambda VI subclass [24, 25]. Compilation of large numbers of fibril protein sequences may provide information to affirm or refute the hypothesis that the structure of certain light chains renders them uniquely amyloidogenic.

PAG represents the 10th reported variable kappa I fibril sequenced. Antiserum produced using the purified fibril protein did not cross-react by immunodiffusion with other fibril proteins of the same immunoglobulin light-chain subtypes.

REFERENCES

1. E. P. Benditt, et al.: Excepta Medica International Congress Series No. 497, XI (1980).
2. G. G. Glenner, W. Terry, M. Harada, C. Isersky, and D. Page, Science, 172:1150 (1971).
3. R. P. Linke, D. Zucker-Franklin, and E. C. Franklin, J. Immunol., 111:10 (1973).
4. J. B. Natvig, et al., Scnad. J. Immunol., 14:89 (1981).
5. T. Shirahama, M. Skinner, A. S. Cohen, Histochemistry, 72:161 (1981).

6. M. D. Benson, M. Skinner, and A. S. Cohen, J. Lab. Clin. Med., 85:650 (1975).
7. C. Isersky, D. Ein, D. Page, M. Harada, and G. G. Glenner, J. Immunol., 108:486 (1972).
8. G. G. Cornwell III, et al., Scand. J. Immunol., 6:1071 (1977).
9. G. G. White II, R. J. Jacobson, R. A. Binder, R. P. Linke, and G. G. Glenner, Blood, 46:713 (1975).
10. M. Skinner, T. Shirahama, A. S. Cohen, and C. L. Deal, Prep. Biochem., 12:461 (1982).
11. A. L. Shapiro, E. Vinuela, J. V. Maisel, Jr., Biochem. Biophys. Res. Commun, 28:815 (1967).
12. D. H. Spackman, W. H. Stein, and S. Moore, Anal. Chem., 31:1190 (1958).
13. P. Edman and G. Begg, Eur. J. Biochem., 1:80 (1967).
14. C. L. Zimmerman, E. Apella, and J. J. Pisnoa, Anal. Biochem., 77:569 (1977).
15. O. Smithies, et al., Biochemistry, 10:4912 (1971).
16. E. A. Kabat, T. T. Wu, H. Biofsky, M. Reid-Miller, and H. Perry, Sequences of Proteins of Immunological Interest. United States Department of Health and Human Services, Public Health Service, National Institutes of Health, Bethesda, Maryland, 14 (1983).
17. A. S. Cohen, T. Shirahama, M. Skinner, M. D. Benson, and E. S. Cathcart, Protides Biol Fluids, 20:73 (1973).
18. J. B. Lian, M. Skinner, M. D. Benson, and A. S. Cohen, Biochem. Biophys. Acta, 491:167 (1977).
19. G. G. Glenner, N. Engl. J. Med., 302:1283 (1981).
20. H. M. Falck and P. Westermark, Clin. Exp. Immunol., 54:259 (1983).
21. P. Westermark, J. B. Natvig, R. F. Anders, K. Sletten, and G. Husby, Scan. J. Immunol., 5:31 (1976).
22. Y. Levo, N. Livni, A. Laufer, Pathol. Res. Pract., 175:373 (1982).
23. P. Westermark, K. Sletten, and J. B. Natvig, Acta Pathol. Microbiol. Scand. (C), 89-C:199 (1981).
24. D. Cohen, M. Pras, E. C. Franklin, and B. Frangione, Am. J. Med., 74:513 (1983).
25. R. A. Kyle, Clin. Haematol., 11:151 (1982).

MOLECULAR HETEROGENEITY AND γ-CARBOXYGLUTAMIC ACID CONTENT OF BENCE-JONES

PROTEINS: POSSIBLE RELEVANCE TO AMYLOIDOGENICITY*

Giampaolo Merlini, Michael Mastanduno, Peggy W. Moy,
Peter V. Hauschka†, and Elliott F. Osserman‡

Department of Medicine and
Cancer Center/Institute of Cancer Research
Columbia University College of Physicians and Surgeons
New York, New York

†Department of Oral Biology
 Harvard School of Dental Medicine
 Boston, Massachusetts

ABSTRACT

Ammonium sulphate precipitated Bence Jones proteins (BJP)** from 33
plasma cell dyscrasia patients with (A+) and without (A-) AL amyloidosis
were analyzed by chromatofocussing (CMF), immunofixation (IF), and SDS-PAGE.
Agarose gel electrophoresis and IF of CMF-separated urinary proteins revealed the presence of 3 to 6 components containing either κ or λ light
chain (LC) determinants. SDS-PAGE after reduction confirmed the expected
molecular weight range (22-28 Kd) of the major consituent. Lower molecular
weight (12-16 Kd) light chain related fragments were found in 15 A+ and in
5 A- cases, but with particularly high concentration (>15% total Bence-
Jones protein) only in A+ cases. We postulate that these LC fragments may
be precursors of the amyloid deposits in these patients.

To investigate the possibility that calcium might be involved in the
polymerization of LC' in the formation of amyloid, we analyzed 32 BJP's
(14 A+: 18 A-) for the presence of γ-carboxyglutamic acid (Gla), a documented mediator of calcium binding by protein. The majority of A+ and A-
BJP's had less than 0.5 Gla per 1000 glutamic acid (Glu) residues. Four
A+ BJκ's had 0.5-1.0 Gla/1000 Glu, and one BJκ had 2.1 Gla/1000 Glu. These
results suggest that the presence of Gla may be associated with the amyloidogenicity of certain kappa BJP's.

---

*Studies supported by a grant (CA 21112) from the National Cancer Institute
 and the Saul Z. and Amy Scheuer Cohen Family Foundation.
‡Dr. Osserman is an American Cencer Society Professor of Medicine.
**Abbreviations used in this paper: A+ and A-, amyloid positive and nega-
   tive; CMF, chromatofocusing; IF, immunofixation; SDS-PAGE, sodium dodecyl
   sulfatepolyacrylamide gel electrophoresis; AgGE, agarose gel electrophoresis; LC, light chain; MJ, Bence Jones; Gla, γ-carboxyglutamic acid;
   Glu, glutamic acid; $β_2μ$, $β_2$-microglobulin; $β_{TR}$, β-trace.

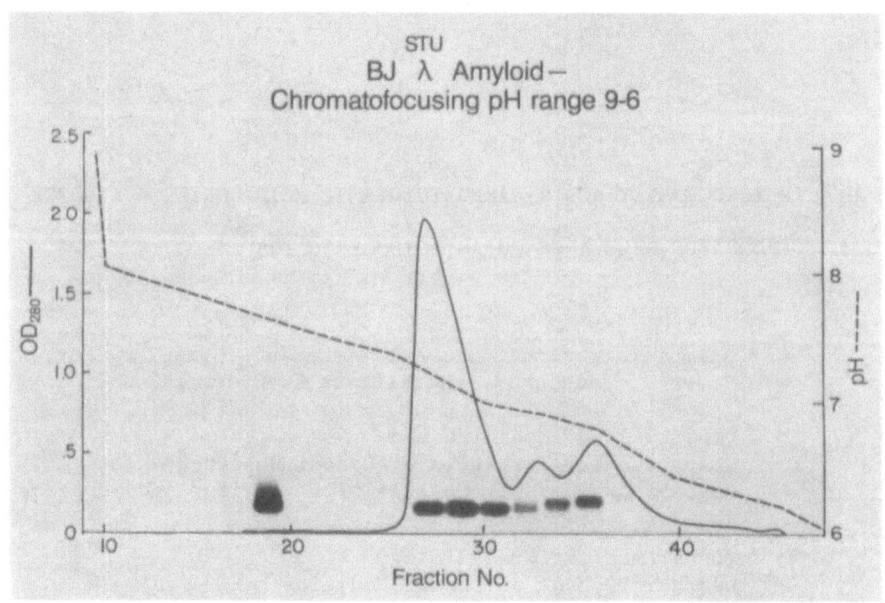

Fig. 1.   Chromatofocusing (pH range 9–6) and AgGE (anode at the
top) patterns of non amyloid BJ$^{STU}\lambda$.   To the left is the
starting material applied to the CMF column; the other
protein bands correspond to the elution peaks.   No residual column-bound protein was eluted with high salt
(1 M NaCl) washing (not shown).

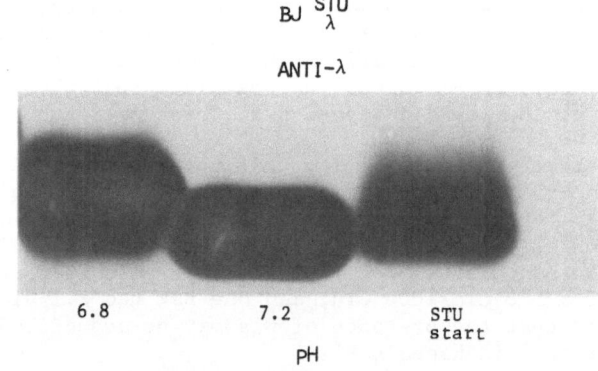

Fig. 2.   Immunofixation with anti-λ antiserum
on agarose gel (anode at the top) of
BJ$^{STU}\lambda$ starting material and of CMF-
separated components at pH 7.2 (main
peak) and pH 6.8 (third peak).

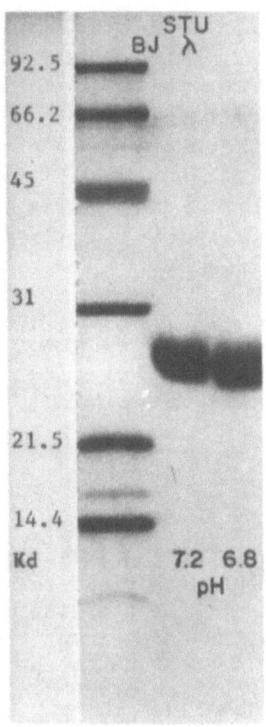

Fig. 3. SDS-PAGE of
the BJ^{STU}λ pH
7.2 and 6.8
CMF fractions.
Molecular
weight stand-
ards to the
left.

INTRODUCTION

The molecular basis of the amyloidogenicity of certain Bence-Jones
proteins (BJP's) is still not clarified. Certain properties which have been
reported for amyloid-related (A+) BJP's, such as a relatively low isoelectric point [1] and the presence of fragments [2, 3] suggests a non-specific
physical-chemical mechanism; however the observed binding of fluorescein-
labelled amyloid-related BJP's to normal tissue [4] and their binding of
dinitrophenyl (DNP) derivatives [5] are suggestive of antibody-like activity.

Since the major component of many AL amyloid fibrils appears to be
derived from the N-terminal (variable V) region of monoclonal immunoglobulin
light chains [6], we have analyzed the molecular heterogeneity of 33 BJP's
from plasma cell dyscrasia patients with and without AL amyloidosis. We
have found that many (∿40%) patients with amyloidosis excrete high concentration of low molecular weight (12-16 Kd) light chain-related polypeptides.

Several lines of evidence suggest an association between amyloid and
calcium, notably the presence of the calcium binding protein P-component
in virtually all amyloids [7], the not-infrequent localization of bone scan
agents, e.g. diphosphonate [8, 9], to soft tissue amyloid, the occasional
observation of calcification in amyloid deposits, and the induction of ex-

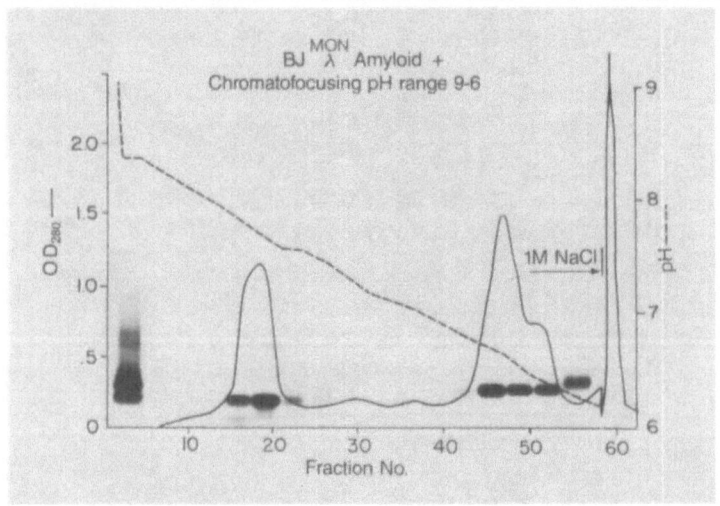

Fig. 4. Chromatofocusing and AgGI (anode at the
top) patterns of amyloid-related BJ$^{MON}\lambda$.
To the left is the starting material
applied to the CMF column, the other protein bands correspond to the elution peaks
with the exception of the last (far right)
protein band which corresponds to the very
first material eluted with high salt concentration solution (1 M NaCl).

B J $^{MON}_\lambda$

IMMUNOFIXATION CMF FRACTIONS

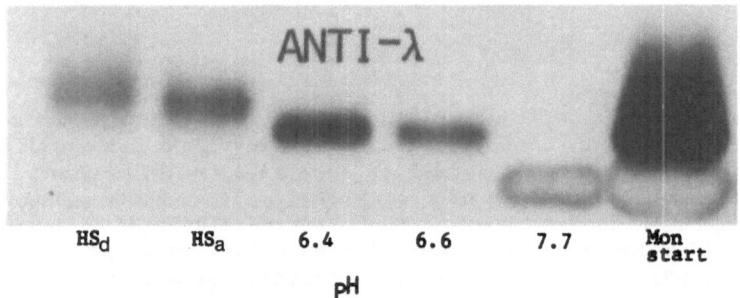

Fig. 5. Immunofixation with anti-λ antiserum on AgGE
(anode at the top) of BJ^{MON} starting material and
of the CMF separated components at pH 7.7 (first
peak), pH 6.6 (second peak), pH 6.4 (second peak
shoulder) and of material from the ascending (HS$_a$)
and descending (HS$_d$) sides of the peak eluted with
high salt concentration solution.

perimental amyloid by casein, the major calcium-binding protein in milk
[10]. Because of the possibility that calcium might be involved in the
polymerization of light chains in the formation of AL amyloid, we have
analyzed 32 BJP for calcium binding activity and for the presence of γ-carb-

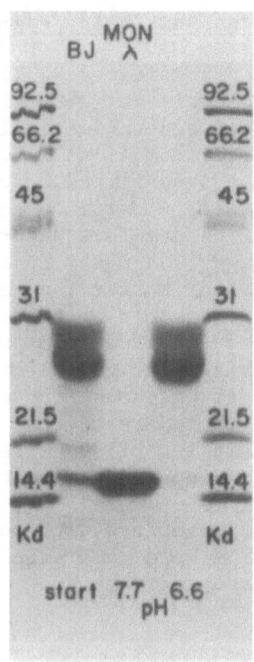

Fig. 6.   SDS-PAGE of BJ^{MON}
starting material and
of chromatofocusing
separated components
at pH 7.7 (first peak)
and pH 6.6 (second
peak). Molecular
weight standards at
the sides.

oxyglutamic acid (Gla), a calcium-binding modified amino acid. Using electrophoretic techniques, we could be detect calcium binding by complete BJP's
or by their fragments. However preliminary analyses indicate the presence
of Gla in some amyloid-related kappa BJP's but not in amyloid-related lambda
BJP's or in BJP's from patients without amyloidosis.

MATERIALS AND METHODS

All chemicals were reagent grade. Buffers were prepared with deionized
water and degassed when used for chromatofocusing.

Analytical electrophoresis was carried out on agarose gels by the
method of Jeppsson et al [12].

Immunofixation was performed on agarose gels according to Ritchie and
Smith [13] using monospecific antisera purchased from DAKO (Santa Barbara,
CA 93103) (anti-NHS, κ, λ, γ, α, μ) or produced in our laboratory ($\beta_2\mu$,
β_{TR}).

The screening for carbohydrate content of BJP's was carried out by
periodic acid, Schiff's reagent (PAS) reaction on agarose gel electrophoresis.

Isolation of Bence-Jones Proteins and Their Fragments

Bence-Jones proteins were precipitated by 1.64 M ammonium sulphate from urine of 15 patients with amyloidosis and 18 patients without amyloidosis. The precipitates were redissolved and exhaustively dialyzed (Spectrapor, tubing, m.w. cutoff 6-8 Kd, Spectrum Medical Ind. Los Angeles, CA 90054) against distilled water and then lyophilized. Fourteen BJP's were further purified by chromatofocusing (CMF), a column chromatographic method for separating proteins in a linear pH gradient according to their isoélectric points (pI) (Pharmacia, Piscataway, NH 08854). The linear pH gradient is formed automatically as the eluting buffer (an amphoteric buffer, Poly-buffer™, PB) titrates the charged groups of the ion exchanger (Polybuffer Exchanger™PBE). The pH interval (maximum of 3 pH units) was chosen so that the pI of the BJP, estimated by agarose gel electrophoresis, fell roughly in the middle of the pH gradient. Although the CMF separation mechanism is based on differences in pI, there are several reasons (displacement effects, solubility of a protein at its pI) to expect that most proteins will not elute at pH's corresponding exactly to their pI.

Since the Polybuffer could interfere with some of the subsequent analyses, the CMF eluted proteins were separated from Polybuffer by precipitation with ammonium sulphate.

Molecular Weight Determination

The molecular weights of the proteins separated by CMF were determined by SDS-polyacrylamide gel electrophoresis in 5% β-mercaptoethanol according to Laemmli [14] using a vertical gel electrophoresis system (Pharmacia). Gels were stained with Coomassie Blue R-250. Low molecular weight protein standards are SDS gel electrophoresis were purchased from Bio-Rad (Richmond, CA 94804). The bands containing BJP's or their fragments were identified by transferring the proteins from SDS-polyacrylamide gels to nitrocellulose sheets (Transblot™, Bio-Rad) and subsequent immunostaining by peroxidase-conjugated antibodies (Towbin et al. [15] with minor modifications).

Screening for Calcium Binding Activity of BJP's

BJP's and their fragments separated by CMF, were screened by two-dimensional ^{45}Ca electrophoresis autoradiography according to Lindgärde et al. [16] with modifications and by comparing their electrophoretic mobility in the presence of 10 mM EDTA or 10 mM $CaCl_2$

Determination of γ-carboxyglutamic acid (Gla) content of BJP's was carried out according to Hauschka [17].

RESULTS

I. Molecular Heterogeneity

Figure 1 shows the CMF and AgGE patterns of a representative control nonamyloid (A-) λ BJP[STU]. The AgGE pattern of the starting material shows a major component of slow γ mobility and a minor anodal component. Chromatofocusing in the pH range 9 to 6 reveals a major protein component at pH 7.2 and two minor components at pH 6.9 and 6.8. Figure 2 shows the reaction of pH 7.2 and 6.8 fractions with anti-λ antiserum; there was no reactivity with any other antiserum (anti κ, γ, α, μ, β_{TR} and $\beta_2\mu$). Figure 3 shows the SDS-PAGE of pH 7.2 and pH 6.8 CMF isolated fractions and confirms their identical molecular weight of 24 Ka.

Figure 4 shows the CMF and AgGE patterns of an amyloid positive (A+) λBJP^MON. Consistent with the AgGE pattern of the starting material, the CMF pattern shows a prominent peak with asymmetrical boundaries in the pH range 7.8-7.6 and a major peak at pH 6.6 followed by a shoulder at pH 6.4. All the residual column bound proteins were finally eluted with 1M NaCl. The immunofixation pattern (Fig. 5) with anti-λ antiserum and the other control antisera confirmed the presence of λ determinants in the pH 7.7 and 6.4 fractions, as well as in the material eluted with high salt concentration. The lesser intensity staining of the pH 7.7 as compared with the pH 6.6 and high salt fractions is evident. Figure 6 shows the SDS-PAGE patterns of the starting material, pH 7.7 and pH 6.6 components. The pH 6.6 CMF fraction has a main component of 27 Kd and a lesser component of 30 Kd; in contrast the pH 7.7 component has a molecular weight of 15.5 Kd.

Amino-N-terminal analysis of the pH 7.7 (15.5 Kd) and the pH 6.6 (30-27 Kd) fractions revealed that both have a blocked amino terminus, thereby lending support to the probability that the 15.5 Kd component is V-related. The fact that the molecular weight of this component is 15.5 Kd compared with the expected molecular weight of approximately 11 Kd for a V region as well as its reactivity with an anti-λ antiserum suggests that this fragment may contain a portion of the C region. The possible presence of carbohydrate in either the intact BJP or the 15.5 Kd fragment was apparently excluded by negative periodic acid Schiff's staining of AgGE of these protein fractions.

Table 1 summarizes the results of our analyses of 33 BJP's (18 A+ and 15 A-). High concentrations (from 50 to 15% of total BJP) of low molecular weight (12-16 Kd) light chain related proteins were found only in association with documented amyloidosis. The majority of amyloid negative cases showed either a trace (<5% of total BJP) or no detectable light chain fragments. It should be noted, however, that 8 of the amyloid positive cases and 5 of non-amyloid cases had low concentrations of fragments (from 15 to 5% of total BJP).

In the patients with high urinary concentrations of low molecular weight components, the presence of kappa or lambda determinants in these fragments was confirmed by immunoblotting of the SDS-polyacrylamide gels. Using this technique, light chain-related fragments corresponding to the urinary fragments were found in the serum of these patients.

II. Studies of Calcium Binding and γ-Carboxyglutamic Acid

Content of BJP's

The ammonium sulphate precipitated BJP's and their CMF purified fractions showed no detectable calcium binding by two-dimensional ^{45}Ca electrophoresis autoradiography or by comparing their electrophoretic mobility in the presence of 10 mM EDTA or 10 mM CaCl$_2$.

Thirty-two BJP's (14 A+ and 18 A-) were analyzed for the presence of γ-carboxyglutamic acid (Gla), the documented mediator of calcium binding in several proteins. As shown in Fig. 7, the majority of A+ and A- BJP's had less than 0.5 residues of Gla per 1000 residues of glutamic acid (Glu). However 4 A+ BJ κ proteins had 0.5 to 1.0 Gla/1000 Glu, and one BJ κ had 2.1 Gla/1000 Glu.

Our efforts to identify the specific Gla-containing component using the CMF fractions were unsuccessful in that no Gla enrichment was found in any CMF fractions despite its confirmed presence in the initial BJ preparations.

TABLE 1. Concentration of Low Molecular Weight-Light Chain Related Protein Relative to Total Bence Jones Protein

Bence Jones	Type	Concentration of Low Molecular Weight-Light Chain Related Protein		
		High*	Low†	Trace or none
Amyloid-related (A+)	κ	3	5	1
	λ	4	3	2
Non-amyloid related (A−)	κ	0	2	5
	λ	0	3	5

*High: 50-15% of total BJP.
†Low: 15-5% of total BJP.

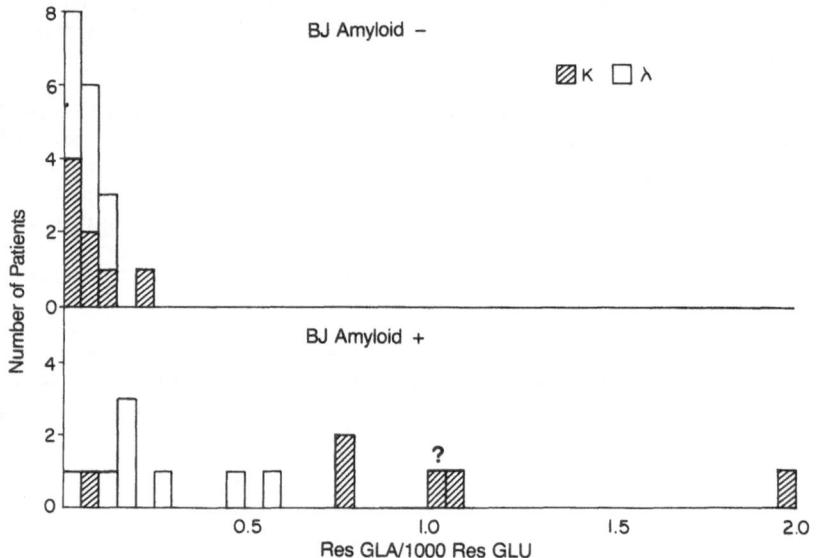

Fig. 7. Gamma-carboxyglutamic acid content, expressed as ratio over 1000 residues of glutamic acid (Res GLA/1000 Res GLU) of 33 Bence Jones proteins, related (amyloid +) or unrelated (amyloid −) to amyloidosis. The question mark refers to a case in which amyloidosis was suspected clinically but not histologically documented.

DISCUSSION

Previous studies have demonstrated the presence of light chain-related polypeptides of lower molecular weight than monomeric Bence-Jones protein in normal urine [18] as well as in the urine of patients with plasma cell dyscrasias [2]. These components more frequently correspond to the N-terminal portion (V_L) than to the C-terminal portion (C_L) of the urinary Bence-Jones protein, and may arise either from *de novo* synthesis or from proteolytic degradation (reviewed in Solomon [19, 20]). Similarly, the majority of proteins extracted from Al amyloid deposits are L-chain fragments of various size, related either to V_L or to V_L plus a portion of C-region [21]. However in at least one case (TEW) the amyloid deposits apparently contained the complete light chain [22].

In the present study, we demonstrated that many, but not all patients with AL amyloidosis excrete high concentrations of low molecular weight (12-16 Kd) light chain related proteins, and that these fragments are present in very low concentrations or are absent from the urine of patients with myeloma without amyloidosis. The finding of light chain fragments in the serum of these patients by immunoblotting suggests that these fragments are synthesized and are not products of proteolysis in the kidney or of degradation during storage. It seems reasonable to postulate that these fragments are related, if not identical, to the amyloid but formal proof is still lacking.

Because of the evidence (*vide supra*) indicating an association between calcium and amyloidosis (7-10), we have investigated calcium binding by Bence-Jones proteins. Using electrophoretic techniques we could not detect calcium binding by complete Bence-Jones proteins or by their CMF-purified fragments. However, our finding of low concentrations of the calcium-binding amino acid γ-carboxyglutamic acid (Gla) in some amyloid-related kappa Bence-Jones proteins suggests that calcium binding may be a factor in the amyloidogenicity of certain kappa Bence-Jones proteins.

ACKNOWLEDGEMENTS

We thank Dr. S. Beychok, Columbia University, for performing the amino-terminal analysis. During the tenure of this study, Dr. Merlini was on leave of absence from the Hospital "Policlinico S. Matteo," Pavia, Italy.

REFERENCES

1. T. Isobe and E. F. Osserman, New Engl. J. Med., 290, 473 (1974).
2. T. Isobe, K. Takatsuki, F. W. Tishendorf, S. Birken, E. F. Osserman, Clin. Immunol. Immunopathol., 19, 55 (1981).
3. J. B. Natvig, P. Westermark, K. Sletten, G. Husby, T. Michaelsen, Scand. J. Immunol., 14, 89 (1981).
4. E. F. Osserman, K. Takatsuki, N. Talal, Sem. Hematol., 1, 3 (1964).
5. J. Bertram, R. J. Gualtieri, E. F. Osserman, in: "Amyloid and Amyloidosis," G. G. Glenner, P. P. Costa, A. F. Freitas, Eds. (Excerpta Medica, Amsterdam, 1980), p. 351.
6. G. G. Glenner, W. Terry, M. Harada, C. Isersky, D. Page, Science, 171, 1150 (1971).
7. M. B. Pepys, Lancet i, 653 (1981).
8. R. W. Kula, W. K. Engel, B. R. Line, Lancet i, 92 (1977).
9. R. A. Yood, M. Skinner, A. S. Cohen, V. W. Lee, Authr. Rheum., 22, 677 (1979).
10. M. H. Kuczynski, Arch. Pathol. Anat. Physiol., 40, 195 (1922).
11. P. M. Gallop, J. B. Lian, P. V. Hauschka, N. Engl. J. Med., 302, 1460 (1980).
12. J. O. Jeppsson, C.-B. Laurell, B. Franzen, Clin. Chem., 25, 629 (1979).
13. R. F. Ritchie and R. Smith, Clin. Chem., 22, 1982 (1976).
14. U. K. Laemmli, Nature (London), 227, 680 (1970).
15. H. Towbin, T. Staehelin, J. Gordon, Proc. Natl. Acad. Sci. USA, 76, 4350 (1979).

16. F. Lindgärde, J. Malmquist, O. Zettervall, Clin. Chim. Acta., 44, 67 (1973).
17. P. V. Hauschka, Anal. Biochem., 80, 212 (1977).
18. I. Berggård and P. Peterson, in: "Gamma Globulins," Nobel Symposium 3, J. Killander, Ed. (Almquist and Wiksell, Stockholm, 1967), p. 71.
19. A. Solomon, N. Engl. J. Med., 294, 17 (1976).
20. A. Solomon, N. Engl. J. Med., 294, 91 (1976).
21. G. G. Glenner, N. Engl. J. Med., 302, 1283 (1980).
22. W. D. Terry, D. L. Page, S. Kimura, T. Isobe, E. F. Osserman, G. G. Glenner, J. Clin. Invest., 52, 1276 (1973).

ABERRANT IMMUNOGLOBULIN SYNTHESIS IN AL AMYLOID

J. Buxbaum* and G. Gallo†

Department of Medicine
New York VA Medical Center*
Departments of Medicine* and Pathology†
New York University Medical Center
New York, New York

ABSTRACT

Bone marrow cells obtained from 13 patients with biopsy documented AL disease were incubated in short term culture with radioactive amino acids. Immunologic precipitation of cytoplasm and secreted material was performed and the precipitates analyzed on SDS containing polyacrylamide gels. All the patients synthesized excess free light chains and light chain dimers. In addition, 8 of 13 patients synthesized molecules smaller than intact light chains which were precipitable with anti-L-chain constant region sera. Two of thirteen patients synthesized heavy chain fragments. These data show that some patients with AL disease synthesize L-chain fragments and suggest that these aberrant synthetic products may play a role in the pathogenesis of AL deposition.

Over the last decade investigation of the amyloidoses has been dominated by the identification and structural analysis of fibrillar material in tissue deposits by either immunologic or biochemical techniques. The rewards of these approaches are apparent with six (at last count) distinct molecules being identified as the major fibrillar components of hereditary acquired and local forms of the disease [1]. In addition, by inference, physiologically soluble proteins which are related to the fibrillar material have been implicated as precursors of the fibrils. Experimentally however, the steps whereby the soluble presumed precursors are transformed into the insoluble fibrillar deposits have been difficult to define. For the moment it appears that both different precursors and different mechanisms of biogenesis may be discovered for each of the amyloid diseases.

In AL disease the major fibrillar component is a monoclonal light chain or a related fragment. Among the 17 AL containing fibrils which have been reported in detail, only 2 appear to represent complete, intact L chains [2]. The remainder are composed of incomplete molecules all of which begin at the amino terminus and contain all or most of the V region and some portion of the constant region. In addition many of these contain multiple components. It is therefore possible that these fragments arise as synthetic products which in part, owe their propensity to tissue deposition to their incomplete protein structure.

MATERIAL AND METHODS

We have carried out an analysis of immunoglobulin biosynthesis by bone marrow cells obtained from 13 patients with biopsy documented AL fibril deposition either in the course of multiple myeloma or primary amyloidosis.

Bone marrow cells were obtained at the time of diagnostic bone marrow aspiration (with the cooperation of a large number of clinicians who were aware of our interest in these patients). The cells were collected in heparinized syringes and suspended in heparinized (5-10 μ/ml) tissue culture medium (Eagle's MEM) which had been depleted of methionine, leucine, and valine (-MLV medium). Cells were spun and the buffy coat separated (although not completely) from the underlying erythrocytes. The predominantly white cell population was washed twice more with the (-MLV) medium, counted and resuspended at a concentration of $(3-5) \times 10^6$ nucleated cells per milliliter. Radioactive ^{35}S methionine (100 μCi/ml) ^{3}H leucine (100 μCi/ml) and ^{3}H valine (100 μCi/ml) were buffered, warmed to 37° and added to the prewarmed cells at time zero. Samples were removed for analysis after various periods of incubation. The number of time points was determined by the total number of cells available. The samples removed at each interval were chilled and made 0.1 M with respect to iodoacetamide. They were centrifuged in the cold and the supernatant fluid removed for analysis as secreted material. The cell pellets were suspended in 9 ml of ice cold distilled water for 60 seconds to lyse the contaminating red blood cells and then brought to isotonicity by the addition of 1 ml of 10× buffered saline. The cells were centrifuged, the hemolyzed supernates removed and the cells washed again in cold tissue culture medium. The pellets were resuspended in 0.9 ml ice cold hypotonic buffer and 0.1 volume 0.5% Non-idet P40 (NP-40) was added to the suspension. The cells were agitated for 30 seconds and placed on ice for 30 min. The NP-40 preparation was then centrifuged at 100,000 G for 30 min at 4°C, the pellet discarded and the supernatant analyzed as cytoplasmic contents.

Portions of both cytoplasm and secreted material were precipitated with a variety of poly and monoclonal antisera specific for various immunoglobulin chains. Many of the sera were obtained commercially while others were made in our own institution or obtained from other investigators.

Immune precipitates were washed in high salt buffer containing 0.5% NP-40 and dissolved in 0.1% SDS prior to gel analysis. Monoclonal antibodies were added to various preparations after they had been cleared with staphylococcal protein A beads (Pharmacia). Additional protein A beads were utilized to harvest the molecules complexed with the monoclonals. The bound labelled molecules were released by boiling the beads (after washing) in 2.0% SDS, 0.5% NP-40 in 0.08 M Tris. Portions of all immune precipitates were counted in a liquid scintillation counter prior to analysis on polyacrylamide slab gels containing SDS.

RESULTS

All the patients studied (none of whom were hyperglobulinemic) synthesized free light chains (Table 1). All but one synthesized and secreted light chain dimers. Nine of the patients produced λ chains while four produced κ. Most of them synthesized relatively small amounts of H_2L_2. One of the patients synthesized a light chain tetramer [3]. Eight patients synthesized molecules which were smaller than light chains and were precipitable with anti-light chain sera.

The sizes of these polypeptides varied considerably. The smallest molecule we could detect was 7500 daltons in patient 1. It was only seen

TABLE 1. Immunoglobulins Synthesized by Bone Marrow Cells from AL Patients

Pt.	H_2L_2	L_2	L	Lf‡	Hf
1	–	λ_4, λ_2	λ	7500	–
2	±	λ_2	λ	13,500† 19,000 20,000	–
3	±	λ_2	λ	12,000†	–
4	–	λ_2	λ	?	–
5	±	λ_2	λ	12,500 17,500 19,000 21,500	–
6		κ_2	κ	19,000 10,000	–
7	+		κ	10,000	–
8	+	λ_2	λ		50,000α
9	+	κ_2	κ		48,000γ
10	+	λ_2	$\pm\lambda$		?
11	+	λ_2	λ		–
12	+	κ_2	κ	22,000	–
13	+	λ_2	λ	13,000† 21,000 22,000	–

*Monoclonal cryoglobulin.
†Identity of 12,000 dalton peptides not yet clear.
‡All sizes of reduced and alkylated immune precipitation.

after reduction and alkylation of the anti light chain precipitate. It appeared to be somewhat heterogeneous in size and might represent a product of degradation as well as aberrant biosynthesis.

Five patients synthesized a molecule with a molecular weight of 10-13,000 daltons which was readily precipitable with some polyclonal anti-light chain sera. Its nature is not yet clear. Experiments utilizing multiple antisera to define antigenic determinants on the peptide have not yet been completed. Four patients synthesized anti-light chain precipitable molecular species with sizes between 15,000 and 21,000 daltons. An example of such a patient is shown in Fig. 1. In some cases the fragments themselves polymerized to yield a disulfide linked dimer which on reduction and alkylation released a fragment monomer (Fig. 2).

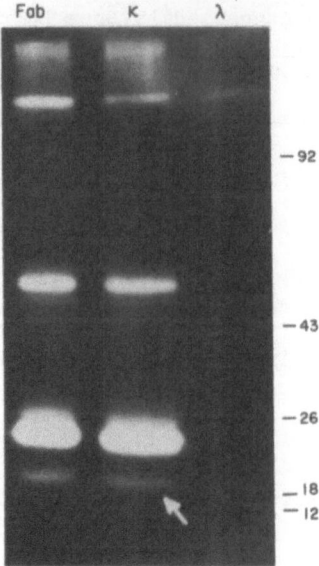

Fig. 1. Immune precipitation of AL peptides
(case 12). Aliquots of cytoplasm
prepared from labelled bone marrow
cells of patient 12 were precipitated with anti Fab, anti-κ and
anti-λ sera. The dissolved precipitates were electrophoresed on
10% polyacrylamide gels containing
0.1% SDS. Radioactive markers with
the molecular weights shown (in Kd)
were electrophoresed on the same
gel. In the lane containing the λ
precipitate a band corresponding
to the position of normal H_2L_2 is
seen. The same band is noted in
the anti Fab and anti-κ precipitates. The latter precipitates
also contain three additional molecular species, a kappa dimer with
a molecular weight of 50,000 daltons,
a kappa monomer of 24,000 daltons and
a protein with a molecular weight of
22,000 daltons which we belive is an
incomplete kappa chain.

Cells from 4 patients showed no synthesis of molecules which had the
antigenic or size characteristics of light chain fragments. However, 3 of
these synthesized peptides which have heavy chain antigenic determinants
and were smaller than intact heavy chains (Fig. 3).

DISCUSSION

These studies clearly show that bone marrow cells obtained from patients with AL disease synthesize both intact heavy and light chains and
fragments. Five of 13 make L-chain antigen containing peptides which are
clearly smaller than the intact molecule. Three patients make polypeptides

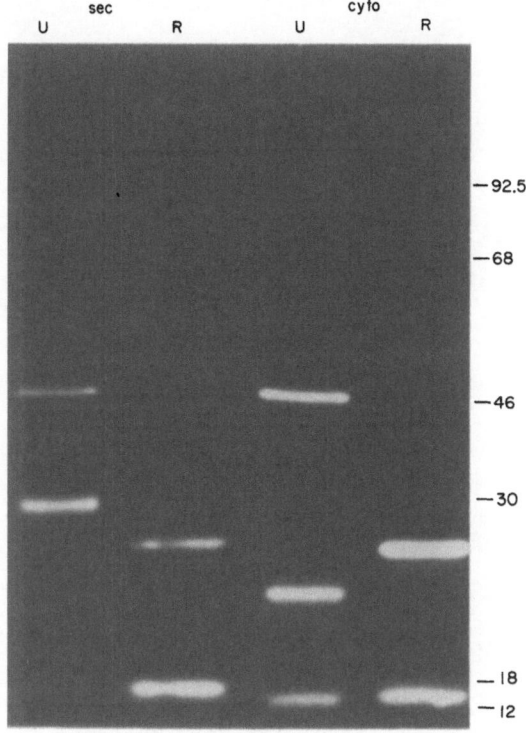

Fig. 2.   Immune precipitation of AL peptides (case
          15). Aliquots of secreted material and
          cytoplasm were precipitated with anti-λ
          serum. Portions of each were reduced and
          alkylated. The unreduced secretions con-
          tain 2 major λ precipitable molecules,
          one of 47,000 daltons and one of 30,000
          daltons. The 30 Kd molecule is not seen
          in the cytoplasm. Reduction yields mole-
          cules of 25,000 and 15,000 daltons. Thus
          it appears that 2 dimers are found in the
          secretions, one composed of 2 normal λ
          monomers while the second is composed of
          2 λ fragment monomers. There is a sug-
          gestion of a mixed dimer in the unreduced
          secretions. The cytoplasm contains λ
          dimer, monomer and fragment, while the re-
          duced cytoplasmic λ precipitate contains
          monomer and fragment. Native L-chain
          monomer and reduced and alkylated L-chain
          monomers frequently do not have the same
          mobility in this gel system.

which bear heavy chain antigenic determinants. In addition, in several
cases we could detect immunologically precipitable polypeptides with molecular weights around 12,000. In at least one case we identified such a molecule as β_2 microglobulin, however, it is not clear if all the proteins of
this molecular weight precipitate with the anti-β_2m serum. We have found
that some anti-light chain sera contain anti-β_2m activity but we have not
yet established whether the precipitation we have seen is due to contamination of the antisera or whether the β_2m is co-precipitated with anti-L chain
sera in an artifactual or biologically significant manner.

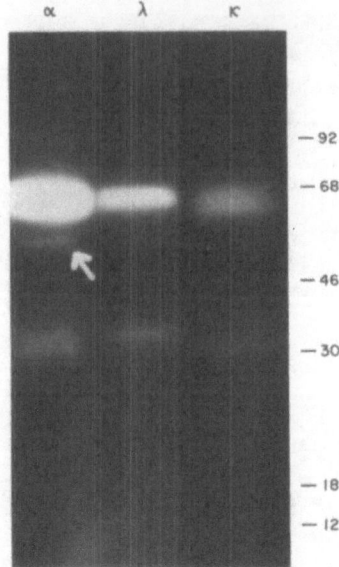

Fig. 3. Immune precipitation AL
peptides (case 8). Cyto-
plasm from patient 8 was
precipitated with anti-α,
anti-λ, and anti-κ sera.
The precipitates were re-
duced and alkylated with
0.1 M dithiothreitol and
0.1 M iodoacetamide. The
κ precipitate shows a
double band in the normal
heavy chain region which
represent normal α and γ
heavy chains bound to κ
in H_2L_2 form synthesized
by the normal plasma cells
in the marrow. Reduction
of the λ precipitate yields
a single λ band and a single
α band. Free λ chains
usually migrate behind κ
chains in this gel system.
Reduction of the anti-α
precipitate shows a heavy α
band of normal size and a
doublet in the light chain
region which contains both
κ and λ. Striking in the α
precipitate (arrow) is a
band with an estimated molecular weight of 50 Kd.
This molecule is also seen
in unreduced anti-α precipitates of cytoplasm (not
shown).

In all the patients reported here only antisera which recognized constant region determinants were utilized, therefore any cells which synthesized only V-region fragments would be scored as producing no fragments unless the fragments were covalently (disulfide) or noncovalently linked to a molecule containing constant region determinants. Patients 4, 10, and 11 fall into this category.

The relevance of the heavy chain fragments in these patients is not clear. To date, no one has shown the presence of Ig heavy chain polypeptide determinants in amyloid fibrils. In other studies we have shown tissue deposition of such fragments in an insoluble but not fibrillar form in monoclonal Ig deposition disease [4]. Hence the existence of such molecules is evident but their significance in AL patients is not.

We feel that the relationship between the synthetic products of the plasma cell and the nature of the deposited fibril must be established. It should be possible in some patients to compare the size and antigenic determinants of the deposited fibril proteins with those synthesized by their bone marrow cells. Should size concordance occur, a strong argument can be made for the predisposition of aberrant fragments toward tissue deposition. Should the sizes and structure be discordant it would suggest either that the aberrantly synthesized peptide must undergo processing prior to deposition, or that the fibrillar material is generated by processing of the intact L-chain.

The presence of multiple peptides could be explained by the presence of a heterogeneous cell population, i.e., AL does not represent a monoclonal disease. We consider this unlikely. While there is strong evidence in in vitro systems supporting the role of proteolysis in the generation of fibrils we believe our data argue against a pure degradative origin [5]. Most interesting of the possibilities is that there may be multiple transcripts from either the same or different genes or different portions of the same genes in these cells. This could reflect different start sites or different termination sites from the same gene, or multiple functional rearrangements. Such aberrant synthetic products have been reported in murine myeloma cells in which both a normal light chain and an aberrant peptide containing the leader sequence derived from another V-gene spliced to the same constant region gene have been found [6].

Our approach to AL disease has suggested an additional mechanism to explain the predisposition of the products of some plasma cell clones to be associated with fibril formation. One must consider that the fibrils may be formed from biosynthetic fragments, from degradative fragments, from intact polymerized proteins, from L-chain proteins with a particular primary structure (e.g., VλVI) or from some combination of these processes. Comparisons of the synthetic products with the deposited material from the same patients should give further insight concerning the relationships among these processes.

ACKNOWLEDGEMENTS

The authors gratefully acknowledge the cooperation and assistance of Doctors E. Amorosi, G. Hellman, B. Rayfield, and H. Mitnick for referral of their patients, Mr. Donald Hauser for his most able technical assistance and Ms. Carol O'Brien for her expert treatment of the manuscript.

This work was supported by research funds from the Veterans Administration.

541

REFERENCES

1. Glenner, G., NEJM, 302:1283-1333 (1980); Sletten, K., et al., Scan. J.
    Immunol., 12:503 (1980); Cohen, D. H., et al., 158:623 (1983).
2. Cohen, A. S., et al., Arthritis and Rheumatism, 21:155 (1978); Pras,
    M., et al., Israel J. Med. Sci., 18:866 (1982); Westermark, P., et al.,
    Molec. Immun., 19:447 (1982).
3. Buxbaum, J., et al., Am. J. Med., 67:867 (1979).
4. Gallo, G., et al., Am. J. Path., 99:621 (1980).
5. Glenner, G. G., et al., Science, 174:712 (1971); Epstein, W. V., et
    al., J. Lab. and Clin. Med., 84:107 (1974); Linke, R. P., et al.,
    J. of Immun., 111:10 (1973).
6. Schnell, H., et al., Nature, 286:170 (1980); Choi, E., et al., Nature,
    286:776 (1980); Alt, F., et al., Cell, 21:1 (1980).

G. CLINICAL STUDIES

PRIMARY SYSTEMIC AMYLOIDOSIS (AL): COMPARISON OF MELPHALAN-PREDNISONE VS. COLCHICINE TREATMENT IN 101 CASES*

Robert A. Kyle, Philip R. Greipp, John P. Garton, and Morie A. Gertz

Division of Hematology and Internal Medicine
Mayo Clinic and Mayo Foundation
Rochester, Minnesota

ABSTRACT

One hundred one patients with primary amyloidosis (AL) were stratified in four groups on the basis of their major clinical features: 1) Nephrotic syndrome or renal insufficiency; 2) congestive heart failure; 3) peripheral neuropathy; and 4) other. The patients were randomized to 1) melphalan (0.15 mg/kg daily) and prednisone (0.8 mg/kg daily) for 7 days every 6 weeks, or 2) colchicine (0.6 mg twice a day). Forty-nine patients were randomized to melphalan-prednisone (M-P) therapy, while 52 were to receive colchicine (C). No important differences were found between the two groups in the history or the initial physical examination and laboratory findings. If there was progressive disease or lack of benefit from therapy, either M-P or C was added to the original therapeutic regimen. Twenty-one of the 40 patients with the nephrotic syndrome who received M-P had >50% reduction in urinary protein. Four patients died of acute nonlymphocytic leukemia. The median survival was 25 months for the M-P group and 18 months for the C group (P = 0.23). When survival was calculated from the onset of randomization to death or progression of disease, the median survival was 16 months for the M-P group and 6 months for the C group (P = 0.0001).

INTRODUCTION

Primary systemic amyloidosis (AL) is an uncommon disease characterized by deposition of a fibrillar protein, often in vital organs (particularly the heart and kidney), resulting in organ dysfunction and death. The median survival was 14.7 months for 132 patients reported from the Mayo Clinic in 1975 [1] and 12 months for 229 patients reported from the same institution in 1983 [2]. Satisfactory treatment for primary amyloidosis (AL) does not exist.

---

*Based on a manuscript currently submitted for consideration by Am. J. Med. (R. A. Kyle, P. R. Greipp, J. P. Garton, and M. A. Gertz, Primary Systemic Amyloidosis (AL): Comparison of Melphalan-Prednisone vs. Colchicine). This investigation was supported in part by Research Grant CA-16835 from the National Institutes of Health, Public Health Service, and by the Toor Myeloma Research Fund.

In 1964, Osserman and colleages [3] emphasized the association of Bence Jones protein and amyloidosis and reported that these amyloid light chains tend to bind to certain normal tissues. Glenner and colleagues in 1971 [4] and Terry et al., 1973 [5] demonstrated that the amyloid fibrils in a patient with AL [6] were virtually identical to the variable portion of the monoclonal light chain (Bence Jones protein). Because monoclonal light chains are synthesized by plasma cells and increased numbers of atypical plasma cells are commonly found on bone marrow examination in AL [7], it is reasonable to attempt treatment with alkylating agents that are effective against diseases characterized by proliferation of neoplastic plasma cells [8]. Melphalan, an alkylating agent, has been reported as beneficially influencing primary amyloidosis [9-18].

In a prospective randomized study of 55 patients with AL comparing melphalan-prednisone therapy with placebo, Kyle and Greipp [19] demonstrating some benefit to patients with the nephrotic syndrome who were treated with melphalan-prednisone but were unable to detect a significant difference in survival.

Colchicine may be helpful in the treatment of amyloidosis. Amyloidosis occurs in more than one-fourth of patients with familial Mediterranean fever and is a major cause of death [20]. Colchicine decreases the attacks of familial Mediterranean fever [21, 22] and has been reported to inhibit casein-induced amyloidosis in mice [23, 24]. Urinary protein excretion decreased significantly in 6 patients with familial Mediterranean fever and proteinuria who were treated with colchicine [25]. In 1976, Nimoityn et al. [26] described a patient with familial Mediterranean fever in whom abdominal pain and proteinuria decreased with colchicine therapy. Suppressor T-cell activity and chemotaxis are decreased in untreated familial Mediterranean fever, but these abnormalities are reversed with colchicine [27]. Colchicine blocks the synthesis and secretion of serum amyloid A protein (SAA) from the hepatocytes of mice [28, 29].

Based on a comparison with historical controls, survival of patients with primary amyloidosis increased with the daily use of colchicine [30]. There has been no prospective study comparing melphalan and colchicine therapies. We are reporting our experience in a prospective randomized study comparing melphalan-prednisone therapy with colchicine therapy.

MATERIALS AND METHODS

Patients

Amyloidosis was confirmed by biopsy in every case. Patients with secondary, familial, or localized amyloidosis; patients with overt symptomatic multiple myeloma or diarrhea; and patients who had received alkylating agents or colchicine were excluded from the study. Each patient was assigned to one of four groups: 1) nephrotic syndrome or renal failure; 2) congestive heart failure; 3) peripheral neuropathy; and 4) other. Patients who had more than one of these features were assigned to the group whose characteristics were most prominent in the patient. By means of a dynamic randomization scheme that assured a balance in the four clinical groups, the patients were assigned to receive: 1) melphalan (0.15 mg/kg) in two divided doses daily and prednisone (0.8 mg/kg) in four divided doses daily for the same 7-day period every 6 weeks; or 2) colchicine (0.6 mg twice a day). The leukocyte and platelet counts were determined every 3 weeks initially, and the melphalan dose was adjusted appropriately. The colchicine dose was increased by 0.6 mg daily each week until abdominal cramps or diarrhea developed. The use of colchicine was then discontinued and resumed in the highest dosage that did not produce side effects. The patient

TABLE 1. Stratification of 101 Patients with Primary Systemic Amyloidosis (AL)

Group	Melphalan-prednisone	Col-chicine	Total No.	%
Nephrotic syndome	23	23	46	45
Congestive heart failure	8	9	17	17
Peripheral neuropathy	7	8	15	15
Others*				
Total	49	52	101	100

*Hepatomegaly (5), macroglossia (4), purpura or other skin lesion (3), ab-
dominal pain (3), myopathy (2), cranial neuropathies (2), pronounced loss
of weight, jaw claudication, joint pains, and proteinuria (1 each).
(From R. A. Kyle et al., Primary systemic amyloidosis (AL): Comparison
of melphalan-prednisone vs. colchicine. Am. J. Med. [Submitted for pub-
lication].)

TABLE 2. Initial Findings of 101 Cases of Primary Systemic Amyloidosis (AL)

	Melphalan-prednisone	Col-chicine	Total group
No. of patients	49	52	101
Age (yr)*	64	62	63
Males (%)	60	57	58
Females (%)	40	43	42
Weight loss:			
% of patients	33	46	40
Amount (lb)*	20	20	20
Hepatomegaly (%)	31	37	34
Macroglossia (%)	8	17	13
Hemoglobin (g/dl)*	14.0	13.5	13.9
Creatinine (mg/dl)*	1.1	1.15	1.1
% >2.0	12	19	15
Alkaline phosphatase (IU)*†	164	174	167
Serum albumin (g/dl)*	3.1	3.0	3.1
Plasma cells in bone marrow (%)*	5	5	5
Serum M-protein present (%)	67	54	60
Serum M-protein (g/dl)*	1.1	1.2	1.1
Urine M-protein present (%)	76	61	73
Urine M-protein (g/24 h)*	0.38	0.30	0.31

*Median.
†Normal >250.
 (From R. A. Kyle et al., Primary systemic amyloidosis (AL): Comparison of
 melphalan-prednisone vs. colchicine. Am. J. Med. [Submitted for publica-
 tion].)

TABLE 3. Serum Immunoelectrophoresis in Primary Systemic Amyloidosis (AL)

| | Percentage of patients | | |
	Melphalan-prednisone	Colchicine	Total
IgG κ	10	6	8
IgG λ	31	15	23
IgA κ	0	4	2
IgA λ	6	6	6
IgM κ	0	0	0
IgM λ	0	2	1
IgD λ	2	0	1
κ only	2	2	2
λ only	16	13	15
Negative	33	52	42
Total	100	100	100

(From R. A. Kyle et al., Primary systemic amyloidosis (AL): Comparison of melphalan-prednisone vs. colchicine. Am. J. Med. [Submitted for publication].)

TABLE 4. Tissue Diagnoses in Primary Systemic Amyloidosis (AL)

| Site | Percentage of biopsies pos. for amyloidosis | | | |
	Tests done	Melphalan-prednisone	Colchicine	Total group
Rectum	76	75	72	74
Kidney	24	100	100	100
Carpal ligament	5	100	50	60
Liver	11	100	72	82
Small intestine	3	100	100	100
Bone marrow	91	43	39	41
Sural nerve	10	80	100	90

(From R. A. Kyle et al., Primary systemic amyloidosis (AL): Comparison of melphalan-prednisone vs. colchicine. Am. J. Med. [Submitted for publication].)

continued on therapy for at least 6 months, unless significant toxicity developed. In the event of progressive disease or lack of benefit from therapy, melphalan-prednisone or colchicine was added to the original therapeutic regimen.

RESULTS

Initial Comparison of Melphalan-Prednisone and Colchicine Groups

One hundred one patients were entered in the study. Forty-nine were randomized to melphalan-prednisone therapy and 52 were randomized to the colchicine regimen (Table 1). No important differences were found between the two groups in the history and initial physical examination or laboratory findings (Table 2). The serum monoclonal proteins were of the λ class in 76% of the colchicine group and in 84% of the melphalan-prednisone group (Table 3). A urinary monoclonal λ light chain was found in 42% of the colchicine group and in 61% of the melphalan-prednisone group. A monoclonal protein was recognized in the serum or urine in 81% of the colchicine group and in 90% of the melphalan-prednisone group.

The prothrombin time was increased (>12 seconds) in only 4 patients. All 4 were receiving melphalan-prednisone. The factor X level was reduced in 3 patients. The serum carotene level was reduced (<48 μg/dl) in only 1 patient. The serum vitamin B_{12} value was <200 ng/liter in 12 patients, but none had evidence of pernicious anemia. Echocardiography (M-mode and two-dimensional) was done in 53 cases. Results of echocardiography revealed abnormalities consistent with amyloid infiltration in 60%. Results were similar in both treatment groups.

Histologic diagnosis of amyloidosis was made in all cases (Table 4). Two patients had a negative carpal tunnel biopsy - in 1, paraffin blocks from the biopsy done elsewhere could not be obtained, and in the other, carpal ligament biopsy was performed after chemotherapy. Two patients had a negative liver biopsy - in 1 of these, the original paraffin blocks from the patient's home hospital had been discarded. Sural nerve biopsy was negative in 1 patient with peripheral neuropathy.

Results of Therapy (Figs. 1-4)

The peripheral neuropathy became worse in all 15 patients. One patient with congestive heart failure was alive at 46 months. However, serial echocardiograms revealed evidence of increased amyloid infiltration. Hepatomegaly developed during therapy in 9 patients in the melphalan-prednisone group and in 10 in the colchicine group. The serum alkaline phosphatase activity increased >50% in 2 patients in the melphalan-prednisone group and in 11 receiving colchicine. Serum alkaline phosphatase decreased in 5 patients receiving melphalan-prednisone and in only 1 on colchicine therapy. The effect of therapy on hemoglobin, serum creatinine, and bone marrow is shown in Table 5. There was a >50% increase in serum creatinine in 17 patients in each group. Hemodialysis was required by 5 patients on the melphalan-prednisone regimen and by 6 patients on the colchicine regimen.

The effect of melphalan-prednisone and colchcicine on the M-protein is seen in Table 6. The nephrotic syndrome was frequently benefitted by melphalan-prednisone but not by colchicine (Table 7). The median interval from the institution of melphalan-prednisone therapy until the urinary protein had decreased >50% was 8 months; however, the decrease in proteinuria did not occur in 7 patients until after 1 year of melphalan-prednisone therapy. Other syndromes that developed during the course of the patient's disease are listed in Table 5. More than two-thirds of patients on the colchicine regime had melphalan-prednisone added because of failure to improve (Table 8). Only 8 patients on melphalan-prednisone therapy received colchicine. Colchicine was not added because gastrointestinal symptoms developed, the patient died, or the amyloidosis stabilized.

Duration and Amount of Therapy

Patients on the melphalan-prednisone regimen received a 1-week course of therapy every 6 weeks for 12 months (median) (range 1-60). The number of 1-week courses of melphalan-prednisone ranged from 1 to 30. The median daily dose of melphalan was 9.8 mg, with a range of 6 to 20 mg. The median total dose of melphalan was 840 mg, with a range of 42 to 2205 mg. Col-

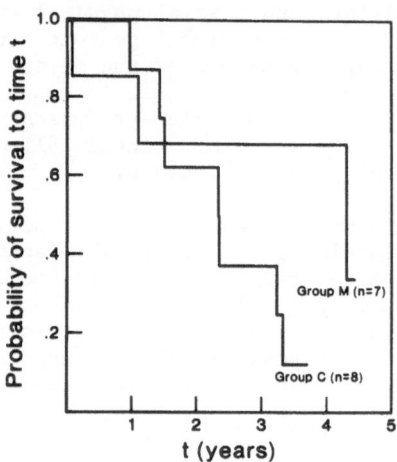

Fig. 1. Probability of survival
of patients with primary
amyloidosis (AL) and pe-
ripheral neuropathy
treated with melphalan-
prednisone (M) or col-
chicine (C). P = 0.19
(logrank).

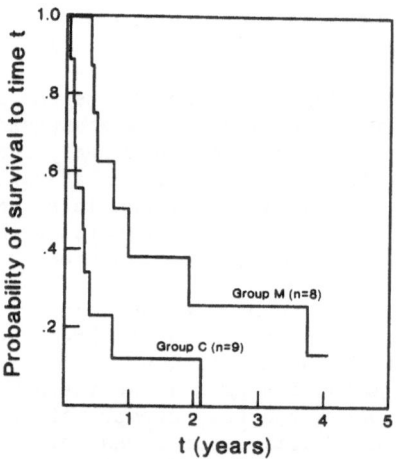

Fig. 2. Probability of survival
of patients with primary
amyloidosis (AL) and con-
gestive heart failure
treated with melphalan-
prednisone (M) or col-
chicine (C). P = 0.02
(logrank).

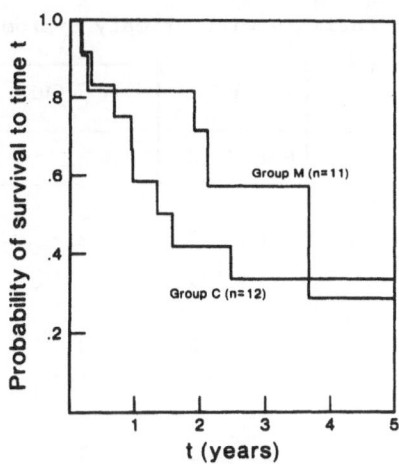

Fig. 3. Probability of survival
of patients with primary
amyloidosis (AL) and
"other" conditions treated
with melphalan-prednisone
(M) or colchicine (C).
P = 0.58 (logrank).

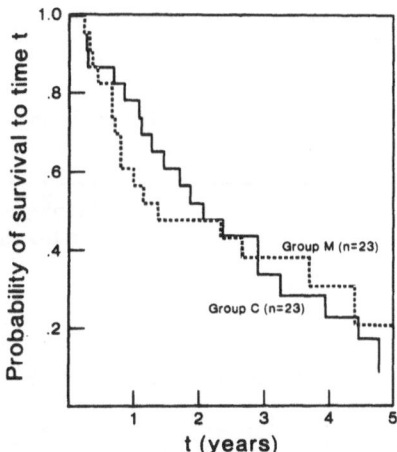

Fig. 4. Probability of survival
of patients with primary
amyloidosis (AL) and
nephrotic syndrome
treated with melphalan-
prednisone (M) or col-
chicine (C). P = 0.98
(logrank).

TABLE 5.   Therapy of Patients with Primary Systemic Amyloidosis (AL)*

	PN		CHF		Other		Neph	
	M–P	C	M–P	C	M–P	C	M–P	C
No. of patients	7	8	8	9	11	12	23	23
Decrease of ≥2 g/dl in Hg†	4	3	2	2	5	4	17	15
Increase of ≥0.5 mg/dl in creatinine†	1	0	0	3	4	1	13	15
Decrease in marrow plasma cells	1	0	0	0	0	0	2	2
Median survival (mo)	52	28	11.5	3	44	18	17	26
Developed (during follow-up)†								
CHF	1	3	0	0	0	2	7	4
CT	0	3	1	3	3	3	4	2
OH	0	0	0	2	0	3	10	6
PN	0	0	0	0	1	0	4	2
MAL	0	1	0	0	0	1	0	0
Neph	0	0	1	1	0	0	0	0

*Abbreviations: CHF = congestive heart failure; CT = carpal tunnel syndrome; MAL = malabsorption; OH = orthostatic hypotension; Neph = nephrotic syndrome; PN = peripheral neuropathy.
†Number of patients involved.
(From R. A. Kyle et al., Primary systemic amyloidosis (AL): Comparison of melphalan-prednisone vs. colchicine. Am. J. Med. [Submitted for publication].)

TABLE 6.   Effects of Therapy on M-Protein in Primary Systemic Amyloidosis (AL)

Result	Melphalan-prednisone	Colchicine
Serum M-protein		
No. of patients	33	38
>50% decrease	5	0
Disappeared	7	0
Urine M-protein		
No. of patients	37	37
>50% decrease	13	0
Disappeared	9	0

(From R. A. Kyle et al., Primary systemic amyloidosis (AL): Comparison of melphalan-prednisone vs. colchicine. Am. J. Med. [Submitted for publication].)

chicine was taken from <I month to 56 months (median 12). The daily dose of colchicine ranged from <0.6 mg to 3.0 mg, with a median dose of 1.5 mg.

Toxicity

Leukopenia (leukocyte count <3000/mm^3) occurred in almost half of the patients receiving melphalan-prednisone. In 9, the leukocyte count decreased to <1500/mm^3. No patient had sepsis related to the leukopenia.

TABLE 7. Results of Therapy on Nephrotic Syndrome in Primary Systemic Amyloidosis (AL)

	Melphalan-prednisone (M-P)	Colchicine (C)	M-P after C failure
No. of patients	23	23	17
Increase of ≥1 g/dl in albumin*	4	1	5
Stable creatinine*	4	1	3
Total urinary protein/24 h*			
Decrease >50%	12	0	9
Stable creatinine	7	0	4

*No. of patients involved.
(From R. A. Kyle et al., Primary systemic amyloidosis (AL): Comparison of melphalan-prednisone vs. colchicine. Am. J. Med. [Submitted for publication].)

TABLE 8. Therapy of Patients with Primary Systemic Amyloidosis

	Melphalan-prednisone (M-P) added			Colchicine (C) added		
	No. of pt.	Months after C (median)	Duration (mo.)	No. of pt.	Months after M-P (median)	Duration (mo.)
Peripheral neuropathy						
M-P	–	–	–	3	10	10
C	8	6	12	–	–	–
Congestive heart failure						
M-P	–	–	–	1	11	34
C	2	6.5	7	–	–	–
Other						
M-P	–	–	–	0	–	–
C	8	6.5	10	–	–	–
Nephrotic syndrome						
M-P	–	–	–	4	17	4
C	17	6	12	–	–	–
Total	35			8		

(From R. A. Kyle et al., Primary systemic amyloidosis (AL): Comparison of melphalan-prednisone vs. colchicine. Am. J. Med. [Submitted for publication].)

Thrombocytopenia occurred in slightly more than half of the patients receiving melphalan-prednisone, and the count decreased to <50,000/mm^3 in 12 patients. There was no serious bleeding related to the thrombocytopenia. Diarrhea, abdominal cramps, or nausea and vomiting occurred temporarily in every patient who received colchicine, because the dosage of the drug was

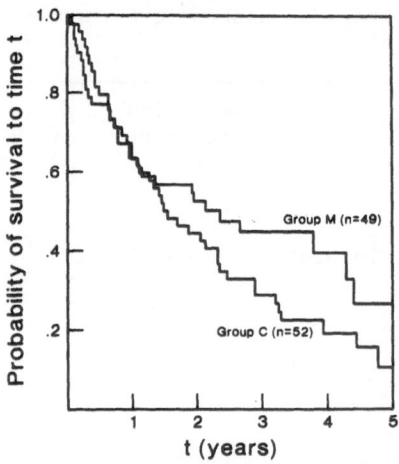

Fig. 5. Probability of survival
of patients with primary
colchicine (C). P = 0.23
(logrank).

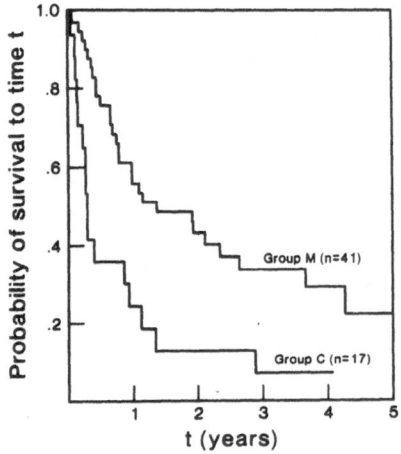

Fig. 6. Probability of survival
of patients with primary
amyloidosis (AL) treated
with a single regimen of
either melphalan-predni-
sone (M) or colchicine
(C). P = 0.001 (log-
rank).

increased until symptoms developed. With a single daily colchicine tablet,
an occasional patient had gastrointestinal symptoms. One patient developed
renal failure after experiencing diarrhea while on colchicine therapy.

Cause of Death

    Cardiac manifestations were the most frequent causes of death in both
groups. Some patients who were reported to have died suddenly with amy-

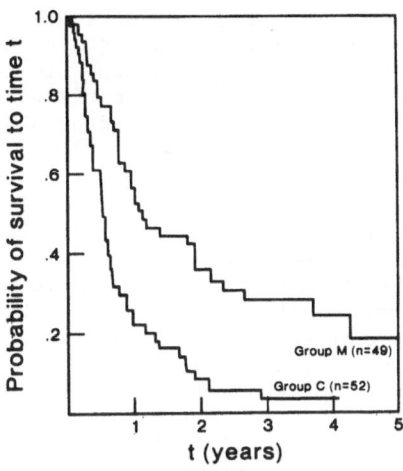

Fig. 7. Probability of survival
of patients with primary
amyloidosis (AL) treated
with melphalan-prednisone
(M) or colchicine (C)
from beginning of therapy
to either death or until
disease progression re-
quired change of therapy.
P = 0.0001 (logrank).

loidosis probably had cardiac arrhythmia as the terminal event. Four patients died of acute nonlymphocytic leukemia. They had received melphalan-
prednisone from 23 to 39 months (median 33) and a median dose of 950 mg
(range 350 to 1316). Three of the 4 had received colchicine – 2 for almost
4 years. Two of the patients had a preleukemia phase characterized by
pancytopenia. One patient had unexpected cytopenias from modest doses of
melphalan and had received only 350 mg of the drug during the 29 months of
chemotherapy.

Survival

The median survival for the 101 patients was 22 months: 25.2 months
for patients randomized to the melphalan-prednisone regimen and 18 months
for those on colchicine therapy (P = 0.23) (Fig. 5).

If survival analysis were limited to patients who had received only a
single regimen, the median survival was significantly different between the
melphalan-prednisone (n = 41) (16 months) and the colchicine (n = 17) (3
months) groups (P = 0.001) (Fig. 6).

Survival was also calculated from the time of study randomization until death or until progression of disease necessitated adding the other
therapeutic regimen. The "progression-free" median survival was 16 months
for the melphalan-prednisone group and 6 months for the colchicine group
(P = 0.0001) (Fig. 7).

DISCUSSION

Treatment for primary systemic amyloidosis (AL) is not satisfactory.
In a double-blind study [19] involving 55 patients with AL, those given

melphalan-prednisone therapy were able to continue on treatment longer and received larger doses than did patients in the placebo group, before the code was broken because of progressive disease. In that study, among 24 patients with the nephrotic syndrome, proteinuria virtually disappeared in 2 and urinary excretion of protein was reduced by 50% in 8 others given melphalan-prednisone therapy.

Six patients with the nephrotic syndrome and histologically proved AL have been reported to have benefitted from chemotherapy [9-13]. Three other patients with histologically proved amyloidosis without the nephrotic syndrome have also benefitted from chemotherapy [16-18]. Spontaneous remissions of the nephrotic syndrome have been noted in 2 patients with amyloidosis [31]. However, 1 of the patients had had pulmonary tuberculosis, and the other had had pulmonary tuberculosis and chronic ulcerative colitis; secondary amyloidosis could not be excluded.

The results of therapy in amyloidosis are difficult to document because the amount of amyloid in a patient cannot be measured accurately. In animals, the redistribution of amyloid deposits from the spleen and liver to the kidneys increases the problem of evaluation [32]. We have described 2 patients with AL and the nephrotic syndrome in whom the administration of melphalan and prednisone was associated with resolution of the nephrotic syndrome [15]. In both patients, however, amyloid deposition was greater in the follow-up renal tissue than in the initial specimen. A simple method is needed for measuring the amount of amyloid in a patient.

Results of therapy were disappointing despite the reduction (>50%) of proteinuria in more than half of the patients with the nephrotic syndrome who received melphalan-prednisone. Peripheral neuropathy became worse in all 15 patients and did not seem to be influenced by either treatment program. Patients with congestive heart failure did not seem to be benefitted objectively, although survival was greater for the melphalan-prednisone group than the colchicine group.

Colchicine was well tolerated, except for the expected gastrointestinal symptoms. Leukopenia and thrombocytopenia did not constitute a serious problem. However, 4 patients receiving melphalan-prednisone developed an acute nonlymphocytic leukemia, presumably from the alkylating agent.

The difference in survival between the total melphalan-prednisone and colchicine groups was not significant. However, survival was significantly longer for the patients treated with melphalan-prednisone when analysis was limited to those receiving only a single regimen or when survival was calculated from the time of randomization to death or to progression of the disease necessitating the addition of the other therapeutic regimen. This suggests that melphalan-prednisone is superior to colchicine. This superiority is also supported by the fact that, in 35 cases, melphalan-prednisone was added to colchicine, while colchicine was added to melphalan-prednisone in only 8 cases. However, colchicine may not have been added because of the presence of gastrointestinal symptoms from amyloidosis or bias on the part of the investigator. In this study, a cross-over design was included because it was considered difficult to withhold another potentially beneficial agent in the presence of progressive amyloidosis. This study suggests that melphalan-prednisone is superior to colchicine, but to confirm this, the agents must be compared in a prospective randomized fashion without a provision for cross-over.

ACKNOWLEDGEMENT

[All illustrations are from: R. A. Kyle, P. R. Greipp, J. P. Garton, and M. A. Gertz, Primary systemic amyloidosis (AL): Comparison of melphalan-prednisone vs. colchicine. Am. J. Med. (submitted for publication).]

REFERENCES

1. R. A. Kyle and E. D. Bayrd, Medicine, Baltimore, 54:271 (1975).
2. R. A. Kyle and P. R. Greipp, Mayo Clin. Proc., 58:665 (1983).
3. E. F. Osserman, et al., Semin. Hematol., 1:3 (1964).
4. G. G. Glenner, et al., Science, 172:1150 (1971).
5. W. D. Terry, et al., J. Clin. Invest., 52:1276 (1973).
6. A. S. Cohen and O. Wegelius, Arthritis Rheum., 23:644 (1980).
7. R. A. Kyle and E. D. Bayrd, Arch. Intern. Med., 107:344 (1961).
8. G. Costa, et al., Am. J. Med., 54:589 (1973).
9. H. J. Cohen, et al., Ann. Intern. Med., 82:466 (1975).
10. N. F. Jones, et al., Lancet, 2:616 (1972).
11. M. K. Horne, III, Ann. Intern. Med., 83:281 (1975).
12. R. S. Schwartz, et al., Arch. Intern. Med., 139:1144 (1979).
13. J. N. Buxbaum, et al., Am. J. Med., 67:867 (1979).
14. R. A. Kyle, et al, Blood, 44:333 (1974).
15. R. A. Kyle, et al., Arch. Intern. Med., 142:1445 (1982).
16. A. D. Mehta, Br. J. Clin. Pract., 32:358 (1978).
17. K. Bradstock, et al., Aust. NZ. J. Med., 8:176 (1978).
18. J. Corkery, et al., Lancet, 2:425 (1978).
19. R. A. Kyle, P. R. Greipp, Blood, 52:818 (1978).
20. E. Sohar, et al., Am. J. Med., 43:227 (1967).
21. S. E. Goldfinger, New Engl. J. Med., 287:1302 (1972).
22. H. A. Reimann, JAMA, 231:64 (1975).
23. T. Shirahama and A. S. Cohen, J. Exp. Med., 140:1102 (1974).
24. I. Kedar (Keizman), et al., Isr. J. Med. Sci., 10:787 (1974).
25. D. Zemer, et al., New Engl. J. Med., 294:170 (1976).
26. P. Nimoityn, et al., Br. Med. J., 2:284 (1976).
27. I. Melamed, et al., Clin. Exp. Immunol., 53:659 (1983).
28. M. J. Selinger, et al., Nature, 285:498 (1980).
29. E. Tatsuta, et al., Arthritis Rheum., 27:349 (1984).
30. A. Rubinow, et al., Arthritis Rheum., 24:S124 (1981).
31. J. Michael and N. F. Jones, Br. Med. J., 1:1592 (1978).
32. T. Shirahama and A. S. Cohen, Am. J. Pathol., 99:539 (1980).

THE LIFE SPAN OF PATIENTS WITH PRIMARY (AL) AMYLOIDOSIS

AND THE EFFECT OF COLCHICINE TREATMENT*

Alan S. Cohen, Alan Rubinow, Herbert Kayne,
Caryn Libbey, Martha Skinner, and John Mason

The Thorndike Memorial Laboratory
and Department of Medicine
Boston City Hospital

Departments of Medicine and Pharmacology

Boston University School of Medicine
Boston, Massachusetts

INTRODUCTION

There is no specific treatment for any variety of amyloidosis [1]. Primary (AL) amyloidosis, now the more commonly seen form of the disorder, usually has a poor prognosis and short life expectancy [2]. Colchicine, which effectively prevents acute fibril attacks in patients with familial Mediterranean fever (FMF), a condition that predisposes to amyloidosis, has been shown to block amyloid production in the mouse model [3, 4]. In addition, reports indicate that patients with FMF receiving colchicine no longer develop amyloidosis and suggest improvement in some amyloidotic patients with this form of AA amyloid [5, 6].

As a referral center for patients with amyloid disease, the decision was therefore made to conduct a therapeutic study with colchicine, a relatively innocuous agent. Our original protocol was a double blind, controlled study in which randomized patients would be treated with colchicine or placebo. Patients with biopsy proven amyloidosis for more than 6 months were to have been excluded from the study since it would be difficult to attribute any measurable differences to the medication (due to rapid mortality noted in literature) [17]. Survival (endpoint death) was to be the essential outcome measurement, for clearly data dependent on this parameter were subject to rigorous analysis. Although reasonably conceived, this study was abandoned for: 1) almost every patient referred had amyloid disease for 6 or more months; 2) the outright refusal of the majority of patients with a potentially fatal disease to accept placebo; and 3) similar

---

*These investigations have been supported by grants from the United States Public Health Service, National Institute of Arthritis, Metabolic and Digestive and Kidney Diseases (AM-04599 and M-07014), Multipurpose Arthritis Center, National Institutes of Health (AM-20613), the General Clinical Research Centers Branch of the Division of Research Resources, National Institutes of Health (RR-533) and from the Arthritis Foundation.

TABLE 1. Survival in Primary (AL) Amyloid Data Base

Eligibility - Original 1976 study

*1. Biopsy proven amyloid (green birefringence on Congo red stain)
 2. Double-blind, random drug allocation
*3. Absence of immature plasma cells in bone marrow
*4. Ineligible if heredofamilial
*5. Ineligible if secondary (AA) amyloid
 6. Biopsy diagnosis not present for over 6 months

Treatment

*1. Informed consent
*2. Colchicine 0.6 mgm bid
*3. Daily colchicine compliance log

Followup

*1. Continuous contact with referring physician
*2. Yearly evaluations at TML-CRC

Analysis

*1. Life table calculation of survival

---

*Factors still in place when study became prospective.

---

unwillingness on the part of the referring physician to allow their patients to enter the study; and 4) the discovery, that whatever protocol we used, referring physicians placed the patient on colchicine (in 4 of the first 6 cases).

An open study, in which all patients were to be offered colchicine, all entrance data would be carefully gathered and compared to our previous experience, appeared to be the realistic alternative. Currently, therefore, the survival of the colchicine treated group is compared with the survival in our own previous experience when no drug therapy was available and only supportive measures were used. All data from prospective patients and from previous experience were gathered in a comparable fashion, by the same investigators.

METHODS

An initial detailed clinical evaluation and classification was carried out on each patient in this study in the Thorndike Memorial Laboratory Clinical Research Center. The presence of amyloid was determined histopathologically by the presence of Congo red positive deposits that showed green birefringence on polarization microscopy. Studies included a search for urinary and plasma M components and κ or λ light chains, bone marrow aspiration or biopsy and skeletal survey. If a diagnosis of multiple myeloma was made (sheets of immature plasma cells in the bone marrow) or if acquired (AA) or heredofamial amyloid was found, the patient was excluded.

All patients, from July 1976 to July 1983 were placed on colchicine 0.5 mgm tablet (1-2 tablets/day) depending upon tolerance. Patients were requested to complete compliance forms and return them on a regulator basis and to return for complete reevaluation in 1-2 years. They also had periodic examinations carried out by local physicians (Table 1).

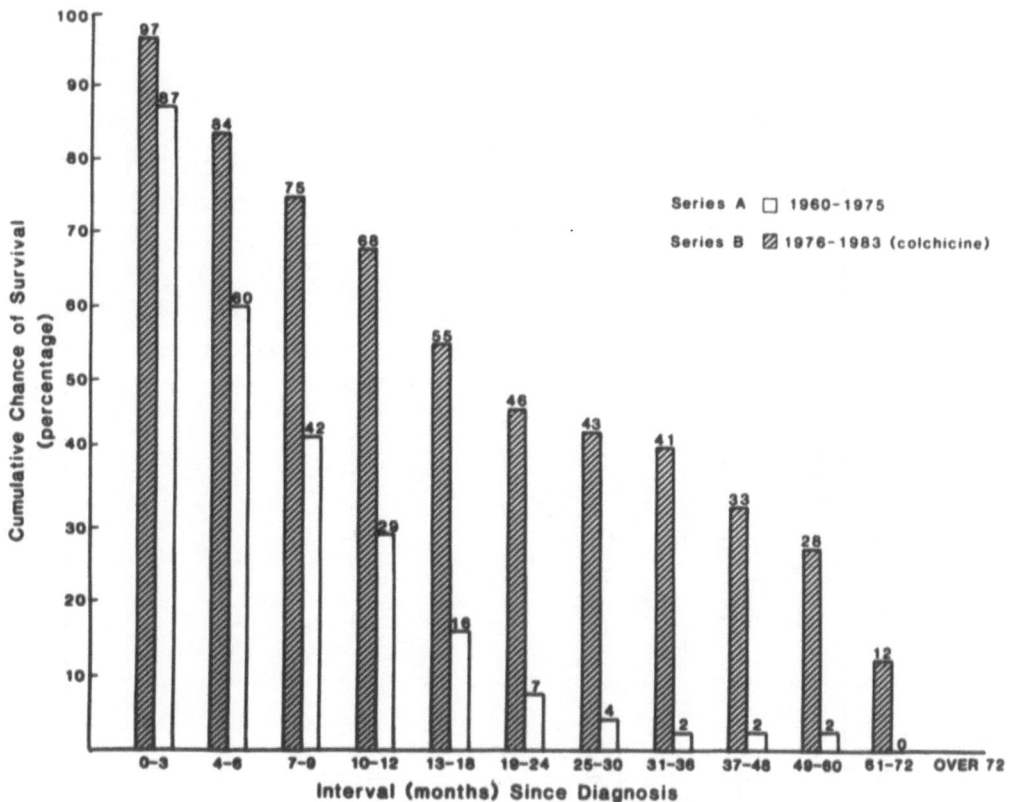

Fig. 1.   Survival rate in Series A (1960-1975) (open bars) and Series B (1976-
1983) (cross hatched bars), demonstrating significantly prolonged
survival in the latter series. Numbers at the top of each column
represent the percent survival at that time interval.

Evaluation included the measurable clinical parameters (congestive
heart failure, nephrotic syndrome, hepatomegaly, splenomegaly and macroglossia) and laboratory tests (e.g., renal, pulmonary and liver function
studies). Note was made of all treatment that the patients had been given,
especially whether they had ever, even for short periods, been on immunosup-
pressive treatment.

RESULTS

There were 45 patients with primary (AL) amyloidosis (series A) from
1961-1975 and 75 patients (series B) from 1976-1983. The mean age was 55
in series A and 59 in series B and 56% were men in both. The mean serum
creatinine at the time of diagnosis and the mean 24 h urine protein showed
no significant differences between the groups. Postural hypotension was
present in 7% in series A and 11% of series B, while congestive heart failure was increased in series A compared to B (28% compared to 11%).

At the end of 72 months all 45 patients in the earlier group had died,
while in the more recent series 53 (71%) had died. The precise time of survival in each series showed in the first 45 cases a rapidly decreasing cumulative chance of surviving with the passage of time. Thus at the end of 6
months the survival was 60%, 9 months 42%, 12 months 29%, and 19 months 16%.
The survival rate at the end of 24 months was down to 7%, 30 months 4% and
2% at 3, 4, and 5 years (Fig. 1).

TABLE 2. Causes of Death in Patients with Primary Amyloidosis

Cause of Death	CONTROL (N = 45)		TREATED (N = 53)		Total
	Post (N = 26)	No Post (N = 19)	Post (N = 21)	No Post (N = 32)	
Cardiac Disorder	10	8	9	15	43
Sudden death	6	6	2	10	
Cong. heart failure	3	2	7	5	
Myocardial infart	1	0	0	0	
Renal Filure	9	2	6	9	26
Liver Failure	1	1	2	2	6
Pulmonary Disorder	2	3	2	2	9
Pulmonary Embolism	0	1	0	0	
Pneumonia	2	2	1	2	
Aspiration	0	0	1	0	
Cerebrovascular Accident	0	0	0	1	1
G. I. Hemorrhage	1	0	0	0	2
Fat Embolus	0	0	1	0	1
Unknown	3	5	0	3	11

Meanwhile at the end of 6 months, the survival was 84% in the 75 patients treated with colchicine, 9 months 75%, 12 months 68% and 18 months 55%. At the end of 12 months, survival was 46%, 24 months 43%, 36 months 41% while the 5 year survival rate was 28% (Fig. 1).

The number of months of survival from the time of diagnosis to death was 10 months for series A and 22 months for the patients followed since 1976 (series B).

The major cause of 'death was cardiac in both groups accounting for 40% in series A and 45% of the later series. Deaths due to renal disease were 24% and 28% respectively, while liver deaths were 4% and 8%, pulmonary 11% and 8% while gastrointestinal bleeding caused 1 death in each series. The precise cause of death could not be determined or was not available to us in 8 (18% of the early and in 3 (6%) of the recent series. The causes of death were comparable whether or not an autopsy was performed (Table 2).

When the cardiac deaths were analyzed, sudden death was found to be responsible for 12 cases in each series, i.e., 27% of total deaths before 1975 and 23% of those after 1976, while intractable congestive heart failure was the cause in 11% of the earlier and 23% of the recent cases, and acute myocardial infarction identified as the cause in only 1 case (in the early series) (Table 2).

In a similar fashion the cause of death was analyzed to determine whether the 2 groups of patients showed any significant differences in the causes of death (cardiac, renal, liver, or pulmonary). None were found, nor were there any differences in outcomes if the patients were on immunosuppresives.

DISCUSSION

The evaluation of the treatment of a chronic disease whose natural history is not well defined poses great problems. Clearly a prospective double blind study with randomized controls should be carried out whenever possible. The use of historical controls is controversial and filled with the possibility of error. It has, however, been pointed out that they are most feasible when the number of patients generally available for study is small and when a reliable historical data base is available from the same institutes [8, 9, 10, 11].

In the present study, the historical controls and the prospective series were followed by the same group of physicians in the same fashion whenever possible. Deficiencies include the possibility of selection by referring physicians in the type of cases sent to us before and after 1976, i.e., if a new treatment is being assessed it is possible that earlier and less severe cases are being referred. Another potential problem, is the possibility that as our knowledge of amyloidosis improves, simple supportive treatment and knowledge about medications causing adverse reactions could be more extensive and favorably affect outcome in this series regardless of the added treatment.

We have previously presented preliminary results that colchicine appears to have a favorable influence on the outcome in primary (AL) amyloidosis [12, 13]. The present study completes this analysis over a longer period of time with a larger number of patients. In this study the life survival of 45 patients seen prior to 1975, 75 followed since 1976 and treated with colchicine, has been assessed. Insofar as could be determined there were no significant clinical or laboratory differences between these groups at the time of diagnosis or entry into the evaluation but for the

TABLE 3. Primary (AL) Amyloidosis Cause of Death

	Boston (1983)	Rochester (1975)	Rochester (1983)	Buffalo (1981)
	98 cases	105 cases	142 cases	20 cases
Cardiac	43%	34%	40%	50%
Renal	27%	16%	11%	35%
Liver	6%	0	0	0
Pulmonary	9%	0	0	0
Gastrointestinal	2%	0	0	10%
Cerebrovascular	1%	5%	3%	0
Infection	0	8%	4%	0
Misc. or unknown	12%	37%*	48%†	5%

*26% were due to "amyloidosis".
†28% were due to "amyloidosis".

higher incidence of congestive heart failure in series A. The number of
months of survival from the time of diagnosis to death averaged 10 in series
A while it was 22 months in series B. This difference is significant at the
P-0012 level. At each time interval (Fig. 1) there was a greater chance of
survival in series B. Several additional statistical analyses evaluated
outcomes in patients with and without congestive heart failure and found
that the aforementioned outcome was unaffected [19].

These results can be compared with the reported survival in several
other modern series. In the Rochester 1960-1972 series of 193 patients [7]
median survival after histologic diagnosis of AL amyloid (nonmeyloma) was
14.7 months. The median survival in their 1970-1980 series of 182 non-
myeloma AL amyloid patients was 13 months [14]. In a differently selected
series (of patients who were autopsied) a mean survival of 24 months (range
4-132 months) was reported in 20 patients from Buffalo [15]. The mean survival in several other smaller series of cases of primary (AL) amyloid has
been 13 months [16], under 12 months [17, 18].

The majority of the patients (over 40%) in both series A and B died of
cardiovascular disease. The second leading cause of death was renal disease (in over 20% of the patitents) while under 10% died of liver or pulmonary disease and 1 or 2 patients of gastrointestinal hemorrage or cerebrovascular disease. These figures are not dissimilar from those reported from
other centers in recent years (Table 3) [7, 14, 15].

Other detailed analyses of the causes of death, of the potential ex-
planations of the varying longevity in series A and B, and of the analytic
methodology are available [19].

SUMMARY

A series of 45 patients with primary (AL) amyloid served as a historical control for 75 similar individuals treated prospectively with colchicine
since 1976. The mean duration of life was significantly longer in the latter series (22 months versus 10 months). The causes of deaths were analyzed in the 45 patients in the first series who succumbed to the disease
and the 53 (of 75) patients in the second series. The major cause of death
was cardiovascular followed by renal disease.

REFERENCES

1. A. S. Cohen, New Engl. J. Med., 277:522, 574, 628 (1967).
2. R. A. Kyle and E. D. Baird, Medicine, 54:271 (1975).
3. I. Kedar, et al., Israel J. Med. Sci., 10:787 (1974).
4. T. Shirahama and A. S. Cohen, J. Exp. Med., 140:1102 (1974).
5. D. Zemer, et al., in: Amyloid and Amyloidosis (G. G. Glenner, P. Costa, and F. Freitas, eds.), Excerpta Medica, pp. 584-586 (1980).
6. D. Zemer et al., New Engl. J. Med., 294:170 (1976).
7. R. A. Kyle and E. D. Baird, Mayo Clin. Proc., 54:271 (1975).
8. E. A. Gehan, Cancer Treatment Reports, 66:1089 (1982).
9. H. Sacks et al., Amer. J. Med., 72:233 (1982).
10. L. E. Moses, New Engl. J. Med., 311:705 (1984).
11. E. A. Gehan and E. J. Freireich, New Engl. J. Med., 290:198 (1974).
12. A. S. Cohen et al., Revue de rhumatisme, XVth International Congress of Rheumatology, June 1981, p. 1171.
13. A. Rubinow et al., Arthritis Rheum., 24:S124 (1981).
14. R. A. Kyle and P. R. Greipp, Mayo Clin. Proc., 58:665 (1983).
15. J. R. Wright and E. Calkins, Medicine, 60:429 (1981).
16. W. F. Barth et al., Amer. J. Med., 47:259 (1969).
17. K. Brandt et al., Amer. J. Med., 44:955 (1968).
18. A. I. Pick et al., Acta Hematol., 66:154 (1981).
19. A. S. Cohen et al., Submitted for publication.

THE IMPACT OF COLCHICINE ON THE AMYLOIDOSIS

OF FAMILIAL MEDITERRANEAN FEVER (FMF)

D. Zemer, E. Sohar,
M. Pras, S. Cabili,
and J. Gafni

Heller Institute for Medical Research
Sheha Medical Center at Tel-Hashomer
and Sackler School of Medicine
Tel-Aviv University
Israel

ABSTRACT

Since Goldfinger's observation in 1972 that daily administration of colchicine may prevent the attacks of familial Mediterranean fever [1], the drug has
become the mainstay of therapy and is recommended to all of our many afflicted.
On a dose of 102 mg/day, 95% of patients experience complete remission or marked
amelioration of their attacks. The remainder do not respond to even higher doses.
Children as a rule respond only to full adult dosage. Side-effects are uncommon
and usually mild but have occasionally required and always responded to desensi-
tization, permitting continuation of the drug. Non-compliance is promptly pun-
ished by renewal of attacks.

INTRODUCTION

In reporting our controlled trial of colchicine we emphasized that "although
their dramatic nature has justifiably made the fibril attacks the clinical hallmark of FMF, it is the insidious development of amyloidosis that causes death,
usually before the age of 40. Since attacks and amyloidosis are independent
phenotypic characters of a pleiotropic gene, it does not follow that an agent
effective in preventing attacks will a priori prevent amyloidosis. One can
cite, cautiously but with hope, that colchicine seems to protect mice from casein-
induced amyloidosis -" (2-4) today, ten years later, we are able to present an over-
view of the amyloidosis of FMF as it appears in the colchicine ERA.

MATERIAL AND METHODS

Since the impact of colchicine was not expected to become apparent
overnight, this survey is based on those 1070 patients who were advised to
begin colchicine from 1973 through 1980, providing a follow-up of at least
4 years and as long as 11. The patients are seen on an ambulatory basis
as a rule at intervals varying from 3 months to 1 year. At each visit, the
urine is examined; when protein is found a 24-h specimen obtained for quantitation of proteinuria and the serum creatinine determined. At each visit
compliance is confirmed by careful questioning and the importance of adhering to the daily prophylactic schedule emphasized.

TABLE 1.   109 Compliant Patients with Renal Disease when Colchicine Started

Stage	No. of pts.	Course		
		Improved	Stable	Deterior.
Proteinuria	85	5	68	12 (9ES*)
Nephorosis	9	–	–	9 (5ES)
Uremia	15	–	–	15 (14ES)

*ES) End–stage renal disease requiring life support by hemodialysis or kidney transplantation.

TABLE 2.   85 Patients in Proteinuric Stage when Colchicine Started

Treat- ment, years	Course		
	Improved No. pts.	Stable No. pts.	Deterior. No. pts.
4		8	
5		10	1
6		5	1
7		5	1
8	1	6	1
9		16	5
10	2	17	3
11	2	1	
	5	68	12

TABLE 3.   Patients Who Developed Proteinuria under Colchicine

Col- chi- cine Age	Pro- tein uria Age	Ethnic origin	Other fea- tures	Rectal biopsy
61	63	Ashk		
49	55	Ashk	DM	neg
45	51	Seph	DM, MI	neg
6	13	Seph	Hen–Sch	

*Abbreviations: DM) Diabetes Mellitus; MI) Myocardial Infarction; Hen-Sch) Henoch-Shoenlein purpura; Ashk) Ashkenazi; Seph) Sepharidi.

Of the 1070 patients, 110 started colchicine when overt renal disease was present. Fifteen evidenced renal insufficiency (serum creatinine $\gtrless$ 1.5 mg/day); 9 were nephrotic (proteinuria $\gtrless$ 3.5 gm/24 h and normal serum creatine): 86 had persistent proteinuria < 3.5 mg/24 h. One of the latter was a non-compliant patient who is now on hemodialysis. Nine hundred and sixty patients had no proteinuria or other evidence of renal disease when

TABLE 4. 960 Patients Without Renal Disease-Colchicine Compliance and
Appearance of Proteinuria

	No. of pts.	Developed proteinuria	
		No.	%
Compliant	906	4	0.44
Non-compliant	54	16	29.6

advised to begin colchicine. Of these non-proteinuria patients, 54 were
admittedly non-compliant. Non compliance was most commonly due to misin-
formation provided by family physicians skeptical of colchicine's efficacy
and reticent regarding its prolonged administration in a young patient population. These 54 non-compliant patient provide an unplanned concurrent control group.

RESULTS

Fourteen of the 15 uremics and 5 of the 9 nephrotics have progressed
to end-stage disease requiring dialysis and or transplantation, and the remainder are in advanced renal failure (Table 1). There is no indication
that the duration of either of these stages has been prolonged by colchicine.

Of the 85 compliant patients in the proteinuric stage of amyloid nephropathy when colichicine was started, 12 have progressed to nephrosis of renal
failure and 5 have improved. The bulk of 68 patients remains stable. Evaluation of this group depends upon knowledge of the duration of the proteinuric stage, appreciating that its onset and termination are often dated from
a fortuitous urine examination that the amount of protein in the urine often
fluctuates and that progression to nephrosis may be almost explosively rapid
or take years. The duration of proteinuria until deterioration to nephrosis
in a series of FMF patients observed before the introduction of colchicine
ranged from 2-9 years, usually 3-5 [5]. The fact that 40 of the 68 patients
who remain stable under colchicine are 8 or more years after the initiation
of therapy - and certainly longer after the onset of proteinuria - strongly
suggests that the proteinuric stage of the disease has been prolonged (Table
2). That this stage may be reversible is indicated by the five patients,
three with positive rectal biopsies, who improved. In all 5, proteinuria
gradually subsided over 1-6 years after colchicine was begun and their urines
remain protein-free since.

Of the 906 compliant patients who had no overt renal disease when starting colchicine, the urine of 902 remains protein-free after 4-11 years of
follow-up. In 4, all of whom enjoy complete remission from attacks, proteinuria has appeared after 2-7 years of treatment. Looking at these patients reveals, that they are not a representative sample of our total patient population (Table 3). Three are older; two of these are of Ashkenazi
extraction (who rarely have FMF and rarely develop amyloidosis) and two have
non-insulin dependent diabetes mellitus (which can also cause proteinuria)
and negative rectal biopsies. In the most representative patient, proteinuria was documented at age 13, three years after a bout of Henoch-Schoenlein.
Accepting proteinuria in all 4 as due to amyloidosis, this is an incompar-
ably better outlook than our pre-colchicine experience.

That this is a lilly in no need of gilding is highlighted dramatically by
the fact of the 54 non-proteinuric patients who formed the unplanned con-

current control group (Table 4). Proteinuria has appeared in 16 of the 54 and advanced to nephrotic proportions in 2. The 16 patients constitute 29.6% of this actively followed-up population sample. This figure is almost exactly that found in a pre-colchicine study of 316 actively followed-up living FMF patients that revealed a 27% prevalence of amyloidosis. The implication is that the administration of colchicine has prevented amyloidosis and overt renal disease in more than 250 of our compliant patients.

COMMENTS

These results are a confirmation in man of the laboratory murine model and indicate that colchicine, by mechanism's not yet known, somehow blocks the formation of AA-amyloid and prevents the development of amyloidosis. This is most clearly brought out by the virtual failure of new cases of amyloidosis to appear in our long-term follow up of over 900 high-risk FMF patients on the drug.

When amyloidosis is clinically manifest, there is a point from which colchicine can provide no return, deterioration of organ function continuing due to amyloid already present. In the kidney, this point has apparently been reached when proteinuria assumes nephrotic proportions, at least in the AA-amyloidosis of FMF with proteinuria of a lesser degree, colchicine seems to prevent deterioration in most cases and makes possible resolution in some.

Since blockage of amyloid formation and accumulation has become the aim of treatment, we recommend colchicine for all FMF patients, even those whose attacks do not respond. Keeping in mind that FMF-amyloidosis is systemic and that renal death can be circumvented, colchicine is administered during all the stages of overt renal disease in order to prevent damage to other organ systems and after renal transplantation, also to prevent involvement of the graft.

REFERENCES

1. Goldfinger, S. E., New Engl. J. Med., 287:1302 (1972).
2. Zemer, D., et al., New Engl. J. Med., 291:932 (1974).
3. Kedar, I., et al., Israel J. Med. Sci., 10:787 (1974).
4. Shirahama, T., and Cohen, A. S., J. Exp. Med., 140:1102 _1974).
5. Sohar, E., et al., Amer. J. Med., 43:227 (1967).
6. Jacob, E. T., et al., Transplantation Proc., 14:41 (1982).

TREATMENT OF SYSTEMIC AA AMYLOIDOSIS

M. H. van Rijswijk, M. A. van Leeuwen,
A. J. M. Donker, and E. Mandema

Department of Medicine
University Hospital Groningen
59 Oostersingle
9713 EX Groningen, The Netherlands

ABSTRACT

The bearing of recent developments in amyloid research on the treatment of amyloidosis is more and more approaching the stage of clinical importance. Illustrated by the data of follow-up studies in systemic AA amyloidosis the following aspects will be discussed.

1. The precursor-product relationship between SAA and AA amyloidosis, and the use of acute-phase reactants for the monitoring of the effect and the adjustment of the dosage of drug treatment.

2. The mechanisms of action of dimethylsulfoxide (DMSO) in the treatment of AA amyloidosis.

3. The recent advances in the maintenance of reduced renal function by adjustment of the dietary protein and phosphate load and its consequences for the interpretation of the course and the prognosis of renal amyloidosis.

INTRODUCTION

Amyloidosis is a disease characterized by organ function disturbances, cuased by the extracellular deposition of amyloid fibrils. The pathogenic effect of amyloid fibril deposition depends on the localization of amyloid, its insolubility under physiologic conditions, its resistance to proteolytic digestion, and probably on its high calcium content by which amyloid fibrils may act like calcium ionophores during phagocytosis.

Differences in the clinical manifestations of amyloid disease appear to be related to differences in the primary structure of amyloid fibril proteins. A summary of the clinico-pathological correlations is shown in Table 1. In most types of amyloidosis distinct precursor proteins have been identified. The way by which such precursor proteins may be or become amyloidogenic obviously comprises different mechanisms, like, e.g., amino acid substitution, incomplete degradation, or oxidative denaturation of the precursor protein. Awaiting the development of methods for selective intervention in, e.g., degradation or denaturation processes _in vivo_, a rational

TABLE 1. Clinico-Pathological Correlations in Amyloidosis

| | Clinical pattern of organ dysfunction | |
	"Typical" distribution nephropathy	"Atypical" distribution nephropathy cardiomyopathy glossopathy neuropathy arthropathy myopathy
ASSOCIATED	Systemic amyloidosis associated with inflammatory diseases.................AA	Systemic amyloidosis associated with multiple myeloma....................AL
IDIOPATHIC	Idiopathic systemic amyloidosis with "typical" distribution..............AA	Idiopathic systemic amyloidosis with "atypical" distribution.............AL
FAMILIAL	Familial systemic amyloidosis associated with – familial Mediterranean fever............AA – urticaria, deafness, and nephropathy.........................AA – fibril attacks and nephropathy	Familial neuropathic amyloidosis........PREALBUMIN Familial cardiopathic amyloidosis Familial amyloidosis with corenal lattice dystrophy and cranial neuropathy
LOCALIZED	Amyloid tumors.....................AL Endocrine tissue related amyloid........PROHORMONE Cutaneous amyloidosis Senile cardiac amyloid...............PREALBUMIN Senile cerebral amyloid	

therapeutic approach would be to reduce the amount of precursor protein. An example of such an approach is, e.g., the steroid and/or cytostatic treatment in myeloma-associated AL amyloidosis in order to reduce the production of the amyloidogenic monoclonal immunoglobulin light chain.

In systemic AA amyloidosis associated with chronic inflammatory disease the precursor protein is an acute-phase reactant, designated SAA. Although it is apparent, that longstanding elevation of SAA levels is a prerequisite for the development of AA amyloidosis [1-4], it seems likely, that an additional predisposing factor must be present to cause the conversion of SAA into AA amyloid fibrils. Such a concept is based on the fact, that only a small percentage of patients with longstanding elevation of SAA levels will develop AA amyloidosis [2]. The question, whether such an amyloid-prone constitution relies on intrinsic precursor abnormalities or on a defective degrading system awaits further elucidation. The approach of reducing the amount of precursor protein has been shown to be particularly useful in the treatment of systemic AA amyloidosis [1-4]. Like we have reported before highly elevated SAA levels are associated with progressive AA amyloidosis, whereas lowering of the SAA levels by anti-inflammatory treatment resulted in a stop of the progression of AA amyloidosis. Such a relationship of SAA levels with the progression of amyloidosis could not be demonstrated for other types of amyloidosis like, e.g., systemic AL amyloidosis [3, 4]. In addition we described the close correlation of SAA and C-reactive protein (CRP) levels with disease activity in chronic inflammatory disorders, both in transverse and longitudinal studies.

Reports indicating, that dimethylsulfoxide (DMSO) could be therapeutically useful by making amyloid soluble [5-8], prompted us to investigate its value in the treatment of systemic AA and AL amyloidosis. Although we did not find any evidence, that DMSO could make amyloid soluble in vivo, it did appear to be effective in the treatment of systemic AA amyloidosis, probably by virtue of its distinct anti-inflammatory action [1-4, 9, 10]. The results of DMSO treatment in systemic AL amyloidosis were inconclusive.

The present paper comprises additional data on the treatment of systemic AA amyloidosis, and a discussion on the mechanism of action of DMSO. An issue that came to our attention during the long-term follow-up of our patients with systemic AA amyloidosis, was the fact that some of them showed a progression to renal failure, despite a significant reduction of SAA and CRP levels. This problem is discussed in view of the recent appreciation of the mechanisms responsible for further progression to renal failure in case of a once developed significant loss of nephrons, even if the causal factor is removed.

PATIENTS AND METHODS

The patients were classified clinically according to Table 1. The associated inflammatory diseases comprised rheumatoid arthritis (6 cases) and Crohn's disease (1 case). In all patients amyloidosis was established by both rectal and renal biopsy. Tissue specimens were stained with Congo red and examined with polarized light for green birefringence. Histochemical and immunohistochemical differentiation was performed by the potassium permanganate method [11] and by immunoperoxidase staining with anti-AA and anti-AP antibodies. Glomerular filtration rate (GFR) and effective renal plasma flow (ERPF) were measured with radioisotopes according to the method described by Donker [12]. Renal tubular function was calculated as the relative clearance of radio-labeled dimercapto-succinic acid (DMSA ratio) according to the method described by Van Luyck [13]. SAA levels were measured according to the method described by Van Rijswijk [2] and Limburg [3]. CRP levels were measured by rate nephelometry (Immunochemistry System,

Beckman). SAP measurements were kindly performed by Dr. M. B. Pepys
(Hammersmith Hospital, London). DMSO was obtained from E. Merk (Darmstadt,
Germany), product No. 2931, and prescribed in the following way: for oral
administration: DMSO 200 grams, distilled water ad 1000 ml, 3 times daily
25 ml; for intravenous administration: DMSO 100 grams, physiologic saline
or glucose ad 1000 ml, 3 times daily 50 ml. Low protein diet (LPD) consisted of 40 grams of protein, with supply of methionine and a multivitamin
preparation, and administration of a phosphate-binder during meals.

RESULTS

    Detailed data of patients IN 11741, IN 36860, IN 26538, and IN A13152
have been reported before [4]. Of particular interest is the follow-up of
patient IN A13152, a woman born in 1951, suffering from severe rheumatoid
arthritis since 1974, treated with gold until proteinuria developed in 1975.
A renal biopsy at that time disclosed membranous glomerulopathy without
evidence of amyloidosis. Renal function was normal and the proteinuria
gradually subsided after discontinuation of gold. In March 1978 she was
hospitalized because of persistently active rheumatoid arthritis, a declining creatinine clearance, proteinuria, and hepatomegaly. Both renal
and liver biopsy revealed extensive deposition of AA amyloid. Treatment
with DMSO was instituted and continued until February 1980. During this
period there was a gradual recovery of renal function and a disappearance
of the proteinuria. Treatment was changed to a combination of prednisolone
and azathioprine. Despite a satisfactory effect on disease activity and an
adequate reduction of SAA and CRP levels, renal function gradually deteriorated from a GFR of 50 ml/min to 13 ml/min (May 1982). Renal biopsy revealed an extensive glomerulosclerosis, whereas the amount of amyloid had
decreased with 50%. This patient was then accepted for primary renal transplantation, which could be realized in December 1982. Since that time she
is in an excellent clinical condition with a stable function of the renal
graft. It should be noticed, that till the moment of transplantation, this
patient had used a protein-enriched diet (instituted at the time of proteinuria).

Patient IN 95403, Male Born 1921 (Fig. 1)

    Seropositive rheumatoid arthritis since 1972, treated with chloroquine
diphosphate and d-penicillamine. The latter drug was discontinued in 1975
because of proteinuria. Recurrent gastric and doudenal ulcers led to a
partial gastrectomy (Billroth II) in 1978. In 1979 he developed a nephrotic
syndrome with selective proteinuria (selectivity index: 11%). Both rectal
and renal biopsy revealed the deposition of AA amyloid. In June 1979 DMSO
treatment was started. Recurrent periods with nausea and vomiting interfered with the regular use of DMSO. In March 1980 DMSO was replaced by
prednisolone (3 × 2 mg/day), which resulted in a satisfactory decrease of
SAA and CRP levels. After an initial period without any particular problems, the patient started again complaining about his stomach. Gastroscopy
revealed anastomositis and bile reflux. Attempts to relieve his symptoms
by dietary adjustments and the prescription of metoclopramide were not successful. At the end of 1980 he started to use prednisolone irregularly and
ultimately decided to reduce the prenisolone dosage to 2 mg/day at his own
responsibility (March 1981). From that moment on his renal function gradually deteriorated from a creatinine clearance of 83 ml/min to 18 ml/min
(December 1982). In January 1983 he was admitted with peritonitis by per-
foration of the sigmoid due to diverticulosis (in our series this is the
second case of such a complication in AA amyloidosis). Surgical intervention was complicated by renal and respiratory failure and the patient succumbed. Our request for autopsy was not granted.

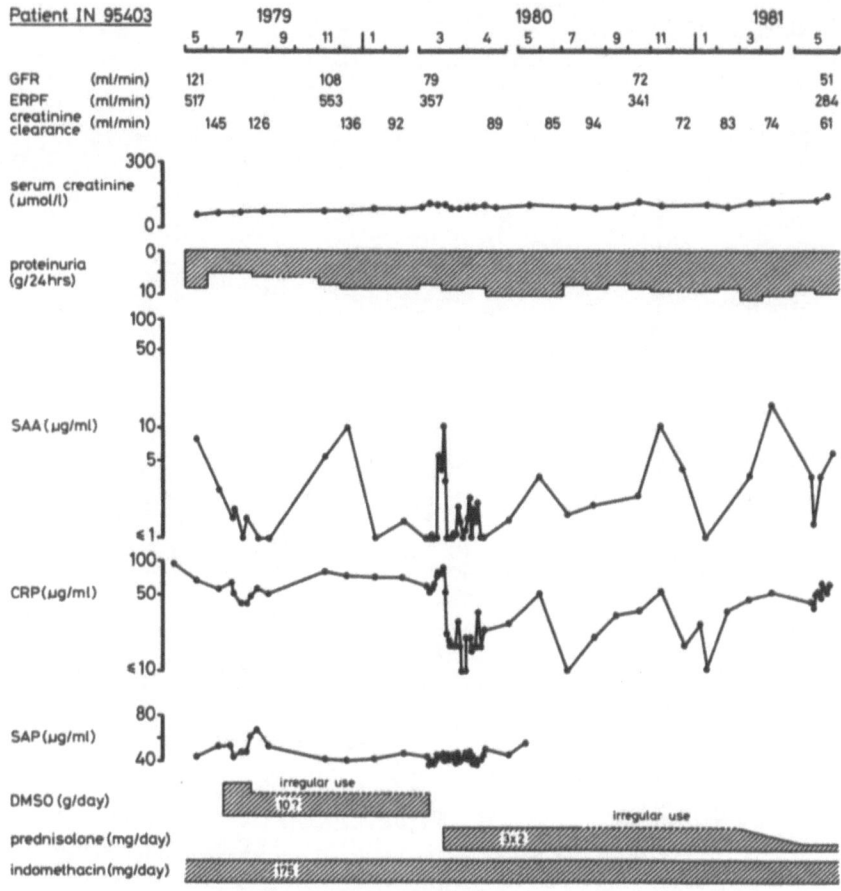

Fig. 1.   Schematic representation of the longitudinal data on
patient IN 95403 (for comments see text).

Patient IN A40533, Male, Born 1942 (Fig. 2)

Seropositive rheumatoid arthritis since 1970, treated with chloroquine diphosphate, gold and d-penicillamine without any effect.   Consequent treatment with prednisolone was discontinued in September 1979.   At
the same time d-penicillamine was discontinued because of proteinuria.   In
December 1979 a total hip arthroplasty was performed without any particular
probelm.   Because of persistent proteinuria, a renal biopsy was performed,
which revealed AA amyloid deposition and treatment was instituted with
prednisolone (7.5 mg divided over 2 gifts/day).   After an initial satisfactory response, SAA and CRP levels started to increase again during a
flare-up of the rheumatoid arthritis.   The prednisolone dosage was adjusted
(4 × 2 mg/day) and azathioprine was added (150 mg/day).   Until now renal
function has been stable and proteinuria has gradually disappeared.   In 1983
this patient has been instituted on a low protein diet.   A repeated renal
biopsy did not reveal amyloid deposits (1984).   The course of the SAP levels
is inconclusive.

Patient IN 92285, Male, Born 1945 (Fig. 3)

Seropositive rheumatoid arthritis since 1966, treated with chloroquine
diphosphate and since 1972 with varying amounts of prednisolone.   In 1977 a

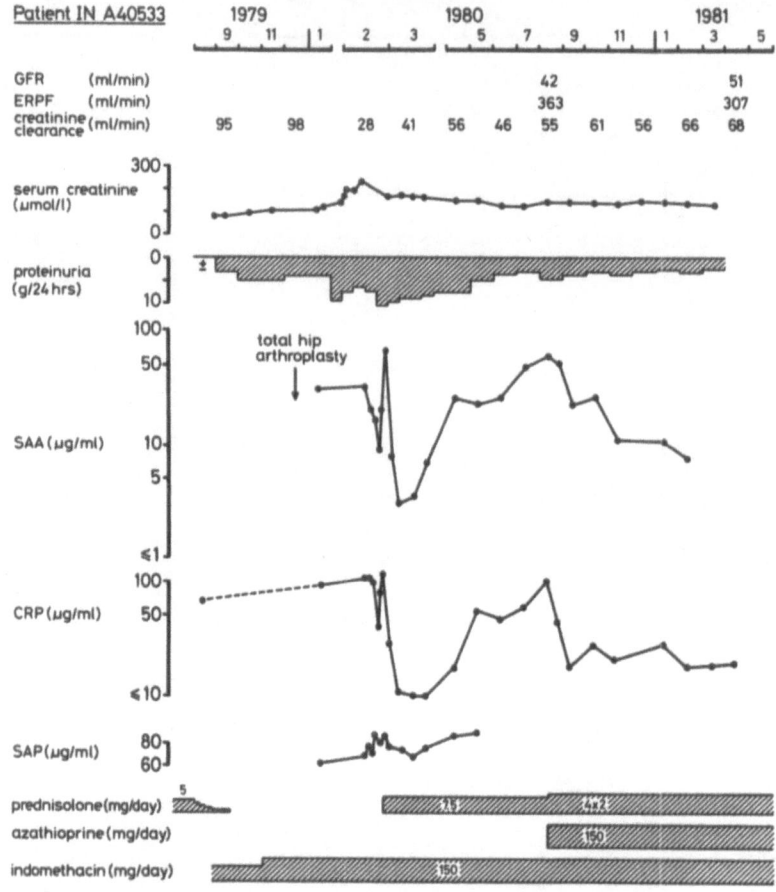

Fig. 2. Schematic representation of the longitudinal data on patient IN A40533 (for comments see text).

decline of renal function was noted without proteinuria. A rectal biopsy at that time revealed AA amyloid deposition. The patient was unwilling to undergo further diagnostic or therapeutic measures, until April 1979 when he agreed to be hospitalized for renal biopsy and adjustment of treatment. At that time GFR had decreased to 27 ml/min and although we advised him to increase his prednisolone dosage he hestiated to do so until August 1979, when he was confronted with a further decline of his renal function. From that moment on his renal function has remained stable. In 1983 he was in-situted on a low protein diet. The course of the SAP levels is inconclusive.

Patient IN 92190, Female, Born 1923 (Fig. 4)

Seropositive rheumatoid arthritis since 1957, treated with chloroquine diphosphate, gold and d-penicillamine. The latter drug was discontinued because of proteinuria. In view of the declining renal function and the persistent proteinuria a renal biopsy was performedin April 1981, which revealed AA amyloid deposition. Treatment with prednisolone was instituted (4 × 2 mg/day) resulting in a satisfactory decrease of CRP levels and a stabilization of renal function. In 1983 this patient was instituted on a low protein diet.

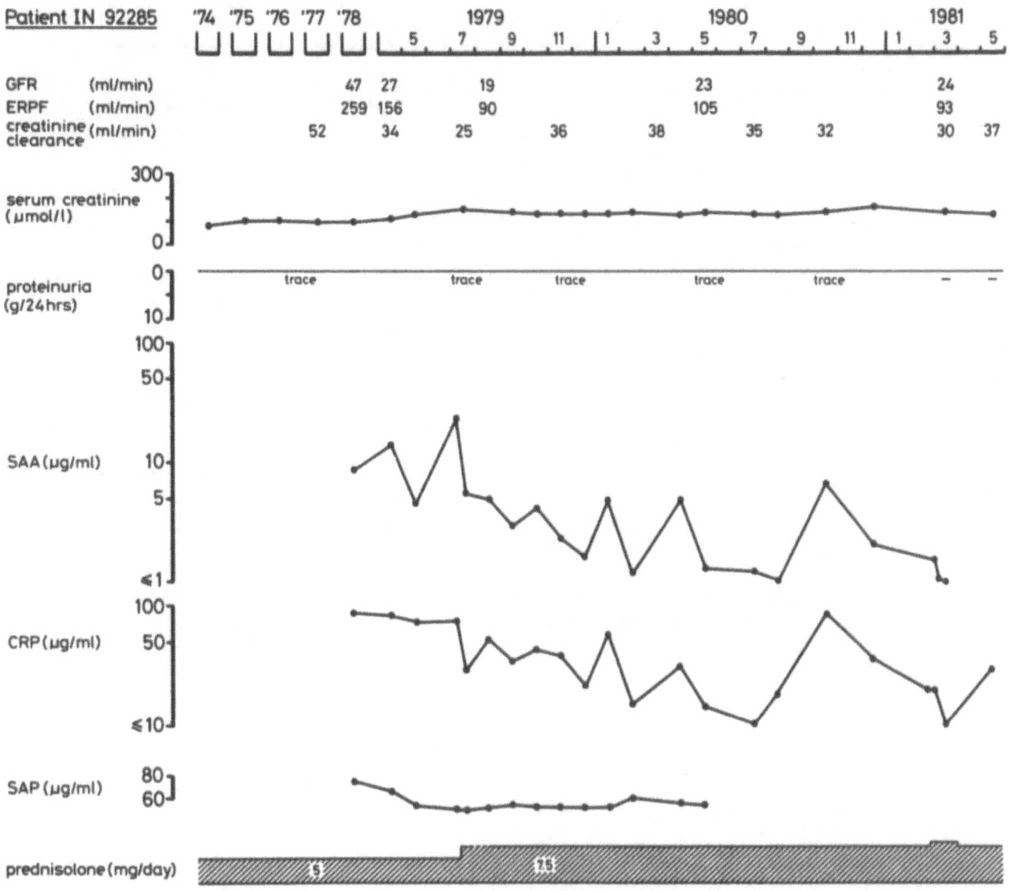

Fig. 3. Schematic representation of the longitudinal data on patient
IN 92285 (for comments see text).

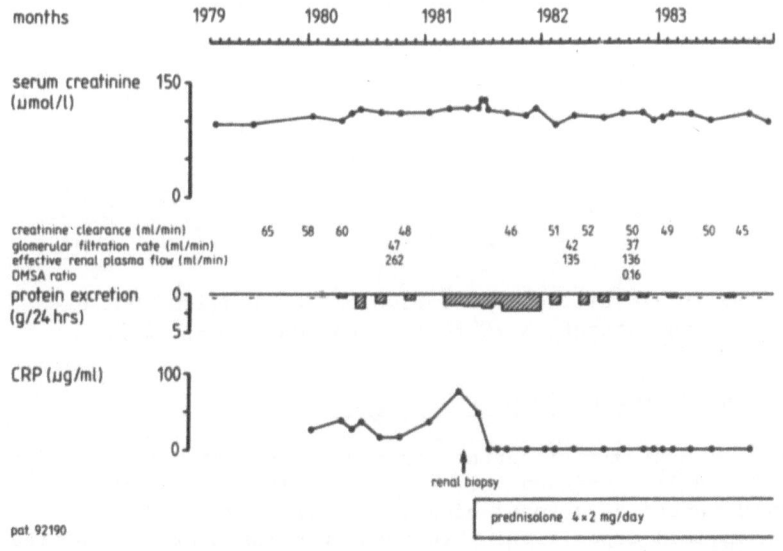

Fig. 4. Schematic representation of the longitudinal data
on patient IN 92190 (for comments see text).

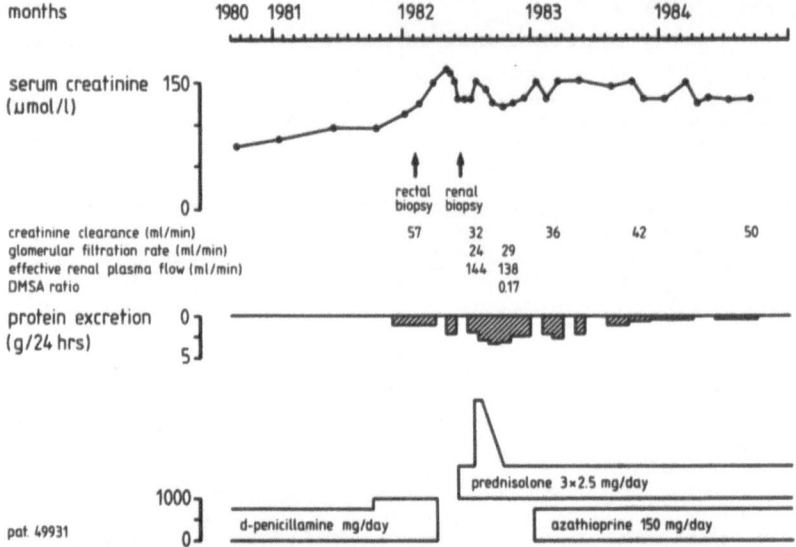

Fig. 5. Schematic representation of the longitudinal data
         on patient IN 49931 (for comments see text).

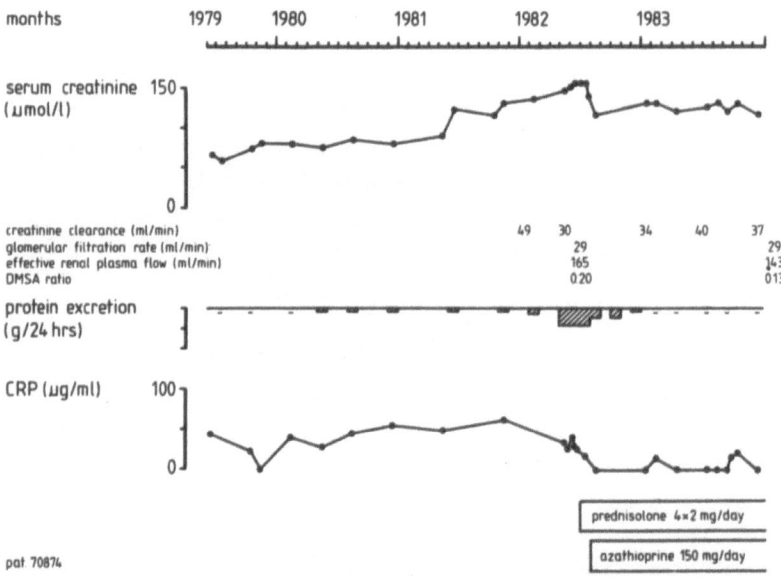

Fig. 6. Schematic representation of the longitudinal data
         on patient IN 70874 (for comments see text).

Patient IN 49931, Female, Born 1913 (Fig. 5)

Seropositive rheumatoid arthritis since 1965, treated with d-penicillamine, which was discontinued because of proteinuria. In view of the declining renal function, a renal biopsy was performed in June 1982, which
revealed AA amyloid deposition. Treatment was instituted with prednisolone
(3 × 2.5 mg/day) and azathioprine (150 mg/day), resulting in a satisfactory
decrease of CRP levels, a stabilization of renal function, and a gradual

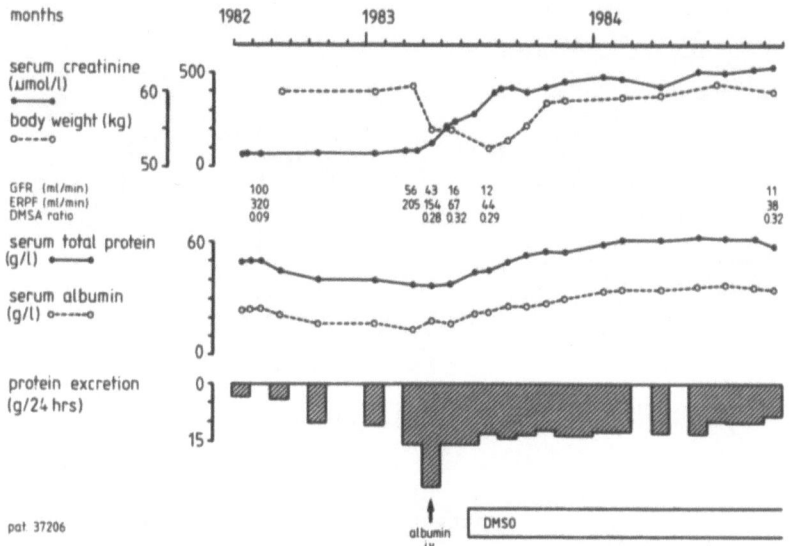

months   1982   1983   1984

serum creatinine (µmol/l) 500
body weight (kg) 60
50

GFR (ml/min)   100   56 43 16   12   11
ERPF (ml/min)   320   205 154 67   44   38
DMSA ratio   009   028 032 029   032

serum total protein (g/l)   60
serum albumin (g/l) 0

protein excretion (g/24 hrs) 0 / 15

pat. 37206   albumin i.v.   DMSO

Fig. 7. Schematic representation of the longitudinal data on patient IN A37206 (for comments see text).

decrease of proteinuria. Note the temporarily increase of serum creatinine levels, due to a short course of high-dose prednisolone treatment, necessary because of intercurrent pulmonary infection.

Patient IN 70874, Female, Born 1924 (Fig. 6)

Seropositive rheumatoid arthritis since 1975, treated with chloroquine diphosphate, gold, and d-penicillamine. The latter drug was discontinued because of declining renal function and the onset of proteinuria. A renal biopsy was performed in June 1982 and revealed AA amyloid deposition. Treatment was instituted with prednisolone (4 × 2 mg/day) and azathioprine (150 mg/day) and a protein restricted diet. Since then renal function has remained stable.

Patient IN A37206, Female, Born 1953 (Fig. 7)

Since 1965 recurrent episodes of diarrhea, in 1979 evolving into a clinically full-blown Crohn's disease, necessitating ileocoecal resection. The onset of proteinuria prompted the gastro-enterologist to perform a rectal biopsy, which revealed AA amyloid deposits. In view of the normal renal function and the clinically inactive bowel disease it was decided to keep her under observation without further treatment. A declining renal function, an increase of proteinuria, together with increasing activity of the bowel disease necessitated hospitalization in March 1983. A renal biopsy revealed AA amyloid deposition. Unfortunately it was decided to try to reduce proteinuria by indomethacin. This attempt necessitated the intravenous administration of albumin in order to restore the circulating volume. During this period renal function further deteriorated and in June 1983 it was decided to start treatment with DMSO (3 × 5 grams/day), and a protein restricted diet. Since that time renal function has remained stable, the activity of the bowel disease has gradually subsided, the patient has returned to an anabolic state and is by now in an excellent clinical condition. Note the increase in body weight and the rise in total serum protein and serum albumin concentration, despite persistent significant proteinuria.

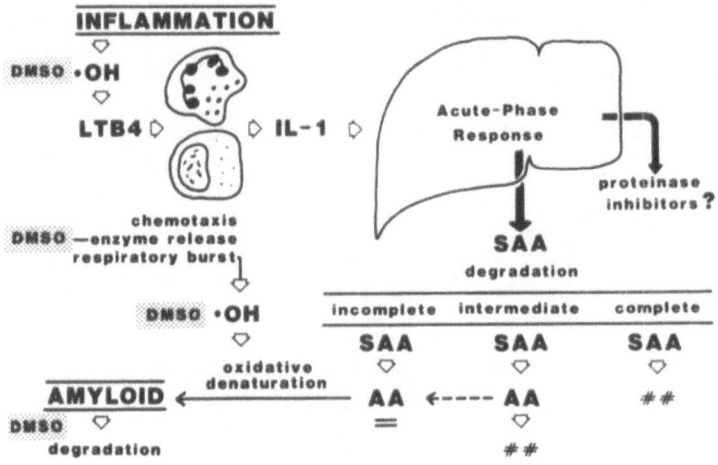

Fig. 8. Schematic representation of the possible
        mechanisms.

DISCUSSION

     The data presented are in accordance with our previously reported ob-
servations, that the reduction of disease activity as measured by the acute-
phase response is at the moment the most practical approach in the treatment
of systemic AA amyloidosis [1-4]. Monitoring of the acute-phase response by
serial measurements of SAA levels provides the means to achieve an optimal
effectiveness of treatment. As CRP and SAA display similar kinetics and a
comparable dynamic range, the monitoring of CRP levels seems to be a good
alternative for routine laboratory use [2, 4].

     DMSO has been shown to exert a distinct anti-inflammatory activity,
both clinically and biochemically. Its effect may rely on a combination of
mechanisms. First of all DMSO is hydroxyl radical scavenger [14]. As such
it may inhibit the release of arachidonic acid from membrane phospholipids,
which is the major initiating event in the synthesis of prostaglandines by
the cyclo-oxygenase pathway and the synthesis of leukotrienes by the lipoxygenase pathway. One of the major products of the lipoxygenase pathway is
leukotriene B4 (LTB4), which is a potent chemotactic substance and a secre-
tagogue [15]. As such it induces the accumulation of neutrophils and the
production of interleukin-1 (IL-1), which is responsible for the generation
of the acute-phase reaction (among which SAA synthesis). This may well account for the biochemical anti-inflammatory effects of DMSO, like reduction
of SAA and CRP levels and the return from a catabolic to an anabolic state,
as protein catabolism during inflammation has been shown to be an IL-1 and
prostagalandin E2 mediated process [16]. The clinical effectiveness, like
reported in rheumatoid arthritis [4], may be explained by the reduction of
both the direct and the IL-1 mediated prostaglandin synthesis in the inflamed joints.

     In addition DMSO has been shown to inhibit the release of neutrophil
granule constituents in a hydroxyl radical independent way [4], and to po-
tentiate the membrane-stabilizing action of other compounds, like cortisol
and chloroquine [17]. Another point that merits consideration is the potential of hydroxyl radicals to induce polymerization of polypeptides, a
common industrial principle in polymer biochemistry [18]. It is conceivable, that oxidative denaturation is of pathogenic importance in fibrillogenesis. As a hydroxyl radical scavenger DMSO would be able to inhibit

precursor oxidation and subsequent polymerization. With regard to the subject of amyloid degradation in vivo, it should be noticed, that in vitro experiments have indicated, that the solubilization of amyloid fibrils is facilitated by DMSO [4]. A major point in the consideration of possible actions of DMSO is the fact, that for this compound virtually no biological barriers exist. A schematic representation of these considerations is given in Fig. 8.

An alternative way of treatment, which is particularly useful in patients with AA amyloidosis associated with rheumatoid arthritis, appears to be prednisolone, alone or in combination with cytostatic drugs. Prednisolone will reduce the acute-phase response by its inhibitory action on phospholipase A2, resulting in a reduction of the LTB4 synthesis and the consequent decrease of IL-1 production. Empirically prednisolone appears to be most effective when administered in three doses, divided over the 24 h. The major disadvantages of prednisolone treatment are its well-known side-effects. Using serial SAA or CRP measurements it has been possible to titrate the optimal individual dosage (usually ranging between 6 and 8 mg/day), thus preventing overtreatment.

As renal disease is the major clinical manifestation of AA amyloidosis, special care must be taken to maintain the remaining renal function. As has been indicated by Mitch [19], in case of a once established loss of nephrons glomerulosclerosis will develop, resulting in a subsequent further progression to renal failure, even if the factor causing the initial loss of nephrons is removed. According to Brenner [20] this phenomenon is due to increased transcapillary ultrafiltration, leading to dysfunction of the glomerular basement membrane, increase of proteinuria, increase of protein reabsorption, increase of mesangial cells and matrix and the occurrence of epithelial cell adhesions. Except for a reduced number of nephrons, the following factors may also lead to increased glomerular pressure and flow: diabetes mellitus, severe anaemia, pregnancy, high dietary protein intake, and increased transmedullary pressure by efferent level of obstruction, afferent level dilation, or an elevated systemic diastolic blood pressure. It has been shown by Maschio [21] and Rosman [22] that protein restriction inhibits the development of glomeruloscerlosis. Preliminary results indicate that such renal function preserving measures also favorably alter the course of renal amyloidosis.

CONCLUSIONS

The treatment of systemic AA amyloidosis should consist of:

1. Reduction of inflammatory activity of the underlying disease with monitoring of SAA or CRP levels.

2. Reduction of the dietary protein intake and addition of phosphate-binder during meals.

3. Adequate control of blood pressure, preferably by efferent level vasodilation (e.g., angiotensin converting enzyme inhibitors).

4. Avoidance of intravenous albumin infusion (probably the use of indomethacin for the reduction of proteinuria is contra-indicated).

REFERENCES

1. M. H. van Rijswikj, C. W. G. J. van Heusden, and L. Ruinen, in: Amyloid and Amyloidosis (G. G. Glenner, P. P. Costa, and A. F. Freitas, eds.), Excerpta Medica, Amsterdam (1980), p. 25.
2. M. H. van Rujswijk, in: Amyloidosis (M. H. van Rijswijk, ed.), University Microfilms Intern., No. 82-70037 (1982).
3. P. C. Limburg, M. H. van Rijswijk, L. Ruinen, H. J. de Jong, J. Marrink, J. J. de Blécourt, and E. Mandema, in: Amyloidosis E.A.R.S. (C. R. Tribe and P. A. Bacon, eds.), J. Wright and Sons, Bristol (1983), p. 108.
4. M. H. van Rijswijk, L. Ruinen, A. J. M. Donker, J. J. de Blécourt, and E. Mandema, Ann. N.Y. Acad. Sci., 411:67 (1983).
5. T. Isobe and E. F. Osserman, in: Amyloid and Amyloidosis (G. G. Glenner, P. P. Costa, and A. F. Freitas, eds.), Excerpta Medica, Amsterdam (1980), p. 247.
6. E. F. Osserman, T. Isobe, and M. Farhangi, in: Amyloid and Amyloidosis (G. G. Glenner, P. P. Costa, and A. F. Freitas, eds.), Excerpta Medica, Amsterdam (1980), p. 553.
7. I. Kedar, M. Greenwald, and M. Ravid, Eur. J. Clin. Invest., 7:149 (1977).
8. M. Ravid, I. Kedar, and E. Sohar, Lancet, 1:730 (1977).
9. M. H. van Rijswijk, A. J. M. Donker, and L. Ruinen, Lancet, 1:207 (1979).
10. M. H. van Rijswijk, A. J. M. Donker, L. Ruinen, and J. Marrink, Proc. Eur. Dialysis Transpl. Assoc., 16:500 (1979).
11. M. H. van Rijswijk and C. W. G. J. van Heusden, Am. J. Pathol., 97:43 (1979).
12. A. J. M. Donker, G. K. van der Hem, W. J. Sluiter, and H. Beekhuis, Neth. J. Med., 20:97 (1977).
13. W. H. J. van Luijk, G. J. Ensing, S. Meijer, A. J. M. Donker, and D. A. Piers, Eur. J. Nucl. Med., 9:439 (1984).
14. J. E. Repine, J. W. Eaton, M. W. Anders, J. R. Hoidal, and R. B. Fox, J. Clin. Invest., 64:1642 (1979).
15. G. Weissmann, C. Sherhan, H. M. Korchak, and J. E. Smolen, Ann. N. Y. Acad. Sci., 389:11 (1982).
16. V. Baracos, H. P. Rodemann, C. A. dinarello, and A. L. Goldberg, New Engl. J. Med., 308:553 (1983).
17. G. Weissman, G. Sessa, and V. Bevans, Ann. N. Y. Acad. Sci., 141:326 (1967).
18. G. W. van Dine and R. G. Shaw, Polym. Prep. (A.C.S.), 12:713 (1971).
19. W. E. Mitch, M. Walser, G. A. Buffington, and J. Lemann, Lancet, 2:1326 (1976).
20. B. M. Brenner, T. W. Meyer, and T. H. Hostetter, New Engl. J. Med., 307:652 (1982).
21. G. Maschio, L. Oldrizzi, N. Tessitore, and A. D'Angelo, Kidney Int., 22:371 (1982).
22. J. B. Rosman, G. Ph. M. Piers-Becht, W. J. Sluiter, S. Meijer, and A. J. M. Donker, Lancet (in press).

SPLENIC FUNCTION IN AMYLOIDOSIS

Marvin J. Stone and Victor J. Hirsch

Charles A. Sammons Cancer Center
Baylor University Medical Center
Dallas, Texas 75246

ABSTRACT

Thirteen of 62 patients (21%) with biopsy-proven amyloidosis seen between 1971 and 1983 had evidence of functional hyposplenism, as defined by
the presence of Howell-Jolly bodies on blood smear and anatomic presence of
the spleen. The latter was established by various imaging procedures, surgery, or autopsy. The patients with functional hyposplenism (9 men, 4
women) ranged between 33 and 79 years of age. Proteinuria, hepatomegaly,
gastrointestinal bleeding, and cardiovascular manifestations were common
presenting findings. Twelve patients exhibited Howell-Jolly bodies initially and 9 were anemic. In no case was there evidence of megaloblastic
dyspoiesis. Eleven patients had a plasma cell dyscrasia; the light chain
component in all was lambda. Marrow plasmacytosis ranged between 3 and 50%;
no patient had lytic bone lesions or hypercalcemia. Surgery or autopsy in
8 patients disclosed spleen weights between 110 and 500 grams; all were extensively replaced with amyloid. Three patients had normal spleen scans
and normal size spleens at autopsy. None of the patients with functional
hyposplenism developed pneumococcal infections and one has survived for 70
months. Although splenic function is generally unaltered or increased in
the presence of infiltrative lesions, amyloidosis occasionally causes
splenic hypofunction which may serve as a useful diagnostic clue. We are
unaware of any instance of functional hypersplenism with amyloidosis.

INTRODUCTION

The spleen is a common site of involvement in patients with systemic
amyloidosis [1, 2]. We first reported functional hyposplenism (FH) in
amyloidosis in 1975 [3]. Subsequently, others have confirmed this association [4-9]. The purpose of this report is to summarize the clinical features encountered in our amyloid patients with FH and to review the literature relating to this subject.

MATERIALS AND METHODS

The hospital and clinic records of patients with biopsy-proven amyloidosis seen between January 1, 1971 and December 31, 1983 were reviewed.
All patients were seen in Dallas at Baylor University Medical Center, Park-

TABLE 1. Clinical and Laboratory Data

Pt	Age/Sex	Clinical Presentation	Dx Amyloid (Site)	M-Protein	% Marrow Plasma Cells	Serum Albumin (g/dl)	Proteinuria (g/24h)	Evidence of Spleen
1	55m	Heart failure Hypotension	Kidney	IgM,λ	20	0.8	14.4	Autopsy 500g
2	60f	GI Bleed Hepatomegly	Liver	λ	24	2.7	3.5	Autopsy 320g
3	43m	GI Bleed Hepatomegly Jaundice	Liver	λ	9	2.1	4.7	Normal Size @ surgery
4	69m	Heart failure Angina	Rectum	λ	11	2.5	9.5	Autopsy 470g
5	55m	GI Bleed	Rectum Stomach	IgG,λ	23	4.1	0.5	Normal Size @ surgery (232g)
6	53m	GI Bleed Heart failure Jaundice	Lymph node GI tract	None	15	3.0	-	Sonogram, radionuclide scan
7	68f	Lymphadenopathy Mediastinal mass	Lymph node	λ	30	3.9	5.1	Sonogram, radionuclide scan
8	72f	Diarrhea Hypotension Macroglossia	Rectum Bone marrow	λ	3	3.3	1.9	Sonogram, radionuclide scan. Autopsy 175g
9	69m	Hepatomegaly Jaundice	Liver Bone marrow	None	10	3.7	1.8	Sonogram, CT scan
10	58f	Carpal tunnel	Carpal ligaments	λ	50	3.6	6.7	Autopsy 150g
11	79m	Intermittent claudication	Liver	λ	8	3.1	3.6	Sonogram, surgery
12	33m	Abd pain weight loss	Liver	λ	7	2.5	2.4	Autopsy 110g
13	59m	Abd pain	Liver Kidney Bone marrow	IgA,λ	5	2.9	6.7	Autopsy 230g

land Memorial Hospital, or the Dallas Veterans Administration Hospital. The diagnosis of amyloidosis required typical histologic features, including green birefringence under polarized light after Congo red staining and/or usual fibrillar appearance by electron microscopy. All available peripheral blood smears and bone marrow were examined. In addition, radionuclide scans, sonograms, and CT scans were reviewed.

Criteria for FH including the following: 1) four or more Howell-Jolly bodies on blood smear in the absence of evidence of megaloblastic anemia, other hemolytic anemia, or early leukemia; and 2) anatomic presence of the spleen as verified by various imaging procedures (radionuclide scan, sonography, CT scan), surgery, or autopsy.

RESULTS

A total of 62 patients with biopsy-proven amyloidosis were identified. Four had "localized" disease, as defined by the presence of amyloid in only one tissue site and no evidence of an M-protein in serum or urine by immunoelectrophoresis. Of the remaining 58 patients, 46 had a plasma cell dyscrasia, as defined by the presence of an M-protein in serum and/or urine. The M-components identified were as follows: κ only-5 patients; λ only-20 patients; IgG,κ-5 patients; IgG,λ-5 patients; IgA,κ-2 patients; IgA,λ-7 patients; and IgM, -2 patients.

Thirteen patients met the criteria for FH; this subset accounted for 21% of the total group, 22% of those with systemic amyloidosis, and 28% of those with plasma cell dyscrasias. Initial clinical and laboratory data on the 13 patients with FH are shown in Table 1; the findings on Patient 2 have been reported in detail previously [3]. Their ages ranged between 33 and 79 years; 9 were men and 4 were women. Initial findings were variable depending on the major sites of amyloid involvement. Hepatomegaly, gastrointestinal bleeding, and cardiovascular abnormalities were common presenting manifestations. Significant proteinuria (0.5-14.4 g/24 h) was present in all patients in whom 24 h urine protein measurements were performed. Electrophoretic and immunoelectrophoretic studies of urine disclosed a nephrotic pattern with or without Bence Jones proteinuria in most patients. Serum creatinine levels were normal in 10 patients and mildly elevated (1.7-1.8 mg/dl) in three.

Anemia (Hgb < 12 g/dl) was present in 9 patients and most often the consequence of gastrointestinal bleeding. Patients 4, 9, 11, and 12 had normal hemoglobin levels at presentation. Twelve patients had Howell-Jolly bodies (Fig. 1) with variable aniso- and poikilocytosis, target cells, and basophilic stippling on blood smear when first seen. Patient 10 initially lacked Howell-Jolly bodies; these subsequently appeared 9 months later and persisted until her demise.

Eleven of the 13 hyposplenic patients had evidence of a plasma cell dyscrasia by virtue of the finding of a monoclonal immunoglobulin component by immunoelectrophoresis of serum and/or urine (Table 1). The light chain component in all was lambda. Patients 1, 5, and 13 had evident serum M-spikes on cellulose acetate electrophoresis associated with IgM, IgG, and IgA monoclonal components, respectively. Patients 6 and 9 had no identifiable M-component in serum or urine on multiple immunoelectrophoretic studies. Hypoalbuminemia (<3 g/dl) was present in 6 patients when initially seen (Table 1).

Bone marrow examinations disclosed variable cellularity with normoblastic erythroid maturation in all patients. The proportion of plasma cells ranged from 3 to 50% of the nucleated marrow cells.

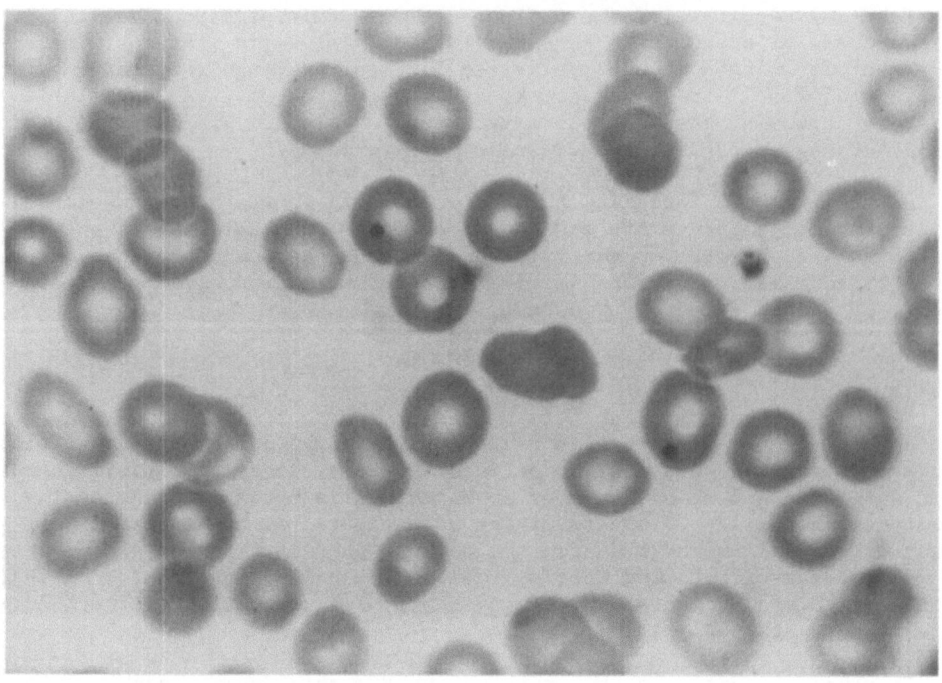

Fig. 1. Blood smear from Patient 4. Two red cells contain Howell-Jolly
bodies (nuclear remnants).

No patient had lytic bone lesions on skeletal roentgenograms, hypercalcemia, or evidence of Factor X deficiency at initial presentation.

All patients with FH had anatomic evidence for the presence of the
spleen by various imaging procedures, surgery, or autopsy. Except for
Patients 1 and 9, all had radionuclide liver-spleen scans performed with
^{99m}Tc-sulfur colloid. Three patients (2, 4, and 12) had no uptake in the
spleen by radionuclide scan but had spleen weights of 320 g, 470 g, and
110 g, respectively, at autopsy. Five patients (3, 6, 7, 8, and 11) were
noted to have decreased splenic uptake on radionuclide scan (Fig. 2). Patients 5, 10, and 13 had normal spleen scans and spleen weights of 232 g,
150 g, and 230 g, respectively, at surgery or autopsy.

Spleens were removed at surgery (1 patient) or autopsy (7 patients).
The organs were normal to moderately enlarged with weights ranging from 110
to 500 g (Table 1, Fig. 3). Histologically, all showed extensive replacement by amyloid.

Most of the patients with FH died within 2 years after diagnosis of
amyloidosis. None developed pneumococcal sepsis or had splenic rupture. Patient 7 remains alive 70 months after first being seen by us and 85 months
since the diagnosis of amyloidosis was initially made by supraclavicular
lymph node biopsy. Amyloid was subsequently demonstrated in mediastinal
lymph nodes and the bone marrow in this patient.

DISCUSSION

We previously described a patient with FH and amyloidosis in a study
of 35 patients with light chain myeloma, 7 of whom had primary systemic

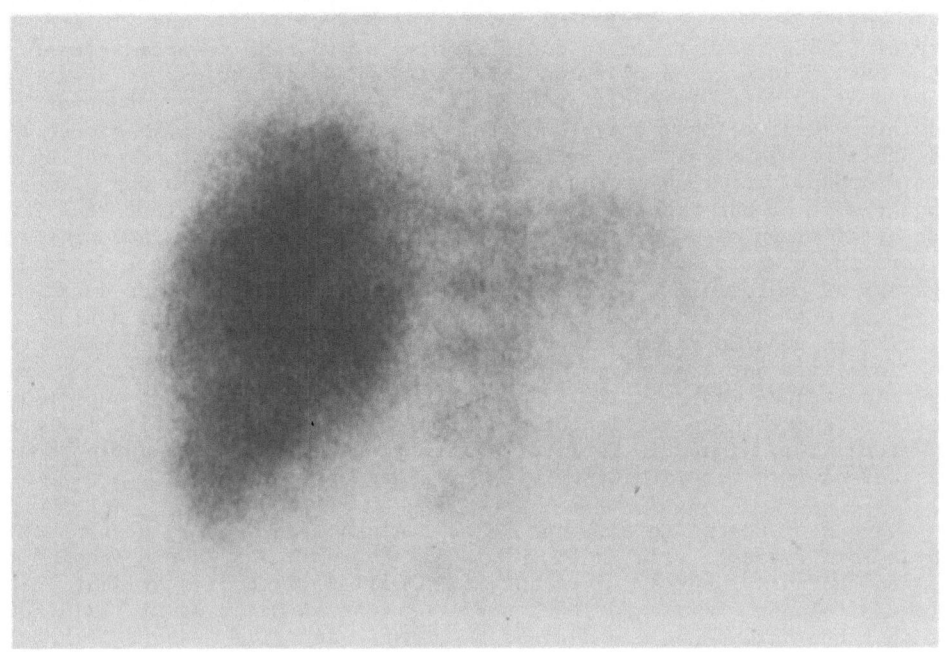

Fig. 2. Radionuclide liver-spleen scan from Patient 7. Note hepatomegaly
with marked reduction of isotope uptake in the spleen.

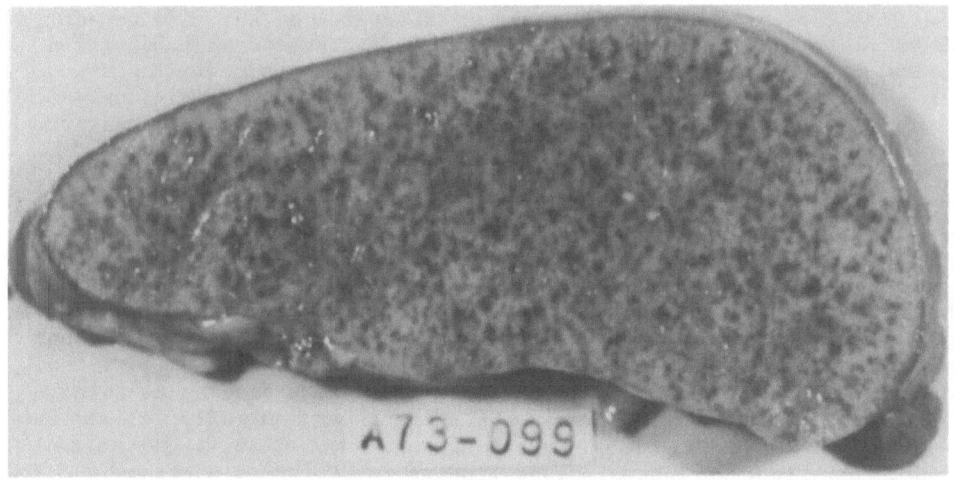

Fig. 3. Spleen from Patient 2. The organ weighed 320 g. Histologically,
splenic tissue was extensively replaced by amyloid.

amyloidosis [3]. In that report, we mentioned that we had seen a second such patient not included in that series. Subsequently, we noted additional hyposplenic amyloid patients [10]. The present report summarizes our experience during the past 13 years. Thirteen of the 62 patients with biopsy-proven amyloidosis seen during that interval have had FH. Our 21% incidence of hyposplenism in amyloidosis is similar to that reported recently by the Mayo Clinic group [7]. We agree with those investigators that the presence of FH in amyloidosis appears to be a measure of the extent of amyloid involvement. Thus, they found that survival of their hyposplenic amyloid patients was significantly reduced as compared with the normosplenic amyloid group. The longest survival in the hyposplenic group was 38 months. Although most of our hyposplenic amyloid patients lived for less than 2 years after diagnosis, Patient 7 has survived for 70 months since we first saw her and established that she had FH, and 85 months since the initial diagnosis of amyloidosis. Although the presence of FH indicates an advanced stage of amyloid involvement in most patients, it should not necessarily be considered an ominous prognostic factor in all. Pneumococcal infections were not a problem in our hyposplenic amyloid patients nor in those reported by Gertz et al. [7]. Nevertheless, pneumococcal sepsis is a well-recognized complication of the post-splenectomy state [11, 12] and of myeloma [10]. Thus, it is likely that hyposplenic amyloid patients are at increased risk for infections with this organism.

Reduced or absent splenic uptake on radionuclide scan is present in most amyloid patients with FH [3, 5-7, 14]. However, 3 of our hyposplenic patients had normal spleen scans but had Howell-Jolly bodies evident in peripheral blood. This experience confirms that of Gertz et al. [7] who feel that the peripheral blood smear is a more sensitive measure of FH than the radionuclide spleen scan. Moreover, the blood smear is certainly simpler and cheaper.

Systemic amyloidosis has a remarkably variable clinical presentation depending on the organ systems most prominently involved [1-3, 9, 13]. We agree with Boyko et al. [6] that the finding of Howell-Jolly bodies in a patient who has a spleen may be a useful clue to the diagnosis of amyloidosis. This circumstance was illustrated in several of the more recently studied patients in the present series; the diagnosis of amyloidosis in Patients 9, 11, 12, and 13 was initially suspected by the finding of Howell-Jolly bodies on blood smear. We have not encountered hyposplenic amyloid patients presenting with Factor X deficiency or splenic rupture. However, these complications do occur rarely [4, 5].

Since the initial description of FH in 1969, a number of conditions have been associated with this entity [15-22]. These are listed in Table 2. In some, such as inflammatory bowel disease, systemic lupus erythematosus, or autoimmune thyroid disease, splenic atrophy occurs. In others, such as sickle cell disease, malignant lymphoma, or amyloidosis, a normal-sized or enlarged spleen is present. Thus, splenic size is an important consideration in differential diagnosis of FH in the adult. All of the disorders associated with FH are characterized by the finding of Howell-Jolly bodies on blood smear. These DNA remnants are normally removed from red cells in the presence of an intact spleen. Howell-Jolly bodies are the most consistent peripheral blood finding following splenectomy and are present in all patients [23]. They appear to be the most sensitive indicator of the asplenic or hyposplenic state.

Splenic function is generally unaltered or increased in the presence of infiltrative lesions such as sarcoidosis [18, 24]. However, we have

TABLE 2. Conditions Associated with
Functional Hyposplenism

Amyloidosis

Neonatal state

Cyanotic congenital heart disease

Torsion of spleen

Sickle cell disease

Ulcerative colitis

Crohn's disease

Adult celiac disease

Dermatitis herpetiformis

Thyrotoxicosis (Graves' disease)

Systemic lupus erythematosus

Malignant lymphoma

Essential thrombocythemia

Thorotrast administration

---

not encountered nor are we aware of any instance of functional hypersplenism with amyloidosis. As noted, the mechanism of FH in amyloidosis appears related to massive replacement of splenic tissue by amyloid. This circumstance may preclude development of the hypersplenic state.

REFERENCES

1. A. S. Cohen, New Engl. J. Med., 277:522, 574, 628 (1967).
2. R. A. Kyle and E. D. Bayrd, Medicine, 54:271 (1975).
3. M. J. Stone and E. P. Frenkel, Am. J. Med., 58:601 (1975).
4. P. R. Greipp, R. A. Kyle, and E. J. W. Bowie, New Engl. J. Med., 301:1050 (1979).
5. W. W. Hurd and R. E. Katholi, Arch. Intern. Med., 140:844 (1980).
6. W. J. Boyko, R. Pratt, and H. Wass, Am. J. Clin. Pathol., 77:745 (1982).
7. M. A. Gerta, R. A. Kyle, and P. R. Greipp, Ann. Intern. Med., 98:475 (1983).
8. I. M. Jacobson and K. J. Isselbacher, Ann. Intern. Med., 99:573 (1983).
9. R. A. Kyle and P. R. Greipp, Mayo Clin. Proc., 58:665 (1983).
10. M. J. Stone, in: Pathology and Immunoglobulins: Diagnostic and Clinical Aspects (S. E. Ritzmann, ed.), Alan R. Liss, Inc., New York, Vol. 2 of Protein Abnormalities, pp. 161-236 (1982).
11. S. W. Hosea, E. J. Brown, M. I. Hamburger, and M. M. Frank, New Engl. J. Med., 304:245 (1981).

12. P. E. Schwartz, S. Sterioff, P. Mucha, L. J. Melton, and K. P. Offord, JAMA, 248:2279 (1982).
13. G. G. Glenner, New Engl. J. Med., 302:1283, 1333 (1980).
14. S. Sostre, N. D. Martin, R. N. Lucas, and H. W. Strauss, Radiology, 115:675 (1975).
15. H. A. Pearson, R. P. Spencer, E. A. Cornelius, New Engl. J. Med., 281: 923 (1969).
16. L. K. Diamond, New Eng. J. Med., 281:958 (1969).
17. H. M. DeBartolo, J. A. van Heerden, H. B. Lynn, and D. G. Norris, Mayo Clin. Proc., 48:783 (1973).
18. E. R. Eichner, Am. J. Med., 66:311 (1979).
19. K. R. Palmer, S. B. Sherriff, C. D. Holdsworth, and F. P. Ryan, Quart. J. Med. NS L, No. 200, 463 (1981).
20. A. M. Dillon, H. B. Stein, and R. A. English, Ann. Intern. Med., 96: 40 (1982).
21. C. N. Coleman, I. R. McDougall, M. O. Dailey, P. Ager, S. Bush, and H. S. Kaplan, Ann. Intern. Med., 96:44 (1982).
22. D. J. Gross, A. J. Braverman, G. Koren, Y. S. Rabinowitz, R. Gordon, and E. Okon, Arch. Intern. Med., 142:2213 (1982).
23. M. M. Wintrobe, Clinical Hematology, edit. 8, Philadelphia: Lea and Febiger (1981), p. 262.
24. J. Bertino and R. M. Myerson, Arch. Intern. Med., 106:213 (1960).

ACKNOWLEDGEMENTS

    We would like to thank Doctors Eugene P. Frankel, Richard G. Sheehan, and J. Wayne Streilein for the helpful discussions and suggestions. This study was supported by the Tri Delta Cancer Research Fund.

DOES THE URINARY PROTEIN PATTERN IN AA-AMYLOID NEPHROPATHY

DIFFER FROM THAT IN OTHER NEPHROPATHIES?

Anna-Maija Teppo and C. P. J. Maury

The Fourth Department of Medicine
University of Helsinki
Helsinki, Finland

ABSTRACT

The urinary excretion of six plasma proteins was determined in reactive (secondary) amyloidosis, in rheumatoid arthritis, in systemic lupus erythematosus, in diabetic patients, in patients with chronic glomerulonephritis and in healthy controls. The type of proteinuria in patients with amyloidosis was compared with that of other patient groups and of nephropathies due to glomerulonephritis or diabetes. In amyloidosis the excretion of lambda light chains was slightly higher and that of kappa chains slightly lower than in other proteinurias, consequently the ratio lambda/kappa chains in patients with reactive amyloidosis was higher (p < 0.01) than in other patient groups or in healthy controls. In patients with moderate/heavy proteinuria the excretion of IgG compared with that of albumin was in reactive amyloidosis as well as in diabetic nephropathy lower than in glomerulonephritis (p < 0.05) and suggest the higher selectivity of protein excretion in these patients than in glomerulonephritis. The finding that the ratio of excreted lambda/kappa chains in reactive amyloidosis exceeds that of normal plasma indicates in these patients either increased plasma concentration and/or decreased reabsorption of lambda light chains.

INTRODUCTION

Nephropathy is a common manifestation in patients with reactive (secondary) amyloidosis and a major cause of death in these patients [1, 2]. Proteinuria is the main sign of amyloid nephropathy. The mechanisms of proteinuria in renal amyloidosis are not well known. Current data suggest that the important factors are the penetrance of the glomerular basement membrane by amyloid fibrils [3-5], the partial detachment of epithelial cells [6], and the distribution but not necessarily the extent of the glomerular amyloid deposition [5, 7].

Since pathological processes in the kidney may affect the urinary output of individual proteins selectively, more useful information of the underlying pathophysiological processes may be obtained by the measurement of the excretion of individual proteins, than by the estimation of the total protein excretion. In this study, the urinary protein pattern in amyloid nephropathy was compared to that in nephropathies of nonamyloid origin.

TABLE 1.   Clinical Data of the Patients

Group	Diagnosis	n	F/M	Mean age years	s-creatinine μmol/l
I Normal renal function, No/slight proteinuria	RA + A	8	7/1	50.0	88 $\pm$ 9
	RA	12	12/0	56.4	72 $\pm$ 6
	SLE	10	9/1	41.9	81 $\pm$ 5
	Healthy controls	15	10/5	32.0	88 $\pm$ 1
II Renal insufficiency, Mild proteinuria	RA + A	8	7/1	40.2	300 $\pm$ 73
	GN	11	2/9	49.5	275 $\pm$ 63
	DM	10	6/4	47.5	325 $\pm$ 51
III Renal insufficiency, Moderate/heavy proteinuria	RA + A	5	3/2	40.8	197 $\pm$ 21
	GN	8	4/4	47.6	455 $\pm$ 129
	DM	10	5/5	33.7	430 $\pm$ 68

PATIENTS AND METHODS

The series consisted of 97 patients as follows: 21 subjects with reactive systemic amyloidosis (RA + A), 20 secondary to rheumatoid arthritis
and one to systemic lupus erythematosus, (17 women, 4 men, mean age 44.1
years); 12 subjects with rheumatoid arthritis without amyloidosis (RA) (all
women, mean age 56.4 years), 10 patients with systemic lupus erythematosus
(SLE) (9 women, 1 man, mean age 41.9 years), 19 patients (6 women, 13 men,
mean age 48.7 years) with chronic glomerulonephritis (GN), none had amyloidosis or diabetes; 20 patients with diabetic nephropathy (DM) (11 women,
9 men, mean age 40.6 years) and 15 healthy persons (10 women, 5 men, mean
age 32.0 years).

According to the renal function and the degree of proteinuria the patients were divided into the following three groups. Group I had normal
renal function (creatinine clearance >84 ml/min/1.73 m^2) and no/slight
proteinuria (urinary excretion of albumin <0.3 g/24 h). Group II had renal
insufficiency (creatinine clearance <84 ml/min/1.73 m^2) and mild proteinuria
(urinary excretion of albumin 0.3-1.0 g/24 h). Group III had renal insufficiency and moderate or heavy proteinuria (urinary excretion of albumin
>1.0 g/h) (Table 1).

METHODS

Aliquots of neutralized (pH = 7.0) 24-urines were stored at -20°C.
Concentrations of albumin, transferrin and IgG were determined by immuno-
turbidimetry [8] by the use of specific antisera (Orion Diagnostica, Espoo,
Finland) and concentrations of free kappa and lambda chains by the same
method by the use of antisera to free kappa or lambda light chains (Dako,
Copenhagen, Denmark). Kappa chains isolated from the urine of a myeloma
patient was used as standard for kappa chains and Lambda Bence Jones Con-
trols^R (Kallestad, Austin, Texas 78701) as standard for lambda chains. β_2-
Microglobulin was measured by radioimmunoassay (Phadebas β_2-microtest,
Phasmacia, Sweden). Sensitivity of the methods was 5 mg/liter for albumin,
transferrin and IgG, 2 mg/liter for kappa and lambda chains, and 0.003 mg/
liter for β_2-microglobulin. All results are expressed as the mean ± SEM.
Student's test for unpaired data was used to evaluate the significance of
between-group differences.

RESULTS

The urinary protein patterns in amyloidosis and in the respective control groups are shown in Table 2. In amyloid patients with renal insufficiency and slight proteinuria (Group II) the excretions of lambda light
chains, transferrin and IgG compared with that of albumin were slightly
higher and the excretion of kappa chains slightly lower than in the respective control groups, whereas in amyloid nephropathy (Group III) the excretion of both lambda and kappa light chains was lower than in patients with
glomerulonephritis or with diabetic nephropathy (Table 2). The excretion
of IgG compared with that of albumin was in reactive amyloidosis lower than
in glomerulonephritis (p < 0.05) and comparable with that in diabetic
nephropathy (Table 2). These findings suggest in amyloidosis and in diabetic patients the higher selectivity of protein excretion than in glomerulonephritis.

The ratios of lambda/albumin and kappa/albumin in amyloidosis were
lower than in diabetic patients (p < 0.01) and comparable with those found
in glomerulonephritis (Table 3). The degree of proteinuria had no effect
on these ratios.

TABLE 2. Daily Urinary Excretion of Plasma Proteins (mg/24 h, Mean ± SEM) in Patients with Reactive Amyloidosis (RA + A) and in Respective Controls

Group	Diagnosis	Daily urinary excretion of plasma proteins (mg/24 hours)					
		Albumin	λ-chains	α-chains	β_2-MG	Transferrin	IgG
I Normal renal function, no/slight proteinuria	RA + A	70 ± 33	6 ± 2	6 ± 2	1.94 ± 1.71	8 ± 4	7 ± 5
	RA	25 ± 13	7 ± 2	5 ± 2	0.11 ± 0.02	< 5	< 5
	SLE	45 ± 28	5 ± 3	14 ± 7	0.35 ± 0.16	5 ± 4	3 ± 2
	Healthy controls	8 ± 1	2 ± 0.1	3 ± 0.1	0.10 ± 0.01	< 5	< 5
II Renal insufficiency, Mild proteinuria	RA + A	644 ± 119	45 ± 6	31 ± 6	15.99 ± 4.64	131 ± 28	133 ± 26
	GN	538 ± 79	27 ± 5	39 ± 7	7.95 ± 2.57	78 ± 16	84 ± 15
	DM	398 ± 91	32 ± 7	49 ± 12	8.16 ± 1.54	54 ± 19	83 ± 26
III Renal insufficiency, Moderate/heavy proteinuria	RA + A	1974 ± 462	128 ± 45	77 ± 29	27.04 ± 11.89	253 ± 49	325 ± 108
	GN	2673 ± 597	181 ± 91	249 ± 64	25.57 ± 6.86	191 ± 40	1549 ± 891
	DM	2798 ± 658	480 ± 139	744 ± 245	87.79 ± 65.19	171 ± 34	321 ± 57

TABLE 3. The Concentration Ratios of Lambda/Albumin, Kappa/Albumin, and Transferrin/Albumin in Patients with Amyloidosis, Glomerulonephritis, and Diabetic Nephropathy (Mean ± SEM)

Diagnosis	n	Concentration ratios x 10		
		Lambda/Albumin	Kappa/Albumin	Transferrin/Albumin
RA + A	21	0.73 ± 0.07	0.47 ± 0.05	1.75 ± 0.11
GN	19	0.57 ± 0.09	0.74 ± 0.12	1.21 ± 0.14
DM	20	1.50 ± 0.33	2.23 ± 0.52	0.99 ± 0.14

TABLE 4. The Ratio of Lambda/Kappa Light Chains in Patients with Amyloidosis and in Respective Controls (Mean ± SEM)

Diagnosis	The ratio of lambda/kappa chains		
	Group I Normal renal function, no/slight proteinuria	Group II Renal insufficiency, mild proteinuria	Group III Renal insufficiency, moderate/heavy proteinuria
RA + A	1.6 ± 0.5	1.6 ± 0.1	1.7 ± 0.3
RA	0.9 ± 0.1		
SLE	0.4 ± 0.1		
GN		0.7 ± 0.1	1.1 ± 0.1
DM		0.6 ± 0.06	0.7 ± 0.03
Healthy controls	0.6 ± 0.02		

In amyloidosis the ratio of lambda/kappa chains was significantly higher than in the other patient groups or in control subjects (Table 4) and independent of the degree of proteinuria.

DISCUSSION

The results show that the urinary excretion pattern of plasma proteins in patients with amyloid nephropathy in some respects differs from that found in other patient groups. The decreased excretion of IgG compared to that of albumin in reactive amyloidosis suggests higher selectivity in these patients than in chronic glomerulonephritis.

The most important finding was that the ratio of lambda/kappa chains was significantly higher in amyloidosis than in the other patient groups or in the healthy controls. Our values of the controls correspond with those reported earlier [9]. The increased ratio of lambda/kappa light chains was evident in patients with normal and impaired glomerular filtration. In rheumatoid arthritis without amyloidosis the mean ratio of lambda/kappa chains is significantly lower than that in amyloidosis. There were, however, 6 of the 12 patients with rheumatoid arthritis with the lambda/kappa ratio ≥1.0.

Circulating, free, immunoglobulin light chains are normally filtered through the glomerulus and catabolized by proximal tubular cells [10]. Increased excretion of light chains has been found in tubular proteinuria [11]. Thus the most likely explanation for the high lambda/kappa ratio in reactive amyloidosis is a disturbed tubular function and/or increased plasma concentration of lambda light chains. Sølling and Sølling [12] reported increased plasma concentrations of both kappa and lambda light chains in reactive amyloidosis, where the increase correlated with impairment of renal function.

Our results agree with those of Isobe and Osserman [13] who found a higher proportion of λ-type Bence-Jones proteins in amyloidosis associated with rheumatoid arthritis. They also showed that these amyloid-related Bence-Jones proteins were relatively more anionic than those found in non-amyloid patients. Eventhough it is suggested [14] that the light chains with a high isoelectric point are more nephrotoxic than the more acid ones, the immunoglobulin light chains in reactive amyloidosis may still possess rather high nephrotoxic activity. In addition, the acid nature may make them less soluble or increase their binding properties. Some light chains have been shown to have antibody activity [16]. Therefore, it is also possible that the light chains in amyloidosis and in amyloid-like deposits may be autoantibodies directed against normal tissue constituents [13, 17].

Since the increased urinary lambda/kappa ratio was evident in patients with reactive amyloidosis already in an early stage of the amyloid nephropathy the reduced ability to reabsorb lambda light chains may be the first sign of tubular dysfunction in reactive amyloidosis and thus of clinical importance.

REFERENCES

1. R. A. Kyle and E. D. Bayard, Medicine, 54:271 (1975).
2. C. L. Pirani, in: Amyloidosis (O. Wegelius and A. Pasternack, eds.), Academic Press, London (1972).
3. H. V. Gise, E. Mikeler, M. Gruber, H. Christ, and A. Boble, Virchows, Arch. Path. Anat. Histol., 379:131 (1978).
4. H. V. Gise, V. V. Gise, B. Stark, and A. Boble, Klin. Wschr., 59:75 (1981).

5. Y. Nakamoto, S. Hamanaka, T. Akihama, A. B. Miura, and Y. Uesaka, Clin. Nephrol., 22:188 (1984).

6. R. Katafuchi, T. Taguchi, S. Takebayashi, and T. Harada, Clin. Nephrol., 22:1 (1984).

7. W. Thoenes and H.-M. Schneider, Klin. Wschr., 58:667 (1980).

8. A.-M. Teppo, Clin. Chem., 28:1359 (1982).

9. E. L. Robinson, E. Gowland, I. D. Ward, and J. H. Scarffe, Clin. Chem., 28:2254 (1982).

10. T. A. Miettinen and M. Kekki, Clin. Chim. Acta, 18:395 (1967).

11. P. A. Peterson and I. Berggård, Europ. J. Clin. Invest., 1:255 (1971).

12. J. Sølling and K. Sølling, Acta Med. Scand., 206:283 (1979).

13. T. Isobe and E. F. Osserman, New Engl. J. Med., 290:473 (1974).

14. R. A. Coward, I. W. Delamore, N. P. Mallick, and E. L. Robinson, Clin. Sci., 66:229 (1984).

15. A. Solomon, New Engl. J. Med., 294:17 (1976).

16. E. F. Osserman, New Engl. J. Med., 304:1110 (1981).

17. C. A. Alpers, J. Hopper, and C. G. Biava, Hum. Pathol., 15:444 (1984).

CLASSIFICATION OF AMYLOID SYNDROMES FROM TISSUE SECTIONS USING

ANTIBODIES AGAINST VARIOUS AMYLOID FIBRIL PROTEINS: REPORT OF 142 CASES**

Reinhold P. Linke*, Walter B. J. Nathrath†,
and Manfred Eulitz‡

*Institut für Immunologie der Universität
 Schillerstrasse 32
 800 Munich 2, Federal Republic of Germany

†Pathologisches Institut der Universität
 Thalkirchnerstrasse 36
 800 Munich 2, Federal Republic of Germany

‡Institut für Hämatologie der Gesellschaft
 für Strahlen- und Umweltforschung
 Landwehrstrasse 61
 800 Munich 2, Federal Republic of Germany

ABBREVIATIONS

AA) Amyloid fibril protein A; Aλ) fibril protein of immunoglobulin λ-light chain origin; Aκ) amyloid fibril protein of κ-chain origin; AF) amyloid fibril protin in familial amyloid polyneuropathy; ASc$_1$) amyloid fibril protein in senile cardiovascular amyloidosis; FMF) familial Mediterranean fever.

ABSTRACT

To identify the chemical nature of amyloid fibril proteins in tissue sections, various formalin-fixed organs from 142 patients with amyloid were investigated with a panel of antisera directed against different purified amyloid fibril proteins from representative generalized amyloid syndromes.

Using anti-AA, Aλ, Aκ, AF, and ASc$_1$ antisera, 112 of 114 generalized amyloidoses (98%) and 120 of all 142 cases (85%) could be identified by either the indirect or the unlabeled immunoperoxidase method. Untypeable cases were usually localized or organ-limited forms of amyloid and may well be amyloid types which have not yet been identified.

The clinical diagnoses correlated well with the immunohistochemical definition of the amyloid type. Most of the 50 identified AA-amyloid syndromes, therefore, were associated with recurrent inflammatory diseases,

---

**This study was supported by Sonderforschungsbereich 0207, LP-12 and LP-13, Munich.

599

predominantly different forms of arthritis. Surprisingly enough, no underlying diseases was found in 7 of the 50 AA cases (14%).

Most of the 41 Aλ and the 11 Aκ cases were B-cell neoplasms or idiopathic amyloidosis with plasma cell dyscrasias. Eight cases with senile
cardiovascular amyloid and 10 with the cross-reacting amyloid polyneuropathy were identified.

Our data, therefore, demonstrate that almost all generalized and some
more localized forms of amyloid can be identified with the panel of antisera against amyloid fibril proteins presented in this study.

INTRODUCTION

The discovery of the chemical heterogeneity of amyloid deposits not
only expanded Virchow's definition [1], which was a misnomer, but it also
formed a new basis for a rational classification of amyloid deposits and
amyloid-induced clinical syndromes [2, 3]. This chemical heterogeneity has
been used to develop a pathogenetically more precise diagnosis of amyloidosis. Techniques have now been employed for routine clinicopathological use.
Differentiation of the various amyloid syndromes on tissue sections, therefore, ought to be possible with immunologic probes for each of the known
amyloid classes. To a certain extent, this has already been achieved with
the immunofluorescence [4, 5] and the more useful immunoperoxidase techniques. The immunoperoxidase method can be performed on paraffin sections
routinely fixed in formalin [6-8].

At present, immunohistochemical typing of amyloid has been carried out
with only a few antisera on a limited number of amyloid-containing samples
[6-8, 13-15, 19]. The results of our 142 cases with a large panel of antisera directed against different amyloid fibril proteins are presented in
this study. Our findings indicate that these antisera are well suited for
the identification and typing of most generalized and some more localized
amyloid syndromes.

MATERIALS AND METHODS

1. Tissues

All specimens were formalin-fixed paraffin sections of biopsy and
autopsy material mounted on glass slides which were sent to us by various
hospitals and pathology institutes, together with the case histories and
laboratory data, for immunohistochemical typing. Diagnosis of amyloid in
the tissue sections was performed by the alkaline Congo red method plus inspection in polarized light [9].

2. Antisera

Isolation as well as immunochemical and chemical identification of
amyloid fibril proteins and the production of antisera in rabbits were performed as cited in Table 1. Antisera not listed in Table 1 were prepared
similarly. Antisera against insulin and glucagon (Nova, Mainz/FRG) were
induced in guinea pigs and one rabbit in our laboratory and tested for specificity on islets of Langerhans by immunohistochemistry. Anticalcitonin
was purchased from Dako, Copenhagen; the anti-γ trace donated by Dr. W.
Machleidt (Munich/FRG).

TABLE 1. Antisera Against Amyloid Fibril Proteins Used for Immunohistochemical Typing of Amyloid

Antigen	Pat.	Ident.	Source of of Antigen	Clinical Diagnosis	Author
AA	BUC	I, S	spleen	rheumatoid arthritis	16
AA	MOS	I, S	spleen	rheumatoid arthritis	
AA	WAL	I, S	spleen * **	Muckle-Wells syndrome	11,16
Aλ	FIS	I, N	spleen	idiopathic amyloidosis	13
Aλ	ULI	I, N	spleen	"secondary" amyloidosis	
Aλ	NEZ	I, N	carpal tunnel	idiopathic amyloidosis	
Aλ	HAR	I, S	spleen	multiple myeloma	17
Aϰ	MEV	I, S	bone marrow	multiple myeloma	12
Aϰ	SIN	I, S	spleen	plasma cell dyscrasia	13
ASc_1	FOL	I, N	heart	senile cardiac amyloidosis	14
AF	TIE	I	vitreous body	familial blindess	13
AF	TAD	I	heart	polyneuropathy	19

S = determination by N-terminal amino acid sequence analysis
I = immunochemical typing by immunodiffusion
N = unreactive N-terminal amino acid
* = monoclonal anti-AA antibody mc1
** = fixed in formalin

3. Immunohistochemistry

The indirect immunoperoxidase method was used with polyclonal rabbit
antibodies; the unlabeled method, with monoclonal antibodies [12, 14-16].

The results were evaluated by rating the staining intensity of the
chromogene 3-amino-9-ethyl-carbazol as 0, +, ++, or +++. When the results
were unclear, the reaction was repeated with additional antisera directed
against an amyloid fibril protein of the same type. Four antisera with
different specificities were routinely used for the Aλ forms. The additional monoclonal anti-AA (mc1) antibody [11] was employed in combination
with the monoclonal peroxidase-antiperoxidase (mc100) complex [16] when the
results for AA syndromes were unclear.

RESULTS AND DISCUSSION

1. General Remarks

An immunochemical classification to different amyloid syndromes was
achieved in 120 of the 142 cases (85%). All but 2 of the 114 generalized
forms (98%) were identified (see Table 3). Clinically, the 2 unidentifiable
cases appeared to belong to the AL forms. One of these patients excreted
a $V\lambda_{VI}$ Bence Jones protein which was identified with a subclass-specific
antiserum supplied by Dr. A. Solomon (Knoxville, Tennessee).

Only 8 of the remaining 27 more localized cases could be typed immunohistochemically: all were AL types. The other nonreactive localized

TABLE 2. Immunohistochemical Typing of Amyloid with Results Obtained on Representative Identified Cases

Case No.	Clinical diagnosis	Immunohistochemical reaction with antisera against					Amyloid type
		AA	Aλ	Aκ	AF	ASc_1	
1	Rheumatoid arthritis	+++	+	−	−	−	AA
2	Idiopathic amyloidosis	+++	−	−	−	−	AA
3	Neuritis	+++	−	−	−	−	AA
4	Osteomyelitis	+++	+	+	−	−	AA
5	Juvenile rheumatoid arthritis	+++	++	+	−	−	AA
6	Idiopathic amyloidosis	−	++	−	−	−	Aλ
7	Multiple myeloma	−	+++	−	−	−	Aλ
8	Local tracheobronchial amyloid	−	+++	−	−	−	Aλ
9	Lung tumor	−	++	+	−	−	Aλ
10	Multiple myeloma	−	+	+++	−	−	Aκ
11	Bence Jones plasmocytoma	−	−	++	−	−	Aκ
12	Idiopathic amyloidosis	−	+	+++	−	−	Aκ
13	Familial blindness	−	−	−	+++	++	AF
14	Polyneuropathy	−	−	−	+++	++	AF
15	Familial polyneuropathy (P)	−	+	−	+++	++	AF_P
16	Familial polyneuropathy (J)	−	+	·+	+++	++	AF_J
17	Cardiovascular amyloidosis	−	+	−	+++	+++	ASc_1
18	Cardiac amyloidosis	−	−	−	++	++	ASc_1

amyloids were probably amyloids with a different chemistry for which no antiserum is currently available. A new amyloid fibril protein was recently reported in Alzheimer's disease [20].

2. Immunohistochemical Diagnosis

The results for the immunohistochemical visualization of amyloid proteins within the different amyloid deposits are presented in Table 2. In each case, the amyloid type was defined by the antiserum with the strongest reaction. One of the 4 noncross-reacting amyloid types, i.e., AA, Aλ, Aκ, or ASc_1/AF, therefore, could be assigned to each case. None of the Aλ, Aκ, or ASc_1/AF amyloids reacted with any of the AA antibodies, not even the monoclonal antibody. A weak reaction with nonrespective antisera, which was previously observed to a certain extent [7], however, occurred in some AA and ASc_1/AF amyloids, especially with anti-Aλ antisera. Addition of purified amyloid-P component did not lead to absorption of the anti-Aλ immunologic reactivity. This weak reaction could be due to cross reactions with immunoglobulins trapped within the amyloid deposits, particularly in inflammatory diseases. Since AF and ASc_1 amyloidosis could be distinguished from the AA and AL forms by immunohistochemistry, but not from each other, the differentiation is based on clinical symptoms, tissue localization, and age distribution [12, 21, 22].

TABLE 3. Clinical Diagnosis of 142 Cases with Immunohistochemical Typing of Amyloid with Reported Antisera

Type	Clinical Diagnosis	Number	Total
AA	rheumatoid arthritis	12	
	idiopathic amyloidosis	7	
	juvenile rheumatoid arthritis	6	
	Crohn's disease	5	
	familial Mediterranean fever	4	
	bronchioectasis	3	
	osteomyelitis	2	
	psoriatic arthritis	2	
	tumors	2	
	recurrent fever of unknown etiology	2	
	tuberculosis	1	
	paraplegia	1	
	sporadic Muckle-Wells syndrome	1	
	Still's disease	1	50
Aλ	idiopathic amyloidosis	16	
	multiple myeloma	6	
	plasmocytoma (without bone lesions)	5	
	Waldenström's disease	3	
	laryngeal and tracheobronchial amyloid	3*	
	Bence Jones plasmocytoma (with bone lesions)	3	
	lung tumor	2*	
	cutaneous amyloidosis	2*	
	osteomyelofibrosis	1	41
A$\varkappa$	multiple myeloma	4	
	plasmocytoma (without bone lesions)	4	
	idiopathic amyloidosis	2	
	tracheal amyloid	1*	11
$ASc_1{}^+$	senile cardiovascular amyloidosis	6	
	senile lung amyloidosis (lung biopsy)	2	8
AF	type I familial amyloid polyneuropathy	4	
	familial polyneuropathy (non-type I)	4	
	sporadic polyneuropathy	2	10
Other**	lichenoid amyloidosis	4*	
	basal cell carcinoma	3*	
	amyloid in seminal vesicles	3*	
	idiopathic generalized amyloidosis (AL?)	2	
	Alzheimer's disease	1*	
	cerebral amyloid angiopathy	1*	
	glucagonoma and amyloid	1*	
	amyloid struma	1*	
	amyloid in medullary carcinoma of thyroid	1*	22
Total			142

*   = not generalized
\+   = cross reaction of ASc_1 and AF (diagnosis based on clinical symptoms)
** = not identifiable with cited antisera

3. Correlation between Chemical Type and Clinical Syndrome

Comparison of immunohistochemical results and clinical diagnoses both confirms and enriches current knowledge concerning the chemical classification of amyloid syndromes [23, 22]. AA amyloid was associated mainly with inflammatory processes, particularly rheumatoid arthritis and related disorders. Only a few cases with chronic bacterial infections, such as tuberculosis and osteomyelitis, so frequent just a few decades ago, were, however, found. Protein AA also occurs in the hereditary syndrome such as FMF and in diseases without any detectable accompanying inflammatory process, i.e., the idiopathic variety of AA-type amyloidosis.

B-cell neoplasias with circulating monoclonal immunoglobulins, with and without bone lesions, are prevalent in Aλ- and Aκ-amyloid syndromes in a more generalized form such as multiple myeloma or in a more localized form such as cutaneous amyloidosis or trachael amyloid deposits [24]. Many of these syndromes are identified as idiopathic without overt monoclonal gammopathy, bone lesions, or signs of neoplasia, but, in many cases, with a certain degree of plasma cell dyscrasia in bone marrow [25].

AF and ASc_1 forms can be reliably distinguished from the other abovementioned forms by appropriate antisera [5, 14, 15]. Since polyneuropathy can be caused by different types of amyloid, the antisera mentioned in this study and by others are essential for differentiating between Aλ- and AF-induced polyneuropathy in cases where little anamnestic and clinical information is available [19].

Most of the more localized amyloid forms cannot be identified because they, in all probability, are types with a chemistry which differs from that of the types analyzed in this study.

Our study demonstrates that the above-mentioned antisera directed against different purified amyloid fibril proteins can be used to differentiate 98% of all generalized amyloid syndromes. Specificity of these antisera was documented by control experiments and correct recognition of all chemically identified amyloid deposits, the amyloid fibril proteins of which were used for immunization. The results obtained in other patients were consistent with the clinical diagnosis and with results obtained by Wright-Calkins modification [21] of the permanganate oxication method introduced by Romhányi on a representative selection of cases with different chemistry (not reported). None of the amyloids listed in Table 3, including the amyloids in Alzheimer's disease, reacted with anti-insulin, antiglucagon, and anti-γ trace or anti-calcitonin antisera, which were applied to try to stain apudamyloid or brain amyloids [2].

Our findings, therefore, demonstrate that the antisera and methodology described in this study are well suited for larger scale clinicopathologic studies and for routine use to obtain a more differentiated chemical diagnosis of amyloidoses and amyloid deposits, a differentiation which is particularly important for therapeutic decisions [6-8, 19, 22, 23].

ACKNOWLEDGEMENTS

We would like to express our appreciation to Ms. Sylvia Wegscheider and K. B. Linke for their expert technical assistance and to the many institutions that supplied the case histories and laboratory data.

REFERENCES

1. R. Virchow, Arch. Path. Anat. Physiol. Klin. Med., 6:135 (1854).
2. E. P. Benditt and N. Eriksen, Amer. J. Pathol., 65:231 (1971).
3. G. G. Glenner, W. Terry, M. Harada, C. Isersky, and D. Page, Science, 172:1150 (1971).
4. G. G. Cornwell, III, G. Husby, P. Westermark, J. B. Natvig, T. E. Michaelson, and B. Skogen, Scand. J. Immunol., 6:1071 (1977).
5. G. G. Cornwell, III, J. B. Natvig, P. Westermark, and G. Husby, J. Immunol., 120:1385 (1978).
6. Y. Levo, N. Livni, and A. Laufer, in: Amyloid and Amyloidosis (G. G. Glenner, P. P. Costa, and F. de Freitas, eds.), Excerpta Medica, Amsterdam, p. 35 (1980).
7. S. Fujihara, J. E. Balow, J. C. Costa, and G. G. Glenner, Lab. Invest.
8. R. P. Linke, O. Geisel, M. Eulitz, and W. B. J. Nathrath, Blut, 41: 465 (1980).
9. H. Puchtler, F. Sweat, and M. Levin, J. Histochem. Cytochem., 10:355 (1962).
10. R. P. Linke, P. R. Hol, E. Gruys, O. Geisel, W. B. J. Nathrath, and G. Trautwein, J. Comp. Path., 94:339 (1984).
11. R. P. Linke, Blut, 45:407 (1982).
12. R. P. Linke and W. B. J. Nathrath, Münch. Med. Wschr., 122:1772 (1980).
13. T. Shirahama, M. Skinner, and A. S. Cohen, Histochemistry, 72:161 (1981).
14. R. P. Linke, Clin. Neuropath., 1:172 (1982).
15. R. P. Linke, in: Cardiology and Ageing (D. Platt, ed.), F. K. Schattauer, Stuttgart-New York, pp. 81 (1983).
16. R. P. Linke, J. Histochem. Cytochem., 32:322 (1984).
17. R. P. Linke, K. L. Heilmann, W. B. J. Nathrath, and M. Eulitz, Lab. Invest., 48:698 (1983).
18. M. Eulitz and R. P. Linke (this symposium).
19. G. E. Feurle, R. P. Linke, E. Kuhn, and A. Wagner, J. Neurol. (in press).
20. G. G. Glenner and C. W. Wong, Biochem. Biophys. Res. Comm., 120:885 (1984).
21. J. R. Wright, E. Calkins, and R. L. Humphrey, Lab. Invest., 36:274 (1977).
22. J. R. Wright and E. Calkins, Medicine, 60:429 (1981).
23. G. G. Glenner, New Engl. J. Med., 302:1283, 1333 (1980).
24. S. Fujihara and G. G. Glenner, Lab. Invest., 44:55 (1981).
25. T. Isobe and E. F. Osserman, New Engl. J. Med., 290:473 (1974).
26. D. H. Cohen, H. Feiner, O. Jensson, and B. Frangione, J. Exp. Med., 158:623 (1983).

CLINICAL, PATHOLOGICAL, AND FUNCTIONAL FINDINGS

IN AMYLOID NEPHROPATHY

S. Janssen, M. H. van Rijswijk
S. Meijer, G. K. van der Hem,
and E. Mandema

Department of Medicine
University Hospital
Groningen, The Netherlands

ABSTRACT

Nephropathy is a major problem in both AA and AL amyloidosis. In 53 patients with amyloidosis we performed a renal biopsy, 50 of which showed amyloid deposits; local focal glomerulonephritis associated with rheumatoid disease was found in 3 patients. In 41 patients the amyloid deposits were potassium permanganate sensitive (AA); 9 patients had potassium permanganate resistant amyloid deposits (AL). No amyloid could be demonstrated in the rectal biopsies of 8 patients in the AA and 2 patients in the AL group.

Hypertension was present in 22% (diastolic blood pressure >90 mm Hg). There was no difference in creatinine clearance between the AA (median 45 ml/min; range <5-175 ml/min) and the AL group (medium 50 ml/min; range 12-106 ml/min) at the time of renal biopsy.

Proteinuria was more massive in the AL (median 9 g/24 h; range <0.5-22 g/24 h) than in the AA group (median 6 g/24 h; range 0.5-20 g/24 h) ($p < 0.02$). There appeared to be a negative correlation between the selectivity of the proteinuria and the creatinine clearance ($r = -0.625$, $p < 0.001$), whereas there was no correlation between the degree of proteinuria and renal function.

Contracted kidneys were a regular finding, particularly in advanced renal failure. Enlarged kidneys were rare. There is a weak positive correlation between kidney size and creatinine clearance ($r = 0.388$, $p < 0.01$).

Renal tubular function has not been studied on any large scale in renal amyloidosis. The clearance of ^{99m}Tc-dimercaptosuccinate, representing (proximal) tubular function, was disturbed (elevated) in 22/24 measurements. There appeared to be a strong negative correlation between the clearance of ^{99m}Tc-dimercaptosuccinate and the glomerular filtration rate ($3 = -0.656$, $p < 0.01$). Renal tubular dysfunction appeared to correlate with the degree of tubular atrophy and interstitial fibrosis.

INTRODUCTION

Nephropathy is a prominent feature in both AA and AL amyloidosis, although the clinical pattern of organ dysfunction is more diverse in the latter (Kyle and Bayrd, 1975). Amyloid nephropathy has no features that are uniquie to it. Therefore the reliance of clinical and laboratory findings is uncertain with regard to renal involvement. The aim of our study was to determine the characteristics of patients with biopsy-proven renal amyloidosis at the time of renal biopsy, with particular emphasis on renal tubular function. ^{99m}Tc-Dimercaptosuccinate (^{99m}Tc-DMSA) is filtrated in the glomerulus and reabsorbed in the proximal tubulus. The clearance of ^{99m}Tc-DMSA represents proximal tubular function and may be disturbed (elevated) in interstitial nephritis or fibrosis (van Luijk et al., 1984). In amyloid nephropathy tubular atrophy and interstitial fibrosis, caused by ischaemic loss of nephrons due to vascular amyloid deposition, parallel the degree and the progression of renal insufficiency (Törnroth et al., 1980). We tried to establish the efficacy of the clearance of ^{99m}Tc-DMSA as a test for the degree of tubulopathy and concomitant interstitial fibrosis in renal amyloidosis.

MATERIAL AND METHODS

Between 1961 and 1983 renal biopsies were performed in 53 patients with systemic non-familial amyloidosis. In 52 of the patients a rectal biopsy specimen was obtained at the same time. All tissue specimens were stained with Congo red and examined in the polarizing microscope for green birefringence. The effect of incubation with potassium permanganate ($KMnO_4$) on the affinity for Congo red was investigated in all patients (van Rijswijk and van Heusden, 1979).

A careful search for the presence of a monoclonal component (MC) included immunoelectrophoresis of serum and concentrated urine and immunofluorescence of bone marrow plasma cells. The data of the investigations mentioned below were obtained at the time of renal biopsy and concern the patients in whom the renal biopsy showed amyloid deposits.

Hypertension is defined as a diastolic blood pressure greater than 90 mm Hg. Both the degree of proteinuria (g/24 h) and the clearance of creatinine (ml/min) were determined over 24 hourly periods (N = 50).

The selectivity of the proteinuria (N = 38) was calculated as the ratio of the immunoglobulin G clearance versus the transferrin or the albumin clearance (×100%).

Kidney size (N - 45) was measured on plain abdominal radiographs or intravenous pyelographs and defined as the sum of the length of right and left kidney divided by 2.

On 24 occasions the clearance of ^{99m}Tc-DMSA and the glomerular filtration rate were determined according to the method described by van Luijk.

RESULTS

The results of renal and rectal biopsies are given in Table 1. Amyloid deposits could be demonstrated in 50/53 renal biopsies, 41 of which were $KMnO_4$-sensitive (AA amyloid) and 9 $KMnO_4$-resistant (non-AA amyloid). In 3 patients with rheumatoid arthritis and a positive rectal biopsy, the renal biopsy did not show amyloid deposits but lesions attributable to the rheumatoid disease (local focal gloermulonephritis). In 8/9 patients with $KMnO_4$-

TABLE 1. Results of Congo Red
         Staining of Rectal and
         Renal Biopsies in 44
         AA and 8 AL Patients

	Rectum pos Kidney pos	Rectum neg Kidney pos	Rectum pos Kidney neg
AA	33 (75%)	8 (18%)	3 (7%)
AL	6 (78%)	2 (22%)	0 (0%)
AA+AL	39 (75%)	10 (19%)	3 (6%)

resistant amyloid deposits the presence of a monclonal gammopathy could be demonstrated (2 × IgGλ, 1 × IgGκ, 1 × IgAκ, 3 × BJλ, 1 × BJκ). In the AA patients no monoclonal component was found.

No amyloid could be demonstrated in the rectal biopsies of 8/41 AA and 2/8 AL patients despite a positive renal biopsy. In 1 AL patient no rectal biopsy material was available.

Hypertension was present in 11/50 patients. The presence or absence of an elevated blood pressure did not correlate with renal function loss (Wilcoxon's rank sum test: $p > 0.05$).

There was no difference in creatinine clearance between the AA (medium 45 ml/min; range <5–175 ml/min) and the AL group (median 50 ml/min; range 12–106 ml/min) (Wilcoxon's rank sum test: $p > 0.05$).

The median proteinuria (AA + AL) was 7 g/24 h (range <0.5–22 g/24 h). The proteinuria tended to be more massive in the AL (median 9 g/24 h; range <0.5–22 g/24 h) than in the AA patients (median 6 g/24 h; range <0.5–20 g/24 h) (Wilcoxon's rank sum test: $p < 0.02$). Nephrotic syndrome was present in 89% of the AL and 59% of the AA group. Two patients presented with no or minimal proteinuria (<0.5 g/24 h).

There was no correlation between the degree of proteinuria and the creatinine clearance (Spearman's rank sum test: $p > 0.05$).

In 14/30 AA and 4/8 AL patients the proteinuria was selective ($\leq 20\%$) at the time of renal biopsy. There appeared to be a negative correlation between the selectivity-index of the proteinuria and the creatinine clearance (Spearman's rank sum test: $r = -0.625$, $p < 0.001$), whereas there was no correlation between the selectivity-index and the degree of proteinuria (Spearman's rank sum test: $p > 0.05$).

Mean kidney size was 12.5 ± 1.4 cm in the AA group (N = 39) and 13.1 ± 0.9 cm in the AL group (Wilcoxon's rank sum test: $p > 0.05$).

Enlarged kidneys (>14 cm) were rare (3/45), while contracted kidneys (<12 cm) were a more regular finding (9/45), especially in advanced renal failure (5/10 patients with creatinine clearance <15 ml/min).

There was a weak positive correlation between kidney size and renal function (Spearman's rank sum test: $r = 0.388$, $p < 0.02$).

The relative clearance of ^{99m}Tc–DMSA was disturbed (>14%) in 22/24 measurements. There appeared to exist a strong negative correlation be-

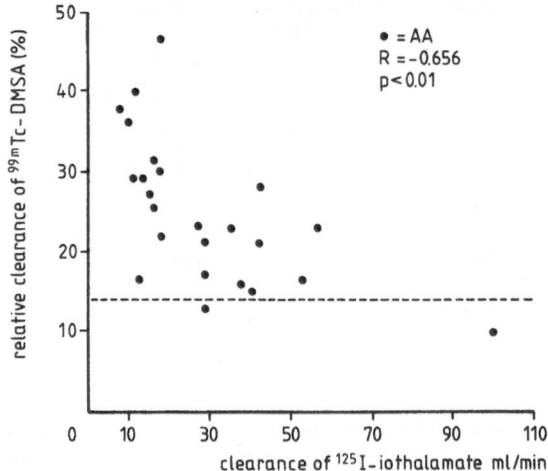

Fig. 1. Correlation between renal tubular
function, measured by the relative
clearance of ^{99m}Tc-dimercaptosuc-
cinate and the glomerular filtration rate of ^{125}I-iothalamate.

tween the relative clearance of ^{99m}Tc-DMSA and renal function, measured by
the glomerular filtration rate of ^{125}I-iothalamate (Spearman's rank sum
test: r = -0.656, p < 0.01) (see Fig. 1).

DISCUSSION

     Diagnosis of amyloidosis requires histological identification of amy-
loid deposits in biopsy specimens. The rectum is considered the best site
for a diagnostic biopsy and is positive in 75-98% of cases (Gafni and Sohar,
1960; Kyle and Bayrd, 1975; Tribe and Mackenzie, 1982). We found an accuracy rate of 80% in 110 patients. The relation between the results of
rectum and kidney biopsy is uncertain (Hamburger et al., 1968). Our results
indicate that the sensitivity of the rectal biopsy as a predictor of renal
involvement is 80%. In 3 patients the results of rectal biopsy may be considered false positive, because the renal biopsy showed no amyloid deposits,
but instead local focal glomerulonephritis, being an extra-articular manifestation of rheumatoid arthritis.

     The absence of hypertension in amyloidotic patients has been overem-
phasized in literature and may be explained by the state of cachexia and
dehydration in patients with tuberculosis, which is the most common cause
of amyloidosis in early series (Dixon, 1934). In addition autonomic neuropathy due to systemic AL amyloidosis may have been responsible for the high
percentage of hypotension. The frequency of hypertension in our patients
(22%) is comparable with the results of later reports (Zuckerbrod et al.,
1956).

     Proteinuria is considered invariable in the course of amyloid disease
and is the presenting feature in 64-72% of cases (Fearnley and Lackner,
1955; Brandt et al., 1968; Triger and Joekes, 1973; Jones, 1974; Kyle and
Bayrd, 1975). Nephrotic syndrome develops in 50-93% of cases (Cohen, 1967;
Brandt, 1968; Triger and Joekes, 1973). In our series 59% of the AA and
89% of the AL patients presented with proteinuria in the range of nephrotic
syndrome; 4% had no significant proteinuria. Falck found predominantly

610

vascular amyloid deposition in renal biopsies of 9 patients with no or minimal proteinuria. There was no correlation between the amount of urinary protein loss and renal function. It should be noticed that even in advanced renal failure proteinuria may be massive. The degree of proteinuria was generally more massive in the AL than in the AA patients, which may be explained as follows: a) regular examination of urine for proteinuria, especially in rheumatoid arthritis, resulting in early diagnosis of amyloidosis; b) amyloid of the AL type is an unexpected finding in 10% of patients with unexplained nephrotic syndrome (Jao, 1973); c) the presence of significant Bence Jones proteinuria.

Proteinuria is considered moderately or poorly selective in renal amyloidosis, although selective proteinuria is reported occasionally (Jones, 1974; Black and Jones, 1979; Brenner, 1981). Our results indicate that proteinuria initially is selective and becomes non-selective with progression of renal function loss.

There still remains disagreement whether kidney size is enlarged in renal amyloid (Heptinstall and Joekes, 1960; Brandt et al., 1968; Ekelung, 1977; Elkin, 1980). In our patients kidney size was correlated with renal function. Contracted kidneys were associated with renal insufficiency, whereas enlarged kidneys were rare.

In one patient the sudden deterioration of renal function was associated with a remarkable increase in kidney size (13-20 cm), which was caused by bilateral renal vein thrombosis.

Amyloid involvement of blood vessels seems to be the primary lesion, causing ischemic loss of nephrons (Törnroth, 1980). Vascular amyloid deposition contributes to tubular atrophy and interstitial fibrosis, which is related to the degree and the progression of renal insufficiency. Renal tubular function has not been studied on any large scale in amyloidosis. Clinical evident tubular dysfunction has been reported in single patients (Bero, 1957; Carone and Epstein, 1960; Lindeman et al., 1961; Dorhout-Mees et al., 1968; Sebastian et al., 1968; Luke et al., 1969). ^{99m}Tc-DMSA is reabsorbed in the proximal tubules after glomerular filtration. An elevated (>14%) clearance of ^{99m}Tc-DMSA represents tubular dysfunction. In the vast majority of our patients the tubular function was impaired, while there appeared to be a strong correlation between tubulopathy and renal function loss, measured by the glomerular filtration rate of ^{125}I-iothalamate.

Although the number of patients is too small to come to definite conclusions, the degree of interstitial fibrosis appears to correlate with the degree of tubular dysfunction, thereby possibly providing a non-invasive test for the extent of interstitial damage.

CONCLUSIONS

   a) The result of rectal biopsy is not conclusive with regard to renal
       involvement.

   b) A renal biopsy should be considered on suspicion of renal amy-
       loidosis, especially in rheumatoid arthritis.

   c) Proteinuria initially is selective and becomes non-selective with
       progression of renal insufficiency.

   d) Kidney size correlates with renal function, enlarged kidneys are
       rare and should raise suspicision for renal vein thrombosis.

e) Disturbance of proximal tubular function (^{99m}Tc—DMSA clearance >14%) is a frequent finding.

f) Renal tubular dysfunction correlates strongly with the degree of renal function loss.

g) Clearance of ^{99m}Tc—DMSA might provide a non-invasive test for the degree of interstitial damage in renal amyloidosis.

REFERENCES

Bero, G. L., Ann. Intern. Med., 46:931 (1957).
Black, D., and Jones, N. F., Renal Disease, Blackwell Scientific Publications, Oxford (1979), p. 713.
Brandt, K., Cathcart, E. S., and Cohen, A. S., Am. J. Med., 44:955 (1968).
Brenner, M. B., and Rector, F. C., The Kidney, W. B. Saunders Company, Philadelphia (1981), p. 1528.
Carone, F. A., and Epstein, F. H., Am. J. Med., 29:539 (1960).
Cohen, A. S., New Engl. J. Med., 277:628 (1967).
Dixon, H. M., Am. J. Med. Sci., 187:401 (1934).
Dorhout-Mees, E. J. de Planque, B. A., Helders, J., and Kooiker, C. J., Nephron., 5:81 (1968).
Ekelung, L., Am. J. Roentgenol., 129:851 (1977).
Elkin, M., RAdiology of the urinary system, Little, Brown, and Company, Boston (1980), p. 1014.
Falck, H. M. Törnroth, T., and Wegelius, O., Clin. Nephrol., 19:137 (1983).
Fearnley, G. F., and Lackner, R., Br. Med. J., 1:1129 (1955).
Gafni, J., and Sohar, E., Am. J. Med. Sci., 240:332 (1960).
Hamburger, J., Richet, G., Crosnier, Funck-Brentano, J. L., Antoine, B., Ducrot, H., Mery, J. P., and de Montera, H., Nephrology, W. B. Saunders Company, Philadelphia (1968).
Heptinstall, R. H., and Joekes, A. M., Ann. Rheum. Dis., 19:126 (1960).
Jao, W., Pollak, V. E., Norris, V. E., Lewy, P., and Pirani, C. L., Medicine, 52:445 (1973).
Jones, N. F., Renal amyloid, in: Advanced Medicine, No. 10 (J. G. G. Ledingham, ed.), Pitman Medical, London, No. 10, 351 (1974).
Kyle, R. A., and Bayrd, E. D., Medicine, 54:271 (1975).
Lindeman, R. D., Scheer, R. L., and Raisz, L. G., Ann. Intern. Med., 54:883 (1961).
Luke, R. G., Allison, M. E. M., Davidson, J. F., and Duguid, W. P., Ann. Intern. Med., 70:1211 (1969).
Luijk, W. H. J. van, Ensing, G. J., Meijer, S., Donker, A. J. M., and Piers, D. A., Eur. J. Nucl. Med. (1984) (in press).
Rijswijk, M. H. van, and Heusden, C. W. G. J. van, Am. J. Pathol., 97:43 (1979).
Sebastian, A., McSherry, E., Ueki, I., and Morris, R. C., Ann. Intern. Med., 69:541 (1968).
Tornroth, T., Falck, H. M., Wafin, F., and Wegelius, O., in: Amyloid and Amyloidosis (G. G. Glenner, ed.), Excerpta Medica, Amsterdam, p. 191 (1980).
Tribe, C. R., and Mackenzie, J. C., Amyloidosis, in: The Kidney and Rheumatic Disease (P. A. Bacon and N. M. Hadler, eds.), Butterworth, London, p. 297 (1982).
Triger, D. R., and Joekes, A. M., Q. J. Med., 42:15 (1973).
Zuckerbrod, M., Rosenberg, B., and Kayden, H. J., Am. J. Med., 21:227 (1956).

FINE NEEDLE ASPIRATION BIOPSY OF ABDOMINAL SUBCUTANEOUS FAT TISSUE FOR

THE DIAGNOSIS AND TYPING OF AMYLOIDOSIS

P. Westermark, L. Benson,
and B.-O. Olofsson

Departments of Pathology and Internal Medicine
University Hospital
Uppsala, Sweden

Department of Internal Medicine
University Hospital
Umeå, Sweden

ABSTRACT

Systemic amyloidosis was diagnosed in 150 patients by fine needle aspiration biopsy of subcutaneous abdominal fat tissue. The method has turned out to be rapid, safe and totally free of complication and is useful in all types of systemic amyloidosis. Subcutaneous abdominal fat tissue can also be used for typing of amyloid.

At the International Symposium in Helsinki 1974 we reported our results with a new method for the diagnosis of systemic amyloidosis, the fine needle aspiration biopsy of subcutaneous fat tissue [1]. The method, which at that time has been used in 10 cases of systemic amyloidosis, promised to be a simple and reliable method. We hereby report our experience of the method in different types of systemic amyloidosis. We now also use abdominal fat tissue for the determination of amyloid type.

METHOD

The method is based on the almost constant appearance of amyloid deposits around fat cells and in the walls of small vessels in the abdominal fat tissue in AL, AA and prealbumin type of systemic amyloidosis. Aspiration biopsy of such fat tissue is easily performed with an ordinary syringe (10-20 ml) equipped with a long needle, which should have a diameter between 0.9 and 1.2 mm. Thicker needles have been used with good result but in that case local anesthesia often is necessary. After aspiration of fat tissue at 1-3 locations of the abdominal subcutis, smears are made. These are allowed to air dry and are then stained with alkaline Congo red without any prior fixation. After mounting in Canada balsam or equal, the smears are examined in a polarization microscope between crossed polars. In cases of systemic amyloidosis, a green birefringence is found, usually in all or most tissue fragments. In rare cases, only a few tissue fragments contain amyloid and therefore a careful examination of all obtained material is recommended.

TABLE 1. Ten Year Material of Patients with Systemic Amyloidosis Diagnosed by Fine Needle Aspiration Biopsy

Clinical type of amyloidosis	Number of patients
Secondary amyloidosis	114
Rheumatoid arthritis 96	
Other causes 18	
Primary amyloidosis	25
Myeloma associated amyloidosis	6
Senile systemic amyloidosis	1
Familial systemic amyloidosis	4

Experience

Since we introduced the method [1, 2] we have been able to diagnose 150 cases of systemic amyloidosis (Table 1). Although developed for secondary amyloidosis, we have found the method equally valuable in AL amyloidosis. The value of the method has been confirmed by others [3] who also found it useful in familial amyloidosis. We have recently tested the method in four patients with known familial systemic amyloidosis, Swedish type, with positive result in all four cases.

During the decade that we used fine needle biopsy of subcutaneous fat tissue, we have seen no falsely positive result. Falsely negative results have occurred in about 5%. These have usually been due to inadequate material or inexperience of the diagnostician. Very rarely, no amyloid is found in an adequate material in spite of a systemic amyloidosis.

Conditions for Good Results

It is almost always easy to get an adequate material for an experienced person. It is necessary to assure that tissue fragments are obtained and not only fat droplets. A reliable Congo red staining is extremely important in this type of biopsy since over-stained specimens easily are judged as positive. A polarization microscope equipped with strong light is also necessary.

Advantages with the Method

The greatest advantages with the method is that it is extremely easy, rapid and free of complications. It can be repeated in one patient as often as wanted. There is no need of preparation of the patient and no special equipments are necessary. Since no embedding and cutting of material is needed, the method can be used and the specimens read by any interested clinicians, provided that he has experience in the microscopic diagnosis of amyloid.

Typing of Amyloid

We use subcutaneous fat tissue also for the typing of amyloid. In local anesthesia about 1 cm3 of fat tissue is removed after a small incision. The specimen tissue specimen is put into normal saline and sent to the laboratory. After that the material has been defatted with acetone and allowed to dry, it is extracted with 6 M guanidine HCl in 0.1 M Tris HCl buffer, pH 8.0 containing 0.1 M dithiothreitol. After centrifugation,

TABLE 2.   Typing of Amyloid Protein from Subcutaneous Fat Tissue
Extract by Double Immunodiffusion

	Type of systemic amyloid					Total
	AA	Aκ	Aλ	Prealbumin	Doubtful	
Number of patients	10	2	12	5*	3	32

*Four patients had familial systemic amyloidosis and one senile
systemic amyloidosis.

the solution is dialyzed against water, lyophilized and redissolved in
0.01 M NaOH and studied in double immunodiffusion against antisera to AA,
ASc_1 and five different AL proteins. The antiserum against protein ASc_1
reacts with both senile systemic amyloid and Swedish type of familial
amyloid. In this way we have been able to classify the amyloid in 29 out
of 32 studied patients (Table 2). In three cases, typing was not possible
due to small amounts of amyloid in the fat tissue.

REFERENCES

1.   P. Westermark, B. Stenkvist, in: Amyloidosis, O. Wegelius, A.
     Paternack, Eds. (Academic Press, New York, 1976), p. 403.
2.   P. Westermark, B. Stenkvist, Arch. Intern. Med., 132, 522, 1973.
3.   C. A. Libbey, M. Skinner, A. S. Cohen, Arch. Intern. Med., 143, 1549,
     1983.

ACKNOWLEDGEMENTS

     Supported by the Swedish Medical Research Council (Project No. 5941)
and the Research Fund of King Gustaf V.

NON-INVASIVE TECHNIQUES FOR DEMONSTRATING CARDIAC INVOLVEMENT IN THE

ACQUIRED FORMS OF SYSTEMIC AMYLOIDOSIS

C. R. K. Hind,* D. G. Gibson,†
J. P. Lavender,‡ and M. B. Pepys*

*MRC Acute Phase Protein Research Group
 Department of Medicine
 Royal Postgraduate Medical School
 London W12 OHS, England

†Department of Radiology
 Royal Postgraduate Medical School
 London W12 OHS, England

‡Department of Cardiology
 Brompton Hospital
 London SW3 6HP, England

ABSTRACT

A prospective study was performed to evaluate the relative efficiency of technetium-99m-pyrophosphate (Tc-99m-PYP) myocardial scanning and M-mode and two dimensional (2D) echocardiography in detecting cardiac involvement in the acquired forms of systemic amyloidosis. Five patients with systemic amyloidosis (AL, 4 cases; AA, 1 case) had characteristic M-mode and 2D echocardiographic features indicative of cardiac involvement, and this was later confirmed histologically. In contrast, Tc-99m-PYP myocardial scanning was negative in all 5 patients. We conclude that echocardiography is a more sensitive and clinically useful investigation than Tc-99m-PYP scanning for detecting cardiac involvement in acquired systemic amyloidosis.

INTRODUCTION

In the acquired forms of systemic amyloidosis cardiac involvement is seen in up to 90% of cases of AL amyloidosis and in 50-60% of the AA form [1-3]. Two methods have been advocated for the non-invasive assessment of the presence and extent of cardiac involvement: (i) technetium-99m-pyro-phosphate (Tc-99-PYP) scanning, which depends on the presence of calcium in amyloid deposits [4], and which is clained to be a specific and sensitive test for diagnosing amyloid heart disease [5-8]; and (II) M-mode and two dimensional (2D) echocardiography [9]. We report here the results of a prospective study to evaluate the relative efficiency of these 2 techniques in detecting cardiac involvement in the acquired forms of systemic amyloido-sis.

PATIENTS AND METHODS

Patients

Between March 1983 and June 1984, 9 consecutive patients with systemic
amyloidosis diagnosed by renal, rectal or gingival biopsy were studied.
The biochemical nature of their amyloid fibril protein was determined by
immunohistochemical staining with specific antisera [10].

Tc-99m-PYP Myocardial Scans

A bolus of 20 m Ci (740 MBq) of Tc-99m-PYP (Amersham International,
Amersham, Bucks, U.K.) was injected intravenously followed by a flush of
10 ml of normal saline. Scintigrams of the upper thorax were recorded
using a Ge 400A gamma camera with parallel-hole low energy all purpose
collimator, and which is on line with a MDS 2 computer. Four supine views
of each patient were obtained: anterior, left anterior oblique 40° and
60°, and left lateral. Imaging was performed between 1-3 h after administration of the radionuclide. Analogue images were recorded on X-ray films
by acquiring 300,000 counts collected at energy peak of 140 KeV with 20%
window, and the same data was recorded on computer with matrix 128 × 128
byte. A negative scan was defined as no activity in the region of the
heart, or activity in the myocardium which is less intense than in adjacent
bond.

M-Mode and 2D Echocardiography

M-mode echocardiograms were recorded with Cambridge equipment at a
paper speed of 100 mm/sec with simultaneous phono-, electro- and apex-
cardiograms. End-diastolic posterior wall and septal thickness were measured along with cavity dimension and shortening fraction. Records were
digitised to demonstrate peak rates of changes of transverse dimension and
posterior wall thickness [11]. 2D echocardiograms were recorded with an
ATL 300 sector scanner using standarized gain settings. Images were color
coded to display echo intensity [12]. Median values of regional pixel intensity were determined in 4 areas of interest in the septum and posterior
wall from stop frame video images [13]. These results were compared with
normal patients.

RESULTS

Six patients had systemic AL amyloidosis and 3 cases had the AA form.
Of these, 5 (AL, 4 cases; AA, 1 case) had characteristic echocardiographic
findings (Figs. 1 and 2) of a small ventricular cavity, with a hypokinetic
and thickened interventricular septum and a thickened posterior wall. More
specifically the amplitude of endocardial movement and the extent of wall
thickening during systole were greatly diminished. In all cases quantitative determination of the 2D echocardiographic intensity was entirely
normal. None showed the appearances of 'sparkling' myocardium [9]. Histological confirmation of cardiac amyloid deposits was made in all 5 patients
(endomyocardial biopsy, 3 cases; autopsy material, 2 cases).

In contrast, Tc-99m-PYP myocardial scanning was negative in all 5
patients.

DISCUSSION

In contrast to previous studies [5-8], there was no myocardial uptake
of Tc-99-PYP in the 5 patients with biopsy-proven cardiac amyloidosis.

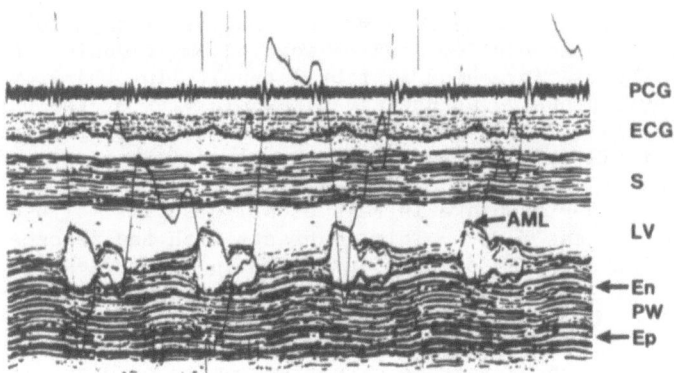

Fig. 1.   M-mode echocardiogram with superimposed phono
(PCG) and apex cardiogram of a patient with
systemic AA amyloidosis.   Note: left Ventricular (LV) cavity size is normal but interventricular septum (S) is hypokinetic and thickened
(2.0 cm; upper limit of normal 1.2 cm).   Posterior wall also thickened at end-diastole (1.5
cm; upper limit of normal 1.2 cm), and amplitude
of endocardial movement and extent of wall
thickening during systole are both greatly
diminished.   (AML = anterior leaflet of the mitral valve.   EN = endocardium.   Ep = epicardium).

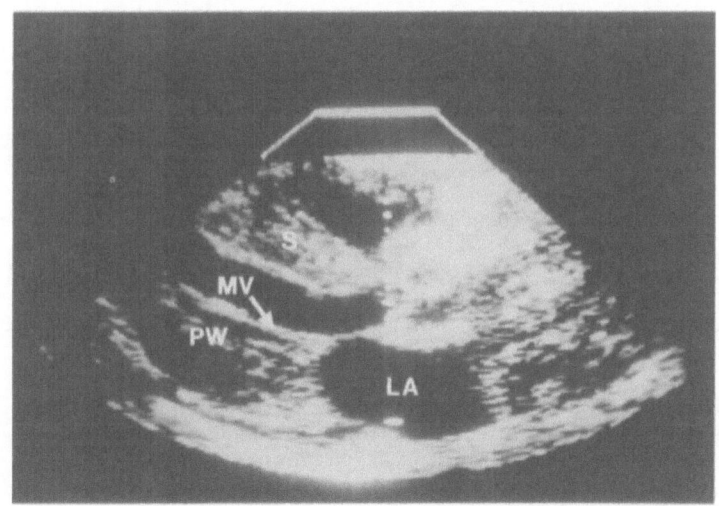

Fig. 2.   3D echocardiogram of a patient with systemic AL
amyloidosis.   There is considerable increase in
septal (S) and posterior wall (PW) thickness
making the left ventricular cavity small.   The
myocardium itself appeared uniformly green on
the display corresponding to a low echo intensity.   Diffuse myocardial fibrosis, the
other main cause of restrictive cardiomyopathy,
reflects ultrasound with considerably greater
amplitude than amyloid (LA = left atrium.   MV =
mitral valve).

This discrepancy is unlikely to be related to the type of amyloid fibril protein since most of these earlier studies were of amyloidosis associated with plasma-cell dyscrasia (presumed AL fibril type). In other reports the type of amyloid fibril protein was not given, and in view of the patients' ages (average 75 years) they may have included some with senile cardiac amyloidosis (ASc_1 fibril type). One possible explanation for this difference is the presence or absence of cardiomegaly on the chest X-ray. Eight of 9 patients with Tc-99-PYP uptake in Falk et al.'s series [8] had cardiomegaly on their chest X-ray. This contrasts with the absence of cardiomegaly on the chest X-ray of the 5 patients in our series.

It was perhaps of interest that using standardized gain settings we failed to demonstrate the 'sparkling' appearance of the myocardium previously reported on 2D echocardiograms of patients with cardiac amyloidosis [9]. It may be significant that previous studies have used phased array equipment stressing the dependence of image texture on machine characteristics.

We concluded that echocardiography is a more sensitive and clinically useful investigation than Tc-99m-PYP scanning for detecting cardiac involvement in acquired systemic amyloidosis.

ACKNOWLEDGEMENTS

This work was supported by Medical Research Council program grant G979/51 to M.B.P. C.R.K.H. is the recipient of a MRC training research fellowship.

REFERENCES

1. K. Brandt, E. S. Cathcart, and A. S. Cohen, Am. J. Med., 44:955 (1968).
2. R. A. Kyle and E. D. Bayrd, Medicine, 54:271 (1975).
3. L. M. Buja, N. B. Khoi, and W. C. Roberts, Am. J. Cardiol., 26:394 (1970).
4. R. W. Kula, W. K. Engel, and B. R. Line, Lancet i, 92 (1977).
5. S. Schiff, T. Bateman, R. Moffatt, R. Davidson, and D. Berman, Am. Heart J., 103:562 (1982).
6. S. M. Sobol, J. M. Brown, S. R. Bunker, J. Patel, and R. J. Lull, Am. Heart J., 103:563 (1982).
7. T. A. Wizenberg, J. Muz, Y. H. Sohn, W. Samlowski, and A. M. Weissler, Am. Heart J., 103:468 (1982).
8. R. H. Falk, V. W. Lee, A. Rubinow, W. B. Hoos, and A. S. Cohen, Am. J. Cardiol., 51:826 (1983).
9. A. G. Siqueiro-Filho, C. L. P. Cunha, A. J. Tajik, J. B. Seward, T. T. Schattenberg, and E. R. Giuliani, Circulation, 63:188 (1981).
10. C. R. K. Hind, G. A. Tennent, D. J. Evans, and M. B. Pepys, J. Pathol., 139:159 (1982).
11. M. T. Upton and D. G. Gibson, Prog. Cardiovasc. Dis., 20:359 (1978).
12. R. Logan-Sinclair, C. M. Wong, D. G. Gibson, Br. Heart J., 45:621 (1981).
13. T. R. D. Shaw, R. B. Logan-Sinclair, C. Surin, R. J. McAnulty, B. Heard, G. J. Laurent, and D. G. Gibson, Br. Heart J., 51:46 (1984).

SOFT-TISSUE UPTAKE OF ^{99m}Tc-DIPHOSPHONATE AND ^{99m}Tc-PYROPHOSPHATE IN SYSTEMIC AA AND AL AMYLOIDOSIS

S. Janssen, D. A. Piers[1],
M. H. van Rijswijk, and E. Mandema

Department of Medicine and

[1]Department of Nuclear Medicine
University Hospital
Groningen, The Netherlands

ABSTRACT

Reviewing the literature it is difficult to assess the significance of soft-tissue uptake on scanning with ^{99m}Tc-labeled phosphates in amyloidosis, because of differences with regard to the radiopharmaceutical and the scanning technique used, and because of lack of information concerning the type of amyloid involved.

A comparative, prospective study was made to determine the efficacy of ^{99m}Tc-methylene-diphosphonate (Tc-MDP) and ^{99m}Tc-pyrophosphate (Tc-PYP) in demonstrating soft-tissue uptake in AA and AL amyloidosis. The results of scintigraphic imaging with Tc-MDP and Tc-PYP were compared with the clinical pattern of organ involvement in 6 patients with systemic AA and 6 patients with systemic AL amyloidosis. Image quality (contrast) was generally better with Tc-MDP than with Tc-PYP, although there was no difference in the extend or the intensity of the soft-tissue uptake. Tc-MDP can play an important role in evaluating amyloid disease with regard to involvement of the thyroid gland, the oropharyngeal region, the nervous system, the liver, the spleen, and the intestinal tract. In contrast with previous reports we found echocardiography to be more sensitive for demonstrating cardiac involvement than scintigraphy. Although nephropathy dominates the clinical scene in AA amyloidosis the scintigraphic pattern of organ involvement was compatible with the histological, multi-systemic, distribution of amyloid.

INTRODUCTION

Clinical manifestations of amyloid disease are variable and depend on the organs involved. The diagnosis of amyloidosis requires histological identification of amyloid material in biopsy specimens. Biopsy procedures are not without risk of hemorrhage. Bleeding may occur in the absence of abnormalities in the coagulation profile and is probably due to amyloid infiltration of the wall of blood vessels (Yood et al., 1983). Non-invasive tests would be helpful to evaluate the extend of organ involvement in cases of suspected or proven amyloidosis. Soft-tissue uptake of ^{99m}Tc-labeled phosphates has been linked with the presence of amyloid in a number of cases of systemic amyloidosis, mainly of the AL type (Janssen et al., 1984). Lee et al. (1983) suggested that ^{99m}Tc-pyrophosphate (Tc-PYP) may be more sensitive in demonstrating cardiac and hepatic amyloidosis than ^{99m}Tc-methylene-diphosphonate (Tc-MDP).

The purpose of our study was 1) to establish the efficacy of whole body scintigraphy with "bone-scanning" agents as a non-invasive screening test for the extend of organ involvement in both AA and AL amyloidosis; 2) to establish the relative efficacy of Tc-MDP versus Tc-PYP.

MATERIAL AND METHODS

Between January 1983 and January 1984, 6 patients with systemic AA and 6 patients with systemic AL amyloidosis were entered into a prospective study. The diagnosis of amyloidosis was confirmed histologically by the apple-green birefringence with polarized light after Congo red staining of biopsy specimens. In all patients the effect of incubation with potassium permanganate ($KMnO_4$) on the affinity for Congo red was investigated.

A careful search for the presence of a monoclonal component was made. Diagnosis of renal amyloidosis was made in the presence of proteinuria and renal function loss. In 7 patients a renal biopsy specimen was obtained, all of which showed amyloid deposits. Diagnosis of cardiac amyloidosis was made if the patient had the typical echocardiographic appearance of amy-loidosis: increased thickness of septum and left ventricular wall with de-creased wall motion. The presence of amyloid neuropathy was established by measurement of nerve conduction velocity. Physical examination revealed the presence or absence of macroglossia and enlargement of the thyroid gland. Thyroid function tests (free thyroxine level; thyroid stimulating hormone) and liver function tests (alkaline phosphatase and transaminases) were made in all patients.

Whole body scintigraphy was performed 4 h after intravenous injection of 500 MBg (13.5 mCi) of Tc-MDP or Tc-PYP at 3 to 5 days intervals; scans were made in random order. Grading of soft-tissue uptake: 0 = normal; 1 = equivocal; 2 = positive with lower intensity than the ribs; 3 = positive with intensity equal to greater than the ribs, but lower than the sternum; 4 = positive and intensity greater than the sternum.

RESULTS

The clinical, laboratory, and scintigraphic data are summarized in Table 1. All patients had biopsy proven amyloidosis; 6 patients presented with systemic amyloidosis associated with overt or covert multiple myeloma ($KMnO_4$-resistant amyloid deposits); amyloidosis was associated with chronic inflammatory diseases in 6 patients ($KMnO_4$-sensitive amyloid deposits).

Tc-MDP images showed a better contrast than Tc-PYP images, although there was no obvious difference in the intensity or the extend of soft-tissue uptake (Chi square test: $p > 0.05$). ^{99m}Tc-labeled phosphates are excreted by the kidneys and this accounts for the visualization of the kid-neys on "bone-scanning." Abnormal soft-tissue uptake in the limbs was ob-served in 4/6 AA and 6/6 AL patients, 2 of whom suffered from severe poly-neuropathy with marked reduction of nervce conduction velocity. Soft-tissue uptake in the limbs was not correlated with renal function loss (Wilcoxon's rank sum test: $p > 0.05$). In both patients with macroglossia the scans showed marked uptake in the oropharyngeal region. Uptake in the thyroid gland was seen in 3 AA and 3 AL patients, all of whom had normal thyroid function tests. In patient 3 the thyroid gland was markedly en-

TABLE 1. Clinical, Laboratory, and Scintographic Findings in 6 Patients with AL and 6 Patients with AA Amyloidosis

PAT NO	SEX AGE	TYPE OF AMYLOID	M-comp	NEPHRO[1] PATHY	KIDNEY MDP	KIDNEY PYP	CARDIO[2] MYOPATHY	HEART MDP	HEART PYP	NEURO[3] PATHY	LIMBS MDP	LIMBS PYP	GLOSSO[4] PATHY	TONGUE MDP	TONGUE PYP	LIVER[5] FUNCTION	LIVER MDP	LIVER PYP	SPLEEN MDP	SPLEEN PYP	THYROID[6] FUNCTION	THYROID MDP	THYROID PYP	MALAB-[7] SORPTION	ABDOMEN MDP	ABDOMEN PYP	MISCELL MDP	MISCELL PYP
1	♂48	AL	BJκ	+			+	4	nd	-	2	nd	-	0	nd	Alk ph↑↑	4	nd	4	nd	N	4	nd	-	4	nd	uterus 4	nd
2	♀74	AL	IgAλ	+			±	2	3	+	2	2	-	0	0	N	1	2	0	0	N	4	4	-	0	0		
3	♂54	AL	BJλ	+		99mTc-labeled phosphates are excreted by the kidneys	+	0	0	+	2	2	-	0	0	N	0	0	0	0	[Goiter]	2	3	+	3	2	skin 3	3
4	♀60	AL	IgGλ	+			+	2	2	-	3	3	-	0	0	N	0	0	0	0	N	0	0	-	0	0		
5	♀60	AL	IgAλ	+			+	0	0	-	2	3	+	2	3	N	0	0	0	0	N	0	0	-	0	0		
6	♂51	AL	BJκ	-			+	0	0	-	2	2	+	2	3	N	0	0	0	0	N	0	0	+	3	3		
7	♂42	AA	-	+			-	0	0	-	0	0	-	0	0	N	0	0	0	0	N	3	3	-	0	0		
8	♀63	AA	-	+			-	0	0	-	2	1	-	0	0	Alk ph↑	3	3	3	3	N	0	0	-	0	0		
9	♀61	AA	-	+			-	3	3	-	3	3	-	0	0	Alk ph↑	3	3	3	4	N	4	4	-	0	0		
10	♂72	AA	-	+			-	0	0	-	2	2	-	0	0	N	0	0	0	0	N	3	3	-	2	2		
11	♀53	AA	-	+			±	4	4	-	2	2	-	0	0	N	3	4	3	4	N	0	0	-	3	3		
12	♀33	AA	-	+			-	0	0	-	0	0	-	0	0	N	0	0	0	0	N	0	0	-	0	0		
Explanation of Indices				1=kidney biopsy			2=echocardiography			3=nerve conduct. veloc.			4=physical examination			5=alkaline phosphatase +transaminases					6=serum free thyroxine level+ thyroid stimulating hormone			7=xylose and Vit A test				

TABLE 2. Soft Tissue Uptake of Bone-Seeking Radiopharmaceuticals in
Amyloidosis; Review of the Literature

Tracer	Abnormal findings	Number of patients	Probable type of amyloid	Reference
Tc-MDP	Periarticular uptake	1	AL	Van Antwerp (1975)
Tc-MDP	Hepatic uptake	1	AL	Vanek (1977)
Tc-MDP	Myocardial uptake Skeletal-muscle uptake	2	1 Heredi-tary and 1 AL	Kula (1977)
Tc-MDP	"Soft tissue" uptake	1	AL	Bada (1977)
Tc-MDP	Myocardial uptake "Soft tissue" uptake	1	AL	Braun (1979)
Tc-MDP	Uptake in skin nodules	1	AL	Moyle (1980)
Tc-PYP	Splenic uptake	1	AL	Rao (1981)
Tc-PYP	Hepatic uptake Splenic uptake Myocardial uptake Periarticular uptake	3	AL	Yood (1981)
Tc-MDP	Hepatic uptake	3	AL	Yood (1981)
Tc-PYP	Skeletal-muscle uptake	1	AL	Johnston (1982)
Tc-PYP	Myocardial uptake	10	AL	Wizenberg (1982)
Tc-PYP	Myocardial uptake	1	AL	Schiff (1982)
Tc-PYP	Myocardial uptake	2	AL	Sobol (1982)
Tc-PYP	Myocardial uptake Hepatic uptake	7	AL	Lee (1983)
Tc-MDP	Myocardial uptake Hepatic uptake	7	AL	Lee (1983)
Tc-PYP	Thyroid uptake	2	1 AL 1 AA	Lee (1984)
Tc-MDP	Uptake in: -salivary glands -thyroid gland -heart -liver/spleen -intestine -uterus	1	AL	Janssen (1984)

larged on palpation. Scintigraphic cardiac uptake was present in 5 patients
(3 AL and 2 AA). There was no difference in septum and posterior wall
thickness on echocardiography between the patients with and without cardiac
uptake (Wilcoxon's rank sum test: p > 0.05). Elevation of alkaline phosphatase, which could not be explained by bone activity or active rheumatoid
arthritis, was present in 3/5 patients with hepatic uptake. 2/5 patients
with diffuse abdominal uptake had signs of malabsorption. Uncommon sites
of soft-tissue uptake include the spleen, the uterus, the salivary glands,
and the skin.

DISCUSSION AND CONCLUSIONS

     Reviewing the published data, it is difficult to assess the true sig-
nificance of soft-tissue uptake on "bone-scanning" in amyloidosis (Table 2).
The case reports and small series published so far differ with regard to
the radiopharmaceutical and the scanning technique used.

     In 63% of the cases there was no information concerning the staining
technique used to confirm the diagnosis. In 79% there were no data on the
type of amyloid. In 79% of the patients attention was focussed mainly on
the heart and liver. Soft-tissue uptake on "bone-scanning" has been reported in 38 cases of systemic amyloidosis, 8 of which can be classified as
AL amyloidosis associated with plasma cell dyscrasia. On clinical grounds
28 of the remaining cases can be classified as AL and 1 as AA amyloidosis.
In 1 patient a diagnosis of heredofamilial amyloidosis was made. It is
possible, however, that some reports, in whom the type of amyloid was not
given, include patients with senile cardiac amyloidosis.

     We tried to establish the efficacy of scanning with ^{99m}Tc-labeled phos-
phates in amyloidosis by comparing the results of scintigraphic imaging with
the clinical pattern of organ involvement in 12 well-defined cases of systemic (AA and AL) amyloidosis. In contrast with previous reports we did
find no difference in the extent or the intensity of soft-tissue uptake between Tc-MDP and Tc-PYP images. Image quality (contrast) was generally
better with Tc-MDP than with Tc-PYP. This may be explained by the biologic
characteristics of the two agents (Rudd et al., 1977). Tc-PYP has slightly
lower bone uptake than Tc-MDP and shows significant red cell labeling,
whereas Tc-MDP is confined primarily to the plasma and has higher urinary
excretion than Tc-PYP.

     Our results clearly show that Tc-MDP scanning can play an important
role in evaluating amyloid disease with regard to involvement of the thyroid
gland, the oropharyngeal region, the nervous system, the liver, the spleen,
and the intestinal tract.

     In contrast, scintigraphy which has been claimed to be a sensitive test
for demonstrating amyloid cardiomyopathy (Wizenberg et al., 1982; Lee et al.,
1983) was negative in 3/7 patients with echocardiographic features of amyloid heart disease and positive in 1 patient with a normal echocardiogram.
A possible explanation for this finding might be a more massive deposition
of amyloid in case of cardiac uptake. There was, however, no difference in
diastolic septum and posterior wall thickness between patients with an
without cardiac uptake on scintigraphy. The precise mechanism of amyloid
affinity for phosphates is not known, but it may be explained by the high
calcium content of amyloid, which is due to the presence of the non-fibrillar protein AP. Protein AP is a common constituent of all types of amyloid
and has been demonstrated to bind in vitro to isolated AA and AL fibrils in
a strictly calcium-dependent way.

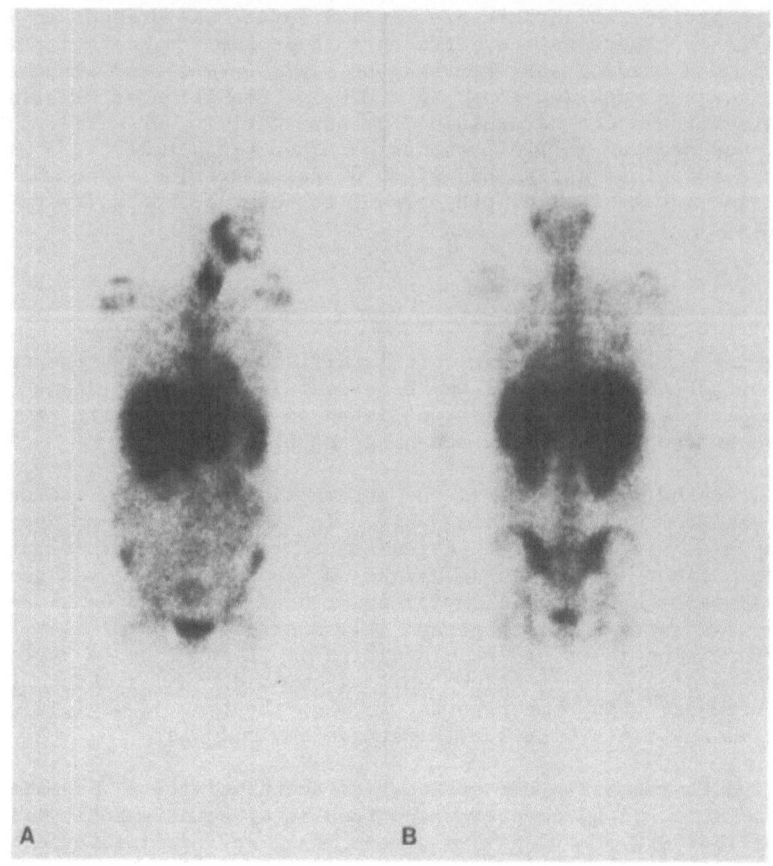

Fig. 1. Whole body scintigraphy with ^{99m}Tc-MDP in patient 1: A = anterior and B = posterior view showing intense uptake in the thyroid, oropharyngeal region, heart, liver, spleen, intestine and uterus.

SUMMARY

1. Scanning with ^{99m}Tc-labeled phosphates is a sensitive non-invasive screening test for the extend or organ involvement in both systemic AA and AL amyloidosis (see Fig. 1).

2. Echocardiography seems to be more sensitive for demonstrating cardiac involvement in systemic amyloidosis than Tc-MDP or Tc-PYP scintigraphy.

3. Tc-MDP images show a better contrast than Tc-PYP images, although there is no obvious difference in the extent or the intensity of soft-tissue uptake.

4. In AA amyloidosis the clinical scene is dominated by nephropathy; the scintigraphic pattern of organ involvement, however, is multisystemic, which is compatible with the histological distribution of amyloid.

REFERENCES

Bada, J. L., Padro, L., and Cervera, C., Lancet, 1:1012 (1977).
Braun, S. D., Lisbona, R., Novalez-Diaz, J. A., and Sniderman, A., Clin. Nucl. Med., 4:244 (1979).

Janssen, S., Van Rijswikj, M. H., Piers, D. A., and De Jong, G. M. Th.,
    Eur. J. Nucl. Med. (1984) (in press).

Johnston, J. B., Rayner, H. L., Trevenen, C., and Greenberg, D., Am. J.
    Hematol., 13:247 (1982).

Kula, R. W., Engel, W. K., and Line, B. R., Lancet, 1:92 (1977).

Lee, V. W., Caldarone, A. G., Falk, R. H., Rubinow, A., and Cohen, A. S.,
    Radiology, 148:239 (1983).

Lee, V. W., Rubinow, A., P-hrson, J., Skinner, M., and Cohen, A. S., J.
    Nucl. Med., 25:468 (1984).

Moyle, J. W., and Spies, S. M., Clin. Nucl. Med., 5:51 (1980).

Rao, B. K., Padmalatha, C., Au Buchon, J., and Lieberman, L. M., Eur. J.
    Nucl. Med., 6:143 (1981).

Rudd, T. G., Allen, D. R., and Harnett, D. E., J. Nucl. Med., 18:872 (1977).

Schiff, S., Bateman, T., Moffatt, R., Davidson, R., and Berman, D., Am.
    Heart J., 103:562 (1982).

Sobol, S. M., Brown, J. M., Bunker, S. R., Patel, J., and Lull, R. J., Am.
    Heart J., 103:563 (1982).

Van Antwerp, J. D., O'Mara, R. E., Pitt, M. J., and Walsh, S., J. Nucl.
    Med., 16:238 (1975).

Vanek, J. A., Cook, S. A., and Bukowski, R. M., J. Nucl. Med., 18:1086
    (1977).

Wizenberg, T. A., Muz, J., Sohn, Y. H., Samlowski, W., and Weissler, A. M.,
    Am. Heart J., 103:468 (1982).

Yood, R. A., Skinner, M., Cohen, A. S., and Lee, V. W., J. Rheumatol., 8:
    760 (1981).

Yood, R. A., Skinner, M., Rubinow, A., Talarico, L., and Cohen, A. S.,
    JAMA, 249:1322 (1983).

PLASMA EXCHANGE IN THE TREATMENT OF PATIENTS

WITH SYSTEMIC AMYLOIDOSIS

C. J. Rosenthal, R. W. Kula,
N. Solomon, and R. DeVita

Departments of Medicine, Neurology, and Radiology
Downstate Medical Center-SUNY
450 Clarkson Avenue
Brooklyn, New York 11203

ABSTRACT

The demonstration of an amyloid degrading activity of human serum
(Kedar et al., 1974) which appears to be defective in patients with amyloidosis led us to assess the possible benefits of plasma exchange through
plasmapheresis in the therapy of advanced systemic amyloidosis. To date,
five patients were enrolled in this program consisting of weekly plasmapheresis of a minimum three units of plasma which were replaced with fresh
frozen plasma. One patient had primary amyloidosis, another one had rapidly
progressing FAP while the other three patients had reactive systemic amyloidosis (RSA) with high SAA levels (11.2, 7.5, 8.3 μg/ml) accompanying
tuberculosis, osteomyelitis, and recurrent tonsillities, respectively. 99m
Technetium-diphosphonate scanning revealed amyloid deposits in the myocardium of three of these patients and in all their liver, spleen, and G.I.
tract.

The exchange procedure was tolerated well by the FAP patient, who underwent 62 exchanges, but was not as well tolerated by the RSA cases who
had an average of only 18.5 exchanges. The major side effects were represented by a sudden drop of their BP at the end of some runs in 7% of cases
and by the development of severe allergic reactions to FFP in 2 cases.
Subjective improvement was significant in the FAP case during the initial
30 exchanges and was modest in the other cases. Objectively, the 99m Tc-
diphosphonate scanning showed a marked decrease of the myocardium labelling
in the FAP patient and one of RSA cases after 10 exchanges. SAA level decreased by 52-65% in all three cases of RSA. Thus, it appears that plasma
exchange could be of some benefit in cases of systemic amyloidosis that do
not develop marked orthostatic hypotension and allergy to plasma.

INTRODUCTION

Despite significant progress during the last three decades in understanding the pathogenesis of systemic amyloidosis, its treatment has re-
amined limited in scope and efficacy.

New agents introduced in the therapy of systemic amyloidosis such as colchicine [1, 2] and DMSO [3] have led only to marginal results.

In an attempt to improve these results we tested the hypothesis that deposition of amyloid in these patients might be due to a deficiency of serum amyloid degrading activity (ADA). Patients were treated with fresh frozen plasma in an attempt to correct this deficiency. The existence of ADA deficiency in systemic amyloidosis was demonstrated by Kedar in 1976 [4] using an agar gel diffusion technique [5] and was confirmed by others [6]. However, since the diffusion technique measuring in vitro enzymatic degradation of amyloid fibrils was found to be somewhat unreliable for monitoring ADA [7], the determination of serum albumin level was instead used for this purpose based on a study showing that it reflected well the variations of the serum ADA in patients with secondary amyloidosis [8].

We attempted to determine if symptomatic and objective improvement could be achieved in patients with systemic amyloidosis through plasma exchange and to establish the best way to monitor the variation of ADA of serum in these patients.

METHODS

Plasma exchange procedure was performed using the Hemonetics (Braintree, MS) plasmapheresis apparatus-model 30, which permitted removal of an average of 500 ml blood its centrifugation, the return of the packed red cells to the patient and concomitant infusion of 250 ml fresh frozen plasma. Four complete cycles were generally performed. ADC anticoagulant (60 ml) was used with each cycle to avoid clotting. All patients with systemic amyloidosis who had evidence of progression of their disease for a period of at least three months were considered eligible for plasma exchange. Significant orthostatic hypotensive (more than 40 mm Hg drop) and a hematocrit lower than the level required to avoid the loss of more than 15% of the plasma volume precluded the performance of plasma exchange. These contraindications were, however, generally correctable. Absolute contraindications included intractable congestive heart failure and known anaphylaxis to plasma or plasma products.

Patients on Study

To date, five patients with systemic amyloidosis, covering almost the whole spectrum of this group of disease, were entered in this study after signing appropriate consent.

- A 38 year old white male with primary amyloidosis (immunocytic dyscrasia not overtly neoplastic) [9] with a lambda light chain in his urine. He presented with diarrhea, evidence of peripheral neuropathy with orthostatic hypotension and documented amyloid involvement of his adrenal glands requiring replacement therapy with gluco- and mineral-cortico steroids. Renal failure developed before he was entered into the plasma exchange program.

- A 29 year old male of Ashkenazi Jewish extraction who presented typical manifestations and course of familial amyloidotic polyneuropathy of the Andrade type (progressive polyneuropathy diarrhea, impotence, vitreous deposition of amyloid); his father died of amyloidosis at age 45; patient received DMSO three months prior to his enrollment in the plasma exchange program.

- A 24 year old white male with reactive systemic amyloidosis (RSA) due to extrapulmonary tuberculosis and chronic glomerulonephritis, who presented with marked hepatomegaly and nephrotic syndrome which resolved when renal failure developed prior to patient's entry in the plasma exchange program.

- A 21 year old white male with RSA apparently caused by frequent recurrent tonsillitis and a limited form of juvenile rheumatoid arthritis, who also presented with marked hepatomegaly and nephrotic syndrome. He developed persistent diarrhea and renal failure requiring hemodialysis, prior to his entry in the plasma exchange program and had also previously received DMSO and colchicine.

- A 67 year old white male with RSA following a 10 year course of rheumatoid arthritis. He presented with marked hepatomegaly and moderate diarrhea at the time of his entry in the exchange transfusion program.

In order to asses patient response to plasma exchange a number of parameters have been followed. The subjective improvement of patients' symptoms and performance status were graded following the Karnofsky's scale [10] before and after treatment. Denistometric measurement of the soft tissue distribution of injected 99 m Technetium diphosphonate including heart, were normally this isotope is not retained [11] was also determined in three of the patients on study before the plasma was started and at the discontinuation of the program or after each 10 exchanges. The localization of this gamma emitting isotope was determined using a light transmission densitometer (Macbeth, N. Y.) for reading of routine scanning radiograms obtained by a Picker 4-15 Auger camera.

The following serum parameters were determined at the patients' entry in this program and after every other exchange: serum albumin, due to its previously demonstrated correlation with ADA [8]; serum prealbumin [11] and serum amyloid A (SAA) which were previously found to monitor disease activity, especially in patients with RSA (as a negative and respectively positive determinant of the acute phase reaction [12]); this serum alkaline phosphatase, lactic dehydrogenase (LDH) and glutanic oxalate transaminase (SGOT) reflecting the liver function before and after several plasma exchanges.

Serum prealbumin was determined by radial immunodiffusion. SAA was quantitated by a liquid phase RIA [13]. The remaining parameters were determined by an automatic processor (Technicon II, Tarrytown, N. Y.).

Statistical Analysis

Coefficients of correlation were determined among the above mentioned parameters, the performance status (PS), and the serum albumin which was previously shown to correlate closely with the variations of the serum ADA. The Pearson product moment correlation coefficient [14] was calculated for five values of each of the parameters followed in each of the five patients. Then the weighted averages of the correlation coefficient were determined and their statistical significance calculated [15].

RESULTS

Tolerance and Side Effects of the Plasma Exchange

To date, 118 plasma exchanges were performed in the five evaluable patients. The procedure was generally well tolerated. The patient with FAP

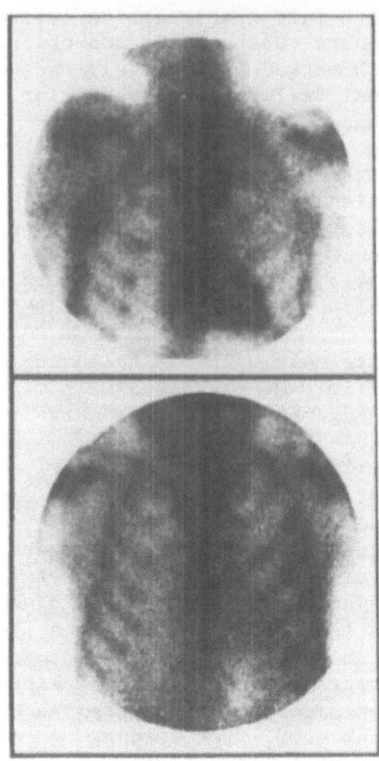

Fig. 1. Comparison of the 99m-
Technetium diphosphon-
ate uptake over the
chest structures in a
patient with FAP before
(upper image) and after
(lower image) 30 plasma
exchanges. The disap-
pearance of the myo-
cardium uptake on the
bottom picture is evi-
dent.

underwent 62 exchanges and is still continuing the program. The patient
with primary amyloidosis underwent 10 exchanges after which the procedure
had to be discontinued due to the persistence of severe orthostatic hypotension despite replacement therapy for his adrenal insufficiency. The patients with reactive systemic amyloidosis underwent an average of 16.5 exchanges. Two of them developed significant allergic reactions to fresh
frozen plasma manifested by urticaria and Quick'es edema which forced us
to discontinue the plasma exchange in one case and to take special precau-
tions in the other case (administration of 50 mg diphenhydramine hydrochloride [Benedryl] i.v. before the plasma infusion).

Side effects of the procedure included, besides the previously mentioned ones: short lasting hypotensive episodes in 7% of all exchanges,
easily correctable by adjusting the flow of the exchange, parasthesias of
the extremities in 11% of exchanges and a cytomegolic virus (CMV) infection
in one case.

Effect of Plasma Exchange on Patients' Amyloid
Deposition and on Their General Conditions

Among the parameters used to determine patient response to therapy, two had independent value and suggested some degree of improvement in all patients. The change in the densitometry of 99 m Technetium diphosphonate localization over soft tissues and especially over the heart showed a significant decrease in the patient with FAP (see Fig. 1) and in one of the patients with RSA (Table 1). Another patient with RSA had only a modest decrease (Table 1). In two patients, no soft tissue scanning studies were performed.

Patient performance status (PA), which correlated less closely with the variation of amyloid deposition and formation, also reflected a moderate improvement in all patients during the duration of the exchange program (Table 1). All patients seemed to improve their physical endurance and to complain less frequently of dizziness. This improvement occurred in patient B.H. with FAP, over the longest period of time (approximately 30 weeks). Beyond this, the serum parameters remained stable with modest irregular fluctuations while the patient's peripheral neuropathy gradually progressed.

In the other cases, no leveling off in improvement was noted although none of them received as many as 30 exchanges. One patient died after 10 exchanges due to causes unrelated to the plasma exchange (bacterial meningitis and pulmonary cryptococcosis). Another two patients developed severe allergic reactions to plasma infusion. The plasma exchange was discontinued in one of them after 26 exchanges at a time when he still showed some benefit and was just recently restarted in the other case after being discontinued at the time of the 18th exchange. Finally, the most recent patient with RSA has reached only his 10th exchange and is still showing signs of improvement.

A third parameter, the serum albumin was shown to closely parallel the ADA of serum and consistently improved in all patients receiving the plasma exchange by an average of 702 mg over the first 10 exchanges.

Among the other serum parameters measured, only serum prealbumin, serum amyloid A and serum lactic dehydrogenase levels appeared to correlate with the variations of the previously mentioned parameters (Table 1). When the Pearson's product moment coefficient of correlation [15] was determined for these parameters it has a fair correlation with the performance status (Table 2). When the weighted averages of the correlation coefficients were compared (Table 2), statistical significant at a $p < 0.01$ was found for the negative correlation of SAA level with patient's performance status and significance at a $p < 0.02$ level was found for the positive correlation of the other parameters (prealbumin, LDH and albumin) with the performance status. The correlation of serum albumin with the other three serum parameters has been at the highest level of significance ($p < 0.01$) for all three parameters.

DISCUSSION

Plasma exchange is a modern version of an old therapeutic modality, which has been increasingly tested as a temporary therapeutic solution in a variety of diseases for which no definitive treatment is available while their pathogenetic events were found either secondary to some deleterious substance circulating in patients' blood or appeared primarily correlated to the deficiency of a degrading enzyme with protective effects. Thrombotic thrombocytopenia purpura (TTP) is the typical example of a disease included

TABLE 1. Variations of the Performance Status (PS), Technetium Scanning Densitometry and of Serum Parameters Presenting Unidirectional Changes in Patients with Amyloidosis Undergoing Plasma Exchange

Name	Age	Type of amyloidosis	Albumin gm/dl	Prealbumin mg/dl	SAA µd/gl	LDH µ/dl	PS	Tc scan densitom.
BH	29	Her. (FAP)	3.3	23.2	.535	199	6	0.86
			3.5	24.5	.515	201	6.	
			3.7	23	.490	202	7	0.30
			3.9	28.5	.525	204	7	
			4.1 (0.7)*	32.1 (+8.9)	.420 (-.115)	220 (+21)	8 (+2)†	0.32 (-2.8)
BM	38	Prim. (AL)	2.8	13.2	.745	172	4	
			2.95	15.8	.720	185	4	
			3.3	18.2	.620	192	4.	
			3.4	21.0	.580	190	5	
			3.45 (+.65)	23.2 (+10)	.585 (-.160)	210 (+38)	5 (+1)	
MP	24	RSA Sec. (AA)	2.4	18.5	11.250	168	8	0.76
			2.7	21.2	8.120	179	8	
			2.9	26.2	5.780	179	8.5	
			3.2	25.8	4.350	188	9	
			3.4 (+1.0)	31.3 (+12.8)	4.980 (-6.971)	190 (+22)	9 (+1)	0.29 (-2.6)
HB	21	RSA Sec. (AA)	2.8	12.4	8.320	202	7	
			2.9	14.7	7.080	204	7	
			3.15	16.2	6.720	204	6	
			3.25	19.4	5.210	215	8	
			3.30 (+0.50)	19.6 (+7.2)	4.250 (-4.071)	220 (+18)	8 (+1)	
SS	67	RSA Sec. (AA)	2.4	11.5	7.550	165	7	0.62
			2.7	13.8	6.700	168	7	
			2.8	16.2	4.350	178	8	
			2.85	16.3	3.820	180	8	
			3.05 (+.65)	18.4 (+6.9)	2.410 (-5.141)	179 (+14)	9 (+2)	0.37 (-1.7)

*The values in parenthesis in the first 5 columns indicate the positive or negative difference between the highest and lowest values.

†The values in parentheses in this column indicate the number by which the ^{32}Technetium radioactive densitometry has decreased during the plasma exchange program.

TABLE 2. Correlation Coefficients of the Variation of Patients' Performance Status and Serum Albumin Level with Other Serum Parameters during Plasma Exchange in Patients with Systemic Amyloidosis

Patient	Performance status vs.				Serum albumin vs.		
	Albumin	Prealbumin	SAA	LDH	Prealbumin	SAA	LDH
BH	.945	.808	-.861	.889	.874	-.763	.840
BM	.775	.875	-.796	.679	.960	-.994	.861
MP	.381	.226	-.615	.402	.950	-.926	.974
HB	.435	.613	-.667	.822	.968	-.933	.847
SS	.891	.940	-.931	.858	.983	-.944	.867
Average*	.770	.778	-.808	.774	.957	-.946	.896
p <	0.02	0.02	0.01	0.01	0.01	0.01	0.01

*Average represents the weight average of the correlation coefficients of each of the analyzed parameters.

in the latter category whose therapy has significantly benefited from plasma exchange. It was for this reason that when Kedar et al. [4] described the deficiency of an amyloid degrading activity in the serum of most patients with systemic amyloidosis, we thought that plasma exchange with the purpose of adding sufficient amounts of plasma with ADA without causing fluid overload could lead to a successful therapeutic approach in amyloidosis. In practice, the efficacy of the plasma exchange trials in the five patients studied, to date, has been less significant than in TTP. Nevertheless, all of them showed some subjective improvement for the duration of at least the first 20 exchanges. In two out of three patients in whome desnitometric determinations of 99m Technetium diphosphonate uptake by soft tissues was measured, a significant decrease localization was clearly noted indicating a decrease in the amount of locally deposited amyloid. This decrease could likely be explained by the persistence of local tissue degradation of the deposited amyloid by macrophages while the deposition of new material is blocked by the infused ADA. If this observation would be confirmed there is hope that by administering agents capable of rapidly and completely destroying or blocking the circulating precursors of amyloid fibrils (enzymes, monoclonal antibodies to the precursor, etc.), amyloidosis could become a curable disease.

From the observations obtained from the patient with FAP who received plasma exchanges for more than one year, it appears that the maximum benefit (subjectively and by 99m Tc-diphosphonate scanning studies) is achieved after 25-30 exchanges. Thereafter, the densitometry of the soft tissues remained unchanged while progression of his peripheral neuropathy was noted. This observation suggests that plasma exchange should be continued for at least 30 exchanges.

The complications of this plasma exchange program have been generally of moderate degree (paraesthesias, occasional transient hypotension, one infestation with cytomegalic virus) and rapidly correctable. However, in two patients, allergic reactions to fresh frozen plasma (FFP) have been severe requiring discontinuation of therapy. The relatively high incidence of these allergic reactions was likely coincidental; they occur in only 5-8% of all cases receiving FFP [17].

One problem that we faced during this study was the quantitation of AA of serum. Preliminary experiments with the agar gel diffusion assay in Petri dishes found this quantitation difficult to reproduce and interpret. For this reason we decided to evaluate the ADA of the serum from the values of serum albumin found by Maury and Teppo [8] to have a close correlation with those of serum ADA. A good correlation of the SAA, albumin, prealbumin and LDH levels in the serum was found with patients' performance status. SAA and prealbumin appear to have a very good correlation with serum albumin in these patients (p < 0.01) which suggest that they could be used interchangeably to monitor patient's response to plasma exchange. These data remain to be confirmed in direct experiments when the ADA of serum will be purified and chemically characterized.

The nature of the serum ADA is not yet fully known and was not the object of this study. It was shown to be related in one study [18] to serine protease which co-migrates with albumin on agarose gel electrophoresis; others have related it primarily to serine proteases associated with the outer membrane of the circulating monocytes [19] and to the neutrophil elastase (Skinner et al., unpublished observation).

Overall, plasma exchange in systemic amyloidosis performed on a limited scale appears to at least delay further deterioration of patients' general conditions and the further deposition of amyloid. For this reason plasma exchange therapy in systemic amyloidosis warrants further study.

REFERENCES AND NOTES

1. S. E. Goldfinger, New Engl. J. Med., 287:1302 (1972).
2. D. Zemer, M. Ravach, et al., New Engl. J. Med., 291:932 (1974).
3. E. F. Osserman, T. Isobe, and M. Farhangi, in: Amyloidosis (O. Wegelius and A. Pasternack, eds.), Academic Press, London (1976), p. 247.
3. I. Kedar, E. Sohar, and J. Gafni, Proc. Soc. Exper. Biol., 145:343 (1974).
5. I. Kedar, M. Ravid, and E. Sohar, in: Amyloid and Amyloidosis (G. G. Glenner, P. P. Costa, and F. Freitas, eds.), Excerpta Media, Amsterdam-Oxford-Princeton (1980), p. 60.
6. O. Wegelius, A. M. Teppo, and C. P. J. Maury, Br. Med. J., 284:617 (1982).
7. D. Caspi, M. I. Baltz, A. Feinstein, E. A. Mann, and M. P. Peppys, unpublished observation.
8. C. P. Maury and A. M. Teppo, Lancet ii, 234 (1982).
9. G. G. Glenner, New Engl. J. Med., 302 (1983).
10. J. Karnofsky, in: Working Conference in Anorexia, Cancer Res., 30: 2816 (1970).
11. R. W. Kula, W. K. Engel, and B. R. Line, Lancet ii, 92 (1977).
12. W. P. Bradley, A. P. Blasco, J. Weiss, et al., Cancer, 40:2264 (1977).
13. C. J. Rosenthal and E. C. Franklin, J. Clin. Inv., 55:746 (1975).
14. G. Snadecor and W. Cochrane, in: Statistical Methods (G. Snadecor and W. Cochrane, eds.), Iowa State Univ. Press (1967), p. 187.
15. A. K. Bahn, in: Basic Medical Statistics (A. K. Bahn, ed.), Grune and Stratton, Inc., New York (1972), p. 178.
16. H. G. Mertens, in: Plasma Exchange Therapy (H. Bomberg and P. Reuther, eds.), Thieme-Verlag-Stratton, Inc., Stuttgart-New York (1981), p. VII.
17. F. R. Seiler, H. Karges, R. Geursen, and H. H. Sedlacek, in: Plasma Therapy (H. Bomberg and R. Reuther, eds.), Thieme-Verlag-Stratton, Inc., Stuttgart-New York, (1981), p. 37.
18. A. M. Teppo, C. P. J. Maury, and O. Wegelius, Scand. J. Immun., 16:309 (1982).
19. G. Lavie, D. Zucker-Franklin, and E. C. Franklin, J. Exp. Med., 148: 1020 (1979).
20. We gratefully acknowledge the excellent assistance of Ms. S. Amrani in preparing this manuscript.

ACKNOWLEDGEMENTS

This study was supported, in part, by NIH Grant No. 5R01AM2008006.

H. AGING AND AMYLOIDOSIS

RESEARCH IN AGING AND AMYLOIDOSIS

Evan Calkins

Division of Geriatrics/Gerontology
Department of Medicine
State University of New York at Buffalo
Buffalo, New York

The relationship of amyloid and aging has received little attention in previous International Conferences on Amyloidosis. With the development of new methodologies, and the increasing recognition, throughout the World, of the importance of research related to aging, this relative void is now being addressed, as attested to by the presentations to follow.

In the design of studies on amyloid and aging investigators are urged to differentiate factors representing the passage of time from those reflecting biological changes of aging. In addition, awareness of recent investigations in the biological changes which characterize the aging process may provide useful perspectives for the study of the nature and pathogenesis of this form of amyloidosis.

RESEARCH IN AGING AND AMYLOIDOSIS

108 years have elapsed since Soyka's initial description of cardiac amyloidosis in aged persons [1]; 57 years have passed since Divry described the birefringence of Congo red stained amyloid in senile plaques [2]. Numerous publications have confirmed the fact that the most frequently encountered forms of amyloid accumulation in humans, and in a number of other species, are those which are related to old age. It is paradoxical, however, that reference to this topic in the earlier International Conferences on Amyloidosis have been exceedingly sparse. Of the 42 presentations at the first Conference, held in Groningen, The Netherlands, in 1968, only two mentioned the relationship of amyloid and aging [3]. Twenty papers on amyloidosis were included in XXth Colloquium on the Protides of the Biological Fluids in Bruges, Belgium, in 1974 [4]; three related to aging. Of the 48 studies presented at the International Conference on Amyloidosis in Helsinki only one made any reference to amyloid and aging.

It was not until 4 years ago, at the Conference at Povoa de Varzim, that this association began to emerge as a significant consideration in this series of Conferences. Presentations at that meeting included differentiation of two types of cardiac amyloidosis, as evidenced by distinctive immunohistologic reactions (Westermark et al. [5]); clinical aspects of senile as differentiated from other forms of cardiac amyloidosis (Wright and Calkins [6]); and the identification of a Congophilic substance in the cartilage of the sternoclavicular joint of most elderly persons (Uchino et al. [7]). Cerebrovascular amyloid was referred to in a single report by Mandybur [8]. The possible importance of senile amyloidosis was recognized, however, by its inclusion within the proposed new classification system [9].

It should be stressed that the paucity of presentations concerning the relationship of amyloid and aging, at these Conferences did not reflect the interest in this topic in the published literature. Over the past 20 years there have been numerous publications of clinical-pathological descriptions of senile cardiac amyloidosis [10-12]. The detailed histologic, histochemical, and immunohistologic studies of Terry, Katzman, Wisniewski and others [13-15] have delineated, further, the presence of amyloid as a component of the anatomical lesions in the brain of many persons of advanced age, especially those with senile dementia of the Alzheimer type. The relative lack of interest in the part of investigators, committed to the study of the nature and pathogenesis of amyloidosis per se, in the age-related forms of amyloid, probably reflects three factors. These are: first, initial failure to recognize the frequency and wide distribution of the senile forms of amyloidosis; second, serious and continuing questions concerning the clinical significance of these amyloid deposits; and third, the fact that senile amyloid accumulations, usually occurring in trace amounts, present an inconvenient model for chemical and structural characterization of amyloid and for study of mechanisms of pathogenesis.

As this IV th International Conference will attest, this relative void is now being addressed. In part this is due to the development of new methodologies and in part to the increasing world wide acceptance of problems related to aging as a topic of major societal importance. Several well established amyloid research groups are now giving increasing attention to the problem of amyloid and aging. We also welcome, at this symposium, the participation of a number of investigators who have not joined in earlier conferences in this series. Additional evidence of the importance of this topic is the encouragement and financial support we have received from the National Institute on Aging, through its award of a grant in partial support for this portion of the Conference.

As the relationship of amyloidosis and, presumably, amyloidogenesis and aging begin to emerge as a topic of interest at this Conference and future Conferences, several perspectives derived from studies of the field of aging per se may prove helpful. The first is the need to differentiate the influence of time from that of aging. Obviously, a disease which requires, for its development, a passage of time which occupies a significant portion of the individual's life will occur with increasing frequency in the elderly members of the species. For example, the impact of a several decades-long history of smoking on the increased incidence of a number of chronic diseases, including emphysema, atherosclerosis and osteoporosis is now recognized. Each of these diseases has, in itself, been associated with advancing age. However, the role of smoking, in the etiology of these conditions, does not appear to represent an age-related phenomenon. There is, to my knowledge, no evidence that smoking is more hazardous in a healthy elderly person than in a young adult. Instead, evidence suggests that it is the decades of exposure to the toxic materials in tobacco smoke that account for the influence of smoking in the genesis of these conditions.

A similar relationship may also be operational in the case of senile cardiac amyloidosis. While the appearance of this disorder among elderly persons may represent a <u>direct</u> association between aging and amyloidogenesis, it should also be born in mind that, in this form of amyloidosis, in contrast to amyloid AL, the small intramyocardial vessels tend to be spared [16]. If one were to postulate that the lethal effects of amyloidosis are related, particularly, to involvement of these small vessels, this relative sparing in senile amyloidosis may explain why the duration of this disorder from its initial symptoms to death is much longer than in the case of amyloidosis AL, and the hearts considerably larger. We are aware of one instance in which a person who ultimately died of senile cardiac amyloidosis with massive amyloid infiltration of the heart initially presented radiologic evidence of cardiac enlargement 40 years previously, during a routine physical examination. Thus, the advanced age of persons with this disorder may reflect the time required for the evolution of the disease process and not specific biological phenomena related to aging.

Depsite the need to differentiate the influence of aging, and that of time, it is likely that several of the so-called senile amyloid syndromes are, indeed, associated with aging per se. It seems reasonable to predict that the pathogenetic mechanisms involved in the development of these syndromes will prove to have a close relationship with the fundamental biological changes associated with aging. As studies of amyloidosis, we should consider, in designing studies of pathogenetic mechanisms operational in this condition, the biological changes that have been identified as having a close relationship with the aging process.

For example, a number of investigators have provided evidence that the biological processes of aging may be mediated, at least in part, by intracellular accumulation of free radicals [17, 18]. A possible relationship of this mechanism to the genesis of amyloidosis was proposed by Denman Harmon [19] in a study which showed that the administration of an antioxidant, Santoquin, to mice during the course of development of casein-induced amyloidosis resulted in an increased life span. Although the autopsy data, presented, are difficult to interpret, the authors concluded that the Santoquin treatment resulted in a decrease in the amount of amyloid formed. The study to be reported by Cathcart, in this symposium, is relevant in this context [20]. The earlier finding of an association between x-ray therapy and subsequent development of amyloidosis [21] may also be explainable on this basis. It is known that a high fat diet leads to increased free radicals [22]. The high incidence of amyloidosis in leprosy patients at Carville, LA, where a high fat diet is the rule, as compared with control patients in Guadalajara, Mexico, may possibly be explainable on this basis [23].

The above studies are cited, not because the data are conclusive, but to illustrate how the study of pathogenetic mechanisms, thought to be operational in aging, may also apply to investigations of pathogenesis of age-related forms of amyloidosis.

Three other mechanisms, which have been regarded as important concomitants if not determinants of the aging process deserve mention. One is the concept that aging is associated with the gradual accumulation, both intracellularly and extracellularly, of complex molecules that undergo cross-linking [24, 25]. With advancing age, there is a gradual disappearance of reversible cross-links between collagen fibrils, and an increase in stable linkage compounds [26]. Coupled with this, is a decreased susceptibility to degradation by a variety of agents.

Advancing age appears to be accompanied by a progressive alteration in immunologic responsiveness, including the development of autoantibodies [27] an increase in helper-inducing T-cells, a diminution of T-cell responsiveness to mitogens and a decrease in the capacity to form certain important mediators, such as Interleuken 1 [28, 29]. The potential interface between these various mechanisms and amyloid formation are currently being explored [30, 31]. Other examples of age-related changes in cell metabolism include the relationship between the longevity of a given species and the ability to repair damage to DMA [32], and also the implications of the so-called Hayflick effect [33, 34]. As greater understanding is achieved concerning the biochemical basis of cell behavior during aging, the potential application of these findings to our understanding of the pathogenesis of age-related diseases [35, 36], including senile amyloidosis, should provide fruitful areas for future investigations.

REFERENCES

1. J. Soyka, Prag. Med. Swchr., 1:165 (1876).
2. P. Divry and M. Florkin, CR Soc. Biol. (Paris), 97:1808 (1927).
3. E. Mandema, L. Ruinen, J. H. S. Scholten, A. S. Cohen, in: Amyloidosis (Excerpta Medica, Amsterdam, 1967).
4. H. Peeters, Protides of the Biological Fluids. XXTh Colloquium (Pergamon Press, Oxford, 1972).
5. P. Westermark, et al., in: Amyloid and Amyloidosis, G. G. Glenner, P. Pe Costa, F. D. Freitas (Excerpta Medica, Amsterdam, 1980), p. 217.
6. J. R. Wright, E. Calkins, A. I. Ozdemir, ibid., p. 17.
7. F. Uchino, H. Nakamura, T. Kamai, T. Nagasawa, ibid., p. 55.
8. T. Mandybur, ibid., p. 231.
9. E. P. Benditt, A. S. Cohen, P. P. Costa, E. C. Franklin, G. G. Glenner, G. Husby, E. Mandema, J. B. Natvig, E. F. Osserman, E. Sohar, O. Wegelius, P. Westermark, ibid., p. XI.
10. L. Buerger and H. Braustein, Am. J. Med., 28:357 (1960).
11. J. R. Wright and E. Calkins, J. Am. Geriat. Soc., 23:97 (1975).
12. G. G. Cornwell, III, W. L. Murdoch, R. A. Kyle, P. Westermark, P. Pitkanen, Am. J. Med., 75:618 (1983).
13. H. M. Wisniewski, A. B. Johnson, C. S. Raine, W. J. Kaye, R. D. Terry, Lab. Invest., 23:287 (1970).
14. H. M. Wisniewski, K. Harash, H. K. Narang, R. D. Terry, J. Neurol. Sci., 27:173 (1976).
15. G. G. Glenner, in: Alzheimer's Disease: Senile Dementia and Related Disorders, R. Katzman, R. D. Terry, K. L. Beck (Raven Press, New York, 1978), p. 493.
16. J. R. Wright and E. Calkins, Medicine, 60:429 (1981).
17. D. Harman, Proc. Nat. Acad. Sci., 78:7124 (1981).
18. R. F. Del Maestro, Acta Physiol. Scand. Suppl., 492:153 (1980).
19. D. Harman, D. E. Eddy, J. Noffsinger, J. Am. Geriat. Soc., 24:203 (1976).
20. E. S. Cathcart, S. Meydani, K. C. Hayes, This Symposium (1984).
21. H. E. Christensen, G. H. Hjort, Acta Path. Microbiol. Scand., 47:410 (1959).
22. C. H. Lea, in: Symposium on Foods: Lipids and their Oxidation, H. H. Schultz, E. A. Day, R. O. Sinnhuber (Avi Publish. Co., Westport, Connecticut, 1962), p. 3.
23. R. C. Williams, Jr., E. S. Cathcart, A. S. Cohen, E. Calkins, J. Barba Rubio, G. L. Fite, Ann. Int. Med., 62:100 (1965).
24. J. Bjorksten, J. Am. Geriat. Sco., 16:408 (1968).
25. D. R. Eyre, Science, 207:1315 (1980).
26. D. Fujimoto, T. Moriguchi, T. Ishida, H. Hayashi, Biochem. Res. Commun., 84:52 (1978).
27. B. Hooper, S. Whittingham, J. Mathews, I. Mackay, D. Curnow, J. Exp. Immunol., 12:79 (1972).
28. M. M. B. Kay, T. Makinodan, Prog. Allergy, 29:134 (1981).

29. G. W. Siskind and M. E. Weksler, in: Annual Review of Geriatrics and Gerontology, C. Eisdorfer, Volume 3 (New York, Springer Publishing Co., 1983), p. 3.
30. J. D. Sipe, S. N. Vogel, M. B. Sztein, M. Skinner, A. S. Cohen, Ann. NY Acad. Sci., 389:131 (1982).
31. A. S. Cohen, T. Shirahama, J. D. Sipe, M. Skinner, Lab. Invest., 48:1 (1983).
32. R. W. Hart and R. B. Setlow, Proc. Nat. Acad. Sci., 71:2169 (1974).
33. L. Hayflick and P. S. Moorehead, Exp. Cell Res., 25:585 (1961).
34. M. Reff and E. L. Schneider, Molec. Cell. Biochem., 36:169 (1981).
35. S. Goldstein, J. Invest. Derm., 73:19 (1979).
36. W. T. Brown, J. B. Little, J. Epstein, J. R. Williams, Birth Defects: Original article Series, 14:417 (1978). The National Foundation.

AMYLOID AND AGING - AN HYPOTHESIS INVOLVING SO-CALLED

AMYLOID DEGRADING ACTIVITY (ADA)

John R. Wright* and Evan Calkins†

*Department of Pathology
 204 Farber Hall
 SUNYAB, Buffalo, New York   14214

†Department of Medicine
 Division of Geriatrics
 Room 602C
 Veterans Administration Medical Center
 3495 Bailey Avenue
 Buffalo, New York   14215

ABSTRACT

Many studies have now documented amyloid accumulation as an almost universal tissue change in aging man. Although this accumulation differs in many respects from that observed in the classic forms of systemic amyloidosis and, with a few notable exceptions, its clinical significance is open to question, an understanding of amyloid deposition in the elderly may advance not only general amyloid research but may provide important insight into the basic biology of aging itself.

In contrast to the other forms of generalized amyloid deposition, this process in the elderly is not only strikingly age-related but the biochemical nature of the major fibril protein appears, at least in many instances, to vary with anatomic site. Also, present evidence suggests that the various forms of age-related amyloid deposits are not associated with significant overproduction of any of the known amyloid-precursor protein species.

Based upon these observations and upon some preliminary experiments, assessing amyloid degrading activity (ADA) in both amyloid agar plates and in tissue sections, we have developed and are exploring an hypothesis which may apply not only to age-related amyloidosis but also may relate to more basic alterations in the physico-chemical properties of aging interstitial and connective tissues.

INTRODUCTION

Over the past 20 years, various investigators [1-4] have recognized amyloid accumulation as a frequent and perhaps universal concomitant of human aging. The major sites of involvement include the cardiovascular system, lungs, central nervous system stem, genitourinary system and the endocrine system [2, 4]. Recently, additional, possibly related, instances of amyloid deposition have been observed in association with degenerating intervertebral disc disease [5] and even in degenerating prosthetic heart valves [6]. In several of these sites, including the cardiovascular and central nervous systems, amyloid deposition is strikingly age related, increasing in frequency with each advancing decade of life. If examined at autopsy, many elderly individuals will exhibit amyloid deposition in multiple organ sites, suggesting a systemic process similar to that regularly observed in AL and AA amyloid protein deposition. There is, however, convincing evidence that these multiple organ deposits are not all directly inter-related. For example, from autopsy population studies, amyloid deposits in the cardiovascular system appear to occur earlier than do cerebral deposits, although after age 75 the latter increase in frequency at a more rapid pace [7]. Furthermore, the presence of cardiovascular amyloid does not correlate with the presence cerebral amyloid deposits. Both genitourinary and endocrine amyloidosis also appear to accumulate at differing time periods. None of these forms of amyloid appear to increase in frequency when associated with disease states, specifically rheumatoid arthritis and multiple myeloma, which are known to predispose to the AL or AA amyloid syndromes [8, 9].

Unfortunately, with the possible exception of senile cardiac amyloid [10, 11], the paucity of amyloid in any given anatomic site has rendered biochemical characterization of the fibril protein involved extremely difficult. To date, much of the evidence for the nature of these amyloid deposits is indirect, and to a large extent based upon immunohistochemical observations [12-15]. The latter, together with the evidence already cited, strongly support the notion that "senile amyloidosis" represents a group of syndromes in which the amyloid proteins are of diverse biochemical origin, each having a propensity to deposit in specific organs or organ system. Whether these amyloid deposits arise from locally produced protein precursors or whether the precursors circulate systemically is unknown, although in all probability both mechanisms are operative. There is certainly no evidence, to date, that any of these amyloid deposits are derived from biologically unique protein species. Since by definition these amyloid proteins represent antiparallel cross-beta-pleated sheets, they are insoluble in biologic environments and once formed they show little tendency to disappear.

In general, amyloid deposition would appear to involve either excessive formation of insoluble beta-pleated sheets, or a defect in the host's ability to dispose of these protein conformations, either as they are formed or once they have been deposited in tissues. In the classic amyloid syndromes, associated with increased monoclonal light chain (AL) or acute phase reactant production (AA), a major component of the problem, obviously, is excess beta-pleated sheet formation. In the elderly, where no obvious overproduction of protein is evident, where the process is almost universal, and where so many different forms of amyloid protein appear to accumulate, the major problem in at least some instances may well be a decreased ability to degrade what might represent an otherwise normal biologic load of beta-pleated sheet protein by-product.

Thus emerges an hypothesis which may explain some of the unique and confounding aspects of amyloid accumulation in the elderly. To have survived the ravages of evolution, biologic organisms, including man must have developed a mechanism for dealing with, and/or disposing of, proteins that become insoluble by virtue of assuming a potentially damaging secondary structure such as a total beta-pleated sheet. If this were not the case, normal catabolism of proteins containing this secondary structure, or otherwise having the propensity to assume such a configuration, would render us all "amyloidotic". This protective process may have developed from rather simple origins - perhaps with the ability of normal serum to denature, and solubilize, circulating beta pleated sheets. Is it possible that a decline in this normal mechanism or process, as a function of age, could explain at least some of the amyloid deposits observed so commonly in the elderly?

That man does have the ability to alter certain beta-pleated sheets has been shown recently by the discovery of a circulating amyloid degrading activity (ADA) and corresponding inhibitors [16-22]. As referred to previously in this symposium, using a technique in which amyloid fibrils are suspended in agar, it can be shown that ADA is present in the sera of normal individuals but is lost or inhibited in some patients suffering from systemic AA (secondary) amyloidosis. To date most investigators have utilized protein AA as the test substrate. Indeed, in the one published instance in which protein AL was used as a substrate serum amyloid degrading activity could not be demonstrated [21].

Using a modification of the method originally described by Kedar et al. [18] we have attempted to assess serum ADA against several AL proteins as well as against protein AA. In addition, a newly devised histochemical method appears to duplicate this phenomenon in tissue sections and may be useful in assessing ADA against small tissue deposits of other forms of amyloid which are unsuitable for the aga-plate method. Preliminary results from these studies form the basis of this report.

METHODS

A. Preparation of Amyloid Agar Plates

Using both the Cohen-Calkin's [23] and the Pras [24] methods, amyloid fibrils were obtained from frozen organ tissues previously determined to contain either AA or AL amyloid on the basis of clinical presentation of the patient, organ distribution of the amyloid deposits and upon potassium permanganate sensitivity [25, 26].

Amyloid agar plates were prepared using a modification of the method described by Kedar et al. [18]. Approximately 200 mgms of fibril protein was dispersed in 100 ml aqueous Noble agar to which thymol was added in order to retard bacterial growth. Ten ml of the mixture was poured into 60 × 15 mm plastic petri dishes, allowed to cool and stored at 4°C. In each agar plate three wells, 5 mm in diameter, were created for introduction of test materials and controls.

To assess serum ADA, 50 µl of test serum was pipetted into one or two of the wells, and, as a control, 0.15 m NaCl was introduced into the remaining well. Plates were incubated at room temperature for 24 h and then flooded with 0.01% aqueous Congo red for two hours. Serum ADA was assessed by measuring the zone of clearing around the wells. Similar experiments were carried out using an appropriately diluted commercial preparation of serum albumen, serial dilutions of both albumen and test serum (Fig. 1), and after attempts to inactive ADA.

Equivalent zones of clearing were observed with both the Cohen-Calkins and the Pras fibril preparations. After the initial experiments, however, the amyloid agar plates were prepared using Pras fibril extracts exclusively.

B. Histochemical Method

Formalin-fixed, paraffin-embedded, histologic sections of amyloid-containing tissue were used as substrate to assess serum amyloid degrading activity (ADA). Identical 6-8 micron sections of amyloid-containing tissue were rimmed with a bead of hot-melt glue using a standard carpenter's glue

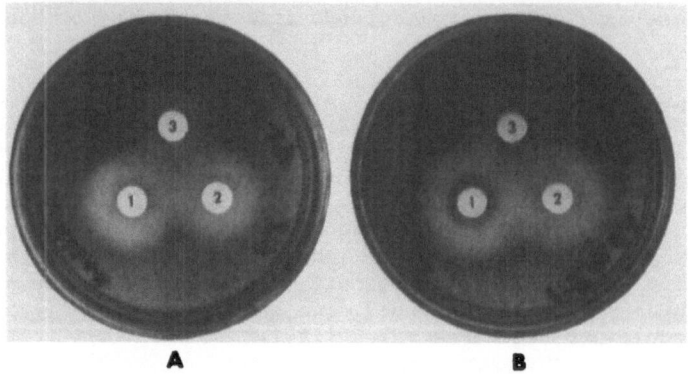

Fig. 1

gun (Sears Model #80508). One of the staining wells thus created was filled with test serum, the other with 0.15 m NaCl. After 18 h incubation, at room temperature, fluid was pipetted from the respective wells and replaced with 0.01% aqueous Congo red for one hour. The rim of glue was then removed with a scalpel (in some instances facilitated by first cooling the slide), the slides were dip-rinsed for 6 seconds in Meyer's hematoxylin and processed through graded alcohols and xylene for permanent mounting. Absence, or significant reduction of appropriate staining with Congo red was taken as evidence of either ADA or of some other significant alteration in the beta-pleated sheets [27].

Sections were prepared from the same tissues used in the amyloid agar plates as well as from a variety of other amyloid-containing tissue sources. The latter included such diverse tissues as brain, pancreas, seminal vesicle and aorta. Also, attempts were made to reverse the process by rinsing the slides with dilute salt solutions prior to application of the Congo red.

C. Test Materials

Serum samples included pooled human serum, serum from non-hospitalized controls, from hospitalized controls and from patients diagnosed as having either AA or AL systemic amyloidosis.

Commercial serum albumen (American National Red Cross Blood Services-25%) was prepared in 0.15 m NaCl to a concentration approximating normal serum albumen levels and was also tested at a number of dilutions.

Cerebrospinal fluid obtained incidental to diagnostic lumbar puncture was also tested using both the agar plates and the slide preparation.

RESULTS

Although our results are very preliminary, several observations can be made:

a) In contrast to previous reports, amyloid-agar plates prepared from either AA or AL amyloid fibrils exhibited identical zones of clearing in response to test sera. To date, three AL and one AA fibril preparations have been used.

b) Serial dilution of test sera resulted in progressively diminished ADA, as measured by the amyloid-agar plates.

c) ADA activity was not affected by heating serum at 50°C for up to 48 h nor by repeatedly freezing or thawing the test serum.

d) Commercial albumin prepared at concentration equivalent to that of normal serum exhibited ADA similar to that of normal serum (Fig. 1).

e) Cleared zones around the wells could be revealed either with the passage of time or with the addition of salt solutions to the well, followed by appropriate incubation and subsequent re-staining with 0.01% Congo red.

f) One patient with AA amyloidosis (and a serum albumen of less than 2 gm/dl) exhibited marked reduction in ADA in the amyloid agar plates while in several patients with AL amyloidosis the ADA of the serum tended to be only mildly subnormal.

g) Cerebrospinal fluid did not exhibit ADA.

h) The histologic method of assessing ADA essentially duplicated all of the findings observed with the amyloid agar plates. Using this method serum from the patient with AA amyloidosis failed to prevent Congo red staining when tested against a variety of different amyloid deposits.

i) In the histologic method, reduced afinity for Congo red occurred within 5-10 minutes of application of active serum; more prolonged incubation was necessary to completely eliminate staining, particularly when large amounts of amyloid were present in the test section.

j) The ability of normal serum to prevent Congo red staining of amyloid deposits appeared to vary little with the type of deposit examined, although cerebral amyloid deposits, pancreatic islet deposits and seminal vesicle amyloid appeared somewhat more resistent to ADA than did senile cardiovascular amyloid deposits. Nevertheless, with sufficient incubation time almost all amyloid deposits appeared to be susceptible.

COMMENT

Whether or not the ADA phenomenon described above is the same process described by others [17, 18, 21] is conjectural at this point. There appear to be significant differences including activity against AL, resistance to heat inactivation, and apparent reversibility. Whether the phenomenon described represents a real or even important step in amyloid biology is also unknown but the observations to date have been consistent and reproducible. Even if the inhibition of Congo red staining proves to represent nothing more than nonspecific adherence of albumen to the amyloid deposits, and not to actual denaturation, this adherence is of sufficient tenacity to withstand up to two hours of bathing in 0.01% aqueous Congo red. Equally unknown is whether or not this phenomenon actually alters solubility of the amyloid fibril protein. Nevertheless it is conceivable, that this mechanism, or one closely related to it, may, indeed, underlie a basic biologic process which protects most of us from accumulating discarded beta-pleated sheets and consequently from developing the clinical syndrome of amyloidosis.

REFERENCES

1. `P. Schwartz, Trans. N.Y. Acad. Sci., 27:393 (1965).
2. J. R. Wright, E. Calkins, W. J. Breen, et al., Medicine, 48:39 (1969).
3. G. G. Cornwell III and P. Westermark, J. Clin. Pathol., 33:1146 (1980).
4. T. Ishii, Y. Hosoda, N. Ikegami, et al., J. Pathol., 139:1 (1983).
5. T. Takeda, H. Sanada, M. Ishu, et al., Arth. and Rheum., 27:1063 (1984).
6. Y. A. Goffin, E. Gruys, G. D. Sorenson, et al., Amer. J. Pathol., 114: 431 (1984).
7. J. R. Wright and E. Calkins, Lab Invest., 30:767 (1974).
8. A. I. Ozdemir, J. R. Wright, and E. Calkins, N. Eng. J. Med., 285:534 (1971).
9. C. Limas, J. R. Wright, M. Matsuzaki, et al., Am. J. Med., 54:166 (1973).
10. K. Sletten, P. Westermark, and J. B. Natvig, Scand. J. Immunol., 12: 503 (1980).
11. P. D. Gorevic, A. B. Cleveland, J. R. Wright, et al., in: Proceedings of the Third International Symposium on Amyloidosis, ed. by G. G. Glenner, P. P. Costa, and A. F. Freitas, Excerpta Medica, Amsterdam, p. 366 (1980).
12. P. Westermark, B. Johansson, and J. B. Natvig, Scand. J. Immunol., 10:303 (1979).
13. G. G. Cornwell III, P. Westermark, W. Murdoch, et al., Am. J. Pathol., 108:135 (1982).
14. P. Pitkanen, P. Westermark, G. G. Cornwell III, et al., Am. J. Pathol., 110:64 (1983).
15. T. Shirahama, M. Skinner, P. Westermark, et al., Am. J. Pathol., 107:41 (1982).
16. I. Kedar, M. Ravid, and E. Sohar, in: Proceedings of the Third International Symposium on Amyloidosis, ed. by G. G. Glenner, P. P. Costa and A. F. Freitas, Excerpta Medica, Amsterdam, p. 60 (1980).
17. Schneller, M. Skinner, and A. S. Cohen, Arth. and Theum., 23:743 (1980) abst.
18. I. Kedar, E. Sohar, and M. Ravid, J. Lab and Clin. Invest., 99:693 (1982).
19. O. Wegelius, A. M. Teppo, and C. P. J. Maury, Brit. Med. J., 284:617 (1982).
20. C. P. J. Maury and A. M. Teppo, Lancet, July 31, 234 (1982).
21. A. M. Teppo, C. P. J. Maury, and O. Wegelius, Scand. J. Immunol., 16: 309 (1982).
22. C. P. J. Maurey, A. M. Teppo, B. Foseth, et al., Clin. Sci., 64:453 (1983).
23. A. S. Cohen and E. Calkina, J. Cell Biol., 21:481 (1964).
24. M. Pras, M. Schubert, D. Zucker-Franklin, et al., J. Clin. Invest., 47:924 (1968).
25. J. R. Wright, E. Calkins, and R. L. Humphrye, Lab Invest., 36:274 (1977).
26. J. R. Wright and E. Calkins, Medicine, 60:429 (1981).
27. G. G. Glenner, E. D. Eanes, and D. L. Page, J. Histochem. Cytochem., 20:821 (1972).

SENILE SYSTEMIC AMYLOIDOSIS

G. G. Cornwell III, P. Westermark,
R. A. Kyle, P. Pitkanen,
L. Benson, and B.-O. Olofsson

Department of Medicine
Dartmouth Medical School
Hanover, New Hampshire

Departments of Pathology and
Clinical Chemistry
University Hospital
Uppsala, Sweden

Department of Medicine
Mayo Clinic
Rochester, Minnesota

Department of Medicine
University Hospital
Umea, Sweden

ABSTRACT

Senile systemic amyloid contains the prealbumin-like fibril protein, AScl,
and is the only known form of systemic age-related amyloid. Although it involves
predominantly the heart, it may be found in a wide range of tissues. Immunologic
studies show that AScl cross reacts with human prealbumin (PA) in binding reactions but not in immunoprecipitation reactions. Protein AScl shows complete
homology with PA in four residues isolated. However, unlike PA, Ascl may have a
blocked N-terminus and is composed of at least three components. Anti-AScl forms
a line of precipitation with sera from patients with familial amyloidosis. A
similar weak reaction has been observed in some elderly patients with senile systemic amyloid.

INTRODUCTION

Senile systemic amyloidosis (SSA) (formerly known as senile cardiac
amyloidosis) is the only known systemic form of age related amyloidosis.
This disease is characterized by the presence of amyloid fibril protein
AScl, a prealbumin-like molecule [1, 2, 3]. It has been found in about 25%
of patients over the age of 80 years. SSA has a predeliction for the
heart, where atria and ventricles are equally involved. The cardiac deposits are generally large and homogenous, strictly extracellular and com-
press heart muscle cells (Fig. 1). The small and medium sized vessels are
usually involved [4]. This appearance is in marked contrast to that of
isolated atrial amyloid. In more than 90% of patients studied, AScl type
amyloid involves extracardiac sites, with deposits generally present in

653

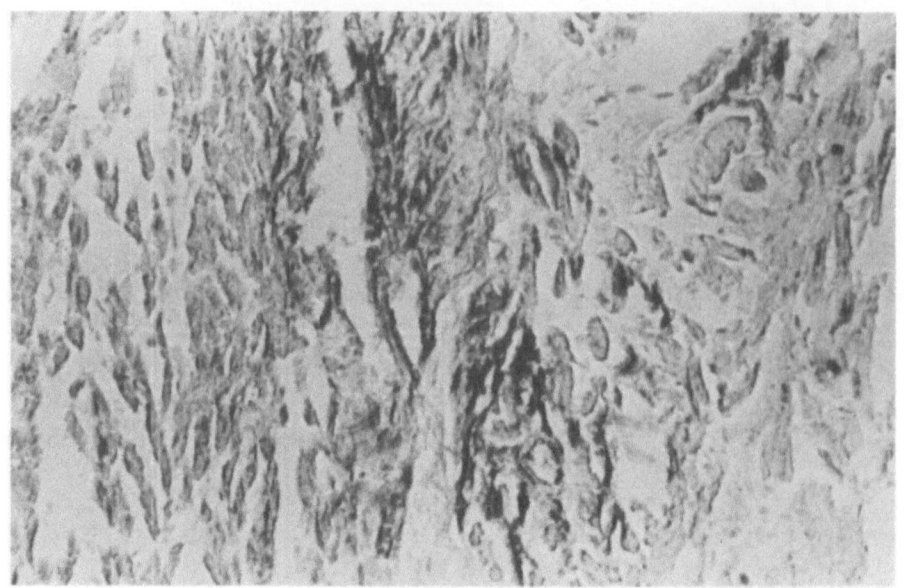

Fig. 1.   Ventricular tissue containing amyloid of the ASc_1 type.   Congo red. Original magnification ×250.

both the parenchyma and vessel walls [4].   Based on the study of 25 different tissues in 13 patients, it appears that the lung, colon/rectum, adrenals and seminal vesicles may be most often involved tissues, but further studies are required.   Every tissue studies, except brain, contained this form of amyloid from at least one patient [5].   In the initial analysis of 86 patients, the renal cortex was not involved in any of the 21 patients with SSA [4], bt subsequent analysis of 12 additional patients demonstrated predominantly renal papillary amyloid in 6 patients [5].

Although SSA is known to cause extreme cardiac enlargement, congestive heart failure and ectopy in some patients, the overall clinical significance of this form of amyloid is not yet clear [4].   Since most patients with ASc1 amyloid of the heart also have isolated atrial amyloid, it is difficult to distinguish the potential clinical effects of these two forms of senile amyloid deposition.

Protein ASc1 has not yet been completely sequenced.   Initial studies by Sletten et al. showed that it may have a blocked N-terminus and that peptic digests from this protein show complete homology with sequences 70–90, 96–107, 109–115, 121–127 in normal human prealbumin (PA) [2].   Antigenic identity of ASc1 to PA has been shown by immunofluorescence studies on tissues, but not by immunoprecipitation reactions on gels [3].   Studies by Felding et al. [6] have demonstrated that ASc1 is not a single protein species but is composed of at least three components: a PA-like protein with a molecular weight identical to normal PA monomer on SDS gels (30% of the total), a somewhat smaller 13K dalton protein (the major component), and still smaller proteins.   The 13K protein reacts with anti-ASc_1 but shows variable reactions with anti-PA.   The absence of detectable cysteinyl residues in this protein indicates that it lacks the N-terminal 10 amino acids of normal PA.

METHODS

Serum PA concentrations were measured in sera from 12 patients with known SSA, utilizing radial immunodiffusion [7].   The mean values were

TABLE 1. Reaction of $aASc_1$ with Sera from Patients with Heredofamilial Amyloidosis

Type	Patient	Reaction with $aASc_1$ (DD)
Swedish	BV	+
	MD	+
	GB	+
	AV	+
	SA	+
	RB	+
	HL	+
	GL	+
	JH	+
Portuguese	JF	+
	JD	+
Indiana	JM	+
	DM (Brother of JM)	+
	PK	+
	WD	?
Unknown	RW	+
Normal	TM (Brother of JM)	+
	RK (Sister of JM)	−
	AM (Daughter of JM)	−
	MK (Daughter of JM)	−
	RM (Son of JM)	−

110.7 ± 14.1 μg/ml (SEM) as compared to a value of 175.1 ± 20.3 μg/ml in 11 age and sec matched controls (p < 0.01). There was a linear correlation between the level of circulating prealbumin and retinol binding protein. SAA in the serum (determined by radioimmunoassay) was significantly higher for the patients with amyloid than in then those without (87.6 μg/ml versus 27.6 μg/ml; p < .05). The concentration of SAA in normal blood donors was less than 1 μg/ml [7]. The significance of these findings is not clear.

Anti-AScl (raised in rabbits) was used in immunoprecipitation reactions to study sera from elderly patients with and without SSA. These sera were collected premortem and studied after postmortem examination of the patient. Preliminary studies showed that three of five patients with known AScl amyloid reacted with anti-AScl whereas seven of eight without detectable amyloid failed to react. The precipitation reactions were very weak and further studies are required before any conclusions regarding these sera can be reached.

RESULTS

In view of the prealbumin-like proteins which have now been identified in a wide range of familial amyloids, attempts to compare AScl with AF proteins have been undertaken. Since AScl has not been completely sequenced, complete comparisons for amino acid substitutions have not yet been pos-

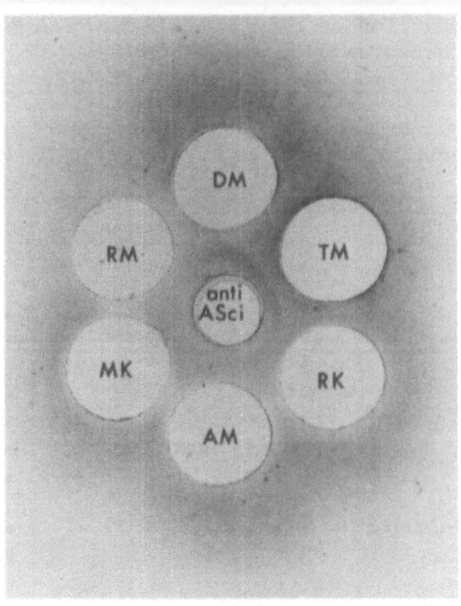

Fig. 2.   Anti-ASc₁ in center well tested
against sera from 6 members of
the family of patient JM with
familial amyloidotic polyneuropathy (FAP). DM (brother) with
FAP; TM (brother), RK (sister),
AM (daughter), MK (daughter),
RM (son) without FAP.

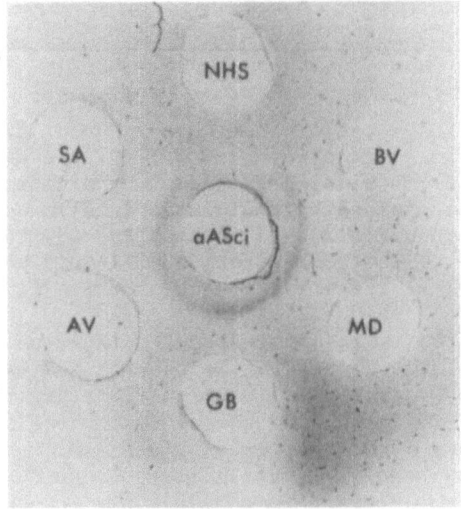

Fig. 3.   Anti-ASc₁ in center well tested
against sera from five Swedish
patients (BV, WD, GB, AV, SA)
with familial amyloidotic polyneuropathy and pool normal human
serum (NHS).

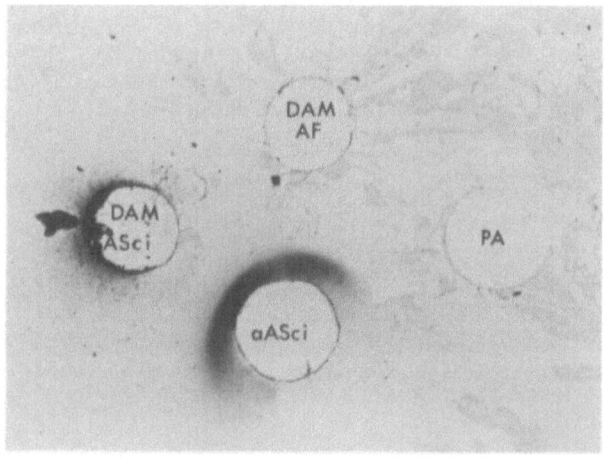

Fig. 4. Anti-ASc₁ in center well tested against
         DAM ASc₁, DAM AF_S and human prealbumin
         (PA).

sible. Indirect comparisons have shown that anti-AScl binds with equal
avidity to amyloid deposits of the AScl type and the AF_S type by immunofluorescence. Both of these reactions can be blocked completely by purified AScl (0.1 mg/ml) or DAM AF_S (3 mg/ml). The use of this same antiserum
to study the sera from patients with varying types of familial amyloidotic
neuropathy (FAP) has shown a high correlation between the presence of
clinical disease and the reactivity of the patient serum in the immunoprecipitation reaction. Table 1 shows the reactivity of sera from 15 patients
with FAP of the Swedish, Portuguese and Indiana types. Sera from seven
members of one family showed that two patients with known disease gave a
positive reaction, whereas four of five patients without evidence of FAP
had nonreactive sera (Table 1; Fig. 2). Lines of identity were present between all sera tested (irrespective of FAP type) (Fig. 3). In addition,
protein ASc₁ formed a line of identity with protein AF_S (Fig. 4).

The prevailing evidence supports the conclusion that SSA is a systemic
disease which results in small amyloid deposits in a wide range of tissues
in more than 25% of elderly patients. Immunologic and biochemical studies
suggest that ASc₁ is composed of several prealbumin variants and that there
may be a prealbumin variant as well as normal prealbumin in the serum of
these patients.

REFERENCES AND NOTES

1. P. Westermark, J. B. Natvig, B. Johansson, J. Exp. Med., 146:631
    (1977).
2. K. Sletten, P. Westermark, J. B. Natvig, Scand. J. Immunol., 12:503
    (1980).
3. G. G. Cornwell III, P. Westermark, J. B. Natvig, W. Murdoch, Immun-
    ology, 44:447 (1981).
4. G. G. Cornwell III, W. L. Murdoch, R. A. Kyle, P. Westermark, P.
    Pitkanen, Am. J. Med., 75:618 (1983).
5. P. Pitkanen, P. Westermark, G. G. Cornwell III, Am. J. Path. (in
    press).
6. P. Felding, G. Fex, P. Westermark, B.-O. Olofsson, P. Pitkanen, L.
    Benson, Scand. J. Immun. (in press).

7. P. Westermark, P. Pitkanen, L. Benson, A. Vahlquist, B-O. Olofsson, G. G. Cornwell III, Lab. Invest. (in press).
8. Supported in part by the Swedish Medical Research Council (Project No. 5941) and the Research Fund of King Gustaf V.

VARIED COMPOSITION AND NATURE OF SENILE LOCALIZED

AMYLOID: IMPLICATIONS FOR VARIED MECHANISMS OF PATHOGENESIS

Per Westermark and Gibbons G. Cornwell III

Department of Pathology
University Hospital
S-751 85 Uppsala, Sweden

Department of Medicine
Dartmouth Medical School
Hanover, New Hampshire   03755

ABSTRACT

    Most forms of senile localized amyloid depositions are very common and
seem almost to be part of normal aging. The fibril proteins typical of
systemic amyloids never occur in the senile localized types. In the latter
groups locally formed secretory proteins often seem to constitute the fibrils. The majority of these secretory proteins are hormone or prohor-
mone-derived. The best studied of the hormone derived amyloids is that in
the islets of Langerhans, which contains insulin B-chain and which is almost
a regular finding in human type 2 diabetes mellitus. The islet amyloid
probably reflects the impaired ability of islet B-cells to secrete insulin
which instead undergoes degradation during which fibrils are formed. Defects in synthesis or release of other hormones might lead to depositions
in different organs. The seminal vesicle amyloid is probably derived from
an excretory protein. The localized cerebrovascular amyloid may be plasma
derived. The nature of most other senile localized amyloid forms is completely unknown. However, the close topographical localization of some
cardiovascular amyloids to elastic structures is evident, and it is possible that structure proteins may also convert to amyloid.

INTRODUCTION

    Amyloid deposits occur in increasing frequency with age. Those types, both
systemic and local, which are so common that they seem to be part of the aging process are called senile amyloidoses. Although not an absolutely adequate term, it
is a very practical one, which was coined in 1876 by Soyka [1] and has been
used since then. The definition excludes rare localized amyloid deposits
of the AL type, which may occur mainly in old persons but which do not show
the clear age relation seen in the senile types.

    Most senile amyloid deposits are small and strictly organ or tissue
restricted. The only exclusion seems to be the senile systemic amyloidosis
[2]. The localized amyloid deposits are easily overlooked and have usually
been regarded as some nonspecific degenerative alteration. In general,
these forms of amyloid have received little scientific attention.

TABLE 1. The Maximal Frequency of Some Forms of Senile Amyloid

	Frequency %	Studied age group	Reference
Cardiovascular			
Atrium	78	≥ 80	4
Senile systemic	25	≥ 80	4
Aorta	100	≥ 80	4
Cerebral			
Vascular	46	≥ 70	35
Endocrine			
Islets of Langerhans	96*	≥ 60	13
Pituitary gland	46	> 70	36
Adrenal cortex	68	≥ 70	26
Articular	77	> 59	37
Seminal vesicle	21	> 75	29

* Much lower frequencies have been found in other materials

The chemical diversity of the senile localized amyloid deposits is now fairly well established. The amyloid fibril proteins found in the AL, AA, AF and ASc_1 forms have not yet been found with certainty in senile localized amyloid deposits. From what we know today, the proteins in senile localized amyloids usually (and perhaps always) are similar or identical to proteins which are normally synthesized in the tissue of deposition. This finding is in contrast to the systemic amyloids, including the senile systemic amyloidosis, in which the main proteins invariably are formed elsewhere but processed in the tissue of deposition.

While the secrets of the systemic amyloidoses are becoming more clear, progresses in our knowledge about the localized forms are more modest. This fact relates, in part, to the lack of scientific studies, but also to the difficulties in working with them. In some forms, such as the tiny deposits of amyloid in joints, it is at present almost impossible to purify enough amounts for biochemical analysis.

There are, however, some exceptions such as the amyloid in the brain, the islet amyloid and the amyloid of the seminal vesicles.

The major senile amyloids are listed in Table 1 as well as their frequencies in some age groups. As is seen, the disorders can be divided into five main groups. Of these, the cardiovascular, the endocrine and the seminal vesicle amyloids will be discussed separately in this paper.

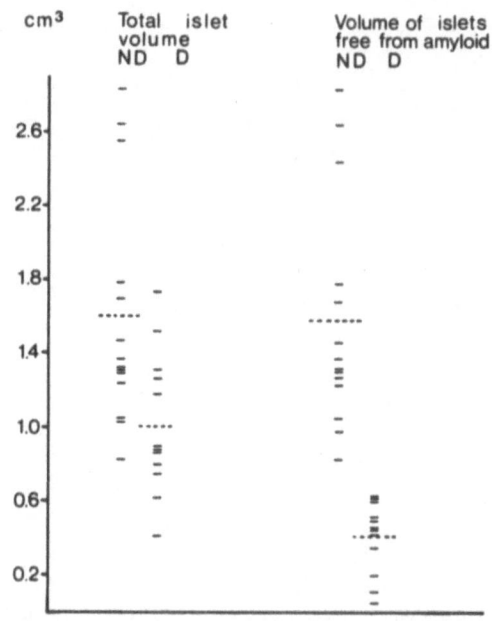

Fig. 1. Comparison of the volume of
pancreatic islets in type 2
diabetes (D) and age matched
non-diabetic patients (ND).
Persons with diabetes have significantly smaller islet volume,
but there is a pronounced overlapping between the two groups.
When the volumes of islets
which are free of amyloid are
compared, the difference between
the two groups is much more pronounced and there is no overlapping. Results from [21].

SENILE LOCALIZED CARDIOVASCULAR AMYLOID

Besides the senile systemic amyloidosis, there is at least one other
age related amyloid type in the heart: the isolated atrial amyloidosis
(IAA) [3]. IAA is strictly limited to the atria. The nature of this
amyloid is not known, but it does not contain protein ASc_1. IAA is very
common and was seen in 78% of patients over 80 years [4].

Small deposits in the wall of the aorta are very common and have been
found in all specimens from 85 patients over 80 years of age [5]. Small
amyloid deposits are often also seen in aortic branches [5]. This type,
designated senile aortic amyloid, occurs mainly in the inner third of the
media and never in the adventitia, in contrast to the systemic forms [6, 7].
The nature of the amyloid is unknown.

SENILE ENDOCRINE AMYLOID

Age-related amyloid deposits in endocrine tissues are common. The
oldest known and perhaps still most well known type is the amyloidosis of

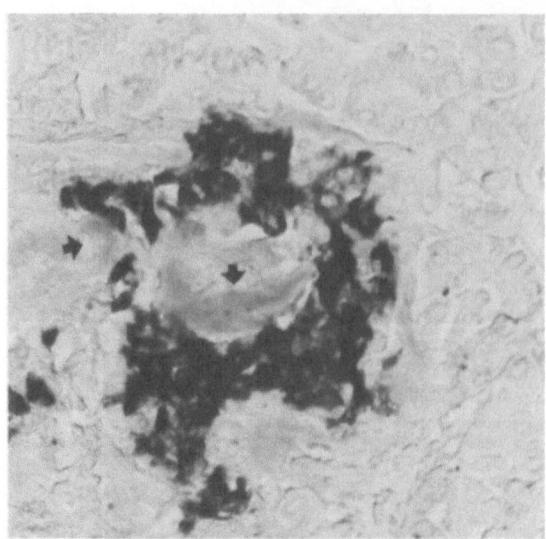

Fig. 2. Immunohistochemical staining (peroxidase-anti peroxidase) of a human
islet with amyloid deposits, using
an antiserum against insulin ß chain
prepared as described in the text.
There is a strong reaction with the
ß cells and a weaker with the amyloid.

the islets of Langerhans, described in 1900 [8]. However, amyloid is also
common in other non-neoplastic endocrine tissues, such as the pituitary
gland and the parathyroid glands. Besides these tissues, some hormone-pro-
ducing tumors contain amyloid. Although the amyloid in such tumors is not
necessarily identical with the amyloid in the non-neoplastic tissue, it
seems very probable that it is closely related. Consequently, studies of
tumor amyloid may give us valuable information about the nature of the
amyloid in endocrine organs.

Correlation studies have shown a definite relationship between the
type of polypeptide hormone produced in tumors and the frequency of amyloid
deposits [9]. Thus, tumors secreting calcitonin, insulin and growth hormone
very often contain amyloid while tumors producing glucagon, gastrin or ACTH
more rarely do [9, 10, 11]. This observation suggests that some polypeptide
hormones, prohormones or hormone degradation products are more apt to form
amyloid fibrils than other. More direct evidence for hormone derivation of
amyloid fibrils was the finding that a 6 kd protein purified from the amyloid of a medullary carcinoma of the thyroid contained a sequence homologous
to calcitonin [12]. This finding provided the first evidence for the
existence of procalcitonin.

Much attention has been paid to the amyloid in the islets of Langerhans
as a result of its interesting connection with type 2 diabetes mellitus.
Although islet amyloid is increasingly common with age in non-diabetic
patients [13], it is even more prevalent and more extensive in patients with
type 2 diabetes [14, 15]. This form of localized amyloid is also found in
spontaneously diabetic cats [16] and monkeys [17]. The islet volume is only
moderately decreased in type 2 diabetes, but electron microscopic studies
have shown that most β-cells in islets with amyloid have signs of injury

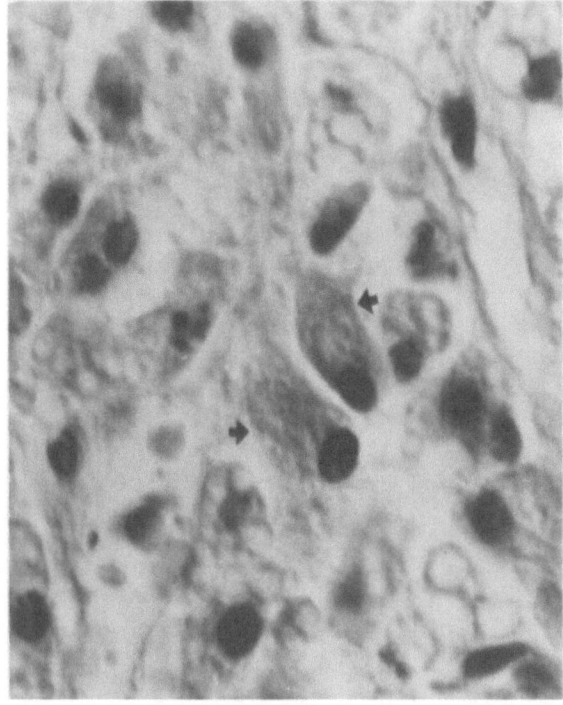

Fig. 3.   Adrenal cortical cells stuffed with
intracytoplasmatic amyloid (arrows).
Congo red, ×1100.

with membrane defects [18]. The volume of islets without any amyloid in
type 2 diabetes is significantly smaller than in age matched controls
(Fig. 1) [19].

The nature of islet amyloid is not definitely known. In humans, electron microscopic studies have shown a close relationship between parallel
bundles of amyloid fibrils and β-cells [18], although studies in cats have
shown a similar relationship between amyloid fibrils and an unidentified
perivascular cell [20]. It has not as yet been possible to purify the protein for amino acid sequence analysis, but immunohistochemical studies
have provided evidence that the amyloid is insulin derived both in man
[21] and cat [22]. In an immunohistochemical study, we found that antibodies to insulin or insulin A-chain did not bind to the amyloid. An
antiserum to insulin B-chain gave a very weak reaction. However, when insulin was cleaved into its two component chains, gel filtered through a
Sephacryl S-300 column and material from the first part of the resulting
double peak containing B-chain mixed with some A-chain was used for immunization, an antiserum was obtained which reacted with the islet amyloid in
both man and cat. The normal mode of degradation of insulin in islet
tissue is of interest in this context. Insulin is first cleaved into its
two component chains, and these are then separately degraded further [23].
During this degradation, there is a spontaneous tendency to form large
aggregates of B and A chains in the proportion 3:1 [24], a situation which
might have been mimicked in the antigen used for immunization. Furthermore, insulinoma, a tumor often containing amyloid, has been associated
with a defect in the second degradation step [25]. From these facts a
hypothesis for the formation of islet amyloid in type 2 diabetes can be
formed. A primary defect in type 2 diabetes is an impaired ability to re-

TABLE 2. Characteristics of Some Senile Localized Amyloids

	Tryptophan	Permanganate	Possible related tissue component	Antigen identified	Protein	Reference
Atrium	-	R	Elastin?	-	nk*	7
Aorta	+	R	Elastin?	-	nk	7
Islets	-	R	B-cells	+	Insulin B-chain	21
Seminal vesicles	-	S	Epithelial cells	+	15 kd	32
Cerebral plaques	-	R	nk	-	Prion?	34
Cerebral vessels	-	R	Plasma protein?	-	4.2 kd	38

*nk = not known

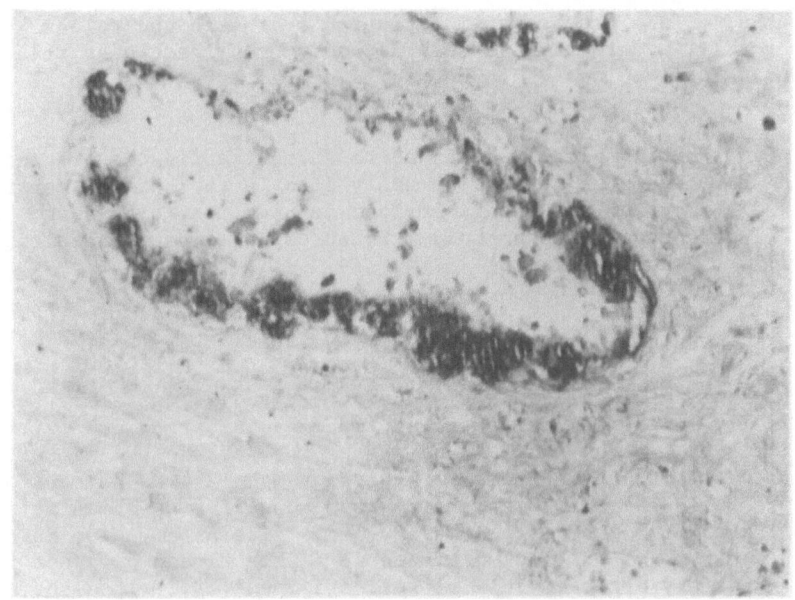

Fig. 4. Seminal vesicle amyloid reacting with an antiserum
against a 15 kd amyloid protein. Peroxidase-anti peroxidase, ×300.

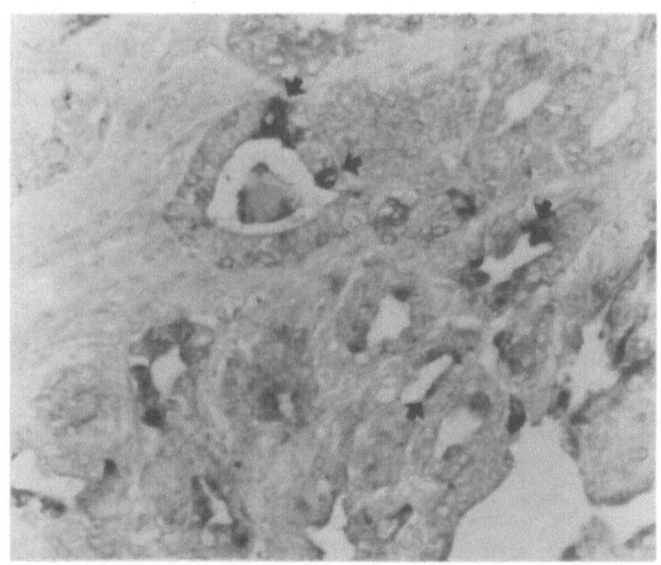

Fig. 5. Seminal vesicle epithelium in a patient without amyloid deposition, stained with the same
antiserum as in Fig. 4. Some epithelial
cells are strongly positive. Peroxidase-anti
peroxidase, ×300.

lease insulin. Since glucose stimulates the synthesis and release of insulin separately, a defective release mechanism can lead to an relative overproduction of insulin, which has to be degraded by the B-cell. During the degradation, aggregates containing mainly B-chain may be formed.

Amyloid is not completely confined to endocrine tissues producing polypeptide hormones, but is also commonly seen in the adrenal cortex [26]. The distribution of adrenal amyloid is peculiar, with accumulations of intracellular needle-like amyloid structures, somewhat resembling the neurofibrillary tangles (Fig. 3).

SENILE SEMINAL VESICLE AMYLOID

In this form of localized amyloidosis, amyloid deposits are found subepithelially in the seminal vesicles, often as a narrow rim [27, 28]. The amyloid is of typical senile type, being rare before the age of 60 but increasing to 21% of patients over 75 years of age [29]. The senile seminal vesicle amyloid (SSVA) has some interesting properties by which it is easily separated from other types of amyloid. Like AA amyloid, SSVA is permanganate sensitive but lacks tryptophan (Table 2) and does not react with anti-AA or any other amyloid fibril antiserum [29]. It also fails to react with anti gammatrace antibodies [30], although gamma trace, which has been shown to be an amyloid fibril protein, has been found in high concentration in seminal plasma [31].

In view of the fairly large amounts of amyloid in some vesicles, a further characterization of SSVA has been possible [32]. A method to concentrate the amyloid was worked out prior to using standard methods for amyloid purification. The resulting material was almost pure amyloid as estimated by light microscopy after staining with Congo red. Gel filtration in 8 M urea, pH 3.0, revealed one typical pattern in all tested cases. A 15 kd protein was purified from the amyloid and two different antisera against this protein showed an immunhistochemical reaction with SSVA (Fig. 4) but with no other tested amyloid of systemic or localized type. Both antisera showed reaction with normal seminal vesicle epithelium (Fig. 5).

These findings favor an epithelial origin of the amyloid in SSVA, and it seems probable that the amyloid fibril protein is derived from a secretory protein. The subepithelial location of the amyloid might appear unexpected. However, it has been shown that the seminal vesicle epithelium not only has the property to reabsorb secretory proteins, but can also transport them transepithelially to the subepithelial space [33]. A disturbance in the transport mechanism might be of importance for the formation of this special amyloid.

CONCLUSIONS

From what we know about the senile localized amyloids, it seems that we can divide them into three groups: one comprising those with an epithelial secretory or incretory origin, i.e. SSVA and the endocrine amyloids, one with possible plasma origin (the amyloid angiopathy), and one comprising the remainder. Perhaps the amyloid of cerebral plaques could make up a fourth group with the very fascinating possibility of prion origin [34]. The islet amyloid in type 2 diabetes mellitus might result from a specific disturbance of the cellular response to a stimulus and reflect a fundamental injury in the B-cell. This alteration therefore deserves much more interest by the diabetes scientists than it has now. Similar, but certainly not identical, disturbances may explain the deposition of amyloid in other epithelial tissues. A prerequisite is that the impaired metabolism affects a protein capable of forming amyloid fibrils. The nature and pathogenesis of the other group of senile localized amyloids is quite obscure. We can only speculate about the nature of the localized cardiovascular amyloids. A fact that might be of importance is that all amyloids in this group favor tissues rich in elastin, but we will have to await further studies to advance our knowledge of this group of amyloids.

REFERENCES

1. J. Soyka, Prag. Med. Wschr., 1:165 (1876).
2. P. Pitkänen, P. Westermark, G. G. Cornwell III, Am. J. Path. (in press).
3. P. Westermark, B. Johansson, J. B. Natvig, Scand., J. Immunol., 10:303 (1979).
4. G. G. Cornwell III, W. L. Murdoch, R. A. Kyle, P. Westermark, P. Pitkänen, Am. J. Med., 75:618 (1983).
5. P. Schwartz, in: Amyloidosis, E. Mandema, L. Ruinen, J. H. Scholten, A. S. Cohen, Eds. (Excerpta Medica, Amsterdam, 1968), p. 400.
6. J. R. Wright, E. Calkins, Lab. Invest., 30:767 (1974).
7. G. G. Cornwell III, P. Westermark, W. Murdoch, P. Pitkänen, Am. J. Pathol., 108:135 (1982).
8. E. L. Opie, J. Exp. Med., 5:397 (1900).
9. P. Westermark, L. Grimelius, J. M. Polak, L.-I. Larsson, S. van Noorden, E. Wilander, A. G. E. Pearse, Lab. Invest., 37:212 (1977).
10. A. Holland, in: Amyloidosis, E. A. R. S., C. R. Tribe, P. A. Bacon, Eds. (John Wright & Sons, Bristol, 1983), p. 201.
11. W. Saeger, C. Gerigh, P. H. Missmahl, D. K. Lüdecke, Pathologie, 4:183 (1983).
12. K. Sletten, P. Westermark, J. B. Natvig, J. Exp. Med., 143:993 (1976).
13. P. Schwartz, Zbl. Allg. Path., 108:169 (1965).
14. P. Westermark, L. Grimelius, Acta Path. Microbiol. Scand. Sect. A., 81:291 (1973).
15. E. T. Bell, Am. J. Pathol., 35:801 (1959).
16. K. H. Johnson, J. B. Stevens, Diabetes, 22:81 (1973).
17. C. F. Howard, Diabetes, 27:357 (1978).
18. P. Westermark, Virshows Arch. Abt. A, 359:1 (1973).
19. P. Westermark, E. Wilander, Diabetologia, 15:417 (1978).
20. B. L. Yano, D. W. Hayden, K. H. Johnson, Lab. Invest., 45:149 (1981).
21. P. Westermark, E. Wilander, Diabetologia, 24:342 (1983).
22. K. H. Johnson, P. Westermark, G. Nilsson, K. Sletten, T. D. O'Brien, D. W. Harden, Manuscript in preparation.
23. K.-D. Kohnert, H. Jahr, S. Schmidt, H.-J. Hahn, H. Zühlke, Biochim. Biophys. Acta, 422:254 (1976).
24. P. T. Varandani, Biochim. Biophys. Acta, 295:630 (1973).
25. P. T. Varandani, Biochim. Biophys. Res. Commun., 60:1119 (1974).
26. Unpublished observation.
27. S. Bursell, Upsala Läkaref. Förh., 47:313 (1942).
28. H. Goldman, Arch. Pathol., 75:94 (1963).
29. P. Pitkänen, P. Westermark, G. G. Cornwell III, W. Murdoch, Am. J. Pathol., 110:64 (1983).
30. Thanks are due to Dr. Anders Grubb, Malmö, Sweden for anti γ trace antiserum.
31. A. Grubb, H. Weiber, H. Löfberg, Scand. J. Clin. Lab. Invest., 43:421 (1983).
32. P. Westermark, P. Pitkänen, L. Eriksson, Manuscript in preparation.
33. L. R. Mata, A. B. Maunsbach, Biol. Cell, 46:65 (1982).
34. S. B. Prusiner, M. P. McKinley, K. A. Bowman, D. C. Bolton, P. E. Bendheim, D. F. Groth, G. G. Glenner, Cell, 35:349 (1983).

35. H. VV. Vinters, J. J. Gilbert, Stroke, 14:924 (1983).
36. W. Saeger, R. Warner, H. P. Missmahl, Pathologie 4, 177 (1983).
37. Y. A. Goffin, Y. Thoua, P. R. Potvliege, Ann. Rheum. Dis., 40:27 (1981).
38. G. G. Glenner, C. W. Wong, Biochem. Biophys. Res. Commun., 120:885 (1984).

ACKNOWLEDGEMENTS

Supported by the Swedish Medical Research Council (Project No. 5941), the Research Fund of King Gustaf V and Nordisk Insulinfond.

A NEW SENILE AMYLOID FIBRIL PROTEIN AND ITS PUTATIVE

PRECURSOR IN SENESCENCE ACCELERATED MOUSE (SAM)

Keiichi Higuchi, Atsuko Matsumura,
Shuji Takeshita, Tomonori Yonezu,
Atsuko Honma, Kayoko Higuchi,
Masanori Hosokawa, and Toshio Takeda

Department of Pathology
Chest Disease Research Institute
Kyoto University
Sakyo-ku, Kyoto, 606, Japan

ABSTRACT

A new amyloid fibril protein was isolated from the livers of Senescence Accelerated Mice (SAM-P), a strain characterized by accelerated senescence and a high incidence of age-associated systemic amyloidosis. This 5,200 dalton amyloid protein "AS_{SAM}" differs in amino acid composition from the amyloid protein of murine secondary amyloidosis. Sequence analysis revealed a blocked N-terminus. Double immunodiffusion tests showed no relationship between AS_{SAM} and murine protein AA or immunoglobulin components.

Sera obtained from normal mice contained a substance that reacted with anti-AS_{SAM} antiserum. This physiological substance, termed "SAS_{SAM}" (Serum AS_{SAM}-related antigenic substance) migrated to the albumin/prealbumin region and stained positively with both protein and lipid stains. Fractionation of lipoprotein from normal mouse serum disclosed that SAS_{SAM} was present mainly in high density lipoprotein (HDL). AS_{SAM} immunoreactivity appeared in the low molecular weight proteins of apo HDL separated through Sephadex G-200. Purified apoprotein of SAS_{SAM} with crossreactivity to anti-AS_{SAM} antiserum was obtained with ion-exchange chromatography of low molecular weight proteins of apo HDL. This apoprotein termed "apo SAS_{SAM}" has about the same molecular weight (5,200) and amino acid composition as AS_{SAM}. Electrophoretic analysis revealed that apo SAS_{SAM} corresponds presumably to apo A-II, a major apolipoprotein of HDL.

INTRODUCTION

Purified amyloid fibril proteins have been obtained from several types of human amyloidosis (Glenner et al., 1983). Specific antisera were produced against these amyloid proteins, and serum amyloid-related substances that reacted with these antisera were investigated. Generally these substances are normal serum proteins and are considered to be precursors of amyloid proteins. To clarify the pathogenesis of amyloidosis and the mechanisms of deposition of amyloid protein, the nature of these precursors has to be determined.

Spontaneous, age-associated amyloidosis in mice has been described in many reports, but there is little information on the biochemical nature of amyloid protein and its precursor protein unique to senile amyloidosis. AA protein has proved to be the age-related amyloidosis in some strains of mice (Westermark et al., 1979; Glenner et al., 1971), but in these cases, amyloid deposition may not reflect age-related phenomena per se.

We have isolated and analyzed a new murine senile amyloid fibril protein in a new inbred strain of mice (SAM-P). A substance with crossreactivity to antiserum against this amyloid protein was found in mouse serum. We proved that this serum substance is apo A-II, a major apolipoprotein in high density lipoproteins.

A New Murine Senile Amyloid Fibril Protein "AS$_{SAM}$"

A murine model of accelerated senescence, Senescence Accelerated Mouse (SAM), was recently developed in our laboratory (Takeda et al., 1981; Hosokawa et al., 1984). Spontaneous, age-associated and systemic amyloidosis is one of the most characteristic findings in these mice (Takeshita et al., 1982). Amyloid fibrils were isolated as a water suspended fraction from the livers of SAM-P by the method of Pras et al. (1969). Further purification was performed by gel filtration through a Sephadex G-100 column equilibrated with 5M guanidine hydrochloride in 1N acetic acid.

Purified amyloid protein migrated as a single protein band on 8M urea-sodium dodecylsulfate(SDS)-polyacrylamide gel electrophoresis (Matsumura et al., 1982), and its molecular weight was calculated to be 5,200 daltons. This molecular weight is lower than the molecular weight of murine protein AA. Its amino acid composition also differs from that of murine protein AA. Sequence analysis of the protein revealed a blocked N-terminus. A specific antiserum against the amyloid protein was produced in rabbits (Higuchi et al., 1983). Double immunodiffusion tests showed no relationship between the amyloid protein and murine protein AA or mouse immunoglobulin components. Thus, we have isolated a new amyloid protein that is distinguishable from previously reported murine amyloid proteins and is not related to immunoglobulin. We termed this new amyloid fibril protein "AS$_{SAM}$", i.e., senile amyloid protein deposits in SAM. Several biological, pathological and biochemical features of AS$_{SAM}$ are summarized in Table 1.

Serum AS$_{SAM}$ Related Antigenic Substance, "SAS$_{SAM}$"

Sera obtained from SAM-P and normal mice of several strains (SAM-R, DDD, CBA/St, C3H/HeN, C57BL/6J, A/J, SJL/J, B10A) gave a single precipitation line when tested by double immunodiffusion against anti-AS$_{SAM}$ antiserum, and this line fused with the precipitation line detected against purified AS$_{SAM}$. Absorption of antiserum with AS$_{SAM}$ (0.05 mg per 1 ml antiserum) eliminated the line between the mouse serum and antiserum (Higuchi et al., 1983). This finding indicates that normal mouse serum has a substance which crossreacts with antiserum against amyloid protein, AS$_{SAM}$, regardless of the strain. We termed this substance "SAS$_{SAM}$" (serum AS$_{SAM}$-related antigenic substance). SAS$_{SAM}$ seems to be a physiological substance in contrast to acute phase reactant protein, SAA (McAdam et al., 1976). SAA was not detected in normal mouse serum in our double immunodiffusion test.

In the immunoelectrophoresis, a single precipitation line was formed at the albumin/prealbumin region between mouse serum and anti-AS$_{SAM}$ anti-

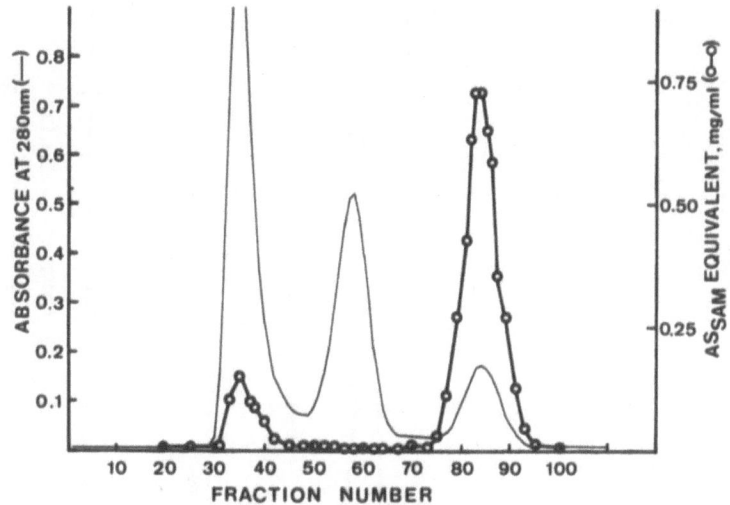

Fig. 1.   Sephadex G-200 gel chromatography in 8M urea,
0.01M Tris HC1, 1mM EDTA, 0.03% NaN₃, pH 8.3 at
22 C, of delipidated HDL fractions from ICR/Slc
mice serum.   Fraction volume, 3.0 ml, column
size, 1.5 cm × 90 cm.   (——), absorbance at
280 nm, (o——o), concentration of apo SAS$_{SAM}$
represented as AS$_{SAM}$ equivalent (mg/ml).
Specially prepared urea (Nakarai Chemicals, Kyoto
Japan) was used and passed through mixed-bed
resin (Bio-Rad Laboratories, Richmond, California) before use.

serum.   This precipitation line stained positively with both Amide Black
10B and Oil Red O/Fat Red 7B solutions.

These data indicate that SAS$_{SAM}$ may be transported in blood as a form
of high density lipoprotein (HDL) in serum.

Lipoprotein fractions of different density classes were prepared by
preparative ultracentrifugation, and the concentration of SAS$_{SAM}$ in each
lipoprotein fraction was measured by a single radial immunodiffusion test
using anti-AS$_{SAM}$ antiserum.   The largest amount of SAS$_{SAM}$, about 60% of
the total, was obtained in the HDL$_2$ fraction (1.063 < d < 1.125), and 30%
of SAS$_{SAM}$ was found in the HDL$_3$ fraction (1.125 < d < 1.210).   Thus about
90% of total SAS$_{SAM}$ was found in HDL fractions, but SAS$_{SAM}$ was very scarce
in very low density lipoprotein (VLDL: d < 1.006) and low density lipoprotein (LDL: 1.006 < d < 1.063).   In our system, the largest amount of
SAA (68%) was detected in HDL$_3$ fractions of CBA mice sera in which SAA
levels were increased by LPS injection.

Purification of apo SAS$_{SAM}$

HDL fractions (1.063 < d < 1.210) were separated from ICR/sln mouse
sera and delipidated with ethanol and ether (3:2) solutions at −10°C.

Sephadex G-200 chromatography in 8M urea, 0.01M Tris, 1 mM EDTA, 0.03%
NaN₃, pH 8.2, of the apolipoproteins of HDL is illustrated in Fig. 1.   Apo
HDL lipoproteins were separated into three distinctly defined ultraviolet
absorbing peaks.   Single radial immunodiffusion tests clearly revealed an

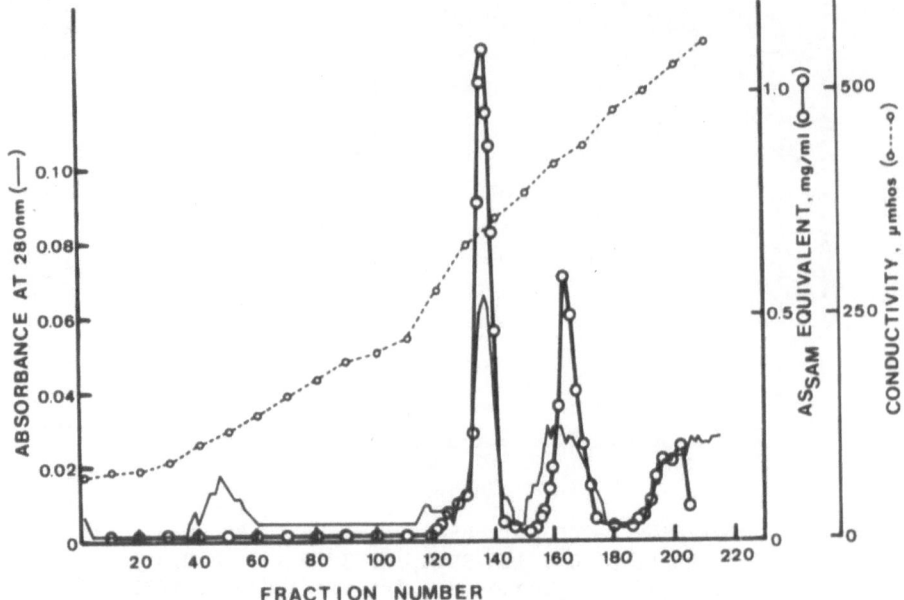

Fig. 2. DEAE-cellulose chromatography of the third peak materials
(10 mg) isolated by gel filtration chromatography of apo HDL
Column size, 1.5 cm × 45 cm, 250 ml volume linear Tris-HCl
gradient in 6M urea, pH 8.2 from 0.01M to 0.1M (total volume
500 ml), flow rate, 7 ml/hr at 4 C. Fraction volume, 2.6 ml.
(———), absorbance at 280 nm, (o———o), concentration of apo
SAS_{SAM} and (------), conductivity (μmho).

SAS_{SAM} peak at the third protein peak. The pooled fractions of the third
peak were dialyzed against 5mM ammonium bicarbonate and lyophilized.

    Ion-exchange chromatography (DEAE-cellulose) of the apoprotein in the
SAS_{SAM} rich third peak in a Tris concentration gradient from 0.01M Tris/6M
urea, pH 8.2 to 0.1M Tris/6M urea, pH 8.2 revealed the bulk of the AS_{SAM}
immunoreactivity to be associated with two protein peaks (Fig. 2). The
fractions in the larger peak were pooled and dialyzed against 5mM ammonium
bicarbonate and lyophilized.

    The electrophoretic analysis of SAS_{SAM} at each step of purification
is shown in Fig. 3. In 8M-urea-SDS-polyacrylamide gel electrophoresis,
with appropriate standards of molecular weight comparison, the apoprotein
purified by DEAE-cellulose migrated as a single band with a molecular weight
estimated to be 5,200. In alkaline-urea polyacrylamide gel electrophoresis
(Davis et al., 1964), apo SAS_{SAM} migrated as a single band purified from
the third peak's protein of Sephadex G-200 chromatography which had three
protein bands. Among the protein bands of apo HCL (A and D in Fig. 3), the
major protein band with a molecular weight of 25,000 is apo A-I, and the
protein band migrating fastest (D in Fig. 3) is apo C; the band of apo
SAS_{SAM} probably corresponds to apo A-II apolipoprotein (Camus et al., 1983;
LeBoeuf et al., 1983).

Comparison of apo SAS_{SAM} with AS_{SAM}

    In 8M-urea-SDS-polyacrylamide gel electrophoresis, apo SAS_{SAM} and AS_{SAM}
migrated to about the same position at a molecular weight of 5,200 (Fig. 4).
This is not the case of SAA and AA. SAA is known to have a 3,000 larger

TABLE 1. Several Features of Amyloidosis in SAM

Biology	Age or senescence associated
Pathology	Severe systemic amyloidosis; high incidence
	KMnO$_4$-resistant
	Tryptophan negative
Bio-immuno Chemistry	AS$_{SAM}$: Amyloid fibril protein in tissue
	Not AA and not related to immunoglobulin
	Molecular weight = 5,200
	Blocked N-terminus
	SAS$_{SAM}$: Serum putative precursor of AS$_{SAM}$
	High density lipoprotein (MW ≢ 200,000)
	apo SAS$_{SAM}$: Apoprotein of SAS$_{SAM}$
	Amino acid composition ≢ AS$_{SAM}$
	MW = 5,200
	Apo A-II?

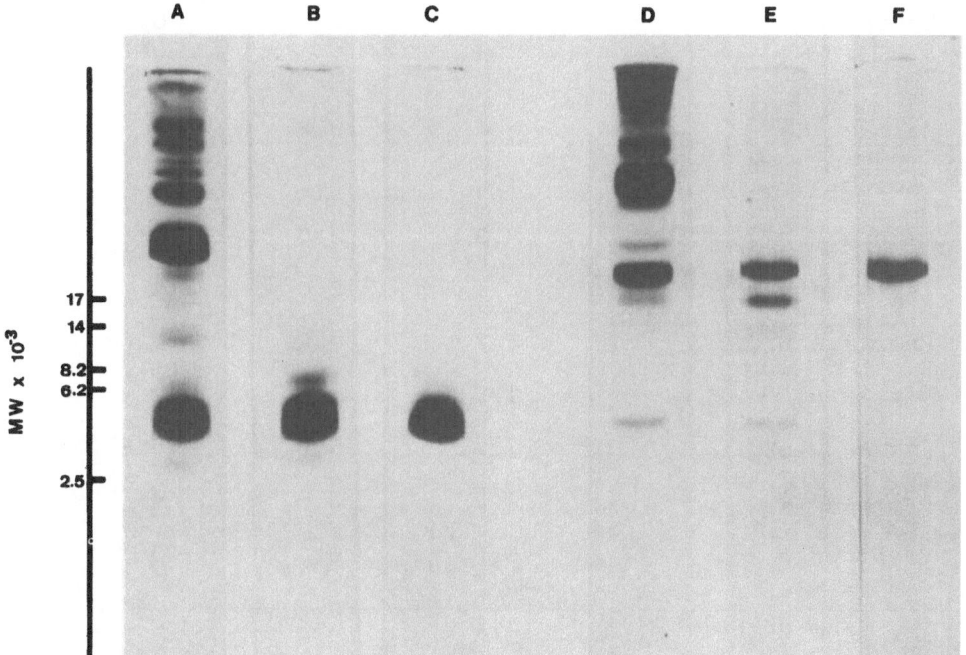

Fig. 3. Gel electrophoresis of apo SAS$_{SAM}$ at each step of purification. 8M urea-SDS-polyacrylamide (12.5%) gel electrophoresis of A) apo HDL, B) the third peak materials isolated by Sephadex G-200 gel chromatography, C) apo SAS SAM purified by DEAE-cellulose chromatography. Molecular weight markers, myoglobin (16,949), and myoglobin I and II (14,400), myoglobin I (8,159), myoglobin II (6,214), myoglobin III (2,512). Alkaline (pH 9.4) 8M urea-polyacrylamide gel (7.5%) electrophoresis of D) apo HDL, E) the third peak materials of apo HDL and F) purified apo SAS$_{SAM}$.

TABLE 2. Amino Acid Compositions of apo SAS$_{SAM}$, AS$_{SAM}$ and Rat apo A-II

Amino acid	Apo SAS$_{SAM}$	AS$_{SAM}$	Rat Apo A-II[a]
	mol/100 mol of amino acid		
Aspartic acid + asparagine	6.7	7.5	9
Threonine	7.1	6.6	7
Serine	11.1	8.2	6
Glutamic acid + glutamine	17.7	17.0	21
Proline	5.5	4.2	6
Glycine	6.8	7.0	3
Alanine	9.5	9.0	12
Cysteine	0	0	0
Valine	3.6	5.1	3
Methionine	3.6	2.8	3
Isoleucine	1.5	3.5	1
Leucine	8.2	9.0	11
Tyrosine	3.1	3.0	4
Phenylalanine	5.7	4.9	5
Histidine	1.2	1.5	0
Lysine	7.2	6.8	5
Arginine	1.2	3.0	4
Tryptophan	N.D.[b]	0	0

a, From Herbert et al., 1974

b, not determined

molecular weight than AA (Benditt et al., 1979). In alkaline-urea-poly-acylamide gel electrophoresis AS$_{SAM}$ exhibited one principal band with the same mobility as apo SAS$_{SAM}$ and four fainter bands.

Those protein bands of apo SAS$_{SAM}$ and AS$_{SAM}$ separated by alkaline-urea-polyacrylamide slub gel electrophoresis were transferred electrophoretically to nitrocellulose paper (Towbin et al., 1979). Protein bands reacting with antisera against apo SAS$_{SAM}$ were detected by the unlabeled immunoperoxidase

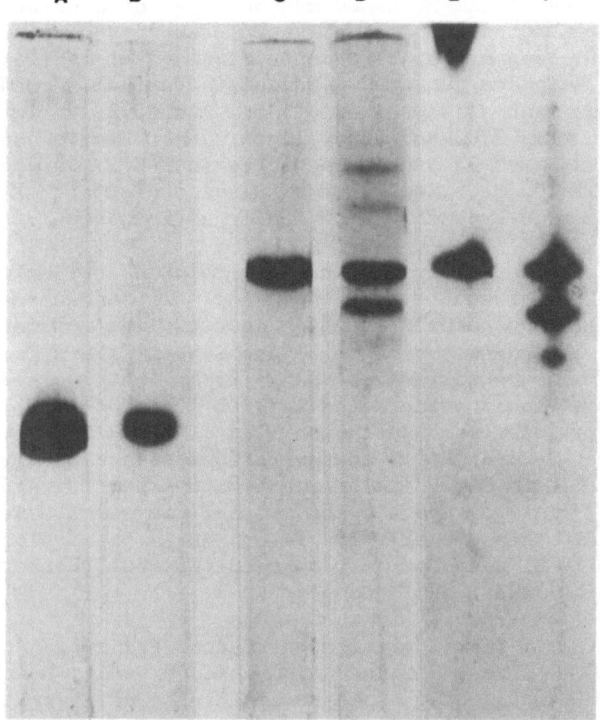

Fig. 4. Comparison of apo SAS$_{SAM}$ with tissue
amyloid fibril protein, AS$_{SAM}$ in gel
electrophoresis (12.5%). A) apo
SAS$_{SAM}$ and B) AS$_{SAM}$. Alkaline 8M urea-
polyacrylamide gel electrophoresis of
C) apo SAS$_{SAM}$ and D) AS$_{SAM}$. Antibody
labeling of E) apo SAS$_{SAM}$ and F) AS$_{SAM}$
separated by alkaline-urea-polyacrylamide slab gel electrophoresis. Protein bands reacting with antiserum
against apo SAS$_{SAM}$ were detected by
the unlabeled immunoperoxidase (PAP)
method after transfer to nitrocellulose
paper.

(PAP) method. Only three protein bands of AS$_{SAM}$ showed immunoreactivity to
anti-SAS$_{SAM}$ antiserum. This finding indicates that the upper bands of AS$_{SAM}$
in alkaline-urea-polyacrylamide gel electrophoresis probably represent contamination. The amino acid composition of apo AS$_{SAM}$ as determined by the
method described (Matsumura et al., 1982) is similar to that of AS$_{SAM}$:
large amounts of glutamic acid and a lack of cystine and tryptophan (Table
2). This amino acid pattern is also similar to that of rat apo A-II apolipoprotein (Herbert et al., 1974).

DISCUSSION

Although senile amyloidosis in mice was described years ago (Thung,
1957; Sheinberg et al., 1976; Chai, 1976), little is known of the pathogenesis of amyloidosis or the biochemical nature of amyloid protein and its
precursor protein. We have isolated a new murine senile amyloid fibril pro-

tein from the livers of SAM-P, a new murine model of accelerated senescence. This amyloid protein is clearly different from murine protein AA and immunoglobulin components. The deposition of this amyloid protein "AS$_{SAM}$" has also been demonstrated immunohistochemically in old mice of some other strains such as SAM-R, A/J, SJL/J and C57BL/6J in addition to SAM-P (Higuchi et al., 1983 and unpublished data). It is conceivable, therefore, that the amyloid protein detected in SAM is unique to murine "Senile amyloidosis." We expect that a human counterpart of AS$_{SAM}$ will soon be detected in various types of human senile amyloidosis.

We found that mouse serum has an AS$_{SAM}$-related antigenic substance, "SAS$_{SAM}$", regardless of the strain. Apo SAS$_{SAM}$ is considered to be apo A-II, a major apolipoprotein in the high density lipoproteins on the basis of the following five observations: 1) Apo SAS$_{SAM}$ exists in physiological concentration in mouse serum, unlike SAA. 2) Apo SAS$_{SAM}$ is present in HDL fractions only and cannot be detected in VLDL fractions. 3) The amino acid composition and gel electrophoretic mobility of apo SAS$_{SAM}$ are similar to those of rat apo A-II. 4) Serum concentrations of apo SAS$_{SAM}$ and apo A-I parallel one another in SAM-P and decrease with advancing age (Higuchi et al., 1984). The levels of apo A-I and apo A-II in serum have been reported to move in parallel (Blum et al., 1977). 5) AS$_{SAM}$ has a blocked N-terminus. Human and rat apo A-II also have a blocked N-terminus (Herbert et al., 1974; Bremer et al., 1972).

AS$_{SAM}$, an amyloid fibril protein in tissue, and apo SAS$_{SAM}$ have the same molecular weight, very similar amino acid composition and the same antigenic properties. Although some heterogeneity of AS$_{SAM}$ was observed in gel electrophoresis, the major component of AS$_{SAM}$ had the same mobility in alkaline-urea-polyacrylamide gel electrophoresis and the same isoelectric point (data now shown) as SAS$_{SAM}$. These findings suggest that AS$_{SAM}$ circulates in serum as apo SAS$_{SAM}$. Amyloid protein "AS$_{SAM}$" appears to be derived from apo A-II. Further studies are under way to determine whether apo SAS$_{SAM}$ is the true precursor of AS$_{SAM}$.

The process of apo A-II (apo SAS$_{SAM}$) transformation to AS$_{SAM}$ has not been elucidated. However, investigation of this amyloid protein and its putative serum precursor in this new murine model will provide significant clues to the pathogenesis of senile amyloidosis and the relationship of senescence and amyloidosis.

ACKNOWLEDGMENTS

Gratitude is extended to Dr. Y. Suzuki, Kyoto University, for pertinent advice and to K. Kogishi, S. Yasuoka, T. Matsushita and T. Tomita for expert technical assistance and to Dr. A. Cary for comments on the manuscript. This work was supported by grants from the Ministry of Education, Culture and Science and Ministry of Health and Welfare.

REFERENCES

1. Benditt, E. P., Eriksen, N., and Hanson, R. H., Proc. Nat. Acad. Sci. U.S.A., 76:4092 (1979).
2. Blum, C. B., Levy, R. I., Eisenberg, S., Hall, III, M., Goebel, R. H., and Berman, M., J. Clin. Invest., 60:795 (1977).
3. Brewer, H. B., Jr., Lux, S. E., Roman, R., and John, K. M., Proc. Nat. Acad. Sci. U.S.A., 69:1304 (1972).
4. Camus, M. C., Chapman, M. J., Forgez, P., and Laplaud, P. M., J. Lipid Res., 24:1210 (1983).

5. Chai, C. K., Am. J. Pathol., 85:49 (1976).
6. Davis, B. J., Ann. N.Y. Acad. Sci., 121:404 (1964).
7. Glenner, G. G., N. Engl. J. Med., 302:1333 (1980).
8. Glenner, G. G., Page, D., Isersky, C., Harada, M., Cuatrecasas, P., Eanes, E. D., DeLellis, R. A., Bladen, N. A., and Keiser, H. R., J. Histochem. Cytochem., 19:16 (1971).
9. Herbert, P. N., Windmueller, H. G., Bersot, T. P., and Shulman, R. S., J. Biol. Chem., 249:5718 (1974).
10. Higuchi, K., Matsumura, A., Hashimoto, K., Honma, A., Takeshita, S., Hosokawa, M., Yasuhira, K., and Takeda, T., J. Exp. Med., 158:1600 (1983).
11. Higuchi, K., Matsumura, A., Honma, A., Takeshita, S., Hashimoto, K., Hosokawa, M., Yasuhira, K., and Takeda, T., Lab. Invest., 48:231 (1983).
12. Higuchi, K., Matsumura, A., Honma, A., Toda, K., Takeshita, S., Matsushita, M., Yonezu, T., Hosokawa, M., and Takeda, T., Mech. Ageing Dev., 26:311 (1984).
13. Hosokawa, M., Kasai, R., Higuchi, K., Takeshita, S., Shimizu, K., Honma, A., Irino, M., Toda, K., Matsumura, A., Matsushita, M., and Takeda, T., Mech. Ageing Dev., 26:91 (1984).
14. LeBoeuf, R. C., Puppione, D. L., Schumaker, V. N., and Lusis, A. J., J. Biol. Chem., 258:5063 (1983).
15. Matsumura, A., Higuchi, K., Shimizu, K., Hosokawa, M., Hashimoto, K., Yasuhira, K., and Takeda, T., Lab. Invest., 47:270 (1982).
16. MacAdam, K. P. W. J., and Sipe, J. D. (1976); J. Exp. Med., 144:1121 (1976).
17. Pras, M., Zucker-Franklin, D., Rimon, A., and Franklin, E. F., J. Exp. Med., 130:777 (1969).
18. Sheinberg, M. A., Cathcart, E. S., Eastcott, J. W., Skinner, M., Benson, M., Shirahama, T., and Bennet, M., Lab. Invest., 35:47 (1976).
19. Takeda, T., Hosokawa, M., Takeshita, S., Irino, M., Higuchi, K., Matsushita, T., Tomita, Y., Yashuhira, K., Hamamoto, H., Shimizu, K., Ishiii, M., and Yamamuro, T., Mech. Ageing Dev., 17:183 (1981).
20. Takeshita, S., Hosokawa, M., Irino, M., Higuchi, K., Shimizu, K., Yasuhira, K., Takeda, T., Mech. Ageing Dev., 20:13 (1982).
21. Towbin, H., Staehelin, T., and Gordon, T., Proc. Nat. Acad. Sci. U.S.A., 76:4350 (1979).
22. Westermark, P., Sletten, K., Naeser, P., and Natvig, J. B., Scand. J. Immunol., 9:193 (1979).

AMYLOID DEPOSITION IN THE ARTICULAR STRUCTURES

OF SENESCENCE ACCELERATED MOUSE (SAM)

Katsuji Shimizu*, Masaharu Ishii*,
Ryuichi Kasai*, Mutsumi Matsushita*,
Takao Yamamuro*, Keiichi Higuchi†,
and Toshio Takeda†

*Department of Orthopaedic Surgery
 Faculty of Medicine and

†Department of Pathology
 Chest Disease Research Institute
 Kyoto University
 Sakyo-ku, Kyoto 606, Japan

INTRODUCTION

Age-associated amyloid deposition in human articular structure has been described in synovial joints (Uchino et al., 1980; Goffin et al., 1981) and in intervertebral discs (Takeda et al., 1984). Although spontaneous or induced amyloidosis can be demonstrated in different species, little is known of amyloid in articular structures. In autopsies of Senescence Accelerated Mouse (SAM), a new inbred strain of mouse raised from AKR strain as an animal model of senescence (Takeda et al., 1981), the high incidences of amyloid deposition was noted and these closely related to aging (Shimizu et al., 1981; Shimizu et al., 1982).

MATERIALS AND METHODS

For histological studies of synovial joints, 48 mice of SAM-P which originate from AKR and show a process of accelerated aging, and 38 mice of SAM-R which also originate from AKR and show a normal aging process were autopsied (Takeda et al., 1981). For histological studies of intervertebral discs, 51 mice of SAM-P and 23 mice of SAM-R were autopsied. Joints of the limbs and spine were fixed in 10% formalin and processed routinely. Sections were stained with hematoxylin and eosin, alkaline Congo red (Puchtler et al., 1962), and Thioflavin-T (Vassar and Culling, 1959). The intertarsal, knee, hip, glenohumeral, elbow, intercarpal, zygapophyseal joints and interverebral disc from cervical to sacral spine were examined histologically. Green birefringence of the Congo red stain under the polarizing microscope was considered to represent amyloid.

Articular cartilage from the knee joint and cervical intervertebral disc were also examined by electron microscopy. After dissection of sacrificed mice, specimens were fixed for 1.5 hours in 3% glutaraldehyde, buffered with 0.1 M cacodylate at pH 7.4, and postfixed with 1% osmium tetroxide for 1 h at 4°C. These specimens were embedded in Epon 812 after dehydration. Ultrathin sections cut with glass knives were stained with uranyl acetate–lead citrate and examined under an electron microscope (JEM-100C) with an accelerated voltage of 80 kV.

Immunohistochemical characterization of the amyloid in articular structures were carried out using peroxidase–anti–peroxidase (PAP) method (Fujihara et al., 1980). A novel amyloid protein AS_{SAM} was obtained by water solubilization followed by Sephadex chromatography (Matsumura et al., 1982). Amyloid AA protein was obtained after serial casein injection of CBA mice and with the same method applied to AS_{SAM}. Anti–serum against AS_{SAM} and AA were raised by foot pad injection of these antigens with complete Freund's adjuvant and absorption with normal liver homogenate (Higuchi et al., 1983).

RESULTS

Amyloid in the synovial joint was located in the capsular attachment of the meniscus and in the joint capsule of the transition zone. Thin layers of amyloid were seen on the surface of the articular cartilage and meniscus, particularly in the contact area and remote from the transition zone. Blood vessels around the joint were frequently infiltrated with amyloid. Annulus fibrosus was the site of amyloid deposition in intervertebral disc. The absence of blood vessels in these lesions was verified in the serial sections stained by H & E because these mice have amyloid deposition in blood vessels systemically (Takeshita et al., 1982).

Electron microscopic studies of the articular cartilage of the knee joint and cervical intervertebral disc revealed an accumulation of fibrils which were rigid and nonbranching. The sizes of the fibrils were about 100 Å in width and 1000–10,000 Å in length in cartilage and about 70 Å in width and 1000–3000 Å in length in annulus fibrosus respectively.

The incidence of amyloid synovial joints was correlated with age in each series of mice. When any tissue of the joint (synovium, fibrous capsule, articular cartilage or meniscus) showed amyloid deposition, a joint was described as amyloid-positive. No positive amyloid joint was found in mice younger than 6 months, and the incidence of amyloide joint was significantly age-related according to Spearman's Rho test ($P < 0.01$) in SAM-P mice. Incidence was equal between both sexes. SAM-P/2 was the most likely to develop amyloid joint, since the incidence in mice over 8 months of age was 88% (7/8). In SAM-R, the incidence was low. None of SAM-R/1 mice had amyloid joints. One positive case was found in each of SAM-R/2 and SAM-R/3 series. Both were old mice, 16 months in SAM-R/2 and 20 months in SAM-R/3. In those animals, no histologic difference was noted with respect to the site or pattern of amyloid deposition.

The incidence of amyloid in intervertebral disc was also found to be closely related with age. No amyloid positive discs were found in mice younger than 6 months, and the incidence of amyloid in discs was significantly related to age in SAM-P series, according to Spearman's Rho test ($P < 0.001$). SAM-P/1 mice were the most likely to develop amyloid in discs; the incidence of amyloid in mice more than 12 months old in this group was 100% (10/10). In SAM-R series, the incidence of amyloid was low, but three older SAM-R/2 mice had amyloid deposition for which no histologic difference was noted in regard to the site or pattern of deposition. The incidence of amyloid was the same for both sexes.

Among the synovial joints examined, the knee joint was the most frequently involved; the glenohumeral, hip, elbow and zygapophyseal joints were less often infiltrated, whereas the intertarsal and intercarpal joints were spared without exception. Among the intervertebral discs from the

cervical to the sacral spine, cervical and upper thoracic intervertebral
discs had amyloid deposition. There was no preference of deposition in
the anterior or posterior part of the annulus.

Immunohistochemical study of the amyloid in articular structures revealed coexistence of two kinds of amyloid simultaneously. The amyloid in
the knee joint and cervical disc reacted both with anti-AS$_{SAM}$ and anti-AA,
whereas control specimen did not react with normal rabbit serum or with
anti-sera absorbed with specific antigens.

DISCUSSION

Amyloid is represented by the green birefringence that is visible in
polarized light after staining with Congo red (Glenner, 1980). Although
the specificity of the green birefringence following Congo red staining has
been questioned by several authors, Carson and Kingsley (1980) noted that
false birefringence is closely related to the excess dye retained in the
tissue and that the technique used is most important. Using their suggestion, the histologic method of Puchtler, Sweat, and Levine (1962) was used
in this study and emphasis was placed on the saturation of the staining reagent with sodium chloride. Although Thioflavin-T stain lacks specificity
for amyloid fibrils, it corroborates the identification of amyloid by its
distinctly brilliant color under fluorescence microscopy. Demonstration
of the characteristic fibrils by electron microscopy in the cartilage and
annulus fibrosus provides a more definite identification of the substance
as amyloid (Cohen and Shirahama, 1972).

These mice show a high incidence of systemic amyloidosis (Takeshita
et al., 1982). The pathologic findings in the liver, spleen, and kidney
of 81 of the 86 mice in the present study were correlated with the lesions
of the synovial joints. The incidence of systemic amyloidosis as denoted
by the presence of amyloid deposition in the liver, spleen or kidney increased with age from as early as 6 months in SAM-P; SAM-P/2 showed an incidence of 100% over the age of 6 months. However, the joints in all the
6-months-old mice were negative for amyloid. The mice without systemic
amyloidosis were free from amyloid joints, but 15 mice with joints negative for amyloid had systemic amyloidosis. These data indicate that articular structures are less prone to develop amyloid deposition than sites such
as the liver, spleen, and kidney.

The relation between amyloid and aging in the absence of any causative
disease has been noted in both humans and laboratory animals (Thung, 1957).
Several recent reports describe age-associated amyloid deposition in human
articular structures (Uchino et al., 1980; Goffin et al., 1981; Takeda et
al., 1984). The amyloid deposition in the articular structures of these
mice seems to have a close relation to aging for two reasons: 1) the age
and the incidence of amyloid deposition in the articular structures showed
a statistically significant correlation in SAM-P series, and 2) several
older mice of SAM-R series showed positive amyloid deposition histologically
identical to the lesion in SAM-P series.

Immunohistochemical study revealed coexistence of two kinds of amyloid
in the articular structures of these mice. PAP method was found to be useful for the study of the amyloid in articular structures. It is provable
that many kinds of amyloid deposit in articular structures as well as in
the typical site of amyloid deposition such as liver, spleen, and kidney.

Amyloid deposition in the articular structures of SAM had a close coincidence with that of human joint in the site and pattern of deposition.

These mice will be an excellent model for the study of aging change of articular structures especially from the viewpoint of amyloid deposition.

REFERENCES

Carson, F. L., and Kingsley, W. B., Arch. Path. Lab. Med., 104:333 (1980).
Cohen, A. S., and Shirahama, T., Amer. J. Path., 68:441 (1972).
Fujihara, S., Balow, J. E., Costa, J. C., and Glenner, G. G., Lab. Invest., 43:358 (1980).
Glenner, G. G., New Engl. J. Med., 302:1283 (1980).
Goffin, Y. A., Thoua, Y., and Potvliege, P. R., Ann. Rheum. Dis., 40:27 (1981).
Higushi, K., Matsumura, A., Honma, A., Takeshita, S., Hashimoto, K., Hosokawa, M., Yasuhira, K., and Takeda, T., Lab. Invest., 48:231 (1983).
Matsumura, A., Higuchi, K., Shimizu, K., Hosokawa, M., Hashimoto, K., Yasuhira, K., and Takeda, T., Lab. Invest., 47:270 (1982).
Puchtler, H., Sweat, F., and Levine, M., J. Histochem. Cytochem., 10:355 (1962).
Shimizu, K., Ishii, M., Yamamuro, T., Takeshita, S., Hosokawa, M., and Takeda, T., Arthr. Rheum., 25:710 (1982).
Shimizu, K., Kasai, R., Yamamuro, T., Hosokawa, M., Takeshita, S., and Takeda, T., Arthr. Rheum., 24:1540 (1981).
Takeda, T., Hosokawa, M., Takeshita, S., Irino, M., Higuchi, K., Matsushita, T., Tomita, Y., Yasuhira, K., Hamamoto, H., Shimizu, K., Ishii, M., and Yamamuro, T., Mech. Ageing Dev., 17:183 (1981).
Takeda, T., Sanada, H., Ishii, M., Matsushita, M., Yamamuro, T., Shimizu, K., and Hosokawa, M., Arthr. Rheum., 27:1063 (1984).
Takeshita, S., Hosokawa, M., Irino, M., HIguchi, K., Shimizu, K., Yasuhira, K., and Takeda, T., Mech. Ageing Dev., 20:13 (1982).
Thung, P. J., Gerontologia, 1:234 (1957).
Uchino, F., Nakamura, H., Kamei, T., and Nagasawa, T., in: Amyloid and Amyloidosis (G. G, Glenner, P. P. Costa, and A. F. Freitas, eds.), Excerpta Medica, Amsterdam (1980), p. 55.
Vassar, P. S., and Culling, C. F. A., AMA Arch. Path., 68:487 (1959).

ANTIOXIDANTS IN EXPERIMENTAL AMYLOIDOSIS OF YOUNG

AND OLD MICE

Simin Nikbin Meydani, Edgar S. Cathcart,
Robert E. Hopkins, Mohsen Meydani,
Kenneth C. Hayes, and Jeffry B. Blumberg

E.N.R.M.V.A. Hospital
Bedford, Massachusetts

USDA Human Nutrition Research Center on Aging
Tufts University
Boston Massachusetts

Boston University School of Medicine
Boston, Massachusetts

ABSTRACT

Santoguin and vitamin E were added to the diets of six week old CBA/J mice that were fed mouse chow and received daily subcutaneous casein (CAS) injections and 24 month old C57BL/6Nia mice fed a casein enriched diet respectively. DNA synthetic responses to Phytohemagglutinin (PHA) and Concanavalin A (ConA) were measured in spleen cell cultures to determine the effects of these potent antioxidants on cellular immune function. The incidence and degree of amyloidosis was measured after Congo red staining of formalin fixed sections.

Fifty seven percent of mice receiving santoguin plus CAS injections developed amyloid, and the mean score of amyloid infiltration was 1.2 × 1.2. In contrast, 95% of mice receiving CAS injections without santoquin developed amyloid, and the score (2.8 ± 1.0) was greater than the santoquin plus CAS group ($p \leqslant 0.05$). None of the old C57BL/6Nia mice receiving 500 ppm vitamin E or young mice (3 month old) receiving 30 ppm vitamin E developed amyloidosis, whereas 40% of old mice receiving 30 ppm vitamin E had amyloid deposits in the kidney. ConA and PHA responses were significantly higher in spleen cell cultures from mice given santoquin or vitamin E versus mice that did not receive antioxidants ($p \leqslant 0.05$). These data clearly show that antioxidants retard or prevent casein induced amyloidosis in young and aged mice. The beneficial effects of these agents may be due to preservation of normal catabolism of serum or tissue amyloid precursors and/or thymus dependent immune function.

INTRODUCTION

Although substantial progress has been made in defining the composition and chemical nature of amyloid deposits, the pathological process(es) leading to their deposition is not well understood. Recent studies indi-

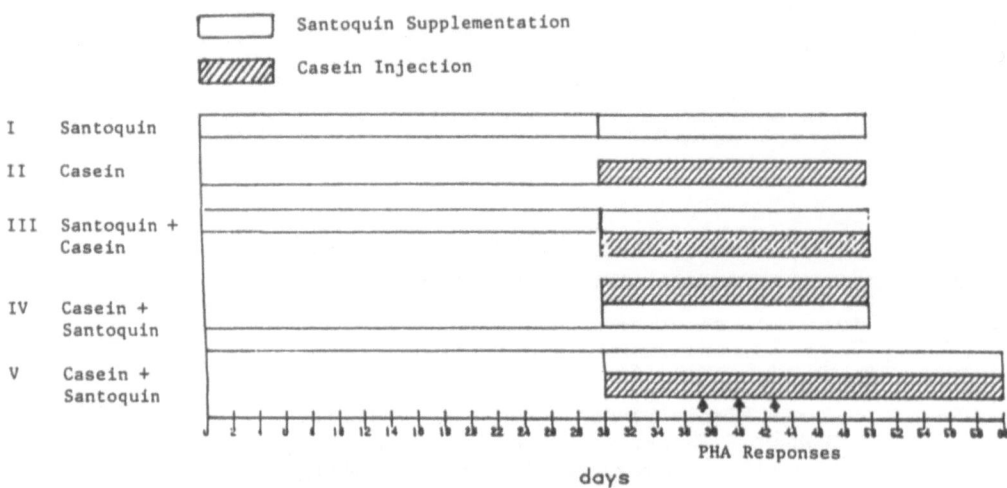

Fig. 1. Experimental design for experiment 1.

cate that proteolysis of a soluble precursor by monocytes [1, 2] and/or
polymorphonuclear leukocytes (PMN) [3] plays a significant role in formation
of fibril of the AA type. Oxidative products of arachidonic acid metabolism, including prostaglandins (PGs), thromboxane and leukotrienes are involved in control of different aspects of monocytes and PMN function including their proteolytic enzyme activity [4] and monokine production.
Furthermore, the immunoregulatory role of prostaglandins is well known
[5, 6]. One of the features associated with both aging and development of
experimentally induced amyloidosis in mice is depressed mitogenic response
of lymphocytes [7, 8]. Free radical formation and lipid peroxidation may
also play a key role in the genesis of amyloidosis [9] and the aging process [10]. Therefore, in the present study, we looked at: 1) The effect
of antioxidant santoquin (1,2-dihydro-6-ethoxy-2,2,4-trimethylquinoline)
on severity and incidence of casein induced amyloidosis in six weel old
CBA/j mice. 2) The effect of vitamin E (dl-α-tocopheryl acetate) on incidence of kidney amyloidosis in 3 and 24 month old C57BL/6Nia mice.

METHODS

Animals and Experimental Design

1) Experiment 1: Six week old CBA/j mice were fed a diet to which
0.25% by weight of santoquin (Monsanto, St. Louis, Missouri) was added.
One month later, daily subcutaneous injections of 5% casein (CAS) solution
were started and the incidence and degree of amyloid deposition measured
at weekly intervals on a scale of 0-4 splenic involvement. Controls included age and sex-matched mice receiving only santoquin or CAS. The overall design of the experiment is shown in Fig. 1. DNA synthetic responses
to phytohemaglutinin (PHA) and Concanavalin-A (ConA), both T-cell mitogens,
were also measured in spleen cell cultures from experimental animals to determine the effect of santoquin on cellular immune function.

2) Experiment 2: Twenty-four month old male C57BL/6Nia mice were fed
a semi-synthetic diet containing 18% by weight of vitamin free casein and
supplemented with either 30 ppm dl-α-tocopheryl acetate (vitE) (control
diet) or 500 ppm vitE (vitE diet) for six weeks. In addition a group of
3 month old mice were fed the control diet. Prior to the start of the ex-

TABLE 1. Composition of the Basal Diet for Experiment 2

Ingredient	% weight
Vitamin free casein	18.00
Fat[a]	7.00
Corn Starch	31.55
Sucrose	31.55
Cellulose	5.00
D-L methionine	0.30
Choline Chloride	0.10
Salt Mix (AIN-76)[b]	3.50
Vitamin Mix[c]	1.00

a - 1.2% stripped corn oil and 3.8% stripped lard

b - The salt mix was supplemented with 0.0023 mg/kg
diet of Na fluoride

c - Composition/kg vitamin mix: vitamin A acetate, 150,000
IU; vitamin D, 15,000 IU; vitamin E, (per experimental
design); vitamin K, 5 mg; biotin, 20 mg; folacin, 200
mg; inositol, 2,380 mg; niacin, 3,000 mg; Ca pantothen-
ate, 1,600 mg; riboflavin, 700 mg; thiamin, 600 mg;
vitamin B_6, 700 mg; vitamin B_{12}, 1 mg.

periments, the mice were fed mice show which contains about 22% mixed protein (combination of ground wheat, soybean meal, ground corn, meat and bone
meal). Incidence of kidney amyloidosis as well as mitogenic response of
splenocytes to ConA was measured at sacrifice.

HISTOLOGY

Parafin-embedded sections were cut at 6 μm and stained with Congo red
by the method of Puchtler, Sweat, and Levine [11], and counterstained with
hematoxylin. On polarization microscopy, amyloid was identified as
amorphous green birefringent material.

LYMPHOCYTE PROLIFERATION

Spleen cells obtained under sterile conditions were washed twice in
RPMI 1640 supplemented with penicillin-streptomycin and then suspended in
RPMI1640 for experiment 1 or RPM1640 supplemented with 10% fetal calf serum
for experiment 2. Cultures were performed in triplicate in falcon tissue
culture plates at 37°C in 5 percent CO_2. Each well contained 2×10^5 cells

TABLE 2. Incidence and Severity of Amyloidosis in Casein Induced Amylosis in CBA/j Mice

Treatment	Group[a]	No. of animals	Amyloid Production (mean score)	(% incidence)
Casein	II	20	2.8 ± 1.0[b]	95[c]
Santoquin + Casein	III	28	1.2 ± 1.2	57
Casein + Santoquin	IV	30	1.7 ± 1.4	70

a - See figure 1,

b - Mean $\pm$ SD, statistically significant at $P < 0.05$.

c - Statistically significant at $P < 0.05$ by chi-squared test.

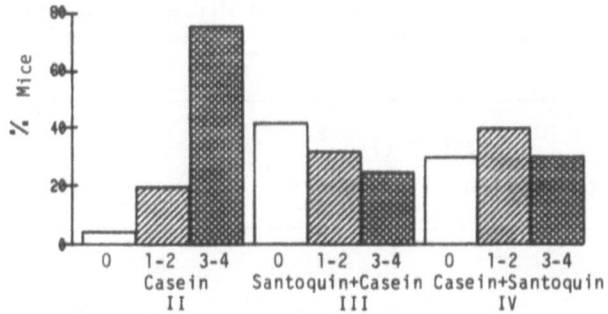

Fig. 2. Effect of santoquin supplementation
on amyloid score distribution in
CMA/J mice.

TABLE 3. Effect of Age and Vitamin E Supplementation on Kidney Amyloidosis in Mice

Age(Mo.)	Dietary vitE(ppm)	% mice with kidney amyloidosis
3	30	0
24	30	40[a]
24	500	0

a - Statistically significant by chi-squared
test at P< 0.05.

in a total of 0.2 ml. For each mitogen dose response curves were determined and optimal concentrations used for all cultures.

Prior to termination of cultures 0.5 μCi of 3H thymidine (NEN specific
activity 6.7 Ci/mmol) was added to each well. Cultures were harvested 72 h
after the start. Means from triplicate cultures were used to calculate the
stimulation index (XI) at each concentration of mitogen: SI = mitogen
stimulated counts/counts in unstimulated cultures.

STATISTICAL ANALYSIS

The data were analyzed by one way analysis of variance or chi-squared
test (per percent indicence) and are reported at mean ±SD.

RESULTS

As seen in Table 2, 95% of the animals receiving casein injection without santoquin developed amyloidosis whereas 57% of the mice supplemented
with santoquin one month prior to injection of casein developed amyloidosis.
The mean score of mice supplemented with santoquin was significantly less
(1.2 ± 1.2) (p < 0.05) than that of mice not supplemented with santoquin
(2.8 ± 1.0). Figure 2 shows the distribution of amyloid score among different groups. As can be seen 75% of the mice receiving casein and no
santoquin supplementation had a score of 3-4, whereas only 25% of santoquin
supplemented mice had a score of 3-4. Santoquin supplementation was most

687

TABLE 4. The Effect of Casein Injection on Mitogenic Response of Splenocytes from Mice Fed Chow or Chow Supplemented with Santoquin
(mean ± SD)

No. of Casein injections	Casein (II) [a]		Casein and Santoquin [a]	
	cpm Control	cpm PHA[b]	cpm Control	cpm PHA
8	1540±500	1490±330	570±400	11650±3470
10	1570±540	4860±876	4280±320	17180±4720
13	3220±710	5260±1020	5480±610	12300±2080
29	980±430	13060±4010	910±320	13420±3110

a - see experimental design, figure 1

b - 10 µg/ml

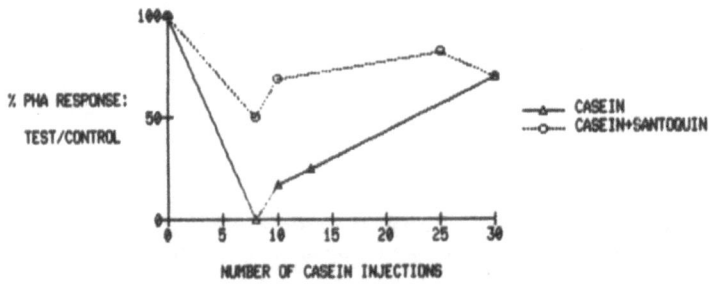

Fig. 3. Effect of casein injection and santoquin supplementation on mitogenic response of splenocytes
to PHA.

effective in preventing amyloidosis if it was given prior to the start of
casein injections (group III vs. IV). On the other hand, 40% of the old
mice fed high casein diet developed kidney amyloidosis, whereas none of the
young mice fed the same diet or old mice fed the same diet supplemented
with vitE developed kidney amyloidosis (see Table 3). As expected, splenocytes from mice given casein alone had marked depression of PHA responses
following 7 and 14 daily injections (see Table 4 and Fig. 3). However,
these responses were not altered in mice given casein injection and santoquin supplement. Figure 4 show mitogenic response of splenocytes from
young and old mice fed control or vitE diet. As can be seen old mice fed
control diet (30 ppm vitE) have significantly less SI than young mice fed
control diet. However, vitamin E supplementation (old mice fed vitE diet)
significantly improved their ConA response ($p < 0.05$).

DISCUSSION

Amyloidosis can be produced in mice by frequent injections of casein
solution [12] or by feeding a casein enriched diet [13, 14]. Recent studies

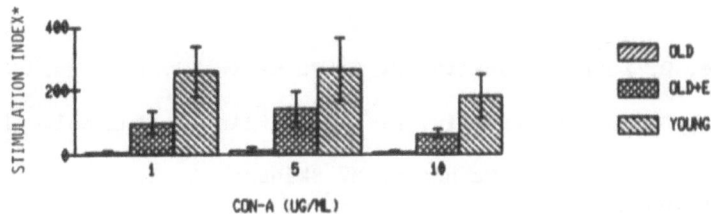

Fig. 4. The effect of age and vitamin E supplementation on proliferative response of splenocytes to CON/A mitogen. (*) Ratio of CPM of stimulated culture to that of non-stimulated culture.

from our laboratory showed that oxidative metabolism of arachidonic acid by monocytes might be important in the casein model [15]. Moreover, the incidence of amyloidosis increases with age and aged mice have altered PG metabolism and depressed immune responsiveness. Therefore, a hypothesis has been entertained that oxidative processes might contribute to the patho-genesis of casein induced amyloidosis in amyloid susceptible as well as in aged mice and that supplementing the diets with antioxidants (santoquin or vitE) might decrease incidence and severity of amyloidosis in both cases. The results of the present study indicate that santoquin decreased inci-dence and severity of casein induced amyloidosis in young CBA/j mice. This is in agreement with a previous report by Harman et al. [9]. In addition vitE, a well known biological antioxidant, prevented induction of kidney amyloidosis in aged mice fed a high casein diet. The effect of santoquin and vitamin E in both cases was associated with improved mitogenic response of lymphocytes.

It is interesting that none of the young mice fed a high casein diet with 30 ppm vitE developed amyloidosis, whereas 40% of old mice fed the same diet showed amyloidosis in their kidneys. This is even more remarkable when it is realized that amyloidosis is a very rare histopathological find-ing associated with aging C57BL/6Nia mice [16]. Since impaired monocytic and/or PMN proteolytic activity seems to play an important role in patho-genesis of amyloidosis [1, 2, 3], decreased proteolytic activity in aged mice might have predisposed them to development of kidney amyloidosis [17].

On the other hand, the beneficial effect of santoquin and vitamin E might be due to their antioxidant dampening of cyclooxygenase (generation of PG) or lipoxygenase (generation of hydroxy fatty acids and leukotriene) pathways or their terminating propagation of lipid peroxidation in general. This, in turn, can affect proteolytic enzyme activity by changing cAMP level. PGs have been shown to change intracellular cAMP level and in aged mice vitamin E decreases PG level in splenocytes [18]. Furthermore, since both santoquin and vitE have immuno-stimulatory effect [19, 20], their beneficial effect in preventing amyloid deposits might be due to preserva-tion of immune function.

ACKNOWLEDGEMENT

Supported by the Veterans Administration and USPHS Grant #AM32588 and USDA Human Nutrition Research Center on Aging at Tufts University.

REFERENCES

1. G. Lavie, D. Zucker-Franklin, E. C. Franklin, J. Exp. Med., 148:1020 (1978).
2. G. Lavie, D. Zucker-Franklin, E. C. Franklin, J. Immunol., 125:175 (1980).
3. S. L. Silverman, E. S. Cathcart, M. Skinner, A. S. Cohen., Immunol., 46:737 (1982).
4. J. B. McCarthy, S. M. Wahl, J. C. Rees, C. E. Olsen, A. L. Sandberg, L. M. Wahl, J. Immunol., 124:2405 (1980).
5. D. R. Webb, T. J. Rogers, I. Nowowiejski, Proc. N.Y. Acad. Sci., 332:260 (1980).
6. J. S. Goodwin, R. P. Messner, G. T. Peake, J. Clin. Invest., 54:368 (1974).
7. E. S. Cathcart, M. Mullarkey, A. S. Cohen, Immunol., 20:1001 (1971).
8. M. A. Scheinberg, M. Bennett, E. S. Cathcart, Lab. Invest., 33:96 (1975).
9. D. Harman, D. E. Eddy, J. Noffsinger, J. Am. Ger. Soc., 24:203 (1975).
10. D. Harman, Proc. Natl. Acad. Sci. U.S.A., 78:7124 (1981).
11. H. Puchtler, E. Sweat, M. Levine, J. Histochem. Cytochem., 10:355 (1964).
12. A. S. Cohen, E. S. Cathcart, Meth. Achievm. Exp. Path., 6:207 (1972).
13. E. Clerici, Path. Microbiol., 28:806 (1965).
14. D. Harman, J. Gerontol., 23:476 (1968).
15. C. Leslie, E. S. Cathcart, A. A. Lazzari, in: Proceedings of the 4th International Amyloid Congress (in press).
16. NIH Rodents: 1980 catalog (NIH Pub. No. 81-606), pp. 26-28 (1980).
17. R. W. Gracy, M. L. Chapman, M. Jhani, H. S. Lu, B. Oray, J. M. Talent, K. Yuksel. Fed. Proc., 43:1671 (1984).
18. S. N. Meydani, M. M. Meydani, C. P. Verdon, J. B. Blumberg, K. C. Hayes, Fed. Proc., 43:578 (1984).
19. D. Harman, Age, 3:64 (1980).
20. R. P. Tangerdy, Basic Clin. Nutr., 1:429 (1980).

I. CEREBRAL AMYLOIDOSIS AND ALZHEIMER'S DISEASE

AMYLOID RESEARCH AS A PARADIGM FOR ALZHEIMER'S DISEASE

George G. Glenner and Caine W. Wong

University of California
San Diego, California

School of Medicine
Department of Pathology
(M-012)
La Jolla, California   92093

ABSTRACT

    Previous studies on amyloidosis have established certain concepts that
can be applied to newer investigations. Staining of tissues with Congo
red and subsequent polarization microscopy detects the β-pleated sheet conformation of proteins. Amyloid diffusely deposited in the walls of vessels
has its origin from an abnormal (variant, isotypic) serum protein. Protein
variants that can be formed into amyloid fibers are operationally defined
as "amyloidogenic". Amyloid fibrils must be solubilized before they become
immunogenic.

    The major diagnostic lesions of Alzheimer's disease (AD) consist of
amyloid fibrils in neuritic plaques, cerebrovascular amyloidosis and Congo
red stained, birefringent, neurofibrillary tangles (composed of paired
helical filaments). These same lesions are present in adult Down's syndrome (DS). The protein component, β-protein, of the cerebrovascular amyloid fibrils from Alzheimer's disease has been purified and amino acid sequence analysis performed with a computer search revealing no homology to
any previously sequenced protein. An homologous protein has been isolated
from the amyloid-laden vessels in Down's syndrome individuals over age 40.
This suggests that Down's syndrome is the first predictable model for
Alzheimer's disease. Previous studies have revealed that vascular amyloid
is derived from an abnormal (variant, isotypic) serum protein. In Alzheimer's disease the detection of such an "amyloidogenic" serum protein
could provide (for the first time) a diagnostic test for Alzheimer's
disease. Immunohistochemical studies not only revealed β-protein reactivity
of cerebrovascular amyloid but also in all neuritic plaques of both Alzheimer's disease and Down's syndrome.

AMYLOID RESEARCH AS A PARADIGM FOR THE STUDY OF
ALZHEIMER'S DISEASE

    In the past amyloidosis was an enigma enveloped in a baffling variety
of clinical manifestations and dramatic pathologic lesions. Once the major

693

fibrillar component was recognized [1, 2] and means were developed to solubilize its resistant protein components [3], and these were chemically defined, much of the mystery peeled away to reveal a disease complex of multiple protein origins that corresponded to the clinically evident nosology, i.e., different clinically defined processes had amyloid fibrils composed of different distinct proteins [4]. The commonality that unified this disease complex was fibrils composed of proteins in a twisted β-pleated sheet conformation [5]. Of all the amyloidotic processes Alzheimer's disease is the most prevalent representing the fourth most common cause of death in the United States and claiming 2.5 million victims. The purpose of this paper is to demonstrate how the principles of amyloid research were applied to Alzheimer's disease and the results of these investigations.

Congo Red Polarization Color

Since its discovery by Bennhold in 1924, Congo red has been found to be relatively selective as a dye for amyloid deposits. Using polarization microscopy following Congo red staining Divry in 1927, showed the distinctive lesions of Alzheimer's disease: the neuritic plaques, neurofibrillary tangles and cerebrovascular amyloidosis were green biregringent and called all "amyloid" [6]. With the advent of the Puchtler et al. [7] staining method greater selectivity for amyloid was achieved, though linear polysaccharides [8] gave the reaction. Its specificity was still questioned [9], usually when improperly employed. The periodic acid Schiff reaction most often was reactive in amyloidotic sites suggesting to some that amyloid was a glycoprotein. The polarization color with Congo red established that an ordered ultrastructure existed [10].

Electron Microscopy

The ordered structure of amyloid was defined by electron microscopy as ribbon-like, non-branching filaments twisted in a helical fashion [11] appearing to represent the major component of the deposits and responsible for the polarization color. Although the fiber was stated "classically" to have dimension of 70-80 Å in width, narrowing to 25 Å these measurements often varied over ±25% depending upon the fibril source studied.

X-Ray Diffraction

Examination of concentrates of amyloid fibrils from many conditions including multiple myeloma, insulinoma, rheumatoid arthritis, medullary carcinoma of the thyroid all revealed a 4.75-6 Å outer and a 9.8-10 Å inner d-spacing [5]. On orientation of the fibers arcing of the 9.8 Å line in the equatorial plane and of the 4.75 Å line in the meridional plane occurred. This pattern is characteristic of the β-pleated sheet configuration of proteins as described by Pauling and Corey [13] and exemplified by the egg-stalk of the silkworm, Chrysopa.

Insolubility

Concentration of the fibrillar component of amyloid by various methods could be used [14, 15]. None were universally effective [16]. Most likely as a result of its β-structure amyloid fibers are resistance to solution in the usual solvents and to enzymic degradation. The use of 6 M guanidine with dithiothreital proved an almost (but not quite-see below) universal solvent for the amyloid fibers [3]. Sephadex chromatography in this solvent (5 M guanidine-1 N acetic acid) provided the first fractionation of the amyloid fibril protein and its subsequent amino acid sequence analysis and characterization.

In Vitro Creation

Proof that fibers with all the characteristics of amyloid fibers could be created from some, but not all, of potential precursor serum proteins by proteolysis [17] indicated that proteolytic cleavage of precursor proteins could be one mechanism for amyloid formation. Enzymes most capable of this function are the lysosomal complement of phagoytic cells.

Amyloidogenic Proteins

From the above findings it appeared that systemic amyloidosis was caused by the proteolytic cleavage of variants (isotypes) of normal serum proteins. This could explain the 25% incidence of AL amyloidosis in light chain disease and the 11% incidence of AA amyloidosis in rheumatoid arthritis. It was predicted that the SAA protein in reactive amyloidosis was a generic eponym for several SAA species, one or more of which were "amyloidogenic" [18]. This was reemphasized [19] and proven by the finding of one of two serum AA isotypes being the protein incorporated in fiber formation in the mouse [20]. It was again confirmed with the isolation of prealbumin variants in clinically distinct familial amyloidotic polyneuropathies [21, 22]. It was predicted that in systemic disease a serum protein was the "amyloidogenic" protein and in tissue localized disease the "amyloidogenic" protein was of epithelical origin.

APPLICATION TO STUDIES IN ALZHEIMER'S DISEASE

Our interest in Alzheimer's disease (AD) was fostered during the composition of a review article on amyloidosis [4]. Our reading on the subject revealed a recurrent, but often contradictory, theme relating cerebrovascular amyloidosis to AD. Often this theme was hidden e.g. in the summary descriptions of cerebrovascular amyloidosis of Pantelakis [23] and Surbeck [24], the former noted that all his patients had plaques, while the latter noted that they were all demented. In order to clarify the relationship one of us (G.G.) spent a year at the Armed Forces Institute of Pathology, Washington, D.C., reviewing cases described as having neuritic plaques, neurofibrillary tangles, cerebral atrophy and dementia. Ninety-two percent of the cases studied by polarization microscopy after Congo red staining had evidence of cerebrovascular amyloidosis [25]. A review of other conditions including Pick's, hypertensive encephalopathy and age-matched normals revealed no cerebrovascular amyloidosis. We realize this is contrary to the reports of several other groups [26, 27] for which we have no ready explanation other than variations in the Congo red staining technique [9] and polarized light visualization. With this study [25] as baseline we then approached the isolation of the cerebrovascular amyloid from cases of AD. First it was necessary to establish the first National-Alzheimer's Disease Brain Bank at the University of California, San Diego in order to obtain sufficient material for isolation purposes.

The Theory

There are six pathologic conditions in which amyloid consistently affects vascular walls. Three are systemic and have an abnormal protein in their sera (AL, AA and AF) which has been isolated. Three are localized only to the cerebral vessels: Alzheimer's disease [25], adult Down's syndrome [28], and hereditary Icelandic cerebrovascular amyloidosis (HCHWA) [29], the nature (normal or abnormal) of their precursor protein is presently unknown (the amyloid fibril protein of HCHWA has, however, been identified as homologous to the serum protein, gamma trace).

Applying the concept of the "amyloidogenic" protein precursor to this problem, we speculated [30] that all of the cerebrovascular amyloidoses derive from an abnormal serum protein precursor. To explain any amyloid was localized to cerebral vessels and not systemically we reasoned that, since cerebral vessels are structurally different (tight-junction epithelia, a single arterial elastic lamella), they would as a consequence probably also be metabolically different. In other words we predicted that the lysosomal enzyme complement of cerebral vessel endothelial cells would differ from that of peripheral vessels. Invoking the proteolytic theory of amyloid fibril pathogenesis, we surmised that an abnormal serum protein normally digested by lysosomal enzymes in peripheral vessels would not be similarily cleaved by the different lysosomal enzymes in cerebral vessels and cerebrovascular amyloid fibril formation would result. Such a theory suggests the abnormal precursor serum protein is encoded by abnormal genes or subjected to abnormal modification (perhaps by an abnormal enzyme or by one that is improperly activated). Since AD is probably not a single disease there are probably several causes [25], but probably only a major single one. This is one of the few amyloidotic processes that has both familial and sporadic components.

Down's syndrome individuals over age 40 are known to have clinical aymptoms of dementia or cerebral dysfunction [30]. They also have all the pathologic cerebral lesions of AD: plaques, tangles and cerebrovascular amyloidosis [28, 32]. No logical explanation for these lesions has been forthcoming except for a gene overdosage due to the trisomy 21 condition. The finding that Down's individuals occur in AD families with an incidence three times that of normal [33] is striking.

Our hypothesis implicated an abnormal serum protein as the precursor of the cerebrovascular amyloid fibrils [30]. This lesion is known to cause hemorrhage [34], or stroke-like episodes in about 30% of AD patients as the result of damage to and rupture of vessel walls [28]. The vascular amyloid deposition would under any circumstances cause leakage of plasma into the cerebrum, a break in the blood-brain barrier [30]. The abnormal or other serum protein would penetrate the neuropil and as the result of pathoclisis attach to the neural receptors of specific pyramidal cells. This would perturb the neuronal environment to cause formation from neurofilament proteins of the paired helical filaments (PHF) composing the tangles. These cells would die and remnants be deposited as plagues, the microglia contributing their lysosomal enzymes to their degradation and amyloid core plaque formation [30]. This hypothesis has since been modified (see below).

The Research: Amyloid Fibril Isolation and Protein Characterization

It was decided that, since a continuum of amyloid deposits extended between leptomeningeal and intracortical vessels, the amyloid was probably of the same composition in both. In order, therefore, to prevent contamination by parenchymal brain tissue the leptomeningeal tissue was stripped from the cortical surface. Only this leptomeningeal tissue was used for amyloid isolation. The concentration of the cerebrovascular amyloid fibers followed previous methods [16]. They were resistant to distilled water suspension [15]. To rid or reduce the leptomeningeal preparation of its large quantity of collagen, collagenase treatment was employed during monitoring with Congo red under polarization optics. X-ray diffraction revealed clear 4.76 Å and 10 Å d-spacings with little background consistent with a relatively clean β-pleated sheet fibril preparation. The concentrate was

TABLE 1. Automated Amino Acid Sequence Analyses of β_2 Protein to Position 28 from Cerebrovascular Amyloid Fibrils Obtained from Alzheimer's Disease (AD) and Adult Down's Syndrome (DS). Variant Residue is Underlined

	1	2	3	4	5	6	7	8	9	10	11	12	13	14
AD	Asp	Ala	Glu	Phe	Arg	His	Asp	Ser	Gly	Tyr	Gln	Val	His	His
DS	Asp	Ala	Glu	Phe	Arg	His	Asp	Ser	Gly	Tyr	Glu	Val	His	His

	15	16	17	18	19	20	21	22	23	24	25	26	27	28
AD	Gln	Lys	Leu	Val	Phe	Phe	Ala	Glu	Asp	Val	Gly	Ser	Asn	Lys
DS	Gln	Lys	Leu	Val	Phe	Phe	Ala	Glu	Asp	Val	Gly	Ser	Asn	Lys

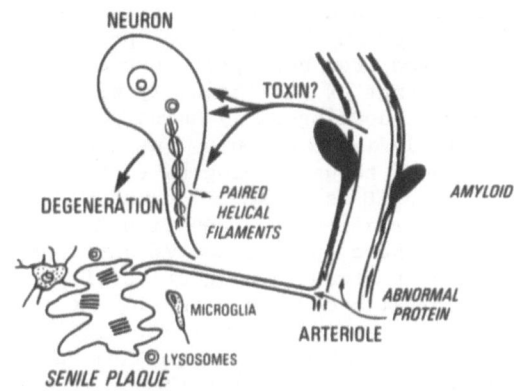

Fig. 1. Diagrammatic representation of the pathogenesis of Alzheimer's disease. An abnormal β protein serum precursor is taken up specifically by cerebrovascular endothelial cells to be proteolytically cleaved by their lysosomal complement to form amyloid fibrils. The amyloid fibril deposition breaks the blood-brain barrier and the (abnormal) serum protein(s) bind to neuronal cell membranes perturbing their environment. These neurons are caused to form abnormal neurofilaments (paired helical filaments) which cause the cells' death. Proteolytic cleavage by microglia of β protein, which has seeped through amyloid-affected capillary walls, produces the amyloid cores of neuritic plaques.

dissolved in guanidine-HCL in the presence of dithiothreitol and centrifuged, the supernatant dialyzed against distilled water and lyophilized. This sediment was dissolved in 1% SDS and applied to a calibrated SDS-urea PAGE gel [35]. A protein band at 4,800 daltons appeared only with amyloid preparations from AD patients and not from normal controls. It was designated β protein. This sediment was redissolved and placed on a calibrated G-100 Sephadex column and the proteins fractionated. Molecular weight determination of the β protein was 4,200 daltons.

We, thus, isolated from leptomeningial amyloidotic vessels a unique, major protein, the standard criteria for the amyloid fibril protein. The β protein was further fractionated by high pressure liquid chromatography (HPLC) in 100% acetonitrile to yield three peaks, β_1, β_2, and β_3. Amino acid sequence analysis of β_2 peak was performed to 28 amino acids (Table 1). Sequence analysis was also performed on the β_1 peak and this was found to be identical. The entire procedure was repeated on leptomeningial amyloidotic tissues from two cases of adult Down's syndrome ages 61 and 62 [35].

The Down's profile revealed a lesser quantity of the β_1 peak. No corresponding peaks were noted in three control preparations. In addition these chromatographs resolved from both protein preparations a β_3 peak, previously obscured within that of β_2 [36]. It was shown that the β_1 protein and the β_2 protein were homologous by amino acid sequence analysis [34]. Since β_3 was initially included in β_2 but did not result in sequencing background, β_3 is assumed to be homologous to β_2. Why β protein appears as a doublet or triplet on HPLC is presently unknown. A lesser amount of protein initiating with the Ala residue (position 2) and having the identical amino acid sequence as above to position 28 was found, however, in both the β_1 and β_2 peaks. This is strongly suggestive of proteolytic cleavage of the β-protein from a larger precursor primarily at the N-terminal Asp but also to a lesser extent at the Ala[2] residue. This situation is identical to that described for the amyloid fibril protein AA [37] in which the majority N-terminal sequence is Arg-Ser-Phe-Phe-Ser-Phe-but a lesser amount is Ser-Phe-Phe-Ser-Phe, presumably derived from a larger serum protein, SAA. The amino acid sequence analysis of the Alzheimer's and Down's β_2 protein fraction to residue 28 is presented in Table 1. Their proteins were found to have identical amino acid sequences through position 28 with the exception of a substitution in the Down's protein of a Glu for Gln residue at position 11. The retention of Gln[15] suggests that Gln[11] may be a true substitution, rather than the result of an artifactual deamidation. The preparation from the second Down's case gave an HPLC profile with an identical major peak at 36% acetonitrile, but inadequate material was available for sequencing. The β_2 protein is not homologous by computer search to the serum protein gamma trace [38] found to compose the cerebrovascular amyloid protein of an Icelandic hereditary amyloid angiopathy [20] nor to any other known sequenced protein [35].

These findings indicate that of the three disease processes most often characterized by cerebrovascular amyloidosis, i.e., Alzheimer's disease [25], adult Down's syndrome [28] and hereditary Icelandic amyloid angiopathy [38], only Alzheimer's disease and adult Down's syndrome share an homologous amyloid protein. This is the first evidence of a chemical relationship between Alzheimer's disease and Down's syndrome.

These findings indicate that of the three disease processes most often characterized by cerebrovascular amyloidosis, i.e., Alzheimer's disease [25], adult Down's syndrome [28] and hereditary Icelandic amyloid angiopathy [38], only Alzheimer's disease and adult Down's syndrome share an homologous amyloid protein. This is the first evidence of a chemical relationship between Alzheimer's disease and Down's syndrome.

Down's Syndrome

There is presently no known spontaneous or experimental animal model for Alzheimer's disease. There are mouse models for Down's syndrome [38], but since the trisomic fetuses do not survive beyond term, their value for the study of Alzheimer's disease is limited. The human familial cases of Alzheimer's disease tend to follow an autosomal dominant pattern of inheritance [33] with the usual statistical prediction of affected progeny. However, the great similarity in the cerebral lesions between adult Down's syndrome and Alzheimer's disease [28, 32] and the demonstration of chemical homology in the pathologic amyloid fibril β protein strongly suggests that Down's syndrome may represent the first truly predictable model for Alzheimer's disease.

The presence of a common amyloid protein and a protein synthetic abnormality in both Down's syndrome (trisomy 21) and Alzheimer's disease suggests the possibility that the genetic defect in Alzheimer's disease (whether acquired or heritable) is localized to chromosome 21. This makes possible alternative approaches to the non-invasive diagnosis of Alzheimer's disease [40, 41]. One intriguing possibility amongst many others is that this chemical evidence may signify that a gene defect in addition to the chromosomal abnormality of the trisomic condition exists in Down's syndrome. Such a defect may signify a specifically labile gene locus on chromosome 21 and might help to explain the statistically significant relationship between familial Alzheimer's disease and Down's syndrome [33].

No specific diagnostic test for Alzheimer's disease short of brain biopsy is presently available during the patient's life. The presence of amyloid fibril deposits in vessel walls is indicative of fibrillar derivation from an "abnormal" serum protein, i.e. a variant or isotype of a normal slerum protein. Several examples can be cited. This has been shown for amyloid fibrils derived from the light polypeptide chain of an immunoglobulin protein [40, 41], a prealbumin (Met[30]) variant [21] and an SAA protein isotype [20]. Therefore, we anticipate that a protein antigenically related to β protein will be detectable in the serum of normal individuals and persons with Alzheimer's disease and in those with adult Down's syndrome. The isotypic variant of the normal serum β-related protein, however, should only be present in Alzheimer's disease and Down's syndrome sera. This should lead to a specific blood serum test (e.g. radioimmunoassay) for the diagnosis of Alzheimer's disease based on the presence of a serum protein sharing antigenic determinants with β protein. Furthermore, Down's syndrome individuals may provide a diagnostic pattern of serum β protein concentration levels during aging that might be predictive of eventual diffuse cerebral dysfunction and/or dementia [31, 43]. Such a pattern might help to detect individuals at risk for Alzheimer's disease and lead to a better understanding of the pathogenesis of the cerebral process common to both Alzheimer's disease and Down's syndrome [28].

Immunohistochemical Localization

Rabbit and murine polyclonal antibodies were raised to the synthetic peptide (Asp-Ala-Glu-Phe-Arg-His-Asp-Ser-Gly-Tyr), corresponding to the N-terminus of β protein, coupled to keyhole limpet hemocyanin. These antibodies were demonstrated to be specific for the synthetic β protein homologue and were used immunohistochemically in the peroxidase-antiperoxidase method of Sternberger [44] on Alzheimer's disease in both conditions were reactive. In addition neuritic plaques of diffuse and compact type throughout the cortex in both Alzheimer's disease and adult Down's syndrome stained. The neurofibrillary tangles were uniformly unreactive. These findings strongly suggest that the amyloid fibers of neuritic plaques are composed of β protein and strengthens the role of the β protein in the pathogenesis of Alzheimer's disease. They also support a serum origin [35] of amyloid in both neuritic plaques and cerebrovascular amyloid, vascular leakage [45] and a close vascular-plaque relationship [46]. These findings do not support the thesis of Prusiner et al. [47] that neuritic plaques in Alzheimer's disease are of viron or "prion" origin.

REFERENCES

1. D. Spiro, Amer. J. Path., 35:47–74 (1959).
2. A. S. Cohen, E. Calkins, Nature (Lond), 183:1202–1203 (1959).
3. G. G. Glenner, P. Cuatrecasas, C. Isersky, H. A. Bladen, E. D. Eanes, J. Histochem. Cytochem., 17:769–780 (1969).
4. G. G. Glenner, New Eng. J. Med., 302:1283, 1333 (1980).
5. E. D. Eanes, G. G. Glenner, J. Histochem. Cytochem., 16:673 (1980).
6. P. Divry, M. Florkin, C. R. Soc. Biol. (Paris), 97:1808–1810 (1927).
7. H. Puchtler, F. Sweat, M. Levine, J. Histochem. Cytochem., 10:333 (1962).
8. R. L. Delellis, M. C. Bowling, Human Path., 1:655 (1970).
9. F. L. Carson, W. B. Kingsley, Arch. Path. Lab. Med., 104 (1980).
10. G. Romhanyi, Schweiz. Z. Path., 12:253–262 (1949).
11. T. Shirahama, A. S. Cohen, J. Chem. Biol., 33:679–708 (1967).
12. G. G. Glenner, E. D. Eanes, H. A. Bladen, R. P. Linke, and J. D. Termine, J. Histochem. Cytochem., 22:1141 (1974).
13. L. Pauling and R. B. Corey, Proc. Nat. Acad. Sci. (Wash.), 37:729–740 (1951).
14. A. S. Cohen, Lab. Invest., 15:66–83 (1966).
15. M. Pras, D. Zucker-Franklin, A. Rimon, and E. C. Franklin, J. Exp. Med., 130:777–791 (1969).
16. M. Harada, C. Isersky, P. Cuatrecases, D. Page, H. A. Bladen, E. D. Eanes, H. R. Keiser, and G. G. Glenner, J. Histochem. Cytochem., 19:1–15 (1971).
17. G. G. Glenner, E. Ein, E. D. Eanes, H. A. Bladen, W. Terry, and D. L. Page, Science, 174:712 (1971).
18. J. D. Sipe, K. P. W. J. McAdam, B. F. Torain, and G. G. Glenner, Br. J. Exp. Path., 57:582 (1976).
19. P. D. Gorevic, C. J. Rosenthal, and E. C. Franklin, Clin. Immunol. Immunopathol., 6:83 (1976).
20. J. Hoffman, L. H. Ericsson, N. Eriksen, K. A. Walsh, and E. P. Benditt, J. Exp. Med., 159:641 (1984).
21. F. E. Dwulet, M. D. Benson, Proc. Nat. Acad. Sci. USA, 81:694 (1984).
22. M. Pras, F. Prelli, E. C. Franklin, and B. Frangione, Proc. Nat. Acad. Sci. USA, 80:539–542 (1983).
23. S. Pantelakis, Monatschr. Psychiat. Neurol., 128:219–256 (1954).
24. B. Surbek, Acta Neuropathol. (Berl), 1:168–197 (1961).
25. G. G. Glenner, J. H. Henry, and S. Fujihara, Ann. Pathol., 1:120 (1981).
26. H. V. Venters, J. J. Gilbert, Stroke, 14:924 (1983).
27. C. T. Vanley, M. J. Aguilar, R. J. Kleinbenz, M. D. Lagios, Human. Pathol., 12:609–616 (1981).
28. G. G. Glenner, Banbury Report 15: Biological Aspects of Alzheimer's Disease (Cold Spring Harbor, New York), 137–144 (1983).
29. D. E. Cohen, H. Feiner, H. O. Jensson, and B. Frangione, J. Exp. Med., 158:623 (1983).
30. G. G. Glenner, Med. Hypotheses, 5:1231 (1979).
31. G. A. Jarvis, Am. J. Psychiatry, 105:102 (1984).
32. W. G. Ellis, J. R. McCulloch, and C. L. Corley, Neurology, 24:101 (1974).
33. L. L. Heston, Science, 196:322 (1976).
34. R. M. Torack, Am. J. Pathol., 81:349 (1975).

35. G. G. Glenner, C. Wong, Biochem. Biophys. Res. Commun., 120:885 (1984).
36. G. G. Glenner, C. Wong, Biochem. Biophys. Res. Commun., 120:1131 (1984).
37. E. P. Benditt, N. Eriksen, M. A. Harmodson, and L. H. Ericsson, FEBS Lett., 19:169 (1971).
38. H. Lofberg, A. O. Grubb, T. Sveger, and J. E. Olsson, J. Neurol., 23: 159 (1980).
39. C. J. Epstein, Banbury Report 15: Biological Aspects of Alzheimer's Disease (Cold Spring Harbor, New York), 169-182 (1983).
40. T. Maniatus, E. F. Fritsch, and J. Sambrook, Molecular Cloning: A Laboratory Manual (Cold Spring Harbor, New York), 545 (1982).
41. J. F. Gusella, N. S. Wexler, and P. M. Conneally, Science, 306:234 (1983).
42. G. G. Glenner, W. Terry, M. Harada, C. Isersky, and D. Page, Science, 172:1150 (1971).
43. D. Owens, J. C. Dawson, and S. Losin, Am. J. Ment. Defic., 75:606 (1971).
44. S. Fujihara, J. E. Balow, J. C. Costa, and G. G. Glenner, Laboratory Investigation, 43 (1980).
45. A. B. Sheibel, Senile Dementia: Outlook for the Future, Alan R. Liss, New York, 137 (1984).
46. T. Miyakawa, A. Shimoji, R. Juramoto, Y. Higuchi, Virchows Arch. (Cell Pathol), 40:121 (1982).

NEUROBIOLOGICAL PROBES FOR SPECIFIC CONSTITUENTS OF SENILE PLAQUES IN AGING AND ALZHEIMER'S DISEASE

Donald L. Price†, Robert G. Struble, Cheryl A. Kitt,
Linda C. Cork*, Lary C. Walker, Manuel F. Casanova,
and Richard E. Powers

Neuropathology Laboratory
Department of Pathology
The Johns Hopkins University
School of Medicine
Baltimore, Maryland

*Division of Comparative Medicine
 The Johns Hopkins University
 School of Medicine
 Baltimore, Maryland

†Departments of Neurology
 and Neuroscience
 The Johns Hopkins University
 School of Medicine
 Baltimore, Maryland

ABSTRACT

Senile plaques are composed of neurites (enlarged axons, nerve terminals, and, possibly, dendrites) associated with focal deposits of amyloid.
Plaques are present in small numbers in the amygdala, hippocampus, and
neocortex in elderly primates and are abundant in these regions in individuals with Alzheimer's disease. Aged macaques provide a model for investigations of plaques. One of the earliest abnormalities identified in
these older animals is multifocal enlargement of individual axons within
the cortex. Later, enlarged neurites appear in clusters (neurite plaques);
in mixed plaques, neurites are associated with amyloid. In the oldest animals, many plaques show relatively greater proportions of amyloid. These
observations are interpreted to indicate that axonal pathology is an early
event and that plaques evolve from the neurite type to the amyloid type.
Using antibody probes, we have identified abnormal axons and neurites derived from cholinergic, monoaminergic, and peptidergic systems. These
axons and neurites also show accumulations of cytoskeletal antigens, including neurofilament peptides. Similarly, in human tissues, these
approaches have identified abnormalities of the cytoskeleton and demonstrated a variety of transmitter-specific antigens in plaques.

INTRODUCTION

As occurs in humans, aged nonhuman primates show cognitive and amnestic abnormalities which have certain parallels in aged humans, including problems with short-term memory, impairments in recognition memory, and difficulty shifting set [1]. At the end of the second decade of life, macaques develop senile plaques, made up of a variety of constituents, i.e., enlarged axons and synaptic terminals (neurites) associated with amyloid [2]. Because, in humans, a correlation exists between the presence of plaques and the presence of cognitive impairment [3], it has been suggested that this type of pathology is related, in ways yet unknown, to behavioral impairments occurring in monkeys and humans. The present review discusses our current understanding of senile plaques in the brains of aged nonhuman primates and the relevance of this research to Alzheimer's disease (AD).

AXONAL PATHOLOGY AND SENILE PLAQUES

In Macaques (>15 years of age), nodular varicosities occur along the course of individual intracortical axons of several transmitter types [4]. In our preliminary analysis, this axonal pathology appears to antedate the presence of detectable amyloid. We suspect that this axonal pathology has been overlooked previously, because the thicker sections used in our work allow excellent visualization of focal abnormalities along the course of individual axons.

Older animals (17-35 years of age) show senile plaques. Individual plaques, which are most common in the prefrontal and temporal cortices of macaques, can be types according to the relative proportions of neurites and amyloid. "Neurite" plaques are rich in enlarged axons/nerve terminals (neurites) and contain little detectable amyloid. Some neurites show acetylcholinesterase (AChE) activity [5]. "Mixed" plaques have an admixture of neurites and amyloid. "Amyloid" plaques show lesser proportions of neurites. In our studies, this nomenclature ("neurite, mixed, and amyloid") was chosen in preference to the terms "immature, mature, and end stage" which presuppose an evolutionary pattern for the formation of senile plaques. When comparing plaque densities to the percentage of different types of plaques, a trend was apparent: as the density of plaques increased, the percent of amyloid plaques increased; moreover, the percentage of neurite and mixed plaques appeared to be inversely related to overall plaque density.

CYTOSKELETAL CONSTITUENTS IN SENILE PLAQUES

Neurites in plaques are enlarged, and many of these neurites contain accumulations of cytoskeletal elements [6]. The nature of these cytoskeletal constituents can be proved by using antibodies directed against epitopes of cytoskeletal antigens [7]. In collaboration with Drs. Ludwig and Nancy Sternberger and Dr. Douglas Murphy, we have begun to investigate with antibody probes, patterns of cytoskeletal constituents in plaques, e.g., tubulin, microtubule-associated protein (MPA2), and phosphorylated and nonphosphorylated neurofilament triplet proteins. Phosphorylated epitopes of neurofilament peptides, normally visualized within axons, are a conspicuous constituent of neurites in plaques — an observation consistent with the concept that axons are a major source of neurites. However, MAP2 immunoreactivity, normally present in dendrites [8] (Cork, Struble, Murphy and Price, personal observation), is present in a few neurites [9] (Cork, Struble, Murphy and Price, personal observation) — a finding which suggests that some neurites may represent altered dendrites. It is possible that, as these neuronal elements degenerate, certain constituents are liberated into the neuropil and, subsequently, these elements (as well as those derived from serum leaking through permeable vessels) may participate in the formation of plaques [10]. Antibody probes, which allow delineation of specific constituents in plaques, should help clarify the evolution of abnormalities in the cytoskeleton and other constituents which eventually lead to the formation of senile plaques.

TRANSMITTER SYSTEMS IN SENILE PLAQUES OF AGED PRIMATES

Basal Forebrain Cholinergic System

To examine the hypothesis that some neurites in plaques are derived from axons of forebrain cholinergic systems, we have used two strategies: anterograde tracing studies and choline acetyltransferase (ChAT) immunochemistry.

Anterograde Tracing Studies

If some neurites in plaques are derived from the basal forebrain cholinergic system, then these neurites should be radiolabeled following injection of [^{3}H] amino acid into the substantia innominata. Preliminary studies in a 20-year old monkey whose substantia innominata was injected with [^{3}H] amino acids revealed irregular, knob-shaped, and linear accumulations of silver grains in axons in proximity to amyloid (Kitt, Mitchell, DeLong, Struble, Cork, and Price, personal observation). This study does not provide conclusive evidence for cholinergic neurites in plaques but does suggest that some of the labeled processes in plaques are derived from neurons whose perikarya are located in the basal forebrain.

Choline Acetyltransferase Immunocytochemistry

Immunocytochemical studies of the brains of several old macaques disclosed ChAT-immunoreactive abnormal axons and neurites; some of the latter were associated with amyloid [11]. Results of this study, similar to those demonstrated by AChE histochemistry [12], provide direct evidence for cholinergic elements in plaques.

Catecholaminergic Systems. In older nonhuman primates, we have also observed some abnormal tyrosine hydroxylase (TH)-like immunoreactive axons which exhibit multiple, greatly enlarged varicosities along their course. Some of these processes appear to be associated with blood vessels. Some immunoreactive neurites are associated with amyloid deposits, while others are seen in regions with no discernable evidence of local amyloid deposition. These catecholaminergic neurites could be derived from dopaminergic neurons located in the substantia nigra and ventral tegmental area and from noradrenergic neurons of the locus coeruleus. Use of antibodies against cholecystokinin and dopamine β-hydroxylase should permit delineation of the contributions of neurons in the ventral tegmental area and locus coeruleus, respectively. This catecholamineric axonal pathology may be related to reductions in cortical catecholaminergic markers which have been demonstrated in older macaques [13].

Serotonergic Systems. Enlarged 5-hydroxytryptamine (5-HT)-containing axons were seen in cortex of two aged animals (Kitt, Struble, Molliver, Walker, Cord and Price, personal observation). Some axons showed multiple enlarged varicosities, and several of these abnormal 5-HT fibers were seen in association with deposits of amyloid.

Peptide Systems. In two old monkeys, abnormal somatostatinergic neurites were present in the amygdala, particularly in the basolateral complex, and some somatostatinergic neurites were associated with deposits of
amyloid [14].

RELATIONSHIP OF BEHAVIORAL CHANGES TO AXONAL PATHOLOGY
AND SENILE PLAQUES IN PRIMATES

In a longitudinal study, monkeys of various ages were extensively
tested on delayed match-to-sample tasks [15]. While older animals had performed better than younger animals, testing years later revealed that there
had been some deterioration in older animals' performance, and younger
animals were performing better than older animals. Just prior to sacrifice, all animals were retested, and statistical differences between the
two groups no longer existed. One of the younger animals performed poorly,
and this animal's poor performance was critical in the lack of statistical
significance. Without knowledge of behavioral data, we had, on neuropathological grounds, also selected this animal as different from his peers.
In our report delaing with these animals [16], we included this 26-year-
old animal with the three 31-year old animals, because it had a large number of senile plaques in cortex, exceeding the density of one of the older
animals. When this animal was included in the older group, analysis for
behavioral deficits almost reached statistical significance [17]. The finding that this animal was identified as different by both neuropathological
examination and by behavioral testing supports the concept that senile
plaques are related to functional deficits expressed in these animals.

RELEVANCE OF THESE INVESTIGATIONS TO ALZHEIMER'S DISEASE

In individuals with AD, the presence of plaques correlates with the
presence of dementia [3]. Moreover, there appears to be a correlation between the presence of plaques and reductions in cholinergic markers [18]
and in somatostatin-like immunoreactivity [19]. These observations suggest
that cholinergic and somatostatinergic axons and terminals may, in some
way, be related to the formation of plaques. Some patients with AD show
abnormal axons and enlarged neurites which stain intensely for AChE (for
review see Perry and Perry [20]), a marker enriched in cholinergic neurons. Other plaques show neurites containing markers with noradrenergic
(dopamine β-hydroxylase) and peptidergic (neurotensin, substance P, and
somatostatin) systems (Struble, Powers, Casanova, Kitt, and Price, personal
observations). Moreover, some of the same cytoskeletal abnormalities observed in monkeys are also seen in plaques in AD (Cork, Sternberger, Sternberger, Struble, Casanova, Murphy, and Price, personal observations). These
observations suggest that the approaches used to examine plaques in aged
nonhuman primates can be used to further clarify the transmitter specificity
and cytoskeletal pathology occurring in AD and related disorders.

REFERENCES AND NOTES

1.   R. T. Bartus, R. L. Dean III, B. Beer, and A. S. Lippa, Science, 217:
      408-417 (1982); R. T. Davis, Exp. Gerontol., 13:237-250 (1978); S. K.
      Presty et al., Soc. Neurosci. Abstr., 10:774 (1984); D. L. Price et
      al., in: Behavior and Pathology of Aging in Rhesus Monkeys, R. T.
      Davis and C. W. Leathers, Eds. (Alan R. Liss, New York, in press).

2. D. L. Price et al., in: Behavior and Pathology of Aging in Rhesus Monkeys, R. T. Davis and C. W. Leathers, Eds. (Alan R. Liss, New York, in press); R. G. Struble, L. C. Cork, P. J. Whitehouse and D. L. Price, Science, 216:413-415 (1982); R. G. Struble, J. C. Hedreen, L. C. Cord, and D. L. Price, Neurobiol. Aging (in press); R. G. Struble, D. L. Price Jr., L. C. Cork, and D. L. Price, Senile plaques in the neocortex of aged monkeys (submitted for publication); H. M. Wisniewski, B. Ghetti and R. D. Terry, J. Neuropathol. Exp. Neurol., 32:566-584 (1973).

3. G. Blessed, B. E. Tomlinson, and M. Roth, Br. J. Psychiatry, 114: 797-811 (1968); B. E. Tomlinson, G. Blessed, and M. Roth, J. Neurol. Sci., 11:205-242 (1970).

4. C. A. Kitt et al., Science (in press); C. A. Kitt et al., Catechol-aminergic neurites in senile plaques in prefrontal cortex of aged nonhuman primates (submitted for publication); R. G. Struble, J. C. Hedreen, L. C. Cord, and D. L. Price, Neurobiol. Aging (in press); R. G. Struble, C. A. Kitt, L. C. Walker, L. C. Cord, and D. L. Price, Brain Pres. (in press).

5. R. G. Struble, L. C. Cork, P. J. Whitehouse, and D. L. Price, Science, 216:413-415 (1982); R. G. Struble, J. C. Hedren, L. C. Cordk, and D. L. Price, Neurobiol. Aging (in press).

6. H. M. Wisniewski and R. D. Terry RD, in: Progress in Neuropathology, H. M. Zimmerman, Ed. (Grune and Stratton, New York, 1973), Vol. II, pp. 1-26.

7. B. H. Anderton et al., Nature, 298:84-86 (1982); L. Autilio-Gambetti, P. Gambetti, and R. C. Crane, Banbury Rep., 15:117-124 (1983); P. Gambetti, G. Shecket, B. Shetti, A. Hirano, and D. Dahl, J. Neuro-pathol. Exp. Neurol., 42:69-79 (1983); D. J. Selkoe, Y. Ihara, and F. J. Salazar, Science, 215:1243-1245 (1982); G. P. Wang, I. Grundke-Iqbal, R. J. Kascsak, K. Iqbal, and H. M. Wisneiwski, Acta Neuro-pathol., 62:268-275 (1984).

8. N. Nukina and Y. Ihara, Proc. Jpn. Acad., 59:284-287 (1983).

9. N. Nukina and Y. Ihara, Proc. Jpn. Acad., 59:288-292 (1983).

10. J. M. Powers, W. W. Schlaepfer, M. C. Willingham, and B. J. Hall, J. Neuropathol. Exp. Neurol., 40:592-612 (1981); D. L. Price et al., Neurosci. Comment., 1, 84-92 (1982).

11. C. A. Kitt, et al., Soc. Neurosci. Abstr., 10:271 (1984).

12. R. G. Struble, J. C. Hedreen, L. C. Cork, and D. L. Price, Neurobiol. Aging (in press).

13. P. S. Goldman-Rakic and R. M. Brown, Neuroscience, 6:177-187 (1981).

14. R. G. Struble, C. A. Kitt, L. C. Walker, L. C. Cork, and D. L. Price, Brain Res. (in press).

15. R. T. Davis, C. L. Bennett, and R. P. Weisenburger, Percept. Motor Skills, 55:703-709 (1982); R. T. Davis, Exp. Gerontol., 13:237-250 (1978).

16. R. G. Struble, L. C. Cork, P. J. Whitehouse, and D. L. Price, Science, 216:413-415 (1982).

17. R. G. Struble, D. L. Price Jr., L. C. Cork, and D. L. Price, Senile plaques in the neocortex of aged monkeys (submitted for publication).

18. E. K. Perry et al., Br. Med. J., 2:1457-1459 (1978).

19. P. Davies, R. Katzman, and R. D. Terry, Nature, 288:279-280 (1980); M. Rossor et al., Brain Res., 201:249-253 (1980); M. N. Rossor, P. C. Emson, L. L. Iversen, C. Q. Mountjoy and M. Roth, in: Alzheimer's Disease: Advances in Basic Research and Therapies. Proceedings of the Third Meeting of the International Study Group on the Treatment of Memory Disorders Associated with Aging, R. J. Wurtman, S. H. Corkin and J. H. Growdon, Eds. (Zurich, 1984), pp. 29-37.

20. E. K. Perry and R. H. Perry, in: Alzheimer's Disease, B. Reisberg, Ed. (The Free Press, New York, 1983), pp. 93-99.

21. The authors gratefully acknowledge discussions with Drs. Peter J. Whitehouse, John C. Hedreen, Mahlon R. DeLong, Susan J. Mitchell, Richard M. Zweig, Juan C. Troncoso, John W. Griffin, and Paul N. Hoffman. Drs. Ludwig Sternberger, Nancy Sternberger, Bruce Wainer, and Douglas Murphy provided antibodies for some of the original studies described in this review. Mr. Richard Altschuler and Mark Becher and Ms. Barbara Holden and Eleanor Brown provided technical assistance. Mrs. Carla Jordon prepared the manuscript. This work was supported by grants from the U.S. Public Health Service (AG 03359, AG05146, NS 20471, NS 10580, NS 15721, NS 07179) and funds from Point of View Inc. and the Hurd Foundation.

BIOCHEMICAL AND STRUCTURAL STUDIES OF PAIRED HELICAL FILAMENTS AND

SENILE PLAQUE AMYLOID IN ALZHEIMER'S DISEASE

Dennis J. Selkoe and Carmela Abraham

Department of Neurology and Neuropathology
Harvard Medical School
Boston, Massachusetts 02115

Mailman Research Center
McLean Hospital
Belmont, Massachusetts 02178

ABSTRACT

During aging of the human brain and particularly in Alzheimer's disease
(AD), abnormal fibers accumulate both inside neurons (in neurofibrillary
tangles and the neurites of senile plaques) and extracellularly (as amyloid
in senile plaque cores and in vessels). Both types of fibers show birefringence with Congo red, but their ultrastructures are distinct. The
principal intraneuronal fibers are paired helical filaments (PHF) with
maximal diameters of 20-24 nm in $situ$. However, we have recently observed
in several cases of AD that both neuronal cell bodies and neurites can display a complex mixture of abnormal fibers including, in addition to an
abundance of PHF, straight filaments varying from 10 to 20 nm in diameter,
most commonly ∿15 nm. The extracellular fibers in the amyloid cores of
senile plaque are generally approximately 10 nm in diameter. We have found
that both PHF and amyloid core fibers are highly insoluble in a variety of
detergents and denaturants including sodium dodecyl sulfate, reducing
agents, urea, and guanidine HCl. The PHF are also resistant to a variety
of specific and non-specific proteases; we have not yet fully determined
the extent of resistance of senile plaque amyloid to these proteases. We
have raised highly specific antibodies to PHF which decorate neurofibrillary
tangles both in AD brain tissue sections and following the isolation and
partial purification of the tangles. We have also raised a polyconal antiserum which immunolabels SDS-isolated senile plaque cores. Taking advantage of the dense spherical nature of the senile plaque core and its intactness following SDS-extraction, we have developed a novel method for
purification of cores from postmortem brain using a combination of sucrose
density centrifugation and fluorescence activated cell sorting. This flow
cytometry technique produces highly purified, intact cores in quantities
suitable for further biochemical and structural analyses. Results of initial analyses of the purified cores are provided. The evidence available
to date suggests that although PHF and extracellular amyloid core fibers
are morphologically distinct, they have similar amino acid compositions
and share major antigenic determinants.

INTRODUCTION

The deposition of protein fibers having the structural and tinctorial properties of amyloid occurs in three principal forms in the brain of patients with Alzheimer's disease (AD). First, abnormal cytoplasmic fibers of 20-24 nm width accumulate intraneuronally in large masses called neurofibrillary tangles (NFT). The vast majority of the fibers comprising these tangles appears to be pairs of helically wound intermediate-sized (10 nm) filaments, referred to as paired helical filaments (PHF) [1-3]. Some of the intracellular fibers in tangle-bearing neurons are straight and display diameters from 10 to 20 nm, usually ∿15 nm [4-7]. PHF and/or straight filaments are also found within the degenerating neurites that form the peripheral rim of so-called senile, or neuritic, plaques, in Alzheimer cerebral cortex. Second, extracellular deposits of amyloid fibers form the central cores of many, but not all, senile plaques. These extracellular fibers appear structurally similar to amyloid fibrils found in non-CNS organs in various systemic amyloidoses: they are ∿7-10 nm in diameter and have a tighter helical periodicity than the 160-nm period of the PHF. Third, amyloid fibrils having similar fine structure to those comprising the senile plaque cores occur as extracellular deposits in the walls of both extracerebral (meningeal) and intracerebral arteries and arterioles, resulting in so-called Congophilic angiopathy [8-10]. This vascular amyloid deposition is present in many but not all cases of AD.

All three of these morphological types of brain amyloid deposits occur less abundantly and in restricted topographical distribution in normal aged human brain. Thus, understanding the cellular origin and molecular pathogenesis of these various tissue deposits in AD may provide clues to certain mechanisms of brain aging in general.

METHODS AND RESULTS

Although numerous hypotheses regarding the cellular and molecular origin of CNS amyloid in AD and other Alzheimer-like degenerative diseases have been put forward, there have been few direct protein chemical analyses of the three principal types of amyloid deposits in this disorder. A considerable number of immunocytochemical studies of both NFT and senile plaques have been carried out with complex and often conflicting results. These studies have not provided a clear understanding of the protein composition and thus the cellular origin of amyloid fibrils in AD. During the past few years, our laboratory has sought to develop methods of isolating and purifying both the NFT and the amyloid cores of senile plaques from AD cerebral cortex and then applying analytical protein chemical techniques to them.

Our initial efforts were directed at isolating first neuronal perikaryal fractions [11, 12] and later cytoskeletal preparations [13] enriched in PHF from frozen postmortem cerebral cortex. Electrophoretic analyses of such fractions in comparison to similarly prepared fractions from control (aged normal) human neocortex free of PHF failed to demonstrate any selectively increased or altered polypeptides. After numerous attempts to identify PHF subunit proteins by SDS-polyacrylamide gel electrophoresis, we concluded that PHF proteins might have unusual molecular properties that prevent their visualization by conventional one- and two-dimensional gel electrophoresis. We then examined the SDS/βME-insoluble residue excluded from such gel sand remaining at the top of the stacking gel. This excluded material contained abundant intact PHF which showed slightly thinner diameters than   (∿17-20 nm vs. ∿20-24 nm) but still retained their typical helical periodicity (∿160 nm) [13]. Numerous additional experiments confirmed that PHF are largely insoluble in detergents and reducing agents. Subsequent attempts to solubilize PHF using urea, guanidine HCl, several other chaotropic salts, and mild acid or base failed to produce evidence of quantitative depolymerization of the PHF fibers [13, 14]. Similarly, several specific or non-specific proteinases did not appear to quantitatively digest the PHF [14]. Such analyses could not exclude the possibility that some portion or associated component of the PHF fibers was solubilized or digested by one or more of the reagents; however, no such released proteins could be detected by gel electrophoresis or immunoblotting with PHF-specific antibodies, and the fibers could be recovered in particulate form after such treatments.

These results indicate that PHF, in contrast to known non-CNS amyloid deposits in other diseases, are not solubilized even in high concentrations of guanidine and other salts. However, certain salts such as saturated guanidine thiocyanate (7 M) produce structural changes in the PHF fibers so that their helical periodicity is no longer recognizable without apparently depolymerizing the fibers quantitatively [14]. It appears from these data as well as recent studies in other laboratories [15, 16] that PHF are assembled by very strong noncovalent forces and may also contain covalent crosslinks. The solubility properties briefly summarized here and detailed elsewhere [13-16] fulfill the initial operational criteria for a crosslinked protein polymer. However, the inability to fully digest PHF to individual amino acids plus intact crosslinks has thus far precluded the identification of any putative crosslinks in the fibers.

In order to carry such analyses further and determine both the polypeptide composition and bonding structure of PHF, we have sought a method of purification of the fibers to homogeneity. Consequently, we have developed both polyclonal and monoclonal antibodies to SDS-isolated PHF fibers. The characterization of these antibodies has been reported in detail elsewhere [17, 18]. The polyclonal PHF antibodies are of particular interest because they appear to show no crossreaction with normal brain fibrous proteins either in tissue sections or by immunoblotting [17]. This apparent specificity of the polyclonal PHF antibodies makes them a useful ligand for various immunopurification strategies.

New Approaches to the Purification of PHF and Amyloid Cores in AD

In considering the problem of purifying a large, insoluble fiber from postmortem human brain, it was apparent that these fibers represented only a minor cytoskeletal constituent of the human cortex even in severe cases of familial AD with large numbers of NFT and senile plaque neurites. Furthermore, their rigid, chemically inert, insoluble structure made them a less than ideal candidate for purification by immunoaffinity chromatographic methods. We have attempted to carry out immunoaffinity chroamtography of sonicated PHF fragments using our polyclonal PHF antibodies. A batch method rather than a column technique was employed in this work. Although considerable further enrichment of the PHF fragments resulted from immunoaffinity chromatography on Affigel-15 using purified IgG from our αPHF serum, particulate contaminants, especially fragments of lipofuscin, remained. In light of our observations that both the entire NFT as well as the amyloid core of the senile plaque remain intact after boiling cerebral cortex in SDS and β-mercaptoethanol (βME), we decided to try to purify the entire fibrous aggregate (i.e., the NFT or the core) using particle sorting by flow cytometry. Such an approach would have several theoretical and practical advantages.

To initiate this new approach, we first attempted to develop a method of purifying amyloid cores by fluorescence-activated cell sorting (FACS).

We determined that SDS-isolated senile plaque cores varied in diameter from 5 to 18 microns, a size range similar to blood-derived cells that are routinely sorted by flow cytometry. Thus, it appeared that senile plaque cores, which were dense and spherical even though not membrane-bound, might be effectively separated from other particulate contaminants by such an approach.

We have now developed a FACS method of purifying amyloid cores starting with large quantities of senile-plaque-rich cerebral cortex from AD cases. Following initial mincing and heating of plaque-rich cortex (50-100 g) in a buffer containing 2% SDS/0.1 M βME, the tissue is sieved through decreasing pore-size Nitex meshes to eliminate large- and medium-sized vessel fragments. The suspension is centrifuged on a discontinuous sucrose gradient. Much of the lipid in the cortical sample remains at the top of this graident. Intact amyloid cores are principally recovered at the 1.6/1.8 M and 1.4/1.6 M sucrose interfaces of the gradient; cores are also found at the 1.2/1.4 M interface. Since the lower two layers are relatively more enriched in cores and contain less lipofuscin granules and microvessel fragments, we have used these layers for further purification by FACS.

In designing a protocol for using FACS to purify amyloid cores, we realized that the major contaminant of post-sucrose gradient core fractions is lipofuscin (LF). The autofluorescent properties of the partially denatured LF granules present in the SDS-extracted fractions suggested that initial immunolabeling of the cores with fluorescent-tagged antibodies might not produce good separation of cores from LF granules. Consequently, we carried out a primary sort without immunolabeling the fraction in an attempt to sort large particles in the fraction (principally cores) from smaller autofluorescent contaminants (principally LF). This first FACS run resulted in marked enrichment of the cores and a marked decrease in both LF granules and the other principal contaminant, microvessel fragments, in the post-FACS fraction. However, the yields of cores following this first FACS run were small, varying from 10% to 25% of the number loaded into the FACS instrument; we are currently examining methods of improving the yield from this FACS run.

The next step involved immunolabeling the cores with antibodies. For this purpose, we have developed an α-amyloid core rat polyclonal antiserum using SDS-extracted, post-sucrose gradient core-enriched fractions as immunogen. Since microvessel fragments are present in the immunogen, the rat serum also contains antibodies to these. We therefore absorbed the α-amyloid core serum with homogenates of SDS-extracted aged human cerebellum (free of senile plaques) at a ratio of serum to absorbant of 1:1000. This resulted in a marked decrease in immunostaning of contaminants in the post-sucrose gradient core fraction, particularly vessel fragments, with persistent immunolabeling of the cores. The labeled cores varied in their immunofluorescence from barely above background (i.e., that seen with non-immune serum) to intensely fluorescent. We then analyzed the immunolabeled sample on the FACS instrument and selected both forward-angle light scattering gates (i.e., particle size) and fluorescence gates that included the labeled cores and excluded contaminating particles. The second FACS run produced better yields, ranging from 15% to 30% of the cores loaded on the instrument. More importantly, the resultant fractions were now very clean by light microscopic analysis, using both Congo red staining and fluorescence microscopy. Throughout the cell-sorting procedure, the cores retained their cohesive, roughly spherical conformation. Their intactness allows one readily to count the number of cores at each step during the procedure, although the apparent hydrophobic nature of the cores make them highly sticky and causes them to self-aggregate during various steps in the procedure. We believe this problem may produce falsely low core counts in the samples. To avoid continuous self-aggregation of the cores, the fractions were dispersed by homogenization and sieving through 35-μ Nitex just prior to each FACS run.

Both light and electron microscopic analyses of the final core fractions prepared by this method reveal highly purified cores which appear identical to those seen *in situ* in brain tissue sections. Some of the cores contain small particles of electron-dense granules suggesting pieces of LF. In addition, a very small number of larger LF aggregates, assuming the approximate size of small cores (and therefore sorted with the cores by FACS), are found. The only other minor contaminant is fragments of fibrous material that by high resolution electron microscopy are entirely composed of homogeneous arrays of 5-10 nm fibrils suggestive of an amyloid deposit. These large fibrous fragments, which range widely in diameter from 2 to 25 μ and have various irregular shapes, appeared to display intense green/red birefringence after Congo red staining by polarization light microscopy. Thus, we believe they represent a kind of tissue deposit of amyloid. We are not certain whether these structures arise from the amyloid-bearing blood vessels or whether they represent cortical tissue deposits that assume a form other than typical senile plaque core morphology. They represent a very minor component of the final fraction as judged by both light and electron microscopy. By far the major constituent is the senile plaque cores; there is virtually no find granular background material in the EM sections of the final FACS-purified pellets.

The development of a method for the high-grade purification of amyloid cores from AD brain tissue will now allow us to begin structural protein chemical studies of the fibrils. We have begun this work by determining the solubility characteristics of cores in comparison to the PHF-containing neurofibrillary tangles. It appears that the amyloid cores are at least as resistant to quantitative solubilization in various strong denaturants as PHF are. For example, 5 M lithium bromide treatment for 20 h at room temperature appears not to dissolve the majority of neurofibrillary tangles in an SDS-isolated NFT fraction and also does not dissolve the amyloid cores that are present to a certain extent in such fractions. After 20 h treatment with 7 M LiBr, however, the number of recognizable NFT is markedly reduced while numerous intact cores remain. At near-saturated concentrations of LiBr (9 M), some cores still remain intact. We are presently repeating these studies using the light-microscopically counted purified cores prepared as above in order to detect changes in core numbers and search for released polypeptides following such treatment in chaotropic salts. Such an analysis could not be carried out heretofore since numerous particulate contaminants were found in core fractions prior to FACS-purification and could represent the source of any soluble protein released by a particular treatment.

We have already exposed isolated cores to treatment in 6 M guanidine HCl for up to 2 weeks and have still observed abundant intact cores which retain their Congo red birefringence. These studies are now being repeated quantitatively. Treatment with 5 M guanidine HCL in L M acetic acid likewise fails to provide evidence of quantitative solubilization of cores. In this regard, AD amyloid cores differ from most amyloid deposits in non-CNS tissues, for which solubilization in guanidine HCl in acetic acid has been used as the initial step for protein analysis. Studies are also being carried out on the susceptibility of the purified cores to digestion, and it will be interesting to determine whether this property is also shared by the amyloid cores. Now that a high degree of purification has been achieved, we hope to be able to find the proper solvent and/or proteinase conditions that will allow separation of polypeptides or generation of peptide fragments from the amyloid fibrils and consequent partial sequence determination.

The new FACS purification method has been used to prepare cores for amino acid analysis. Initial analyses demonstrate a reproducible composition from fraction to fraction by this method. The most abundant amino acid is glycine, followed by aspartic acid and glutamic acid. A relatively high proportion of non-polar residues is found, as might be expected for an amyloid fibril protein. Of particular interest is the fact that our initial amino acid analyses of purified senile plaque amyloid show considerable similarity to earlier analyses we carried out on partially purified PHF from Alzheimer cortex. We are currently modifying the FACS purification protocol for cores in order to obtain highly purified intact NFT rather than cores. Several strategies are being tried to modify the method both as to the cell-sorting parameters and as to the initial preparation of NFT-rich cortical tissue.

Immunocytochemical Studies of Amyloid Cores in AD

The SDS-isolated, FACS-purified amyloid cores present an attractive substrate for immunocytochemical studies of constituent proteins. Since all adsorbed soluble proteins that might be present on the cores either in vivo or as a result of postmortem conditions would presumably be removed by the SDS/βME extraction, one can better determine the antigenic cross-reactivities of the amyloid fibrils themselves. We have carried out staining with several antibodies. In general, non-immune serum as well as secondary antibodies (anti-IgG) alone produce a light-to-medium brown staining using the indirect peroxidase technique. It appears that, as has been postulated from immunocytochemical studies in tissue sections [19], the amyloid fibril proteins of senile plaque cores may readily adsorb proteins. However, this staining is relatively low in intensity. In contrast, PHF polyclonal antibodies [17] produce an intense dark brown/black peroxidase reaction product. Virtually all SDS-isolated plaque cores are intensely labeled. For reasons that are not yet clear, the PHF antibodies label amyloid cores in tissue sections very weakly or not at all. This result suggests that there may be some exposure or modification of antigenic sites on the amyloid fibers that results from their isolation and allows their reactivity with PHF antibodies.

DISCUSSION

The structural and biochemical evidence presently available indicates that the intraneuronal PHF and the extraneuronal amyloid fibers in AD brain have both shared and distinct properties. The most obvious difference between these two types of amyloid deposits is the ultrastructure of the fibers. The amyloid types of amyloid deposits is the ultrastructure of the fibers. The amyloid fibrils comprising the senile plaque cores are approximately half the diameter of PHF or less. On the other hand, we have recently carried out studies that indicate that the fibrous cytopathy of NFT and senile plaque neurites in AD is more complex than generally stated. We found straight filaments having a spectrum of diameters between 10 and 20 nm in addition to PHF in certain degenerating neurons or neurites in three cases of light microscopically typical AD that we have studied [7]. Furthermore, the PHF polyconal antibodies we have produced, which do not react intensely with the Pick bodies that are the characteristic intraneuronal inclusions in degenerating neurons in Pick's disease. By electron microscopy, these Pick bodies are composed of a randomly oriented meshwork of straight filaments with diameters between 10 and 20 nm (principally ∿15 nm) and usually contain only rare PHF of unconventional morphology. This finding, as well as the heterogeneity of filaments seen within αPHF-reactive NFT in AD, suggests that fibers with different fine structure may share antigenic determinants. Thus, the ultrastructural distinctions between PHF and senile plaque core amyloid fibrils could represent a different organization of certain shared protein precursors. This hypothesis is supported both by our preliminary amino acid analyses of FACS-purified amyloid cores in comparison to partially purified PHF fractions as well as by the immuno-cytochemical evidence that PHF antibodies label isolated amyloid cores.

The two types of amyloid deposits in AD brain tissue also share certain biochemical properties in that the fibrils are highly insoluble in detergents, reducing agents, and chaotropic salts. In contrast to most other organ deposits of amyloid that have been studied, both PHF and amyloid core fibrils are not quantitatively solubilized by guanidine HCl. This fact complicates the further compositional analysis of AD amyloid deposits. We are currently investigating a series of solvents, chemical cleavage reagents and proteolytic enzymes as regards their ability to depolymerize or partially break down both PHF and amyloid core fibrils.

The development of a method for the quantitative, high-grade purification of amyloid cores by fluorescence-activated cell sorting which we are now also applying to NFT should allow the determination of the precise molecular relationship of the intraneuronal and extraneuronal amyloid fibers that accumulate progressively in AD.

REFERENCES

1. M. Kidd, Nature, 197:192 (1963).
2. R. D. Terry, J. Neuropath. Exp. Neurol., 22:629 (1963).
3. H. M. Wisniewski, H. K. Narang, R. D. Terry, J. Neurol. Sci., 27:173 (1976).
4. S. Oyanagi, Brain Nerve (Tokyo), 26:637 (1974).
5. H. Shibayam, J. Kitoh, Acta Neuropathol. (Berlin), 41:229 (1978).
6. S. Yagashita, Y. Itoh, W. Nan, and N. Amano, Acta Neuropathol. (Berlin), 54:239 (1981).
7. D. J. Selkoe, Neuroscience, Abstracts, Vol. 10 (in press, 1984).
8. G. G. Glenner, in: Banbury Report 15: Biological Aspects of Alzheimer's Disease, R. Katzman, Ed. (Cold Spring Harbor Laboratory, Cold Spring Harbor, N.Y., 1983), p. 137.
9. C. T. Vanley, M. J. Aguilar, R. J. Kleinhenz, and M. D. Lagios, Human Pathology, 12:609 (1981).
10. G. G. Glenner, and C. Wong, Biochem. Biophys. Res. Common., 120:885 (1984).
11. D. J. Selkoe, Ann. Neurol., 5:468 (1980).
12. D. J. Selkoe, B. A. Brown, F. J. Salazar, and C. A. Marotta, Ann. Neurol., 10:429 (1981).
13. D. J. Selkoe, Y. Ihara, and F. J. Salazar, Science, 215:1243 (1982).
14. D. J. Selkoe, Y. Ihara, C. Abraham, C. G. Rasool, and A. H. McCluskey, in: Banbury Report 15: Biological Aspects of Alzheimer's Disease, R. Katzman, Ed. (Cold Spring Harbor Laboratory, Cold Spring Harbor, N.Y., 1983), p. 155.
15. S.-H. Yen, Y. Kress, in: Banbury Report 15: Biological Aspects of Alzheimer's Disease, R. Katzman, Ed. (Cold Spring Harbor Laboratory, Cold Spring Harbor, N.Y., 1983), p. 155.
16. B. Pons-Estel, F. Goni, F. Alvarez, P. Gorevic, and B. Frangione, in this volume.
17. Y. Ihara, C. Abraham, and D. J. Selkoe, Nature, 304:727 (1983).
18. D. J. Selkoe, C. Abraham, C. G. Rasool, A. McCluskey, and L. K. Duffy, Ann. N.Y. Acad. Sci. (1984, in press).
19. J. M. Powers, W. W. Schlaepfer, M. C. Willingham, and B. L. J. Hall, J. Neuropath. Exp. Neurol., 40:592 (1981).

ALZHEIMER NEUROFIBRILLARY TANGLE AND ITS RELATIONSHIP

WITH PLAQUE CORE AMYLOID

Khalid Iqbal, Inge Brundke-Iqbal,
and Henry M. Wisniewski

New York State Office of Mental
Retardation and Developmental Disabilities
Institute for Basic Research in
Developmental Disabilities
1050 Forest Hill Road
Staten Island, New York 10314

ABSTRACT

Alzheimer neurofibrillary tangles and senile plaques are the two most characteristic lesions of Alzheimer disease/senile dementia of the Alzheimer type. Methods for the isolation of both the tangles and the plaque core amyloid have been only recently developed and therefore their biochemistry is still in its infancy. In this communication the isolation of the paired helical filaments of the tangles, their solubility characteristics, polypeptide composition and relationship with the plaque core amyloid are discussed.

Alzheimer disease/senile dementia of the Alzheimer type (AD/SDAT) is diagnosed histopathologically by the presence of numerous neurofibrillary tangles and senile plaques in the cerebral cortex especially the hippocampus [1]. The Alzheimer neurofibrillary tangles (ANT) are composed of paired helical filaments (PHF) [2]. The senile plaques consist of many dystrophic and degenerating neurites intermixed with one or more microglia and or astroglia as reactive cells often surrounding a central core of amyloid [3]. The concentration of ANT and senile plaques, both of which are also present in small numbers in normal aged humans, correlates strongly with the degree of dementia [4], but their origin and role in disease are not understood. The number of tangles and plaques does not appear to be interdependent because in some cases there are numerous tangles and very few plaques and vice versa (our unpublished observation). Therefore each of these lesions are of importance on their own and the understanding of their pathogenetic mechanisms should enhance our understanding of the disease.

Although ANT are strictly intraneuronal and amyloid is extraneuronal, both when stained with Congo red and viewed through polarized light produce red-green birefringence. This Congo red birefringence is believed to be characteristic of polypeptides in β-pleated sheet conformation [5]. Because of this common property ANT have been referred at times in the literature as amyloid. In this chapter we will discuss ANT and their relationship with plaque amyloid.

A) General

PHF are morphologically unlike any of the normal neurofibrils. Each
PHF is a pair of filaments, 10-13 nm in diameter wound helically around
each other at regular intervals of 80 nm [6]. PHF is made up of 8 protofilaments [7]; in longitudinal section only four protofilaments are seen,
the other four are hidden behind [8]. The substructure of PHF is different
from normal neurofilaments in that the globules making the PHF protofilaments are larger ($35°A \pm 4$ vs $20°A \pm 3$) and the longitudinal bars are
longer ($47°A \pm 6$ vs $27°A \pm 3$) than those in neurofilaments [9]. In addition to ANT, PHF are found as bundles in the dystrophic neurites of the
senile plaques and less frequently as individual fibrils in myelinated
axons. ANT are found mostly in cerebral cortex, especially in the hippocampal pyramidal neurons of Sommers sector and in small pyramidal neurons
in the outer laminae of fronto-temporal cortex. They have not been observed in cerebellum, spinal cord, peripheral nervous system or extraneuronal tissues.

In addition to AD/SDAT, ANT are also found in great abundance in the
Guam Parkinsonism dementia complex, dementia pugilistica, postencephalitic
Parkinsonism and adults with Down's syndrome (for review see 10). ANT have
also been reported in small numbers in several cases of subacute sclerosing panencephalitis (SSPE) and in rare cases of Hallerworden-Spatz disease
and juvenile neurovisceral lipid storage disease. However, ANT have never
been observed in any aged animal species or have they been produced experimentally in animals. The neurofibrillary changes of straight filament type
are also seen in some human disorders. For instance, in progressive supra-
nuclear palsy (PSP) some of the same neurons which contain ANT in Alzheimer
brain have neurofibrillary tangles of 15 nm straight filaments [11] which
are sometimes admixed with PHF [12]. Occasionally either tangles of 15 nm
straight filaments or these filaments admixed with PHF have been observed
in AD/SAT [13]. In sporadic motor neuron disease, vincristine neuropathy
and infantile neuroaxonal dystrophy in humans, the neurofibrillary changes
are of the 10 nm intermediate neurofilament type.

B) Biochemistry

Normal neurofibrils are made up of proteins. The subunit protein of
microtubules is tubulin, of neurofilaments is a triplet of polypeptides
of around 200 kDa, 160 kDa and 70 kDa, and of microfilament is actin. The
polypeptide composition of PHF is still under investigation. Employing
preparations of neuronal cell bodies isolated from the affected areas of
Alzheimer brains and a PHF enriched fraction prepared under nondenaturing
conditions the first identification of a 50 kDa PHA polypeptide in SDS-
polyacrylamide gel (SDS-PAG) was made in 1974 in our laboratory [14]. Subsequently we showed the localization of this 50 kDa polypeptide to PHF
[15] and its chemical characterization [16]. Immunochemical crossreactivity
of this 50 kDa PHF polypeptide with brain microtubule enriched preparations
led to the discovery of a PHF crossreacting polypeptide/s present normally
in brain [17]; this PHF crossreactive polypeptide in normal brain copuri-
fies with but is not tubulin [17, 18].

The PHF isolated under nondenaturing conditions were not highly purified and the recovery was low. Therefore, recently we developed a new
method for the bulk isolation of highly purified ANT [19]. In this method
the isolation of PHF is achieved by a combination of tissue disaggregation
by sieving through nylon bolting cloth, sucrose density gradient centrifugation and SDS treatment. ANT isolated by this method are highly purified

as determined by light microscopy of Congo red stained preparations in polarized light and by electron microscopic examination. Counts of ANT treated with or without 2% SDS at room temperature for 3-5 minutes, the treatment employed for the isolation of purified PHF, revealed that there are two populations of ANT. A population of ANT (ANT I) are readily soluble by the above treatment and are thus lost during the detergent treatment in the isolation procedure. The second population of ANT (ANT II) are not soluble by this treatment and are thus the type isolated by the method involving the detergent treatment. The proportion of these two populations of ANT varies considerably from Alzheimer brain to brain. The isolated PHF (ANT II) are, however, solubilized either by about 6-10 repeated extractions in SDS-β-mercaptoethanol solution at 100°C for 10 minutes or considerably easily by ultrasonication followed by heating at 100°C in SDS-β-mercaptoethanol for 3-5 minutes; almost all of the PHF are solubilized by a single treatment with the latter method.

The solubility of isolated PHF in SDS-β-mercaptoethanol solution was monitored by the loss of PHF as determined by negative stain electron microscopy and by the loss of the 130,000 × g residue, the fraction which normally contains PHF. SDS-PAGE pattern of PHF extract consisted of major polypeptides in the 45 kDa - 62 kDa region and about 30-40% of the material at the top of the gel; the material not entering the gel did not contain any fibrils as determined by negative stain electron microscopy. On re-electrophoresis the 45 kDa-62kDa PHF polypeptides and the protein not entering the gel in part generated each other. Both the 45 kDa-62 kDa polypeptides and the protein aggregate at the top of the gel were labelled on immunoblots with rabbit antisera to isolated PHF which labeled both ANT and neurites of the neuritic (senile) plaque in sections of Alzheimer hippocampus [20]. Furthermore the PHF staining antibodies in the anti PHF sera were absorbed with the PHF polypeptides cut out and extracted both from the resolving gel and the top of the SDS-PAGE. The neurofilament polypeptides identically extracted from the gel did not absorb the ANT staining antibodies in the anti-PHF sera.

Recently we have generated several different hybridomas which produce antibodies to PHF [21]. Like polyclonal antibodies to PHF reported previously, the monoclonal antibodies (mAb) to PHF from two hybridomas tested label on immunoblots both the 45 kDa-62 kDa PHF polypeptides and the protein aggregates at the top of the gel; none of the polypeptides were labelled with these mAb in a neurofilament enriched preparation used as antigen control. These findings clearly show that PHF isolated by our method [19] are soluble in SDS and that the apparent size of the major PHF polypeptides by SDS-PAGE is 45 kDa-62 kDa. Contrary to our findings, Selkoe and his colleagues have recently reported that the PHF are insoluble in SDS, urea and other denaturing agents and are resistant to protease digestion [22]. Furthermore, based on this contention these investigators have concluded that PHF are polymers of polypeptides covalently crosslinked possibly by γ-glutamyl-ε-lysine linkages and thus cannot be identified by SDS-PAGE or immunoblots [22]. However, this discrepancy between Selkoe's and our findings is due to the differences in the PHF isolation method employed by the two labs. Selkoe's method for isolation of PHF involves treating the whole brain homogenate with SDS and β-mercaptoethanol in Tris buffer for 5 minutes at 100°C and for about 6-8 hours at room temp. This treatment not only selects relatively insoluble population of ANT but probably also increases their insolubility artifactually [23].

C) Relationship with Plaque Amyloid

Relationship between ANT and plaque amyloid is summarized in Table 1. Both ANT and amyloid are Congophilic and because of this common stain-

TABLE 1. Relationship between Alzheimer Neuro-
          fibrillary Tangles and Senile Plaque
          Core Amyloid

Characteristic	Tangles	Amyloid
Nervous tissue	Intraneuronal	Extraneuronal
Extraneuronal tissue	-	+
Fibril diameter	10 - 22 nm	7 nm
Congophilia	+	+
Thioflavin S	+	+
Argentophilia	+	-
PAS	-	+
Solubility in SDS	+	-
Anti PHF sera	+	rare
Anti prealbumin	-	few

ing property a close relationship between the two lesions have been suggested by some investigators. It has been shown that this property is
most likely due to β-pleated sheet structure [5] and this conformation can
be induced in many unrelated polypeptides which will then in turn become
Congophilic. PHF and amyloid fibrils are different ultrastructurally and
in several staining properties other than with Congo red and thioflavin S.
Anti PHF sera which label ANT do not by and large label plaque amyloid.
To date we have observed immunostaining of plaque amyloid in only 1/17
AD/SDAT cases studied. Recently Shirahama, et al. [24] reported immunostaining of both ANT and plaque amyloid with a commercially available anti
prealbumin serum. We have in our lab been able to observe no staining of
ANT and staining of only a few plaque amyloid cores with anti prealbumin
sera obtained from several commercial sources.

D) Summary and Conclusions

    1. PHF isolated by our method are indeed soluble in SDS and their
major polypeptides are in the 45 kDa-62 kDa region by SDS-PAGE.

    2. The discrepancy between Selkoe's and our data regarding the solu-
bility of PHF is due to different methods used for the isolation of PHF.
The PHF isolated by Selkoe's procedure are insoluble in SDS.

    3. In situ PHF and plaque core amyloid in most of the Alzheimer cases
do not cross react; chemically isolated amyloid cores might be labelled with
antibodies to PHF. However, pending characterization of individual polypeptides making the two types of fibrils the exact relationship between
these lesions remains to be determined.

ACKNOWLEDGEMENTS

We thank Drs. Gian Ping Wand and Nasim Ali, Ms. Tanweer Zaidi, and Ms.Chyn Yunn Tung for carrying out some of the studies review in this article, and Ms. Patricia Calimano for typing the manuscript. Our labs are supported in part by NIH grants NS 17487, NS 18105 and P01 04220.

REFERENCES

1. A. Brun, L. Gustafson, Arch. Psychiatr. Nervenkr., 223:15 (1976); H. M. Wisniewski and R. D. Terry, in: Neurobiology of Aging, R. D. Terry, S. Gershon, Ed. (Raven Press, New York, 1976); pp. 256-280.

2. K. Iqbal and H. M. Wisniewski, in: Alzheimer's Disease: The Standard Reference, B. Reisberg, Ed. (Free Press, New York 1983), pp. 48-56.

3. H. M. Wisniewski, in: Alzheimer's Disease: The Standard Reference, B. Reisberg, Ed. (Free Press, New York 1983), pp. 57-61.

4. M. Roth, B. E. Tomlinson, G. Blessed, Nature (London), 209:190 (1966); B. E. Tomlinson, G. Blessed, and M. Roth, J. Neurol. Sci., 11:205 (1970).

5. G. G. Glenner, E. D. Eanes, H. A. Bladen, R. P. Linke, and J. D. Termine, J. Histochem Cytochem., 22:1141 (1974).

6. M. Kidd, Nau-re (London), 197:192 (1963); H. M. Wisniewski, H. K. Narang, and R. D. Terry, J. Neurol. Sci., 27:173 (1976).

7. H. M. Wisniewski, G. Y. Wen, Acta Neuropathol. (Berl) in press.

8. H. M. Wisniewski, P. A. Merz, and K. Iqbal, J. Neuropathol. Exp. Neurol (in press).

9. G. Y. Wen and H. M. Wisniewski, Acta Neuropathol. (Berl), 64:339 (1984).

10. K. Iqbal, H. M. Wisniewski, I. Grundke-Iqbal, and R. D. Terry, in: The Aging Brain and Senile Dementia Nandy K, Sherwin I. Eds. (Plenum Press, New York 1977), pp. 209-227; K. Wisniewski, G. A. Jervis, R. C. Moretz, and H. M. Wisniewski, Ann. Neurol., 5:288 (1979).

11. I. Tellez-Nagel and H. M. Wisniewski, Archs. Neurol. (Chicago), 29:324 (1973).

12. N. R. Ghatak, D. Nochlin, and M. G. Hadfield, Acta Neuropathol, 52:73 (1980).

13. H. Shibayama, J. Kitoh, Acta Neuropathol. (Berl), 41:229 (1978); S. Yagishita, Y. Itoh, W. Nan, and N. Amano, Acta Neuropathol. (Berl), 54:239 (1981).

14. K. Iqbal, H. M. Wisniewski, M. L. Shelanski, S. Brostoff, B. H. Liwnicz, and R. D. Terry, Brain Res., 77:337 (1974).

15. I. Grundke-Iqbal, A. B. Johnson, R. D. Terry, H. M. Wisniewski, and K. Iqbal, Ann. Neurol, 6:532 (1979).

16. K. Iqbal, I. Grundke-Iqbal, H. M. Wisniewski, and R. D. Terry, Brain Res., 142:321 (1978).

17. I. Grundke-Iqgal, A. B. Johnson, H. M. Wisniewski, R. D. Terry, and K. Iqbal, Lancet I, 578 (1979); I. Grundke Iqbal, Acta Neuropathol. (Berl) In press (1984).

18. K. Iqbal, I. Grundke-Iqbal, A. B. Johnson, H. M. Wisniewski, in: Aging of the Brain and Dementia, Vol. 13, L. Amaducci, A. N. Davison, and P. Antuono, Eds. (Raven Press, New York 1980), pp. 39-48; S. H. Yen, F. Gaskin, and R. D. Terry, Am. J. Pathol., 104:77 (1981).

19. I. Grundke-Iqbal, K. Iqbal, P. Merz, and H. M. Wisniewski, J. Neuropath. Exp. Neurol., 40:312 (1981); K. Iqbal, T. Zaidi, C. H. Thompson, P. A. Merz, H. M. Wisneiwski, Acta Neuropathol. (Berl), 62:167 (1984).

20. I. Grundke-Iqbal, K. Iqbal, Y. C. Tung, and H. M. Wisniewski, Acta Neuropathol. (Berl0, 62:259 (1984).

21. G. P. Wang, I. Grundke-Iqbal, R. J. Kascsak, K. Iqbal, and H. M. Wisniewski, Acta Neuropathol (Berl), 62:268 (1984).

22. D. J. Selkoe, Y. Ihara, F. J. Salazar, Science, 215:1243 (1982);
    I. Ihara, C. Abraham, and D. J. Selkoe, Nature, 304:727 (1983).
23. K. Iqbal, I. Grundke-Iqbal, H. M. Wisniewski, T. Zaidi, and N. Ali,
    in preparation.
24. T. Shirahama, M. Skinner, P. Westermark, A. Rubinow, A. S. Cohen,
    A. Brun, and T. L. Kemper, Am. J. Pathol, 107:41 (1982).

CEREBRAL AMYLOID AND ALZHEIMER'S SYNDROME

D. Allsop, M. Landon,
and M. Kidd*

Department of Biochemistry
University of Nottingham Medical School
Queen's Medical Centre
Nottingham NG7 2UH, England

*Department of Human Morphology
 University of Nottingham Medical School
 Queen's Medical Centre
 Nottingham MG7 2UH, England

ABSTRACT

In 'Alzheimer's syndrome' cerebral amyloid is deposited as the central cores of senile plaques; in the neurons in the form of tangles; and often in the blood vessel walls. A spectrum of diseases exhibiting this syndrome ranges from scrapie (no tangles) through Alzheimer's disease and Down's syndrome to dementia pugilistica (no plaques).

Intact plaque cores were isolated from both Alzheimer and Down's syndrome brains. It was noted in the case of Down's syndrome that some of the amyloid cores had a strikingly different morphology from those previously observed for AD. The isolated Alzheimer plaque cores were resistant to solution in SDS, SDS/urea and guanidine and were poorly immunogenic in mice. Amino acid analyses of Alzheimer and Down's syndrome plaque cores were characteristically unusual and remarkably similar to analyses published recently for β protein isolated from cerebrovascular amyloid [7, 8].

The amino acid composition of a preparation of isolated PHF's also showed interesting similarities to that of plaque amyloid. Previous work has shown that the plaque amyloid fibril in AD is composed of two 4-8 nm protofilaments [33, 34]. Our own observations suggest that the PHF consists of two pairs of 3.5-4.5 nm protofilaments.

It is concluded that plaque amyloid and cerebrovascular amyloid are the same protein. The possibility must also be considered that PHFs are a different form of this protein.

INTRODUCTION

It has become apparent over the last 15 years or so that material described as 'amyloid' can be deposited in a variety of organs as the result

TABLE 1.   Chemical Classes of Amyloid

Fibril Protein	Clinical Condition
1. IgG light chain (or fragment) (1,2)	'Primary' amyloidosis
2. Amyloid A protein (1,3)	'Secondary' amyloidosis
3. Prealbumin (or variant) (4)	Familial amyloid polyneuropathy and senile cardiac amyloidosis
4. Procalcitonin fragment (5)	Medullary carcinoma of thyroid
5. Gamma trace fragment (6)	Hereditary cerebral haemorrhage with amyloidosis
6. β protein (7,8)	Cerebrovascular amyloid in Alzheimer's Disease and Down's Syndrome

This Table includes only biochemical classes for which partial or complete amino acid sequence information is available.

of a number of different disease processes. Amyloid has shown a surprising degree of biochemical diversity with six different biochemical classes so far defined by partial or complete amino acid sequence analysis (Table 1). This number will certainly increase as the less well defined amyloids (such as the secretory amyloids) are more fully characterized. Some of the general properties of amyloid (such as the characteristic Congophilia with birefringence, and the relative resistance to proteolysis and to solution) have been ascribed to an anti-parallel beta-pleated sheet structure of the protein in the fibrils [1].

The most common cause of amyloid deposition in man is Alzheimer's disease (AD) which is currently said to afflict around 1.5 million people in the United States [9]. In AD amyloid in the brain is associated with two identifying histopathological lesions; the senile plaque and the neurofibriallary tangle [10, 11]. Frequently, though not invariably, amyloid is also deposited in the blood vessels of the brain parenchyma and the adjacent leptomeningeal vessels (Congophilic angiopathy or cerebrovascular amyloid) [12]. The classical senile plaques of AD, which are found in the neuropil, consist of a central core of radially arranged amyloid fibrils

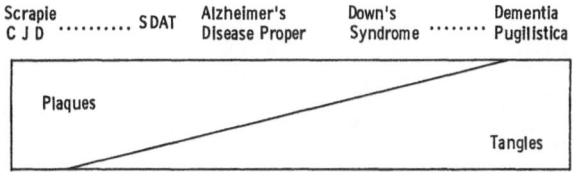

Fig. 1. Concept of 'Alzheimer's Syndrome'.

surrounded by a pale-staining 'hof' of non-degenerate glial processes, which is in turn surrounded by a rim of degenerating neurites and synapses with some associated microglial cells [11]. In contrast, the tangles are intracellular bundles of parallel fibres which swirl around the nucleus and often enter the neuronal processes. After Congo red staining the tangles exhibit the characteristic green birefringence typical of amyloid. However, at the level of the electron microscope they have been shown to be formed from paired helical filaments (PHFs); pairs of approximately 10 nm filaments wound around each other to form a double helix [13, 14]. The numbers of plaques and tangles correlate with the extent of cognitive impairment [15]; and also with the reduction in cholinergic function associated with AD [16].

Amyloid-containing plaques are also found in varying numbers in some transmissible encephalopathies (scrapie in animals [17] and Creutzfeld-Jacob disease [18], Gerstman-Sträussler syndrome [19] and Kuru [20] in man); plaques and PHFs are both found in the majority in cases of Down's syndrome surviving to middle age [21]; while PHFs alone occur in dementia pugilistica, the dementia of 'punch drunk' boxers [22]: the term 'Alzheimer's syndrome' has been used [23] to refer collectively to this group of conditions which share a common histopathology (Fig. 1).

Thus infection by an as yet undefined agent, genetic factors, and also cerebral trauma can all be involved in the pathogenesis of cerebral amyloid, although at present the sequence of events leading to amyloid deposition is obscure, and very little is known about the biochemistry of the amyloid involved. The recent isolation by Glenner and Wong of β protein from the cerebrovascular amyloid found in AD [7] and Down's syndrome [8] (included in Table 1) represents a significant advance. Our own work has been largely concerned with the isolation and characterization of plaque amyloid from Alzheimer brain, and more recently from cases of Down's syndrome, and suggests that this amyloid is similar to cerebrovascular amyloid. This work is discussed below, together with some observations on the nature of PHFs.

ISOLATION OF INTACT PLAQUE CORES FROM ALZHEIMER AND
DOWN'S SYNDROME BRAINS

The development in the 1960s of methods for the separation of neuronal cell bodies, based on gentle disruption of brain tissue by passage through stainless steel or nylon meshes followed by isolation of a neuronal fraction on a sucrose density gradient, provided a new tool for the study of pathological neurons [24]. In the initial stages of our work we applied such methods to unfixed, frozen Alzheimer brain and found that amyloid (in the form of plaque amyloid, PHFs or vascular amyloid) could be readily detected in the neuronal preparations by its characteristic staining properties with Congo red [25]. The amyloid cores of the senile plaques were freed from any surrounding degenerating neuritic material and remained intact. These cores proved to be resistant to proteolysis, and a purifica-

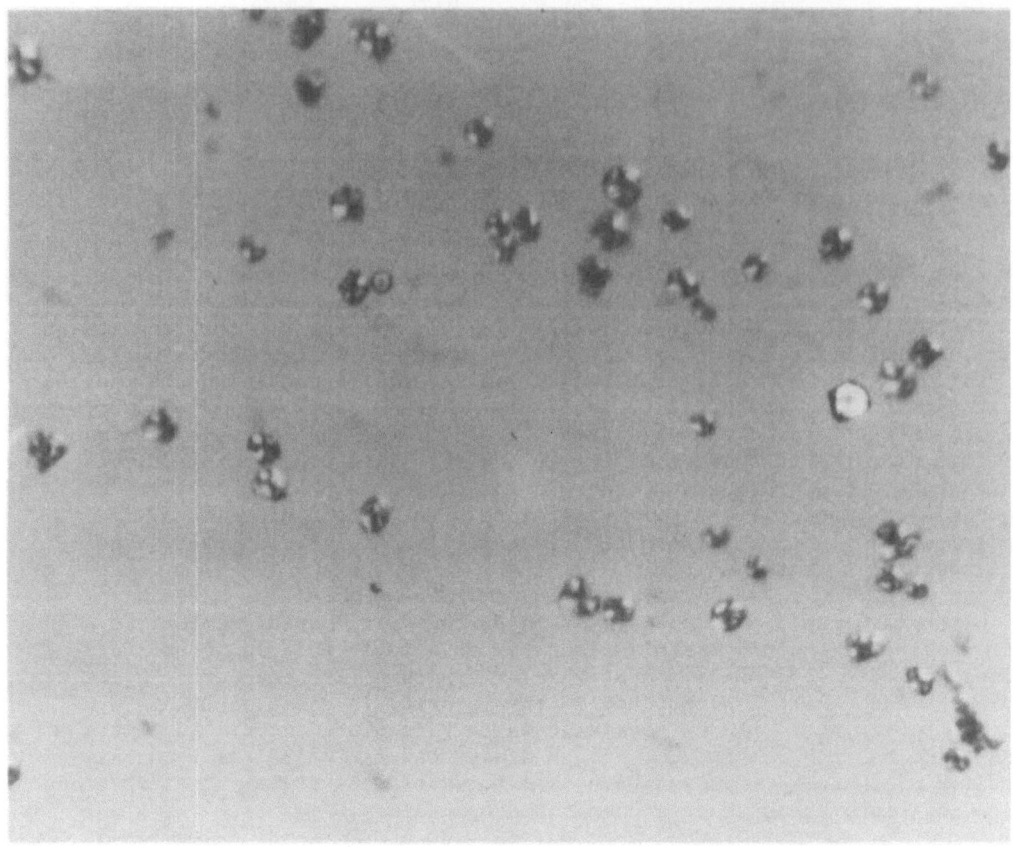

Fig. 2. Isolated Alzheimer senile plaque cores. The isolated cores were
suspended in 0.25% aq. Congo red and photographed under a polarizing microscope with the polarizers set near to 90° (×300).

tion scheme based treatment of neuronal preparations with subtilisin,
followed by final purification on a sucrose density gradient was developed
[25]. This scheme was later modified to include removal of contaminating
blood vessel fragments on a glass bead column [23]. A preparation of purified plaque cores is shown in Fig. 2.

The maximum yield of cores in any neuronal fraction to date has been
1.2×10^5 per g combined frontal/temporal cortex from an Alzheimer brain
estimated by counts carried out on Congo red-stained cryostat sections to
contain an average of 1.1×10^5 amyloid cores/cm³ starting material. This
is a low number when compared with published plaque counts estimated from
silver-stained sections; however, may argyrophilic senile plaques in AD
contain only wisps of amyloid and lack discrete amyloid cores [26]. It is
reasonable, then, to suppose that our yields are in fact a true reflection
of the starting material.

Of the cores present in the neuronal fractions 45-65% are routinely
recovered in the final preparation. Estimates of protein based on amino
acid analysis suggest that 10^6 cores contain about 100 μg protein.

More recently we have used this same method for the preparation of
amyloid cores from two cases of Down's syndrome. Yields of 0.015 and
0.050 cores/g frozen cortex were obtained in the two neuronal fractions.

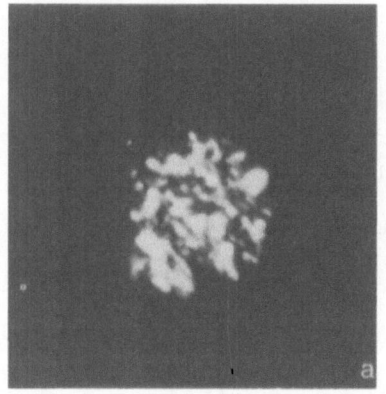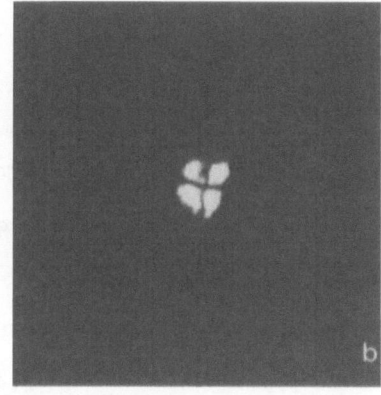

Fig. 3. Isolated Down's syndrome plaque cores. The isolated cores were suspended in 0.25% aq. Congo red
and examined between crossed polarizers (×450).
(a) Isolated plaque core of unusual morphology.
Note the lack of any distinct polarization cross.
(b) Isolated plaque core with the more typical appearance of those prepared from Alzheimer brain.

Surprisingly, it was noted in both cases that a significant proportion of
the isolated amyloid cores had a different morphology under the polarizing
microscope (after staining with Congo red) to that observed previously from
Alzheimer brains (Fig. 3). These unusual Down's syndrome plaque cores
were on the whole larger (up to 50 µm in diameter ranther than the more
usual 10-20 µm) and although intensely birefringent showed poorly distinguishable or non-existent polarization crosses.

Some Characteristics of Plaque Core Protein

     Analysis of plaque core protein by the conventional methods associated
with protein chemistry has been hampered by the small amounts obtained
coupled with difficulties experienced in solubilizing this material in SDS,
SDS/urea and also guanidine-containing solvents [23, 25]. After polyacrylamide gel electrophoresis (PAGE) in the presence of SDS or SDS/urea,
for example, the bulk of material extracted with these solvents invariably
failed to enter the gel. Treatment of plaque cores with 0.02 M NaOH,
followed by PAGE at high pH did yield a single, very broad protein band
centering on a molecular weight of about 9,000 but the significance of this
observation is uncertain since only 20% of the material was solubilized
[23].

     Recently we have suspended isolated plaque cores in 98/100% formic
acid, 25 mM DTT. After sonication (6 × 10 second bursts at 75 W with a
Branson microprobe) followed by centrifugation at 12,000 xg for 15 min only
5% of the original protein remained in the pellet. We are currently engaged in HPLC analysis of the supernatant fraction.

     Isolated plaque cores have proved to be poorly immunogenic. In an
attempt to raise a polyvalent antiserum, and subsequently develop monoclonal
antibodies, several mice have been injected with a plaque core suspension
sonicated in the presence of 98/100% formic acid. After drying off the
formic acid and resuspending in adjuvant or saline a total of 100-550 µg
protein was injected intra-peritoneally into each mouse. In all cases a
first injection of 50 µg protein in Freund's complete adjuvent followed by
a second injection a month later of 50 µg protein in incomplete adjuvant

TABLE 2. Amino Acid Composition of Cerebral Amyloid

	Alzheimer Plaque Core Protein (23, 25) (F, age 94)	Down's Syndrome Core Protein (F, age 59)	Alzheimer's Disease β Protein (7)	PHF Preparation (F, age 64)
Asp	7.8	8.0	11.1	8.0
Thr	1.5	2.4	1.4	3.5
Ser	4.8	5.9	5.4	6.4
Glu	11.2	10.2	11.2	10.4
Pro	2.0	5.4	trace	7.9
Gly	15.0	17.8	15.2	17.6
Ala	9.0	8.5	7.9	6.1
Cys	ND	ND	trace	ND
Val	12.8	9.8	11.7	9.3
Met	1.9	1.2	2.5	1.1
Ile	6.7	4.6	3.9	5.1
Leu	6.6	6.4	6.3	6.3
Tyr	2.4	1.7	2.1	1.5
Phe	5.4	4.8	7.0	3.4
His	5.2	4.7	5.9	3.6
Lys	5.3	4.9	5.4	6.6
Arg	2.3	3.8	2.9	3.0
Trp	ND	ND	ND	ND

The Down's syndrome core protein and PHF analyses were carried out after hydrolysis in vacuo for 24 h in 6 M HCl at $110^{\circ}C$ as described previously (23,25). ND = not determined. The figures are expressed as moles %. Serine was increased by 10% and threonine by 5% to compensate for destruction. The PHF preparation is that shown in Fig. 4.

was given. This was followed by up to three injections of 150 µg protein in saline at monthly intervals. So far no reactivity to plaque amyloid has been detected in either mouse serum, or in the tissue culture supernatants produced by spleen cell × NS1 myeloma cell hybridomas, using an indirect peroxidase-antiperoxidase staining method on cryostat sections of Alzheimer brain.

Amino acid analyses of plaque core protein from cases of AD have been consistent and unusual with a characteristic high level of valine and glycine, and low level of threonine [23, 25]. A typical analysis is given in Table 2 together with a composition recently obtained from a case of Down's syndrome. It is notable that this analysis is similar to previous analyses from Alzheimer brain, apart from the level of proline which is significantly greater in the case of Down's syndrome. These compositions are remarkably similar to those obtained by Glenner and Wong [7, 8] for the β proteins isolated from cerebrovascular amyloid, and show large discrepancies when compared with the compositions of other known amyloid proteins. Glenner and Wong have shown by automated sequence analysis that β protein from Down's syndrome [8] is identical up to position 24 (apart from one variant residue at position 11) to β protein from AD. A computer search by the latter workers revealed no homology between β protein and any known protein sequence. Our compositional data strongly suggest that the plaque amyloid in both AD and Down's syndrome is similar to the cerebrovascular amyloid. Thus it appears more likely that in Alzheimer's syndrome both plaque amyloid and cerebrovascular amyloid are derived from an unknown circulating serum precursor (analagous to amyloid fibrils derived from IgG, SAA protein and prealbumin) rather than from a protein secreted locally in the brain. Although the morphological relationship between senile plaques and blood vessels has been controversial, it is interesting to note in this context that Miyakawa et al. [27] observed at least one degenerate capillary with Congophilic angiopathy in close relation with each senile plaque after electron microscopy of serial-sectioned material.

Are PHFs and Plaque Amyloid Different Forms of the Same Protein?

It has been widely assumed that PHFs are formed from pairs of neurofilaments. This assumption was strengthened by the observation that monoclonal antibodies directed against epitopes on the 155 Kd and 210 Kd neurofilament polypeptides strongly stained PHFs in tissue sections [28]. Subseuqent work, however, has shown that these monoclonals will not stain the majority of isolated PHFs prepared by extraction with solvents containing SDS [29]. Furthermore, both monoclonal [30] and conventional antibodies [29] raised to the PHFs themselves have failed to react with any neurofilament components. Reports concerning the staining of PHFs using conventional polyvalent antisera to neurofilament polypeptides have been conflicting [31]. Thus there is at present no convincing evidence relating PHFs to neurofilaments.

It is interesting to speculate on the possibility that plaque amyloid and PHFs are, in fact, derived from the same protein as originally suggested by Divry [10]. We have carried out a number of PHF preparations, by the method of Selkoe [32], from several Alzheimer brains. The amino acid analysis of the least contaminated preparation (as judged by negative-stain electron microscopy), which was produced from an area of cortex in which around 7% of the neurons contained tangles, is included in Table 2. This analysis shows some intriguing similarities to those produced from plaque core protein, including a low level of threonine and high levels of glycine and valine. The only large difference is the higher level of proline in the PHF preparation, and this could be due to contaminating collagen which we have invariably observed amongst isolated PHFs.

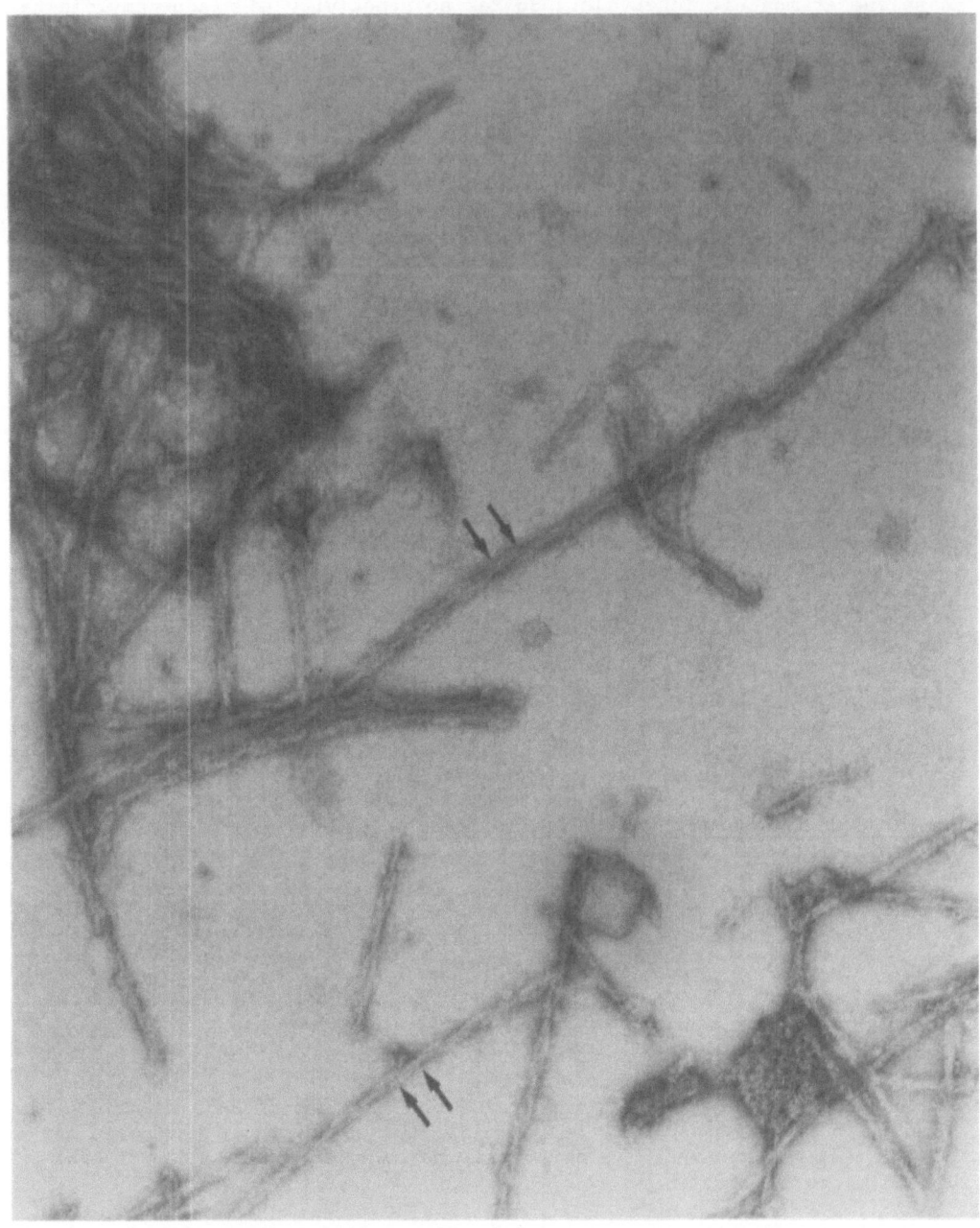

Fig. 4. Negatively-stained electron microscope appearance of isolated paired
         helical filaments. The PHFs were isolated from an Alzheimer brain
         (F, age 64) by the method of Ihara et al. [32]. The isolated PHFs
         were dried onto a carbon film, stained for 2 min with 1% uranyl
         acetate, and examined under a Philips 300 electron microscope.
         The PHF s are seen to consist of a pair of 8 nm filaments arranged
         in the form of a double helix. In certain regions (marked by
         arrows) it is apparent that each 8 nm filament consists of two
         3.5-4.5 nm protofilaments (×143,000).

Obviously the ultrastructural morphology of plaque amyloid and PHFs is different. By means of tilt-stage electron microscopy of positively-stained ruthenium red-impregnated sections, Narang [33] observed that plaque amyloid fibrils are composed of a pair of 6 nm protofilaments arranged in the form of a bifilar helix. The double-helical nature of plaque amyloid was confirmed by Merz et al. [34] who described the plaque amyloid fibrils from AD, on the basis of negative-stain electron microscopy, as two helically-intertwined 4-8 nm protofilaments. Our own observations on negatively stained PHFs (Fig. 4) suggest that they consist of two filaments with an average diameter of 8 nm arranged in the form of a double helix, completing one half turn in approximately 80 nm as originally described by Kidd [13]. In certain areas of the photograph in Fig. 4 it appears that each of these 8 nm filaments in fact consists of two protofilaments each with a diameter of 3.5-4.5 nm. Thus the whole PHF is apparently built up from four protofilaments. It is not impossible for the PHF protofilaments (3.5-4.5 nm) to be the same as the plaque amyloid protofilaments (408 nm) although this is speculative, and is in contradiction with the observation that antibodies to PHFs fail to react with plaque amyloid [29, 30].

Definitive amino acid sequence information is required to resolve this suggestion on PHF composition, and to confirm our conclusion, based on amino acid analysis, that plaque amyloid and cerebrovascular amyloid are the same substance.

REFERENCES

1. G. G. Glenner, N. Engl. J. Med., 302:1283 (1980).
2. K. Sletten et al., Biochem. J., 195:561 (1981).
3. E. P. Benditt et al., FEBS Lett., 19:169 (1971); K. Sletten and G. Husby, Eur. J. Biochem., 41:117 (1974).
4. M. D. Benson, J. Clin. Invest., 67:1035 (1981); M. Skinner and A. S. Cohen, Biochem. Biophys. Res. Commun., 99:1326 (1981); K. Sletten, P. Westermark, and J. B. Natvig, Scand. J. Immunol., 12:503 (1980); S. Tawara et al., Biochem. Biophys. Res. Commun., 116:880 (1983).
5. K. Sletten, P. Westermark, and J. B. Natvig, J. Exp. Med., 143:993 (1976).
6. D. H. Cohen et al., J. Exp. Med., 158:623 (1983).
7. G. G. Glenner and C. Wong, Biochem. Biophys. Res. Commun., 120:885 (1984).
8. G. G. Glenner and C. Wong, Biochem. Biophys. Res. Commun., 122:1131 (1984).
9. R. D. Terry, Fed. Proc., 37:2837 (1978).
10. P. J. Divry, J. Belge Neurol., 27:643 (1927).
11. M. Kidd, Brain, 87:307 (1964); R. D. Terry, H. K. Gonatas, and M. Weiss, Am. J. Pathol., 44:269 (1964).
12. T. I. Mandybur and S. R. D. Bates, Arch. Neurol., 35:246 (1978).
13. M. Kidd, Nature (Lond.), 197:192 (1963).
14. H. M. Wisniewski, H. K. Narang, and R. D. Terry, J. Neurol. Sci., 27:173 (1976).
15. G. Blessed, B. E. Tomlinson, and M. Roth, Br. J. Psychiatry, 114:797 (1968); G. K. Wilcock and M. M. Esiri, J. Neurol. Sci., 56:343 (1982).
16. E. K. Perry et al., Br. Med. J., 2:1457 (1978); G. K. Wilcock et al., J. Neurol. Sci., 57:407 (1982).
17. M. E. Bruce and H. Fraser, Neuropathol. Appl. Neurobiol., 1:189 (1975).
18. S. M. Chou and J. D. Martin, Acta Neuropathol. (Berl.), 17:150 (1971).
19. C. L. Masters, D. C. Gajdusek, and C. J. Gibbs, Brain, 104:559 (1981).

20. J. Klatzo, D. C. Gajdusek, and V. Zigas, Lab. Invest., 8:799 (1959).
21. P. C. Burger and F. S. Vogel, Am. J. Pathol., 73:457 (1973); M. I. Olson and C. Shaw, Brain, 92:147 (1969).
22. H. M. Wisniewski, H. K. Narang, and J. A. N. Corsellis, J. Neuropathol. Exp. Neurol., 35:367 (1976).
23. M. Kidd, D. Allsop and M. Landon, in: Interdiscipl. Topics Geront., Vol. 19, ed. F. C. Rose, Karger, Basel, Switzerland, in press.
24. V. Bocci, Nature (Lond.), 212:826 (1966); S. P. R. Rose, Nature (Lond.), 206:621 (1965); M. Satake and S. Abe, J. Biochem. (Tokyo), 59:72 (1966).
25. D. Allsop, M. Landon, and M. Kidd, Brain Res., 259:348 (1983).
26. P. H. Gibson, Neuropathol. Appl. Neurobiol., 9:379 (1983); H. M. Wisniewski and R. D. Terry, in: Progress in Neuropathology, Vol. 2, ed. H. M. Zimmerman, pp. 1-26, Grune and Stratton, N.Y.
27. T. Miyakawa et al., Virchows Arch. (Cell Pathol.), 40:121 (1982).
28. B. M. Anderton et al., Nature, 298:84 (1982).
29. C. G. Rasool et al., Brain Res., 310:249 (1984).
30. G. P. Wang et al., Acta Neuropathol. (Berl.), 62:268 (1984).
31. P. Gambetti et al., Lab. Invest., 49:430 (1983); J. M. Powers et al., J. Neuropathol. Exp. Neurol., 40:592 (1981); S-H. C. Yen, F. Gaskin, and R. D. Terry, Am. J. Pathol., 104, 7 (1981).
32. Y. Ihara, C. Abraham and D. J. Selkoe, Nature, 304:727 (1980).
33. H. K. Narang, J. Neuropathol. Exp. Neurol.. 39:621 (1980).
34. P. A. Merz et al., Acta Neuropathol. (Berl.), 60:113 (1983).

ACKNOWLEDGEMENTS

We are grateful to Mrs. A. Tomlonson for assistance with electron microscopy and photography; Miss G. Rumford and Miss W. Tomlinson for technical assistance; Miss K. Ayres for the work on PHF purification; the MRC Brain Bank, Cambridge for the supply of Alzheimer and Down's syndrome brains; and Professor B. E. Tomlinson and Dr. R. H. Perry of the Neuroendocrinology Unit, Newcastle, Dr. I. A. Ansell, Professor T. H. D. Arie and Dr. R. G. Jones of the Nottinghom City Hospital, Professor J. A. N. Corsellis and Dr. L. H. Carasco of Runwell Hospital, Essex for the supply of Alzheimer brains. This work was supported by a project grant from the Wellcome Trust.

PRION AMYLOIDS IN SCRAPIE AND CREUTZFELDT-JAKOB DISEASE

Stanley B. Prusiner*†, Ronald A. Barry*,
Michael P. McKinley*, Stephen J. DeArmond‡,
and David T. Kingsbury†**

Departments of *Neurology, *Biochemistry and
Biophysics, and ‡Pathology
University of California
San Francisco, California 94143

†Department of Biomedical and Environmental
 Sciences
 School of Public Health
 University of California
 Berkeley, California 94720

**Naval Biosciences Laboratory
 Naval Supply Center
 Oakland, California 94625

ABSTRACT

Amyloid has been found in a limited number of diseases of the central
nervous system. Amyloid plaques have been observed in some cases of both
natural and experimental scrapie, but the relationship of these plaques
to the scrapie agent or prion was not appreciated until recently. A protocol has been developed for the purification of scrapie prions 3,000- to
10,000-fold from infected hamster brains. Extensively purified preparations of scrapie prions contain only one major protein (PrP 27-30) and rod-
shaped particles. PrP 27-30 is a sialoglycoprotein and has an apparent
molecular weight of 27,000 to 30,000 as determined by sodium dodecyl sulfate polyacrylamide gel electrophoresis. The rods measure 10-20 nm in
diameter and 100-200 nm in length by negative staining. The rods appear
to represent a polymeric form of the scrapie prion and each rod may contain as many as 1,000 PrP 27-30 molecules. Arrays of prion rods resemble
ultrastructurally and histochemically many purified amyloids; antiserum
to PrP 27-30 decorates filaments within amyloid plaques of scrapie-infected
hamster brain. Our findings for scrapie suggest that amyloid plaques found
in similar human transmissible disorders - kuru, Creutzfeldt-Jakob disease,
Gerstmann-Sträussler syndrome - may also represent paracrystalline arrays
of prions. In addition, our observations raise the possibility that the
amyloid proteins in Alzheimer's disease may also play an etiologic role.

INTRODUCTION

The most common form of cerebral amyloidosis is Alzheimer's disease.
This dementing disorder afflicts primarily older people and its cause is
unknown. For many decades, the presence of amyloid proteins within senile

733

plaques and neurofibrillary tangles in the brains of patients with Alzheimer's disease has been appreciated. Generally, these amyloid accumulations have been considered a consequence of the disease process [1]. Experimental studies with the scrapie agent have shown that amyloid deposits in scrapie-infected brains are composed of causative molecules. These observations raise the possibility that amyloid molecules might also play a causative role in nontransmissible disorders of the central nervous system such as Alzheimer's disease.

Scrapie and Creutzfeldt-Jakob disease are both caused by prions which can be distinguished from both viruses and viroids. Aggregates of the prions are ultrastructurally and histochemically identical to amyloid. Extracellular collections of prion proteins form amyloid plaques within scrapie-infected brain. Prion amyloid plaques seem analogous to some viral inclusion bodies in that they are composed of causative infectious pathogens.

Purification of the Scrapie Agent

Progress in purification of the infectious particles causing scrapie is leading to an understanding of their chemical structure. Numerous attempts have been made to purify the scrapie agent over the past three decades [2-8]. Few advances in this area of investigation were made until a relatively rapid and economical bioassay was developed [9, 10]. Over a period spanning nearly a decade, our investigations of the molecular properties of the scrapie agent have been oriented toward developing effective procedures for purification. We began our studies by determining the sedimentation properties of the scrapie agent in fixed angle rotors and sucrose gradients [11-13]. Subsequent work extended those findings and demonstrated the efficacy of nuclease and protease digestions as well as sodium dodecyl sarcosinate gel electrophoresis in the development of purification protocols [14, 15]. Once a 100-fold purification was achieved, convincing evidence demonstrating that a protein is required for infectivity was obtained [16, 17].

Even before the scrapie protein was identified, we began an intensive search for the putative nucleic acid genome of the scrapie agent. To date, we have failed to find this elusive nucleic acid [18-21]; indeed, our results are consistent with those reported by Alper and her colleagues nearly two decades earlier [22-24]. The requirement of a protein for infectivity and the extraordinary resistance of the scrapie agent to inactivation by procedures that modify or hydrolyze nucleic acids led to the introduction of the term "prion" to denote these infectious particles [18].

Scrapie Priors Contain a Sialoglycoprotein

In our search for a scrapie-specific protein, it became necessary to substitute discontinuous sucrose gradients in vertical rotors for gel electrophoresis [25]. The resulting purification scheme led to the first identification of a macromolecule within the scrapie prion [26-30]. This molecule is a sialoglycoprotein designated PrP 27-30 with an apparent molecular weight of 27,000-30,000 (Table 1) [31]. Hydrolysis or selective chemical modification of PrP 27-30 resulted in a loss of scrapie infectivity. The development of a large scale purification protocol has allowed us to determine the N-terminal sequence of PrP 27-30 and to raise antibodies against the protein [29, 32, 33]. Other investigators using purification steps similar to those developed by us seem to have demonstrated the presence of this protein in their preparations [34, 35].

TABLE 1.   Properties of Hamster Scrapie PrP 27-30

Composition: Sialoglycoprotein

Molecular Weight: 27,000-30,000 sodium dodecyl sulfate
                              polyacrylamide gel electrophoresis
                          19,500 sodium dodecyl sulfate HPLC

Properties: Size and charge heterogeneity
                          Protease-resistant in native state

Biological Function: Native conformation required for prion
                              infectivity
                          Reversible inactivation by chemical
                              modification with diethylpyrocarbonate

Structure: N-X_n-Trp-Gly-Gln-Gly-Gly-Gly-Thr-His-
                              Asn-Gln-Trp-Asn-Lys-Pro-Ser-Lys-
                          Polymerizes into amyloid rods

Occurrence: Scrapie hamster brain
                          Similar proteins in mouse scrapie as well
                              as human, guinea pig and mouse CJD

Search for a Prion Genome

    The size of the smallest infectious unit remains controversial due
largely to the extreme heterogeneity and apparent hydrophobicity of the
scrapie prion [18, 19, 36, 37]. Early studies of Alper and her colleagues
suggested a molecular weight of 60,000 to 150,000 [22]. While an alternate
interpretation of that data has been proposed [37], there is no firm evidence to suggest that Alper's molecular weight calculations are incorrect.
In fact, sucrose gradient sedimentation, molecular sieve chromatography
and membrane filtration studies all suggest that a significant portion of
the infectious particles may be considerably smaller than the smallest
known viruses [18, 37]. However, the propensity of the scrapie agent to
aggregate makes molecular weight determinations by each of these methods
subject to artefact.

TABLE 2. Characteristics of Hamster Scrapie Prion Rods

Dimensions:	10–20 nm diameter, 100–200 nm length
Morphology:	Flattened rods, no unit structure, resemble purified amyloids
Substructure:	A few twisted suggesting protofilaments
Composition:	500–1,000 PrP 27-30 sialoglycoprotein molecules per rod N-X$_n$-Trp-Gly-Gln-Gly-Gly-Gly-Thr-His-Asn-Gln-Trp-Asn-Lys-Pro-Ser-Lys
Infectivity:	Aggregate of prions – sonication produces spheres 19 nm in diameter and rods 60 nm long without altering titers
Histochemistry:	Bind Congo red dye and exhibit green–gold birefringence
Occurrence:	Purified fractions from scrapie hamster and mouse, and CJD human, guinea pig and mouse

To date, no experimental data has been accumulated which indicates that scrapie infectivity depends upon a nucleic acid within the particle. Attempts to inactivate scrapie prions with nucleases, ultraviolet irradiation at 254 nm, Zn^{++} catalyzed hydrolysis, psoralen photoinactivation and chemical modification by hydroxylamine have all been negative [18, 20, 21] even using preparations which contain one major protein as determined by amino acid sequencing [38]. While these negative results do not establish the absence of a nucleic acid genome within the prion, they make this possibility seem likely. Attempts to identify a nucleic acid in purified prion preparations by silver staining and [^{32}P]-end-labeling have been unsuccessful to date [39].

Ultrastructural Identification of Prion Aggregates

Many investigators have used the electron microscope to search for a scrapie-specific particle. Spheres, rods, fibrils and tubules have been described in scrapie, kuru and Creutzfeldt-Jakob disease (CJD)-infected brain tissue [40-47]. Notable amongst the early studies are reports of filamentous virus-like particles in human CJD brain measuring 15 nm in diameter [45] and rod-shaped particles in sheep, rat and mouse scrapie brain measuring 15-26 nm in diameter and 60-75 nm in length [46, 47]. Studies with ruthenium red and lanthanum nitrate suggested that the rod-shaped particles possessed polysaccharides on their surface; these findings are of special interest since PrP 27-30 has been shown to be a sialoglyco-protein [31].

In purified fractions prepared from scrapie-infected brains, rod-shaped particles were found measuring 10-20 nm in diameter and 100-200 nm in length (Table 2) [25, 28]. Although no unit morphologic structure could be identified, most of the rods exhibited a relatively uniform diameter and appeared as flattened cylinders. Some of the rods had a twisted structure suggesting that they might be composed of protofilaments. In the fractions containing rods, one major protein (PrP 27-30) and $\sim 10^{9.5}$ ID_{50} units of prions per ml were also found. The high degree of purity of our prepara-tions demonstrated by radiolabeling and sodium dodecyl sulfate polyacryl-amide gel electrophoresis allowed us to establish that the rods are com-posed of PrP 27-30 molecules. Since PrP 27-30 had already been shown to be required for and inseparable from infectivity [27], we concluded that the rods must be a form of the prion [28]. In earlier studies with less puri-fied fractions, we could not determine whether the rods were a pathologic product of infection or an aggregate of the prion [25]. Subsequently, others faced the same dilemma because their preparations lacked sufficient purity due to protein contaminants [34]. Recent immunoelectron microscopic studies using antibodies raised against PrP 27-30 have confirmed that the rods are composed of PrP 27-30 molecules [48]. Sonication of the prion rods reduced their mean length to 60 nm and generated many spherical parti-cles without altering infectivity titers [49]. In contrast, fragmentation of M-13 filamentous bacteriophage by brief sonication reduced infectivity significantly [50].

Amyloid Plaques in Prion Diseases

The presence of amyloid plaques in natural and experimental scrapie was reported more than two decades ago [51]. Studies with inbred mice have shown that amyloid deposition in scrapie depends upon the genetic back-ground of the host as well as the isolate of the scrapie prion [52]. Be-sides scrapie, amyloid plaques have been found in four other transmissible disorders: CJD, kuru and Gerstmann-Sträussler syndrome of humans as well as chronic wasting disease of mule deer and elk [53-55].

Prion Rods and Filaments are Amyloid

The ultrastructure of the prion rods is indistinguishable from many purified amyloids [28]. Histochemical studies with Congo red dye have ex-tended this analogy to purified preparations of prions [28] as well as to scrapie-infected brain where amyloid plaques have been shown to stain with antibodies to PrP 27-30 (Table 3) [32]. In addition, PrP 27-30 has been found to stain with periodic acid Schiff reagent [31]; amyloid plaques in tissue sections readily bind this reagent.

Recent immunocytochemical studies with antibodies to PrP 27-30 have shown that filaments measuring approximately 16 nm in diameter and up to

TABLE 3. Some Comparative Properties of Prions and Amyloids in Scrapie-Infected Hamster Brains

Properties	Purified Prions	Amyloid Plaques
Ultrastructure	Aggregate into rod-shaped particles	Composed of filaments with uniform diameter
Polysaccharides	PrP 27-30 is a sialoglycoprotein	Stain with periodic acid Schiff
Congophilia	Green-gold birefringence	Green-gold birefringence
Antigenicity	α-PrP 27-30 decorates prion rods	α-PrP 27-30 stains plaques and component filaments

1,500 nm in length within amyloid plaques of scrapie-infected hamster brain are composed of prion proteins [56]. The antibodies to PrP 27-30 did not react with neurofilaments, glial filaments, microtubules and microfilaments in brain tissue. The prion filaments have a relatively uniform diameter, rarely show narrowings and possess all the morphologic features of amyloid. Except for their length, the prion filaments appear to be identical ultrastructurally with the rods which are found in purified fractions of prions.

In extracts of scrapie-infected rodent brains, abnormal structures were found by electron microscopy and labeled scrapie-associatedfibrils [57]. These abnormal fibrils were distinguished from other filamentous structures by their characteristic and well defined morphology. Published electron micrographs of the scrapie-associated fibrils consistently show helically wound structures measuring 300 to 800 nm in length. Based on their ultrastructural characteristics, the fibrils have been reported repeatedly to be different from amyloid [57-59]. Attempts to stain scrapie-associated fibrils with Congo red dye have yielded negative results; however, even a positive result would have been uninterpretable due to impurities in the extracts.

No structures with the ultrastructural morphology of scrapie-associated fibrils have been found in thin sections of scrapie-infected brain specimens. If scrapie-associated fibrils in brain extracts are eventually found to be composed of PrP 27-30 molecules, then the possibility that these fibrils are an artefact of the preparative extraction procedure must be en-

TABLE 4. The Prion Hypothesis

	Nucleic Acid	Template for PrP 27-30
1.	Prions contain a genomic nucleic acid (prions are viruses)	PrP 27-30 is encoded within the prion nucleic acid
2.	Prions contain a small, nongenomic nucleic acid	PrP 27-30 is encoded within the host
3.	Prions are devoid of nucleic acid	PrP 27-30 is encoded within the host or PrP 27-30 serves as a template for its own reproduction

tertained. This may well be the case in view of the folloiwng observations: 1) filaments within scrapie-infected brain are composed of PrP 27-30 molecules; 2) these filaments have a uniform diameter and rarely twist; 3) they are morphologically and histochemically identical to amyloid; and 4) they possess the same ultrastructural and antigenic characteristics as the rods found in purified fractions of prions except for length. Clearly, both the prion filaments and rods are indistinguishable from amyloids, but can be readily differentiated morphologically from scrapie-associated fibrils.

Prion Morphology

It seems doubtful that electron microscopic studies to date have been able to demonstrate the smallest infectious unit or fundamental particle of the scrapie prion. Certainly, the morphology of the unit structure has not been defined. The extreme morphologic heterogeneity of the rods is inconsistent with the hypothesis that prions are filamentous viruses. Based upon the morphology of scrapie-associated fibrils, several investigators have suggested that the scrapie agent is a filamentous virus [58].

Spherical particles have been found within postsynaptic evaginations of the brains of scrapie sheep and mice as well as CJD humans and chimpanzees [40-43]. These particles measured 23-35 nm in diameter. Since sonication fragmented prior rods and generated spheres measuring 10-30 nm in diameter, the question arises whether or not the spherical particles in brain tissues are related to the sonicated spheres.

Creutzfeldt-Jakob Disease Prions

Investigations of scrapie prions have recently been extended to studies on CJD. The CJD agent has been partially purified using procedures developed for scrapie prions [33, 60]. The CJD agents from humans, mice and guinea pigs contain protease-resistant proteins that exhibit cross-immunoreactivity with PrP 27-30 antisera. By electron microscopy the CJD preparations contain rod-shaped particles of similar dimensions as those found in scrapie prion preparations. Furthermore, the CJD prion rods stain with Congo red dye and exhibit green-gold birefringence. It is noteworthy that long helically twisted fibrils have been reported in extracts from human, mouse and guinea pig CJD brains and called scrapie-associated fibrils [61]; however, our results with purified preparations of CJD prions show that structures with the morphology of these fibrils are not required for infectivity.

The Prion Hypothesis

New knowledge about the molecular structure of the scrapie agent has allowed us to elaborate upon the prion hypothesis (Table 4) [18]. If prions are viruses, then they contain a genomic nucleic acid which encodes PrP 27-30. This possibility is increasingly unlikely. Alternatively, prions may contain a small, nongenomic nucleic acid which does not encode PrP 27-30. There is no chemical or physical evidence to indicate the presence of such a nucleic acid, but the biological diversity of prions could readily be explained by such a model. The third possibility is that prions are devoid of nucleic acid. In this case, information for the synthesis of new PrP 27-30 molecules is encoded either within the host genome or PrP itself. The former is more likely than the latter. Knowledge of the amino acid sequence of PrP 27-30 as well as antibodies to the protein provide new tools with which to extend our investigations of the chemical structure and genetic origin of prions.

The discovery that scrapie prions aggregate into rod-shaped particles which are histochemically and ultrastructurally identical to many purified amyloids, may be important in understanding the pathogenesis of other cerebral amyloidoses. Antibodies to the scrapie prion protein, PrP 27-30, have demonstrated that amyloid plaques in scrapie-infected hamster brain are composed of PrP 27-30 polymers. Whether or not the prion remains infectious when its protein polymerizes into amyloid filaments and is deposited into the extracellular space remains to be determined. Indeed, studies on scrapie prion amyloid have forced a reconsideration of the role of amyloid proteins in both the transmissible and nontransmissible cerebral amyloidoses. In scrapie, amyloid deposits are composed of causative molecules - prion amyloid is not a mere consequence of the disease.

REFERENCES

1. S. B. Prusiner, N. Engl. J. Med., 310:661 (1984).
2. G. D. Hunter, J. Infect. Dis., 125:427 (1972).
3. G. C. Millson, G. D. Hunter, R. H. Kimberlin, in: Slow Virus Diseases of Animals and Man, R. H. Kimberlin, Ed. (American Elsevier, New York 1976), pp. 243-266.
4. A. N. Siakotos, D. C. Gajdusek, C. J. Gibbs, Jr., R. D. Traub, and C. Bucana, Virology, 70:230 (1976).
5. D. L. Mould, W. Smith, and A. M. Dawson, J. Gen. Microbiol.,40:71 (1965).
6. H. Diringer, H. Hilmert, D. Simon, E. Werner, and B. Ehlers, Eur. J. Biochem., 134:555 (1983).

7. R. F. Marsh, C. Dees, B. E. Castle, W. F. Wade, and T. L. German, J. Gen. Virol., 65:415 (1984).

8. P. Brown, E. M. Green, D. C. Gajdusek, Proc. Soc. Exp. Biol. Med., 158: 513 (1978).

9. S. B. Prusiner, D. F. Groth, S. P. Cochran, F. R. Masiarz, M. P. McKinley, and H. M. Martinez, Biochemistry, 19:4883 (1980).

10. S. B. Prusiner, S. P. Cochran, D. F. Groth, D. E. Downey, K. A. Bowman, and H. M. Martinez, Ann. Neurol., 11:353 (1982).

11. S. B. Prusiner, W. J. Hadlow, C. M. Eklund, and R. E. Race, Proc. Natl. Acad. Sci. USA, 74:4656 (1977).

12. S. B. Prusiner, W. J. Hadlow, C. M. Eklund, R. E. Race, and S. P. Cochran, Biochemistry, 17:4987 (1978).

13. S. B. Prusiner, W. J. Hadlow, D. E. Garfin, S. P. Cochran, J. R. Baringer, R. E. Race, and C. M. Eklund, Biochemistry, 17:4993 (1978).

14. S. B. Prusiner, D. F. Groth, C. Bildstein, F. R. Masiarz, M. P. McKinley, and S. P. Cochran, Proc. Natl. Acad. Sci. USA, 77:2984 (1980).

15. S. B. Prusiner, D. F. Groth, S. P. Cochran, M. P. McKinley, and F. R. Masiarz, Biochemistry, 19:4892 (1980).

16. S. B. Prusiner, M. P. McKinley, D. F. Groth, K. A. Bowman, N. I. Mock, S. P. Cochran, and F. R. Masiarz, Proc. Natl. Acad. Sci. USA, 78:6675 (1981).

17. M. P. McKinely, F. R. Masiarz, and S. B. Prusiner, Science, 214:1259 (1981).

18. S. B. Prusiner, Science, 216:136 (1982).

19. S. B. Prusiner, Adv. Virus Res., in press (1984).

20. T. O. Diener, M. P. McKinley, and S. B. Prusiner, Proc. Natl. Acad. Sci. USA, 79:5220 (1982).

21. M. P. McKinley, F. R. Masiarz, S. T. Isaacs, J. E. Hearst, and S. B. Prusiner, Photochem. Photobiol., 37:539 (1983).

22. T. Alper, D. A. Haig, M. C. Clarke, Biochem. Biophys. Res. Commun., 22:278 (1966).

23. T. Alper, W. A. Cramp, D. A. Haig, and M. C. Clarke, Nature, 214:764 (1967).

24. T. Alper, D. A. Haig, and M. C. Clarke, J. Gen. Virol., 41:503 (1978).

25. S. B. Prusiner, D. C. Bolton, D. F. Groth, K. A. Bowman, S. P. Cochran, and M. P. McKinley, Biochemistry, 21:6942 (1982).

26. D. C. Bolton, M. P. McKinely, S. B. Prusiner, Science, 218:1309 (1982).

27. M. P. McKinley, D. C. Bolton, and S. B. Prusiner, Cell, 35:57 (1983).

28. S. B. Prusiner, M. P. McKinley, K. A. Bowman, D. C. Bolton, P. E. Bendheim, D. C. Groth, and G. G. Glenner, Cell, 35:349 (1983).

29. S. B. Prusiner, D. F. Groth, D. C. Bolton, S. B. Kent, and L. E. Hood, Cell, 38:127 (1984).

30. D. C. Bolton, M. P. McKinley, and S. B. Prusiner, Biochemistry, in press (1984).

31. D. C. Bolton, R. K. Meyer, S. B. Prusiner, J. Virol., in press (1985).

32. P. E. Bendheim, R. A. Barry, S. J. DeArmond, D. P. Stites, and S. P. Prusiner, Nature, 310:418 (1984).

33. P. E. Bendheim, J. M. Bockman, M. P. McKinely, D. T. Kingsbury, S. B. Prusiner, Proc. Natl. Acad. Sci. USA, in press (1985).

34. H. Diringer, H. Gelderblom, H. Hilmert, M. Özel, C. Edelbluth, and R. H. Kimberlin, Nature, 306:476 (1983).

35. H. Hilmert, H. Diringer, Biosci. Rep., 4:165 (1984).

36. H. Diringer, R. H. Kimberlin, Biosci. Rep., 3:563 (1983).

37. R. G. Rohwer, Nature, 308:658 (1984).

38. C. G. Bellinger, J. E. Cleaver, S. B. Prusiner, in preparation.

39. C. G. Bellinger, M. P. McKinley, R. K. Meyer, and S. B. Prusiner, in preparation.

40. J. F. David-Ferriera, K. L. David-Ferreira, C. J. Gibbs, Jr., and J. A. Morris, Proc. Soc. Exp. Biol. Med., 127:313 (1968).
41. A. Bignami, H. B. Parry, Science, 171:389 (1971).
42. P. W. Lampert, D. C. Gajdusek, and C. J. Gibbs, Jr., J. Neurol. Sci., 30:20 (1971).
43. J. R. Baringer and S. B. Prusiner, Ann. Neurol., 4:205 (1978).
44. E. J. Field, J. D. Mathews, and C. S. Raine, J. Neurol. Sci., 8:209 (1969).
45. M. L. Vernon, L. Horta-Barbosa, D. A. Fuccillo, J. L. Sever, J. R. Baringer, and G. Birnbaum, Lancet, 1:964 (1970).
46. E. J. Field and H. K. Narang, J. Neurol. Sci., 17:347 (1972).
47. H. K. Narang, Acta Neuropathol. (Berl.), 28:317 (1974).
48. R. A. Barry, M. P. McKinley, P. E. Bandheim, G. K. Lewis, and S. B. Prusiner, submitted for publication.
49. M. P. McKinley, M. B. Braunfeld, S. B. Prusiner, submitted for publication.
50. C. G. Bellinger, M. P. McKinely, and S. B. Prusiner, in preparation.
51. E. Beck, P. M. Daniel, in: Slow, Latent and Temperate Virus Infections, D. C. Gajdusek, C. J. Gibbs, Jr., M. Alpers, Eds. (U.S. Government Printing Office, Washington, D.C., 1965), pp. 203–206.
52. M. E. Bruce, A. G. Dickinson, and H. Fraser, Neuropathol. Appl. Neurobiol., 2:471 (1976).
53. I. Klatzo, D. C. Gajdusek, and V. Zigas, Lab. Invest., 8:799 (1959).
54. C. L. Masters, D. C. Gajdusek, C. J. Gibbs, Jr., Brain, 104:559 (1981).
55. S. Bahmanjar, E. S. Williams, F. Johnson, S. Young, and D. C. Gajdusek, personal communication.
56. S. A. DeArmond, M. P. McKinley, R. A. Barry, M. B. Braunfeld, J. R. McColloch, and S. B. Prusiner, submitted for publication.
57. P. A. Merz, R. A. Somerville, H. M. Wisneiwski, and K. Iqbal, Acta Neuropathol. (Berl.), 54:63 (1981).
58. P. A. Merz, R. G. Rohwer, R. Kascsak, H. M. Wisniewski, R. A. Somerville, C. J. Gibbs, Jr., and D. C. Gajdusek, Science, 225:437 (1984).
59. P. A. Merz, H. M. Wisniewski, R. A. Somerville, S. A. Bobin, C. L. Masters, K. Iqbal, Acta Neuropathol. (Berl.), 60:113 (1983).
60. J. M. Bockman, D. T. Kingsbury, M. P. McKinley, P. E. Bendheim, and S. B. Prusiner, submitted for publication.
61. P. A. Merz, R. A. Somerville, H. M. Wisniewski, L. Manuelidis, and E. E. Manuelidis, Nature, 306:474 (1983).

ACKNOWLEDGEMENTS

Collaborative studies with Drs. L. Hood, S. Kent, T. Diener, J. Cleaver, G. Glenner and W. Hadlow have been important to the progression of these studies. The authors thank D. Gorth, K. Bowman, P. Cochran and B. Hennessey for technical assistance as well as L. Gallagher and F. Elvin for editorial and administrative assistance. Helpful discussions with Drs. S. Stites, G. Lewis, C. Bellinger, R. Meyer, P. Bendheim and D. Bolton are acknowledged. M. P. M. is the recipient of an Alzheimer's Disease and Related Disorders Associateion Award. This work was supported by research grants from the National Institutes of Health (AG02132 and NS14069) as well as by gifts from R. J. Reynolds Industries, Inc., Sherman Fairchild Foundation and W. M. Keck Foundation. Portions of this manuscript are adapted from a review published in Microbiological Sciences.

SENILE CEREBRAL AMYLOID - EVIDENCE FOR A NEURONAL

ORIGIN OF THE FIBRIL PROTEIN

James M. Powers

Department of Pathology
Medical University of South Carolina
171 Ashley Avenue
Charleston, South Carolina

ABSTRACT

AS_c of pre-senile and senile Alzheimer's disease and asymptomatic senile patients are morphologically indistinguishable with the histochemical and immunoperoxidase techniques utilized. Core and dyshoric amyloid stains similarly. Congophilic angiopathy amyloid of ten stains differently from core and dyshoric amyloid with histologic and histochemical stains, but possesses similar antigenic determinants. GAGS and a large variety of serum glycoproteins are present in AS_c; the IgG noted morphologically in AS_c does not appear to be bound to brain or vascular components. AS_c is distinct from AA. Our data support a local source for the fibrillar protein of AS_c. Neurofilament protein is the only local protein to be identified in AS_c; many of its physicochemical properties suggest an amyloidogenic potential.

INTRODUCTION

The pathogenesis of senile cerebral amyloidosis (AS_c), particularly neuritic plaque amyloid of Alzheimer's disease, has been a major inveistigative effort of mine for the past 13 years. Since this type of amyloid has proven to be extremely resistant to biochemical analysis, I attempted to learn about this lesion through a systematic evaluation of AS_c with a variety of morphologic techniques. I would like to review this morphologic data and present some new findings which relate to this significant pathologic process. Before this presentation, however, a definition of terms seems appropriate. For the sake of the present discussion, AS_c (of Alzheimer's pre-senile or senile cerebral disease and of "normal" aged humans) is divided into three forms: 1) core amyloid of neuritic or senile plaque, 2) dyshoric angiopathy of Morel & Wildi, and 3) Congophilic angiopathy of Pantelakis. Amyloid may be found within the majority of, if not all, neuritic plaques as linear to globoid to stellate cores surrounded by a corona of degenerate neurites and reactive glia. In the setting of dyshoric angiopathy, amyloid is found within and adjacent to cortical blood vessels, usually small arterioles and capillaries, and often appears to flow from blood vessels into neuropil. The final form, Congophilic angiopathy of Pantelakis, is characterized by amyloid deposits within leptomeningeal and cortical small arteries and arterioles. Both dyshoric angiopathy and Congophilic angiopathy represent amyloidotic involvement of cerebral blood vessels and, therefore, are examples of senile cerebrovascular amyloidosis. The last item, which needs clarification, is that of amyloid itself. The pathologic term, amyloid, has traditionally been used to describe amorphous to slightly fibrillar extracellular deposits which bind certain dyes (e.g., Congo red, eosin, alcian blue, periodic acid-Schiff, thioflavine), display green birefringence in polarized light and have a ∿10 nm filamentous ultrastructure. Although the fibrillar protein may constitute most of the amyloid mass and certainly has dominated recent investigative efforts, it is important to emphasize that other substances (e.g., glycosaminoglycans (CAGS) and serum glycoproteins) may also be integral components of amyloid. Therefore, it appears improper to refer to intracellular collections of proteinaceous intermediate filaments as "amyloid", irregardless of whether they are, or will ultimately become, the extracellular fibril of amyloid. It also seems capricious to equate Congophilia or β-pleated sheet conformation with a pathologic conundrum, amyloid. Consequently, my findings and comments will not relate to the intraneuronal paired helical filaments of Alzheimer's disease, which exhibit many features of classical amyloid fibrils. To minimize false positive reactions, I have considered a core or dyshoric deposit as amyloid only if it had a stellate appearance. Most specimens have been collected prospectively in order to promote brief fixation in 10% neutral formaldehyde (1-6 hours) and to retard autolysis by short postmortem intervals (usually 1-6 hours).

Based upon the prevailing concept of amyloidogenesis in 1971, my original hypothesis was that the fibrillar protein of AS_c was of vascular origin and that the blood-brain-barrier (BBB) played a significant role in its formation. Some doubt about the validity of this hypothesis quickly arise, when I was unable to detect amyloid around hyperpermeable BBB lesions (abscesses, infarcts, biopsy sites) from patients with cerebral amyloidosis of Alzheimer's disease or senility (Powers, unpublished observations). I was also unable to elicit cerebral amyloid in amyloidotic mice (natural-KK strain; induced-casein or Mycobacterium butyricum) by focally destructive lesions (Powers, unpublished observations). These negative experiences, coupled with the identification of the distinctive apudamyloid (AE), suggested that the fibril protein of AS_c might be derived from a local brain source. In order to test this hypothesis, a comparison of various types of amyloids was undertaken.

The results of routine histochemical staining showed that core and dyshoric amyloid were similar and most closely resembled AE, particularly that of medullary cercinoma of the thyroid [1]. The amyloid of Congophilic angiopathy resembled systemic amyloids (Table 1).

AS_c was next compared to other amyloids for its resistance to oxidation with potassium permanganate-sulfuric acid (Table 2). This data proved difficult to interpret, since AE (insular and medullary carcinoma) was resistant or variably affected. Core and dyshoric amyloid was variably affected and again most closely resembled the amyloid of medullary carcinoma of the thyroid. Congophilic angiopathy was essentially resistant to oxidation and, hence, behaved like AL. In view of these perplexing findings, it became necessary to look for AA protein by utilizing specific antisera in an immunoperoxidase bridge (Table 2). AA immunoreactivity was noted only in AA amyloid, although an evanescent, weak reactivity was noted in very briefly fixed core and dyshoric amyloids [2].

These observations showed that AS_c was different from AA and seemed to indicate that AS_c was most closely related to AE, which implicated a local protein source. The recent period of immunologic explosiveness did not spare AS_c. A major, if not the prevailing, hypothesis was that the amyloid protein of AS_c was of immunoglobulin (IgG) origin. AS_c was believed to be similar to AL primarily because IgG was detected morphologically in AS_c. Consequently, an immunoperoxidase search of AS_c for a variety of plasma proteins, including IgG, was undertaken (Table 3).

744

TABLE 1. Histochemical REsults

Reaction or Stain	AL (3)	AA (1)	AE (2)	ASb (3) C-DA	CA
Congo red	2+	2+	2+	2+	2+
Tryptophan	4+	3+	+/-	+/- → +	3+
Tyrosine	3+	3+	+/-	+/- → +	3+
Alcian blue 2.5	2+	2+	3+	4+	3+
PAS	3+	2+	2+	2+	2+

TABLE 2

	Potassium Permanganate - Sulfuric Acid Congo Red		AA Immunoperoxidase
AL	Lung, Heart (6)	Resistant	Negative
AA	Adrenal, Liver (2)	Sensitive	Positive
AE$_t$	Thyroid (3)	Variable	Negative
AE$_p$	Pancreas (2)	Resistant	Negative
AS$_c$	Heart (2)	Sensitive, Resistant	Negative
AS$_{b(C-DA)}$	Brain (6)	Variable	Negative
AS$_{b(CA)}$	Brain (2)	Resistant	Negative

All plasma proteins, which were looked for, could be identified [3, 4]. Generally, smaller and more stable proteins were easiest to detect. We could not assign a primary pathogenetic importance to the IgG, since there appeared to be a rather non-specific leakage of serum proteins into amyloid. Consequently, we began to look for the presence of local brain proteins in AS$_c$ in the same samples and with the same immunoperoxidase technique [4]. Recently, we have investigated two additional local proteins in core and dyshoric amyloid: S100 (Fig. 1) and laminin (Fig. 2), which are located within astrocytes and blood vessel basement membranes, respectively. Only neurofilament (NF) protein, and slight S100, reactivity was noted. When S100 was present, it was usually located around the periphery of the core. Since S100 appears to be secreted into the extracellular space by astrocytes [5], I interpret S100 immunoreactivity as due to non-specific adherence of an extracellular protein to amyloid. This data is summarized in Table 4. It should be noted that the same antigenic determinants were identified in core and dyshoric amyloid as in the amyloid of Congophilic angiopathy.

Considerable controversy ensured over the specificity of the polyclonal pooled and monospecific NF antibodies used in our original study. The NF antibodies consistently stained axons in tissue samples. All monospecific antibodies were raised against double-electroporesed, gel-excised immunogen. NF immunoreactivity was still observed in AS$_c$ after adsorption with normal human serum; it was abolished by adsorption with neurofilament protein or serial dilution of the antibodies. Cross reaction with a non-vascular, single contaminating protein was also unlikely, because the gel-excised immunogens had separate origins (68, 150, 200 kd) [4]. Additional lots of monospecific polyclonal antibodies were used in another immunoperoxidase technique (avidin-biotin complex ABC) and continued to reveal the presence of NF protein (Fig. 3). A few reports utilizing monoclonal

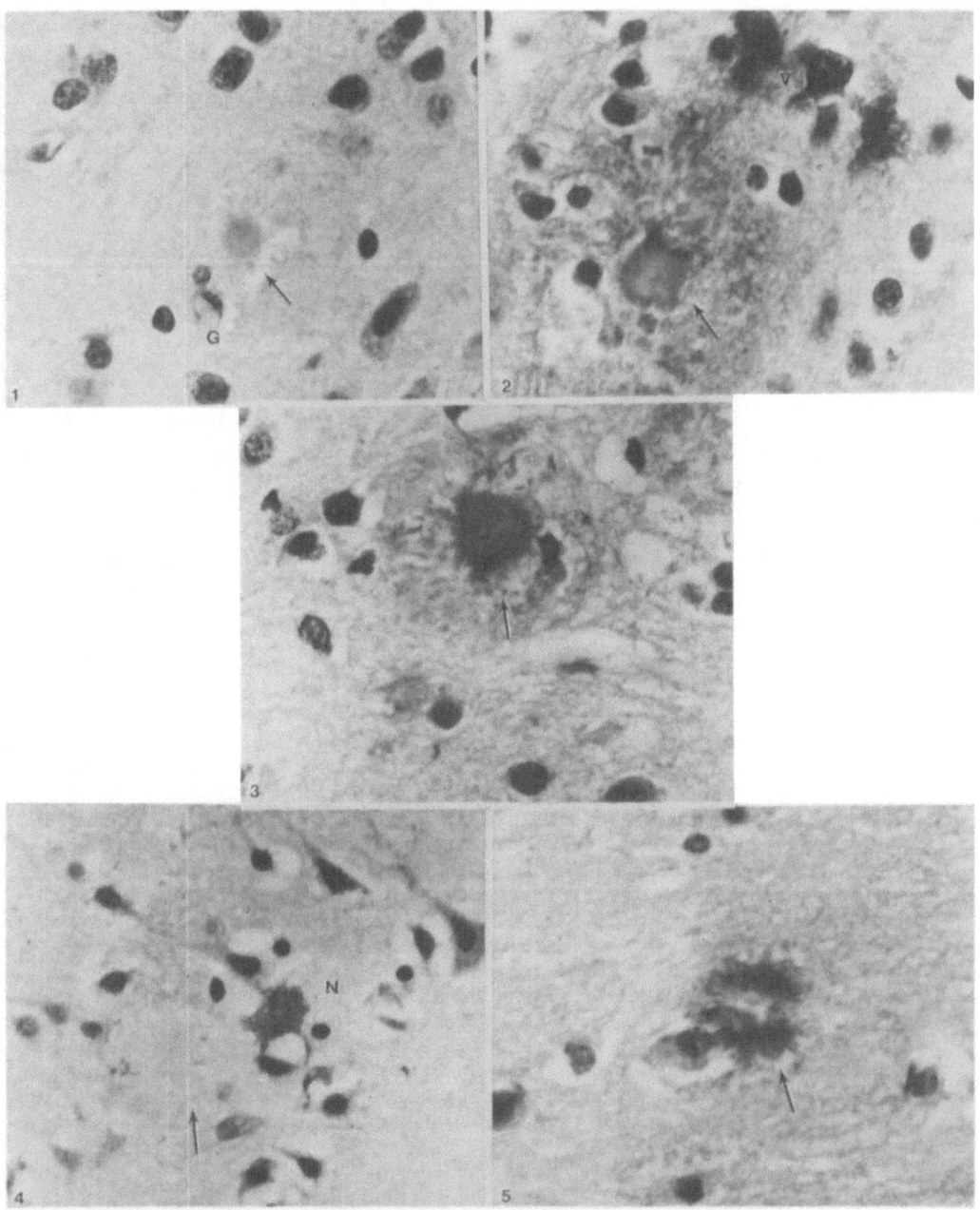

Figs. 1-5. Immunoreactivity of AS$_c$ (arrows). ABC immunoperoxidase technique ×800. Fig. 1; anti-S100, 1:200; slightly reactive per-
ripheral core and background of plaque, strongly reactive glial
cells (G). Fig. 2; anti-laminin, 1:200; negative core, reactive
blood vessel (V). Fig. 3; anti-68 kd neurofilament, 1:200; core
intensely reactive, background of plaque slightly reactive.
Fig. 4; monoclonal anti-200 kd neurofilament, undiluted; negative core, strongly positive neuron (N). Fig. 5; anti-200 kd
neurofilament, 1:200; strongly positive dyshoric amyloid.

TABLE 3

Immunoperoxidase - Plasma Proteins		
(3+ Strong, 2+ Weak, + Trace, 0 Negative)		
Core & Dyshoric (12)	IgG, Kappa, Lambda	3+
Congophilic Angiopathy (3)	IgA, IgM, Fib, Alb	2+
	Macroglobulin, Microglobulin	+
	Haptoglobin, C_3	+
	Lysozyme, Fe, $F(ab')_2$	+

TABLE 4

Immunoperoxidase - Local Proteins			
(3+ Strong, 2+ Weak, + Trace, 0 Negative)			
Core (15) and Dyshoric (6) Congophilic Angiopathy (3)	Astrocyte	GFAP (brain)	0
		S100 (brain)	0 → +
	Blood Vessel	Laminin (murine tumor)	0
	Neuron	Tubulin (brain)	0
		Actin (skeletal)	0
		Cholinergic vesicle (electric organ)	0
		Neurofilament (brain)	2+ → 3+

200 kd NF antibodies have failed to detect NF protein in core amyloid. We have also been unable to detect NF protein in core or dyshoric amyloid with a monoclonal 200 kd antibody (Fig. 4), which was raised in the same laboratory as the polyclonal NF antibodies (Schlaepfer et al., University of Pennsylvania). This, in itself, does not weaken the positive polyclonal findings, since monoclonal antibodies only react to a single antigenic determinant (epitope) usually consisting of a amall number of amino acid residues. We have recently acquired another polyclonal 200 kd monospecific antibody from a different laboratory (Dr. Chiu, Albert Einstein College of Medicine). This NF antibody also stained core and dyshoric amyloid (Fig. 5) in one briefly fixed autopsy sample with a short postmortem interval. However, it failed to stain two other samples, fixed briefly with formalin or B4-glutaraldehyde, which were taken from a pre-senile Alzheimer's patient 12 h after death. Our current NF data are summarized in Table 5. The duration and type of fixation and the extent of autolysis appear to be important limiting factors.

I should emphasize that uniform staining of all AS_c in a sample was never observed. This may indicate that most antigenic sites recognized by the NF antibodies are hidden in, or have been destroyed in the genesis of, the amyloid deposits. Alternatively, this finding may indicate that small amounts of neurofilament proteins are occasionally trapped within the amyloid. Although we have not resolved this dilemma, we have performed certain experiments which may begin to answer the question. We have been unable to uncover reactive sites by prior treatment with trypsin or pepsin, but the antigenic sites in core amyloid can be greatly reduced by prior oxidation with potassium permanganate-sulfuric acid. This latter response mimicked the response of core amyloid Congophilia to oxidation, while the

TABLE 5

Polyclonal pooled (Schlaepfer)	+(4)
Polyclonal 68, 150, 200 kd monospecific	+(4)
Polyclonal 200 kd monospecific (Chiu)	+(1); −(2)
Monoclonal 200 kd monospecific (Schlaepfer)	−(5)

PAS (serum glycoproteins) and alcian blue (glycosaminoglycans) positively was essentially unaffected. These observations support the notion that AS_c may be derived from neurofilament protein and, if so, that many NF antigenic sites are destroyed or rendered inaccessible during amyloidogenesis. We found that isolated bovine neurofilament protein exhibited Congophilia by microscopic and spectrophotometric examination. Finally, the weak birefringence of partially denatured Congophilic, neurofilament protein could be augmented and changed to apple-green by paraformaldehyde treatment [4].

In addition to our experimental evidence, there are several other lines of evidence which support the candidacy of neurofilaments for the fibrillar protein of AS_c. Neurofilaments are 10 nm intermediate filaments with a protofilamentous substructure and a central core [6]. Neurofilaments are capable of disassembly - reassembly; as a matter of fact, the 68 kd component can self-assemble its polypeptides into 10 nm filaments [7]. Thus, the original and reconstituted size and infrastructure of NF closely approximates amyloid filaments. Second, the insolubility of neurofilament protein and amyloid is similar. Third, in contrast to the former belief that NF is highly alpha helical, recent information indicates that the triplet NF proteins contain many highly acidic and highly basic non-alpha helical domains [8]. Beta domains may also be present in the portions of the molecule not yet sequenced.

The significance of IgG observed in ASc remained unclear. Was this a secondary, non-specific leakage or could this have an immunopathogenetic basis? All of the available data was purely morphologic (static) and incapable of assessing the activity of that IgG. We attempted to circumvent this limitation by utilizing standard immunologic and electrophoretic techniques to characterize the IgG eluted from brains with AS_c [9]. We found that the vast majority of brain-associated IgG were polyclonal could be eluted at neutral pH. The trace quantities of acid-elutable IgG were derived from cortex and white matter with and without amyloid. This indicates that most of the IgG identified in AS_c morphologically is not bound to brain or blood vessels and probably represents a non-specific deposition of this serum protein in amyloid. Our results do not exclude a possible role for soluble, neurotoxic immune complexes in the pathogenesis of AS_c.

We have most recently attempted to characterize AS_c by studying its lectin-binding properties. Preliminary data indicates the presence of a sialoglycoconjugate and N-linked glycosidic side chains as evidenced by positive staining with certain lectins: RCA I (Ricinus communis agglutinin), LCA (Lens culinaris agglutinin), and PSA (Pisum sativum agglutinin).

CONCLUSIONS

We believe that the fibrillar protein and GAGS of AS_c are most likely derived from local neurons; its glycoproteins are probably of serum origin.

Observed morphologic differences between core-dyshoric amyloid and Congo-philic angiopathic amyloid probably reflect variations in secondary components (e.g., GAGS and serum glycoproteins), not the fibrillar protein. An intraparenchymal immunopathogenetic mechanism in AS_C formation is implausible. Degraded neurofilament protein, perhaps the 68 kd component, appears to be a good candidate for the AS_C fibril. Valid and reproducible biochemical information, especially amino acid seequence data, is needed.

REFERENCE

1. J. M. Powers and S. S. Spicer, Virchows Arch. (Path. Anat.), 376:107 (1977). D. Stiller and D. Katenkamp, Exp. Pathol. Suppl., 1:1 (1975).
2. J. M. Powers et al., Acta Neuropathol., 58:275 (1982). R. P. Linke, Clin. Neuropathol., 1:172 (1982).
3. J. M. Powers and J. T. Skeen, J. Neuropathol. Exp. Neurol., 39:385 (1980). D. M. A. Mann, Neuropathol. Appl. Neurobiol., 8:55 (1982).
4. J. M. Powers et al., J. Neuropathol. Exp. Neurol., 40:592 (1981).
5. V. E. Shashoua et al., J. Neurochem., 42:1536 (1984).
6. W. W. Schlaepfer, in: Progress in Neuropathology, H. M. Zimmerman, Ed. (Raven, New York, 1979), p. 101.
7. R. V. Zackroff and R. D. Goldman, Science, 208:1152 (1980). N. Geisler and K. Weber, J. Mol. Biol., 151:565 (1981).
8. N. Geisler et al., EMBO J., 2:1295 (1983).
9. Goust et al., J. Neuropathol. Exp. Neurol., 43:481 (1984).

ACKNOWLEDGEMENTS

I thank Drs. Schlaepfer, Lee and Chiu for their generous gifts of neurofilament antibodies. I also thank Ms. Virginia R. Sincuya for preparing the manuscript, and Ms. Carol Moskos and our Photography Laboratory for photographic assistance.

ISOLATION AND PARTIAL CHARACTERIZATION OF ALZHEIMER

NEUROFIBRILLARY TANGLES

Fernando Goñi, Bernardo Pons-Estel,
Fernando Alvarez*, Peter D. Gorevic†,
and Blas Frangione

*Departments of Pathology and Cell Biology
New York University Medical Center
550 First Avenue
New York, N.Y. 10016

†State University of New York
Stonybrook, N.Y. 11794

ABSTRACT

Neurofibrillary tangles (NFT) were isolated from cerebral cortex of three cases of Alzheimer's disease (AD) by SDS-βME treatment followed by sucrose gradient ultracentrifugation. This material was predominantly NFT by electron microscopy and was excluded from all pore-sized polyacrylamide gels. It remained insoluble in strong acid and basic conditions, chaotropic and reducing agents. It resisted digestion by trypsin, chymotrypsin, subtilisin, urea-pepsin, collagenase, pronase, hyaluronidase, lipases and phospholipases but yielded a consistent amino acid analysis showing the presence of cysteine and methionine, more than 20% hydrophobic residues and 12% basic residues. Subjected to automated Edman degradation presented a non-reactive amino terminus. Under electron microscopy NFT appeared to be composed mainly by single and double filaments. Single filaments can turn and intertwine with themselves to make the regular arrangement of the double filaments. Purified NFT have been used to raise high titered polyclonal antisera for immunohistological studies. It specifically reacted with isolated NFT, affected neurons in cases of AD, aging brains, postencephalitic Parkinson's disease, Down's syndrome and dementia pugilistica but no reaction was observed with normal brain, cerebrovascular amyloid angiopathy, or the amyloid core from neuritic plaques.

INTRODUCTION

The main neuropathological features of Senile Dementia of the Alzheimer's type (SDAT) are: intraneuronal neurofibrillary tangles (NFT) and neuritic amyloid plaques. Ultrastructurally, NFT are composed of abnormal single and double filaments that also surround the amyloid core in the neutritic plaques [1-3]. NFT also occurs in aging brain, postencephalitic Parkinson's disease, Guam-Parkinson, dementia pugilistica, Down's syndrome and subacute sclerosing panencephalitis [4, 5]. Similar structure have been induced in experimental animals following aluminum intoxication and in vitro following exposure to agents such as colchicine [6, 7].

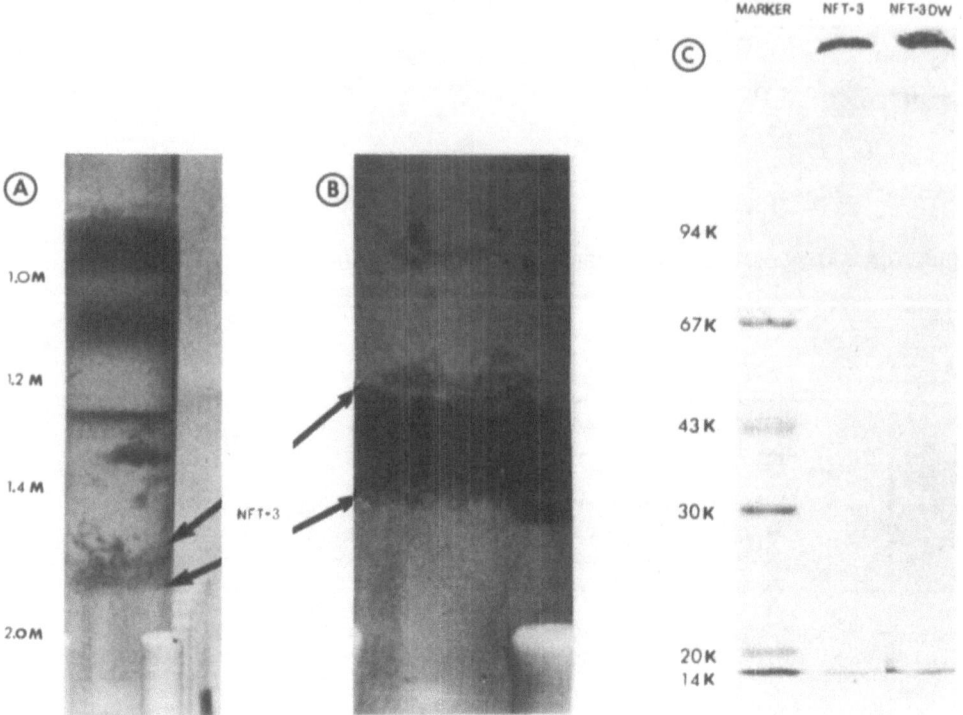

Fig. 1.   A) Discontinuous sucrose gradient after ultracentrifugation at
          220,000 g for 3 h at 25°C. Macroscopically, fibrillar material is
          seen in the 1.4–2.0 M sucrose interface. B) Close up of the 1.4–
          2.0 M interface. C) 10% SDS–PAGE of the NFT-enriched fraction ob-
          tained from the 1.4–2.0 M interface (NFT–3) and after sonication
          and recentrifugation in distilled water (NFT-3 DW).

Difficulties in obtaining pure and homogeneous NFT preparations have
so far precluded complete detailed biochemical and ultrastructural characterization [8-10].

In an attempt to gain some insight into the nature of the NFT we have
obtained an enriched NFT fraction from three AD brains. Biochemical and
ultrastructural studies were initiated, and a polyclonal anti-NFT antisera
was developed.

MATERIALS AND METHODS

Isolation of NFT

Dissected cerebral cortex from three cases of AD were extracted by
the procedure described by Selkoe and collaborators with minor modifications
[9]. The obtained material was repeatedly resuspended in small volume of
distilled water, sonicated for several hours and centrifuged at 140,000 g
for 60 min each time. Pellets were checked both by electron microscopy
following negative staining with 1% aqueous uranyl acetate pH 6.0 and 3%,
5%, 7.5%, 10%, 15% and 15%-6 M urea, SDS-polyacrylamide (SDS-PAGE) gels.
Samples were run both under reducing and nonreducing conditions as well as
in denaturing and non-denaturing sample buffers.

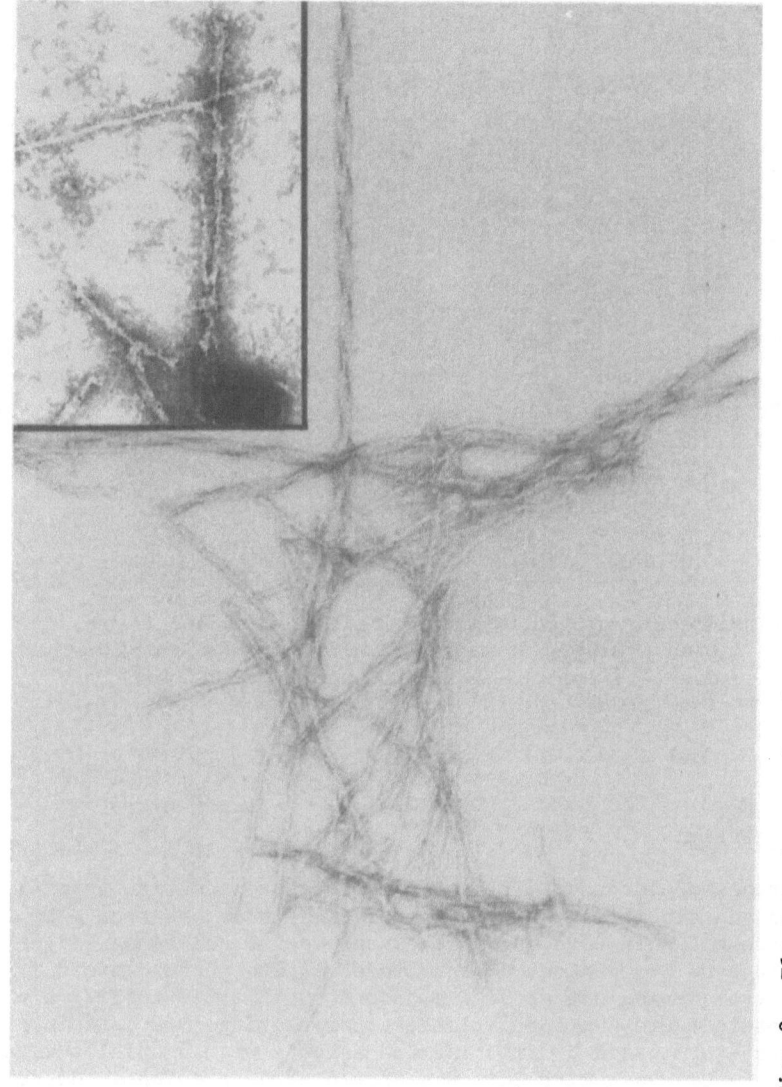

Fig. 2. Electronmicrography of a neurofibrillary tangle from the enriched fraction (×177,500). Inert - NFT-enriched fraction treated with the polyclonal anti-NFT, 1:50 dilution, and revealed by the immunogold technique. Gold particles are seen on the double filaments but not on the single filaments (×112,500).

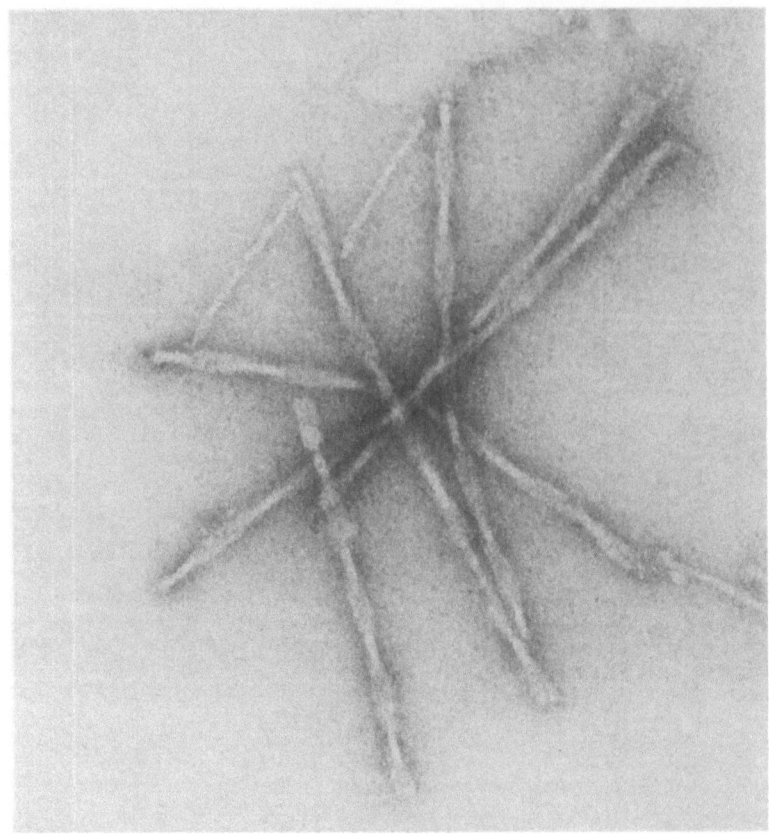

Fig. 3. Electronmicrography from the NFT-enriched frac-
         tion. Single straight filaments appear to make the
         double filaments when intertwined with themselves
         (×177,500).

Enzymatic Digestions

Suspensions of enriched NFT fractions were treated with trypsin,
chymotrypsin and subtilisin both separately and in combination. Experiments were run with elastase, pronase, urea-pepsin, collagenase type III,
hyaluronidase type IV, lipase, phospholipase A_2 and phospholipase C. All
digestions were carried out at 37°C and/or 60°C at 1:100 to 1:25 w/w
enzyme: protein ratio and for variable times ranging from 1 to 16 h. All
reactions were terminated by diluting the samples with distilled water and
freeze-drying. Cleavage with CNBr was attempted as previously described
[11]. Reduction with dithiothreitol (DTT) and alkylation with iodoacetic
acid (IAA) was performed in distilled water or denaturing solutions brought
to pH 11.5 with NH_4OH.

Amino Acid Analysis and Sequence Studies

Performic acid oxidized or unoxidized samples were hydrolyzed under
vacuum with 6N HCl, 0.1% phenol for 24 h at 110°C and analyzed on a Durrum
D-500 automated amino acid analyzer. Automated amino acid sequence analysis was carried out on a Beckman 890C sequencer with a 0.1 M Quadrol program as previously described [12].

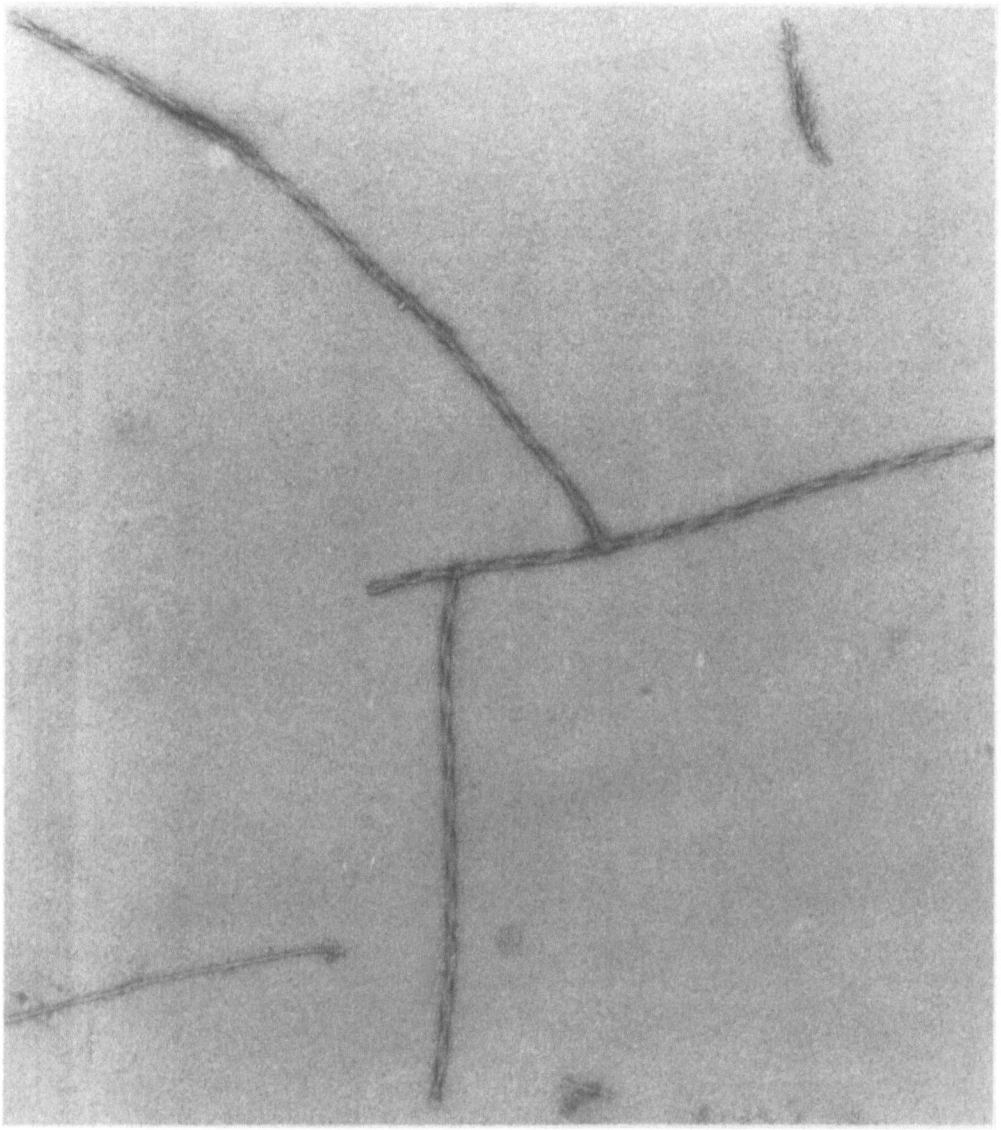

Fig. 4. Typical double filament made of a single filament intertwined with itself. Termination in tight hairpin loops are clearly seen (×112,500).

Antisera and Immunohistological Studies

NZW rabbits were injected weekly subcutaneously with NFT-enriched fractions in complete Freund's adjuvant. Antisera were checked by the immunoperoxidase method [13] on tissue sections of known cases of AD hippocampus. The immunogold technique [14] was used to visualize reaction with isolated NFT under EM.

RESULTS AND DISCUSSION

Following homogenization in 2% SDS [9], NFT could be isolated from an insoluble pellet on a discontinuous sucrose ultracentrifugation. The

1.4–2.0 M sucrose interface, considerably enriched in NFT, was subsequently recentrifuged after dilution and sonication in distilled water (Fig. 1). This procedure succeeded in removing significant contaminants, though with some small loss of tangles from the preparation.

This latter NFT fraction was assayed for DNA and RNA by both the ethidium bromide reaction under UV (shortwave) and the toluidine blue staining of NFT spotted onto cellulose acetate. By both methods negative results were obtained. No effect was produced by enzymatic digestion with hyaluronidase, lipases, phospholipase A_2 and phospholipase C. Nevertheless, the presence of small amounts of lipids or carbohydrates cannot be ruled out.

When run on various concentrations SDS–PAGE gels (7.5%, 10%, 12.5%, 15%, 15%–6 M urea gel; with 3% and 5% stacking gels) with and without reducing and denaturing conditions, most of the material remained on top of the gel and after fixation was revealed by both the Coomassie brilliant blue and the silver stain. Bands were not consistently seen in the medium to low MW range (Fig. 1). When removed from the top of the gel with a Pasteur pipette and centrifuged, the resuspended pellet was still found to contain unaltered NFT by electron microscopy (EM).

Purified NFT was hydrolyzed and an amino acid analysis was obtained that showed 12% Gly, 10% Glu, 9% Ala and 8% Asp as dominant amino acids. The presence of 1% cysteine, detected as half-Cys and after oxidation as cysteic acid, and 2% Met was observed; 12% of the material was accounted by basic residues and 23% by hydrophobic ones (9% Leu).

The original material was subjected to automated Edman degradation and consistently yielded a non-reactive amino terminus. Whether this was due to the presence of a blocked amino terminus or insolubility in the Quadrol buffer could not be determined.

Attempts were made to dissolve the NFT enriched fraction in 1% or 2% SDS, reducing agents (DTT; 2-mercaptoethanol), chaotropic agents (6 M urea, 5 M guanidine), acids (88% formic acid, 1N HAc, 1N HCl, 2% trifluoroacetic acid), bases (1N NaOH, 6% NH$_4$OH) and organic solvents (ethanol, methanol, chloroform, ether, propylene oxide). Only very dilute solutions could be obtained in distilled water.

Knowing the insoluble nature of the NFT several enzymatic protease digestions and chemical treatments were carried out on suspensions in the appropriate buffers under continuous agitation. Trypsin, chymotrypsin, subtilisin, both separately and in combination, urea-pepsin, pronase, elastase and collagenase treatments did not result in new bands entering gels when the digestions were analyzed by SDS–PAGE. Although no chemically detectable changes were observed, some of the digestons did yield macroscopically altered fibrillar material that ultrastructurally appeared as disaggregation of the characteristic tangles. Attempts to produce amino acid Edman degradation after enzymatic digestions also resulted in the presence of non-reactive amino terminus.

Based on the finding of methionine by amino acid analysis, NFT fractions were subjected to CNBr cleavage. This procedure resulted in the appearance of an ill-defined smear on a 15%–6 M urea polyacrylamide gel of MW range 3–12,000 daltons. Further characterization of this material is currently in progress.

Radiolabelling was only achieved after reduction and alkylation under strong denaturing conditions at pH 11.5; however, it is not certain wheter cysteine or methionine were labelled because of the high pH used.

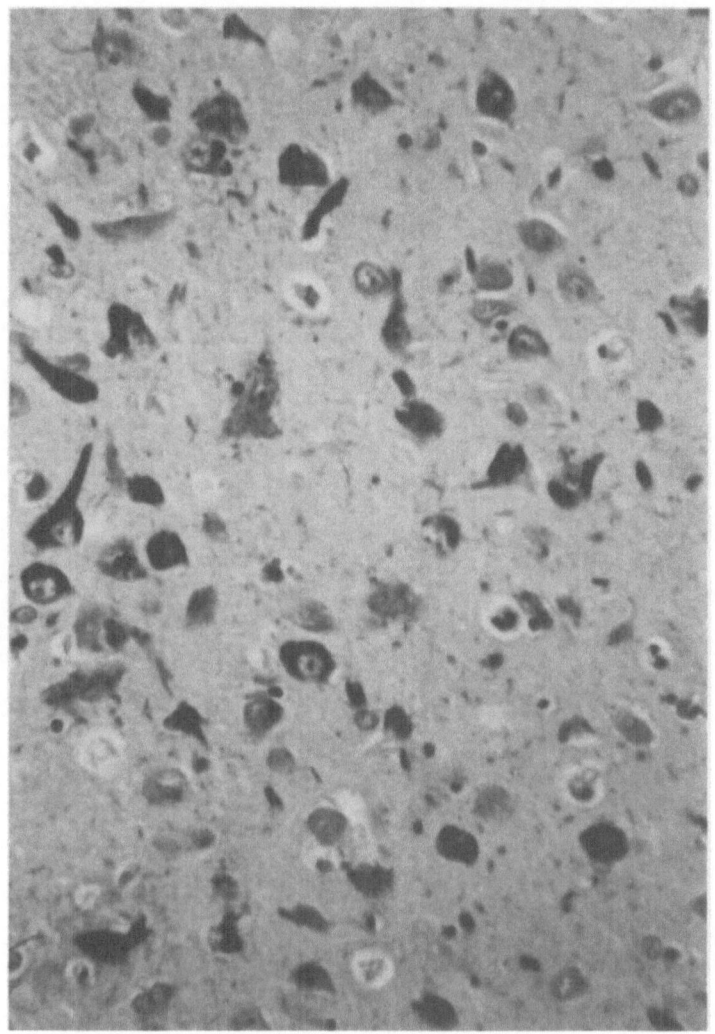

Fig. 5. Immunoperoxidase stain of hippocampal cortex,
developed with rabbit anti-NFT serum, 1:250 dilution, showing several neurons with intracellular neurofibrillary pathology (×200).
Specific staining was completely abolished NFT
(approximately 1 mg/ml) overnight at room temperature.

Electromicroscopically, the enriched fractions contained abundant
NFT as the major constituent, as well as some amorphous material. Ultrastructurally NFT appears to be composed of single and double filaments (Fig.
2a). A single filament can turn and intertwince with itself to form the
regular arrangement of the double filament (Fig. 3). This phenomenon can
apparently occur at any point along a single strand and in fact, one filament can be involved in several of these structures, each terminating in a
tight hairpin loop (Fig. 4). Double filaments have apparent periodic
crosses at an average 66.5 nm with a maximum width between 17 to 18 nm and
a minimum at the "crossing points" of 9 to 9.5 nm. When observed alone
single filaments are twisted over themselves with average diameters ranging

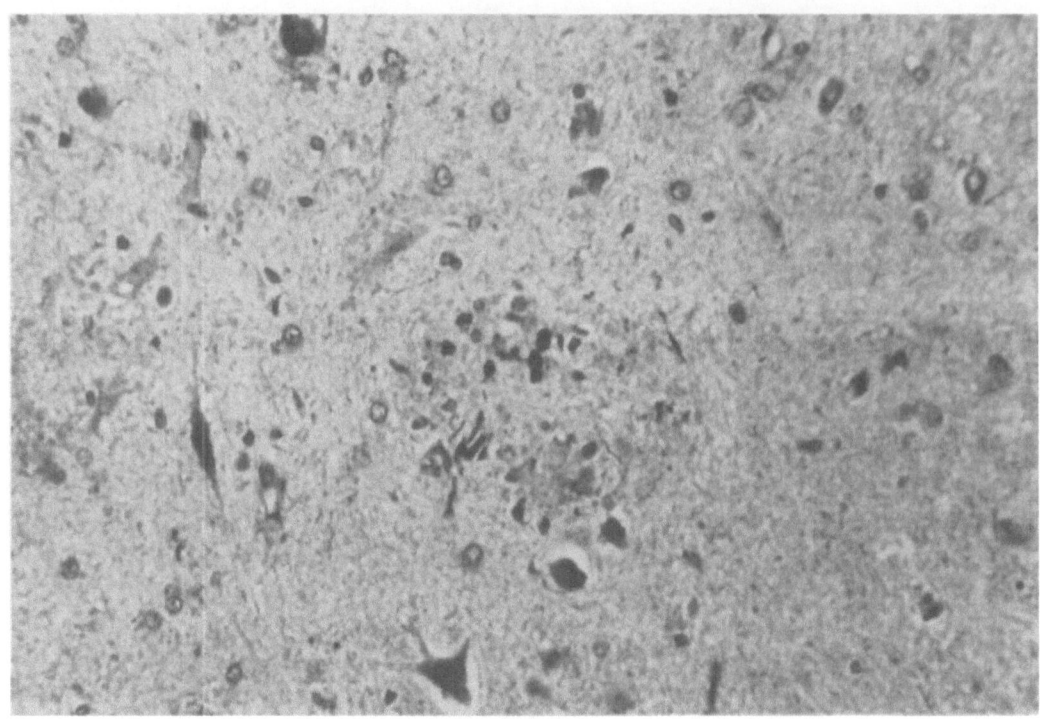

Fig. 6. Neurofibrillary degeneration of neuritic end processes in a mature senile plaque seen under high power (×500) stained with anti-PHF serum at 1:500 dilution. Anti-NFT did not react with the amyloid core.

from 6.5 nm at the narrowest part to 9.3 nm at the widest part. This particular arrangement seen in single and double filaments resembles the configuration of a "corkscrew" and is characteristic of NFT fibrils.

A comparable NFT-enriched fraction was used to raise a polyclonal antisera in rabbits. Preliminary Western blots were positive with the material excluded on top of the polyacrylamide gels, although results cannot be conclusive due to the insoluble nature of the NFT.

Reaction of this polyclonal antisera with isolated NFT was demonstrated by EM using the immunogold technique. Positive antibody binding was seen with double filaments while single filaments appeared to be negative (Fig. 2b). The specificity of the antisera was also determined by immunoperoxidase staining of sections of cerebral cortex from cases of SDAT showing specific reactivity with intraneuronal masses confirmed to be NFT by Bodian staining of parallel sections (Fig. 5), as well as with fibrillar material surrounding the amyloid core in neuritic plaques (Fig. 6). Positivity was consistently removed by preabsorption of the antiserum with the native NFT preparation. Similar reactivity was found on tissue sections from aging brains showing senile pathology, as well as known cases of postencephalitic Parkinson's disease, Down's syndrome and dementia pugilistica. No staining was seen of tissue sections of normal human brain, sporadic and hereditary cerebrovascular amyloid angiopathy, and the amyloid core from neuritic plaques.

These findings show a major specificity of the antisera for NFT as well as activity that appears to be directed towards some quaternary struc-

ture on double filaments. Although useful for the definition of isolated
NFT and as an immunohistological reagent, activity of our antisera with
dissociated subunits or NFT precursor proteins remains to be established.

ACKNOWLEDGEMENTS

    The authors would like to thank Dr. D. Sabatini for fruitful discussions and Dr. Nancy Peress for her assistance with the neuropathology.

    This work was supported by USPHS Grants #AM 01431 (BF) and FM 31866 and the HOR Foundation (PG).

REFERENCES

1. M. Kidd, Nature, 197:192 (1963).
2. K. Iqbal, H. M. Wisniewski, I. Grundke-Igbal, J. K. Korthals, and R. D. Terry, J. Histochem. Cytochem., 23:563 (1975).
3. H. K. Narang, J. Neuropathol. Exp. Neurology, 34:621 (1980).
4. A. Hirano, in: Alzheimer's Disease and Related Conditions, London, Churhill, 185 (1970).
5. K. Wisniewski, G. A. Jervis, R. C. Moretz, and H. M. Wisniewski, Ann. Neurol., 5:288 (1979).
6. H. Wisniewski, M. L. Shelanski, and R. D. Terry, J. Cell. Biol., 38: 224 (1968).
7. D. J. Selkoe, R. K. H. Liem, S. H. Yen, and M. L. Shelanski, Brain. Res., 163:235 (1979).
8. K. Iqbal, T. Zaidi, C. H. Thompson, P. A. Merz, and H. M. Wisniewski, Acta Neuropathol. (Berlin), 62:167 (1984).
9. P. Selkoe, Y. Ihara, and F. Salazar, Science, 215:1243 (1982).
10. S. H. Yen and Y. Kress, in: Biological Aspects of Alzheimer's Disease, Cold Spring Press, 155 (1983).
11. F. Goni and B. Frangione, Proc. Natl. Acad. Sci., 80:4837 (1983).
12. B. Frangione, E. Rosenwasser, H. Penefsky, and M. E. Pullman, Proc. Natl. Acad. Sci., 78:7403 (1981).
13. J-L. Guesdon, T. Ternynck, and F. Aurameas, J. Histochem. Cytochem., 27:1131 (1979).
14. J. W. Slot and H. J. Geuze, J. Cell Biol., 90:533 (1981).

AMYLOID FIBRILS IN HEREDITARY CEREBRAL HEMORRHAGE WITH AMYLOIDOSIS (HCHWAS) IS RELATED TO CYSTATIN (GAMMA TRACE)

Daniel H. Cohen, Helen Feiner,
Olafur Jensson*, and Blas Frangione

New York University Medical Center
Department of Pathology
550 First Avenue
New York, N. Y. 10016

*The Blood Bank
 Genetical Division
 University Hospital of Iceland
 Reykjavik, Iceland

ABSTRACT

Amyloid fibrils were isolated from the leptomeningeal blood vessels obtained at autopsy from three Icelandic patients dying of Hereditary Cerebral Hemorrhage with Amyloidosis (HCHWA) and verified by Congo red staining and electron microscopy. Gel filtration on Sephadex and Ultrogel columns yielded predominantly one component (molecular weight 11,500 daltons) and also another minor component (molecular weight 15,800 daltons). Automated amino terminal sequencing showed these proteins to be similar (36 residues) to a recently described human protein, gamma trace, beginning at its eleventh amino terminal residue. The amyloid deposits in all three patients stained with rabbit anti-gamma trace antiserum. Although the function of gamma trace is not known, it appears to have structural homology with, and in vitro activity similar to, several systeine proteinase in-hibitors and has been localized to the brain, pancreas and pituitary. Furthermore, gamma trace may; like endorphins, belong to a family of pro-teins derived from polycistronic RNA, which are cleaved at the site of ac-tion to peptides of different biological functions. The amyloid fibril subunits seem to have polymerized after cleavage of the amino terminal decapeptide from gamma trace-related proteins.

INTRODUCTION

Hereditary Cerebral Hemorrhage with Amyloidosis (HCHWA) is an auto-somal dominant form of amyloidosis isolated to the cerebral vasculature which leads to hemorrhagic and thrombotic strokes causing death before the age of 40 years. In eight families originating from one geographical area in Iceland 130 affected family members have been identified [1]. Since the description of these families a similar autosomal dominant cerebral amyloid angiopathy has been described in The Netherlands [2]. The genetic and clinical aspects of the Icelandic form were presented in detail by Dr. Jensson at this meeting.

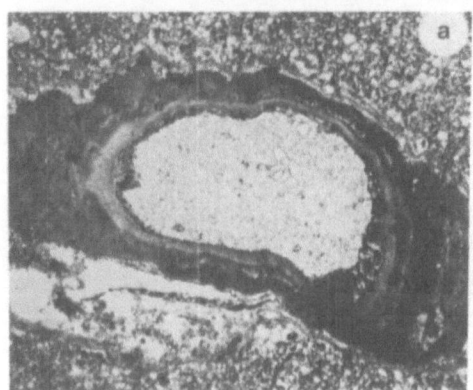 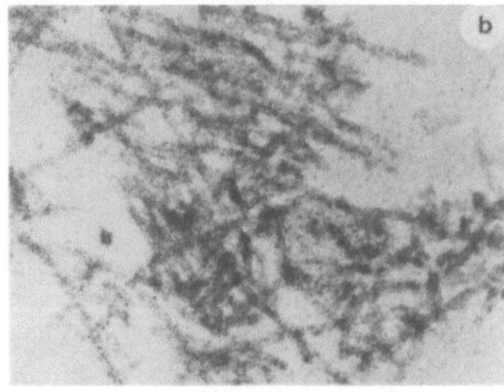

Fig. 1.   a) Electron photomicrograph of a small intracerebral artery show-
          ing thickening of the vessel wall and obliteration of normal land-
          marks by fibrillar material characteristic of amyloid (×1,400).
          b) Electron photomicrograph of extract from pooled meninges showing
          fibrils characteristic of amyloid (×187,500).

The histopathology of HCHWA brains is similar to that of the congophilic angiopathy associated with some cases of Alzheimer's disease and to
that of cases of cerebral hemorrhage caused by sporadic Congophilic angiopathy. In HCHWA there are no plaques or neurofibrillary tangles and the
amount of vascular amyloid is quantitatively much greater than in the two
other forms of cerebral amyloid angiopathy mentioned above [3, 4] making
chemical extraction of the amyloid fibrils feasible.

Because of extensive unsuccessful experience with attempts at extraction of pure amyloid fibrils from the parenchyma of HCHWA brains (which
could be attributed to the quantitatively huge ratio of brain lipids to
amyloid proteins), it was decided to first isolate the leptomeninges with
their blood vessels and discard the brain parenchyma prior to beginning the
classical fibril extraction procedure. There was also a greater likelihood
of success with HCHWA brains because of the extremely large quantity of
vascular amyloid (Fig. 1a). The leptomeninges from three brains were
pooled and distilled water extraction carried out according to the method
of Pras et al. [5]. After several differential centrifugations in saline
and distilled water, a relatively pure fibril preparation was harvested
from the supernatant (Fig. 1b). The fibrils were dissolved in guanidine
HCl and reduced to break cross links and thereafter gel filtered on Sephadex
and Ultrogel columns. After gel filtration in Sephadex a single retarded
peak contained the two amyloid protein fragments (Fig. 2a). The subsequent
filtration of this peak on Ultrogel yielded a major amount of one species of
MW 11,500 daltons and a minor amount of another of 15,800 daltons (as shown
in Figs. 2b and c). These proteins were subjected to automated amino
terminal sequencing revealing that they were identical amongst themselves
[5]. A computerized search for homologies to known proteins revealed that
the HCHWA amyloid proteins were homologous to a recently described protein,
gamma trace starting at position 11 [6] (Fig. 3).

To confirm these findings immunofluorescence on brain sections using
antigamma trace provided by Dr. Anders Grubb and standardized anti-AA, anti-
IgG, A, M anti-κ, anti-λ, anti-prealbumin and anti-P component, was performed [5, 7]. There was bright localization of gamma trace in the walls
of leptomeningeal and intracerebral arteries of all three patients with
HCHWA as well as vascular localization of amyloid P component in two cases

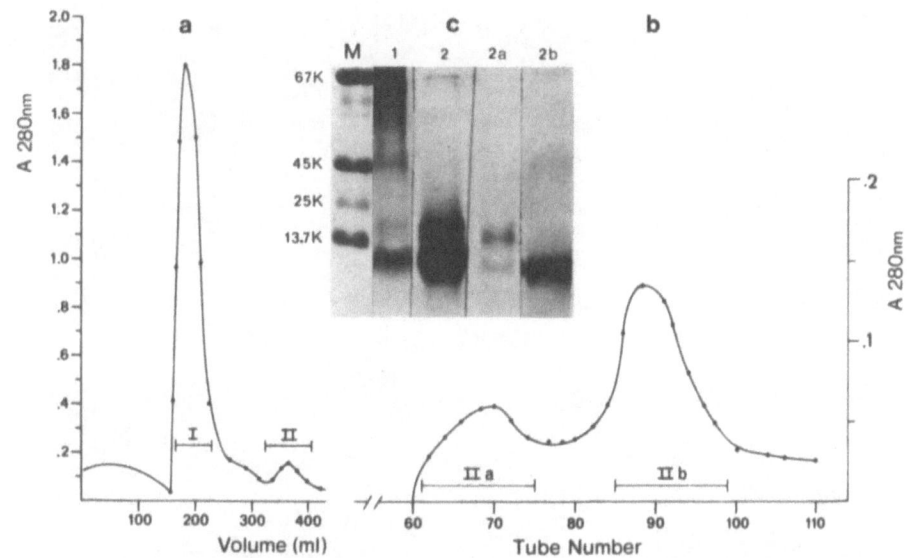

Fig. 2.   a) Fractionation of HCHWA amyloid fibrils on 2.5 × 180 cm
          Sephadex G-100 column equilibrated in 5 M guanidine 1 M acetic
          acid. b) Rechromatography of peak II on 2.5 × 180 cm Ultrogel
          AcA 54 column equilibrated in 3 M guanidine 2 M NH₄HCO₃. c)
          SDS-Page 17% slab gel of unfractionated amyloid fibrils ex-
          tracted from leptomeninges (lane 1). Lanes 2, 2a, and 2b
          are purified components from Fig. 2a and b. M, markers; 67K,
          bovine serum albumin 67,000 mol. wt.; 45K, ovalbumin 45,000
          mol. wt.; 25K, chymotrypsinogen A 25,000 mol. wt.; 13.7K ribo-
          nuclease A 13,700 mol. wt. All samples were reduced in 0.1M
          dithiothreitol before application.

                                           10   20
Human γ trace   Ser-Ser-Pro-Gly-Lys-Pro-Pro-Arg-Leu-Val-Gly-Gly-Pro-Met-Asp-Ala-Ser-Val-Glu-Glu-Glu-Gly-Val-Arg-Arg

HCHWA amyloid peak II   _____

HCHWA amyloid peak IIa   _____

HCHWA amyloid peak IIb   _____

                                           30   40
Human γ trace   Ala-Leu-Asp-Phe-Ala-Val-Gly-Glu-Tyr-Asn-Lys-Ala-Ser-Asn-Asp-Met-Tyr-His-Ser-Arg-Ala

HCHWA amyloid peak II _____

HCHWA amyloid peak IIa _____

HCHWA amyloid peak IIb _____

Fig. 3.   The amino terminal sequence of peaks II, IIa, and IIb from Fig. 2
          compared with that of gamma trace. The solid lines indicate iden-
          tical residues.

(Fig. 4). A negative result was obtained with antisera to prealbumin, AA
protein κ or λ light chain IgG, IgA and IgM. Control brains from patients
without neurologic disease and from five patients with Alzheimer's disease
were also negative for gamma trace.

     Human gamma trace is a basic serum and cerebrospinal fluid protein of
MW 13,260 daltons with gamma electrophoretic mobilicy that has been local-

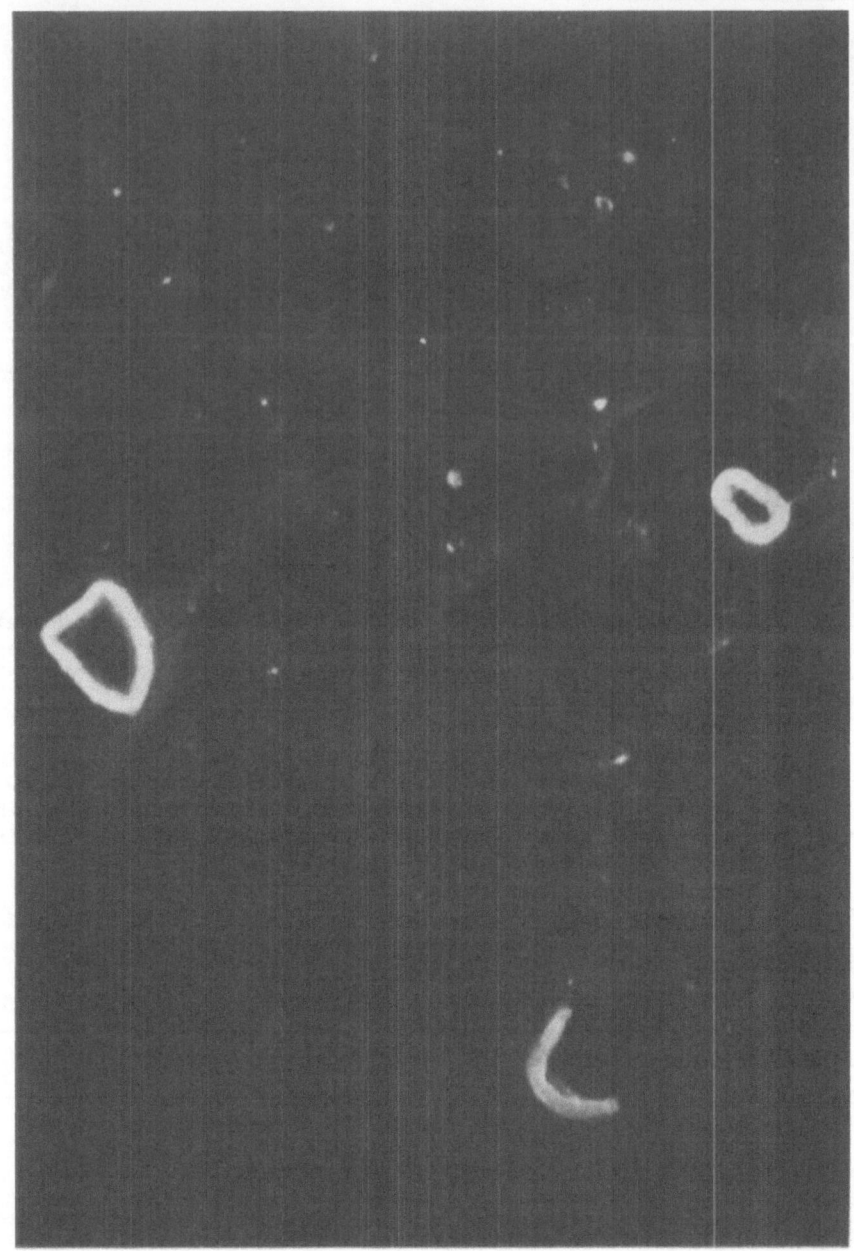

Fig. 4. Immunofluorescence photomicrograph showing bright locali-
         zation of gamma trace in three intracerebral arteries.
         Similar localization was present in meningeal vessels.
         Rabbit anti-human gamma trace and fluorescein-labeled goat.
         anti-rabbit IgG were used (×225).

ized immunocytochemically to the anterior pituitary, pancreatic A cells and
certain cortical neurons. Its concentration in cerebrospinal fluid is five-
fold that in serum and CSF concentrations are extremely low in patients dying from HCHWA [8]. As evident in Fig. 3, the HCHWA amyloid proteins seem
to represent cleavage products of the gamma trace sequence as they begin
at its position 11. This fact fits with the general tendency of amyloid
fibril subunit proteins to appear to be degradation products of soluble

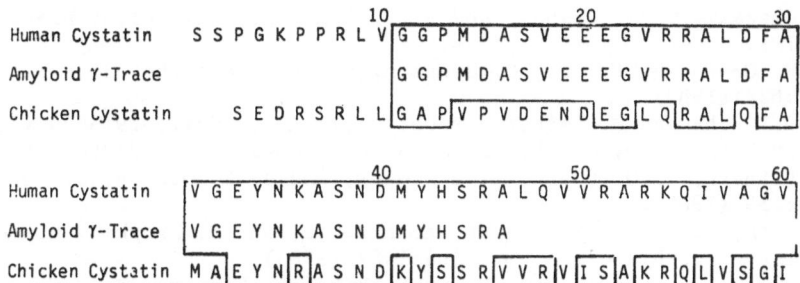

Fig. 5. Amino terminal sequences of human cystatin C, chicken
cystatin and HCHWA amyloid fibril protein, gamma trace
(cystatin).

precursor proteins. It remains to be determined whether these cleavages
merely reflect the chance action of tissue proteases after deposition or
whether they are necessary for precipitation or polymerization of amyloid
from the extracellular fluid.

In 1982 Grubb indicated the homology of gamma trace with glucagon and
corticotropin [6]. Because of this and localization of the protein by
immune techniques in hypophysis, adrenal cortex, thyroid brain and GI
tract, its function was believed to be related to a diffuse peptidergic
neuroendocrine system. However, since very recently two groups [9-11] have
indicated that gamma trace may function as an inhibitor of cysteine proteinases and have suggested it be called cystatin C by relation to the
other chicken and human cysteine proteinase inhibitors (cystatins A and
B). This assertion is based on sequence homology between gamma trace and
the cysteine proteinase inhibitors (Fig. 5) from granulocytes (stefin) and
egg white, as well as the *in vitro* demonstration that gamma trace is a
potent inhibitor of papain, ficin and human cathepsins B, H and L [10, 11].
The structure of gamma trace shows aspects which are reminiscent of neuroendocrine peptides such as the endorphins. The gamma trace like endorphine
precursors has a cluster of basic residues every 25 residues from both ends.
This suggests that gamma trace could belong to a family of proteins initially translated from polycistronic RNA and subsequently cleaved at the
tissue site of action to peptides with different biological functions.
This line of reasoning is supported by the recent finding that a salivary
form of gamma trace is not identical to the serum or urine forms but shares
at least 50% sequence homology with them [12]. The function of all cystatin or gamma trace-related proteins as well as the specific deposition of
gamma trace in the cerebral vasculature of patients with HCHWA remains to
be elucidated.

ACKNOWLEDGEMENTS

This work was supported by USPHS Grants #AM 01431 and 02594.

REFERENCES

1. G. Gudmundsson, J. Hallgrimsson, T. A. Jonasson, and O. Bjornason,
    Brain, 95:387 (1972).
2. A. F. Wattendord, G. Th. A. M. Bots, L. N. Wents, and L. J. Edntz, J.
    Neurol. Sci., 55:121 (1982).
3. T. I. Mandybur, Neurology, 25:120 (1975).

4. H. Okazaki, T. J. Reasan, and R. J. Campbell, Mayo Clin. Proc., 54:22 (1979).
5. D. H. Cohen, H. Feiner, O. Jensson, and B. Frangione, J. Exp. Med., 158:623 (1983).
6. A. O. Grubb and H. Lofberg, Proc. Natl. Acad. Sci., 79:3024 (1982).
7. H. Lofberg, A. O. Grubb, and A. Brun, Biomed. Res., 2:298 (1981).
8. H. Lofberg, A. O. Grubb, T. S. Veger, and J. E. Olsson, J. Neurol., 223:159 (1980).
9. V. Turk, J. Brzin, M. Louger, A. Ritonja, and M. Eropkin, Hoppe-Seyler's Z. Physiol. Chem., 364:1487 (1983).
10. J. Brzin, T. Popovic, and V. Turk, Biochem. Biophys. Res. Comm., 118:103 (1984).
11. A. J. Barrett, M. E. Davies, and A. O. Grubb, Biochem. Biophys. Res. Comm., 120:631 (1984).
12. S. Isemira, E. Saitoh, and K. Sanada, J. Biochem., 96:489 (1984).

CEREBRAL AMYLOID ANGIOPATHY CAUSING INTRACRANIAL HEMORRHAGE

A CLINICOPATHOLOGICAL STUDY OF 12 CASES

Uma P. Kalyan-Raman* and
Krishna Kalyan-Raman†

*Associate Professor of Clinical Pathology
 University of Illinois
 College of Medicine at Peoria, and
 Neuropathologist,
 Saint Francis Hospital-Medical Center,
 Peoria, Illinois

†Professor of Clinical Neurology
 University of Illinois College of Medicine at Peoria
 Peoria, Illinois

ABSTRACT

A clinicopathologic study of 12 cases of sporadic cerebral amyloid angiopathy (CAA) presenting as intracranial hemorrhage (ICH) was presented. CAA was seen as a stroke or catastrophic ICH in all cases. Eleven of 12 patients died in spite of aggressive medical or surgical treatment. CAA was diagnosed in 4 of 12 cases from surgical material and from autopsy in 8 cases. Senile dementia of Alzheimer's type was present in only 1 patient. Computerized tomographic scanning in 4 patients initially was not diagnostic for hemorrhage. Lambda chains and amyloid P protein were demonstrated in the areas of amyloid angiopathy immunocytochemically. The pathogenesis of hemorrhage in CAA could be either increased fragility of amyloid-laden blood vessels or rupture of microaneurysms due to CAA. We feel surgical treatment of ICH in CAA should be undertaken with caution.

INTRODUCTION

Cerebral amyloid angiopathy (CAA) is a disorder characterized by deposits of amyloid in the media and intima of the arteries and arterioles of the brain and meninges. Recent reviews that discuss the classification, pathogenesis, and composition of amyloidosis including CAA [1, 2, 3, 4] emphasize that CAA seldom accompanies systemic amyloidosis [5]. Nonhereditary sporadic forms of CAA, however, do appear to cause intracranial hemorrhage [6, 7, 8, 9, 10]. Some authorities have concluded dementia is considered to be common in CAA [7, 10, 11]. This is debatable. As association of CAA with senile (neuritic) plaques is well established [12]. It is unclear, however, whether there is an association of clinically apparent senile dementia of Alzheimer's type (SDAT) and CAA [11].

This study presents the clinical features and neuropathology of 12 cases of sporadic nonhereditary CAA first seen with intracranial hemorrhage; 8 patients were diagnosed at postmortem examination and 4 by surgical biopsy. Immunocytochemical studies for presence of immunoglobulins and amyloid P

TABLE 1. Summary of Clinical Features of Cerebral Amyloid Angiopathy

Patient No.	Age, sex	Presenting symptoms	Associated illness	Precipitating factors	Findings on admission and course of illness	CT Scan findings on admission
1	67, M	Sudden severe headache and vomiting, followed by coma	Diabetes, mellitus, on tolbutamide therapy, and ? hypertension	None	Comatose with decerebrate posturing; pupils midsize and fixed; left leg weakness; BP 220/60 mm Hg; EKG: left ventricular hypertrophy; died 24 h after admission	Right ganglionic hemorrhage with rupture into ventricules
2	68, M	Sudden onset of left hemiplegia and dysphasia, preceded by head trauma 10 days before admission	2 year history of dementia	Head trauma	Conscious, globally dysphasic with left hemiplegia and spasticity; lapsed into coma and died 4 weeks after admission	Low density lesion in right parietal lobe area with ring enhancement; improved after 2 weeks
3	64, M	Found unresponsive in his living room, duration ? 24–36 h	Chronic alcoholism	None	Comatose with hyperventilation and left upper extremity weakness; died 2 weeks after admission without regaining consciousness	Symmetrical dilation of 3rd and lateral ventricles; one week later an area of increased absorption in the right putamen, suggesting a resolving hematoma
4	61, M	Confusion and disorientation of one week's duration before admission	? Diabetes mellitus	None	Conscious, with fluent paraphasic speech and neologism; hematoma evacuated surgically, with recovery; readmitted 14 months later with sudden onset of coma and left hemiplegia; died 12 days after reganining consciousness after surgical evacuation of clot	Right temporal mass with slight enhancement; right frontoparietal lobar hematoma on second admission

5	79, F	Sudden onset of headache, nausea, vomiting and dizziness followed by coma	Deep venous thrombosis; ? occlusion, right posterior inferior cerebellar artery 2 years earlier	Sodium warfarin therapy	Comatose on ventilator, with small pupils; died 48 h after admission	Large left cerebrellar hemorrhage with extension into 4th and 3rd ventricles and obstructive hydrocephalus
6	83, M	Sudden onset of coma	Akinetic spells for 5-6 years	Head trauma	Comatose, with contusion of left occipital area and and ecchymoses of orbits; left pupil larger than right; leftsided decerebration; died 1 month later in spite of prompt surgical treatment	Large left subdural and temporal lobe hematoma
7	54, F	Sudden onset of dysphasia and headache	2-month history of dull bifrontal headaches relieved by aspirin	None	Lethargic, nonfluent dysphasia and mild weakness of right grip; BP: 200/120 mm Hg; died 3 days later in spite of surgical treatment	Large left temporal hematoma with mass effect
8	88, F	Weakness of legs in the evening; next morning became confused and disoriented and bumped into the furniture; onset suggesting stroke in evolution	Breast carcinoma, Stage I, 4 years before present illness	? Head trauma	Right orbital ecchymoses; confused, disorineted, and agitated with no focal signs; became comatose 2 days later and died 17 days after admission	Large right frontal lobe hematoma; small left frontal lobe hematoma

(continued)

TABLE 1 (continued)

Patient No.	Age, sex	Presenting symptoms	Associated illness	Precipitating factors	Findings on admission and course of illness	CT Scan findings on admission
9	62, F	Sudden onset of severe headache and vomiting, progressing to coma	Hypertension	None	Comatose on ventilator, with dilated fixed pupils; died with 24 h	Severe diffuse subarachnoid hemorrhage; left frontal and temporal subdural hematoma with mass effect
10	66, F	First admission, sudden onset of right temporal headache and personality change	Mild hypertension	None	No focal signs	Right posterior frontal lobe low-density lesion with ring enhancement
		Second admission, 6 weeks later, no new complaints				On operation an organized intracerebral clot was found
		Third admission, 3 months later, severe occipital headache			Lethargic and ataxic	No change
		Fourth admission, 6.5 years later, sudden onset of inability to read and frontal headache with nausea	BP: 200/100 mm Hg in emergency room, falling spontaneously to normal		Conscious, oriented; mild neck stiffness; left hemianopsia	Recent right occipital lobe hematoma; old infarct, right frontal area

| 11 | 81, M | Found unconscious at home | Old MI, aortic aneurysm | None | Unconscious, but stable. Operated 2 days later for left subdural; 2 days later developed seizure, another bleed on left occipital area and expired 8 days later | Right intracerebral and left subdural hematoma on admission; later – left occipital lobe hemorrhage |
| 12 | 77, M | Difficulty seeing in right eye and speech difficulty | Remote MI | None | Lethargic with right hemiparesis and right homonymous hemianopsia; hematoma surgically evacuated; expired 4 days later without regaining consciousness | Left parietooccipital hematoma |

component (AP protein) in the area of amyloid deposition in the vessels were done in 4 and 7 cases, respectively.

MATERIALS AND METHODS

These 12 cases of CAA were collected over a period of 7 years. CAA was diagnosed in 4 cases by surgical biopsy and in 8 cases on autopsy. In the 8 autopsied patients, sections were taken from frontal, parietal, temporal, and occipital areas, hippocampus, basal ganglia, midbrain, pons, medulla, cerebellum at the level of the dentate nucleus, and several regions around the areas of hemorrhage. Sections were stained with hematoxylin and eosin (H&E), Gomori's trichrome, Verhoeff-Van Gieson's elastic, and Bielschowsky stains. Ultrastructural study was done in all cases by standard procedure using a JEM 100C transmission electron microscope. The diagnosis of CAA was suspected by the presence of hyaline thickening of smaller arteries and arterioles of cerebral parenchyma and/or meninges in H&E sections and confirmed by positive staining on Congo red with birefringence, fluorescence with thioflavin T staining, and ultrastructural demonstration of amyloid fibrils.

The modified indirect immunoperoxidase technique of Sternberger [13] was used on paraffin sections to demonstrate the presence of AP protein as well as immunoglobulins IgG, IgA, IgM, Kappa and Lambda in the amyloid-laden blood vessels. The reagents were mostly obtained from Dako Corp, Santa Barbara, California, and Sigma, St. Louis, Missouri. Gils Hematoxylin Formula 2 was used for counterstaining.

A grading system of 0, +, ++, +++, and ++++ was used to denote the intensity of the brown reaction on the immunoperoxidase staining. Fifty leptomeningeal and cortical blood vessels were studied in each case, and if more than 60% of the vessels showed positive reaction, it was taken to indicate positivity for the substance studied. Neuritic plaques were judged based on the intensity of staining as either strongly positive or faintly positive.

The following modification of the cirteria of McCormick and Rosenfield [14] was used in defining "hypertensive brain hemorrhage": 1) clinical documentation of blood pressure recordings of usually at least 140 to 150/90 to 100 mm Hg before the onset of hemorrhage; 2) electrocardiographic (EKG) changes consistent with hypertension in the absence of cardiac disease; 3) increased left ventricular thickness (more than 1.5 cm) and increased heart weight (over 375 gm) at postmortem examination in the absence of any nonhypertensive cardiovascular cause; 4) evidence of hypertensive vascular disease in the retina or other organs such as kidneys. At least two of these four criteria were required for the diagnosis.

RESULTS

Table 1 summarizes the clinical findings. The ages ranged from 54 to 88 years (mean, 70.6 years). Seven patients were men and 5 were women. Five patients were seen with sudden onset of headache and vomiting followed by coma; a stroke-like onset with motor weakness and/or dysphasia occurred in 5 patients. Two patients were comatose at the time of admission, and events preceding the onset were unclear.

At the time of admission to the hospital, 5 patients were comatose with focal signs and/or brainstem dysfunction and 5 were conscious with focal signs, motor weakness, disorientation and/or dysphasia. One was confused and disoriented, and another was neurologically normal.

TABLE 2. Gross Postmortem Neuropathological Findings in 8 Patients with
Cerebral Amyloid Angiopathy

Location of hemorrhage	No. of patients
Right basal ganglia with ventricular rupture	1
Right frontoparietal and basal ganglia with ventricular rupture	1
Left putamen, vermis, and left cerebellum	1
Left temporal lobe	1
Left cerebrellum and vermis	1
Left subdural hematoma with subarachnoid hemorrhage	1
Right frontal lobe	1
Bilateral occipital with left subdural hematoma	1

Hypertension was present in 3 patients. Only 1 of the 3 had evidence
of left ventricular hypertrophy on EKG to suggest that the hypertension was
long standing. Diabetes with mild hypertension was present in 1 patient,
and another was a chronic alcoholic. Two patients gave a history of recurrent headaches before admission, and another had a history of deep vein
thrmobosis and possible stroke and was receiving sodium warfarin. Two patients had a history of head trauma, one of whom had akinetic falling
spells. Only 1 patient had a history of dementia suspected to be SDAT.

Computed tomographic (CT) scan of head was done in all patients on or
immediately after admission. The location and type of lesions were varied
and were as given in Table 1. One patient had symmtrical dilatation of the
third and fourth ventricules on admission; on a repeat scan a week later,
he had evidence of a resolving hematoma in the right basal ganglia area.
Three of the 12 patients had recurrent hemorrhages by CT scan, one 2 days
after admission, one after a year, and the other after 6.5 years.

Table 2 summarizes the gross postmortem findings. Eight patients had
a complete postmortem examination at which no systemic evidence of amyloidosis or hypertension was found. Hemorrhages were present in the right
putamen; right frontoparietal and basal ganglia areas with ventricular
rupture (Fig. 1), left putamen, vermis, and left cerebellum; left temporal
lobe; left cerebellum and vermis; left subdural hematoma with subarachnoid
hemorrhage; right frontal lobe, and occipital lobes bilaterally and left
subdural hemorrhage.

Microscopic Findings

Amyloid angiopathy was diagnosed by the following criteria in all 12
patients: hyaline thickening of the wall of the arteries and arterioles on
H&E, positive Congo red staining with birefringence (Fig. 2A and B), birefringence with thioflavin T, and amyloid fibrins observed on electron microscopy (Fig. 3). In the 8 patients examined postmortem, amyloid angiopathy
was found mostly in the cortex and overlying meninges of the frontal parietal, and temporal areas. A moderate amount of amyloid angiopathy was noted
in the hippocampus in 4; in the cerebellum in 5; in the basal ganglia in
7; and in the brainstem in 3 of the 8 patients. Scattered neuritic plaques
were present in the frontal, parietal, temporal and hippocampal areas in 6
of 8 patients. In the 1 patient clinically suspected of having SDAT, neuritic plaques were abundant in the frontal and hippocampal areas. This
patient also had a moderate number of neurofibrillary tangles in the hippo-

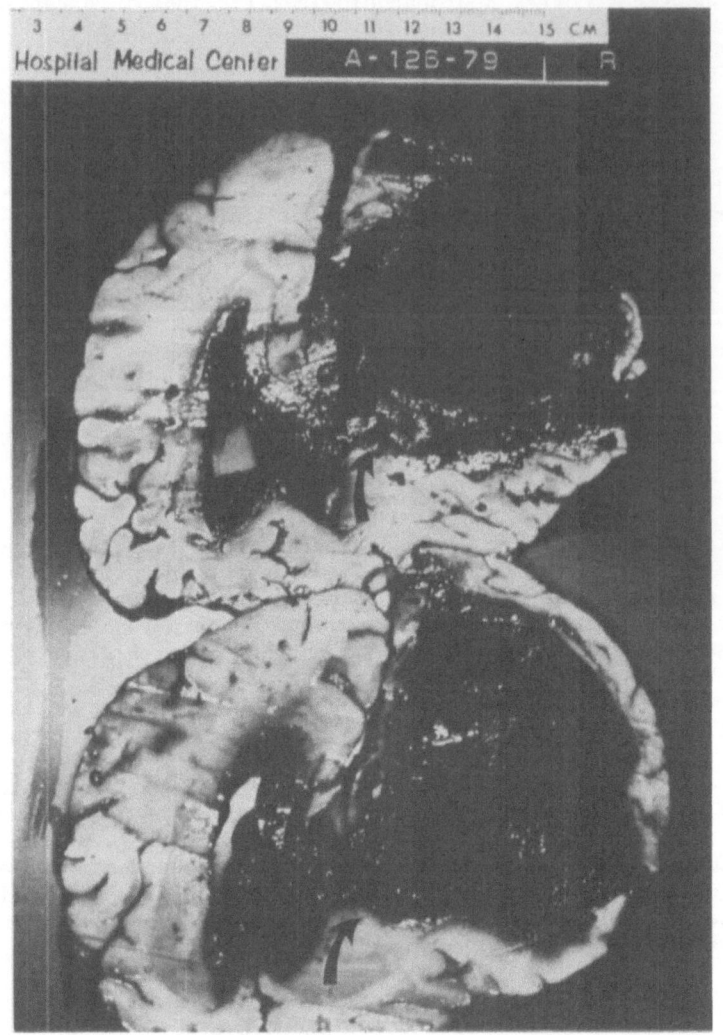

Fig. 1. Gross photograph of coronal sections of brain
from patient 2, showing massive intracerebral
hemorrhage in the frontal white matter and
basal ganglia with rupture into the right
lateral ventricle (arrow).

campal area. Microaneurysm formation of blood vessels with amyloid deposition was observed in 2 patients, in the basal ganglia in 1 (Fig. 4) and
in the cerebral cortex and overlying meninges in the other.

Results of Immunocytochemistry

AP protein was strongly positive in the area of CAA in all 7 patients
studied (Fig. 5A). Four of these 7 were studied for the presence of IgG,
IgA, IgM, and kappa and lambda chains. All 4 were positive for lambda
(Fig. 5B) and one was positive for IgM. The central core of the senile
plaque and neurofibrillary tangles (see only in the patient with dementia)
showed mild positivity with the AP protein.

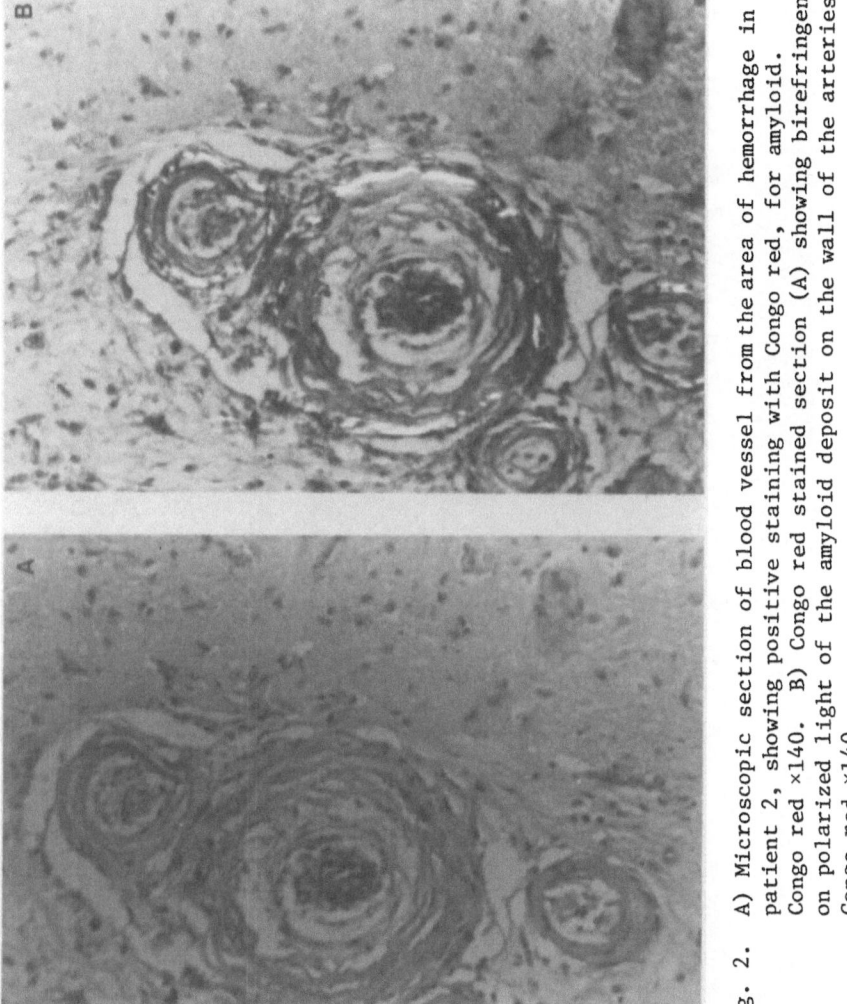

Fig. 2.   A) Microscopic section of blood vessel from the area of hemorrhage in
patient 2, showing positive staining with Congo red, for amyloid.
Congo red ×140. B) Congo red stained section (A) showing birefringence
on polarized light of the amyloid deposit on the wall of the arteries.
Congo red ×140.

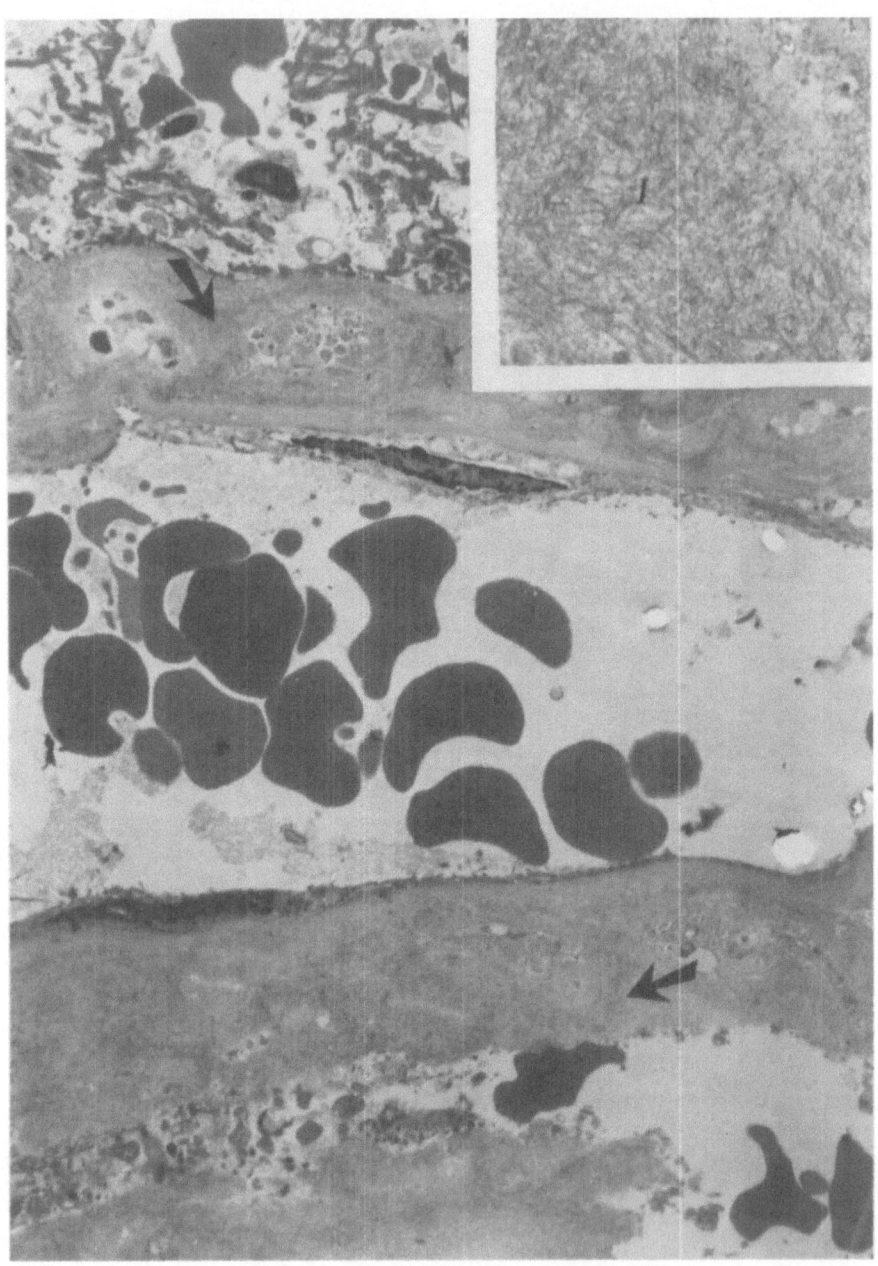

Fig. 3.   Blood vessel with amyloid showing the presence of characteristic amyloid fibrils (arrows) ultrastructurally: inset (I) showing higher magnification of the fibrils.
(Uranyl acetate–lead citrate ×4000: inset ×26,000.)

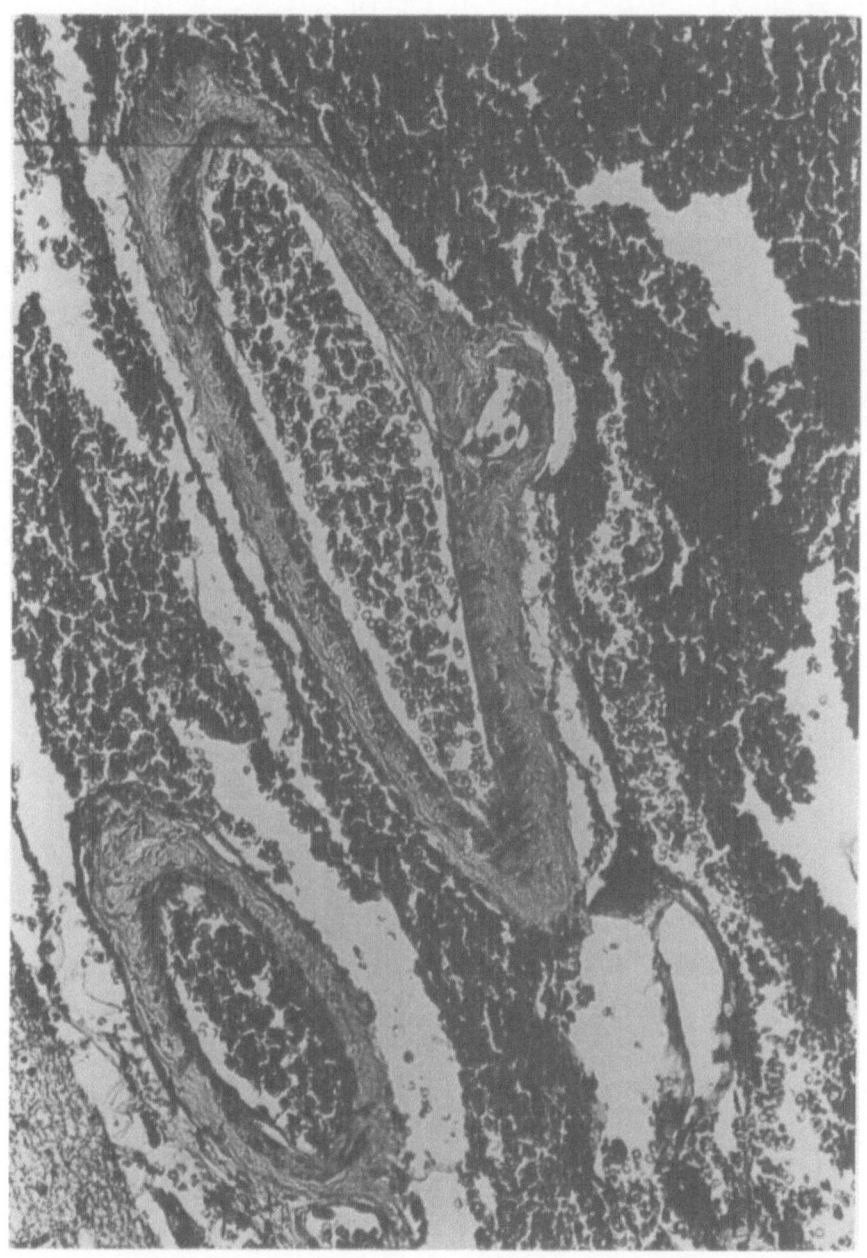

Fig. 4. Section from basal ganglia area from patient 1 showing an amyloid-deposited vessel with microaneurysm formation. Arrow points to the neck. Note the thin wall of aneurysm made of connective tissue. Trichrome ×200.

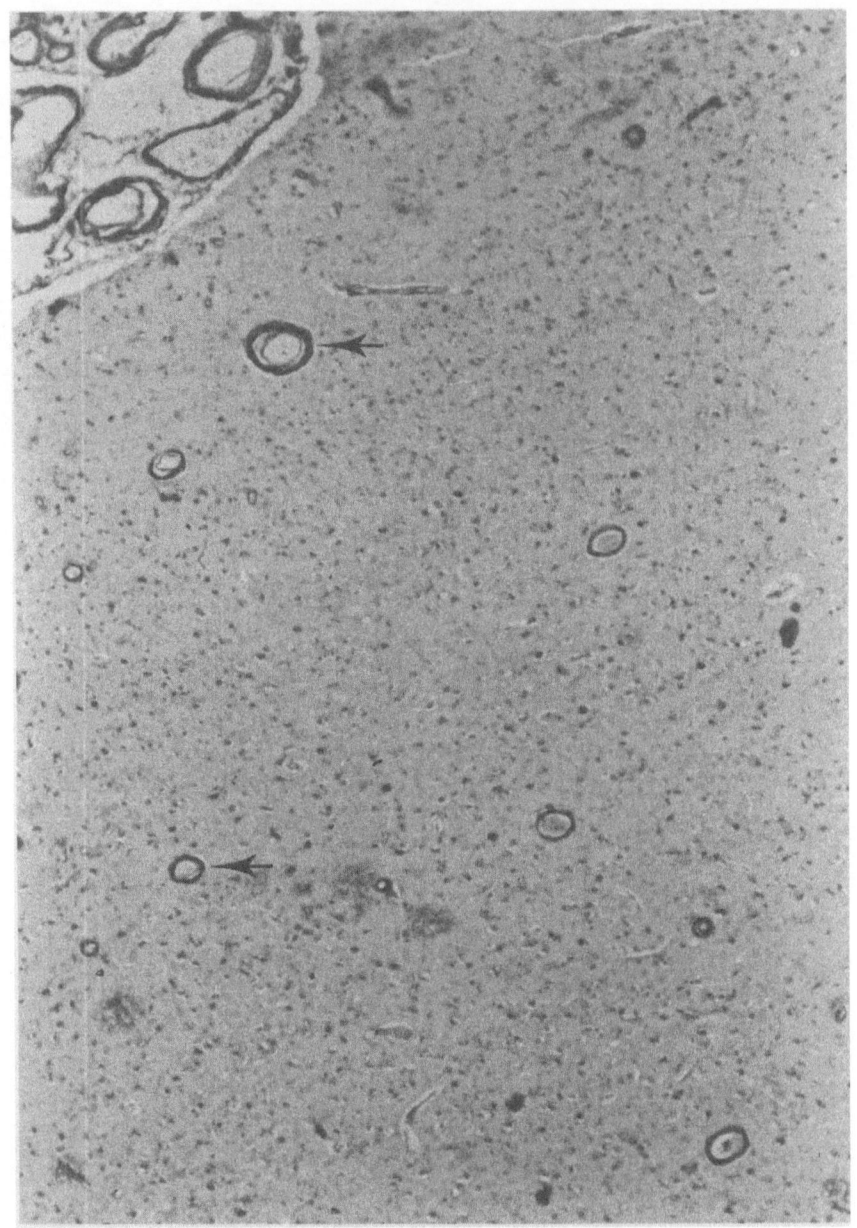

Fig. 5A

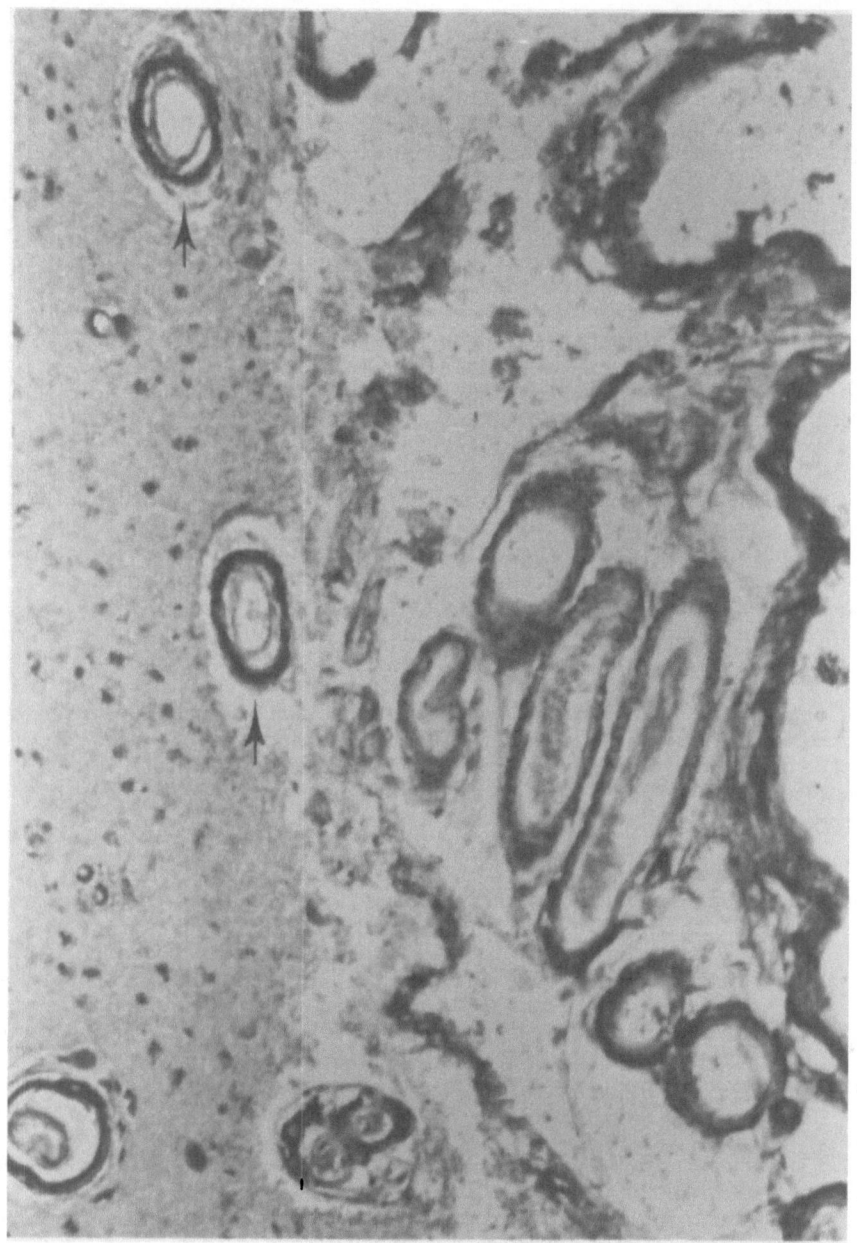

Fig. 5B

Fig. 5. A) Section of cerebral cortex from patient 1 showing blood
        vessels with amyloid, staining positive for amyloid P com-
        ponent (arrows). Peroxidase-antiperoxidase method for
        amyloid P component – ×140. B) Section from patient 1
        showing cortical blood vessels with amyloid deposits
        staining positive for lambda chains. Peroxidase-anti-
        peroxidase staining for immunoglobulin (lambda) ×50.

DISCUSSION

CAA causing intracranial hemorrhage is not rare. Our study indicates
that with a high index of suspicion it was demonstrated by appropriate
staining methods to be the cause of nontraumatic intracranial hemorrhage,
in 4 surgically treated patients and in 8 patients at the time of autopsy.

CAA with intracranial hemorrhage occurred in persons over the age of
50 years, especially in the sixth decade of life. Our findings differ from
Okazaki and co-workers [10] in the following ways: 11 of 12 patients in
our series suffered from massive intracerebral hemorrhage. In Okazaki's
series only 9 of 23 had large hemorrhages, and they encountered regularly
multiple, small, cortical infarcts which were conspicuously absent in our
series. Incidence of dementia was again less in our series. Lee and Stem-
mermann [8] also found a lower incidence of large intracerebral hemorrhages
and a strong correlation between CAA and compact plaques.

CAA and neuritic plaques in the brain are considered to be a phenomenon of aging [15, 16, 17, 18]. In our series the maximum incidence of
CAA was in the sixth decade and not in the eighth. We, therefore, believe
that CAA producing intracranial hemorrhage is probably no solely a phenomenon of aging. Neuritic plaques were present in all 8 patients in our
series who were examined postmortem; however, clinical dementia was present
in only 1. Moderate amounts of neurofibrillary tangles and granulovacuolar
degeneration were present in the hippocampal area in the 1 patient with
dementia, whereas they were absent in all other patients. Also, neuritic
plaques in the cortex were profuse in the patient with dementia, whereas in
all other patients they were minimal. In our series, therefore, only 1 patient had the clinical and neuropathological criteria for SDAT. These
findings differ considerably from those of Okazaki and associates [10] and
Lee and Stemmerman [8].

Our immunocytochemical findings in CAA are important. Neuritic plaques
and CAA have both been shown to contain immunoglobulins [19, 20]. Glenner
[2] has established that amyloid fibrils are composed of the aminoterminal
end of either light or heavy chains. The immunocytochemical demonstration
of lambda chains in our patients is not, therefore, surprising. Powers and
Skeen [20, 21] and Torack and Lynch [20] observed positive reactions in the
angiopathic lesions and neuritic plaques against antiserum to IgG, immunoglobulin light chains, IgM, IgA, fibrinogen, albumin, C_3, lysozyme, and
glial fibrillary acidic protein. They interpreted their findings as evidence of a breakdown of the vacular blood brain barrier, leading to amyloid
deposition. In a later study of senile cerebral amyloidosis, Powers and
co-workers [21] showed that in 3 patients with Congophilic angiopathy (CAA),
the affected blood vessels were positive for all plasma proteins (especially
IgG, fibrinogen, and albumin) and for neurofilament proteins. Neurofilament staining in CAA, although variable, revealed a peripheral or adven-
titial distribution, whereas plasma proteins tended to be localized in the
media for the vessel wall. The distribution of Congo red and neurofilament
positivity was often identical. Powers and associates postulated that
neurofilament proteins are liberated from degenerating neuritic plaques
that combine with glycoproteins and glycosaminoglycans to form amyloid. In
CAA this reaction occurs in superficial arteries and may depend on focal increase of vascular permeability. Shirahama and associates [22] have demonstrated immunocytochemically that all three characteristic histological
lesions of SDAT consisting of CAA, neuritic plaques, and neurofibrillary
tangles react with antihuman prealbumin serum. Westermark and associates
[23] have demonstrated in SDAT the presence of AP protein in the blood
vessels with amyloid, but not in the neuritic plaques or tangles. Our
findings in the 1 patient with SDAT are similar. Westermark and co-workers,
however, postulated that failure to find AP protein in neuritic plaques and

tangles is due to their inability to pass the blood-brain barrier, a conclusion that directly contradicts the suggestion by Powers and Skeen [21] and Torack and Lynch [20] of increased vascular permeability in CAA. The contradiction remains unresolved. Meanwhile, Okoye and Watanabe [24], in a recent study of ultrastructural pathology of CAA, found that amyloid deposition occurs after degeneration of the vascular basement membrane. They concluded that the deposition of the amyloid from the vascular wall into the brain parenchyma is due to a disarrangement of the perivascular astroglial end-feet, resulting in increased permeability of the vessel wall and an overflow of amyloid.

Recurrent intracerebral hemorrhages affected 3 of our patients, as reported by others as well [6]. Vasculature of the brain infiltrated by amyloid can lead to microangiopathy and aneurysm formation [10]. This result was seen in 2 of our 12 patients. Yood et al. [25] have pointed to the common occurrence of focal or generalized hemorrhage in systemic amyloidosis due to amyloid angiopathy.

Efforts to evacuate an intracerebral clot or extracerebral collection of blood are difficult in the presence of CAA, as the bleeding is often profuse and difficult to control, presumably because of friability of blood vessels infiltrated with amyloid [6]. The occurrence of massive fatal cerebral hemorrhage in CAA after intracranial surgery has been reported [26]. It is, therefore, doubtful that surgical treatment would improve outcome in CAA. In our series, 3 of 4 patients who underwent surgery for evacuation of intracranial hemorrhage died. One survived the initial surgery when a small localized clot in the temporal lobe was evacuated, but a subsequent surgical attempt to evacuate a recurrent larger hematoma was fatal. The patient who survived surgery had a delayed evacuation of the hematoma 6 weeks after its onset.

The importance of head trauma as the cause of intracranial hemorrhage in 2 of our patients is uncertain. In view of the friability of blood vessels in CAA, it is possible that head trauma could have precipitated the catastrophic intracranial hemorrhage. Hypertension by history was found in 3 patients. However, as per our previously outlined criteria, only 1 of the 3 patients with CAA complicated by intracranial hemorrhage had documented hypertensive vascular disease. This differs considerably from the findings of Jellinger [7]. However, Jellinger's criteria for diagnosis of hypertension were not clearly defined.

ACKNOWLEDGEMENTS

The authors thank Martha Skinner, M.D., Boston University School of Medicine, for the antihuman AP protein antiserum; Linda Kroesen for technical assistance with immunocytochemistry; Robert Caughey for technical assistance with electron microscopy; and Larry Crossett for illustrations.

REFERENCES

1. A. S. Cohen, T. Shirahama, J. D. Sipe, and M. Skinner, Lab. Invest., 48:1 (1983).
2. G. G. Glenner, Ann. Clin. Lab. Sci., 5:257 (1975).
3. G. G. Glenner, 30:1283, 1333 (1980).
4. C. T. Vanley, M. J. Aguilar, R. J. Kleinhenz, and M. D. Lagios, Hum. Pathol., 12:609 (1981).
5. C. Haberland, J. Neuropathol. Exp. Neurol., 23:135 (1964).
6. Case Records of the Massachusetts General Hospital (Case 49-1982), New Engl. J. Med., 307:1507 (1982).

7. K. Jellinger, J. Neurol., 214:195 (1977).
8. S. S.Lee and G. N. Stemmerman, Arch. Pathol. Lab. Med., 102:317 (1978).
9. T. I. Mandybur and S. R. D. Bates, Arch. Neurol., 35:246 (1978).
10. H. Okazaki, T. J. Reagan, and R. J. Campbell, Mayo Clin. Proc., 54:22 (1979).
11. T. I. Mandybur, Neurology, 25:120 (1975).
12. M. A. Neumann, J. Neuropathol. Exp. Neurol., 19:370 (1960).
13. L. A. Sternberger, Immunocytochemistry, Prentice-Hall, Englewood Cliffs, New Jersey (1974).
14. W. F. McCormick and D. B. Rosenfield, Stroke, 4:946 (1973).
15. J. Bruni, J. M. Bilbao, and K. P. Pritzker, Can. J. Neurol. Sci., 4:239 (1977).
16. J. M. Powers, W. W. Schlaepfer, M. C. Willingham, et al., J. Neuro-pathol. Exp. Neurol., 40:592 (1981).
17. P. Schwartz, Trans. New York Acad. Sci., 27:393 (1965).
18. J. R. Wright, E. Calkins, W. J. Breen, et al., Medicine, 48:239 (1977).
19. T. Ishu and S. Hoga, Acta Neuropathol., 32:157 (1975).
20. R. M. Torack and R. G. Lynch, Acta Neuropathol., 53:189 (1981).
21. J. M. Powers, J. T. Skeen, J. Neuropathol. Exp. Neurol., 39:385 (1980).
22. T. Shirahama, M. Skinner, P. Westermark, et al., Am. J. Pathol., 107:41 (1982).
23. P. Westermark, T. Shirahama, M. Skinner, et al., Lab. Invest., 46:457 (1982).
24. M. I. Okoye, I. Watanabe, Hum. Pathol., 13:1127 (1982).
25. R. A. Yood, M. Skinner, A. Rubinow, and L. Talarico, JAMA, 249:1322 (1983).
26. R. M. Torack, Am. J. Pathol., 81:349 (1975).

THE ROLE OF CEREBRAL AMYLOID ANGIOPATHY IN DEMENTIA OF ALZHEIMER'S TYPE (Preliminary Results)

T. I. Mandybur

Department of Pathology and Laboratory Medicine
University of Cincinnati College of Medicine
Cincinnati, Ohio

ABSTRACT

Material of 35 autopsy cases showing any degree, type, or distribution of CAA was divided into two groups: cases with a history of dementia (18 cases) and cases with no history of dementia (17 cases). The first group included 10 cases clinically diagnosed as Alzheimer's disease, the remaining 7 cases had a history of slight to mild cognitive deterioration. The two groups were compared as to the degree of involvement, morphological patterns, and distribution of the CAA. No significant difference was found. Specifically, the cases of clinical Alzheimer's dementia (10 cases of 35 did not differ from the others in the involvement by the CAA); severe CAA was encountered in two of these cases only. Of both groups together, in five cases, moderate or severe CAA was possibly responsible for cerebral hemorrhage, and in 11 for small to medium sized infarcts.

It was concluded that whatever the role of CAA in the pathogenesis of Alzheimer's disease is, it does not contribute significantly to the basic dementia. Lack of ischemic cortical change in non-infarcted, non-hemorrhagic areas affected by CAA indicated that the exchange between the parenchyma and the blood vessels was not significantly impaired. Cortical areas with abundant CAA were not particularly rich in Alzheimer's neurofibrillary tangles and parenchymal neuritic plaques, except for perivascular plaques. Similarly, as in arteriosclerosis, the vascular change in CAA seems to be important principally to the degree that it leads either to severe narrowing of the lumen, occlusion or rupture and hemorrhage. Cases with widespread neuritic plaques and Alzheimer's neurofibrillary tangles and granulovacuolar degeneration were more common in the Demented Group. These features might have more "dementogenic impact" as the CAA.

INTRODUCTION

The role of Alzheimer's neurofibrillary tables (ANT), neuritic plaques (NP) and cerebral amyloid angiopathy (DAA) in "inducing" dementia or contribution to dementia in Alzheimer's disease and related disorders is not precisely known. It has been postulated that patients showing abundant NP develop the severest dementia; on the other hand, those having ANT only or ANT with infrequent NP may display a milder course or manifest no symptoms of dementia [1].

TABLE 1. Patients with CAA - Age and Sex Distribution

Decades	Demented (18)		Non-demented (17)	
	M	F	M	F
40–49				
50–59	1			
60–69	1	2	2	
70–79	8	2	5	2
80–89	3	1	7	1
90–100				
Total	13	5	14	3

TABLES 2. Cases with Hemorrhage, Infarcts and CAA

	Demented (18)	Non-demented (17)
Cases with any CVD	8	12
Cases with massive hemorrhage	1	4
Cases with small hemorrhage	1	0
Cases with small infarcts	8	3
Cases with large infarcts	0	6

TABLE 3. CAA - Types - Distribution

CAA - Type	Demented (18)	Non-demented (17)
1. Occipital lobe only (plaque-like degen.)	7	6
2. Diffuse leptomeningeal + cortical CAA	8	7
3. Diffuse leptomeningeal + cortical CAA + obliterative changes, etc.	3	4

The contribution of CAA to the dementing process remains most controversial. It has been reported that in cases in which CAA appears as a "solo" morphological change, dementia may be absent. Also, in the Icelandic CAA (due to deposition of gamma-trace proteins) in which no NP and ANT appear, there is typically no dementia [2]. At this time, to seek direct proof of the role of CAA in dementia is unrealistic, but looking for circumstantial evidence by means of correlation of features is possible.

In the study, the correlation between CAA and dementia has been evaluated in 35 cases showing any type or degree of CAA. The degree of involvement (severity), the morphological patterns and the distribution of the CAA were investigated.

TABLE 4. Alzheimer Changes, Lewy Bodies, and ALS with CAA

	No. of cases demented (18)	No. of cases non-demented (17)
Neuritic plaques: any distribution	18	18
diff. neocortex and hippocampus	12	4
occip. cortex cortex only	2	10
temporal only	0	2
temporal + occipital cortex	4	1
Alzheimer's tangles:		
any distribution	14	6
diff. neocortex and hippocampus	6	2
temporal cortex only	7	4
brain stem	5	2
Granulovacuolar deg. hippocampus	8	3
Lewy Bodies	2	0
ALS	1	0

Of the 35 cases, 17 had no history of psychiatric illness. Among the remaining 18, there were 11 cases diagnosed clinically as Alzheimer's disease, the 7 remaining were at the 2-4 stage of the global cognitive deterioration scale.

In this presentation, I will refer to all 18 patients with any degree of cognitive decline as demented, and discuss them basically as one group [DG]. The aim of this study is to compare the brain pathology in the non-demented group (NDG) with the demented group (DG).

Firstly, the sex and age distribution will be reviewed (Table 1).

On the basis of Table 1 of sex and age distribution, at least three observations can be made.

1. In the present material, there is a tendency for the DG to develop CAA slightly earlier than the NDG.

2. Both in DG and NDG, the relationship of males to females was almost 3:1.

3. The first case was observed in the age as early as the fifties, then with progression of age, the disease became more frequent.

It has been reported that the risk of hemorrhage or infarct in people with CAA is substantial.

In the present material, 20 cases had severe CVD. Fifteen of these had cerebrovascular disease which could have resulted from CAA. Six patients had large cerebral infarcts, which were related to occlusion of a major cerebral artery and attributed either to embolism or atherosclerosis, not to the CAA. The latter infarcts were seen only in cases of NDG.

In comparing the cerebrovascular disease in the two groups, it can be stated that:

1. More CVD cases were seen in the NDG.

2. Massive hemorrhage was more frequent in the NDG (age factor?).

3. Small infarcts were more common in the DG.

4. Large atherosclerotic infarcts were more frequent in the NDG (slightly older patients).

The comparison of CAA in DG and NGD was not easy, because the histometrical evaluation of CAA is difficult. Not only counting the number of vessels with amyloidosis is important, but also the intensity of the amyloid stain, the degree of thickening of the vessels wall, also the degree of involvement of the brain. Moreover, in the severest form of CAA, complicated by obliterative change or hyaline degeneration, there is actually less amyloid in the previously amyloid infiltrated vessel, because the infiltrated coat (usually the media) had already degenerated.

For these reasons, I have used a qualitative evaluation of the CAA. I have distinguished three grades of CAA, which, in reality, correspond to the three most commonly observed patterns of CAA:

1. With CAA being represented mainly by plaque-like degeneration of the cortical vessels, usually involving only the occipital cortex (one lobe, lowest grade).

2. With simple CAA involving leptomeningeal and cortical vessels in more than one lobe (medium grade).

3. The CAA complicated by obliterative and hyaline vascular changes (severe grade).

Using this classification, the groups showed the distribution of the CAA types (Table 3).

Table 3 shows a surprising lack of different between the two groups. All three types of CAA show about the same incidence in the DG and the NDG. Specifically in cases clinically diagnosed as Alzheimer's dementia (11 cases of 35) the complicated CAA (severe) was encountered in two cases only.

The 25 patients with no clinical Alzheimer's disease (mentally normal or with minimal mental deterioration only) included five cases with complicated (most severe) CAA.

There are also other morphological features of Alzheimer's dementia and cerebral ageing than CAA. There are the neuritic plaques (NP), Alzheimer's neurofibrillary tangles (ANT), the granulovacuolar degeneration (GVD), the Lewy bodies, etc.

Table 4 indicates that:

1. All cases of both groups showed NP.

2. The major difference was that more cases in the DG showed ANT.

3. Granulovacuolar change was seen more often in cases of the DG.

4. Lewy bodies were seen only in the DG.

5. ALS present in one of our cases, I believe, was more or less co-incidental.

In summary, both groups show the following similarities.

1. Similar types of CAA with approximately the same case frequency.

2. Frequent cerebrovascular complications of the CAA (small infarcts, small and large hemorrhages).

3. Amyloid containing plaques (NP) (all cases).

4. Both in DG and NDG, the CAA was seen predominantly in males (this differs from literature).

The differences were as follows.

1. CAA seemed to appear slightly later in NDG than in the DG.

2. More cases with more ANT were present in the DG versus the NDG group.

3. Granulovacuolar degeneration was more often noted in the DG.

4. Widespread NP in the cerebral cortex were more frequently observed in the DG.

5. Hemorrhages and large (atherosclerotic) infarcts were more common in NDG; small infarcts predominated in the DG.

DISCUSSION

Comparing present results with data of the literature is not possible because this subject has never been systematically studied the way it was presently done.

In a paper of 1975, by Mandybur [3] in a series of 15 cases of Alzheimer's disease, 80% showed CAA, but its degree was very variable. Only four cases showed complicated (severe) CAA. No non-demented controls were studied.

In a publication 1982, Mountjoy, et al. [4], reported no significant correlation between the amount of vascular amyloid and the clinical severity of the dementia. I wish to expand this statement (with which I agree entirely), to many cases with no dementia. Two of their cases (I presume controls, with no dementia), had CAA without NP. This, I have never seen so far, but indeed, sometimes the NP were extremely scant. Of numerous cases reported of cerebral hemorrhage due to CAA (review literature, Gilbert, et al., 1983 [5]) some were demented, but most were not. The degree of the CAA was evaluated only in some of these publications. For these reasons, these cases are not proper for a comparison.

CONCLUSION

1. This study confirms previous reports that patients can harbor CAA to a severe degree without manifesting dementia.

2. It is impossible to assess the contribution of amyloid angiopathy in dementia in cases also showing NP or NP and ANT (a "synergistic" effect?). All cases showed NP although often only a few.

3. Similarly, as in arteriosclerosis, the vascular change in CAA seems to be important principally in that it could lead either to severe narrowing of the lumen, ischemia, occlusion and infarct, or rupture and hemorrhage.

4. Recently published cases of cerebral hemorrhage due to CAA (also the present study) indicate that this cause of cerebral hemorrhages has been previously underestimated.

5. No significant qualitative differences of CAA were observed between the DG and NDG. Actually cases with severe CAA were common in the NDG and low grade dementia cases.

6. The vascular complications related to CAA qualitatively were also not different in both groups.

7. Lack of ischemic cortical change, gliosis, etc., in the non-infarcted, non-hemorrhagic areas affected by CAA indicate that the exchange between the parenchyma and the affected blood vessels was not significantly impaired to cause morphological changes. Cortical areas with abundant CAA were not particularly rich in ANT and parenchymal NP, except for perivascular NP.

8. The clinical presentation of dementia in cases of Alzheimer's disease, with severe CAA, did not differ significantly from those showing slight to mild CAA.

9. It appears that whatever the role of CAA in the pathogenesis of Alzheimer's disease is, it probably does not "as such" contribute significantly to the basic dementia. At least hypothetically, however, it could contribute to dementia by the means of multi-infarct dementia factor, and mult-small hemorrhage factor.

10. It appears that cases with widespread ANT and NP were more common in the DG, also, those with GVD were more common in that group.

REFERENCES

1. G. Blessed, B. E. Tomlinson, and M. Roth, Br. J. Psychiatry, 114:797-811 (1968).
2. G. Gudmundsson, J. Hallgrimsson, T. A. Jonasson, et al., Brain, 95:387-404 (1972).
3. T. I. Mandybur, Neurology (Minneapolis), 25:120-6 (1975).
4. C. Q. Mountjoy, B. E. Tomlinson, and P. H. Gibson, J. Neurol. Sci., 57:89-103 (1982).
5. J. J. Gilbert and H. V. Vinters, Cerebral hemorrhage, Stroke, 14:915-923 (1983).

HEREDITARY CENTRAL NERVOUS SYSTEM γ-TRACE AMYLOID ANGIOPATHY AND STROKE IN ICELANDIC FAMILIES

Olafur Jensson*, Gunnar Gudmundsson†,
Alfred Arnason*, Hanes Blöndal‡,
Anders Grugg**, and Helge Löfberg††

*Blood Bank, Genetic Division

Departments of †Neurology and ‡Pathology
National Hospital
University of Iceland, Reykjavik, Iceland, and

Departments of Clinical **Chemistry and ††Pathology
University of Lund, Malmo General Hospital
Malmö, Sweden

ABSTRACT

Hereditary central nervous system amyloid angiopathy occurring in Icelanders is the first human disease known to be caused by selective deposition of fragments of the alkaline microprotein γ-trace forming amyloid fibrils in the walls of the brain and spinal cord arteries. This causes single or multiple strokes ending fatally in most cases. A regulation of cysteine proteinase activity has been suggested as the function of γ-trace. Studies of 128 affected members in eight families from the same geographical area, indicate transmission of an autosomal dominant gene over two centuries. About 90% of those who died of this disorder were less than 50 years. The studies indicate, that in few members the carrier state is compatible with reaching old age. This CNS angiopathy is characterized by an abnormally low value of γ-trace in the CSF or one third of the mean value found in comparable normal adults. Estimation of γ-trace in the CSF is presently the only test available for supporting diagnosis of the disorder and differentiating it from other types of cerebral hemorrhage. This test will significantly improve genetic counseling and make search for genetic linkage possible.

INTRODUCTION

In the last two years significant progress has been made in the investigation of the hereditary cerebral hemorrhage with amyloidosis (HCHWA) occurring in Icelandic families and causing untimely fatal brain hemorrhage in family members.

A new landmark in the study of HCHWA was made when its amyloid protein was identified [2] and found to be related to the γ-trace microprotein [3]. Furthermore, it was demonstrated recently, that the γ-trace in the cerebrospinal fluid of patients suffering from HCHWA and in the CSF of some of

789

their asymptomatic sibs and children, was significantly reduced [4]. The mean level of γ-trace in the CSF of HCHWA patients was only one third of the mean value found in healthy subjects with an overlap in less than 1%. Estimation of γ-trace in the CSF could therefore be used as diagnostic test

1	10	20	30	40	50	60

SSPGKPPRLVGGPMDASVEEEGVRRALDFAVGEYNKASNDMYHSRALQVVRARKQIVAGV

61	70	80	90	100	110	120

NYFLDVELGRTTCTKTQPNLDNCPFHDQPHLKRKAFCSFQIYAVPSQGTMTLSKSTCQDA

Fig. 1. γ-Trace (Cystatin) molecule.

for HCHWA and also to identify carriers amongst asymptomatic family members.

Very recently, the γ-trace microprotein was shown to be a potent inhibitor of several human cysteine proteinases [5, 6].

The genetic studies of HCHWA reported in this paper are supported by estimation of γ-trace in several family members.

METHODS

Family Studies

In the present survey only families are included in which the diagnosis of HCHWA in one or more family members is based on post-mortem examination and positive Congo red staining of blood vessels on sections of brain and spinal cord.

Classification of sibs into affected versus unaffected was made by assigning any sib as normal who had lived to be 50 years of age or more. This applies to approximate 90% of sibs forming the group with early onset age of 15-50 years. For those relatively few members with late onset, or after the age of 50, we have arbitrarily classified their sibs as unaffected, if they lived to be at least 5 years older than their eldest affected sib. One hundred and twenty eight affected members have been included in this survey. Of these 52 have been investigated in the Department of Neurology, the National Hospital of Iceland. In 76 of the affected family members ascertainment is based on the diagnosis recorded on their death certificates available since 1911.

Post-Mortem Examination

Post-mortem examination was carried out on thirty family members. From nineteen of these formalin fixed brain tissue sections were stained for amyloid by the Congo red technique [7] and examined under polarized light to produce apple-green birefringence. Congo red positive and negative brain tissue was used as control.

TABLE 1. Number and Percentage of Symptoms and
Signs in 52 Male and Female Patients
with Hereditary CNS Amyloid Angiopathy

Signs	Males		Females	
	N.	%	N	%
Motor	25/25	100	27/27	100
Sensory	18/22	82	20/26	77
Mental	14/20	70	15/19	79
Dysphasia	12/17	71	16/20	80
BP NORMAL	16/16	100	22/23	96

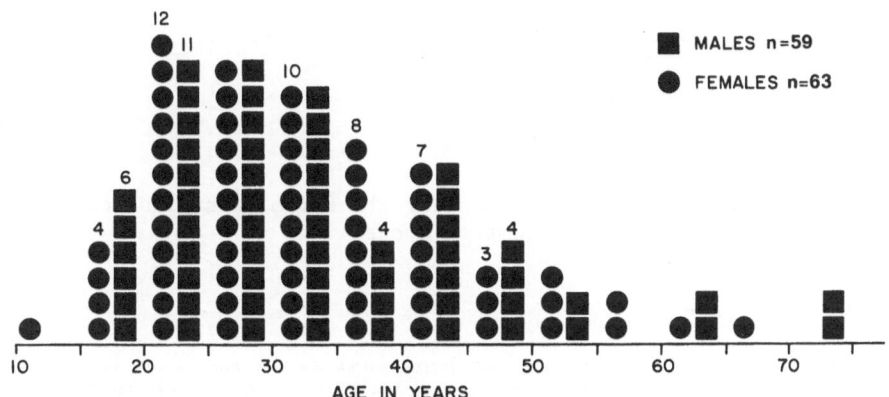

Fig. 2. Age of death of patients with hereditary CNS amyloid angiopathy.

Electronmicroscopy

Brain tissue for EM was obtained from autopsy material within one hour
after death. The tissue was fixed in 1% glutaraldehyde buffered with 0.1
M sodium cacodylate buffer at pH 7.4 and postfixed in 2% OsO_4. Tissue
blocks were dehydrated in an ascending series of ethanol and embedded in
Spurr resin [15]. Ultrathin sections were stained with uranyl acetate and
lead citrate and examined with a Philips EM 300 electron microscope.

Immunohistochemistry

Indirect immunofluorescence staining was done on autopsy tissue sections from the cerebral cortex and leptomeningeal arteries using rabbit
antigamma trace, normal rabbit serum and fluorescein labelled sheep anti-
rabbit IgG × 160.

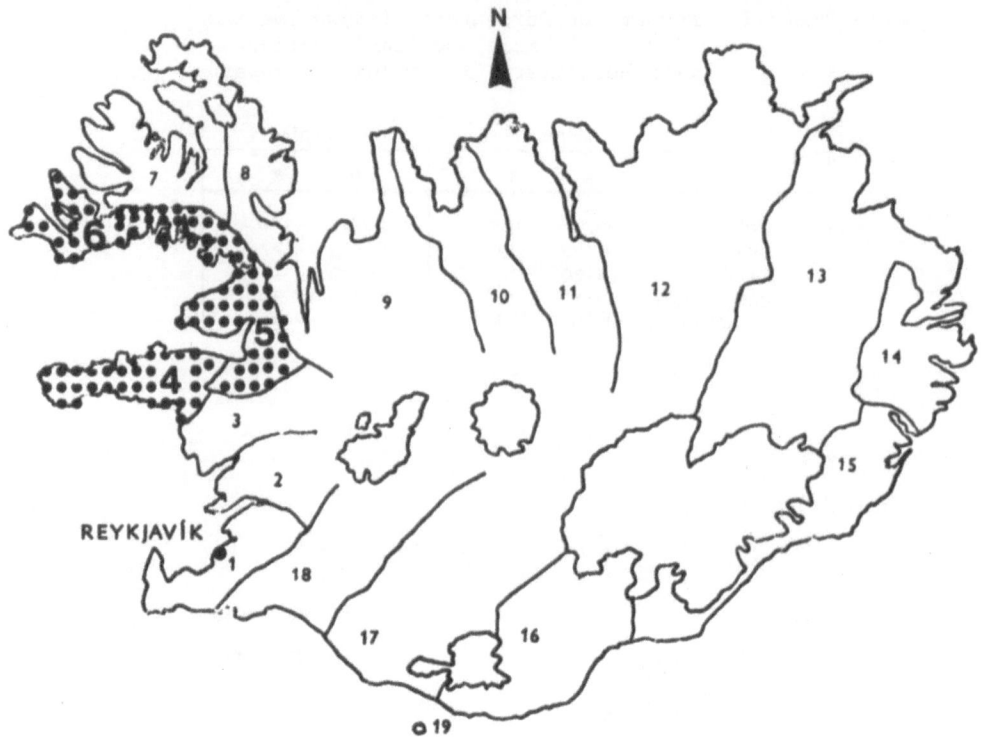

Fig. 3.   Map of Iceland.   The homestead of the 8 families with hereditary
          CNS amyloid angiopathy (dotted areas).

Estimation of γ-Trace

     Estimation of γ-trace in the cerebrospinal fluid was made in 28 family
members, 10 patients and 18 of their asymptomatic sibs and children by
methods previously described [8].

Genetic Markers

     Over 20 genetic marker systems were investigated.   These included HLA
(A, B, C), BF, GLO-1, Gc, C_3 and 13 blood group systems [9].

RESULTS

     The main symptoms and signs of 52 patients, of whom 46 had died and 6
were alive, are summarized in Table 1.   The age of death from HCHWA of 122
family members is shown in Fig. 2.   The values of γ-trace in the cerebrospinal fluid of 28 members of five families are shown in Fig. 4.   The analysis of the pedigree data is recorded in Table 2.

Morbid Anatomy and Histopathology

     Macroscopically, hemorrhagic lesions in the brain are most common in
the basal ganglia region although not infrequent in other locations.   Areas
of infarction are found occasionally.   Light microscopy shows hyalinization
and thickening of the walls of small arteries and arterioles in the meninges
and within the brain tissue itself.   Similar changes are found in the spinal
cord.   The hyalinization extends generally and thickening of the walls of

TABLE 2. Analysis of the Pedigree Data. Genetic and Sex Ratios
         in 221 Members, Including 128 Affected Members, of 8
         Families with Hereditary CNS Amyloid Angiopathy

Sibs	Females	Males	Total
Affected	67	59	126
Unaffected	47	49	95
Total	113	108	221

Segregation ratio   126/221 = 57%   (P > 0.05)
Sex ratio of affected   59/126 = 47% male (P > 0.05)
Sex ratio of unaffected   49/95 = 52% male (P > 0.05)

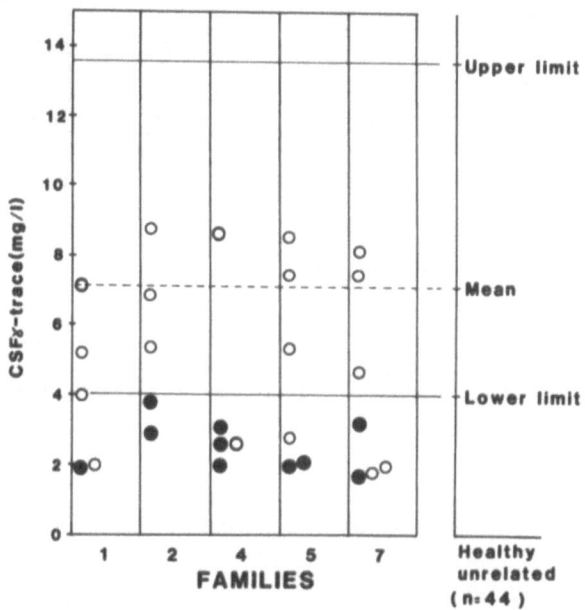

Fig. 4. Estimation of γ-trace in 28 family members, 10 patients with symp-
         toms of HCHWA and 18 of their asymptomatic sibs and children.

small arteries and arterioles in the meninges and within the brain tissue
itself. Similar changes are found in the spinal cord. The hyalinization
extends generally through the entire vessel wall. Commonly the intima is
separated from the rest of the wall by a definite space. This space is
empty except for delicate strands and an occasional macrophage. The hyaline
change is characterized by Congophilia and a greenish birefringency under
polarized light.

Electron microscopy

     Electronmicroscopy showed a dense feltwork of fibrillar material
throughout the media of the vessel walls (Fig. 7). This material is made

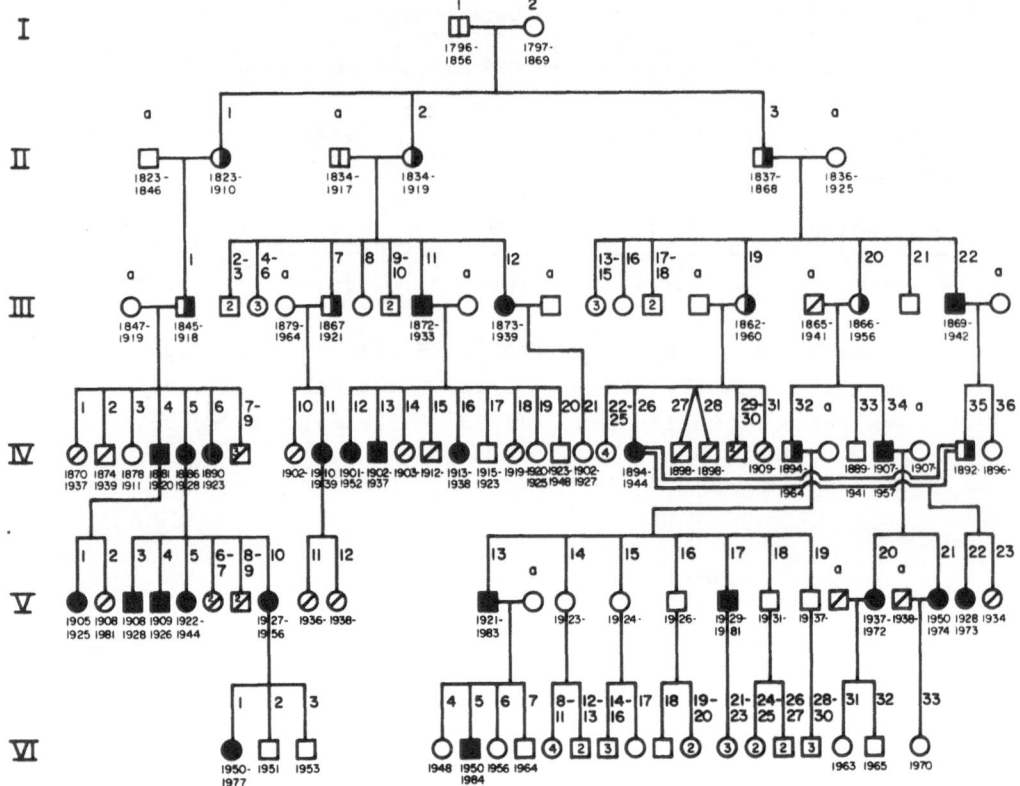

Fig. 5. Family 3.

of randomly arranged nonbranching fibrils (Fig. 7a) interspersed with particles made of five subunits (Fig. 7b). These particles (Fig. 8) are
identical in size and appearance to tissue amyloid P-component [16].

Immunohistochemistry

Fluorescent labelled anti- gamma trace reacted strongly with the amyloid
deposits in the brain and leptomeningeal vessels (Fig. 9a and 9b).

Genetic Studies

The transmission of the gene causing HCHWA is illustrated in two of
the 8 families studied (Figs. 5 and 6). In these 2 families transmission
in different family branches from a common progenitor demonstrates that the
mutant gene has been present in the kindred for at least 200 years. The
autosomal dominant mode of inheritance is confirmed by the segregation and
sex ratios (Table 2) and by the uninterrupted transmission from one generation to the next (Figs. 5 and 6).

DISCUSSION

Genetics

The present genetic survey shows that the HCHWA is an autosomal dominant disease and confirms previous results regarding its genetic transmission [1, 13].

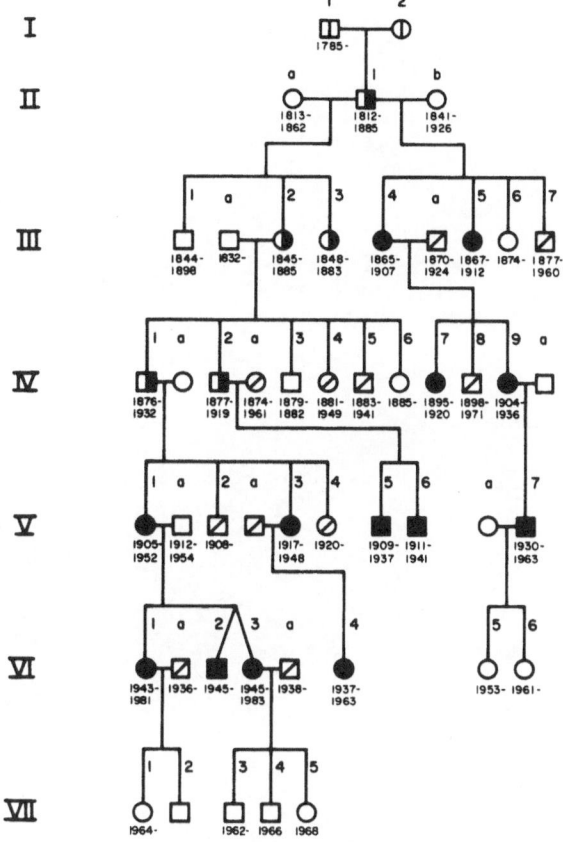

Fig. 6.   Family 5.

In seven of the 8 HCHWA families transmission lines through two or more family branches extend back from affected members ascertained in the last 70 years to progenitors born 150-200 years ago. A common progenitor, who initially transmitted this mutant gene to his descendants has probably lived in this area, as indicated by the founder effect amply illustrated by the family studied (Fig. 5). The geographical area, in which all these families and their progenitors are found, surrounds a large by in the west of Iceland (Fig. 3).

The continuous transmission, characteristic of a dominant gene with full pentrance, was occasionally broken by premature death of the carrier parent due to different causes; in some cases an asymptomatic carrier state prevailing to old age is probable. The latter possibility is supported somewhat by the age distribution of confirmed cases and by unascertained probable parental carriers, especially female carriers.

The preponderance of affected members (Table 2) is mostly explained by bias towards entering affected members aged 20-50, while leaving out the few unaffected members, who died at this age due to causes unrelated to HCHWA.

Relatively few cases of cerebral hemorrhage due to HCHWA have been re-liably diagnosed in family members dying after 50 years of age. However, in addition to such cases, elderly patients who are in the line of genetic

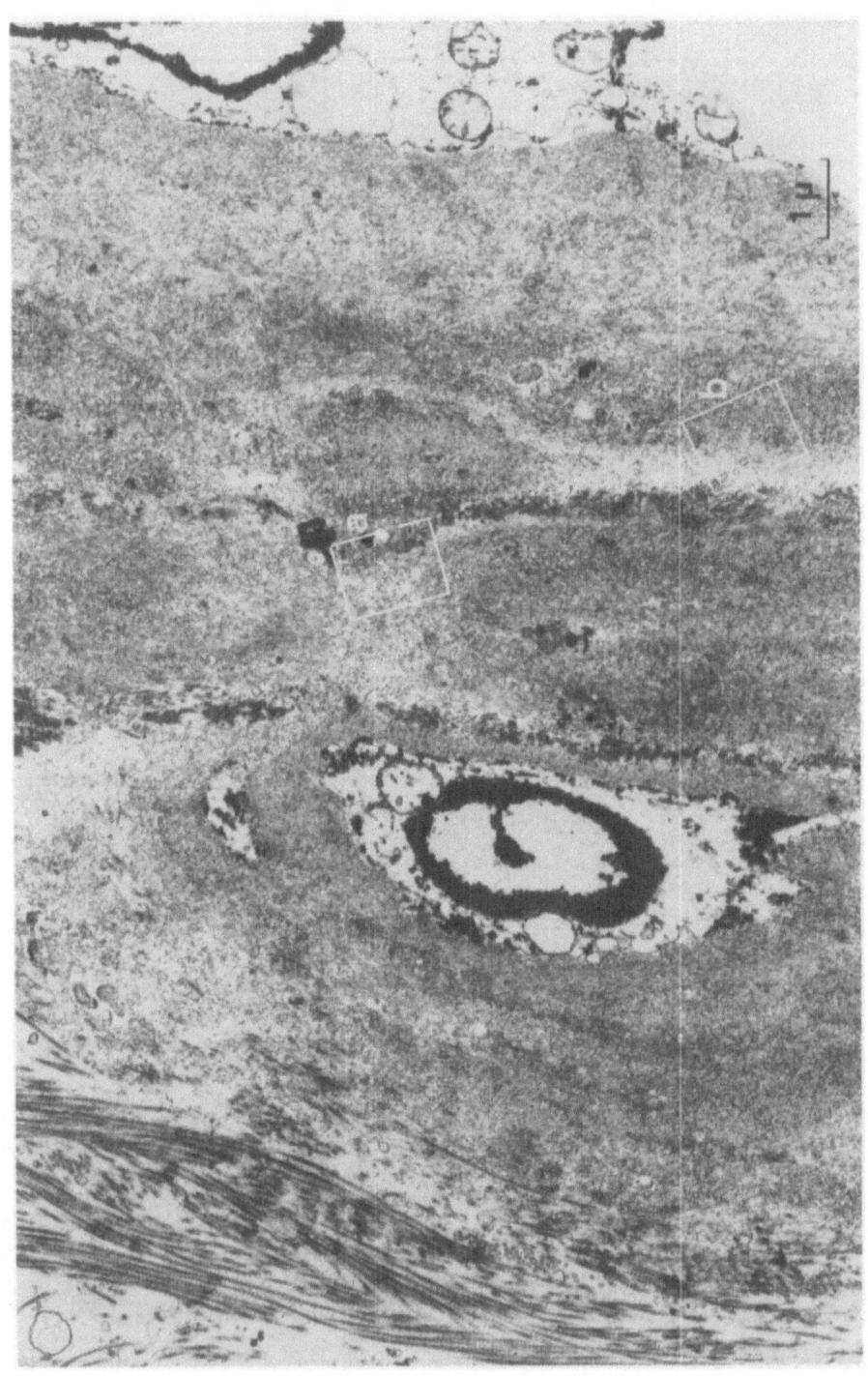

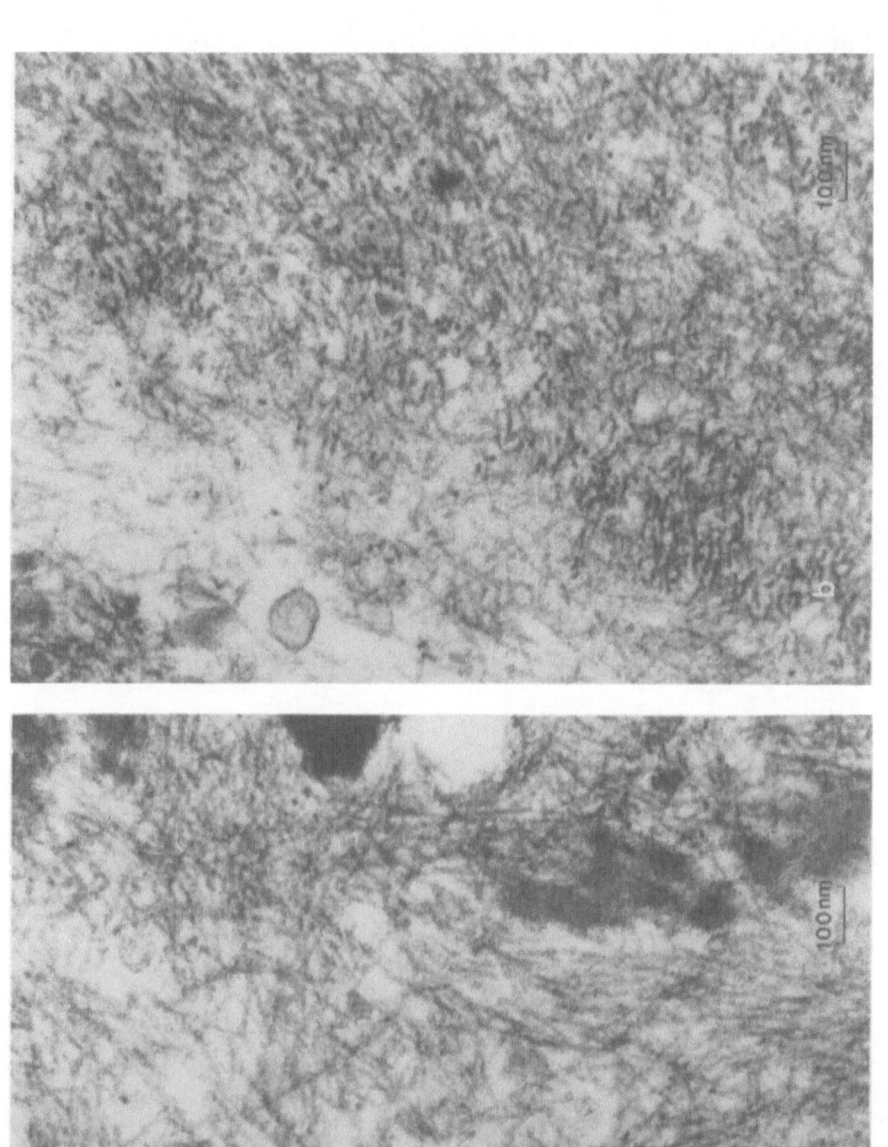

Fig. 7. Electron micrograph showing an arteriole from the depth of a sulcus in the temporal lobe. The media is extensively infiltrated by amyloid material (× 10,000). a) Higher power view of area a in the same arteriole showing the fibrils and their disposition (× 100,000). b) Higher power view of area b in the same arteriole showing fibrils and scattered particles (amyloid P-component) (× 100,000).

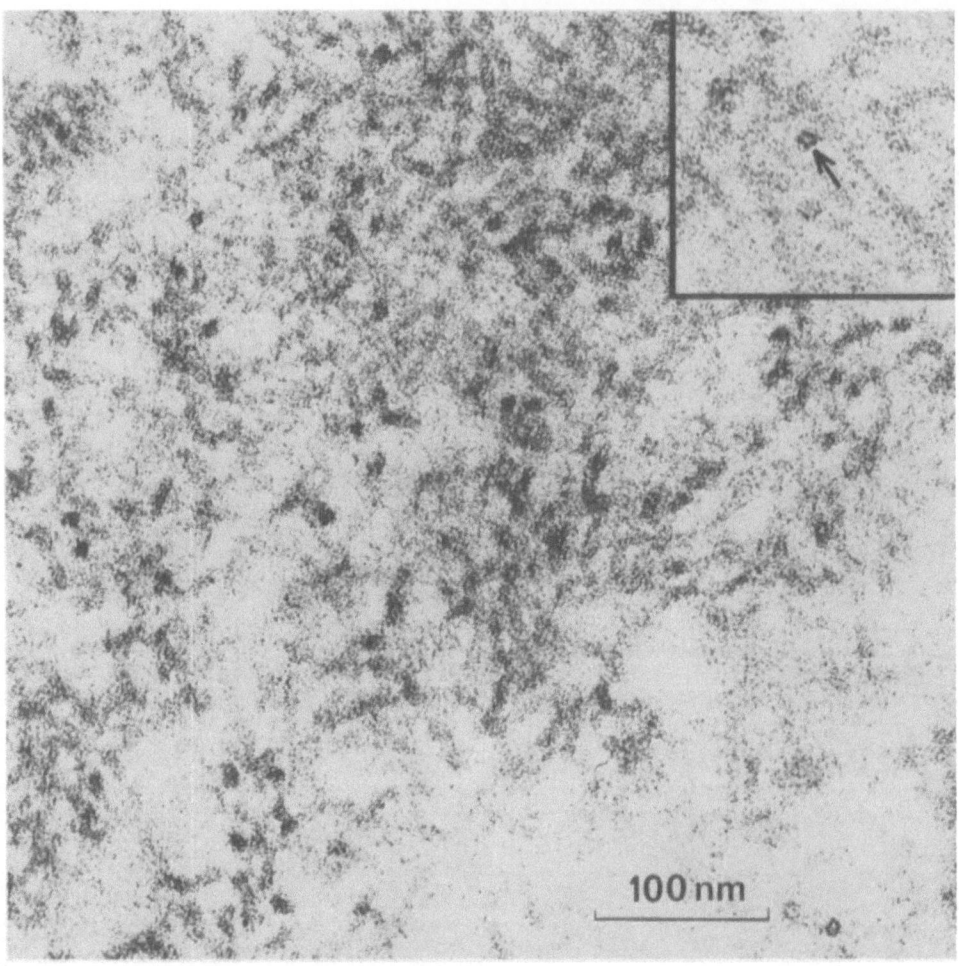

Fig. 8.   Electron micrograph showing particles some of which (inset) show
          subunits with pentagonal arrangement (× 100,000).

transmission, indicate that HCHWA is compatible with old age in a small proportion of family members. This "form fruste" is likely to occur also in
some of the elderly sibs belonging to sibships in which late onset is a
characteristic feature. How much this form of cerebral angiopathy contributes to the incidence of death from stroke in the elderly and morbidity in
the aging brain is presently unknown.

Clinical and Post Mortem Findings

     The clinical manifestations of HCHWA range from dying immediately or
after few days or weeks following the first stroke to living for many years
crippled by multiple strokes of varying severity. The latter is much more
common and leads to motor signs of different severity in all 52 patients examined and sensory signs in most (Table 1). Mental signs are common, showing a gradual deterioration over a number of years. In a few patients these
have been the dominant type of signs and sometimes lead to long stays in
psychiatric wards. In 96-100% of the patients blood pressure was normal
(Table 1).

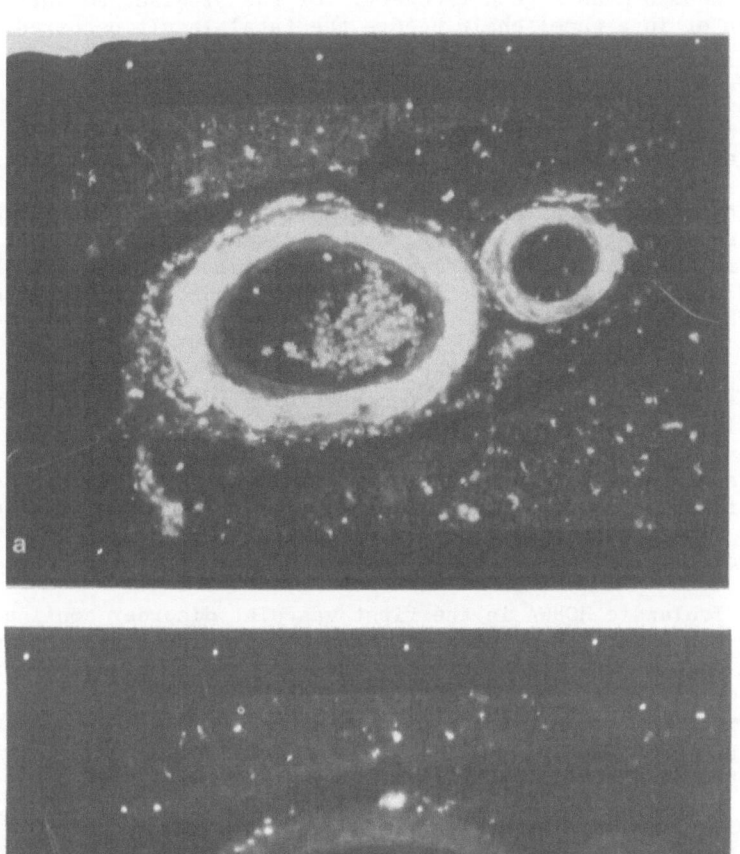

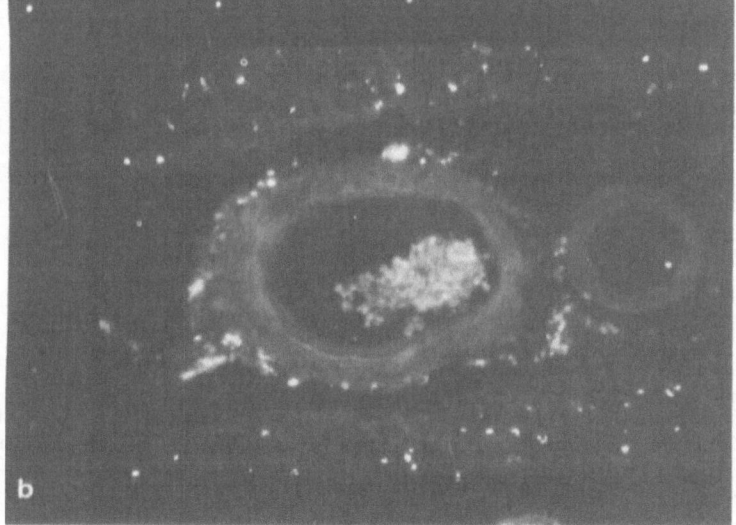

Fig. 9. Immunohistochemical reactivity of gamma trace in two leptomeningeal arteries (a) of a patient with HCHWA and control (b).

In some cases the disease seems to be in a stable or non-progressive state for long periods of up to several years. Exceptionally there has been one or two small strokes with apparent full recovery lasting for a number of years. Of 42 patients, 28 made some recovery after the first insult, of whom 6 made a good recovery. Of the 37 diseased patients, 24 were bedridden or in a wheel chair before the fatal insult occurred.

The brains examined most commonly show multiple lesions of different ages, which is consistent with the usual clinical course of the disease. Exceptionally the first insult proves fatal. Apparently the vascular changes are most pronounced in leptomeningeal and cortical arterioles.

Electronmicroscopy has demonstrated the two components of amyloid: fibrils and pentagonal particles, to be present in the media of these vessels. Presumably these particles are identical to the amyloid P-component. Detailed analysis of the distribution and morphology of the vascular changes is in progress [16].

The amyloid P component (AP) was found in the brain vessel walls of HCHWA patients but not in the intracerebral plaques in tissue from patients with senile amyloidosis [12].

A condition similar to the γ-trace related HCHWA has been described in several families in the Netherlands [10, 11]. The Dutch HCHWA can now be compared with the Icelandic one by estimating γ-trace in the CSF and testing for γ-trace amyloid in the brain vessels of the Dutch patients [13].

The Icelandic HCHWA is the first vascular disorder confined to the central nervous system that has been shown to occur on the background of a biochemical defect that can be easily detected in a small volume of CSF [4]. Estimation of γ-trace in the CSF is presently the only test available for supporting diagnosis of γ-trace related HCHWA and differentiating it from other types of cerebral hemorrhage. Ascertainment of HCHWA in asymptomatic family members by this test will significantly improve possibilities for genetic counseling in HCHWA families and also make search for genetic linkage considerably more promising.

REFERENCES

1. G. Gudmundsson, J. Hallgrimsson, T. A. Jonasson, and O. Bjarnason, Brain, 95, 387 (1972).
2. D. H. Cohen, H. Feiner, O. Jensson, and B. Frangione, J. Exp. Med., 158, 623 (1984).
3. A. Grubb and H. Löfberg, Proc. Natl. Acad. Sci., 79, 3024 (1982).
4. A. Grubb, O. Jennson, G. Gudmundsson, A. Arnason, H. Löfberg, and J. Malm, New Engl. J. Med. (in press) (1984).
5. J. Brzin, T. Popovic, V. Turk, U. Borchart, and W. Machledit, Biochem. Biophys. Res. Commun., 118, 203 (1984).
6. A. J. Barrett, M. E. Davies, and A. Grubb, Biochemical and Biophysical Research Communications, 120, 631 (1984).
7. M. I. Stokes and R. J. Trickey, J. Clin. Path., 26, 241 (1973).
8. H. Löfberg and A. O. Grubb, Scand. J. Clin. Lab. Invest., 39, 619 (1979).
9. A. Arnason, O. Jennson, et al., Unpublished observation (1984).
10. W. Luyendijk and G. T. A. M. Bots, in: Advances in Diagnosis Therapy (H. W. Pia, C. Langmaid, and J. Zierski, eds.), Springer Verlag, Berlin (1980), pp. 50-56.
11. A. R. Wattendorff, G. T. A. M. Bots, L. N. Went, and L. J. Endtz, J. Neurol. Sci., 55, 121 (1982).
12. I. F. Rowe, O. Jensson, P. D. Lewis, J. Candy, G. A. Tennent, and M. B. Pepys, Neuropathol. and Applied. Neurobiol., 10, 53 (1984).

13. O. Jensson, W. Luyendijk, et al., Unpublished observations (1984).
14. A. R. Spurr, J. Ultrastruct. Res., $\underline{26}$, 31 (1969).
15. M. Skinner, J. D. Sipe, R. A. Yood, T. Shirahama, and A. S. Cohen, in: C-Reactive Protein and the Plasma Protein Response to Tissue Injury (J. Kushner, J. E. Volanakis, and H. Gequrz, eds.), Ann. N.Y. Acad. Sci., $\underline{389}$, 190-198 (1982).
16. H. Blondal, et al., Unpublished observations (1984).

ACKNOWLEDGEMENTS

Supported in part by the Icelandic Science Foundation and the U.S. Department of Energy (Contract No. DE-AC02-76EV03214) the the Genetical Committee of the University of Iceland.

J. OTHER TYPES OF AMYLOIDOSIS

AMYLOID ASSOCIATED WITH CALCIFYING EPITHELIAL ODONTOGENIC TUMOR -

A NEW TYPE OF AMYLOID FIBRIL PROTEIN CEOT

Takashi Isobe, Takanori Miki,
Fuyuki Kametani,* and Tomotaka Shinoda*

Department of Medicine and Oral Surgery
Kobe University School of Medicine
Kobe, Japan

*Department of Chemistry
Tokyo Metropolitan University
Tokyo, Japan

ABSTRACT

A 55 year old Japanese female was found to have calcifying epithelial odontogenic tumor (CEOT), which is known to be an amyloid producing neoplasm. Amyloid deposits are resistant to permanganate reaction for Congored, green birefringent, and of characteristic fibrillar structure. CEOT tissue was purified by water extraction, followed by column chromatography. The amino acid composition of the major component of the CEOT-amyloid proteins is unique and different from those of any amyloid fibril proteins preveiously reported.

INTRODUCTION

The variability of the nature of the amyloid proteins have been clarified in the past 15 years, which is in part dependent on the accompanying clinical disorders [1]. Differences of amyloid protein have also provided a reclassification of amyloid that is dependent on the nature of protein deposited. In the present paper, we present a new type of amyloid fibril protein from a case with calcifying epithelial odontogenic tumor (CEOT). Since CEOT is an amyloid-producing tumor, the clarification of the nature of amyloid protein may give some insights into pathogenesis of amyloidosis [2].

CASE PRESENTATION

M. Tan, 55 year old female, started to notice swelling of the right jaw with occasional toothache. Within 6 months, the swelling gradually increased. Her family and past history is not contributory. On admission, she was found to be thinly built, having diffuse swelling of right-sided buccal area. Intraoral findings were diffuse swelling of gingiva, around the right premolar regions. X-ray and computed tomography (CT) disclosed partial bone defect of the maxilla, suggestive of some malignant process in

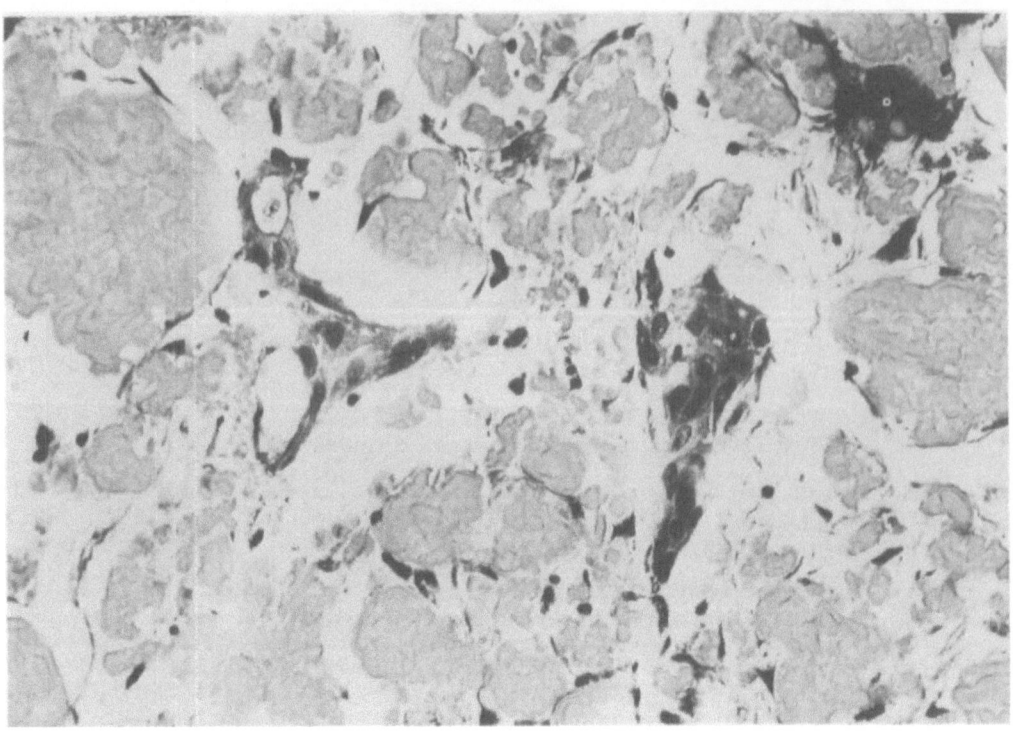

Fig. 1. Acidophilic amyloid associated with sheets of polygonal epithelial
         cell. (H-E original magnification ×100).

the involved area. There was no abnormality of physical findings on cardio-
pulmonary, abdominal and neurological examinations. Laboratory data included red blood cells $436 \times 10^4/mm^3$, hemoglobin 12.6 g/dl, white cell
counts $2400/mm^3$ including neutrophils $720/mm^3$, platelet $7.0 \times 10^4/mm^3$, serum
total protein 8.0 g/dl consisting of albumin 5.0 g/dl α_1-0.2, α_2-0.4, β-0.6
and γ-globulin 1.8, serum IgG 2222 mg/dl, IgA 298 mg/dl, IgM 222 mg/dl,
negative urinary protein, CRP (-), RA (+2), serum calcium 9.3 mg/dl and
phosphorus 3.9 mg/dl. There was no abnormality for liver kidney and thyroid
function tests.

Pathological Study

    Biopsy specimen revealed tumor clusters composing of polygonal epi-
thelial cells with eosinophilic cytoplasm. Amyloid, associated with neoplastic cells, was observed abundantly in stromal portions (Fig. 1). Histological diagnosis was calcifying epithelial odontogenic tumor (CEOT). Subsequently, a surgical operation was done for the removal of the tumor with
the lateral one half of the right maxilla, all of which were involved by
the tumor. Histologically, the tumor was composed of polygonal epithelial
cells, often with prominent intercellular bridges, arranged in sheets or
strands in a fibrous stroma by HE-stained sections. The epithelial cells
were sometimes multinucleated, and also showed nuclear polymorphism. Acidophilic homogenous materials revealed strongly positive reactions and birefringence under polarization microscopy, suggesting amyloid, where permanganate reaction was resistent to Congo red. Calcification was scarcely
seen. Electron microscopically, large, polygonal cells were characterized
by large numbers of microvilli (cytoplasmic processes), either finger-like
or often rounded. Desmosomal connections between tumor cells were asso-

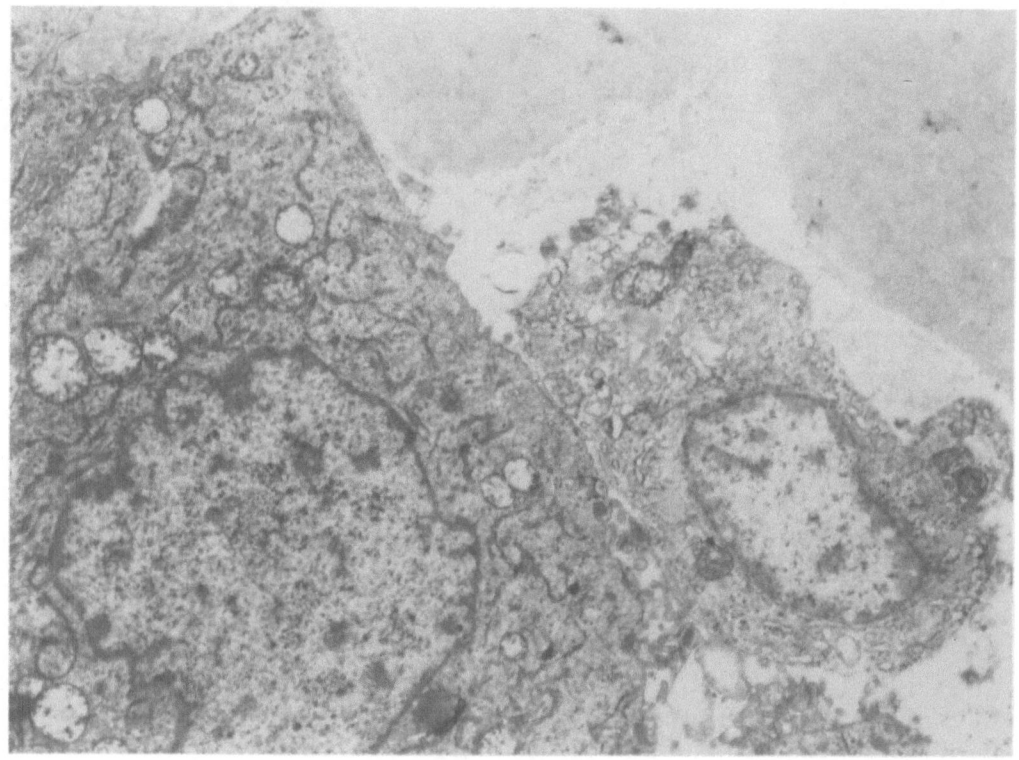

Fig. 2. Electronmicroscopy revealing amyloid fibrils (right upper) with two
epithelial cells, with desmosomal connections (original magnification ×5000).

ciated with bundles of tonofilaments. Rigid, nonbranching fibrils 70–150
A° in diameter were characteristic of amyloid (Fig. 2). Some collagen
fibrils and fibroblastic processes were also present.

In summary, the present case exhibited histological findings of calcifying epithelial odontogenic tumor (CEOT) associated with amyloid deposits
and low-grade calcification.

Materials and Methods for Biochemistry and Immunochemistry

Amyloid-laden tissues of mandibular regions (1.6 gm) dissected by
knife, then were homogenized in 100 ml of phosphate buffered saline (PBS)
in a universal homogenizer at full speed for 5 min. The homogenate was
centrifuged in a No. 30 rotor at 13,000 rpm for 30 min in a Spinco Model L
ultracentrifuge (Beckman, USA). The supernatant was monitored for protein
contents at 280 mm. The extraction with PBS was repeated 4 times to remove
soluble protein fractions. As to water extraction, 100 ml of distilled
water were added to the final pellet, rehomogenized and centrifuged. This
procedure was repeated for 7 times until the protein contents in the super-
natents reduced to 0.05 at 280 mm. Fractionations of the water-extracted
materials were done through Sephadex G-100 column (2.5 × 100 cm) equilibrated with 5M guanidine in 1N acetic Acid [3]. Further fractionations
were done by high performance liquid chromatography (HPLC) with Hitachi
3013-0 resin (0.4 × 25 cm, 20–75% CH_3CN gradient, 0.1% trifluoroacetic acid,
pH 2.5).

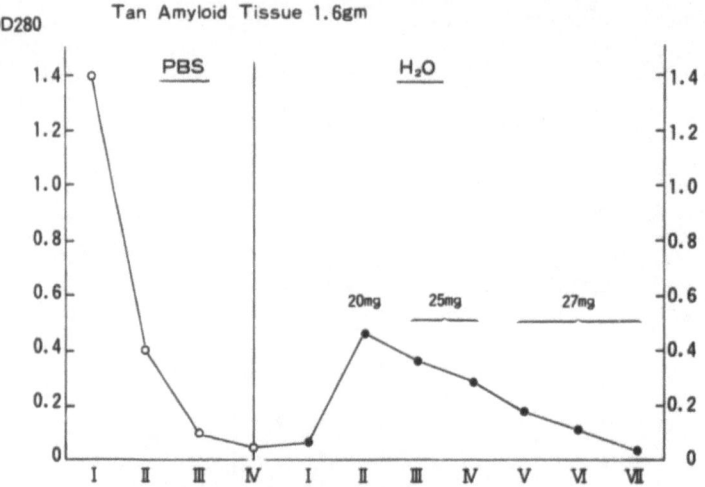

Fig. 3. Initial crude extraction profile of CEOT amyloid
         by PBS washing and water extraction.

TABLE 1. Amino Acid Analysis of Amy-
          loid Fibril Protein CEOT,
          Compared to the Data from
          Other Amyloid Proteins

Amino acid	CEOT (Tan)	AA (Kub)	AL (Tew) Vk II	AL (Kor) Vλ I	AF j (Am-16)
Lysine	1.0	4.5	5.0	5.5	6.3
Histidine	1.8	3.2	1.4	1.9	3.1
Arginine	1.8	9.0	3.7	1.5	3.1
Aspartic Acid	5.9	13.9	8.2	6.7	6.3
Threonine	3.0	1.4	6.4	9.2	9.4
Serine	6.9	8.6	14.1	14.2	8.7
Glutamic Acid	21.0	8.0	11.4	10.2	9.4
Proline	12.2	1.5	5.9	8.9	6.3
Glycine	8.4	12.6	6.4	8.2	7.9
Alanine	6.4	15.6	5.9	8.6	9.4
Half Cystine	1.8	0.1	2.3	2.1	0.8
Valine	2.4	1.3	7.3	7.6	9.4
Methionine	1.5	1.5	0.9	0	0.8
Isoleucine	4.3	2.5	3.2	2.2	3.9
Leucine	13.1	3.7	9.1	6.0	5.5
Tyrosine	1.8	5.2	4.1	3.3	3.9
Phenylalanine	4.9	7.3	3.7	1.9	3.9
Tryptophan	1.8	nd	0.9	1.9	1.9
	100.0	99.9	99.9	99.9	100.0

Rechromatography was done after the material was reduced and amino-
ethylated in 6M guanidine hydrochloride, 0.1M DTT in 0.5M Tris.HCl, pH 8.5
[3]. For amino acid analysis, purified protein was hydrolyzed with 6N
HCl at 110°C for 24 h. Analysis was performed with an automatic amino
acid analyzer (Hitachi KLA-5). Tryptophan contents were determined by
amino acid analysis after hydrolysis with 3N mercaptoethane-sulfonic acid.

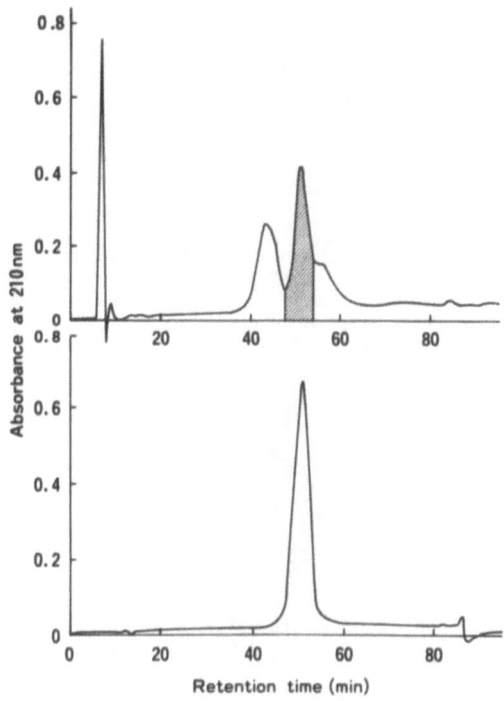

Fig. 4. Purification by reverse phase
HPLC of amyloid protein CEOT;
elution profile of low-molecu-
lar weight components of Sephadex G-100 fraction (upper) and
rechromatography by reverse
phase HPLC of the second peak
(hatched) in the lower panel.

Half cystine contents were determined as AEC by amino acid analysis of the
AE-protein as described previously [3].

    Sequence analysis by the manual Edman degradation was carried out as
previously described. SDS-urea disc electrophoresis of the purified protein was carried out as described previously [3].

    Antiserum against the purified protein (Tan) was raised in the rabbits
by repeated immunization of degraded amyloid protein with 0.1N NaOH emulsified with an equal volume of complete Freund's adjuvant. Immunodiffusion
analysis was done between the antiserum and antigens including degraded
antigens off AA (kub), AL (3 kappa and 5 lambda), AE (medullary carcinoma
of the thyroid) studied in our laboratory [3]. Normal pooled sera (NS$_1$ and
NS$_2$) was also used.

Biochemical Study

    Figure 3 shows the yield at each extraction step of crude amyloid
fibril proteins by distilled water. The decrease in the PBS-soluble proteins is shown on the left side, and the profile of the extraction of the
water-soluble fractions on the right side of the figure. The amount of
the extract protein is indicated as dry weight of the proteins.

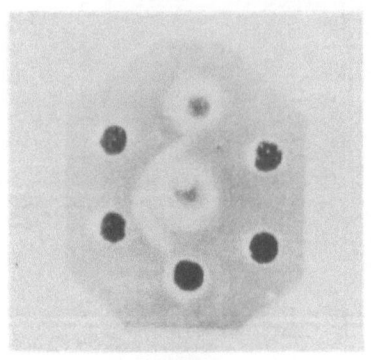

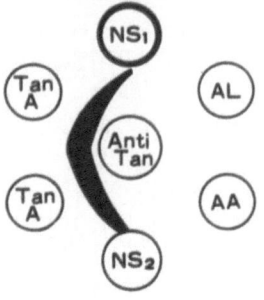

Fig. 5. Positive immune pre-
         cipiration of CEOT
         amyloid protein
         against anti CEOT,
         with no cross-reac-
         tions with other pro-
         teins by Ouchterlony.

        Through Sephadex G-100 column, crude amyloid proteins were fraction-
ated into two peaks, the void volume and another major peak containing low
molecular weight. The latter material was then applied to HPLC, where
two peaks were recorded as shown in the upper panel of Fig. 4. Further
purification was obtained by rechromatography with the same column, yielding a symmetrical peak in the lower panel of Fig. 4, which was designated
as the major component of amyloid protein CEOT from a patient Tan. Table
1 summarizes an amino acid analysis of amyloid protein CEOT, compared with
those of AA (kub), AL (Tew and Kor) and AFj (prealbumin, Am-16), all of
which have already been worked up in our laboratory. The composition of
the major component of CEOT is unique and is quite different from those of
the other amyloid proteins or precursor proteins. Especially noteworthy
is that CEOT protein has high contents in glutamic acid, proline and leucine together with low contents in basic amino acids. The molecular weight
was estimated by SDS-PAGE, giving a smear-like spot on repeated trials,
despite several trials in varying conditions, probably due to insolubility
property of this protein. An extimated Mw of the major component of CEOT
is approximately 30,000 daltons, although further clarification is to be
required. The N-terminus is rather heterogeneous, but a Ser-Gly- sequence
is to be deduced as its N-terminal positions on the basis of recoveries of
PTH-amino acid at each step.

Immunochemical Study

Figure 5 demonstrated the immunodiffusion profile by Ouchterlony method, in which a center well filled with the antiserum against CEOT (anti Tan). The antiserum reacted with the homologous antigen (Tan A), without any evidence of cross-reactions with two batches of normal pooled sera (NS$_1$ and NS$_2$), or with two types of amyloid degraded antigens (AL and AA). Other 5 AL's and AE studied in our laboratory were also negative. These findings suggest that the CEOT amyloid has antigenic determinants different from those of the other amyloid materials and normal serum components.

DISCUSSION

Calcifying epithelian odontogenic tumor (CEOT), first described by Pindborg in 1958, is now recognized as a distinctive entity among the epithelial odontogenic tumors, although the incidences of the cases are still limited [2]. The tumor invades the mandible and the maxilla, usually in the premolar-molar region. Histologically, the tumor consists of sheets of polyhedral cells in a connective tissue stroma. They tend to be closely packed and their nuclei considerably vary in shape and in size. This paper shows the light and electron microscopic findings most of which were consistent with those of the cases previously reported [2]. Associations of amyloid deposits and calcification are characteristic of this tumor and thus CEOT is one of the amyloid-producing tumors [2].

The presented data on the biochemical and immunochemical analyses of the amyloid fibril protein CEOT (Tan) demonstrate that it is a unique protein species which has not been described. Although further clarifications are required, we propose that it is a new type of amyloid fibril protein. Since the close association of the deposition of amyloid materials and calcification is generally observed, it should be a good example to study not only for the pathogenesis of this disease, but also for amyloidogenesis in general.

REFERENCES

1. A. L. Cohen, E. S. Cathcart, M. Skinner, Arth. Rheum., 21:153 (1978); G. G. Glenner, Néw Engl. d. Med., 302:1283 (1980).
2. J. J. Pindborg, Cancer, 11:838 (1958); D. G. Gardner, L. Michaels, M. C. Path, E. Piepa, Oral Pathology, 26:812 (1969); D. L. Page, J. W. Weiss, J. C. Eggleston, Cancer, 36:1426 (1975); G. Chomette, M. Auriol., F. Guilbert, Virchows Arch (Pathol. Anat.), 403:67 (1984).
3. T. Shinoda, K. Titani, F. W. Putnum, J. Biol. Chem., 245:4463 (1970); T. Isobe, Acta Haem. Jap., 41:757 (1978); T. Shinoda, T. Takahashi, T. Takayasu, T. Okuyama, A. Shimizu, Proc. Natl. Acad, Sci. USA, 78: 785 (1980).

IMMUNOLOGICAL HOMOLOGY OF THE AMYLOID OF INSULINOMA AND THE ISLET AMYLOID

OF THE AGED: BIOCHEMICAL CHARACTERIZATION OF THE INSULINOMA AMYLOID

Takako Iwata*, Shigeyoshi Fujihara†,
Yoshimi Yamashita†, and Fumiya Uchino†

*Yamaguchi University
 School of Allied Health Sciences
 Ube, Yamagushi, 755, Japan

†First Department of Pathology
 Yamaguchi University School of Medicine
 Ube, Yamaguchi, 755, Japan

ABSTRACT

Amyloid fibril protein was isolated from the insulinoma which was revealed by frequent hypoglycemic attacks clinically. In the tumor the
large quantities of amyloid was found between the tumor cells. About 235
mg (dry weight) of crude material (Insul 'A') was isolated from 7.5 gm of
the frozen tumor tissue. The estimated molecular weight of Insul'A' was
about 12,000 daltons. The amino acid composition of the protein was different from any of insulin, C-peptide and proinsulin. Rabbits were immunized and the antiserum against Insul'A' was obtained. By indirect immunoperoxidase (PAP) method, these amyloid deposits showed negative reaction
to any of antisera against AA, Aκ, Aλ, prealbumin, insulin, glucagon,
gastrin and somatostatin. Anti-Insul'A' reacted positively with the insulinoma amyloid as well as all of 23 cases of islet amyloid of the aged but negatively with other control amyloid tissues, such as AA, Aκ, Aλ, AF_j, AS_c, AMC_t.
The cytoplasm of the insulinoma cells reacted positively with anti-insulin but
gave negative reaction with anti-Insul'A' or other hormones. The results
suggested the homology of the insulinoma amyloid and the islet amyloids of the
aged.

INTRODUCTION

It is well-known that some endocrine tumors such as thyroid medullary
carcinoma often contain amyloid, which has been called apudamyloid by
Pearse et al. [1]. Insulinoma is also frequently accompanied by amyloid
deposits like a thyroid medullary carcinoma. Whereas in medullary carcinoma amyloid protein appears to be established as procalcitonin origin [2],
the nature of the amyloid in the insulinoma is still unclear.

Deposition of amyloid in the islets of Langerhans of patients with
diabetes or the aged is a well known phenomenon, too, and insulin or proinsulin has been presumed as an important constituent of islet amyloid
[3], but the origin of the amyloid protein is yet obscured.

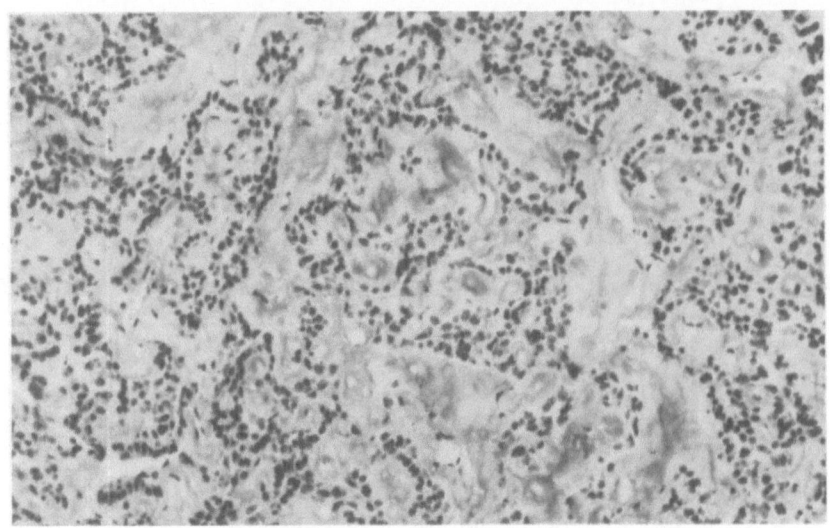

Fig. 1. Massive amyloid deposition is found in the interstitium
of insulinoma. Congo red stain.

Recently we examined a case of insulinoma with abundant amyloid deposits. Amyloid fibril protein was isolated from the tumor and antiserum
against it was obtained. The analysis of its amino acid composition was
performed.

In this paper, amyloid protein of insulinoma was compared with that
of systemic or localized amyloidosis using the obtained antiserum immunohistochemically. The homology of the antigenisity between the insulinoma
amyloid and the islet amyloid of the aged was shown.

MATERIALS AND METHODS

Case Report

A 56-year old male had been suffered from frequent attacks of con-
vulsion and unconsciousness preparedially for two years. Fasting blood sugar
ranged 12 to 127 (mean: 43) mg/dl and the radioimmunoassay showed increased plasma insulin level of 82 (normal 5-23) μm/ml. The symptoms were
improved by intravenous injection of glucose. Under the diagnosis of
insulinoma, the pancreatic tail tumor was resected surgically. It was
yellow in color, elastic soft in consistency and 6 × 6 × 4 cm in size.
Histopathologically massive amyloid deposition was recognized in the interstitium of the insulinoma (Fig. 1). After operation his blood glucose
level turned to normal.

Materials

About seven grams of resected tumor tissue was kept frozen at −80°C
and the remaining was fixed in buffered formalin or 3% glutaraldehyde for
histological examination. Paraffin sections were stained with hematoxylin-
eosin, alkalin Congo-red with or without potassium permanganate pretreatment [4], and studied immunohistochemically as described below. Electron-
microscopic findings were described elsewhere [5].

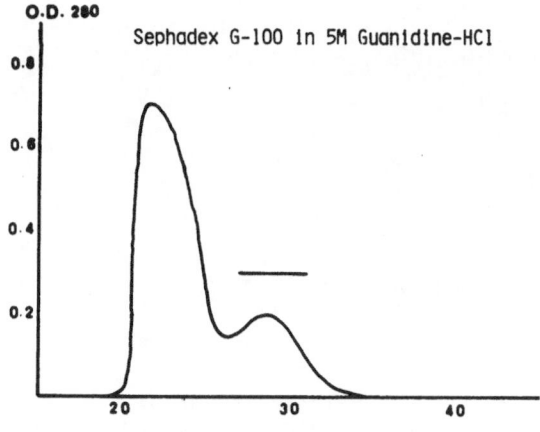

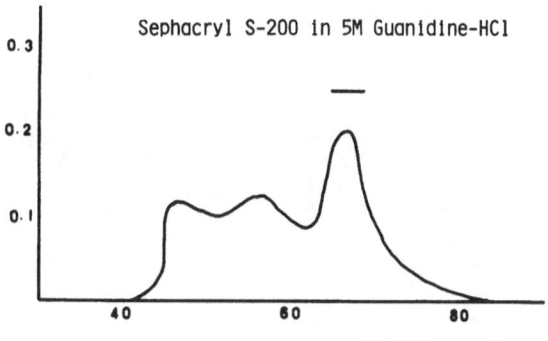

Fig. 2. A) Chromatogram of insulinoma extract from a column of Sephadex
G-100. B) Rechromatogram from a
column of Sephacryl S-200.

Purification of Amyloid

Amyloid fibrils were isolated from the frozen tumor tissue by the
method of Pras et al. [6] and Glenner et al. [7]. Amyloid was recovered
mainly in the sediment of distilled water extraction. This crude fibril
protein, Insul'A', was solubilized in 6M guanidine HCl 0,1M Tris-buffer
pH 8.2 and purified by gel filtration with the Sephadex G-100 column
equilibrilated with 5M guanidine HCl, of which pooled peak fractions were
rechromatographed with the Sephacryl S-200 column equilibrilated with 5M
guanidine HCl, followed by exhaustive dialysis to distilled water and
lyophilization. This purified protein was used for further biochemical analysis, for absorption of antiserum and for examination of antigenicity of
insulin and insulin C chain with radioimmunoassay.

SDS Polyacrylamide Gel Electrophoresis (PAGE)

For molecular weight determination, 10% SDS PAGE was performed [7]
with molecular weight markers such as, bovine albumin, cytochrome C,
chymotripsinogen A, myoglobin, and insulin commercially obtained from
Sigma.

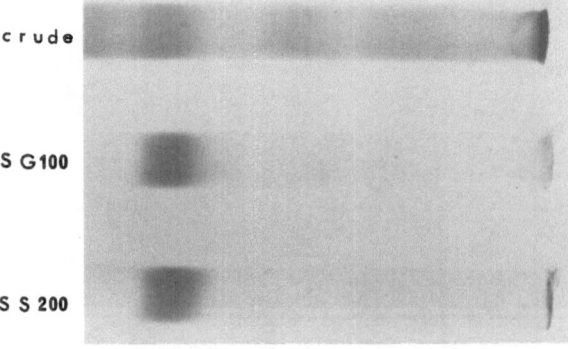

Fig. 3. By SDS polyacrylamide gel electrophoresis (PAGE) estimated molecular
weight of Insul'A' is about 12,000
daltons.

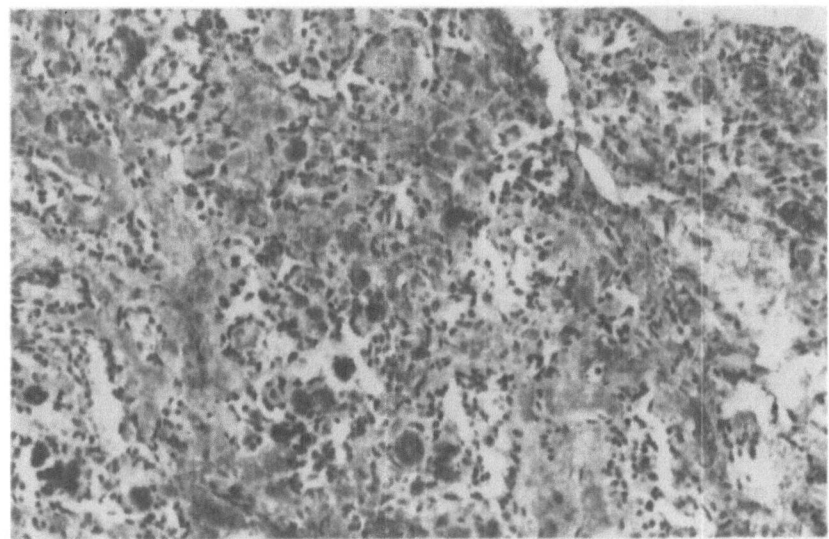

Fig. 4. By PAP method amyloid deposits in the tumor show strongly
positive reaction with anti-Insul'A' serum.

Analysis of Amino Acid Composition

The amino acid analysis of the purified protein was performed with
Hihon Denshi 200A under standard condition.

Preparation of Anti-Insul'A' Antiserum

Two rabbits were immunized with the unfractionated protein of Insul'A'
denatured with 6M guanidine HCl 0.1M Tris-buffered pH 8.2 and emulsified
in complete Freund's adjuvant. They were boosted triweekly and bled one
week after the booster injection.

TABLE 1.   Amino Acid Composition of
Purified Insul'A'

	Conc. (mg/g)	Molar ratio(%)
Asp	59.8	9.0
Thr	30.8	5.3
Ser	31.7	6.2
Glu	58.1	8.1
Pro	26.3	4.7
Gly	33.0	9.0
Ala	60.5	3.9
Cysteine	+	—
Val	55.0	9.6
Met	6.4	0.9
I-Leu	4.2	0.7
Leu	72.4	11.3
Tyr	13.2	1.5
Phe	42.7	5.3
His	38.2	5.0
Lys	52.1	7.3
Arg	22.8	2.7
Total	606.2	100

+ : under 3mg

Immunohistochemistry

Unlabeled immunoperoxidase (PAP) method for characterization of amyloid was described previously [8]. In this study the anti-prealbumin was
used in addition to anti-AA, Aλ, Aκ, antisera. Some anti-sera (DAKO,
Copenhagen) against the hormones produced by pancreatic islet cells such
as, insulin, glucagon, somatostatin, and gastrin were applied.

Control Studies

The amyloid tissues of known amyloid fibril proteins such as AA, Aλ,
Aκ, and prealbumin were examined as well as localized amyloid of the senile
heart, medullary carcinoma of the thyroid, senile plaques of the brain, and
of the senile pancreatic islets. The last were obtained from 23 autopsied
patients over 65 years old, of which three cases had clinically evident
diabetes mellitus. In order to check the specificity of the reaction of
the anti-Insul'A' antiserum, one ml of the anti-serum was absorbed with
one mg of the Insul'A' protein purified through the repeated gel filtration.

TABLE 2. Results of PAP I

Antisera / Tissues	AA	A κ	A λ	Prealb.	Insul'A'
Insul'A'	−	−	−	−	+
AA	+	−	−	−	−
A κ	−	+	−	−	−
A λ	−	−	+	−	−
AFj (Arao)	−	−	−	+	−
ASc	−	−	−	+	−
AMCt	−	−	−	−	−
Islet amyloid	−	−	−	−	+

TABLE 3. Results of PAP II

Antisera / Tissues	insulin	glucagon	gastrin	somatos.	Insul'A'
Insulinoma cells	+ +	−	−	−	−
Insulinoma amyloid	−	−	−	−	+
Islet amyloid	−	−	−	−	+

RESULTS

Purification of Amyloid Fibril Protein

About 235 mg (dry weight) of crude material (Insul'A') was isolated from 7.5 gm of the frozen tumor tissue. By the gel filtration with Sephadex G-100, following the void volume peak, the second peak was observed (Fig. 2A). By the SDS PAGE this second peak fractions were composed of two bands. One is the main band of molecular weight of about 12,000, which is also seen as the predominant band of the crude protein, unfractionated Insul'A'. Another is a faint band at the position of estimated molecular weight as about 27,000 (Fig. 3). Rechromatogram with Sephacryl S-200 of the pooled peak fractions showed the highest peak corresponding to the second peak of the Sephadex G-100 column chromatogram (Fig. 2B). The SDS PAGE of the peak fractions showed a single band with estimated molecular weight of about 12,000 (Fig. 3).

By the radio-immunoassay this purified protein was negative for insulin and insulin C-peptide.

Amino Acid Composition

The results of amino acid analysis of Insul'A' are shown in Table 1. Tryptophan was absent.

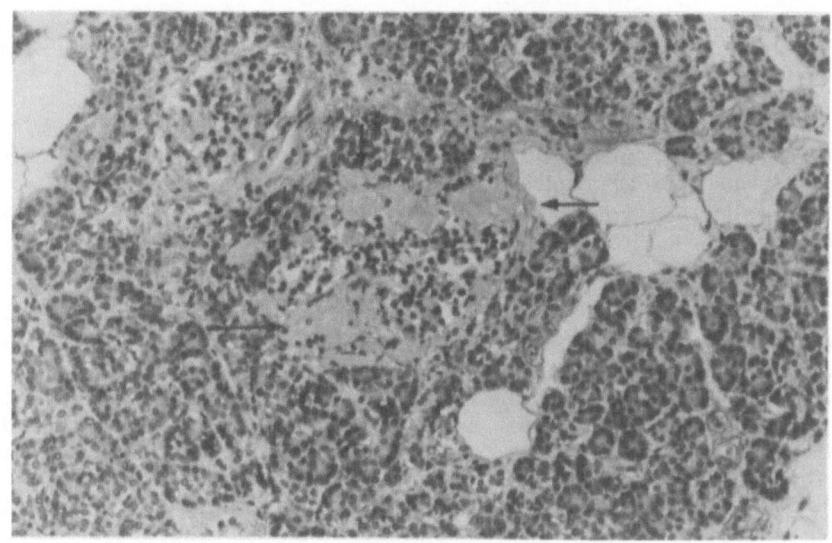

Fig. 5. Islet amyloid of the aged (arrows) is positively stained with anti-Insul'A' by PAP method.

Immunohistochemistry

The amyloid deposition in the interstitium of insulinoma and the control tissues except for those of AA protein showed resistance to the potassium permanganate treatment. The results of PAP are summarized as shown in Tables 2 and 3. Briefly, this insulinoma amyloid reacted only with the anti-Insul'A' (Fig. 4), and negative with the antisera against AA, Aλ, Aκ or prealbumin, which reacted specifically with the corresponding tissues. On the other hand, besides the insulinoma amyloid anti-Insul'A' reacted with all of the 23 cases of islet amyloid of the aged (Fig. 5). These reactions of the anti-Insul'A' were blocked by the absorption of the antiserum with the purified Insul'A' protein.

The cytoplasm of the insulinoma cells were stained positively with anti-insulin but negative for the antisera against the other hormones or anti-Insul'A'. The insulinoma amyloid and the islet amyloid of the aged reacted negatively with the antisera against insulin and other hormones.

DISCUSSION

Many investigators have tried to become clear the genesis of apud-amyloid. Morphological studies of the insulinoma indicated that the tumor cells were involved in the formation of amyloid [3, 6, 9, 10]. In 1972 Pearse et al. [1] studied endocrine polypeptide tumors histochemically and revealed the absence of tryptophan and tyrosin in apudamyloid. They also suggested that amyloid protein of insulinoma was derived from C-peptide chains.

On the other hand Westermark [11] isolated islet amyloid of Langerhans from the pancreases of patients with diabetes mellitus and said that C-peptide, insulin or ordinary insulin chains did not seem to constitute any major component of islet amyloid.

Schneider et al. [13] studied, however, islet amyloid of Langerhans and insulinoma immunocytologically, and considered insulin or proinsulin as a component of amyloid proteins.

In this study the amino acid composition of the isolated amyloid protein from insulinoma, Insul'A', was analyzed and it revealed that though tyrosine was found, no tryptophan was contained. The amino-acid composition was different from that of insulin, C-peptide or proinsulin. According to this result, insulin, C-peptide or proinsulin could not be considered as a major component of Insul'A'.

By the PAP method the antiserum against Insul'A' only reacted with the Insul'A' and the islet amyloid of the aged, and did not reveal any reaction with insulinoma cells. On the contrary, both amyloid deposits showed negative reaction to the antisera of insulin as well as all of the other peptide hormones and other amyloid protein examined, even though the insulinoma cells showed strongly positive reaction with the antinsulin serum. These results mean that the insulinoma cells are producing insulin, but the associated amyloid around the tumor cells is not the same product as insulin antigenetically, and that the Insul'A' and the islet amyloid of the aged have the same antigenesity.

Considering the above results of the amino acid analysis and the immunohistochemical studies, the homology of the insulinoma amyloid and the islet amyloid of the aged is suggested, and insulin, C-peptide or proinsul-proinsulin would not be a major component of their amyloid protein.

REFERENCES

1. J. E. Pearse, S. W. B. Ewen, J. M. Polak, Virchows Arch. Abt. B. Zellpathol., 10:93 (1972).
2. K. Sletten, P. Westermark, J. B. Natvig, J. Exp. Med., 143:993 (1976).
3. H.-M. Schneider, F. S. Storkel, W. Will, Path. Res. Pract., 170:180 (1980).
4. J. R. Wright, E. Calkins, R. L. Humphrey, Lab. Invest., 36:274 (1977).
5. Y. Yamashita, J. Clin. Electron Microscopy, 15:915 (1982).
6. M. Pras, M. Schubert, D. Zucker-Franklin, A. Rimon, E. C. Franklin, J. Clin. Invest., 47:924 (1968).
7. G. G. Glenner, M. Harada, C. Isersky, Prep. Biochem., 2:39 (1972).
8. S. Fujihara, J. E. Balow, J. C. Costa, G. G. Glenner, Lab. Invest., 43:358 (1980).
9. P. Westermark, L. Grimelius, J. M. Polak, L.-I. Larsson, S. V. Nourden, E. Wilander, A. G. E. Pearse, Lab. Invest., 37:212 (1977).
10. T. An, G. I. Kaye, Arch. Pathol. Lab. Med., 102:227 (1978).
11. P. Westermark, Acta Path. Microbiol. Scand. Sect. C, 83:439 (1975).

ACKNOWLEDGEMENT

We express our thanks to Prof. G. G. Glenner who supplied us with his antisera generously. This work was supported by a Grant-in-Aid for Scientific Research of the Minstry of Education.

HISTOPATHOLOGY OF CUTANEOUS AMYLOID: A COMPARATIVE STUDY ON 144 CASES OF LOCALIZED CUTANEOUS AMYLOIDOSIS AND 20 CASES OF SYSTEMIC AMYLOIDOSIS

Yoshiko Okuzono, Toshikazu Gondoh,
Hiroo Kawano, Takaaki Nagasawa, and
and Fumiya Uchino

First Department of Pathology
Yamaguchi University School of Medicine
Ube, Yamaguchi, 755, Japan

ABSTRACT

Skin specimens from 164 patients were studied, including 20 cases of systemic and 144 cases of localized cutaneous amyloidosis.

In localized cutaneous amyloidosis, subepidermal amyloid deposits were noted only in the papillae (136/144), the subpapillary layer (75/144) and the uppermost part of the reticular layer (2/144). Mesenchymal cells in the amyloid deposits, intraepidermal amyloid fragments and pigmentary incontinence were detected in 102, 43 and 121 cases respectively.

In systemic amyloidosis, amyloid deposits were detected in 17 of the 20 cases, whose protein was identified by PAP method as Aλ (4/17), AA (6/17), AA + Aκ (2/17) and was unidentifiable in the rest. They were discerned in the papillae (2/17), the subpapillary layer (5/17), the reticular layer (4/17), the subcutaneous fatty tissue (6/17), around the appendages (7/17) and on the walls of vessels (16/17). Intraepidermal amyloid fragments (2/17), mesenchymal cells in amyloid (4/17) and pigmentary incontinence (2/17) were noted less frequently than in localized cutaneous amyloidosis.

It would appear that in systemic amyloidosis, skin involvement bears no reference to the property of amyloid protein and that the manner in which amyloid is deposited is not relevant in distinguishing localized cutaneous amyloidosis from systemic amyloidosis, except for the different distribution of the substances.

INTRODUCTION

Amyloidosis of the skin is divided into two main categories; which are localized cutaneous amyldosis and skin involvement by systemic amyloidosis. Although amyloid deposits are often found in the deeper dermis in systemic amyloidosis, we may sometimes find the materials in the papillae or the subpapillary dermis where amyloid substances are usually seen in primary localized cutaneous amyloidosis. The authors analyzed 164 skin specimens

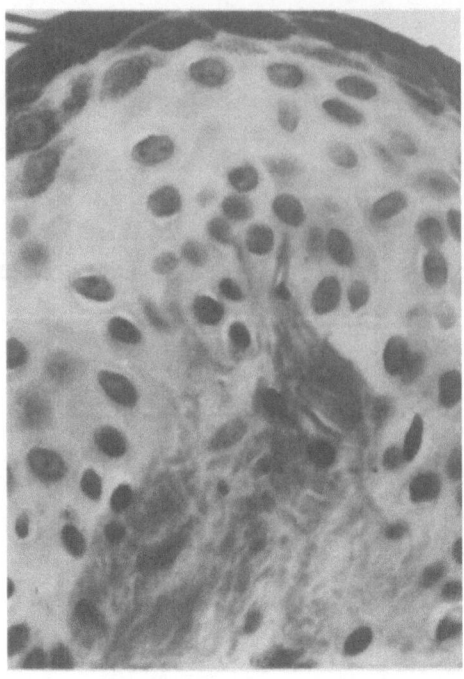

Fig. 1.   Amyloid seems to be interposed
between the basal cell layer.
Dylon multi stain, ×400.

obtained from 144 cases of primary localized cutaneous amyloidosis and 20
cases of systemic amyloidosis, and histopathologically compared the findings.

MATERIALS AND METHODS

144 biopsied skin specimens from localized cutaneous amyloidosis, all
of which were clinically regarded as primary type — lichen amyloidosus and
macular amyloidosis — and 20 skin specimens from systemic amyloidosis (one
biopsied case and 19 autopsied cases), were analyzed by light microscopy
with H.E. stain, Congo red stain, Dylon multi stain and Direct fast scarlet
stain.   They were further examined under polarized light after staining
with Congo red.   In order to certify the types of amyloid proteins, PAP
methods were applied on the specimens from all systemic cases and on several
specimens from localized cases.   The antisera used were anti-AA antiserum,
anti-Aλ antiserum, anti-Aκ antiserum, anti-prealbumin antiserum and anti-
keratin antiserum.   The anti-AL antisera were supplied by Dr. G. G. Glenner
generously.

RESULTS

Primary Localized Cutaneous Amyloidosis

In cases of this type, amyloid deposits were shown in the dermal
papillae (136 out of 144 cases), in the dermal subpapillary layer (75 out
of 144) and in the dermal reticular layer (only 2 out of 144).   We could
not find any deposits around the appendages, on the blood vessel walls
or in the subcutaneous fatty tissues.

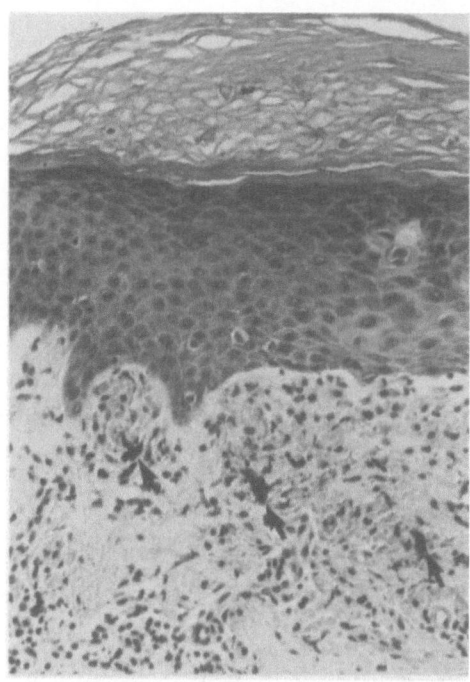

Fig. 2. Some mesenchymal cells within
the amyloid deposits. Some
such cells have melanin pigment in their cytoplasm (arrow).
Congo red stain, ×400.

There were various amounts of amyloid deposits in the dermal papillary
portion. Some contained so much that we were able to recognize them only
by H.E. stain; however, in many cases amyloid deposits were too small to
be recognized in the specimens stained without Congo red or other special
stainings for amyloid substances. They were composed of some particles
very close to the basal cell layer of the epidermis. In some places,
liquefactive degeneration of the basal cells was observed where amyloid
substances seemed to be interposed between the basal cells (Fig. 1). Even
in the two instances in which we found amyloid substances in the dermal
reticular layer, they were very close to the hair follicles. Liquefactive
degeneration was revealed in 62 out of 144 cases and amyloid substances
within the epidermis were shown in 43 out of 144 cases. Infrequently we
indeed found the Congo-red positive particles within not only the basal
cell layer but also within the squamous cell layer. These particles exhibited bright green birefringence under the polarized light.

One common finding, seen in many cases, was the occurrence of some
mesenchymal cells within the amyloid deposits. Some such cells had long,
slender projections and within their cytoplasm melanin pigment was observed (Fig. 2). Other common findings were pigmentary incontinence and
inflammatory cell infiltration in the dermal subpapillary and reticular
layers. We observed mesenchymal cells within the amyloid deposits in 102
out of 144 cases, pigmentary incontinence in 121 out of 144 and inflammatory cell infiltration in 82 out of 144 cases respectively.

In 85 out of 144 cases, the overlying epidermis showed hyperkeratosis,
and the rete ridges were flattened in 65 out of 144 cases-these cases

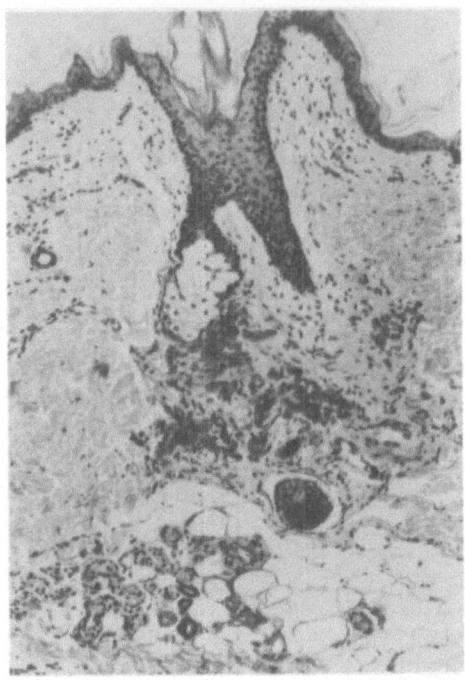

Fig. 3.   Amyloid deposits observed in
deep portion of the skin.
Congo red stain, ×100.

might be regarded as lichen amyloidosis (Fig. 2). These findings were
not revealed when the amounts of amyloid substances deposited were small.
Dyskeratosis was relatively common (33 out of 144); however, parakeratosis
was seldom found (3 cases only).

We examined several specimens by PAP method to certify the properties
of the amyloid protein. However, we failed to find reactive products with
any one of the antisera used.

Systemic Amyloidosis

In 17 out of 20 systemic cases, in which amyloid proteins had been
identified by PAP methods (AA in 6, Aλ in 4, AA with small amounts of Aκ
in 2 and with no reaction to any antisera in the rest), skin involvement
was demonstrated. The amyloid deposits were shown in the dermal papillae
(only two out of 17 cases), in the dermal subpapillary layer (5 out of 17),
in the dermal reticular layer (4 out of 17), around the appendages (7 out
of 17), on the vessel walls (16 out of 17) and in the subcutaneous fatty
tissues (6 out 17). In contrast with primary localized cutaneous amyloidosis, these tend to be deposited in the deeper portion of the skin (Fig. 3).

Concerning five cases that showed the substances in the dermal
papillary portion (in the dermal papillae and in the dermal subpapillary
layer), the configuration of the deposits was very similar to that seen
in the primary localized type (Fig. 4). In three cases the deposits were
separated from the epidermis by a narrow zone and arranged in corpuscular
figures, but in two cases these were obviously in contact with the epi-
dermal basal cell layer. In these cases small amounts of amyloid interposed between the cells were observed and liquefactive degeneration of the

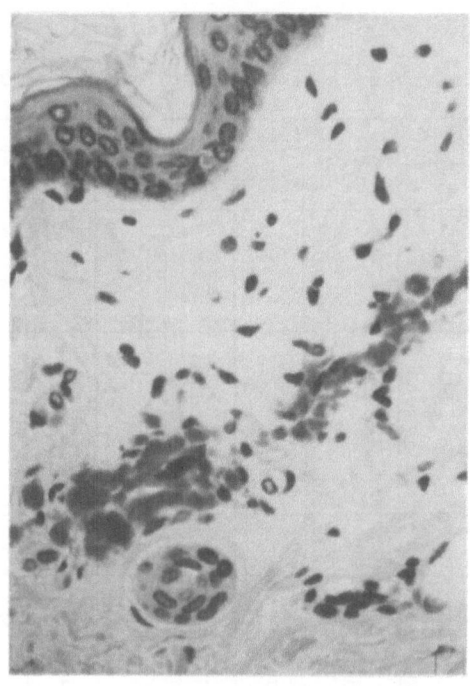

Fig. 4.   Amyloid deposited in a simi-
          lar manner as in primary
          localized cutaneous amyloidosis.
          Congo red stain, ×400.

basal cells was also found in one of them as in the case of primary localized cutaneous amyloidosis. Properties of amyloid proteins in both cases
were identified as Aλ. One of them was the autopsied case of a patient referred for primary systemic amyloidosis. This property of amyloid protein
was demonstrated to be the same as that in the deeper portion of the skin
such as around the appendages, on the vessel walls, in the subcutaneous
fatty tissues.

The mesenchymal cells were infiltrated in the deposits in 4 out of 5
cases mentioned above as in the cases of primary localized cutaneous
amyloidosis. Pigmentary incontinence was revealed in two cases that were
the same as those in which intraepidermal amyloid depositions were found.
However, it was slighter than in the cases of primary localized cutaneous
amyloidosis.

In conclusion, we found liquefactive degeneration in 1 out of 5 cases,
intraepidermal amyloid substances in 2 out of 5, mesenchymal cell infiltration within the deposits in all, and pigmentary incontinence in 2 out of
5 cases. The overlying epidermis showed neither hyperkeratosis nor dyskeratosis in systemic cases. These findings are summarized in Table 1,
and the compared frequencies of some typical findings between systemic and
localized cutanous amyloidosis are shown in Table 2.

DISCUSSION

In the present study we analyzed 164 cases of cutaneous amyloidosis
including 144 cases of primary localized type and 20 cases of systemic
amyloidosis and compared them histopathologically.

TABLE 1. Distribution of Amyloid in Systemic Amyloidosis

No.	SEX	AMYLOID PROTEIN		AMYLOID DEPOSITS IN THE SKIN							*DISTRIBUTION
		AA	A L	VOLUME	*DISTRIBUTION						
					PAP	RET	APP	VESS	FAT		
77-A-7	M	−	+ (Aλ)	3 +	−	−	−	3 +	−		PAP:
79-A-3	M	−	+ (Aλ)	3 +	−	−	−	3 +	/		Papillary portion
83-A-3	M	−	+ (Aλ)	3 +	+	2 +	+	2 +	3 +		RET:
84-B-1	F	−	+ (Aλ)	2 +	2 +	+	−	/	/		Reticular layer
78-A-1	F	+	−	+	−	−	−	+	−		APP:
78-A-2	M	+	−	2 +	−	−	+	3 +	−		Appendages
79-A-1	F	+	−	−							VESS:
79-A-4	F	+	−	2 +	−	−	2 +	+	+		Vessel walls
80-A-1	M	+	−	+	−	+	+	2 +	+		FAT:
82-A-1	F	+	−	2 +	+	+	3 +	2 +	+		Fatty tissues
75-A-1	F	+	+ (Aκ)	2 +	−	−	−	2 +	−		
79-A-2	F	+	+ (Aκ)	+	+	+	+	+	+		
69-A-2	F	−	−	+	−	−	−	+	−		
70-A-1	M	−	−	3 +	+	−	−	+	3 +		
70-A-2	M	−	−	+	−	−	+	+	−		
76-A-1	F	−	−	+	−	−	−	+	−		
77-A-1	M	−	−	+	−	−	−	+	−		
77-A-6	M	−	−	−							
81-A-1	F	−	−	−							
76-A-2	F	/	/	2 +	−	−	−	3 +	−		

TABLE 2. Comparative Frequencies of Common Findings

		SYSTEMIC AMYLOIDOSIS					*P L C A
		A L		A A			
		A λ		A A	AA+Aκ	TOTAL	
CASES ANALYZED		4	8	6	2	2 0	1 4 4
CASES WITH AMYLOID		4	6	5	2	1 7	1 4 4
DISTRIBUTION	PAPILLAE	2	0	0	0	2	1 3 6
	SUBPAPILLARY LAYER	2	1	1	1	4	7 5
	RETICULAR LAYER	2	0	2	1	4	2
	AROUND THE APPENDAGES	1	1	4	1	7	0
	VESSEL WALLS	3	6	5	2	1 6	0
	FATTY TISSUES	1	1	3	1	6	0
LIQUEFACTIVE DEGENERATION		1	0	0	0	1	6 2
INTRAEPIDERMAL AMYLOID		2	0	0	0	2	4 3
MESENCHYMAL CELLS WITHIN THE DEPOSITS		1	1	1	1	4	1 0 2
PIGMENTARY INCONTINENCE		2	0	0	0	2	1 2 1
HYPERKERATOSIS		0	0	0	0	0	8 5
DYSKERATOSIS		0	0	0	0	0	3 3
RETE RIDGE FLATTENING		0	0	0	0	0	6 5

*P L C A : Primary Localized Cutaneous Amyloidosis

We found skin involvement in 17 out of 20 cases of systemic amyloidosis. The properties confirmed by PAP method of amyloid proteins deposited in the skin were the same as those in the other organs. These were identified as AA in 7 cases (coexistent with small amounts of Aκ revealed in 2 cases), Aλ in 4 cases, and nonreactive with any antisera in the rest, which might be regarded as different subgrouped AL proteins. Some authors have pronounced that skin involvement was a more common finding in primary and myeloma-associated systemic amyloidosis, but even if found in secondary systemic amyloidosis, the amyloid is usually found only in the deep dermis [1, 2]. In the present study we showed that every type of amyloid protein was deposited in the skin, even in the dermal papillary portion. Thus it would appear that in systemic amyloidosis, skin involvement bore no reference to the properties of amyloid proteins.

The most important difference between primary localized cutaneous amyloidosis and skin involvement by systemic amyloidosis might be supposed to be the distribution of the substances. In primary localized cutaneous amyloidosis we found amyloid deposits only in the upper dermal portion; that is only in the dermal papillae, dermal subpapillary layer and in the uppermost part of the dermal reticular layer. However, in systemic amyloidosis we observed them besides, around the appendages, on the vessel walls and in the subcutaneous fatty tissues. Thus when amyloid substances are encountered in the deeper portion such as mentioned above in a biopsied skin specimen obtained from a patient clinically referred for primary localized cutaneous amyloidosis, systemic amyloidosis should be suspected and further examinations such as biopsies of the alimentary tract should be performed.

Concerning amyloid deposits in the dermal papillary portion (the dermal papillae and the dermal subpapillary layer), obvious histopathological differences were not shown between the primary localized type and the systemic type. Westermark previously proposed that pigmentary incontinence and liquefactive degeneration of the basal cells were specific findings of primary localized cutaneous amyloidosis [3]. We observed similar findings as mentioned by him in cases of systemic amyloidosis. Thus, we should conclude that liquefactive degeneration and/or pigmentary incontinence are not indications for primary localized cutaneous amyloidosis.

Hashimoto et al. and Maeda et al. have proposed the possibilities of epithelial cell degeneration and transformation of tonofilaments or microfilaments into amyloid fibrils in primary localized cutaneous amyloidosis [4, 5, 6]. We are not quite sure about pathogenesis in the present study but it might suggest the possible epithelial origin of amyloid in primary localized cutaneous amyloidosis in that liquefactive degeneration of the basal cells was often shown and small amyloid particles were observed even in the squamous cell layer.

CONCLUSION

1) Skin involvement by systemic amyloidosis was revealed in 17 out of 20 cases which we analyzed. By PAP method their amyloid proteins were identified as AA in 5 cases, AA + Aκ in 2 cases and Aλ in 4 cases. Although the rest could not be identified because they were non-reactive to any antisera, they may in fact be some different subgroups AL proteins.

2) In the cases of systemic amyloidosis, amyloid deposits were found in the dermal papillae (2/17), in the dermal subpapillary layer (5/17), in the dermal reticular layer (4/17), around the appendages (7/16), on the vessel walls (16/17) and in the subcutaneous fatty tissue (6/16). On the

other hand, in the cases of primary localized cutaneous amyloidosis we could find them only in the dermal papillae (136/144), in the dermal sub-papillary layer (75/144) and in the uppermost part of the dermal reticular layer (2/144).

3) Concerning the amyloid deposits in the dermal papillary portion, any obvious differences were not demonstrated histopathologically between primary localized cutaneous amyloidosis and systemic amyloidosis. In both of them common findings were observed; including mesenchymal cell infiltration into the deposits (102/144) in the former and 4/5 in the later), amyloid fragments interposed between the basal cells (43/144 in the former and 2/5 in the later) and pigmentary incontinence (121/144 in the former and 2/5 in the later).

4) When amyloid deposits are encountered around the appendages, on the vessel walls and/or in the subcutaneous fatty tissues in the biopsied skin specimens, further examinations such as biopsies of the alimentary tract should be performed on the patient. The most importnat difference between primary localized cutaneous amyloidosis and skin involvement by systemic amyloidosis, might be in the distribution of the amyloid substances.

REFERENCES

1. A. Rubinov and A. S. Cohen, Ann. Intren. Med., 88:781 (1978).
2. P. Westermark, Acta Pthol. Microbiol. Sand. (A), 81:718 (1972).
3. P. Westermark, Acta Dermatvener (Stockholm), 59:341 (1979).
4. K. Hashimoto and H. Kobayashi, in: Amyloid and Amyloidosis. G. G. Glenner, P. P. e Costa and A. F. de Freitas Eds. (Excerpta Medica, 426, 1980. Amsterdam-Oxford-Princeton, in press).
5. H. Maeda et al., Brut. J. Dermatol., 106:345 (1982).
6. K. Hashimoto and H. Kobayashi, Am. J. Dermatopathol., 2:165 (1983).

ACKNOWLEDGEMENTS

We express our thanks to Professors Fukushiro, Oohashi and many other doctors who sent their specimens to us and allowed us to analyze them, and Dr. G. G. Glenner who generously supplied us with his antiserum. This work was supported by a Grant-in-Aid for Scientific Research of the Ministry of Education.

HISTOLOGICAL EVIDENCE OF AMYLOID DEPOSITION IN OLD THROMBOTIC LESIONS AND
IN LONGTERM BIOPROSTHETIC CARDIAC VALVE IMPLANTS IN MAN: TWO RECENTLY
OBSERVED AND POSSIBLY RELATED FORMS OF LOCALIZED AMYLOIDOSIS OF THE
CARDIOVASCULAR SYSTEM

Yves A. Goffin, Fabienne Rickaert,
George D. Sorensen, and Erick Gruys

Department of Pathology,
Hôpital Brugmann and Hôpital Erasme
Free University of Brussels,
Brussels, Belgium

Department of Pathology
Dartmouth Medical School
Hanover, New Hampshire, U.S.A.

Department of Pathology
Institute of Vterinary Medicine
State University of Utrecht
New Utrecht, The Netherlands

ABSTRACT

In a series of old thrombotic lesions, amyloid deposition is shown in
sclerotic heart valves, a thrombus of the left atrium, a post-infarction
aneurysm of the left ventricle, two arterial aneurysms and an encapsulated
scalp hematoma. The deposits are permanganate-resistant and contain tryptophan. Electron microscopy demonstrates typical fibrils in three cases. No
patient showed evidence of systemic amyloidosis.

The natural history of sclerocalcific valvulopathies and present observations favor the following pathogenesis: ageing of the thrombus with degradation of a coagulation-related amyloid precursor protein and its transformation into amyloid fibrils; inclusion of amyloid in replacement sclero-
sis.

In a parallel study of bioprosthetic cardiac valve explants, amyloid
microdeposits were demonstrated in a fascia lata valve and 23 porcine aortic
valves (PAV) (47% of all longterm implants): Electron microscopy confirmed
this finding in 3 PAV. All positive PAV had been implanted for at least 33
months and all except 5 presented dysfunction and/or severe cusp degradation. In most cases, amyloid was permanganate-resistant and tryptophan-
positive.

The pathogenesis of this new form of amyloidosis might consist in penetration of human macrophages in deteriorated cusps and their interaction
with blood-borne precursors. One of these may be identical to the precursor involved in thrombus-related amyloidosis.

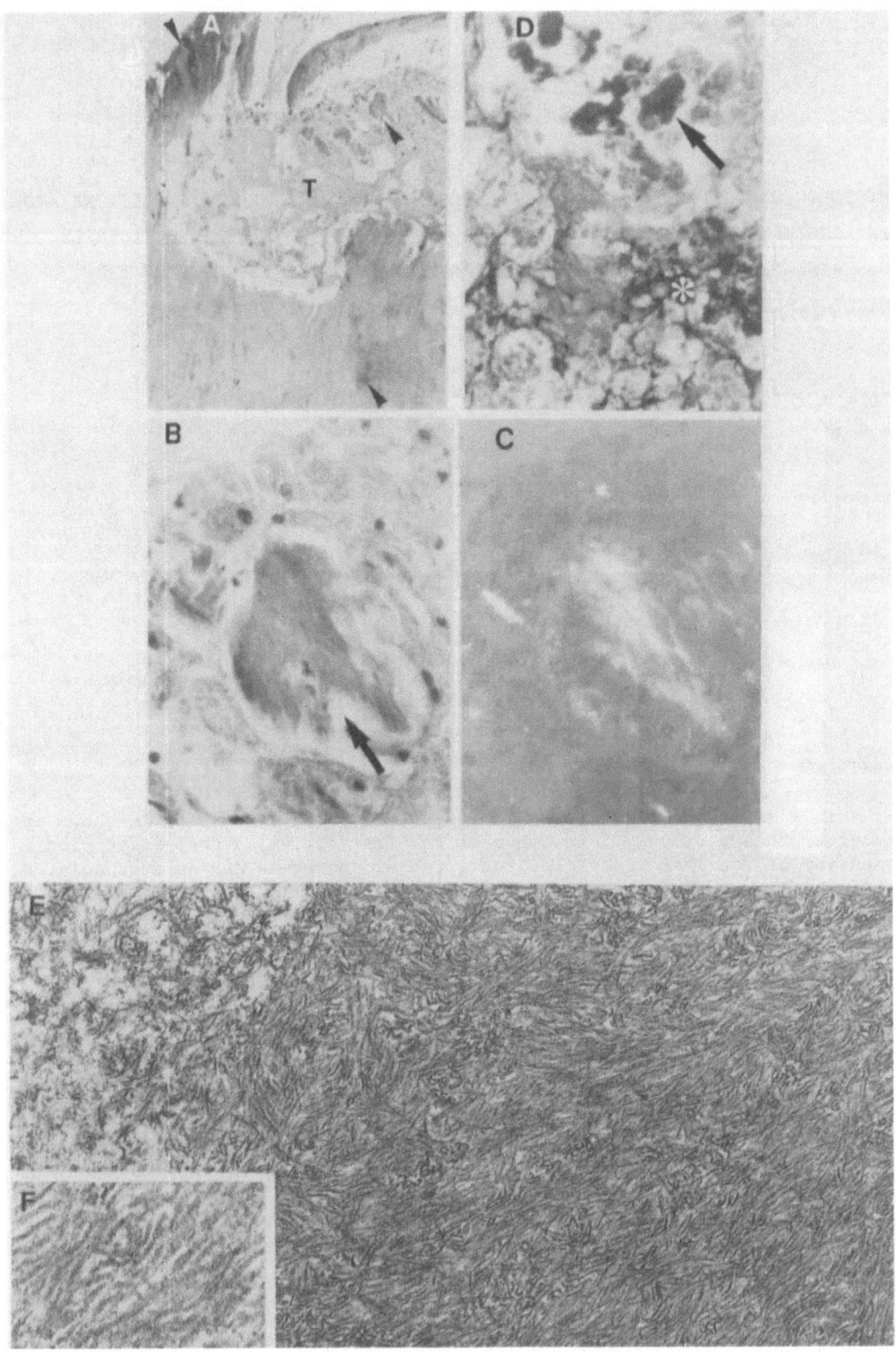

INTRODUCTION

Deposition of amyloid in human sclero-calcific heart valves has been reported recently, as a localized age-independent and dystrophic form of amyloidosis [2]. Histochemical studies have shown that the deposits are permanganate-resistant, contain tryptophan and P-component and are immunologically unrelated to any known type of amyloid fibril protein [2].

METHODS AND RESULTS

In our study, histological observations from a series of four selected sclerotic heart valves show amyloid deposition in old thrombotic material covering fusing commissures of appositional collagen on the body of the leaflets. Similar cases from extravalvular sites have been added to the series: a partly hyalinized thrombus of the left atrium, a thrombotic aneurysm of the left ventricle, two thrombotic atherosclerotic aneurysms of the aorta and popliteal artery respectively and an encapsulated hematoma of the scalp (Table 1).

Samples were fixed in 10% formalin and embedded in paraffin; 6 μm sections were stained with hematoxylin-eosin-saffron, alkaline Congo red, orcein-Van Gieson and phosphotungstic acid hematoxylin for fibrin. Sections were treated with potassium permanganate prior to Congo red staining and the DMAB method for tryptophan. The Congo red stained sections were mounted in arabic gum-sucrose in order to prevent unspecific greenish birefringence of dense collagen bundles. The diagnosis of amyloid was made on the basis of its selective affinity for alkaline Congo red and subsequent apple green birefringence under polarized light.

For transmission electron microscopy (TEM), paraffin embedded tissues were deparaffinized, postfixed in 2.5% GTD and 2% O_SO_4 and embedded in epon. Thin sections were stained with lead citrate and examined on a Philips EM 400 T.

The deposits are Congo red positive with typical green dichroism in polarized light, permanganate resistant and contain tryptophan. Electron microscopy displays small fibrils which are consistent with amyloid (Fig. 1). No patient showed evidence of systemic amyloidosis.

The natural history of sclero-calcific valvulopathies and present observations favor the following pathogenesis: first, recurrent thrombotic disposition on thickened and fibrotic endocardium: second, degradation of a coagulation-related protein with B-potential during the ageing of the clot with tranformation into amyloid fibrils; finally, inclusion of the amyloid in sclerotic replacement tissue.

In a parallel study, Congo red staining with microscopic examination under polarized light was performed in 81 porcine bioprosthetic cardiac valves and one autologous fascia lata valve explanted from 78 patients in order to detect the presence of amyloid.

Fig. 1. Fusing commissure of a sclerotic postrheumatic aortic stenosis in a 53 year-old female (case 6). A) Low magnification showing an area of replacement fibrosis covered by thrombotic material (T): amyloid deposits (arrows) are present both in the thrombus and sclerotic tissues; B, C, and D) high magnification of the thrombus showing macrophages and fibrin streaks (×) around the deposits (arrow). Typical birefringence of amyloid in C. (A - Congo red ×12.5, B and C - Congo red ×125, D - HPTA - ×125.) Electron micrographs of Congo-red positive material show nonbranching fibrils disposed at random (mean width: 11 nm) E, ×42.500, F, 115000.

TABLE 1. Clinical and Histopathological Data* in 10 Cases of Coagulation – Related Amyloid

Cases	Age (Y) and sex	Site of amyloid deposition	Clinical diagnosis	Histological findings*
1	75 m	Left atrium	Large mural thrombosis, chronic rheumatic carditis	Partly hyalinized thrombus attached to sclerotic endocardium
2	62 f	Mitral valve	Sclerotic stenosis, chronic rheumatic endocarditis	Old thrombotic deposits partly replaced by sclerotic tissue
3	49 m	Mitral valve	Sclerotic stenosis, chronic rheumatic endocarditis	Sclerotic adhesion of commissure covered by thrombotic deposits
4	39 f	Mitral valve	Sclerotic stenosis, chronic rheumatic endocarditis	Sclerotic adhesion of commissure covered by thrombotic deposits
5	56 m	Left ventricle	Ventricular aneurysm with thromobosis, resulting from myocardial infarction	Old scar of transmural myocardia with partly hyalinized thrombus
6	53 f	Aortic valve	Sclerotic stenosis, chronic rheumatic endocarditis	Fibrotic infiltration of ventricularis covered by thrombotic deposits sclerotic adhesion of the 3 commissures
7	77 m	Abdominal aorta	Atherosclerotic aneurysm	Ulcerated calcified atheroma covered by thrombotic deposits
8	73 m	Femoral	Atherosclerotic aneurysm with thromobisis	Ulcerated atheroma with micro-calcifica-tion; covered by hyalinized thrombus
9	76 m	Popliteal artery	Atherosclerotic aneurysm with thrombosis	Ulcerated atheroma with micro-calcifica-tions, old intraparietal hemorrhage and hyalinized thrombus
10	60 m	Scalp	Old encapsulated hematoma	Old hematoma surrounded by sclerotic tissue

*Exclusive of amyloid.

TABLE 2. Comparative Clinical Data in a Series of Amyloid Positive and Amyloid Negative Porcine Aortic Valve Bioprotheses

	Age (years)	Sex		Implantation site		Implantation duration (months)	Valve function		Type	
		M	F	Mitral	Aortic		N	AN	C.E.	Hancock
Amyloid Positive valves (27 cases)	9-74 Mean: 47	14	13	13	14	33-101 Mean: $70^{1}/_{3}$	5	22	12	15
Amyloid Negative valves (35 cases)	11-69 Mean: 41	14	21	26	9	30-130 Mean: 64	9	26	11	24
Total 62 cases	9-74 Mean: 44	28	34	39	23	30-130 Mean: 67	14	48	23	39

N = Normal.
AN = Abnormal.
C.E. = Carpentier-Edwards.

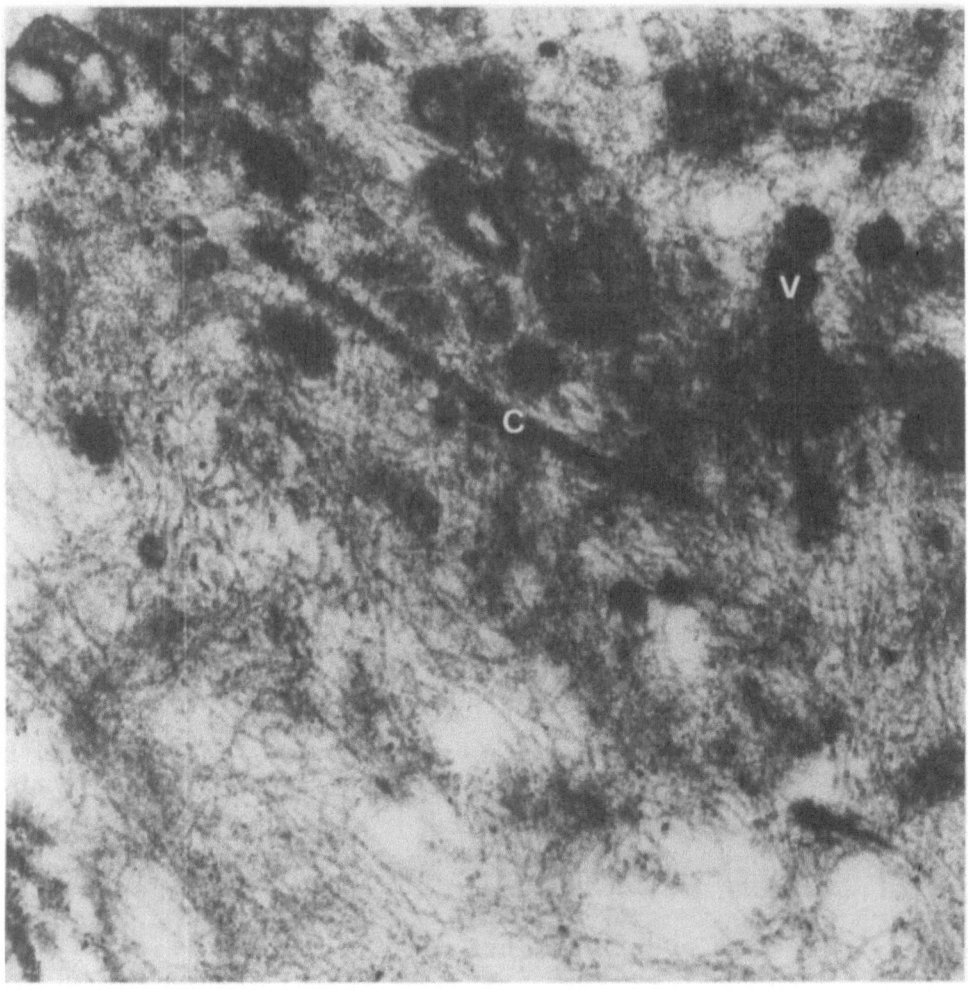

Fig. 2. Electron micrograph of the superficial area of a Carpentier-
Edwards porcine aortic valve implanted for 82 months in mitral
position in a 63-year old woman. Masses of criss-crossed non-
branching amyloid fibrils are seen together with a collagen fiber
(C) and remnants of electron dense membrane-bound vessels (V)
(lead citrate × 102,000).

The same histological and histochemical methods were used as for the
thrombus study. The blocks for TEM were postfixed in one percent buffered
osmium tetroxide, contrasted with uranyl acetate and embedded in epon.
Thin sections were contrasted with lead acetate and analyzed on a Philips
201 electron microscope. Chi squared and Student t tests were applied for
statistical analyses of the results.

Microdeposits of amyloid were present in the sewing ring of the fascia
lata valve and in 33 porcine bioprostheses: This finding was confirmed by
transmission electron microscopy in three porcine bioprostheses (Fig. 2).
All amyloid-laden porcine valves had been implanted for at least 33 months
before removal and all except five showed dysfunction and/or severe degeneration of cuspal tissues (Table 2, Fig. 3). All patients over the age of
70, except one, had positive valve although statistical analyses failed to

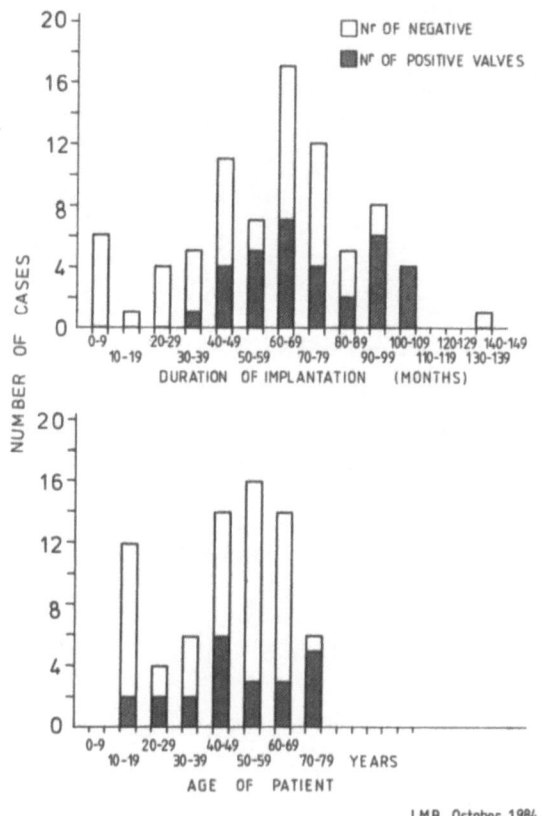

Fig. 3. Histograms displaying total numbers of cases and numbers of cases and numbers of amyloid positive cases per month of implantation decade (top) and patients age decade (bottom).

establish any correlation between the presence of amyloid and patient-related factors. The amyloid was permanganate-resistant in the fascia lata valve, while in a vast majority of porcine bioprostheses the deposits were tryptophan-positive as well.

The pathogenesis of this new form of heart valve amyloidosis might consist in penetration of human macrophages in deteriorated bioprosthetic cusps and their interaction with blood-borne amyloid precursors [3].

One of these precursors may be identical to the one involved in thrombus-related amyloidosis.

REFERENCES

1. Y. Goffin, J. Clin. Pathol., 33, 262–268 (1980).
2. Y. Goffin, W. Murdoch, G. Cornwell, III, and G. Sorensen, J. Clin.. 36, 1342–1349 (1983).
3. Y. Goffin, E. Gruys, G. Sorensen, and F. Wellens, Am. J. Pathol., 114, 431–442 (1984).

CONTRIBUTORS

Dr. D. Allsop, The University of Nottingham, Nottingham, England.

Professor Corino de Andrade, Centro de Estudios de Paramiloidose, Servico de Medicina 2, Faculdade de Med., Hospital de S. Joao, Porto, Portugal.

Nobuyuki Anzai, M.D., Department of Cardiology and Cardiac Surgery, Higashi Nagano national Hospital, 2-477 Uwano Nagano City, Nagano 380, Japan.

Professor Shukuro Araki - Chairman, Dept. of Neurology, First Dept. Internal Medicine, Kumamoto Univ. Medical School, 1-1-1 Honjo, Kumamoto 860, Japan.

Dr. Marilyn L. Baltz, Immunological Medicine Unit, Department of Medicine, Royal Postgraduate Medical School, London W12 OHS, England.

Linda L. Bausserman, Ph.D., Asst. Prof. of Med. (Research), Brown Univ. Prog.-in-Medicine, The Miriam Hospital, 164 Summitt Ave., Providence, R. I. 02906.

Earl P. Benditt, M.D., Professor and Chairman, Department of Pathology, University of Washington, Seattle, WA. 98195.

Merrill D. Benson, M.D., Professor and Director, Division of Rheumatology, Indiana University School of Medicine, 11 West Michigan St., Indianapolis, IN. 46202.

Sydney R. Brandwein, M.D., Asst. Professor of Medicine, McGill University, Division of Rheumatology, Montreal General Hospital, 1650 Cedar Av., Montreal, Que., Canada H3G 1B4.

Vincent P. Butler, Jr., M.D., Professor of Medicine, Columbia University, College of Phys. & Surg., 630 West 168the St., New York, N. Y. 10032.

Joel Buxbaum, M.D., Professor of Medicine, Veterans Admin. Medical Center, First Ave. & 24th St., New York, N. Y., 10010.

Evan Calkins, M.D., Professor and Head, Division of Geriatrics & Gerontology, Department of Medicine SUNY at Buffalo, Buffalo, N. Y. 14215.

Ronald I. Carr, Ph.D., Assoc. Prof. of Medicine & Assoc. Prof. of Microbiology, Dalhousie University, Div. of Rheumatology, Halifax Civic Hospital, 5938 University Ave., Halifax, N.S., Canada, B3H 1V9.

Dr. Dan Caspi, MRC Research Fellow, Immunological Medicine Unit, Department of Medicine, Royal Postgraduate Medical School, London W12 OHS, England.

Edgar S. Cathcart, D.Sc., M.D., Direct, G.R.E.C.C., Professor of Medicine, Boston Univ. School of Medicine, E.N.R.M. Veterans Admin. Hospital, Bedford, MA 01730.

Dr. Larry K. Chaney, Post-doctoral Fellow, Arthritis Section, Boston Univ. School of Medicine, 71 East Concord St., Boston, MA 02118.

Alan S. Cohen, M.D., Director, Thorndike Memorial Laboratory, Chief of Medicine, Boston City Hospital, Thorndike 314, Boston, MA 02118.

Daniel H. Cohen, M.D., 200 Haven Ave., Apt. #3G, New York, N. Y. 10033

Ms. Lawreen Heller Connors, Graduate Student/Biochemistry, Boston Univ. School of Medicine, 71 East Concord St., Boston, MA 02118.

J. H. Cooper M. D., The Victoria General Hospital, Department of Pathology, 5788 University Ave., Halifax, N.S., Canada B3H 1V8.

Dr. Gibbons G. Cornwell, III, Professor of Medicine, Chief, Section on Hematology and Oncology, Dartmouth-Hitchcock Medical Center, Hanover, N. J. 03756.

Gerhard A. Coetzee, Ph.D., Senior Lecturer, Department of Medical Bio-chemistry, University of Cape Town Medical School, Observatory 7925, Cape Town, South Africa.

Dr. Pedro P. Costa, Chief, Laboratorio de Neuroquimica, Centro de Estodos de Paramiloidose, Hospital Geral de Santo Antonio, Porto, Portugal.

Dr. Frederick C. deBeer, Resident Coordinator, Consultant Physician, De-partment of Internal Medicine, University of Stellenbosch, P. O. Box 63, Medical School, Tygerberg, 7505, South Africa.

Stephen P. DiBartola, D.V.M., Asst. Professor of Medicine, College of Veterinary Medicine, Ohio State University, 1935 Coffey Road, Columbus, OH 43210.

Brian G. M. Durie, M.D., Professor of Medicine, Dept. of Hematology & Oncology, University of Arizona Health Sciences Center, Internal Medicine, Room 6324, Tucson, AZ 85724.

Francis E. Dwulet, Ph.D., Asst. Professor of Medicine, Indiana Univ. School of Medicien, Rheumatology Div. Clin. Bldg. 492, 541 Clinical Drive, Indianapolis, IN 46223.

Peter Ebbeson, M.D., Head, The Institute of Cancer Research, Radiumstationen Nörrebrogade 44, DK-8000, Aarhus, Denmark.

Nils Eriksen, Ph.D., Research Assitant Professor, Department of Pathology SM-30, University of Washington, Seattle, WA 98195.

M. Eulitz, M.D., Institut für Hämatologie, Gesellschaft fur Strahlen und Umweltforschung MBH, München Landwehrstrasse 61, 8000 München 2, West Germany.

Hans M. Falck, M.D., Fourth Dept. of Medicine, Helsinki University General Hospital, Unioninkatu 38, SF-00170, Helsinki 17, Finland.

Mehdi Farhangi, M.D., Associate Professor of Medicine, School of Medicine, University of Missouri-Columbia, N408 Medical Sciences Building, One Hospital Drive, Columbia, MO 65212.

Blas Frangione, M.D., Ph.D., Professor of Pathology, Department of Pathology, NYU Medical Center, 550 First Ave., New York, N. Y. 10016.

Dr. Shigeyoshi Fujihara, Department of Pathology, Yamaguchi University School of Medicine, Ube, Yamaguchi 755, Japan.

Joseph Gafni, M.D., Professor of Medicine, Heller Institute of Medical Research, Sheba Medical Center, Tel-Hashomer 52621, Israel.

Morie A. Gertz, M.D., Asst. Professor of Medicine, Department of Hematology, Mayo Medical School, Rochester, MN 55905.

George G. Glenner, M.D., Professor of Pathology, School of Medicine, University of California — San Diego, La Jolla, CA 92093.

Robert M. Glickman, M.D., Professor of Medicine, Columbia University, College of Physicians & Surgeons, 630 West 168th St., New York, N. Y. 10032.

Yves A. Goffin, M.D., Hôpital Universitaire, Brugmann Service Anatomie Pathologie, 4, Place van Gehuchten, B 1020 Brussels, Belgium.

DeWitt S. Goodman, M.D., Professor of Medicine, Columbia University, College of Physicians & Surgeons, 630 West. 168th St., New York, N. Y. 10032.

Peter D. Gorevic, M.D., Associate Professor of Medicine and Pathology, SUNY, Health Sciences Center 16T 030, Stony Brook, N. Y. 11724.

Professor E. Gruys, D.V.M., Ph.D., Institute of Veterinary Pathology, State University Utrecht, Yalelaan 1 - Postbus 80.158, de Ulthof - 3508 TD, Utrecht, The Netherlands.

Dr. Evan Hadley, National Institute on Aging, National Institutes of Health, Building 31, 2C06, Bethesda, MD 20205.

Reid R. Heffner, M.D., Department of Pathology, University of Buffalo and Erie County Medical Center, 462 Grider St., Buffalo, N. Y. 14215.

Peter N. Herbert, M.D., Professor of Medicine, Brown Univ. Program-in-Medicine, The Miriam Hospital, 164 Summitt Ave., Providence, R. I. 02906.

Keiichi Higuchi, Ph.D., Asst. Prof., Dept. of Pathology, Chest Disease Research Inst., Kyoto University, 53 Kawara-cho, Shogoin, Sakyo-ku, Kyoto 606, Japan.

Charles R. K. Hind, M.D., MRC Training Fellow, Immunological Medicine Unit, Royal Postgraduate Medical School, Du Cane Road, London W12, OHS, England.

Gunnar Husby, M.D., Professor and Director, Department of Rheumatology, Institute of Clinical Medicine, University of Tromsø, 9001 Tromsø, Norway.

Anne Husebekk, Research Fellow, Department of Rheumatology, University of Tromsø, Institute of Medicine, 9001 Tromsø, Norway.

Shu-ichi Ikeda, M.D., Department of Med. (Neurology), Shinshu University School of Medicine, Matsumoto, 390, Japan.

Shinichi Ikegawa, M.D., Postgraduate Student, First Dept. of Internal Medicine, Kumamoto Univ. Medical School, 1-1-1 Honjo, Kumamoto 860, Japan.

Masae Inokawa, M.D., Third Dept. of Internal Med., Hiroshima Univ. School of Medicine, 1-2-3 Kasumi, Minami-ku, Hiroshima 734, Japan.

Khalid Iqbal, Ph.D., N.Y.S. Institute for Basic Research in Developmental Disabilities, 1050 Forest Hill Road, Staten Island, N. Y. 10314.

Takashi Isobe, M.D., Professor, Department of Applied Medical Science, c/o Department of Medicine, Kobe University, Kusunokicho, Chuo-ku, Kobe City, Japan.

Takako Iwata, M.D., Professor, The School of Allied Health Sciences, Yamaguchi University, Ube, Yamaguchi 755, Japan.

Sven Janssen, M. D., Department of Medicine, University Hospital, Groningen, 59 Oostersingel, 9713, EZ, Groningen, The Netherlands.

Olafur Jensson, M.D., Director of the Blood Bank, National Hospital, University of Iceland, P. O. Box 1408, Reykjavik, Iceland.

Uma P. Kalyan-Raman, M. D., Assoc. Prof. Clin. Pathology, Dept. of Neurosciences, Univ. of Illinois, Coll. of Medicine, 530 N. E. Glen Oak Ave., Peoria, IL 61637.

Igal Kedar, M.D., Building 10, 8S South 243, NIA DDK, National Institutes of Health, Bethesda, MD 20205.

Koichi Kimura, M.D., Third Dept. of Internal Med., Kuramoto-cho 3, Tokushima, 770, Japan.

Yoshihiro Kimura, M.D., Postgraduate Student, First Dept. of Int. Med. & Second Dept. of Pathology, Kumamoto Univ. Medical School, 1-1-1 Honjo, Kumamoto 860, Japan.

Robert Kisilevsky, M.D., Ph.D., Professor, Departments of Pathology & Biochemistry, Queen's University, Kingston, Ontario, Canada, K7L 3N6.

Professor Shozo Kito, Professor of Internal Medicine, Third Dept. of Internal Med., Hiroshima University School of Medicine, 1-2-3 Kasumi, Minamiku, Hiroshima 734, Japan.

Robert A. Kyle, M.D., Division of Hematology & Internal Medicine, Mayo Clinic and Mayo Medical School, Rochester, MN 55905.

Dr. Gad Lavie, Director, Bloodbank and Center of Transfusion, Beilinson Medical Center, Tel-Aviv University, 59 100 Petah-Tiqva, Israel.

Jenny J. Li, Ph.D., Instructor of Surgery, Shriners Burn Institute, Mass. General Hospital, Harvard Medical School, Department of Surgery, Boston, MA 02114.

Caryn Libbey, M.D., 19 Tyler St., Nashua, NH 03060.

Dr. Reinhold P. Linke, Institüt fur Immunologie, Schillerstrasse 42, 8000 München - 2 West Germany.

Prof. Enno Mandema, Department of Medicine, University Hospital, Groningen, The Netherlands.

Thaddeus I. Mandybur, M.D., Ph.D., Professor of Pathology and Neurology, Director, Laboratory of Neuropathology, College of Medicine, University of Cincinnati School of Medicine, Cincinnati, OH 45267-0533.

Gudmund Marhaug, M.D., Assistant Professor, Department of Pediatrics, Institute of Clinical Medicine, University of Tromsø, N-9000 Tromsø, Norway.

Dr. Jan Marrink, Immunochemistry Laboratory, Department of Internal Medicine, University Hospital, 59 Oostersingle, 9713 EZ Groningen, The Netherlands.

Ms. Mary Ellen Martin, Assistant Clinical Instructor, Downstate Medical Center, 450 Clarkson Ave., Box 20, Brooklyn, N. Y. 11203.

Michael Mastranduno, M.D., Department of Medicine, Columbia University, Institute of Cancer Research, 701 West 169 St., New York, N. Y. 10032.

Dr. C. P. J. Maury, Assistant Professor of Medicine, Fourth Department of Medicine, University of Helsinki, Unioninkatu 38, SF-00170 Helsinki 17, Finland.

Dr. Keith P. W. J. McAdam, Professor of Clinical Tropical Medicine, London School of Hygiene & Tropical Medicine, Keppel St., Gower St., London WCIE, 7HT, England.

Rick Meek, Ph.D., Department of Pathology SM-30, University of Washington, Seattle, WA 98195.

Giampaolo Merlini, M.D., Institute of Cancer Research, Columbia University, 701 West 168 St., New York, N. Y. 10032.

George S. Merz, Ph.D., Head, Nerve Tissue Culture Lab., N. Y. State Institute for Basic Research in Developmental Disabilities, 1050 Forest Hill Road, Staten Island, N. Y. 10314.

Professor Shunsuke Migita, Department of Molecular Immunology, Cancer Research Institute, Kanazawa University, Takara-machi, Kanazawa 920, Japan.

Jane Morse, M.D., Assoc. Prof. Clinical Medicine, Department of Medicine, Columbia University, 630 West 169 St., New York, N. Y. 10032.

Thomas J. Muckle, M.D., Director of Laboratories, Chedoke McMaster Hospitals, McMaster Univ. School of Medicine, P. O. Box 2000, Station A, Hamilton, Ontario, Canada L8N 325.

Masamitsu Nakazato, M.D., Third Dept. of Internal Medicine, Miyazaki Medical College, 5200 Kiyotake, Miyazaki 889-16, Japan.

Prof. Jacob B. Natvig, Institute of Immunology and Rheumatology, Rikshospitalet University Hospital, Oslo 1, Norway.

Yoshiko Okuzono, M.D., Director, Department of Pathology, Yamaguchi University School of Medicine, Ube, Yamaguchi 755, Japan.

Elliott F. Osserman, M. D., Professor of Medicine, Columbia University, Institute of Cancer Research, 701 West 168 St., New York, N. Y. 10032.

Professor Mark B. Pepys, Head, MRC Acute Phase Protein Research Gr., Immunological Medicine Unit, Department of Medicine, Royal Postgraduate Medical School, Du Cane Road, London W12, OHS, England.

J. M. Powers, M. D., Department of Pathology, Medical University of South Medical University of South Carolina, Charleston, SC 29403.

Mordechai Pras, M. D., Professor of Medicine, Tel-Aviv University, Heller Institute of Medical Research, Sheba Medical Center, Tel-Hashomer 52621, Israel.

Dr. Donald L. Price, Professor of Neurology & Pathology, Deparrment of Neuropathology, The Johns Hopkins Hospital, Baltimore, MD 21205.

Stanley B. Prusiner, M. D., Associate Professor, Department of Neurology, University of California M-794, San Francisco, CA 94143.

Moti Ravid, M. D., Head, Department of Medicine, Meir Hospital, Kfar Saba, Israel.

C. Julian Rosenthal, M. D., Associate Professor of Medicine, Department of Medicine, Downstate Medical Center, State University of New York, Brooklyn, N. Y. 11203.

Ian F. Rowe, M. D., MRC Training Fellow, Immunological Medicine Unit, Department of Medicine, Royal Postgraduate Medical School, Du Cane Road, London W12 OHS, England.

Alan S. Rubinow, M.D., Chief, Rheumatology, Hadassah Medical Center, Department of Medicine "A", Ein Kerm, Jerusalem, Israel.

George H. Sack, Jr., M.D., Ph.D., Assoc. Professor of Medicine Pediatrics & Biol. Chemistry, Joseph Earle Moore Clinic, The Johns Hopkins Hospital, Department of Medicine, Baltimore, MD 21205.

Saburo Sakoda, M.D., Research Fellow, The Third Department of Internal Medicine, Osaka University Hospital, Fukushima-ku, Osaka 553, Japan.

Dr. Maria João Saraiva, Department of Bioquimica, Instituto de Ciencias Biomedicas, Universidade do Porto, Largo da Escola Medica, 4000 Porto, Portugal.

Dr. Edward L. Schneider, National Institute on Aging, National Institutes of Health, Bethesda, MD 20205.

Morton A. Scheinberg, M.D., Ph.D., Head of Immunology, Instituto do Cancer Arnaldo, Vieria de Carvalho, Rua Cesario Motta Jr. 112, Sao Paolo, Brazil.

Dennis J. Selkoe, M.D., Ralpha Lowell Laboratories, Mailman Research Center, McLean Hospital Belmont, MA 02178.

William H. Sherman, M.D., Assistant Professor of Medicine, Department of Medicine, Columbia University, 161 Ft. Washington Ave., New York, N. Y. 10032.

Katsuji Shimizu, M.D., Chief, Department of Orthopaedic Surgery, 1-1 Kifunemachi, Koburakitaku, Kitakyushi 802, Japan.

Tomotaka Shinoda, Ph.D., Associate Professor, Department of Biochemistry, Tokyo Metropolitan University, Setagaya-ku, Tokyo 158, Japan.

Tsuranobu Shirahama, M.D., Dept. of Medicine (Arthritis), Boston University School of Medicine, Thorndike Memorial Laboratory, Boston, MA 02118.

Dr. Jean D. Sipe, Arthritis Section, Division of Medicine, E337, Boston University School of Medicine, 75 East Newton St., Boston, MA 02118.

Martha Skinner, M.D., Director of Research, Arthritis Section, Boston University School of Medicine, 75 East Newton St., Boston, MA 02118.

Bjørn Skogen, M.D., Institute of Immunology and Rheumatology, Rikshopitalet University Hospital, Fr. Qvamsgt 1, Oslo 1, Norway.

Knut Sletten, Ph.D., Institute of Immunology and Rheumatology, Rikshopitalet University Hospital, Department of Biochemistry, University of Oslo, Oslo, Norway.

Ezra Sohar, M.D., Professor of Medicine, Heller Institute of Medical Research, Sheba Medical Center, Tel Hashomer 52621, Israel.

Alan Solomon, M.D., Department of Medicine, University of Tennessee, Center for Health Sciences, 1924 Alcoa Highway, Knoxville, TN 37920.

Marvin J. Stone, M.D., Chief of Oncology, Internal Medicine, Sammons Cancer Center, Baylor Univ. Medical Center, 3500 Gaston Ave., Dallas, TX 75246.

Dr. A. F. Strachan, Dept. of Internal Medicine, University of Stellenbosch, P. O. Box 63, Tygerberg 7505, South Africa.

Tomokazu Suzuki, M.D., Assistant Professor, Third Dept. of Internal Medicine, Osaka University Hospital, Fukushima-ku, Osaka 553, Japan.

Mutsuo Takahashi, M.D., Direct, Department of Pathology, Yamaguchi University School of Medicine, Ube, Yamaguchi 755, Japan.

Emiko Tatsuta, M.D., Department 3rd Medicine, University O.E.H. School of Medicine, 1-1 Iseioaoka, Yahatahishiku, Kitakyushu, 807, Japan.

Satoru Tawara, M.D., Instructor of the Third Department of Int. Medicine, Yamaga City Hospital, Kumamoto Ken, 861-05, Japan.

Dr. A. M. Teppo, Fourth Department of Medicine, Helsinki University Central Hospital, Helsinki, Finland.

Eiro Tsubura, M.D., Director, Toneyama National Hospital, Toneyama 5-1-1 Toyonaka, Osaka 560, Japan.

Dr. Fumiya Uchino, Department of Pathology, Yamaguchi University School of Medicine, Ube, Yamaguchi, Japan.

Dr. M. H. van Rijswijk, Division of Rheumatology, Department of Medicine, University Hospital, Groningen, The Netherlands.

Professor Jan Waldenström, Department of Medicine, General Hospital, S-214 01, Malmö, Sweden.

Professor Otto Wegelius, Helsinki University Central Hospital, Fourth Department of Medicine, Helsinki, Finland.

Dr. P. Westermark, Department of Pathology, University of Uppsala, Uppsala, Sweden.

843

Dr. Frank Williams, Director, National Institute on Aging, National Institutes of Health, Building 31, 2C06, Bethesda, MD 20205.

Henryk M. Wisniewski, M.D., Department of Pathological Neurobiology, Institute for Basic Research in Developmental Disabilities, Staten Island, N. Y. 10314.

John R. Wright, M.D., Professor and Chairman, Department of Pathology, SUNY at Buffalo, 204 Farber Hall, Albany, N. Y. 14214.

Dr. Yasuhiro Yamamura, Third Dept. of Internal Medicine, Hiroshima Univ. School of Medicine, 1-2-3 Kasumi, Minami-ku, Hiroshima, 734 Japan.

Tadaaki Yokota, M.D., Director, Department of Pathology, Yamaguchi University School of Medicine, Ube, Yamaguchi 755, Japan.

Dorothea Zucker-Franklin, M.D., Professor, Department of Medicine, New York University School of Medicine, 550 First Ave., New York, N. Y. 10016.